Advance Concepts of
NURSING PRACTICE

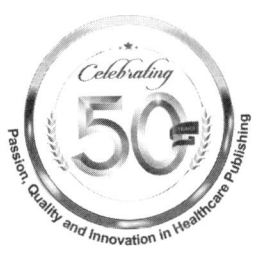

Advance Concepts of NURSING PRACTICE

As per INC Syllabus for MSc Students

Reddamma GG MSc(N), PhD Scholar
Lecturer, OBG Nursing Department
Government College of Nursing
Fort, Bengaluru, India

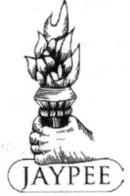

JAYPEE BROTHERS MEDICAL PUBLISHERS
The Health Sciences Publisher
New Delhi | London

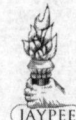

Jaypee Brothers Medical Publishers (P) Ltd

Headquarters
Jaypee Brothers Medical Publishers (P) Ltd
EMCA House, 23/23-B
Ansari Road, Daryaganj
New Delhi - 110 002, INDIA
Landline: +91-11-23272143,+91-11-23272703, +91-11-23282021,+91-11-23245672
Head Office : 011-43574357
Email: jaypee@jaypeebrothers.com

Corporate Office
Jaypee Brothers Medical Publishers (P) Ltd
4838/24, Ansari Road, Daryaganj
New Delhi 110 002, India
Phone: +91-11-43574357
Fax: +91-11-43574314
Email: jaypee@jaypeebrothers.com

Website: www.jaypeebrothers.com
Website: www.jaypeedigital.com

Overseas Office
J.P. Medical Ltd
83 Victoria Street, London
SW1H 0HW (UK)
Phone: +44 20 3170 8910
Fax: +44 (0)20 3008 6180
Email: info@jpmedpub.com

© 2021, Jaypee Brothers Medical Publishers

The views and opinions expressed in this book are solely those of the original contributor (s)/author (s) and do not necessarily represent those of editor (s) of the book.

All rights reserved. No part of this publication may be reproduced, stored or transmitted in any form or by any means, electronic, mechanical, photocopying, recording or otherwise, without the prior permission in writing of the publishers/editors.

All brand names and product names used in this book are trade names, service marks, trademarks or registered trademarks of their respective owners. The publisher is not associated with any product or vendor mentioned in this book.

Medical knowledge and practice change constantly. This book is designed to provide accurate, authoritative information about the subject matter in question. However, readers are advised to check the most current information available on procedures included and check information from the manufacturer of each product to be administered, to verify the recommended dose, formula, method and duration of administration, adverse effects and contraindications. It is the responsibility of the practitioner to take all appropriate safety precautions. Neither the publisher nor the author (s)/editor (s) assume any liability for any injury and/or damage to persons or property arising from or related to use of material in this book.

This book is sold on the understanding that the publisher is not engaged in providing professional medical services. If such advice or services are required, the services of a competent medical professional should be sought.

Every effort has been made where necessary to contact holders of copyright to obtain permission to reproduce copyright material. If any have been inadvertently overlooked, the publisher will be pleased to make the necessary arrangements at the first opportunity. The **CD/ DVD-ROM** (if any) provided in the sealed envelope with this book is complimentary and free of cost. **Not meant for sale**.

Inquiries for bulk sales may be solicited at: jaypee@jaypeebrothers.com

Advance Concepts of Nursing Practice

First Edition: **2021**

ISBN: 978-93-90020-95-9

Printed at Sanat Printers

Dedicated to

The revered memory of
My Parents and Mother-in-Law

Success is the result of perfection, hard work, learning from failure, loyalty, and persistence.

— **Colin Powell**

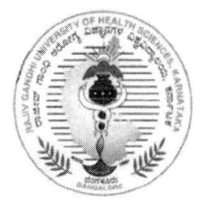

ರಾಜೀವ್ ಗಾಂಧಿ ಆರೋಗ್ಯ ವಿಜ್ಞಾನಗಳ ವಿಶ್ವವಿದ್ಯಾಲಯ, ಕರ್ನಾಟಕ, ಬೆಂಗಳೂರು
Rajiv Gandhi University of Health Sciences, Karnataka, Bengaluru

Dr. S. Sacchidanand
MD, DVD, DHA, FRCP (Glasgow)
VICE-CHANCELLOR

No. PS/ 85 / 2018-19

Foreword

It is my pleasure to pen a foreword to this book to the fraternity of Nursing Profession aimed especially to the students of MSc Nursing.

This book is helpful in gaining essential knowledge about different concepts and their application in Nursing Practice.

The author has translated her vast clinical/teaching experience into this book, which I hope will become an essential book for the students of nursing profession.

I am sure that this book will be widely used and will contribute significantly in the dissemination of knowledge among the student community of Nursing Profession.

I congratulate the author for such a contribution in field of **"Advance Concepts of Nursing Practice"**.

Dr S Sacchidanand
Vice-Chancellor

Preface

Master of Science in Nursing programs have increased over the last 5 years, to maintain accreditation, standards and changing needs of the society, review of the curriculum was done in the year 2009-10 by INC and adopted by RGUHS, Bengaluru. To meet the requirements of the changed syllabus, an integration of all concepts on the recent advances in Nursing Practice is done. This book was developed based on author's experience and student's desire. It has all the core content for advanced nursing practice that is brought together into one source. The idea was based on the core curriculum content which is very broad and difficult to address all areas. But there are no books which include all these topic areas of the syllabus. This book also helpful for Graduates to explore their attitudes and make decisions regarding the incorporation of Professional value systems. This text is based on Indian Nursing Council Syllabus and the outline of curriculum in Advance Concepts of Nursing Practice is as follows:

Section 1: Nursing as a Profession: The objective is to prepare professional nurses, to take up advanced roles and work in different settings of nursing practice, education, research, administration, etc.

Section 2: Healthcare Delivery: Provides an understanding of hospital and community based healthcare and health delivery system.

Section 3: Genetics: Involves the concepts of genes, chromosomes and genetic testing and practical application of genetics in nursing.

Section 4: Epidemiology: Provides an understanding of epidemiological concepts of disease, causation and health surveillance.

Section 5: Biopsychosocial Pathology: Describes common problems of life processes, infection prevention and treatment aspects.

Section 6: Philosophy and Theories of Nursing: Knowledge about theory helps an Advance Practice Nurse be prepared to evaluate and utilize appropriate theory, critique to apply his or her practice.

Section 7: Nursing Process Approach: Knowledge about how advance practice nurse utilizes the systematic steps of health assessment and methods of data collection through nursing process approach.

Section 8: Psychological Aspects and Human Relations: Understands human behavior, personality development, growth and development from conception to older adult.

Section 9: Nursing Practice: Information related to health promotion, models of prevention, extended and expanded roles, evidenced-based nursing practice and innovations in nursing.

Section 10: Computer Application for Patient Care Delivery Systems and Nursing Practice: Includes use of computers in teaching, learning, research and nursing practice and hospital management information system.

I hope that this book will serve the MSc Nursing Students to understand the milestones of Advance Nursing Practice, Referral text for Postgraduate MSc Nursing Students and will also be useful for Nursing Professionals working in practice areas. Thus make a positive contribution to the field of nursing education and practice.

I invite constructive comments and suggestions from the students, teachers and all the readers to further improve this book in future revised editions.

With good wishes!

Reddamma GG

Acknowledgments

I thank Almighty God for His abundant blessings, honor and commitment in every effort, which led the completion of this work.

No endeavors are completed in isolation and this project too is a product of efforts and contribution of many noble persons around me. I express deep and sincere gratitude to all the reviewers for their suggestions.

My sincere appreciation to my family for their constant cooperation throughout the endeavours of my work.

My sincere gratitude to all my teachers, colleagues and friends who have helped me for the successful completion of my work. My great respect and Sincere thanks to Dr S Sachidanand, Vice Chancellor, RGUHS for consenting foreword.

Special thanks to Dr Clement Irudhyanathan, Principal, Columbia Asia College of Nursing, Bengaluru and Chief Editor RGUHS. This wouldn't have been possible without his assistance.

I would like to acknowledge the encouragement and support received from Dr Sukanya, Principal, Govt. College of Nursing, Bengaluru to complete this book.

I extend my sincere thanks to Mr Venugopal (Branch Manager), Mr Santosh Kumar (Commissing Editor), Bengaluru, India and the entire team of M/s Jaypee Brothers Medical Publishers, New Delhi for making my dream a reality.

Reviewers List

Girjiamba Devi
Principal cum Dean/Secretary
TNAI Karnataka State Branch
AECS Maruthi College of Nursing
Bengaluru

Hemalatha R
Princpal
Universal College of Nursing
Bengaluru

Jyothi B
Principal
Government College of Nursing
VIMS, Bellary

Thresa Mendonca
Vice Principal
Lakshmi Memorial College of Nursing
Mangaluru

Saroja Jayakumar
Chief of Nursing Service
Columbia Asia Hospital-Whitefield (CAHW)
Bangalore

Shilpa N
2nd year MSc Nursing (Ex student)
OBG Nursing Speciality
Government College of Nursing
Bengaluru

Thabasum MS
2nd year MSc Nursing (Ex student)
OBG Nursing Speciality
Government College of Nursing
Bengaluru

Anand
2nd year MSc Nursing (Ex student)
Medical Surgical Nursing Speciality
Government College of Nursing
Bengaluru

Contents

Section 1: Nursing as a Profession

1. History and Development of Nursing Profession, Characteristics and Criteria of the Profession, Perspectives of Nursing Profession—National and Global — 3
- Definitions of Nursing 3
- Overview of History and Development of Nursing Practice 3
- Prehistoric Period 4
- Ancient Period (Period of Early Civilization) 4
- Middle Ages (Period of Christianity) 4
- Dark Age (Renaissance Period) (1500–1700 AD) 4
- Colonial American Period 4
- Nursing in the 19th Century 5
- Nursing in the 20th Century 5
- Nursing in the 21st Century 5
- Development of Nursing Education in India 6
- Characteristics of Nursing Profession 7
- Criteria of the Profession 8
- Perspectives of Nursing Profession 9

2. Code of Ethics and Code of Professional Conduct — 13
- Ethics 13
- Morals 13
- Values 13
- Code of Ethics 14
- Code of Ethics in Nursing 14
- Ethical Principles 17
- Ethical Philosophical Theories 18
- Ethical Dilemmas 19

3. Autonomy, Accountability, Assertiveness and Visibility of Nurses — 20
- Autonomy in Nursing 20
- Meaning 20
- Definitions 20
- Different Aspects of Autonomy 20
- Barriers of Autonomy 20
- Evolution of Professional Autonomy 21
- Methods to Achieve Autonomy 21
- Accountability 22
- Assertiveness 23
- Visibility of Nurses 23

4. Legal Considerations in Nursing — 24
- Meaning 24
- Definition 24
- Sources of Law for Nursing Practice 24
- Values of Law in Nursing 25
- Legal Safeguards In Nursing Practice 25
- Legal Responsibilities of a Nurse 27
- Legal Liability in Nursing 27
- Legal Aspects of Charting Techniques 28
- List of Do's and Don'ts as Guidelines for Safe Practice 29

5. Role of Regulatory Bodies — 30
- Definition of Regulatory Bodies 30
- Vital Role of Regulatory Bodies 30
- Major Regulatory Bodies 30
- Important Professional Regulatory Bodies 32

6. Professional Organizations — 40
- Definition of Organization 40
- Meaning of Professional Organization 40
- Major National Professional Organizations 40
- Trained Nurses Association of India 41
- National Students Nurses Association 43
- Health Visitors League 44
- Midwives and Auxiliary Nurse Midwives Association 44
- Nursing Research Society of India 45
- International Professional Organizations 46
- Other Associations 49

7. Unions, Individual and Collective Bargaining — 51
- Collective Bargaining 51
- Definition of Unions 51
- Types of Unions 51
- Labor Unions 51
- Unions/Labor Organization 51
- Nurses Unions and Associations 51
- Meaning of Collective Bargaining 52
- Definition of Collective Bargaining 52
- Objectives of Collective Bargaining 52
- Characteristics of Collective Bargaining 52
- Principles of Collective Bargaining 53
- Types of Bargaining 53
- Preparation for Collective Bargaining 53

- Process of Collective Bargaining 53
- Steps of Collective Bargaining 54
- Types of Strikes 55
- Levels of Collective Bargaining 56
- Importance of Collective Bargaining 56
- Advantages of Collective Bargaining 56
- Disadvantages of Collective Bargaining 56
- Research Abstract 57

8. **Educational Preparations, Continuing Education and Career Opportunities—Professional Advancement, Role and Scope of Nursing Education**   **58**
    - Educational Preparations 58
    - Meaning of Educational Preparation 58
    - Need for Educational Preparations in Nursing 58
    - Problems Associated with Changing Educational Requirements for Licensure 62
    - Concept of Nursing Education 62
    - Continuing Education Program 64
    - Preceptorship Model of Clinical Teaching (Burns and Paterson 2005) 67
    - Professional Advancement and Role and Scope of Nursing Education 68
    - Professional Advancement System for Nurse Clinicians 69
    - Role of Nursing Educator in Teaching 70

9. **Role of Research, Leadership and Management**   **71**
    - Role of Research in Nursing Profession 71
    - Research Process 74
    - Research Utilization 77
    - Barriers Related to Research 78
    - Strategies to Promote Research 78
    - Nurse Researcher Roles 79
    - Current and Future Strategies for Research Utilization 79
    - Introduction to Leadership and Management 80
    - Types of Leadership 81
    - Styles of Leadership 81
    - Roles of Leadership 82
    - Techniques of Leadership 83
    - Role of Management in Nursing Profession 83
    - Common Management Functions 83
    - Time Management Principles 84
    - Five Rights of Delegation 84
    - Responsibilities of Manager 84
    - Research Abstract 84

10. **Quality Assurance in Nursing**   **85**
    - Terminologies 85
    - Meaning of Quality Assurance 85
    - Definition of Quality Assurance 85
    - Historical Development of Quality Assurance in Nursing and Healthcare 86
    - Concept of Quality Assurance in the Nursing Profession 86
    - Quality Assurance of Nursing in India 86
    - Goals of Quality Assurance 87
    - Criteria in Quality Assurance System 87
    - Frames of References for Evaluation of Nursing Care 88
    - Definition of Standards 88
    - Nursing Standards 89
    - Techniques of Quality Assurance in Nursing 90
    - Components of Quality Assurance Program 90
    - Audit 90
    - Nursing Audit 91
    - Factors Affecting Quality Nursing Care 93
    - Measurable Initiatives for Continuous Quality Improvement in Nursing 93

11. **Futuristic Nursing**   **95**
    - Nursing Future Challenges 95
    - Challenges in Nursing Practice 96
    - Challenges in Nursing Education 97
    - Trends of Nursing Education for Future 97
    - Variation on Traditional Roles in Nursing 99
    - New Millennium Nurses 100

Section 2: Healthcare Delivery

12. **Healthcare Environment, Economics, Constraints, Planning Process, Policies, Political Process vis-a-vis Nursing Profession**   **105**
    - Health for All in the 21st Century 105
    - Definition of Health 105
    - Health Care Environment 106
    - Environmental Protectional Agency 107
    - Health Economics 108
    - Problems of Resources and Personnel in Health Care Services 108
    - Problems of the General Structure of Health Services 109
    - Health Planning Process 111
    - Politics and Policy Making 112
    - Role of Nurse in Politics 115

13. **Healthcare Delivery System in National, State, District and Local Level**   **117**
    - Definitions 117
    - History of Healthcare System 117
    - Healthcare Delivery System in India 119
    - Organization of Health Service at District Level 124

14. **Major Stakeholders in the Healthcare System: Government, Nongovernment, Industry and Other Professionals**   **129**
    - Stakeholders in Healthcare System 129
    - Employees State Insurance Scheme 131
    - Other Agencies 131
    - Voluntary Health Agencies 131
    - National Health Programs in India 132

15. Patterns of Nursing Care Delivery in India 133
- Health 133
- Nursing 133
- Dimensions of Nursing Care 134
- Patterns of Nursing Care Delivery 134
- Comprehensive Nursing Care/ Total Patient Care 134
- Progressive Patient Care Concept 135
- Team Nursing Concept 137
- Functional Method 138
- Case Method 138
- Primary Nursing Concept 138
- Self-Care Concept 139
- Palliative Care Concepts 139
- Other Concepts of Nursing Care 139

16. Healthcare Delivery Concerns, National Health and Family Welfare Programmes—Intersectoral Coordination, Role of Nongovernmental Agencies 141
- National Health and Family Welfare Programmes 141
- Organization For Family Welfare Services 150
- Intersectoral Coordination 153

17. Information, Education and Communication in Healthcare Delivery 156
- Definition of Information, Education and Communication 156
- Objectives of Information, Education and Communication 156
- Principles to Follow in Planning Information, Education and Communication Initiative 156
- Advantages 157
- Information, Education and Communication Tools 157
- Importance of Information, Education and Communication 157
- Training 159
- Need of Information, Education and Communication Specific Areas 159
- Gender Considerations 160

18. Telemedicine/Telenursing 161
- Definition 161
- History 161
- Electronic Health and Telehealth 162
- Applications in Different Forms 162
- Types of Telemedicine 162
- Benefits and Uses of Telemedicine 162
- First Interactive Telemedicine System 163
- Teletransmission of ECG Using Indigenous Methods 163
- Teleradiology 163
- Specialties 163
- Telemedicine in India 164
- Telenursing 165

Section 3: Genetics

19. Review of Cellular Division, Mutation and Law of Inheritance, Human Genome Project, Genomic Era 169
- Cell Structure 169
- Cell Membrane 170
- Cytoplasm 170
- Cell Organelles 170
- Cell Division 170
- Mitosis 170
- Meiosis 171
- Spermatogenesis 172
- Oogenesis 172
- Mutations 173
- Law of Inheritance 174
- Human Genome Project, Genomic Era 174
- Human Genome Project (HGP) 175
- Techniques and Analysis 180
- Ethical, Legal and Social Issues 180
- Genomic Era 180

20. Basic Concepts of Genes, Chromosomes and DNA 182
- Genes 182
- Concepts of Genetics 182
- Chemistry of a Gene 183
- Deoxyribonucleic Acid 183
- Chromosomes 183

21. Approaches to Common Genetic Disorders 185
- Definition of Genetics 185
- Incidence of Genetic Disorders 185
- Types of Genetic Disorders 185
- Management of Genetic Disorders 191

22. Genetic Testing: Basis of Genetic Diagnosis, Presymptomatic and Predisposition Testing, Prenatal Diagnosis and Screening 192
- Types of Genetic Tests 193
- Indications for Prenatal Screening and Diagnostic Testing 193
- Goals of Genetic Screening 194
- Preventive and Social Measures 196
- Other Preventive Measures 196
- Reproductive Alternatives 197
- Ethical, Legal and Psychosocial Issues in Genetic Testing 197

23. Genetic Counseling 200
- Definition 200
- Aims and Objectives 200
- Types of Genetic Counseling 200
- Purposes 201
- Clients Seeking Genetic Counseling 201
- Genetic Counseling Team 201

- Principles of Genetic Counseling 201
- Process of Genetic Counseling 202

24. **Practical Application of Genetics in Nursing** 203
    - Nurses Role in Genetic Counseling 203
    - Role of Nurse in Diagnostic Tests and Procedures 204
    - Follow-Up Care 204
    - Role of the Administrator in Genetic Services 204

Section 4: Epidemiology

25. **History, Scope, Aim, Epidemiological Approach and Methods** 209
    - History of Epidemiology 209
    - Definitions and Modern Concepts of Epidemiology 209
    - Scope of Epidemiology 210
    - Aims of Epidemiology 210
    - Epidemiological Approach 210
    - Epidemiological Methods 211
    - Case Control Study 212
    - Cohort Study 214
    - Experimental Epidemiology 218
    - Association and Causation 222
    - Epidemiological Investigation Process 223

26. **Mortality and Morbidity** 224
    - Basic Measurements of Epidemiology 224
    - Tools of Measurement 224
    - Mortality Rate (Death Rate) 225
    - Morbidity Rates 226

27. **Concepts of Causation of Diseases and their Screening** 229
    - Concept and Theories of Disease Causation 229
    - Natural History of Disease 232
    - Conclusion 233

28. **Application of Epidemiology in Healthcare Delivery, Health Surveillance and Health Informatics, Uses of Epidemiology** 234
    - Concepts of Prevention 234
    - Modes of Intervention 234
    - Levels of Prevention 234
    - Measures of Preventive Epidemiology 239
    - Uses of Epidemiology 244

29. **Role of Nurse in Epidemiology** 245

Section 5: Biopsychosocial Pathology

30. **Pathophysiology and Psychodynamics of Disease Causation** 249
    - Psychobiology 249
    - Neuroanatomy 250
    - Neuroregulation 252
    - Diagnosis of Psychobiological Disorders 253
    - Psychobiology and Nursing 253

31. **Life Process, Homeostatic Mechanism, Biological and Psychosocial Dynamics in Causation of Disease and Lifestyle** 255
    - Life Processes 255
    - Definition of Life Processes 255
    - Homeostatic Mechanism 259
    - Biological and Psychosocial Dynamics in Causation of Disease 260
    - Terminologies 260
    - Factors Influencing the Health Beliefs and Practices 260
    - Variables Influencing Illness Behavior 261
    - Psychological Stages of Illness 262
    - Kinds of Emotions 262
    - Health-Illness States: Interaction Between the Mind and Body 265
    - Role of Emotion in Health and Disease 265
    - Illness with Negative Progresses 266
    - Role of a Nurse 267
    - Healthcare has become increasingly Focused on Health Promotion, Wellness and Illness Prevention 267

32. **Common Problems** 268
    - Oxygen Insufficiency 268
    - Oxygen Therapy 269
    - Fluid and Electrolyte Balance 270
    - Fluid Imbalance 272
    - Electrolyte Imbalance 274
    - Nutritional Problems 277
    - Client with Obesity 278
    - Malnutrition 280
    - Client with an Eating Disorder 282
    - Hemorrhage and Shock 282
    - Altered Body Temperature 288
    - Unconsciousness 290
    - Sleep Pattern and its Disturbances 294
    - Physiology of Sleep and Arousal 295
    - Stages of Sleep 295
    - Pain 300
    - Sensory Deprivation 305
    - Stress of Immobility or Confinement 307
    - Social Isolation 308

33. **Treatment Aspects: Pharmacological, Pre- and Postoperative Care Aspects** 312
    - Definition 312
    - Concept of Perioperative Nursing 312
    - History of Surgical Nursing 312
    - Types of Surgery According to Urgency 313
    - Purpose of Surgery 313
    - Variables Affecting Surgical Problem Status 313
    - Factors Influencing Surgical Outcomes 314
    - Preoperative Nursing Care 314

- Preoperative Patient Admission 314
- Preparation of the Patient for Surgery 314
- Preoperative Phase 316
- Intraoperative Phase 316
- Postoperative Phase 317
- Anesthesia 317

34. Cardiopulmonary Resuscitation 320
- Resuscitation 320
- Cardiopulmonary Resuscitation 320
- Aftercare 323
- Risks 323
- Neonatal Resuscitation 323

35. End-of-Life Care 326
- Terminologies 326
- Concept of Death and Dying 326
- Changes in Healthcare Related to Dying and Death 326
- Standard for Healthcare in Providing End-of-life Care 327
- States of Awareness Manifested by Client and Family 328
- Common Fears and Concern of the Dying 328
- Journey Toward Death 328
- 1–2 Weeks Prior to Death 329
- Journey's End: A Couple of Days to Hours Prior to Death 329
- Stages of Death and Dying 329

36. Infection Prevention (Including HIV) and Standard Safety Measures 331
- Definition 331
- Hand Hygiene 331
- Key Points 335
- Infection Control and Standard Safety Measures 335
- Control Measures 336

37. Biomedical Waste Management 339
- Types of Hospital Waste 339
- Treatment and Disposal 341
- Biomedical Waste Management and Handling Rules 342
- Nurse's Role 343

Section 6: Philosophy and Theories of Nursing

38. Values, Conceptual Models and Approaches 349
- Terminologies 349
- Introduction 350
- Model 350
- Theory 352

39. Nursing Theories 356
- Nightingale's Theory 356
- Henderson's Theory 359
- Rogers' Theory 361
- Two Derived Theories 363
- Peplau's Theory 366
- Abdellah's Theory 369
- Conservation Model 372
- Dorothea E Orem 374
- Dorothy E Johnson 377
- Imogene King Theory 380
- Betty Neuman's System Theory 384
- Roy's Adaptation Theory 389
- Watson's Theory 394

40. A Health Belief Model 401
- Health Belief Model [Becker and Maiman's (1975)] 401
- Advantages 402

41. Concept of Self-health 403
- Definitions 403
- Self-Care in Health 403
- Nurses' Role in Self-care Health of People 404

42. Evidence-based Practice Model 405
- Definition 405
- Features of Evidence-based Practice 405
- Purposes 405
- Examples of Real Life Situation 405
- Barriers in Evidence-based Practice 405
- Types of Evidence and Evidence Hierarchies 406
- Strategies and Steps for Individual Clinicians 406

Section 7: Nursing Process Approach

43. Health Assessment 411
- Definition 411
- Equipment Needed 411
- Techniques 411
- Psychological Consequences of Illness 420

44. Methods of Collection, Analysis and Utilization of Data Relevant to Nursing Process 426
- Definitions 426
- Steps of Nursing Process 426
- Purposes of the Nursing Process 427
- Characteristics of Nursing Process 427
- Advantages of Nursing Process 427
- Nursing Assessment 428

45. Nursing Diagnosis 431
- Definition 431
- Use of Nursing Diagnosis 431
- Diagnostic Process 431
- Nursing Diagnosis and Medical Diagnosis 434

46. Planning 436
- Definition 436
- Purpose 436
- Types of Planning 436
- Elements of Planning 436

47. Formulation of Nursing Care Plans, Health Goals, Implementation, Modification, and Evaluation of Care 440
- Formulation of Nursing Care Plans 440
- Implementation 443
- Evaluation 445
- Documentation 446

48. Theory Application in Nursing Process 449
- Application of Nursing Theory into Practice 449
- Johnson's Behavioral System and the Nursing Process 449
- Application of Theory 451

Section 8: Psychological Aspects and Human Relations

49. Human Behavior, Life Process, Growth and Development, Personality Development, and Defense Mechanisms 455
- Definition of Psychology 455
- Application of Psychology 455
- Human Behavior 455
- Overview of Human Development 456
- Personality 461
- Defense Mechanisms 469

50. Communication, Interpersonal Relationships, Individual and Group, Group Dynamics and Organizational Behavior 472
- Definition 472
- Factors Influencing Communication 472
- Types of Communication 473
- Components of Communication 473
- Barriers of Communication 473
- Techniques to Improve Therapeutic Communication 473
- Theories of Communication 474
- Characteristics of Therapeutic Communication 475
- Levels of Communication 475
- Interpersonal (Therapeutic) Relationship 475
- Development of a Therapeutic Relationship 477
- Phases of Therapeutic Relationship 477
- Group Dynamics 480
- Organizational Behavior 482

51. Basic Human Needs, Growth and Development (Conception Through Preschool, School Age Through Adolescence, Young and Middle Adult, and Older Adult) 484
- Abraham Maslow (1954) Basic "Human Needs" 484
- Growth and Development from Conception to Old Age 484

52. Sexuality and Sexual Health 489
- Development of Sexual Identity 489
- Adolescent Sexuality 492
- Adult Sexuality 493

53. Stress and Adaptation, Crisis and its Intervention 495
- Definition of Stress 495
- Definition of Adaptation 495
- Stressors 496
- Mediating Processes 496
- Physiologic Response to Stress 497
- Stress Theories 499
- Models of Illness 500
- Adaptive Coping Strategies (Methods) 500
- Nursing Management of Stress Assessment 501

54. Coping with Loss, Death and Grief 504
- Loss 504
- Grief and Bereavement 506

55. Principles and Techniques of Counseling 512
- Guidance and Counseling 512
- Guidance 512
- Counseling 513
- Relationship Between Guidance and Counseling 514
- Principles of Guidance and Counseling 514

Section 9: Nursing Practice

56. Framework, Scope and Trends 523
- Definition 523
- Framework 523
- Trends/Scope in Nursing Practice 523
- Trends in Nursing Practice 525
- Models of Quality Management 526

57. Alternative Modalities of Care, Alternative Systems of Health and Complimentary Therapies 529
- Alternative Medicine 529
- Alternative Modalities of Care 530
- Alternative Systems of Health 532

58. Extended and Expanded Role of the Nurse in Promotive, Preventive, Curative and Restorative Healthcare Delivery System in Community and Institutions 537
- Extended Roles of the Nurse 537
- Extended Care Facilities 537
- Common Expanded Roles of Nursing 539
- The Roles of Nurse Related to Medical Surgical Nursing Area 541
- Expanded Roles of Nurse in Child Health Nursing Area 545
- Expanded Roles in Community Health Nursing 545
- Expanded Roles in Psychiatric Nursing 546

59. Health Promotion and Primary Healthcare 548
- Health Promotion Model 548
- Promotion of Health Through Pender Model in Nursing Practice 549
- Nurses' Role in Health Promotion 551

- Primary Healthcare 551
- Concept of Health for All 551
- Indian Health System Infrastructure for Primary Healthcare Institutions and Tiers of Delivery 556

60. **Independent Practice Issues—Independent Nurse Midwifery Practitioner** 558
    - Independent Nursing Practice 558

61. **Collaboration Issues and Models Within and Outside Nursing Models of Prevention** 561
    - Health 561

62. **Family Nursing, Home Nursing** 569
    - Use of Coping Index and Family Process 569
    - Family Nursing Process 570
    - Home Nursing 572

63. **Gender Sensitive Issues and Women Empowerment** 575
    - Women Empowerment 578
    - Men in Nursing 581

64. **Disaster Nursing** 583
    - Definition 583
    - Phases of Disaster Management 583
    - Disaster Syndrome 585
    - Rehabilitation 586

65. **Geriatric Considerations in Nursing** 588
    - Concepts of Aging 588
    - Demography: Myths and Realities 589
    - Theories of Aging 590
    - Age-related Body System Changes 591
    - Pharamacokinetics 594
    - Common Health Problems and Nursing Management; Concept of Old Age 595
    - Disorders More Common in Older People 597
    - Geriatric People Problems 600
    - Psychosocial and Sexual Changes 600
    - Abuse 601
    - Role of Nurse for Caregivers of Elderly 602
    - Use of Aids and Prosthesis (Hearing Aids/Dentures) 603
    - Provisions and Programs for Elderly: Privileges, Community Programs, and Health Services 606
    - Home and Institutional Care 607

66. **Evidence-based Nursing Practice: Best Practice** 609
    - Definitions 609
    - What is Evidence? 609

67. **Transcultural Nursing** 613
    - Terminologies Used 613
    - Concept of Culture 613
    - Definitions 613
    - Historical Perspectives 614
    - Goals of Transcultural Nursing 614
    - Transcultural Nursing Model or Sunrise Model 614
- Role of Nurse In Transculture Nursing 617
- Research Abstract 618

68. **Innovations in Nursing** 619
    - Steps in Innovation 619
    - Factors Preventing to Attempt Innovation 619
    - Factors Needed for Innovation 619
    - Factors Leading to Change 619
    - Factors in Organizational Change 620

Section 10: Computer Application for Patient Care Delivery Systems and Nursing Practice

69. **Use of Computers in Teaching, Learning, Research, and Nursing Practice** 627
    - Uses of Computers 627

70. **Windows, MS Office, Word, Excel, Powerpoint/ Operating Systems of a Computer** 629
    - Microsoft Windows 629
    - History of Microsoft Windows 629
    - Future of Windows 630
    - Microsoft Office (Ms Office) 630
    - Microsoft Office Excel 633
    - Microsoft Powerpoint 635

71. **Internet Literatures Search** 638
    - Definition 638
    - Types of Computer Networks 638
    - Sources of Internet Medical Literature 638
    - World Wide Web 638

72. **Statistical Packages** 640
    - Major Statistical Software Packages 640
    - Using a Packaged Program 641

73. **Hospital Management Information System Software** 642
    - Objectives 642
    - Computerization of Hospital and Nursing Homes 642
    - Electronic Hospital Management Software 644
    - Computers in Medicine and Health Care 647
    - Hospital Information System 648

Annexures

1. **Health Assessment Format** 653
    - History Taking 653
    - Physical Examination/Assessment 653
    - Lab Investigations 655
    - Medical Treatment 655
    - Surgical Management 656
    - Nursing Management 656

2. **Community Health Assessment Format** 657
    - Baseline Survey Data 657

Index 661

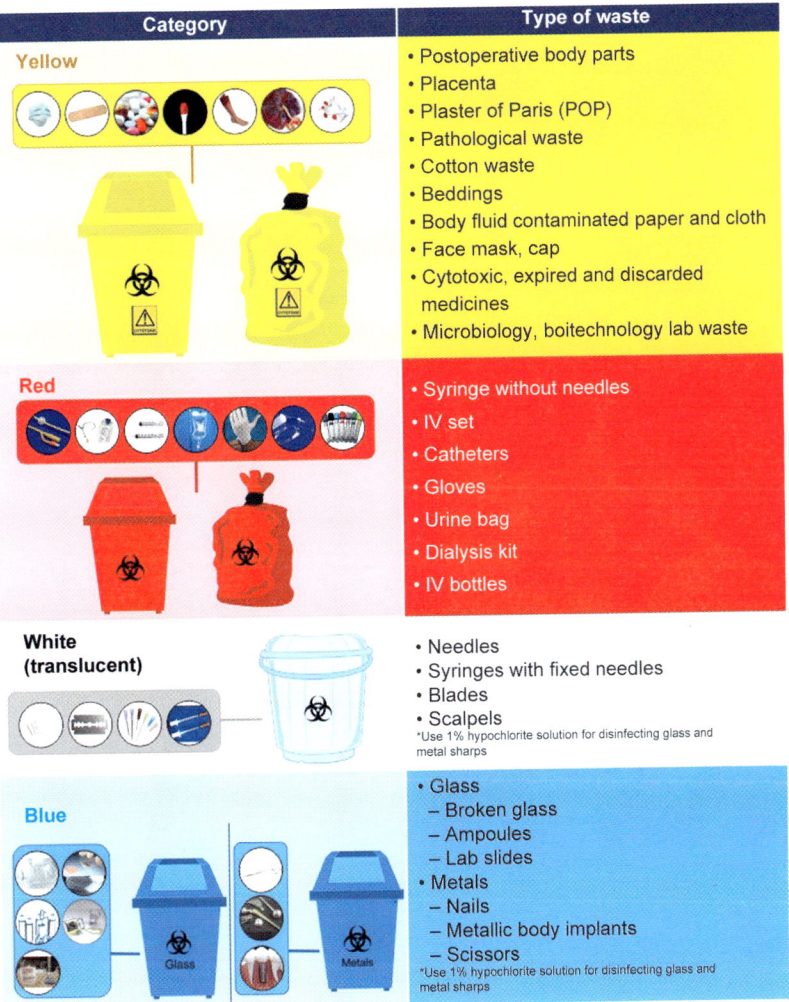

Fig. 37.5: Segregation of the waste.

(IV: intravenous)

Plate 2

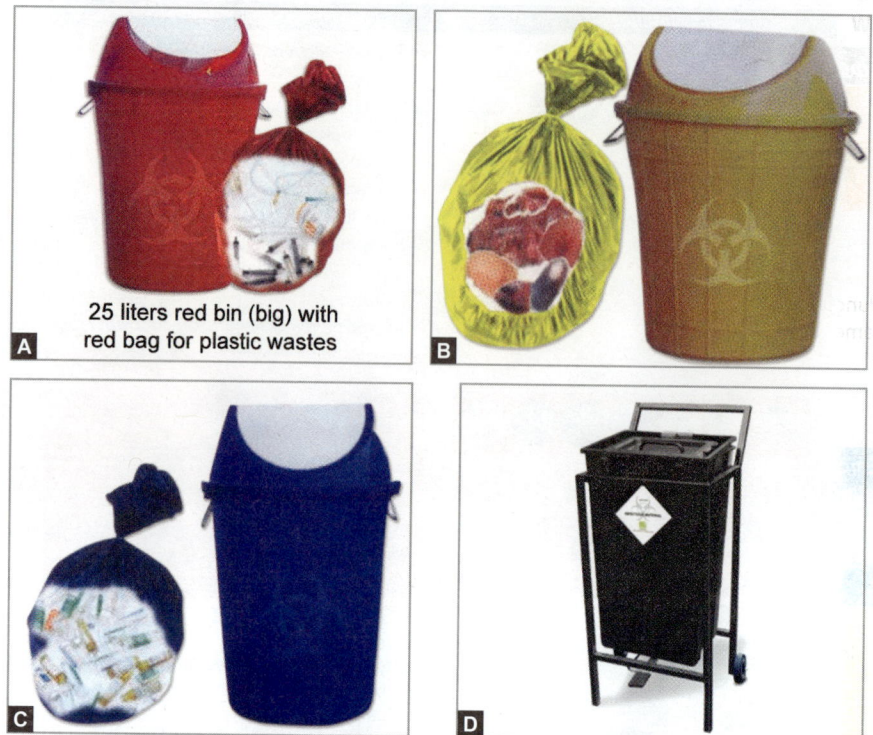

Figs. 37.6A to D: (A) Red; (B) Yellow; (C) Blue; (D) Black.

Plate 3

Categories of BMW

Color code	Type of bag/container	Type of waste	Treatment options
Red	Red colored non-chlorinated plastic bags or containers	Contaminated waste (recyclable)	Autoclaving or micro-waving/hydroclaving followed by shredding or mutilation or combination of sterilization and shredding treated Waste to be sent to registered or authorized recyclers
White (Translucent)	Puncture proof, leak proof, tamer proof containers	Waste sharps including metals	Autoclaving or Dry Heat sterilization folowed by shredding
Blue	Cardboard boxes with blue colored marking	a. Glassware b. Metalic body implants	Disinfection and then sent for recycling.
Yellow	Yellow coloured non-chlorinated plastic bags	a. Human anatomical waste b. Animal anatomical waste c. Soiled waste	Incineration or plasma pyrolysis or deep burial
		d. Expired or discarded medicines	Returned back to the manufacturer or supplier for incineration
		e. Chemical waste	Disposed of by incineration or plasma mixing with other wastewater
	Separate collection system leading to effluent treatment system	f. Chemical liquid waste	Chemical liquid waste shall be pre-treated before mixing with other wastewater
	Non-chlorinated yellow plastic bags or suitable packing material	g. Discarded linen, mattresses, beddings contaminated with blood or body fluid	Non-chlorinated chemical disinfection followed by incineration or plazma Pyrolysis or for energy recovery
	Autoclave safe plastic bags or containers	h. Microbiology, biotechnology and other clinical laboratory waste	Pre-treat to sterilize with nonchlorinated chemicals on-site

Fig. 37.8: Categories of waste.

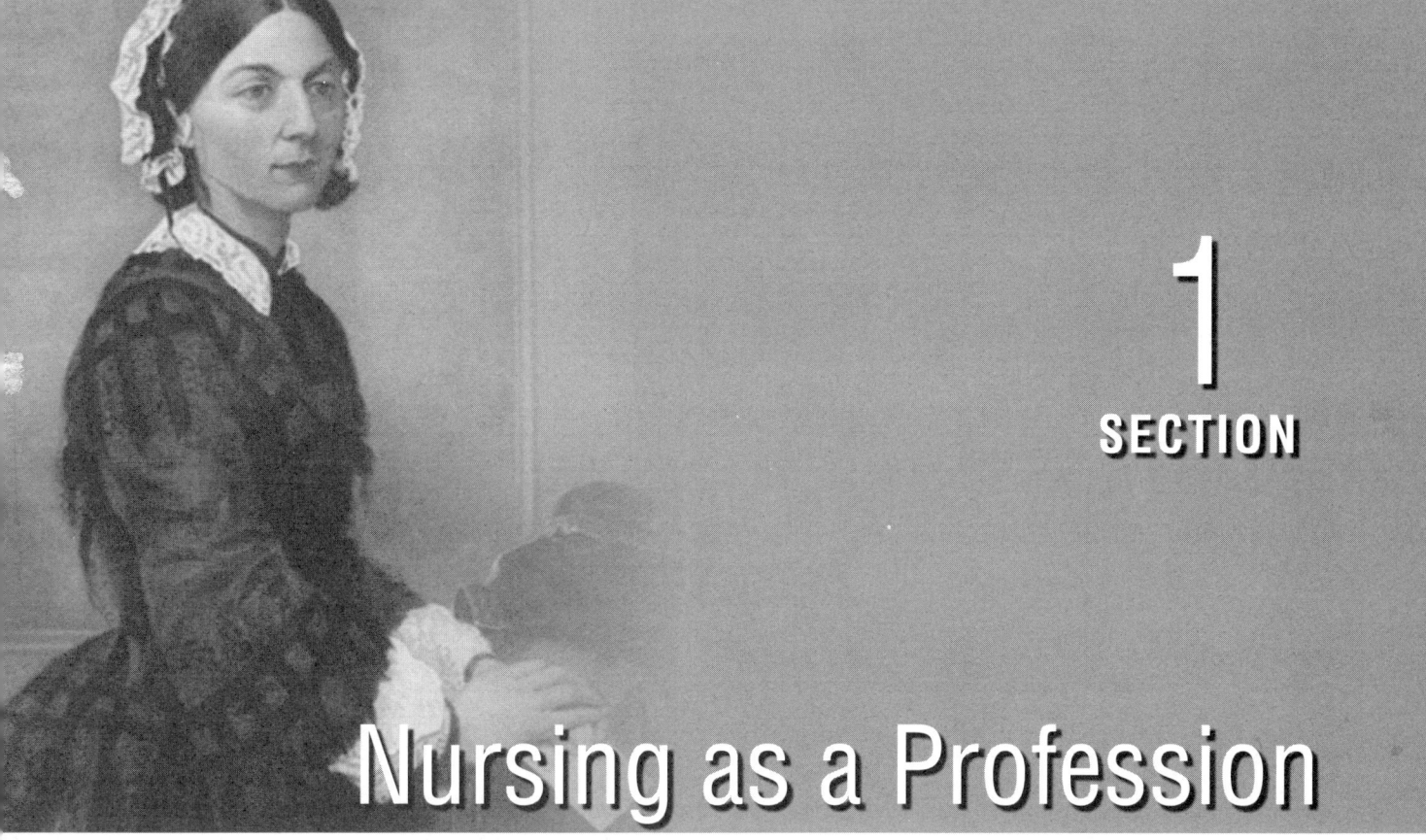

SECTION 1
Nursing as a Profession

Section Outline

1. History and Development of Nursing Profession, Characteristics and Criteria of the Profession, Perspectives of Nursing Profession—National and Global
2. Code of Ethics and Code of Professional Conduct
3. Autonomy, Accountability, Assertiveness and Visibility of Nurses
4. Legal Considerations in Nursing
5. Role of Regulatory Bodies
6. Professional Organizations
7. Unions, Individual and Collective Bargaining
8. Educational Preparations, Continuing Education and Career Opportunities—Professional Advancement, Role and Scope of Nursing Education
9. Role of Research, Leadership and Management
10. Quality Assurance in Nursing
11. Futuristic Nursing

CHAPTER 1

History and Development of Nursing Profession, Characteristics and Criteria of the Profession, Perspectives of Nursing Profession—National and Global

CHAPTER OUTLINE

- Overview of History and Development of Nursing Practice
- Prehistoric Period
- Ancient Period (Period of Early Civilization)
- Middle Ages (Period of Christianity)
- Dark Age (Renaissance Period)
- Colonial American Period
- Nursing in the 19th Century
- Nursing in the 20th Century
- Nursing in the 21st Century
- Development of Nursing Education in India
- Characteristics of Nursing Profession
- Criteria of the Profession
- Perspectives of Nursing Profession

INTRODUCTION

Nursing is an art and a science involving many activities, concepts and skills related to social sciences, physical science, ethics, contemporary issues and other areas. Nursing is a unique profession and a professional registered nurse (RN) provides a specified service according to the standards of practice and follows a code of ethics. The foundation for professional practice arises from theories of nursing relevant to basic social values, education, motivation, autonomy, a sense of commitment and a code of ethics. Nursing has passed through many phases. Many changes were necessary to meet the changing needs of society. As we embark on a career in nursing, we can best appreciate the role and responsibilities we are learning to assume, if we have an understanding of the history of development of the profession.

DEFINITIONS OF NURSING

Nursing has developed many philosophies and definitions. The following definition, written by Virginia Henderson (1996) and adopted by the International Council of Nurses (ICN) in 1973, is a concise, mutually agreed on statement, "The unique function of the nurse is to assist the individual, sick or well, in the performance of those activities contributing to health, its recovery, or to a peaceful death that the client would perform unaided if they had the necessary strength, will or knowledge. And to do this in such a way as to help the clients gain independence as rapidly as possible."

1. *According to American Nurses Association (ANA), 1965:* Nursing practice is a direct service, goal-directed and adaptable to the needs of the individual, the family and community during health and illness.
2. *According to Dorothy E Johnson (1968):* Nursing is an external force acting to preserve the organization of patient behaviors, while the patient is under stress by means of imposing regularity mechanism or by providing resources.

OVERVIEW OF HISTORY AND DEVELOPMENT OF NURSING PRACTICE

When exploring the pages of history, it becomes apparent that nursing has always existed and functioned within a framework of human caring and has progressed in response to the needs of society and scientific advances. Through the competence, commitment and struggle of nurses, past and present, nursing has evolved from primitive roles as bedside attendants to advanced practice nurses. The evolution of nursing practice is a reflection of the social, cultural, economic and political events that have shaped our world history. The important periods in the development of nursing are listed below:

- Prehistoric period
- Ancient period (period of early civilization)
- Middle ages (period of Christianity)
- Dark age (renaissance period)
- Colonial American period
- Nursing in the 19th century
- Nursing in the 20th century
- Nursing in the 21st century.

PREHISTORIC PERIOD

In this era, image of the nurse was folk image.

The art of healing began thousands of years ago with the primitive man trying to provide relief in sickness and suffering, motivated by feelings of sympathy and kindness. The causes of disease were thought to be the wrath of God, the invasion of the body by evil spirits, etc. The medicine he/she practices consisted of pleasing Gods by prayers and rituals, driving out evil spirits from the human body by noise or violence, etc.

Since the time of the first mother, women carried the major responsibility of nourishing and nurturing of children, and caring for the aging members of the family. During times of need, women, who demonstrated aptness and interest in meeting the needs of the sick and injured, would come forward. Training these women was largely by trial and error, and nursing skills evolved from intuition.

ANCIENT PERIOD (PERIOD OF EARLY CIVILIZATION)

In ancient times, people often attributed illness to punishment for sins or to possession by evil spirits. For the medicine, man performed rituals using various plants, herbs and other materials to heal the sick. Women were not involved except for assistance in childbirth.

Egypt: The oldest records date back to the 16th century BC credited as one of the healthiest societies of the ancient times, and the Egyptians valued personal health and practiced preventive medicine to please the Gods and spirits of the dead. It is known that women were hired by families of privileged aristocracy to provide care to the sick and elderly, and to assist with childbirth.

Palestine: Hebrew priests selected women, usually widows and maidens, for assistance in the care of the infirm, mainly at home.

Greece: Attendants who were referred to as "basket healers" assisted the temple priests and physicians. These "basket healers" often traveled with the physicians from town to town offering their services.

India: The Vedas were used as the source of information about health practices. Public hospitals were constructed from 274 to 236 BC and were staffed by male nurses with qualification and duties similar to those of the 20th century. Women were primarily responsible for the caring of the home and family.

Rome: As a military dictatorship, they adopted medical practices from the countries they conquered. The first military hospital was established in Rome. Female and male attendants assisted trained physicians in the care of the sick and injured.

MIDDLE AGES (PERIOD OF CHRISTIANITY)

The first developments in the history of nursing began with Christianity. Most of the changes made in health care were based on the Christian concepts of charity and sanctity of human life.

With the establishment of churches, groups were organized whose primary concern was care of the sick, poor, orphans and widows. They had three orders, namely deaconesses, widows and virgins—all concerned with care of the needy.

The first recorded history of nursing begins with biblical women, who cared for the sick and injured. Phobe, mentioned in the epistle to the Romans in the Bible, is known as the visiting nurse and deaconess. Fabiola influenced and paid for the construction of the first free hospital in Rome in 390 AD. St Marcella, considered the first nursing educator, converted her home into a monastery, where she taught nursing skills. She is the first person to teach nursing as an art rather than a service. St Helena, the mother of Roman Emperor Constantine, is credited with establishing the first geriatric facility.

Monasteries became the centers for education, medical attention and nursing care for travelers and the poor and needy.

In this period, image of the nurse was a religious image.

This era finds women from high society and of high intellect responding to the needs of society in times of war, epidemics and persecution.

DARK AGE (RENAISSANCE PERIOD) (1500–1700 AD)

During renaissance period, as a result of tremendous dissension between the Roman Catholic Church and growing Protestant sects, the role of women changed. The Reformation, a religious movement started with the work of Martin Luther, in Germany.

In this period, image of the nurse was servant image.

The role of women changed after the Reformation. Many monasteries closed down and the work of women in religious orders nearly ended. Hospital care was relegated to "uncommon women" (prisoners, prostitutes and drunks). Nursing was considered the most menial of all tasks, and thus became the least desirable. This period is called the "Dark Age" and women were forced to work as servants.

COLONIAL AMERICAN PERIOD

Health care in the American colonies was sadly deficient. Almshouses or pesthouses were established to isolate people with infectious diseases. The first hospital in America was started in Philadelphia in 1751. The early hospitals were seen as places for immoral unfortunate people, who needed medical care. They were staffed by people who had some nursing or housekeeping experience.

In this period, image of the nurse was servant image.

NURSING IN THE 19TH CENTURY

Apart from the contributions of Florence Nightingale, the 19th century, also called period of the industrial revolution, saw Europe being devastated by poverty, famine and plague. Many groups sought to minister to the sick and poor during the crisis.

Florence Nightingale (1820–1910)

In the latter half of the 19th century, Florence Nightingale changed the form and direction of nursing, and made it a respected field of endeavor.

Born on May 12th, 1820, into a wealthy family, she was well-educated and well-cultured. Through the influence of the people she met, she desired to become a nurse.

In 1853, she started working with an establishment. She assisted with nursing care during the Crimean war with her group of 38 nurses. She was awarded the Order of Merit in 1907 by the Queen of England for her achievements.

In 1860, she devoted her efforts to the creation of a school of nursing at St Thomas Hospital in London. Florence Nightingale wrote extensively about nursing, hospitals, sanitation, health and nursing education until her death in 1910. Her work was a catapult for the reorganization and advancement of professional nursing. So she is honored as the founder of professional nursing. The Sisters of Charity of St Vincent de Paul attended to the sick and needy during the periods of crisis in Europe.

Kaiserswerth and his wife established the Deaconess Institute at Kaiserswerth, Germany, where Florence Nightingale trained for 3 months.

The International Red Cross was established in 1864.

During this period, image of the nurse was a respectable image/angel image.

NURSING IN THE 20TH CENTURY

Nurses gained a position of power in the health care industry during this period. Economic pressure to reform the health care system promised to improve the stature and opportunities for nurses in advanced practice roles. Nursing attained the status of a profession. Many educational institutions were started during this period. Graduate and postgraduate training programs in nursing were started. Statutory bodies for registration of qualified nurses came into being. Various organizations took birth. These organizations released publications as the official voice for nurses and nursing education. By 1990, certified nurse practitioners and nurse specialists worked independently and in joint practice with physicians.

During this period, the image of the nurse was a professional image.

During the 1970s and 1980s, a great deal of time and energy was invested in the study of the image of nursing. Since the 1970s the popular image of the nurse has not only failed to reflect changing professional conduct but also assumed derogatory traits that have underlined public confidence in and respect for the professional nurse.

Development of Organizations

- 1886—Visiting Nurses Association (Philadelphia)
- 1897—American Nurses Association
- 1900—Established American Journal of Nursing
- 1902—School of Nursing established in New York City by Linda Rogers
- 1903—The first Nurse Practice Acts were passed and registration of nurses implemented
- 1908—The Trained Nurses Association of India was established
- 1912—National League for Nursing (NLN)
- 1916—Cincinnati School of Nursing established a 5-year bachelor's degree program
- 1920—Founded Student Nurses Association of India
- 1922—Six nurses founded Sigma Theta Tau International Honor Society of Nursing
- 1941—Nurse Training Act passed
- 1946—Nurses were classified as professional by the US Civil Service Commission, and Hospital Survey and Construction (Hill-Burton) is passed
- 1973—Founded Commonwealth Nurses Federation and founded ICN

NURSING IN THE 21ST CENTURY

As nursing moves into the 21st century, it faces enormous challenges. The major health-related problems of this century are:
- An ongoing epidemic of blood borne diseases
- Civil war and related illnesses
- Substance abuse
- Poverty
- Homelessness
- Threat to public health and personal safety.

These challenges present opportunities to nursing as never before. While holding onto its commitment to care, nursing can meet these challenges by applying the intellectual energy, technical skill, organizational ability, clinical competence and ethical standards that typify the profession.

In the 21st century, major shifts have occurred in the health care delivery system. They are:
- Emphasis on community-based nursing
- Focus on health promotion and risk reduction
- Increased severity of illness in patient facilities coupled with major cost reductions and restructuring
- Increased incidents of chronic illnesses, especially in the growing number of the elderly

- Growth of integrated health care system using managed care approaches across multiple types of health care systems
- Increased need for a diverse compliment of health care providers to assure access to high quality care and positive outcomes.

These health care trends in many countries provide additional opportunities for nurses and nurse practitioners to contribute in new roles and settings.

DEVELOPMENT OF NURSING EDUCATION IN INDIA

The origin of nursing is from the history of Ayurveda and is as old as humans came into existence. Ayurveda gives nursing a significant place by making it one of the four legs on which therapeutics stands. The four legs are the physician, drugs, attendant and patient. Thus, the nurse was considered as important as the physician, medicine and patient.

Though there are scattered references to the art of nursing in ancient literature, no definite systematic practice of nursing is described before the period of Charaka and Sushruta. By the time of Charaka, nursing had already become an acknowledged part of therapy. It has been well said that, "nursing is an art: the master of an art has no end, you can always be a better nurse." Sushruta also defines the qualities of a nurse as "knowledgeable" devoted to helping patients "clever" and "pure" in body and mind.

The art of nursing attained a well-developed form during the reign of Emperor Ashoka. The Kashyapa Samhita bears ample testimony to the advance for this purpose in 1859. In 1857, the British East India Company turned Miss Nightingale's interest to the health of the army in India. A Royal Commission was appointed for this purpose in 1859. A group of 10 qualified nurses arrived in India in 1888 for the service of the British army. In 1905, nurses came to India as members of the Missionary Medical Association. This marked the start of formalized nursing service. The INC Act was passed by the Parliament in 1947.

Major Milestones of Nursing Education in India

Major milestones are as follows:
- 1871—School of Nursing started in a general hospital at Madras.
- 1886—School of Nursing, in a full-fledged form, was started in J J Hospital, Bombay.
- 1892—Many hospitals in Bombay started nursing associations which were intended to provide additional facilities for the training of local nurses.
- 1908—Trained Nurses Association of India (TNAI) was established.
- 1909—Bombay Presidency Nursing Association was formed.
- 1910—United Board of Examination for Nurses was organized.
- 1913—South India Board was organized.
- 1918—Lady Reading Health School was started in Delhi offering Health Visitors Course.
- 1926—First Nurse's Registration Act passed in Madras.
- 1931—Madras State first attempted to replace dais by qualified personnel such as midwives and nurse midwives.
- 1933—Training course started in the All India Institute of Hygiene and Public Health, Calcutta, women doctors for a diploma in Maternity and Child Welfare.
- 1935—Madras and Bombay Nursing Councils were established.
- 1942—ANM program started.
- 1943—School of Nursing, and in 1946, BSc Nursing Program was started at RAK College, New Delhi and in CMC, Vellore, and Diploma Program in Nursing Administration started in New Delhi.
- 1946—Bhore Committee (1943) submitted a report in which recommendations were made for the improvement of various aspects of nursing profession, nursing education and nursing research, working conditions, and nursing services in both hospitals and community, sending nurses for higher education abroad, etc.
- 1947—As per the recommendations of Bhore Committee, the central government granted approval for the establishment of two colleges of nursing in Delhi (1946) and Vellore (1947). These institutions provided university-level degree courses. Over the decades, there has been an improvement in the availability of nursing education in India. This has raised the level of Indian nurses to International Standards, and hence becoming the largest provider of trained nurses to various countries around the world.
- 1947—Indian Nursing Council Act, 1947 of Indian Parliament passed.
- 1953—Ms Edith Buchanan, Vice Principal, Rajkumari Amrit Kaur (RAK) College of Nursing, New Delhi, was the first nurse from India, who went to Columbia University to earn her Doctorate of Education (DEd) under the World Health Organization (WHO) fellowship program.
- 1959—Master of Nursing program was started at RAK College.
- 1960—First 2 years' master degree program in nursing was started by RAK College of Nursing, New Delhi, which included nursing research as a full subject with a thesis work on nursing topic.
- 1963—A study of health services was carried out in connection with the religion of syllabus of general nursing and midwifery by the INC.
- 1971—Post Basic of Bachelor Nursing (after GNM—2 years) and Bachelor of Nursing (BN—after general

degree—2 years) degree was started by Health Department as an experimental basis at the Government College of Nursing, Bangalore, and in 1977, the degree was renamed as PBBSc Nursing and Basic BSc Nursing. This is the Pioneer Institute of Nursing in Karnataka State and it is 5 decades old.

- 1986—For the first time, MPhil program in nursing started at RAK College of Nursing, University of Delhi, New Delhi.
- 1986—Curriculum changes took place for GNM program from 3.5 years to 3 years.
- 1987—MSc Nursing started in Kerala.
- 1987—Separate Directorate of Nursing was created in Karnataka State.
- 1988—MSc Nursing started in NIMHANS, Bangalore.
- 1992—PhD started in RAK College, New Delhi.
- 1992—Post BSc program started under IGNOU.
- 1994—MSc Nursing started in MAHE, Manipal.
- 1994—Basic BSc Nursing program under School of Medical Education at Mahatma Gandhi University, Kottayam.
- 1996—MPhil and PhD at MAHE, Manipal and Kottayam.
- 2000—MSc Nursing program started in Government College of Nursing under RGUHS.
- 2001—PhD Nursing started in NIMHANS, Bangalore.
- 2005—National PhD Nursing has been constituted by INC under the leadership of Shri T Dileep Kumar, President of INC, New Delhi in collaboration with RGUHS, Bangalore, six centers of College of Nursing designated as study centers, i.e. CMC-Ludhiana, Trivandrum, SNDT Women's University in Mumbai, CMC-Vellore, RAK College at New Delhi and St Johns Medical College Hospital, Bangalore. These centers are connected by video conferencing facilities to impart the education.
- 2005—INC revised syllabus for general nursing and midwifery course from 3 years to 3.5 years and Post Basic BSc Nursing.
- 2006 to 2007—ANM syllabus was revised.
- 2009—IGNOU started PhD Nursing programs.
- 2009—Revision of BSc and MSc Nursing course regulations and curriculum is done by INC and adapted in all states of India.
- 2010—Faculty of Nursing Sciences, Baba Farid University of Health Sciences, Faridkot, Punjab started PhD in Nursing.
- 2015 to 2016—Revision of GNM syllabus and decreased the duration from 3.5 years to 3 years by INC.

Recently in the 21st century, many private organizations and universities have started with PhD in Nursing in India.

CHARACTERISTICS OF NURSING PROFESSION

Greenwood (1957) and Etzioni (1961) also describe a classic work on professionalism in which the proposed five characteristics of a profession are as follows:

- A profession requires an extended education of its members as well as a basic liberal foundation.
- A profession has a theoretical body of knowledge leading to defined skills, abilities and norms.
- Profession provides a specific service.
- Members of a profession have autonomy in decision-making and practice.
- The profession as a whole has code of ethics for practice.

Education

As a profession, nursing requires that its members possess a significant amount of education. The issues of standardization of nursing education are major and demand for increase in education and services; professional organizations such as ANA and NLN also support a purpose that associate and diploma graduates take one licensing examinations. Every state implemented a policy that state board has authority to discrete, that only associate and baccalaureate degree graduates may set for practical and registered nursing licenses examinations, respectively.

Theory

As nursing emerged as a profession, a theory is the way of understanding a reality and all practicing nurses use the theories they have learned. Several approaches described on definitions and philosophies are artfully developed nursing theories.

Service

Nursing has been a service profession; although in the past, service was usually viewed as a charitable one. Today, nursing is a vital component of the health care delivery system.

Autonomy

Autonomy means that a person is reasonably independent and self-governing in decision-making and practice. It has been difficult for nurses to attain the degree of autonomy enjoyed by other professionals. In the past, gaining autonomy in health care delivery system was difficult. But because of greater educational preparation and clinical competence, nurses are increasingly taking on independent roles, collaborative practice and advanced nursing careers. With increased autonomy comes greater responsibility and accountability. The type and quality of nursing care is required to be legal, and the nurse is accountable for keeping abreast of technical skills and knowledge needed to perform nursing care provided. The nursing profession itself regulates accountability and standards of practice.

Code of Ethics

Nursing has a code of ethics, which defines the principles by which nurses function. In addition, nurses incorporate their own values and ethics into practice.

Regulation

Profession has their regulatory bodies, whose functions are to define, promote, oversee, support and regulate the affairs of its members. There may be several such bodies, e.g. state nursing councils.

Status, Prestige and Power

The most successful professions achieve high status, public prestige and rewards for their members and have clear legal authority over same activities. All professions require having technical, specialised, highly skilled work and need professional expertise. All professions have power. This power is used to control its own members, and also its area of expertise and interests. A profession is characterized by the power and high prestige it has in society as a whole.

CRITERIA OF THE PROFESSION

Many writers have listed the criteria of profession. The following are the prerequisite or criteria for a profession:

In General

- It should have fundamental truth that will make one free to think and act
- It should have the ability to apply truth in dealing with new problems
- It should have suitable techniques
- A profession should have an impressive body of knowledge
- It should concern with those that are relevant to human activities
- Profession should have relevant traditions
- It should be scholarly
- It should be able to meet the perplexities of changing knowledge, demands and social conditions wisely.

William Shephard (1948)

William Shephard listed the following criteria of profession:
- A profession must satisfy the social need, and based on well-established and socially accepted scientific principles, must have the responsibility for determining its own role and the society which is in need for its service
- It must give evidence of needed skills and practice
- It must have developed scientific techniques
- It must require the exercise of discretion and judgment as to time and manner of performance of duty
- It must be a type of beneficial work
- Profession must have group consciousness designed to extend scientific knowledge in technical language
- It must have sufficient self-impelling power to retain the members throughout life and it must not be used as a mere stepping stone to other occupation
- It must recognize the obligation to society by instituting that its members live up to an established code of ethics.

Kelly's Dimensions of Profession

According to Kelly, profession should have the following criteria:
- The work should be intellectual and distinguished by a substantial body of knowledge
- There should be provision of unique service to society
- It should have an expanded body of knowledge
- Personal responsibility to the public for services provided
- A long period of education including both theory and practice
- Autonomy and the ability to develop policy about the discipline and control of one's members
- Members share a common identity, values and attitudes
- Career choice of its members is motivated by altruism and reflects a long-term commitment to public
- A code of ethics to which its members adhere.

Is Nursing a Profession?

There have been many debates about whether nursing is a profession rather than an occupation. However, for nursing to be recognized as a profession by the society it serves, nursing meets the criteria of a profession. **Following are the criteria that support nursing as a profession:**
- Nursing requires knowledge, judgment and skills based on biological, sociological, psychological and other allied sciences including medical and nursing sciences.
- Nursing education is both theory and practical based, and more emphasis is given to practical skills and abilities.
- Nursing is having knowledge base. Nursing research, nursing theory, nursing publications and accreditation of schools and colleges of nursing have contributed the development of a nursing body of knowledge.
- Nurses are providing unique service to public through hospitals, community and in other settings.
- The RN is accountable for their negligence in care and thus accountable for the public through legal regulations and licenses.
- Professional nursing organizations have existed since the beginning of the 20th century in India. TNAI shares common values.
- Today both men and other background groups are entering nursing. RN and employed nurses are appointed on a regular basis such as other government employees.
- INC has published its code of ethics for nurses. Many of the values are identified within the codes thus establishing them as legal requirements.

- The aim of the nursing community is to develop the profession guided by continuing education based on nursing research and to regulate standards of competency and ethics. Nursing theorists and nurse researchers contribute to the knowledge base and thus provide the evidence-based nursing.
- The authority for the practice of nursing is based upon a social contract that delineates professional rights and responsibilities as well as public accountability.
- Each nurse irrespective of her qualification or position has a definite part to play as the member of nursing profession. Professional nurses provide health services to the individuals, families, the community and society as a whole. They coordinate their services with members of other health team or profession.

PERSPECTIVES OF NURSING PROFESSION

Introduction

Nursing is not a static, mechanizing profession but is continuously growing and evolving as society changes, as health care emphasis and methods change, and as lifestyles change. The current philosophers and definitions of nursing demonstrate the holistic bend in nursing to address a whole person in all dimensions in health and illness and in interaction with the family and community. Nursing continues to draw on the social sciences and other fields at the focus of nursing care expands. A trend is a general direction to follow in the field of nursing education or practice. Several changing perspectives which are apparent in the nursing profession are subtle and emerge slowly, where others are obvious and seem to surface quickly. A number of perspectives are apparent today. Perspective of nursing profession has been discussed in the history and development of nursing profession. Some of the national and global perspectives are as follows.

At the National Level

Nursing profession prepares nurses to practice in a variety of settings. There are tremendous changes in nursing education due to modernization, globalization and liberalization of the society. Significant trends in modern education changes teaching, learning process and advanced educational technology.
- The scientific and technological advances in medicine along with social changes resulted in emergence of specialists and superspecialties. Advanced nursing practice enables to practice in new roles from traditional roles. For example, nurse practitioners, clinical nurse specialists, etc.
- Nursing profession ensures a promising career in India with good job opportunities in abroad.
- Increase in number of educational institutions with postgraduate education programs.
- The rapidly changing health care system requires nurses to possess increasing knowledge, clinical competency, greater independence and anatomy in clinical judgments.
- Trends towards community-based nursing centers, private case management, complexity of measuring homecare, all are rapidly raising the educational needs of nurses.
- Issues and trends in nursing education challenge the student and nurse educators to bring changes in curriculum, numerous types of education programs and address the need for increased man power.

Issues of Nursing Profession

- Nursing shortage
- Mushrooming of nursing schools and colleges have led to fall in standards of education
- Increase in distance learning programs
- Evidence-based practice
- Culturally competent nursing
- Decreased length of hospital stay
- Aging population
- More chronic health needs
- Independent practitioner roles
- Emerging of newer diseases—communicable and non-communicable diseases
- Alternate curriculum plans such as in-service education programs, continuing education and distance education for students who seek higher qualifications
- With large number of graduates passing out every year, it is a challenge to maintain quality in nursing education and completely in the job
- Faculty of nursing institutions play an important role, which is being a role model for the future generations of nursing fraternity in showing the philosophy, ethics and standards of nursing profession
- In developed countries, great emphasis is given on preparing nurses with critical thinking and problem solving skills.

Role of Nurse Educator in the 21st Century

These are many national reports indicating the need for change in health care and in the education of health care professionals in particular.

Emphasis on Student Centered Teaching

Over the past decade, education has shifted from a teacher centered to student centered approach.
- Always focus on the outcomes of leaving rather than on understanding the process involved in learning.
- Research aimed at understanding how students learn results in the development of best practices in teaching. For example, use concept of critical thinking

exercises and skillful assessment of student learning outcomes.

Promotion of Evidence-based Practice

- ❖ The primary focus of health care institution. Today, there is number of provision of quality care within cost effective framework.
- ❖ Movement toward evidence-based practice requires that educators and practitioners engage in collaborative research.

Emphasis on Authentic Student–Teacher Relationship

There is evidence to suggest that a good, thoughtful student-teacher relationship is essential for students to develop and grow. There should be change in traditional behaviorist model of teaching to humanistic approach that recognizes students have their own experiences that enrich learning by their participation in learning.

Confidence

The ability to teach in a student centered way requires considerable confidence in one's professional knowledge and teaching skills. The teacher should develop confidence in a firm grounding in the pedagogy/andragogy of the teaching-learning experience.

Focusing on Student Needs

Student centered teaching should focus on student needs, rather than imposing what teacher believes in essential to learn as "letting learn," explore and discover what they want and need to know.

Critical Reflecting

An underlying assumption in much of the relevant literature in nursing education is that of a critically reflective teacher who is committed in engaging students in reflection and on achieving pre-determined goals.

Learning Partnership

Student centered teaching occurs within a community of partnership of learners. The process of learning within partnership transcends mere content knowledge.

The Learning Setting

Different learning settings pose challenges to nurse educators' intension to use student centered teaching approaches.

Some vital recommendations of the Bhore Committee relevant to nursing profession are given below:

- ❖ **Stipend for nursing students**: In order to prevent economic barrier in the way of suitable persons entering the nursing profession, the committee suggested the provision of Rs. 60/student nurses, but now it is the concept laid by Bhore.
- ❖ **Nurses, midwives and dais**: The committee suggested that by 1971 the number of trained nurses available in country should be raised to 740,000. As an essential step towards the requirements of this objective was the removal of the existing, unsatisfied factor candidates of training and service. The committee made a proposal to improve the situation.
- ❖ **Training of nurses and midwives**: In view of the extreme storage of nursing personnel, the committee recommended that the first group of 100 training centers, each taking 50 pupils, should be started 2 years before the health organization began to be established and that another set of 100 training centers should be created during the first 2 years of the schemes, and that a third group of the same number of training centers should be established before the third year of the second quinquennium (5-year plan).
- ❖ **Male nurses**: Male nurses should be trained and employed in large numbers in the male wards and male outpatient departments of public hospitals, thus releasing women workers for other work.
- ❖ **Public health nurses**: The committee also made specific proposals with regard to the training of the public health nurses. This should be fully qualified nurses with training in midwifery as well.
- ❖ **Midwives**: The number of midwives actually available for midwifery duties in the country was probably 5,000. The committee let down certain fundamental requirements which should be met before an institution could be organized as a training center for midwives.
- ❖ **Dais**: The continued employment of women as dais was inevitable. The committee advocated the training of dais as an interior measure until an adequate number of midwives would become available.
- ❖ **Nursing staff**: The report recommended to produce another category of nursing health personnel called auxiliary personnel. Auxiliary nurse midwives training was started to meet the health needs of the country.

At Global Level

A global perspective is defined as a personnel outlook that considers situations from a broader view point and more critical consideration of experiences. A global perspective incorporates personnel knowledge to enable global issues and the role of the individual country in the developing global economic technological and communicative networks; global perspective of nursing education is discussed below:

"It is nurses—of every stripe—who will deliver, coordinate and direct care in hospital, civil and physician's office, and it is this same most necessary nurses who act in Short Slipp until the pipeline for advanced education in nursing is flowing freely, the nation's nurses work force will have difficulty achieving its potential"

—Barron McBride

- Changes in professional roles and movement of people across national and international boundaries make it important to understand health care and nursing issues in a global context.
- As students travel abroad to receive their education, study abroad programs broaden students' perspectives as students learn about difficult cultures and the values make them to accept cultural difficulties in patients and co-workers.
- While studying abroad gives students an opportunity to understand nursing practice and education in different cultures brings cultural diversity and experiences to one's door step, it challenges us to adapt a global perspective.
- International collaboration brings together nurses with similar research interests who share their knowledge and talents, resources to address the common areas of concern.
- Teaching faculties are collaborating with international researchers in the areas of chronic disease, technology and genetics.
- Many Indian universities have tie-ups with foreign universities; there is student re-change program and facility development program which enrich the academic environment to bring new ideas and perspective to their work.
- The institution collaborates in scholarly exchange and research collaboration among facility information and teaching methods.
- Social media has been used globally as a key vehicle for communication. As members of an innovative profession, many nurses have embraced social media and are actively utilizing its potential to enhance practice and improve health. The ubiquity of the Internet provides social media with the potential to improve both access to health information and services and equity in health care. Thus, there are a number of successful nurse-led initiatives. However, the open and democratizing nature of social media creates a number of potential risks, both individual and organizational.

Global Pattern of Nursing Education

- **Baccalaureate education**: The degree program usually encompasses 4 years of study in a college/university; the program focuses on basic sciences and on theoretical and chemical causes as well as courses in social science, arts and humanities to support the nursing theory. In Canada, BSc in Nursing or BN is equivalent to the degree of Bachelors of Science in Nursing (BSN) in the United States. RN completion programs are available at many colleges and universities, and these programs are designed to assist the practicing RN in obtaining a baccalaureate degree in nursing.
- **Diploma education**: The diploma program in the United States is a 2–3 years' hospital-based program; diploma programs focused on the basic sciences and on theoretical and clinical census related to nursing practice with a substantial clinical component.
- **Associate degree education**: In the United States, it is a 2-year program that is usually offered by a university or junior college; this program focuses on the basic sciences, theoretical and chemical courses related to the practice of nursing.
- **Master degree preparation**: A person completing a graduate program can receive the Degree of Masters in Arts, MA in Nursing or Master of Science in nursing, and this provides the advanced clinical with strong skills in nursing sciences and research based on clinical practice. They can be valuable for nurses seeking roles of nursing education. Chemical nurse specialist nurse administration and practitioners.
- **Doctoral preparation**: The first nursing doctoral program was started in 1953 at the University of Pittsburgh. Other programs emphasized on basic research and theory and awarded the Degree of Doctor of Philosophy (PhD).
- **Licensed practical nurse education**: A licensed practical or occasional nurse is trained in basic nursing techniques and direct client care. The licensed practical nurse (LPN) or licensed vocational nurse (LVN) practices under the supervision of a RN in a hospital or community health practice setting.
- **Accreditation and licensure**: To be accredited, the nursing program must meet certain criteria established by the National League for Nursing Accrediting Commission (NLNAC). This voluntary accreditation is available for basic nursing education programs and Master degree programs in nursing.
  In the United States, RN candidates must pass the National Council Licensure Examination for Registered Nurses (NCLEX-RN), which is administrated by the individual State Board of nursing. Regardless of educational preparation, the examination for RN Licensure is same in every state in the United States.
- **Certification**: Beyond the NCLEX-RN, National Nursing Organization, such as ANA, has many types of certification that a nurse can work towards. After passing the initial examination, the nurse maintains certification by continuing education and clinical administrative practice.
- **Continuing education and in-service education**: Continuing education involves formal organized and educational programs preferred by State Nurses Associations and Educational Healthcare institutions. Other goals including helping nurses become specialized in particular areas of practice and teaching nurses new skills and techniques.

CONCLUSION

As a developing profession, nursing has transitioned from the prehistoric era to the present through four phases, i.e. complacency, constraint, change and challenge.

Each of these phases represents the various periods discussed in the development of nursing. From the phase of complacency during the prehistoric and ancient periods, to the Dark Ages when women and nurses were constrained by the rules of the prevailing society, to the period of Florence Nightingale, when the most dramatic changes were brought about to the present day state, when nursing has become a profession with all its challenges and definitions. As a profession, nursing has made tremendous advancements in the areas of education, practice, and research and technology development. Today nurses continue to be challenged to expand their role and explore newer areas of practice and leadership. Presently, professional nurses are in a key position to promote health and advance the well-being of individuals, families, communities and the nation.

Perspectives of nursing professions are very broad concerned to the field of nursing education and practice; some of the perspectives are discussed.

CHAPTER 2

Code of Ethics and Code of Professional Conduct

CHAPTER OUTLINE

- Ethics
- Morals
- Values
- Code of Ethics
- Code of Ethics in Nursing
  - Indian Nursing Council Code of Ethics
- American Nurses Association (ANA)
- International Council of Nurses (ICN)
- Canadian Nurses Association (CNA)
- Ethical Principles
- Ethical Philosophical Theories
- Ethical Dilemmas

INTRODUCTION

Ethics is a science relating to moral actions and one's value system. Ethics is the study of standards for professional behavior related to right and wrong professional conduct. Concern with ethical issues in health care has increased dramatically in the last two decades. Nursing ethics is a system of principles concerning the actions of the nurse in his/her relationship with clients, clients' family members, other healthcare providers and society as a whole or the code governing a nurse's behavior with patients and their relatives and with colleagues.

ETHICS

Meaning

The word ethics comes from the Greek word "ethos" meaning custom or guiding beliefs.

Definitions

- Ethics is the study of standards for professional behavior related to right and wrong professional conduct.
  —**Potter and Perry**
- Ethics are the rules or principles that deal with what is good and bad with moral duty and obligations. Ethics are designed to protect the rights to human beings.
- A broader conceptual definition of ethics is that concerned with motives and attitudes, and the relationship of these attitudes to the good of the individual.
- Ethics reflects the principles or standards that govern proper conduct related to professional behaviors. The values of the client, nurse and society interact to set the environment for ethical behavior (Table 2.1).

Table 2.1: Distinguish between law and ethics.

Ethics	Law
Ethics is the study of standards for professional behavior related to right and wrong professional conduct	The law comprised of rules and regulations pertinent to society as a whole, and is external to one self and concerns one's actions and conduct
Ethics concerns the good of an individual within society	Law concerns society as a whole as opposed to the individual in society
Ethics are enforced via ethics committees and professional codes	Law can be enforced through the courts on statutes

MORALS

A moral belief is the personal conviction that something is absolutely right or wrong in all situations. A person is generally unwilling to change personal opinions on issues of moral nature. To one person, for example, abortion may be an absolute moral; in other words, there are no acceptable reasons for a woman to end a pregnancy prematurely. A moral issue becomes an ethical one when the choice is no longer clear between right and wrong.

VALUES

Values are interwoven with ethics; values are personal beliefs about the truth and worth of thoughts, objects and behavior. Values are based on experience, religion, education and culture. Values are the building blocks for the development of morals (personal conduct) and ethics (professional conduct). Changes in values produce changes in attitude and behaviors.

Values vary among people, and understanding one's own value system and assessing others value system helps to facilitate decision-making and ensures respect for client autonomy.

CODE OF ETHICS

Ethics are characteristics of a profession and are called "codes." The code of ethics will state what kind of conduct is expected from the members of a profession, and the responsibilities towards the people they serve, their co-workers, their profession and the society as a whole. When a person becomes a member of a profession he/she accepts the responsibility of living up to the code of ethics of that profession. In nursing, code of ethics provides professional standards for nursing activities, which protects the nurse and the patient (see Table 2.1).

CODE OF ETHICS IN NURSING

Nursing has a code of ethics that defines the principles by which nurses function. Nursing ethics states the duties and obligations of nurses to their clients, other health professional, the profession and the community; ethics promotes the philosophical and theological study of morality, moral judgments and moral problems.

A code of ethics is a set of ethical principles that are accepted by all members of a profession. Codes serve as guidelines to assist nurses and other professional groups when conflict or disagreement arises about correct practice or behavior. There are several codes for professional nurses, which are:
1. Indian Nursing Council Code of Ethics
2. American Nurses Association (ANA)
3. International Council of Nurses (ICN)
4. Canadian Nurses Association (CNA)

They have established widely accepted codes that professional nurses attempt to follow.

Indian Nursing Council Code of Ethics

Code of Ethics for Nurses in India

❖ **The nurse respects the uniqueness of individual in provision of care**
  ➢ Provides care for individuals without consideration of caste, creed, religion, culture, ethnicity, gender, socioeconomic and political status, personal attributes, or any other grounds.
  ➢ Individualizes the care considering the beliefs, values and cultural sensitivities.
  ➢ Appreciates the place of individual in the family and community and facilitates participation of significant others in the care.
  ➢ Develops and promotes trustful relationship with individual(s).
  ➢ Recognizes uniqueness of response of individuals to interventions and adapts accordingly.

❖ **The nurse respects the rights of individuals as partner in care and helps in making informed choice**
  ➢ Appreciates individual's right to make decisions about their care and therefore gives adequate and accurate information for enabling them to make informed choices.
  ➢ Respects the decisions made by individual(s) regarding their care.
  ➢ Protects public from misinformation and misinterpretations.
  ➢ Advocates special provision to protect vulnerable individuals/groups.

❖ **The nurse respects individual's right to privacy, maintains confidentiality and shares information judiciously**
  ➢ Respects the individual's right to privacy of their personal information.
  ➢ Maintains confidentiality of privileged information except in life threatening situations and uses discretion in sharing information.
  ➢ Takes informed consent and maintains anonymity when information is required for quality assurance/academic/legal reasons.
  ➢ Limits the access to all personal records written and computerized to authorized persons only.

❖ **Nurse maintains competence in order to render quality nursing care**
  ➢ Nursing care must be provided only by registered nurse.
  ➢ Nurse strives to maintain quality nursing care and upholds the standards of care.
  ➢ Nurse values continuing education, initiates and utilizes all opportunities for self-development.
  ➢ Nurses value research as a means of development of nursing profession and participate in nursing research adhering to ethical principles.

❖ **The nurse if obliged to practice within the framework of ethical, professional and legal boundaries**
  ➢ Adheres to code of ethics and code of professional conduct for nurses in India developed by Indian Nursing Council.
  ➢ Familiarizes with relevant laws and practices in accordance with the law of the state.

❖ **Nurse is obliged to work harmoniously with members of the health team**
  ➢ Appreciates the team efforts in rendering care.
  ➢ Cooperates, coordinates and collaborates with members of the health team to meet the needs of people.

❖ **Nurse commits to reciprocate the trust invested in nursing profession by society**
  ➢ Demonstrates personal etiquettes in all dealings.
  ➢ Demonstrates professional attributes in all dealings.

Chapter 2: Code of Ethics and Code of Professional Conduct

Code of Professional Conduct for Nurses in India

- **Professional responsibility and accountability**
  - Appreciates sense of self-worth and nurtures it.
  - Maintains standards of personal conduct reflecting credit upon the profession.
  - Carries out responsibilities within the framework of the professional boundaries.
  - Is accountable for maintaining practice standards set by Indian Nursing Council.
  - Is accountable for own decisions and actions.
  - Is compassionate.
  - Is responsible for continuous improvement of current practices.
  - Provides adequate information to individuals, which allows them informed choices, and practices healthful behavior.

- **Nursing practice**
  - Provides care in accordance with set standards of practice.
  - Treats all individuals and families with human dignity in providing physical, psychological, emotional, social and spiritual aspects of care.
  - Respects individuals and families in the context of traditional and cultural practices, promoting healthy practices and discouraging harmful practices.
  - Presents realistic picture truthfully in all situations for facilitating autonomous decision-making by individuals and families.
  - Promotes participation of individuals and significant others in the care.
  - Ensures safe practice.
  - Consults, coordinates, collaborates and follows up appropriately when individuals care needs exceed the nurse's competence.

- **Communication and interpersonal relationships**
  - Establishes and maintains effective interpersonal relationships with individuals, families and communities
  - Upholds the dignity of team members and maintains effective interpersonal relationship with them.
  - Appreciates and nurtures professional role of team members.
  - Cooperates with other health professional to meet the needs of the individuals, families and communities.

- **Valuing human being**
  - Takes appropriate action to protect individuals from harmful unethical practice.
  - Considers relevant facts while taking conscience decisions in the best interest of individuals.
  - Encourages and supports individuals in their right to speak for themselves on issues affecting their health and welfare.
  - Respects and supports choices made by individuals.

- **Management**
  - Ensures appropriate allocation and utilization of available resources.
  - Participates in supervision and education of students and other formal care providers.
  - Uses judgment in relation to individual competence while accepting and delegating responsibility.
  - Facilitates conductive work culture in order to achieve institutional objectives.
  - Communicates effectively following appropriate channels of communication.
  - Participates in performance appraisal.
  - Participates in evaluation of nursing services.
  - Participates in policy decisions, following the principle of equity and accessibility of services.
  - Works with individuals to identify their needs and sensitizes policy-makers and funding agencies for resource allocation.

- **Professional advancement**
  - Ensures the protection of the human rights while pursuing the advancement of knowledge.
  - Contributes to the development of nursing practice.
  - Participates in determining and implementing quality care.
  - Takes responsibility for updating own knowledge and competencies.
  - Contributes to the core of professional knowledge by conducting and participating in research.

American Nurses Association: Code of Ethics

The need of a code of ethics was expressed by the nurses associated alumnae (fore runner of the ANA as early as 1897). A written code was actually adopted in 1950. During that 53-year span, nursing was emerging as a profession.

The 1950 code consisted of 17 short statements depicting the nurse in action. In 1958, the ANA's committee on ethical standards began reviewing the entire code and in 1960, major revisions were suggested. The 1960 code also contained 17 statements that addressed nurses' responsibilities to participate in the professional organization and the necessity of identifying and upholding professional organizational standards. The next major revision of the code which was completed in 1976 resulted in 11 statements. The emphasis of the 1976 code was the nurse's relationship to the client. No longer was the word patient used, client was adopted in the belief that it was a more inclusive term than patient.

In 1985, the code was again reviewed. All 11 statements remained the same, but the interpretations were updated. In particular, more emphasis was placed on clients' rights. The 1985 code for nurses is the latest version of nursing's ethical code.

The following are the ANA code of ethics:
1. The nurse provides services with respect for human dignity and the uniqueness of the client unrestricted by

considerations of social or economic status, personal attributes or the nature of health problems. Protecting information of a confidential nature.
2. The nurse acts to safeguard the client and the public when health care and safety are affected by the incompetent unethical or illegal practice of any person.
3. The nurse assumes responsibility and accountability for individual nursing judgments and actions.
4. The nurse maintains competence in nursing.
5. The nurse exercises informed judgment, and uses individual competence and qualifications as criteria in seeking consultation accepting responsibilities, and delegating nursing activities to others.
6. The nurse participates in activities that contribute to the ongoing development of the profession's efforts to implement and improve standards of nursing.
7. The nurse participates in the profession's efforts to establish and maintain conditions of employment conducive to high-quality nursing care.
8. The nurse participates in the profession's effort to protect the public form misinformation and misrepresentation and to maintain the integrity of nursing.
9. The nurse collaborates with members of the health professionals and other citizens in promoting community and national efforts to meet the health needs of the public.

International Council of Nurses (ICN): Code for Nurses

The ICN (1973) also has published a code of ethics for the profession. This document discusses the rights and responsibilities of a nurse related to people, practice, society, co-workers and the profession. The ICN first adopted a code of ethics in 1953. Its last revision in 1973 represents agreement by more than 80 national nursing associations that participate in the international association. Inherent in the ICN code for nurses is nursing's respect for the life, dignity and integrity of all people unmindful of nationality, race, creed, color, age, sex and political affiliation or status.

—Mitchell and Grippando, 1993

Preamble

Fundamental responsibilities of nurses includes the following:
- Promote health, to prevent illness, to restore health and to alleviate suffering.
- The need for nursing is universal. Inherent in nursing is respect of life, dignity and rights of man. It is unrestricted by considerations of nationality, race, creed, color, age, sex, politics or social status.
- Nurses render health services to the individuals, the family and the community, and coordinate their services with those of related groups.

Elements of the Code

The ICN code of ethics for nurses has elements that outline the standards of ethics conduct.
1. **Nurses and people:**
    - The nurse's primary responsibility is to those people who require nursing care.
    - The nurse, in providing care, promotes an environment in which the values, customs and spiritual beliefs of the individual are respected.
    - The nurse holds in confidence personal information and uses judgment in sharing this information.
2. **Nurses and practice:**
    - The nurse carries responsibility for nursing practice and for maintaining competence by continual learning. The nurse maintains the highest standards of nursing care possible within the reality of a specific situation.
    - The nurse uses judgment in relation to individual competence when accepting and delegating responsibilities.
    - The nurses when acting in a professional capacity should at all times maintain standards of personal conduct, which reflect credit upon the profession.
3. **Nurses and society:** The nurse shares with other citizens, the responsibility for initiating and supporting action to meet the health and social needs of the public.
4. **Nurses and co-workers:** The nurse sustains a cooperative relationship with co-workers in nursing and other fields. The nurse takes appropriate action to safeguard the individual when his/her care is endangered by a co-worker or any other person.
5. **Nurses and the profession:** The nurse plays the major role in determining and implementing desirable standards of nursing practice and nursing education. Ethical problems require them to think, and reason in making decisions, judgments and choices.

Canadian Nurses Association: Code of Ethics

Health and Well-being

Nurses value health and well-being, and assist persons to achieve their optimum level of health in situations of normal health illness, injury or in the process of dying:
1. **Choice:** Nurses respect and promote autonomy of clients, and help them to express their health needs and values, and to obtain appropriate information and services.
2. **Dignity:** Nurses value and advocate the dignity of self-respect of human beings.
3. **Confidentiality:** Nurses safeguard the trust of clients so that information learned in the context of professional relationship is shared outside the health care team only with the client's permission or as legally required.

4. **Fairness:** Nurses apply and promote principles of equity and fairness to assist clients in receiving unbiased treatment and a share of health services, and resumes proportionate to their needs.
5. **Accountability:** Nurses act in a manner consistent with their professional responsibilities and standards of practice.
6. **Practice environments:** Conducive to safe, competent and ethical care, nurses advocate practice environments that have the organizational and human support systems, and the resource allocations necessary for sale, competent, ethical nursing care, etc.

ETHICAL PRINCIPLES

A set of ethical principles that all members of a profession generally accept are:
- Respect for persons is the most fundamental human right (Aroskar 1995). It requires that each person be respected as a unique individual that is equal to all others. This means valuing every aspect of a person's life not just the parts that are easy to value because they are congruent with your own values. Respect for persons is the foundation for all ethical principles.
- The ethical principles within the ANA code provide a foundation for nursing practice. Beauchamp and Childress also identify respect for autonomy, beneficence, non-maleficence and justice as the basic ethical principles (Flowchart 2.1).

Primary Principles of Ethics

1. *Autonomy:* Autonomy refers to a person's independence. As a standard in ethics, autonomy represents an agreement to respect another's right to determine a course of action.

   Autonomy is fundamental to the practice of health care. It serves to justify the inclusion of clients in all aspects of decision-making regarding their health care. The agreement to respect autonomy involves the recognition that clients are in charge of their own destiny in matters of health and illness.

   For example, the purpose of the preoperative consent that clients must read and sign before surgery is the assurance in writing that the health care team respects the client's independence by obtaining permission to proceed. The consent process implies that a client may refuse treatment, and in most cases, the health care team must agree to follow the client's wishes. Health care professionals agree to abide by a standard of respect for the client's autonomy.

2. *Beneficence:* Beneficence is commonly defined as doing good. It refers to taking positive actions to help others. The principle of beneficence has four components. Inflict no harm or evil, prevent harm and evil, remove harm and evil, and promote good. As nurses, we are morally obligated to protect the patient from harm. In clinical situations, however, it is often difficult to draw the line between not inflicting harm and preventing or removing harmful situations. For example, the nurse at the well-baby clinic who immunizes children for diphtheria, whooping cough and tetanus inflicts some degree of harm or pain, however, the benefit of being protected against whooping cough is more important. Another example is the case of the client who must receive surgical treatment. Surgery for cancer of the bowel can be seen as inflicting harm, however, the benefit of removing the tumor for the client generally outweighs the harm related to the risk of surgery.

   It requires the balancing of harms and benefits. Benefits promote the client's welfare and health, whereas harms or risks detract from the client's health or welfare. Nurses and physicians must consider the risks and benefits when making decisions related to treatment and research.

3. *Non-maleficence:* Non-maleficence refers to harm or hurt, and thus no maleficence refers to avoidance of harm or hurt. In health care ethics, it is important to remember that ethical practice involves not only the will to do good but also the equal commitment to do no harm. The health care professional tries to balance the risks and benefits of a plan of care while striving to do the least harm possible. The principles of beneficence and no maleficence direct nurses to promote good and avoid causing harm.

4. *Justice:* Justice refers to fairness. The principle of justice holds that a person should be treated according to what is fair, given what is due or owed. This implies that patients with the same diagnosis should receive the same level of care. The term often is used during discussions about resources. What constitutes a fair distribution of resources may not always be clear. In these cases, national discussion about just distribution of resources often helps to clarify methods for achieving fairness. For example, the number of candidates awaiting liver transplants is approximately three times larger than the number of available organs for transplantation. Decisions about who should receive available organs are always difficult. Criteria set by a national multidisciplinary committee strive for profit, which would favor recipients

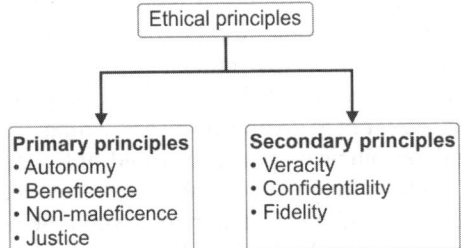

Flowchart 2.1: Types of ethical principles.

with the most money and preferable to distributing without regard to justice. To ensure that all individuals are treated equally—each person considered an equal share, each person according to individual effort, each person according to societal contribution and each person according to merit.

Secondary Principles of Ethics

The secondary principles of ethical conduct outlined in the ANA code of nurses include veracity, confidentiality and fidelity.

1. *Veracity:* Veracity is defined as truth telling the basis for effective communication. As a part of the nursing code of ethics, veracity guides nurses to practice truthfulness. Patients are not always truthful in their disclosure of health histories or practices and some providers may withhold the truth on the basis of "beneficence" feeling that full disclosure may do more harm than good.
2. *Confidentiality:* Confidentiality is a basic ethical principle that ensures a client's privacy. Nurses avoid discussing the condition of a client with anyone who is not involved in the client's care. Often a dilemma arises when a client chooses to keep confidential information that places the client or others at risk. An example is the client who is suffering from acquired immunodeficiency syndrome (AIDS) and chooses not to reveal the diagnosis to family members. If family members will assume the health information of the client, the nurse may believe that they have the right to be properly informed.
3. *Fidelity:* Fidelity refers to the agreement to keep promises. For example, if a nurse assesses a client for pain and then offers a plan to manage the pain, the standard of fidelity encourages the nurse to monitor the client's response to the plan. Professional behavior by the nurse includes revision of the plan as necessary to try to keep the promise to reduce pain.

ETHICAL PHILOSOPHICAL THEORIES

- A theory in any field is an organized explanation of particular phenomena. Explanation in a theory is accomplished by principles or basic premises assumed to be true based on evidence.
- Ethical theories are ethical principles and their corresponding rules to explain what constitutes ethical behavior.
- Ethical theory is a system of principles by which a person can determine what ought and ought not to be done.

There are two main theories proposed in ethics, which are utilitarianism and deontology.

Utilitarianism

Utilitarianism theory was first described by David Hume (1711-1779) and was developed further by many notable philosophers including Jeremy Bentham (1748-1826) and John Staurt Mill (1806-1873). Mill had a significant influence on utilitarian ethics as we know it today.

According to Mill (1985, originally published in 1863) a "right action" conforms to the "greatest happiness principle." In other words, it is the right to maximize the greatest good for the happiness or pleasure of the greatest number of people. It is a pragmatic approach that is concerned with the consequences of actions more than the actual actions themselves. If the outcome is positive, the method of arriving at that outcome is less important.

A utilitarian system of ethics proposes that the value of something is determined by its usefulness. This philosophy may also be known as consequentialism, since its main emphasis is on the outcome or consequence of action. A third term associated with this philosophy is teleology, from the Greek word telos, meaning "end," or the study of ends or final causes. The greatest good for the greatest number of people is the guiding principle for determining right action in this system. As with deontology, this theory relies on the application of a certain principle, namely, measures of "good" and "greatest" (Beauchamp and Childress, 1989). The difference between utilitarianism and deontology is in the focus on consequences or outcomes.

Utilitarianism measures the effect that an act will have; deontology looks into the presence of principle regardless of outcome.

Individuals or groups of individuals may have conflicting definitions of "greatest good." For example, research suggests that education regarding safe sex practices may reduce the spread of human immunodeficiency virus (HIV). But some argue that education about sex should be provided in the family and that sex education in public schools diminishes the role and the value of family. For some, the greater good is defined as educating the greatest number of people in the most effective way possible. For others, the greater good is the preservation of family values and the protection of individual choices regarding sex education of children. The concepts of utilitarianism provide guidance, but they do not inevitably provide answers with universal agreement.

Deontology

The major proponent of deontology was Immanuel Kant (1724-1804). Kant (1985; originally translated in 1959) believed that the tightness or wrongness of an action depends on the inherent moral significance of the action. He believed that an act was moral if it originated from good will. Ethical action consisted in doing one's duty. To do one's duty was right; not to do one's duty was wrong.

The deontological approach would not consider the quality of life or weigh the use of scarce resources against the likelihood that the life maintained would be normal.

Deontology can be further divided into either act or rule:

1. ***Act deontologists:*** Determine the right thing to do by gathering the facts and then making a decision. Much time and energy are needed to judge each situation carefully in and of itself. Once a decision is made, there is commitment to universalizing it. In other words, if one makes a moral judgment in one situation, the same judgment will be made in any similar situation.
2. ***Rule deontologists:*** Emphasize that principles guide the actions. Examples of rules might be "always keep a promise" or "never tell a lie." In all situations, the rule is to be followed. Deontologists are not concerned with the consequences of always following certain rules or actions. If the principle believed in is "always keep a promise," the deontologist will keep promises, even if circumstances have changed. For example, if a father has promised that he will take his son to a baseball game and then a close family member becomes critically ill, the baseball game promise will be kept regardless of the changed circumstances.

In nursing, there are many rules and duties that nurses follow. One such rule is "Do No Harm" (beneficence). Another justifiable rule is "the patient should be allowed to make his or her own decisions" (autonomy). Consider the situation of a severely depressed young man who wishes to end his life by committing suicide and asks the nurse's assistance clearly the rule about doing no harm conflicts with allowing the young man to make his own decision. You can see that dilemmas cannot always be resolved using theoretical approaches alone.

ETHICAL DILEMMAS

Nurses are the largest group of caregivers in healthcare industry. We provide the majority of care on a day-to-day, minute-to-minute basis. The nurse is the most accessible health care provider and even the nature of the nurse–patient relationship is of respect and dignity. That nurses would be confronted with frequent ethical dilemmas. In fact, 79% of the 934 nurses responded to a survey conducted by the Center for Ethics and Human Rights the ANA convention in June 1994 reported confronting ethical problems on either a daily or weekly basis. Ethical dilemmas most frequently involved one of the following.

Each ethical dilemma will be different. However, the nurse in any setting can follow a model for ethical decision-making to increase the probability that all factors are weighed equally.

Process for an Ethical Decision-Making Model (Resolution of Ethical Dilemma) (Flowchart 2.2)

When faced with an ethical dilemma, the following steps should help you determine a course of action. Osteoporosis is a tendency to wander and with a history of falls. Ms Smith has an intravenous (IV) in her left forearm, which was difficult to establish. Concerned that Ms Smith might pull out her IV, wander off the floor or fall, the staff believes it would be best to restrain her. Ms Smith, however, repeatedly declares that she does not want to be restrained:

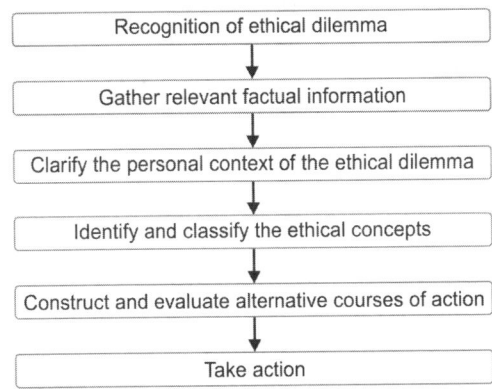

Flowchart 2.2: Process of an ethical decision-making model dilemma.

- ❖ ***Clarify the ethical dilemma:*** This scenario presents a common ethical dilemma. As the nurse responsible for Ms Smith, you need to decide whether to act on the basis of beneficence (specifically, no maleficence—avoiding the possibility of a fall) or on the basis of autonomy (supporting the patient's decision or request).
- ❖ ***Gather additional data:*** Your course of action depends on the additional information you gather.
  Is Ms Smith able to understand that she could harm herself by getting out of bed without assistance? How does the family feel about restraints? What hospital policies relate to this situation?
- ❖ ***Identify options:*** Have all other attempts to help Ms Smith maintain her independence failed? For example, has the staff tried keeping the bed's four side rails up and the call bell within reach? Are they making frequent checks and reminding her to call for assistance? Is there staff available to perform checks every half-hour? Could a sitter be provided? Are there available family friends who might be able to stay with Ms Smith? How long will IV be necessary.
- ❖ ***Make a decision:*** The family says they can stay with Ms Smith as long as she needs the IV. When the IV is no longer necessary, it is hoped that Ms Smith can be discharged to more familiar surroundings.
- ❖ ***Act:*** In this situation, it is essential for the staff and family members to work together to provide patient safeguard and be sure the family members are available to stay with Ms Smith around the clock.

CONCLUSION

Code of ethics are principles by which nurses' function. Different professional organizations laid their view on the code of ethics. The code of ethics acts as a general guide for the nurses in their practice. Ethical problems require to think and reason to make decisions, judgment and choices.

3

CHAPTER

Autonomy, Accountability, Assertiveness and Visibility of Nurses

CHAPTER OUTLINE

- Autonomy in Nursing
- Meaning/Definitions of Autonomy
- Different Aspects of Autonomy
- Barriers of Autonomy
- Evolution of Professional Autonomy
- Methods to Achieve Autonomy
- Accountability
  - Areas of Accountability in a Nursing Unit
- Assertiveness
  - Characteristics, Benefits and Techniques of Assertiveness
  - Strategies for Improving Assertiveness
- Visibility of Nurses

AUTONOMY IN NURSING

The traditional arrangement of most organized health care facilities, places, nurses in a subordinate position to administration as well as physicians. The role of a nurse has developed in a far more fundamental way than he/she taking on or previously medical tasks. Over the past two decades, the nursing profession has begun to develop a knowledge base, which is its own. In order to develop nursing into an occupation deserving the title profession. Nurses need to achieve autonomy in nursing which consists of making unconstrained decisions and being able to act in those decisions. Autonomy is essential to professional nursing.

MEANING

The word autonomy is derived from the Greek word "*autos*," which means "self" and "*nomos*" referring to "rule or law." So autonomy is the right of self-determination, independence and freedom.

Autonomy means that a person is reasonably independent and self-governing in decision-making and practice. You reach autonomy through experience, advanced education and the support of an organization that values the independent role of the nurse. With used autonomy comes greater responsibility and accountability for the performance of nursing care activities.

DEFINITIONS

- Autonomy as the ability to absorb information comprehend it, make a choice and carry out that choice.
  —**Sander J Smith**
- Personal autonomy as personal rule of the self that is free from both controlling interference by others and from personal limitations that prevent meaningful choice. —**Beauchamp and Childress, 1991**
- Autonomy describes each person's experience of being himself. —**Husted and Huted, 1995**

DIFFERENT ASPECTS OF AUTONOMY

There are two main aspects of autonomy:
1. Descriptive aspect
2. Prescriptive aspect

Descriptive autonomy is the capacity for self-governance; prescriptively, autonomy means not interfering with persons' control over their own lives and perhaps taking active steps to facilitate such control. Both these aspects are interrelated.

BARRIERS OF AUTONOMY

- **Historical background**:
  - *Concepts of authority:* Florence nightingale derived the foundation for concept of autonomy from the military tradition, which emphasizes the concept of authority. The authorial system of training was different to the development of autonomy.
  - *Concepts of vocation:* In the past, nursing was considered as a vocation. Thompson (1968) wrote that a vocation leads to blind devotion, which slows progress in a given field.
  - *Traditional submissive role of women:* Ten Brink (1975) contented that one of the greatest reasons for nursing not attaining independent roles is related to the traditional submissive role of women.
  - *Apprenticeship nature of nursing:* The slow growth of nursing probably stemmed from the

apprenticeship nature of nursing and the Victorian attitude that men rather than women should pursue intellectual activities.

- ❖ **Other barriers in the health care system**:
  - ➢ Organized medicine.
  - ➢ *Health service administration:* Organized medicine and health care administration are attempting to maintain control of nursing. Because they believed that it is in their best interest to keep nurses dependent on them. Both are well organized and have powerful influence at state and national level.
  - ➢ *Organized nursing:* Organized nursing promotes independence and autonomy, but its power is fragmented by subgroups and dissension. Rivalry between diploma-educated and BSc-educated nurses saps the energy of the profession. The proliferation of nursing organizations and competition among them also diminishes nurses' potential.
  - ➢ *Lack of theoretical knowledge:* Practice of nursing without using theory does not give a scientific rational or directional for nursing.
  - ➢ *Lack of governmental support:* Nursing has attempted to take back some control over government in regulating its own practice through certification of specialty practices. However, no uniform standards exist in nursing certifications, and the qualifications to certification usually consist of merely passing an exam.
  - ➢ *Hospitals' policy of hiring unlicensed personnel:* Hospitals have also taken away autonomy from nursing with the increased hiring of unlicensed personnel to take over nursing tasks. Having personal autonomy includes controlling entry in the profession, establishing the standard for entry and training, and influencing law makers through professional organizations. Taking a stand for autonomy begins with education.

▮ EVOLUTION OF PROFESSIONAL AUTONOMY

A professional is a member of a self-regulating occupational group granted usually by legislation of the exclusive right to practice in a particular field. Nurses have not always been members of a "profession" in the sense intended here; hence, they have not always accorded professional autonomy. During the American civil war, for example, the word nurse could be used to describe a wide range of trained and untrained care givers. During the early years of professionalization, nurses were often told to think of the physician-nurse. Patient trained as a family, with the physician as the head of the family and nurse playing a watchful supportive role. As nursing roles and educational experiences have become standardized, their recognition as a profession has grown. In the most modern health care systems, nursing is a licensed self-regulating profession. Today, nurses have their own professional standards, which imply art and wrong way of doing things, and no physician's order has sufficient moral weight to override those.

Professional Autonomy

Autonomy is a notion that applies to more than just patients; it also applies to health professionals. Respect for professional autonomy means allowing professionals to have substantial control over professional practices including significant room for exercise of their judgment. Professional autonomy is of two types:
1. Autonomy of the profession nursing.
2. Autonomy of the professional nurse.

Autonomy of the Profession Nursing

The term autonomy in the profession of nursing used to indicate the privilege of self-governance. It depends on legislation—an external enabling factor for its very existence. Nurses, similar to other professions such as medicine, law and engineering, are given the freedom to set, within broad limits, their own standards and to enforce those standards among their members. Today, in modern health care system, the members of the group are given by society the privilege of setting their own standards of both technical and ethical excellence. But this constitutes only partial freedom.

Autonomy of the Professional Nurse

When autonomy applies to individual nurses, the notion of professional autonomy has to do with the ability of particular nurses to make at least some decisions that are not subjective to authoritative review by those outside the profession. Professional implies the right to exercise professional judgment in adherence to professional standards in the face of countervailing pressures from institutional authorities, disagreement with members with other professions or in appropriate demands on the part of patients or clients or the general public.

Example: Professional autonomy provides justification for nurses acting according to their own professional judgment rather than simply being told by physicians what to do. When a physician's order conflict with nursing standards or with a nurse's expert judgment, the nurse's professional autonomy implies the right to object.

▮ METHODS TO ACHIEVE AUTONOMY

Individual nurse's capacity for autonomous action depends on a number of features of the health care institution within which they practice and a number of other factors also.

Factors within the health care institution:
- ❖ **Good practice environment:** This supports autonomy nursing, giving nurses the opportunity to the authority and the accountability to identify and solve practice-related problems.
- ❖ **Adequate staffing:** Without adequate staffing, nurses may find their freedom; their ability is difficult to meet the demands of the professional standards:

- Providing auxiliary personnel to assist nurses with such non-nursing tasks such as laundry, food tray pickup, bed making, checking vital signs, etc.
- Supporting collaborative practices through monthly meetings between unit nurses and the physicians.
- Use the collective personnel power.
- ***Legislations:*** Law and legislations has an important role in facilitating and limiting individual nurse's autonomy. They do not have the autonomy, e.g. to engage in the range of practices granted by legislation to physicians. As a particular example, Cullen notes that nurses' decisions-making autonomy is inhibited by the restrictions on nurses' prescribing.
- Increased standard of nursing education.
- Increased research.
- ***Increased pay packets:*** Since the society is used to judge the merit of any profession by the pay packets allotted, the first and foremost task before the nursing profession is the equality in pay allocation. This will automatically elevate the position and status of the nursing profession in the society.

Autonomy and Independent Practice Roles in India

In India, nursing professionals are the most widely distributed group and they have the most diverse roles, functions and responsibilities. Nurses provide health promotion and disease prevention as well as treatment of common diseases and rehabilitation to individuals, families and groups. There are many advanced practice roles that support autonomy for nurses, which include case manager, clinical educator, clinical researcher, clinical consultant, corporate practitioner, nurse generalist, nurse clinician, nurse practitioner, nurse specialist, etc.

In India, private nurse practitioner is quite unheard by the general public. There can be "a practicing medical man," but a practicing nurse is a highly controversial issue not only in the health community, curiously enough the nursing community doubtful views about the scope and prospects of independent nursing practices.

However, in India, given the limited authority and autonomy, the ability to independently adopt and expand nursing practice remains unlimited.

ACCOUNTABILITY

Definition

Accountability refers to individuals being answerable to oneself and others for one's judgmental actions in the course of nursing practice irrespective of health care organizations, policies or provides directives.

According to ANA, 2001: In concept analysis, professional nurse autonomy is believed to be important to the client when making responsible discretionary decisions, both dependently and independently reflecting advocacy for the client.

Accountability also extended to the broader population as the profession demonstrates involvement in social policy. The concept of accountability has two major attributes: answerable and responsibility. Primary nurse delegates responsibility, but is accountable for his/her patients' outcomes. By using authority in bringing the nursing team together, the primary nurse determines if collaboration was successful. If continuity in teaching occurred, and if the patient and family understand and relate the information, a successful decentralized nursing unit exercises the three elements of decision-making in an ongoing basis. An effective manager sets the same expectations for the staff in how to make decision staff does this, while recognizing their own responsibility, authority and accountability. Ultimately, decentralized decision-making is the way to realize nursing units' visions of what professional care should be.

Areas of Accountability in a Nursing Unit

- Delivering care
- Case management
- Primary nursing, team nursing, comprehensive care, etc.
- Providing safe and therapeutic environment
- Maintaining adequate supplies of material and equipment for the unit
- Maintaining good interpersonal relationships
- Protecting clients' legal rights and privacy
- Working within ethical and legal boundaries
- Delegating responsibility appropriately, e.g. decentralized decision-making
- Keeping pace with changing needs of health and developing technology
- Delivering care as per standards laid down by profession, statutory body and institution.

Role of Accountability in Nursing

Each registered nurse:

- Practices in accordance with the Registered Nurses Act, regulation and by laws of Indian Nursing Council, Code of Ethics and Professional Conduct of Nurses in India.
- Makes nurses responsible for their own actions and decisions at all times.
- Takes action in situations, where client safety and well-being is potentially or actually compromised.
- Understands, promotes and compiles with the values and believes in the Code of Ethics for Registered Nurses.
- Seeks assistance appropriately and in a timely manner.
- Supports policies and practices consistent with the college's standards for Nursing Practice and Education.
- Contributes to a safe, supportive and professional practice environment.
- Recognizes and reports errors and takes all necessary action to prevent and minimize harm arising from an adverse event.
- **The nurse administrator** promotes a practice environment that supports professional accountability and a quality practice environment that supports a

nurse's ability to provide safe, effective and ethical nursing practice.
- **The nurse educator** promotes a learning environment that supports professional accountability and provides appropriate supervision to learners that support their ability to provide effective and ethical nursing education.

ASSERTIVENESS

Introduction
- Confirming confidently and a way of saying yes or no in an appropriate way. It is considered as a healthy behavior for all people against personal powerlessness and results in personal empowerment.
- Assertiveness is one of the important elements of professional communications.

Definition of Assertiveness
Assertiveness is standing up for one's rights without violating those of others.
— **Stanhope and Lancaster**

Characteristics of Assertiveness
Assertive responses are characterized by:
- Feeling of security
- Competence
- Power
- Optimism
- Professionalism

Benefits of Assertiveness in Nursing Practice
- More likely to advocate for clients and peers who are valuable, afraid or experiencing a threat to their human rights.
- Nurses can also teach assertiveness skills to others as a means for promoting personal health.
- Assertive people express feelings and emotions confidently, spontaneously and honestly.
- They make decisions and control their lives more effectively than non-assertive individuals.
- Helps to deal with criticism and manipulation by others and learn to say no, and set limits.
- They are good tools dealing with criticism, change, negative conditions in personal or professional life.
- Reduces conflict or stress in relationship.

Techniques of Assertiveness
- Identify the personal rights, wants and needs.
- Identify how you feel about a particular situation.
- Be direct, deliver the message to the person for whom it is intended.
- Own your message: In describing your feelings use "I" message as "I" statements.
- To express the feelings instead of evaluating.
- Avoid assumptions about others thinking or feeling about what their motives are.
- Ask for feedback.
- Stop apologizing all the time.
- Learn to take a compliment.
- Act confident even if you do not feel confident.
- Feel free to say no, I do not know, I do not understand, etc.
- Evaluate your expectation, i.e. be willing to compromise.

Strategies for Improving Assertiveness at Work
- Ask what are the issues? What I need to communicate effectively?
- Bring energy to the job. Do not go to work, tired or sick with personal issues getting in the way.
- Get the emotions under control.
- Find a good place to talk if possible.
- Decide whether to speak up at that time or to wait until a mere conducive moment.
- Effective assertion requires a listener.
- Help patients every day when they are confronted with challenges such as communication issues, horizontal hostility and high stress levels.
- Maintaining diaries and role playing help us to become more assertive.
- Use diaries to track situations you have encountered where you did not behave assertively.
- You can role play with the family and friends or alone.
- Identify the situation and describe in detail what happened and the level of anxiety during the encounter.
- To make it effective, choose a situation you may have to deal with.

VISIBILITY OF NURSES

Meaning
The act or faculty of seeing, sight—imaginative insight, ability to plan or form policy in a farsighted way.

Visibility of Nursing Care
- Social representation of nurses and nursing profession by communication professions. Since they are intermediate in decoding the images and written representations about society, method, ignorance about nurse's field of work. It is the perception of social media towards nurse's work and nursing profession.
- **Nurses' invisibility**: Before the media and society, nurses' own responsibility to obtain professional recognition.

CONCLUSION

As nurses work in different situations, they have to be assertive in order to meet the challenges in the health care delivery and to win cooperation from others.

CHAPTER 4

Legal Considerations in Nursing

CHAPTER OUTLINE

- Meaning and Definition
- Sources of Law for Nursing Practice
- Values of Law in Nursing
- Legal Safeguards in Nursing Practice
- Legal Responsibilities of a Nurse
- Legal Liability in Nursing
- Legal Aspects of Charting Techniques
- List of Do's and Don'ts as Guidelines for Safe Practice

INTRODUCTION

The term law is derived from its tentoric root "lag," which means something that lies fixed or evenly. Laws which govern motives and internal actions of persons are known as moral laws, and those which regulate external human conduct are known as political laws or positive laws. The former is enforced by the force of moral sense of the people, but they later enjoy the sanctions of the authority of the state.

MEANING

Law means a body of rules to guide human actions.

DEFINITION

"Law is that portion of the established thought and habit, which has gained distinct and formal recognition in the shape of uniform rules backed by the authority and power of the government." —Wilson

SOURCES OF LAW FOR NURSING PRACTICE

Law originates from three sources, which includes constitutional law, common laws and administrative laws (Fig. 4.1).

Constitutional Law (Statutory Law)

Constitutional law is the judgmental law of the country. It is the law that governs the state. It represents the will of the ultimate sovereignty of the people. It determines the structure of the state, its power and duties, and it also determines the form of government and its relationship with various organizations of the government and created by elected legislators, e.g. nurse practice law.

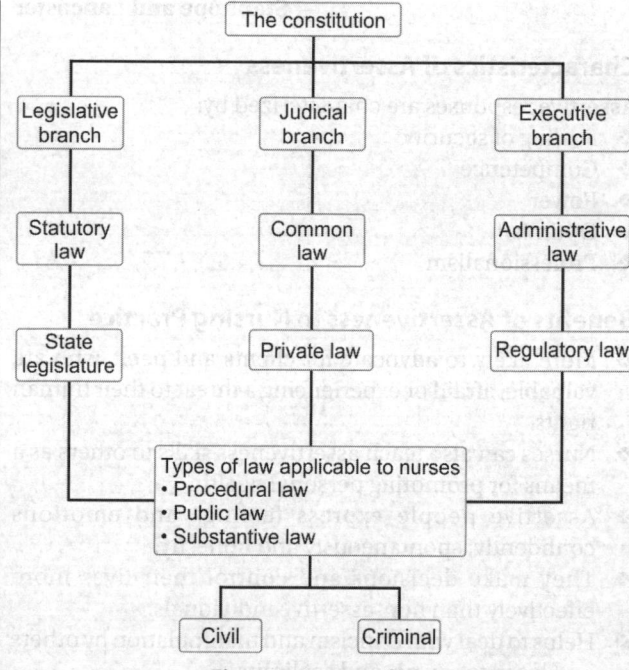

Fig. 4.1: Sources of law.

Common Law

Common law is a body of legal principles which has evolved from court decisions. In other words, it is created by judicial decisions made in courts, where cases are decided.

Administrative Law (Regulatory Law)

Administrative law consists of the rules and regulations established by administrative agencies that have been made of the branches of government (President or Governor). It is the part of public law, which regulates the conduct of public officials and discharge of their duties. It determines the mutual rights and duties of public officials and citizens, e.g. state regulatory body such as Karnataka Nursing Council (KNC).

Criminal Law
Others include criminal law offenses that affect the public welfare and security.

Civil Law
Civil law includes rules and regulations that specify the required course of action and protection of a person's rights.

VALUES OF LAW IN NURSING
The law has many valuable functions when applied to nursing practice. It differentiates nursing practice from the practice of other health care professions. It also describes and protects the right of clients and nurses.

With the increased emphasis on clients' rights, nurses today must understand the legal obligations and responsibilities to clients. Now many clients are knowledgeable about their right related to their health and illness. So nurses should take it as a challenge to become an advocate for clients.

Patient's Bill of Rights (According to Consumer Protection Act 1986):
- Right to considerate and respectful care
- Right to obtain details
- Right to refuse treatment
- Right to confidentiality
- Right to know the name of treating persons
- Right to refuse to participate in research
- Right to privacy
- Right to know the hospital rules and regulations.

LEGAL SAFEGUARDS IN NURSING PRACTICE

Licensure
All nurses who are in nursing practice have to possess a valid licensure. Indian nursing possession of license to practice, which is her/his sole authority.

The purpose of the professional licensure on the one hand is to secure society the benefit, which comes from the services of a highly skilled group and on the other hand to protect society from those who are not highly skilled.

Good Samaritan Laws
"Good Samaritan laws" that exempt doctors and nurses from liability when they render first aid during emergency.

These laws limit liability and offer legal immunity for people helping in an emergency.

Good Rapport
Developing good rapport with the client is very important to prevent malpractice.

Standard of Care
All professionals practicing in the medical field adhere to certain standards when administering standards of care come from several sources including laws, organizational standards and institutional practice and procedures.

Standing Orders
Although a nurse may not legally diagnose illness or prescribe treatment, he/she may, after assessing patient's condition, apply standing orders or treatment guidance that have been established by the physician/doctor as appropriate for certain problems and conditions.

Contracts
Section 13 of the Indian Contract Act defines the word saying that two or more persons are said to consent, which they agree upon the same thing in the same sense. Treating a patient without obtaining proper consent can lead to a change of assault and or batter. Informed consent is a well-recognized doctrine based on the client's right to autonomy.

Consent for Operation and Other Procedures
Any investigation as treatment of a serious nature or an operation in which anesthetic is used requires written consent of the patient. Patients may give their own consent if they are of full age, i.e. has attained the age of 18 years, or is a minor who has attained the age of 16 years from before he has full understanding, requires consent from the client's parent/guardian.

Correct Identity
The nurse has a great responsibility to make sure that at no time they are placing the patient in wrong bed and care is provided to the wrong patient.

All patients in general hospitals wear identity bands in order that mistakes may be avoided. It is very important that the correct band is given to each patient and these are normally checked as part of the admission procedure. With young children and unconscious patients, even greater care must be taken to ensure correct identity.

Counting of Sponge, Lost Instruments and Needles
Nurses advocate that the sponges, instruments and needles counts be performed for all surgical procedures. If an instrument or needle is accidently left in a patient's body during surgery, the operating room nurse will probably be liable for any patient's injury which is caused by the presence of foreign body. It is the responsibility of nurse and nurse administrator to establish policies and procedures

for sponge, instrument and needle counts in the nursing units for surgical procedure, and also minor diagnostics and treatment procedure involving instruments.

During operation, the scrubbed nurse must check the number of all instruments, needles, swabs and packs on her trolley, and as the operation proceeds, check that each item used is returned to her. She will then have to carry out a final check before the body cavity is closed. If any doubt arises, she must inform the surgeon who should delay the final closure until a recount has taken place.

Drug Maintenance

The two acts which control the use of poisons in medicine are:
1. *Misuse of Drugs Act, 1971:* The act aims at checking the unlawful use of the drugs liable to produce dependence or cause harm if misused.
2. *Dangerous Drug Act, 1965 and 1967:* The common drugs controlled under the Dangerous Drug Act include cocaine, diamorphine (heroin), levorphanol, methadone, morphine, opium, pethidine and others.

Medical practitioners and registered dentists may prescribe preparations containing these poisons. A prescription must bear:
- Patient name and address
- Date
- Signature of prescriber
- Total quantity to be supplied in words or figures.

Every general practitioner is required to keep a record of all purchases of these drugs and of the amount issued to individual patients. In hospitals, the use of these drugs is under strict control although minor variations in detail may occur if in individual institutions:
- A special cupboard is used for storing such drugs
- The cupboard is kept locked and the key is carried by the person of the state registered nurse in charge
- Renewal of supplies can only be obtained by an order signed by a medical officer and the drugs can only be given under the written instructions
- Each dose of these drugs administered must be entered into a special register provided for the purpose with the date, patients name and time of giving.

Accidents and Injuries

If a patient sustains injury, while in hospital's authority or against a person (member of a medical nursing or ancillary staff) to whom he/she attributes the injury, he/she may be a member of a medical nursing or ancillary staff. The hospital has a certain degree of responsibility for the actions of its staff. Accidents can arise to visitors or employees of the hospitals through negligence in matters such as cleaning equipment placed on stairways, polish or grease left on the floor, faulty electrical equipment or on furnishings.

Self-discharge of Patient

When the patient demands to discharge, the nurse on duty should try to dissuade patient and should inform the medical officer concerned with patient care. If the patient is adamant, each hospital will follow its own procedure. It is probable that a senior administrative officer will see the patient and ask him/her to sign a written statement to the effect that he/she is discharging against medical advice [discharge against medical advice (DAMA)/leave against medical advice (LAMA)]. If he/she refuses to sign, a note to this effect will have to be made and signed by two witnesses, one of whom is usually the administrative officer concerned and the other is the nurse-in-charge at the time.

Professional Confidence

Guarding the confidence of the patient is an ethical duty of the medical and nursing profession.

Documentation

The medical record is a legal document and is admissible in the court as evidence; the nurse should give themselves credit for care they provided, thoroughly documenting it in the medical record.

Patient Property

In the department of health social security requires hospital to inform all patients under its care that the hospital cannot accept responsibility for valuable or money unless they have been handed over for safekeeping. Money of an unconscious patient admitted as an emergency should be listed and checked by two nurses and put in safe keeping.

While a patient is in hospital, the nurse has no right to go through their locker or personal property without their consent.

Making of Wills and Signing of Legal Documents

Most hospitals have a rule against or discourage nurses from signing legal documents or witnessing signature during their professional duties. This is to protect the nurse lest any document to be challenged later on the grounds of the unfitness of the patient.

Restraining Order

Restraints for clients/children should be used by the nurse according to the doctor's orders. It should not be done without the orders, if any injuries/accidents are to be reported immediately.

Laws that affect nursing practice:
- Responsibilities towards patient
- Responsibilities as an employee
- Relationship with other professionals
- Records keeping and reporting.

LEGAL RESPONSIBILITIES OF A NURSE

Responsibilities of Appointing and Assigning

Nursing administration is expected to be aware of legal restrictions affecting personal appointment and assignment. The nurse administrators have the responsibility for staffing and supervising nursing units to ensure safe and effective patient care. Therefore, they have the authority to temporarily reassign a nursing employee from one unit to another to compensate for emergency staff shortages. In shifting an employee to compensate for personnel shortage, a supervisor or manager must take into consideration the nurse's capability to discharge duties of the temporary position.

Responsibility in Quality Control

The nursing administrator and the authority of the agency at all levels have a legal obligation to ensure nursing care quality. Usually the head nurse or ward-in-charge is responsible for the quality of patient care given by all personnel including medical or the nursing unit.

Responsibility for Equipment

To protect patients and employees from injury, a nurse manager must ensure that all patient care equipment are fully functional and that defective equipment is promptly repaired or replaced. He/she must ensure that the nursing personnel know how to operate sophisticated equipment so that he/she is expected to provide instructions for proper care and storage of patient care equipment.

Responsibility for Observation and Reporting

Nursing personnel have more frequent and prolonged patient contact than other caregivers. Nurses are trained to detect significant symptoms and reactions; consequently, nurses have a legal duty to observe patients frequently and report findings that have diagnostic or treatment value for the patient's physician and other members of the patient's treatment team. Infants, children, aged, disoriented, psychiatric and critically ill patients require more frequent observations than other patients with no evidence of expanding respiratory or cardiac emergency.

The nurse has a duty to record and report observations of a patient's condition promptly, so that the physician can base treatment decisions with up-to-date information about the patient's health needs.

Responsibility to Protect Public

The nurse has a legal duty to protect the public from injury by dangerous patients.

Responsibility for Record Keeping and Reporting

Nurses have legal responsibility for accurately reporting and recording patient conditions, treatment and responses to care. The medical record is a written or computerized account of a patient illness and treatment that includes information submitted by all members of the patients in the health care team. The medical record is an information source document that should be used to plan care, evaluate care, allocate costs, educate personnel, research care measure and substantiate legal claim.

Responsibility for Death and Dying

Nurses must be aware of legal definitions of death because they must document all events that happen when the patient is in their care.

There are many issues that surround the events of death. Sometimes, there will be issues of euthanasia which is defined as intentional homicide, e.g. intentionally administering a lethal dose of morphine to a patient to cause death. An example of passive euthanasia including removing breathing support or withholding blood transfusion from a terminally ill patient with irreversible brain damage may raise legal questions.

Knowledge regarding institutional rules and policies: Institutional rules and policies act as a legal guide to the legal responsibilities of a nurse. Professional conduct can be stated by the institution regarding the employment.

Responsibility for Medicolegal Case

An responsibility for medicolegal case (MLC) is a client who is admitted to the hospital with some unnatural pathology and has to be taken care in concurrence with the police and/or court.

Types of clients which are categorized as MLC in a hospital are:
- Road traffic accidents
- Injuries inflicted during brawls/fights, shooting, bomb blasts, etc.
- Suicide, burns, poisoning, rape victim, assault, etc.

Nurses' role in MLC:
- Obtain complete history from patient or significant others
- Inform the police officer/constable on duty, in the hospital through the **Chief Medical Officer** (CMO)
- When a patient is discharged, inform the CMO after clearance from them
- No patient can leave against medical advise
- Document the care given, timely and accurately
- Records should be kept safely over to the authorized person in the hospital.

LEGAL LIABILITY IN NURSING

Areas of potential liability for nurses:
- Failure to monitor and assess
- Failure to ensure safety
- Medication errors
- Improper implementation of skills or procedures
- Documentation errors.

Tort

Tort is a wrongful act committed against a person or his property independent of a contracts. The word 'tort' is derived from the Latin word 'tortus' means 'twisted', French-injury/wrong. They may be classified as intentional or unintentional (Box 4.1).

Unintentional Torts

Unintentional tort is an act of omission.

Negligence: Neglecting to do something that a reasonably prudent person would do during something that he/she would not do. **For example**, malpractice, common cases of negligence include foreign object (such as sponges) left inside a patient, burns caused by equipment or solutions, falls that caused by injury to a patient, serious inaccuracies in administration of medications and failure to exercise reasonable judgment.

Malpractice: It is professional misconduct, unreasonable lack of skill or infidelity in professional duties, evil practice or illegal immoral conduct. Problems for which nurses are found negligent:
- Failure to use aseptic technique
- Leaving a foreign object in a patient's body during surgery
- Failing to protect and inform patient from falling, which may result in injury
- Administration of wrong medicine, wrong dose and wrong route
- Administrating any care in a wrong manner, which may harm the patient.

Intentional Torts

Intentional torts are useful acts that isolate another's rights.

Assault and battery: The most common suit brought against nurses is assault and battery. Assault is conduct that causes threat and produces a reasonable apprehension of harm, e.g. nurse threatens a child for not taking medication.

Battery is the actual carrying out of such a threat. Battery is any intentional touching of another's body without his/her consent. For example, if the client gives consent for tonsillectomy and surgeon preforms laryngectomy.

Defamation of character: Defamation of character includes false communication or communication resulting in injury to a person's reputation by means of speech.

Box 4.1: Types of torts.

Unintentional torts	Intentional torts
Negligence	Assault and battery
Malpractice	Invasion of privacy
	Quasi-intentional laws—Defamation of character
	False imprisonment
	Conversion of property
	Trespass to land

1. **Slander defamation:** It is in the form of spoken words that could damage a person's reputation or property. For example, if a nurse tells a client that his/her doctor is incompetent, for which the nurse could be held liable for slander.
2. **Libel defamation:** If the damage of a person's reputation or property is done in the form of a written statement, it could be liable for libel.
3. **Fraud:** This is also called quasi-intentional torts. It may be a combination of both the defamations, i.e. slander and libel.

It is the willful, purposeful misinterpretation of self or an act that may cause harm to a person or property. A nurse who misrepresents the outcome of a procedure commits fraud.

Invasion of privacy: The fourth amendment of the United States (US) constitution protects every citizen's right to privacy. Disclosing confidential information to an inappropriate third party subjects the nurse to a possible slander charge or liability. Another form of invasion of privacy is the release of information to an unauthorized person such as a member of the press or the client's employer.

False imprisonment: It is the unjustifiable detentions of a person without legal warrant to confine a person. Nurses falsely imprison the patient when they confine the patient or restrain the patient in a bounded area with the intention to prevent the patient from freedom. The confined area maybe a patient's room or bed.

Conversion of property: When the health care practitioner interferes with the right to possession of the patient's property, either by interfering in something that is not the nurse's concern or by disposing the person's property.

Example: A client cannot be forced to remain in the health care facility.

Trespass to land: This is the tort of unlawful interference with another's possession of land, and may occur either intentionally or as a result of negligent action. This tort occurs when a person intrudes into another's property, fails to leave the property when so requested, places something on the property or causes a third person to enter the property.

LEGAL ASPECTS OF CHARTING TECHNIQUES

The patient's chart has become the determining factor in 80–85% of all malpractice lawsuits involving patient care. A strong record can be an effective defense for the nurse accused of malpractice.

Charting techniques and strategies to improve documentation:
- Sign every entry
- Write neatly and intelligibly

- Use proper spelling and grammar
- Document in blue or black ink
- Use authorized abbreviations
- Use graphic representation to record install signs
- Record patient's name on every page
- Avoid taking verbal or orders over phone
- Document should be complete with full information about medications
- Chart promptly
- Avoid block charting
- Chart after delivery care
- Correctly identify late entries
- Rectify mistaken entries properly
- Do no tamper with records

LIST OF DO'S AND DON'TS AS GUIDELINES FOR SAFE PRACTICE

Do's:
- Documentation of all unusual incidences
- Report all unusual incidences
- Know your job description
- Follow policies and procedures as established by your employing agency
- Keep your registration updated
- Perform procedures that you have been taught that are within the standard scope of your practice
- Establish and maintain rapport with patients and family
- Practice safety with the physician's verbal orders
- Seek and clarify orders when the patient's medical condition changes.

Don'ts:
- Accept money or gifts from patients
- Allow patients to leave the hospital or nursing home unless there is an order or signed release
- Attempt to practice medicine
- Work as a licensed practical/vocational nurse in a state in which you are not licensed
- Take medication that belongs to patients.

The laws summarized for medical practitioners including nurses are as given below (English law):
- The right to refuse to treat a patient in an emergency situation.
- The right to sue for fees (Applicable only to private duty nurse or private practitioners; other nurses are salaried)
- The right to add a title description to one's name—Any title, description, abbreviation or letter which implies holding a degree, diploma, license or certificate showing particular qualifications may be added (Improper use of these is often prohibited by State Nurses Registration Acts). The right to wear the Red Cross Emblem is given only to members of the army medical service.
- Unregistered practitioners are not allowed to hold positions or appointments in public and local hospitals.
- *Fundamental duties:*
  - To exercise a reasonable degree of skill and knowledge in treating patients. The standard held is that exercised by other reputable members of the same profession in similar circumstances.
  - Once a relationship to a patient has been established, there is an obligation to attend the patient as long as necessary unless the patient requests withdrawal or a notice is given of intention to withdraw.
  - A practitioner must give personal attention to his cases and answer calls with reasonable promptness.
  - Children must be protected from harming themselves.
  - Special precautions must be taken in the case of adults who are incapable of taking care of themselves.
- The Indian Penal Code demands that poisonous drugs be kept in separate containers properly labeled and marked. Care must be taken not to mix with nonpoisonous drugs.
- There is a duty of secrecy to the patients. Records must be treated as confidential unless the practitioner is called upon to give evidence in court.
- Dangerous diseases must be reported (These will vary in different parts of the country).

CONCLUSION

Nurses who are aware of legal rights and obligations are better prepared to take good care of patients. Nurses are responsible for knowing the laws that apply to their areas of nursing practice.

CHAPTER 5: Role of Regulatory Bodies

CHAPTER OUTLINE

- Definition of Regulatory Bodies
- Vital Role of Regulatory Bodies
- Major Regulatory Bodies
  - Central Government
  - State Government
  - Institutional Rules
- Important Professional Regulatory Bodies
  - Indian Nursing Council
  - State Registration Councils
  - Universities
  - State Nursing Boards

INTRODUCTION

Health professionals such as nurses, doctors, pharmacist and many others are regulated and licensed by regulatory bodies as required by provincial legislation. All nurses are required to be licensed to practice with their designated provincial nursing regulatory body. Legal responsibility in nursing practice is becoming of greater importance as each year passes. In order to provide safe and competent nursing care, an understanding of legal boundaries is very essential. It is important to know the law in one state and the authorities enforcing these laws.

DEFINITION OF REGULATORY BODIES

- A regulatory body is a public authority or government agency responsible for exercising autonomous authority over some area of human activity in regulatory or supervisory capacity.
- An independent regulatory agency is a regulatory agency that is independent from other branches or arms of the government, and it deals in the areas of administrative law, regulatory law, secondary legislation and rule making for the benefit of the public at large.

VITAL ROLE OF REGULATORY BODIES

- To ensure the public's right to quality health care service
- Set and enforce standards of nursing practice
- To support and assist professional members
- Monitor and enforce standards for nursing education and nursing practice
- Set the requirements for registration of nursing professionals
- Nursing regulatory bodies are also known as colleges or associations, and are responsible for the licensing of nurses within their respective provinces territory. The nursing regulatory bodies receive their authority from legislation.

MAJOR REGULATORY BODIES (TABLE 5.1)

- Central government
- State government
- Institutional rule.

Role of Central Government

The central is a source of regulatory bodies in three ways, which are:
- Government service conduct rules
- Indian Nursing Council Act
- English law.

Government Service Conduct Rules

These are detailed rules of conduct for government employees. Examples of these are the requirement to maintain absolute integrity, devotion to duty and high standards of moral behavior. Only a few are applicable to the nursing practice, but all would be applicable to the practice of a nurse employed by the government.

Official Organization of Health System at the National Level

- The Directorate General of Health Service
- Ministry of Health and Family Welfare
- The Central Council of Health and Family Welfare.

Table 5.1: Regulatory bodies in nursing profession.

Professional regulatory bodies (nursing education)	Some of the regulatory bodies concerned to clinical practice
Government bodies: The central and state government and institutional rules control both the field of nursing education and nursing practice	State Registration Council
Indian Nursing Council	State Nurses Association of India
State Nursing Council	Clinical Establishment Act
Universities	National Accrediting Board for Hospitals and Health Care Providers (NABH)
State Nursing Boards	Joint Commission on Accreditation of Health Care Organization (JCAHO)
International Council of Nurses	National Association for Healthcare Quality (NAHQ)
National League of Nursing	Institute of Health Care Improvement (IHI) Agency for Health Care Research and Quality (AHRQ) Environment Protection Act, 1986—BMW Management Rules, 1998 Trade License Act, Labor Laws Consumer Protection Act, Medico-Legal Case Act Prenatal diagnostic techniques (Regulation and Prevention of Misuse Act, 1994) and in 2003, Pre-Conception and Pre-Natal Diagnostic Techniques (PCPNDT) Act to improve the regulation of the technology used in sex selection. Employees State Insurance Act Drugs and Cosmetics Act Prenatal Diagnostic Technique

Functions of Ministry of Health and Family Welfare

International health relation promotion of health; quarantine of the central institute such as All India Institute of Hygiene and Public Health, Kolkata, National Institute for the Control of Communicable Disease, Delhi; promotion and development of medical, pharmaceutical, dental and nursing profession; establishment and maintenance of drug standards; dental and nursing profession census; collections and publication of other statistical data; regulation of labor in the working of mines and oil fields; migration; nursing professions and emigration. Census, collections and publication of other statistical data by the Indian Nursing Council (INC), the state nurse coordination with states and other ministry for promotion of health.

Concurrent list:
The functions listed under this are the responsibility of both central and state governments:

- Prevention of extension of communicable disease from one unit to another
- Prevention of adulteration of foodstuffs
- Control of drugs and poisons
- Vital statistics
- Labor welfare
- Ports other than major
- Economic and social planning
- Population control and family planning.

Functions of Directorate General of Health Service

- International health relations and quarantine of all major ports in the country and international airport
- Control of drug standards
- Medical store depots are maintained
- Administration of postgraduate training programs
- Administration of certain medical colleges in India
- Conducting medical research through Indian Council of Medical Research
- Central government health schemes
- Implementation of national health programs
- Maintaining the central health education bureau
- Health intelligence to centralize collection compilation, analysis, evaluation and dissemination of all information on health statistics for the nation as a whole
- Maintaining and administering the National Medical Library.

Functions of Central Council of Health

- To consider and recommend broad outline of policy with regard to matters concerning health such as environmental hygiene, nutrition and health education, and provision of remedial and preventive care
- To make proposals for legislation relating to medical and public health matters
- To make recommendation to the central government regarding distribution of available grants-in-aid for health purpose.

Role of State Government

The state government controls nursing practice through the State Nurses Registration Acts. The State Nurses Registration Councils have authority to prescribe rules of conduct, to take disciplinary action and to maintain registers of nurses. The uniform standards given by the Indian Nursing Council, the state nurse practice act is the important law affecting one nursing practice act that protects the public by broadly defining the legal scope of nursing practice.

Functions

- It registers nurses' midwives
- It serves as legal protections to the nurse
- It protects the public from incompetent nursing practice or poor nursing care
- It accredits and inspects schools of nursing and college of nursing

❖ It prescribes the rules of conduct, and take disciplinary action
❖ It takes united efforts to elevate the standards of nursing
❖ It works for the welfare of the members.

Unethical Practices Commonly Prohibited by State

❖ Procuring registration by false means
❖ Dishonest use of certificate
❖ Representation of registration by an unrecognized person
❖ Falsification of the register
❖ Representation of a registrant as a medical practitioner
❖ Many states prohibit an unregistered person from holding a nursing position in an institution wholly or partially supported by government funds
❖ Some states prohibit practice of any unregistered nurse.

A fine is the usual penalty imposed for disobeying the laws stated above although imprisonment is also possible. In actual practice, the state council often delegates responsibility for the supervision of nurses to local authorities such as the District Civil Surgeon or a board appointed for this purpose.

The Trained Nurses Association of India (TNAI) bases its standards for conduct of professional nurses upon the International Code for nurses.

Institution Rules

Institution acts as a regulatory body for all employees by formulating some rules and regulation. Professional rules of conduct may be stated by the institution regarding conditions of agreement for employment such as periods of time needed when giving notification of registration.

IMPORTANT PROFESSIONAL REGULATORY BODIES

Indian Nursing Council

The INC is an autonomous body under the Government of India, Ministry of Health and Family Welfare which was constituted by the Central Government under Section 3(1) of the Indian Nursing Council Act enacted on 31st December in 1947 (no. 48) of Parliament and established in 1949 with a uniform standard of training for nurses, midwives and health visitors. It is enacted with 17 sections and each section points out the specific legislative role of the Council.

Act Objective

It is an act to constitute an INC, whereas it is expedient to constitute an INC in order to establish a uniform standard of training for nurses, midwives and health visitors.

Purpose

The purpose of INC establishment is to formulate a national policy for training and practice of nursing depending mainly on the culture and philosophy of the country (India).

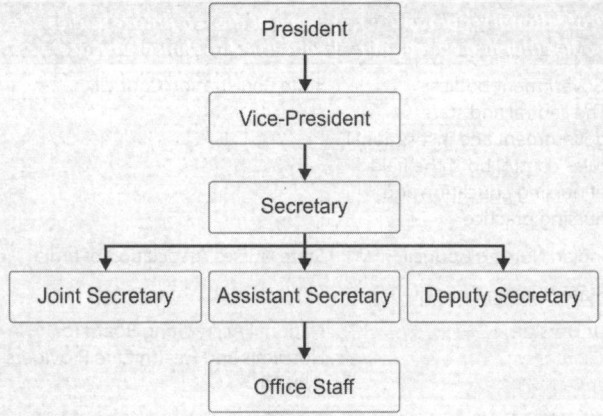

Organization structure of INC.

Composition of INC

The council is composed of the following representatives:
❖ State Registration Council
❖ Central Registration Council
❖ Military Nursing Council
❖ Indian Red Cross Society
❖ Colleges and schools of nursing
❖ Health schools of post-certificate schools
❖ Trained Nurses Association of India
❖ Medical Council of India
❖ Indian Medical Association
❖ Members of Parliament

Constitution and Composition of the Council

The central government shall as soon as may be constitute a council consisting of the following members, namely:

Power to Make Regulations

The Council may make regulations not inconsistent with this Act, such regulations may provide for:
❖ Property of the council
❖ Elections
❖ The meetings
❖ Prescribing the functions of the Executive Committee
❖ Prescribing the powers and duties of the President and the Vice-President
❖ Prescribing the tenure of office and the powers and duties of the Secretary and other officers
❖ Prescribing the standard curriculum
❖ Prescribing the conditions for admission to courses of training
❖ Prescribing the standards of examination and any other matter.

Committees

❖ **Executive Committee**: To function on the issues related to maintenance of standards of nursing programs.
❖ **Equivalence committee**: To control and implement the issues of recognition of foreign qualifications which is essential for the purpose of registration under Section

Chapter 5: Role of Regulatory Bodies

Constitution and composition of the council.

Representation of personnel	Number	Elected by
Nurse	1	From state register by each state council
Nurse with MSc/PPBSc qualification	2	Head of institutions recognized by the Council in teaching and in nursing administration
Health visitors	1	Head of the institution in which health visitors are trained
–	1	By the Medical Council of India
–	1	Elected by the Council of TNAI
Midwife/ANM	1	By each of the state councils in the four groups of states being taken in rotation namely: i. Kerala, Madhya Pradesh, Uttar Pradesh and Haryana ii. Andhra Pradesh, Bihar, Maharashtra and Rajasthan iii. Karnataka, Punjab and West Bengal iv. Assam, Gujarat, Tamil Nadu and Odisha
The Director	1	The Director General of Health Services: ex officio
The Chief Principal Matron	1	Medical Directorate, General Headquarters
The Chief Nursing Superintendent	1	Office of the Director-General of Health Services
The Director	1	The Director of Maternity and Child Welfare, Indian Red Cross Society
The Chief Administrative Medical Officer	1	By whatever name called of each state other than a union territory
The Superintendent of Nursing Services	1	Services by whatever name called, from each of the states in the two groups mentioned below, namely: i. Andhra Pradesh, Assam, Maharashtra, Madhya Pradesh, Tamil Nadu, Uttar Pradesh, West Bengal and Haryana ii. Bihar, Gujarat, Himachal Pradesh, Kerala, Karnataka, Odisha, Punjab and Rajasthan
Nurses, midwives or health visitors	4	By the central government—who are enrolled in a state register and shall be experienced educationist
Parliament members	3	Parliament: Two members by the House of the People One member by the Council of States from among its members

II (2) (a) or (b) of the Indian Nursing Council Act, 1947, as amended.

❖ **The Nursing Education Committee**: Concerned on the issues mainly with nursing education and policy aspects related to nursing education.

❖ **Finance Committee**: This is another important committee of the Council which decides upon the matters pertaining to finances of the Council in terms of budget, expenditure, implementation of central government orders with respect to service conditions, etc.

Amendments in INC Act, 1947

The Act was amended in November 1957 to provide for the following things:

❖ **Foreign qualification:**
  ➢ A citizen of India holding a qualification which entitles him or her to be registered with any registering body may, by the approval of the council, be enrolled in any state register.
  ➢ A person who is not an Indian citizen but who is employed as a nurse, midwife, auxiliary nursing and midwifery (ANM), teacher or administrator in any hospital or institution in any state, by approval of the President of Council, is enrolled temporarily in state register. In such cases, foreign qualifications are recognized temporarily for a period of 5 years. If one continues to practice in India, an extension of recognition should be sort from INC.

❖ **Indian Nurses Register:**
  ➢ The council shall cause to be maintained in the prescribed manner a register of nurses, midwives, ANM and health visitors to be known as the Indian Nurses Register, which shall contain the names of all persons who are for the time being enrolled on any state register.
  ➢ Such register shall be deemed to be a public document within the meaning of the Indian Evidence Act, 1872.

Programs under INC

❖ Auxiliary nurse midwife training
❖ Diploma in general nursing and midwifery (GNM)
❖ Post-basic BSc nursing
❖ BSc nursing
❖ MSc nursing
❖ MPhil in nursing
❖ Doctoral degree in nursing.

Functions of INC

The main purpose of the council is to set standards and to regulate the education and practice of nurses, midwives, auxiliary nurse midwives, health visitors and public health nurses in the country. The Council's regulations specify the minimum requirements for qualifying for a particular course of study in nursing. Thus, the major functions of the council are:

❖ Prescribing and revising syllabi for various courses in nursing:
  ➢ **School program**:
    ♦ ANM
    ♦ GNM

- **College program:**
  - BSc nursing
  - MSc nursing
  - MPhil in nursing
  - PhD in nursing
- **Post-basic diploma courses (1-year specialty courses):**
  - Diploma in nursing education and administration
  - Diploma in public health nursing
  - Other fellowship courses of 3–10 months' duration in various specialty areas such as cardiothoracic nursing, operation theatre, neonatal nursing, ophthalmic nursing, etc.
- Inspecting, monitoring and regulating nursing educational institutions initially and periodically for the purpose of granting recognition for conducting the prescribed courses in nursing
- Evaluating the syllabus implemented by various schools and colleges of nursing through inspection reports
- Prescribing the standards of examination for qualifying in courses
- Recognition of examining bodies an inspection of examination centers
- Withdrawal of recognition from defaulting institutions and examining bodies
- Maintenance of Indian Nurses Register in a prescribed manner for registering to names of nurses, midwives and auxiliary nurses midwives, etc. in the country
- Recognition of qualifications in nursing
- Collection of data from training and educational institutions of nursing
- Maintaining reciprocity in relation to the recognition of foreign qualifications in working out equivalence.

Besides these, the INC also has an advisory role with the State Nursing Councils (SNCs), schools and colleges of nursing in matters other than those mentioned under normal activities relating nursing education in states. They carry on the functions the INC, schools and colleges of nursing and examination board.

Nature of Inspections

There are three types of inspections by INC since 1996.
- **First inspection:** Institutions are inspected by the INC when they apply for starting a course in nursing. This is the first step towards INC recognition. The schools that seek recognition are required to submit:
  - Permission letter of state government
  - Permission letter of SNCs
  - A copy of the inspection report of the SNC
  - A bank draft of fee towards inspection as prescribed by INC
- **Re-inspection:** These are done for those institutions, which are found unsuitable on first or subsequent inspection by INC. The institutions are informed about

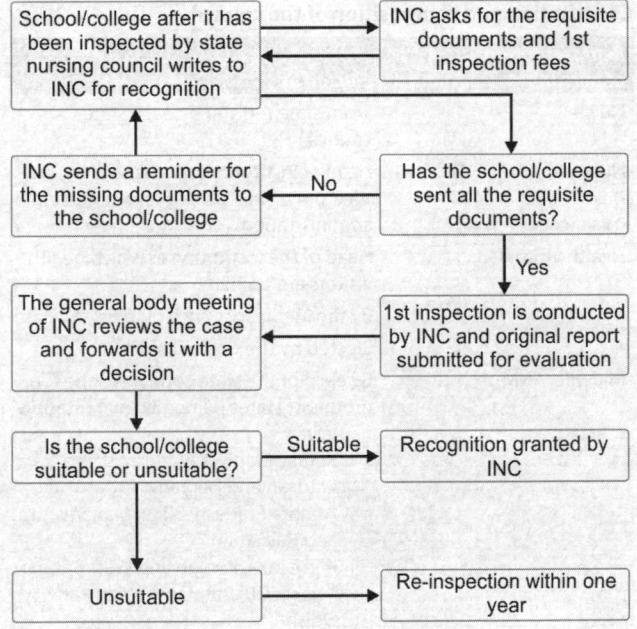

Fig. 5.1: Nature of inspections conducted by Indian Nursing Council.

the deficiencies and are advised to improve upon them. Once the institution takes necessary steps to remove the deficiencies and informs the INCs, re-inspection is done within 1 year or earlier after receiving a re-inspection fee from schools or colleges.
- **Periodic inspections:** Once an institution is given recognition by INC, the institute is required to send an annual inspection fee regularly. The INC inspects the institute generally after 3 years (periodic inspection). An institute with irregular payment pattern falls under defaulter category. The inspections are conducted by a team of voluntary inspectors, who fulfill the criteria for inspectors of INC (Fig. 5.1).

Withdrawal of Recognition

- When, upon report by the Executive Committee, it appears to the Council:
  - Any institution falls short of standard by the council
  - Any institution falls short of standard by a state council may send information to the INC and an intimation sent for the period within which the institution or authority have to submit its explanation to the state government.
- On the receipt of the explanation or where no explanation is submitted within the period fixed, the state government shall make its recommendations to the Council.
- The Council, after such further inquiry, may/can withdraw the recognition.

Resolutions

- Maximum period for students to complete revised ANM and GNM course is 3 years and 6 years, respectively.

Chapter 5: Role of Regulatory Bodies

- INC resolved that maximum age for teaching faculty is 70 years subject to the condition that he/she should be physically and mentally fit.
- Admission to married candidates for the entire nursing program allowed subject to the conditions that they should produce medical fitness certificate.
- Relaxation of norms to establish MSc (N) program: As per INC norm, only those institutions can start MSc Nursing program where at least one batch of students has qualified BSc (N) program. INC resolved that apart from these institutions the super specialty hospitals can also open the MSc (N) program. Even though the institutions are not having BSc (N) program.
- Relaxation of student–patient ratio for clinical practice: 1:3 student–patient ratios instead of 1:5 student–patient ratios.
- Relaxation of teaching faculty qualification to start a BSc (N) program. At least two MSc (N) qualified teaching faculties to be available to start BSc (N) program for the next 4 years in order to combat acute shortage of nursing and teachers till the position of MSc (N) qualified teaching faculty improves.
- To maintain quality of postgraduate in nursing, INC resolved not to have MSc (N) program through distance education.
- Institution should have its own building within 2 years of establishments.
- Maximum number of 60 seats can be sanctioned to those institutions which are having less than 500-bedded hospital, and 100 seats can be sanctioned to those having 500-bedded hospitals.

Recent Trends of INC

Educational role and responsibility:
- INC initiates, prescribes, guides and supervises the different levels of nursing education
- It laid down the qualification for the admission, registration and employment
- It recognizes and approves various institutions for conducting different nursing educational programs
- INC sets educational activities in different occasions like Nurses Day, Breastfeeding Week, AIDS Day, etc.
- It regulates the course duration
- Prescribes the syllabus for all levels of nursing education.

Registration of additional qualification initiatives by INC:
1. **Teaching material for Quality Assurance Model (QAM) prepared:** QAM in nursing is the set of elements that are related to each other and comprises of planning for quality, development of objectives setting and actively communicating standards, developing indicators, setting thresholds, collecting data to monitor compliance with set standards for nursing practice and applying solutions to improve care.

   INC has developed a quality assurance program for nurses in India. The project was implemented in two hospitals in New Delhi and post graduate institute (PGI), Chandigarh for 3 months' duration. The impact of QAM model adopted in Chandigarh can be seen in the paper cutting which was published in Tribune on April 19th 2004.
2. **Princess Srinagarindra Award:** Mrs Sulochana Krishnan, Ex-Principal of RAK College of Nursing was awarded Princess Srinagarindra Award, Thailand, which is an international award to individual(s) registered nurse(s) in honor of Princess Srinagarindra, her Royal Highness. And in recognition for her exemplary contribution towards progress and advancement in the field of nursing and social services, Mrs Sulochana Krishnan's name was proposed by INC from India.
3. **Development of curriculum for HIV/AIDS and training for nurses:** INC, in collaboration with National AIDS Control Organization (NACO) and Clinton Foundation, is developing a curriculum for training of nurses in HIV/AIDS areas. It will be a 6-day training program. The pilot study was conducted in Mumbai and Hyderabad.
4. **National consortium for PhD in Nursing constituted six study centers recognized under national consortium for PhD in Nursing:** Memorandum of Understanding (MOU) has been signed between INC, World Health Organization (WHO) and Rajiv Gandhi University of Health Sciences (RGUHS) National consortium for PhD in Nursing, which has been constituted by INC in collaboration with RGUHS and WHO, under the Faculty of Nursing to promote doctoral education in various fields of nursing. Applications for enrolment in PhD in Nursing were invited for eligible candidates by advertising in the national leading dailies from all over the country by the RGUHS. One hundred and twenty-five candidates appeared for the entrance test conducted on 7th January 2007.
5. **Memorandum of understanding** signed between INC and Sir Edward Dunlop Hospitals Ltd. for advancing standards of nursing education and practices in India to meet challenges currently faced by nursing.

   MOU is entered at New Delhi on 11th April 2006 between INC and Sir Edward Dunlop Hospitals (I) Ltd. with the following **objectives**:
   - Provides training
   - Graduate, postgraduate and PhD courses
   - Organizing research activities
   - To help fill gaps in India and internationally benchmarked standards of nursing education and practice, including credentialing, etc., so that Indian nurses can directly be accepted to meet international standards
   - Train the faculty so as to provide high quality teaching staff to training institutes in the country.
6. **Steps taken up to enter into mutual recognition agreement (MRA) under the Comprehensive**

Economic Cooperation Agreement (CECA) between India and Singapore: This was signed in June 2005 and has come into force from 1st August 2005. In that, it has been agreed that India and Singapore would enter into MRAs in medical, dental and nursing services in the health care sector.
7. **All state registrars were invited to attend the two days' meeting:** The objective was to ensure the uniformity and to maintain the quality of nursing education in the country. It was also aimed to understand the problems/issues of each SNC and evolve consensus between INC and state nursing registration councils (SNRC).
8. **The Indian Nursing Council:** Initiated the live register in the state of Tamil Nadu. The primary objective of the project is to conduct nurses' census, i.e. to collect the data regarding number of working nurses as defined by INC. INC decided to conduct the pilot study in the Sivaganga District of Tamil Nadu.

Problems of regulation and equivalence India:
- Field and clinical practice areas are inadequately equipped in large number of states.
- Clinical supervision and teaching present a major problem. Various schools are not complying with 1:10 teacher–student ratio. This situation puts constraints on the quality of training. Due to lack of qualified teachers, the schools and colleges are not able to maintain the required standards.
- Inadequate clinical experiences are given by many schools/colleges of nursing due to overloading of students and non-adherence to INC norms.
- Quality of training is not uniform.
- Some state councils do not abide by INC guidelines or instructions.
- Problems related to political, economic and commercial issues resulting in proliferation of institutes by government permission dilute the quality of education and service.
- Minimum entry to GNM has been made 10 + 2 but is still not followed by many states.

How does the council become aware of non-adherence to INC norms?
- The inspection reports submitted by the inspectors provide very good data and information regarding e-resources and standards of training. These reports are carefully analyzed and evaluated to reach an objective conclusion regarding the training provided.
- The INC often receives complaints from interested groups and individuals who would like the INC to improve its function and control over the nature of training plight of students, etc.
- Observations and reports by committees appointed by the government, i.e. Bhore Committee, Shetty Committee, High Power Committee on Nursing Profession, etc. not only record their observations, but also provide recommendations.
- Reports received from professional associations such as the TNAI and its state branches provide insights.
- Reports received from central and state ministries of health and family welfare and departments give feedback about the relevance of training to health policies and programs.

State Nursing Councils

State Nursing Councils (SNCs) are formed since 1926 to control the training and practice within the state and issue licenses for qualified nurses. A license issued by a council provides assurance to the public that the nurse has met pre-determined standards.

The major functions of SNCs are:
- Recognition of nursing institution within the state
- Registration and renewal of licenses for the qualified nursing personnel
- Reworking of license
- In India, few SNCs act as qualification conferring body for diploma courses.

State Registration Council

The State Nurses and Midwives Council was established in 1948 under the provisions of Nurses and Midwives Act with the purpose of "Better training of nurses, midwives and health visitors." It works as an autonomous body under the government of respective states, Department of Health and Family Welfare.
- Registration in SNC is very necessary for every nurse. It is necessary to be registered in order to function officially as a professional nurse. Registration councils are functioning in all states of India and they are affiliated to INC.
- A register of names of professional nurses is maintained by each State Nurses Registration Council. These names are also maintained in the Indian Nurses Register by INC. Nurses, midwives, auxiliary nurse midwives and health visitors are registered. All degree-holding nurses also have to get the registration in state council.

Structure:
- Each state determines the specific administrative responsibility and oversight of the council of nursing
- The governor of the state
- The state health directorate
- Nursing directorate
- Another state official or organization.

The salient features of State Registration Council:
- Provision of an autonomous body, comprising majority of nurses, endowed with decision-making powers
- Compulsory registration for all nurses, midwives practicing within the state. Provision of nurses,

midwives, and public health nurses to elect their own representatives to the respective state
- Powers to regulate nursing education prescribe curriculum and enunciate examination policies
- Provision to have a nurse registrar to carry out the functions of the SNC. Provision for recognition of educational institutions of nursing and withdrawal of such recognition, if necessary.

The Karnataka State Nursing Council

The Karnataka State Nursing Council was established in the year 1971 under the authority of Karnataka Nurses, Midwives and Health Visitors Act of 1961. The first council was nominated by the Government with different members representing various constituencies under Section 3 of the Act, all together consisting of 22 members. The Council is an autonomous statutory registration body of qualified nurses, midwives, ANMs and health visitors.

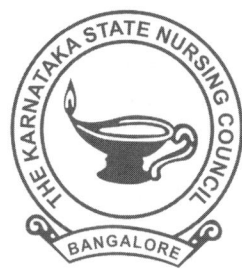

Nursing Council Act

The state government under their letter no. HFW 202 MSN84, dated 27th August 1991, has approved the bylaws.

These bylaws may be called the Karnataka State Nursing Council Bylaws.

Functions of Karnataka State Nursing Council

- Regulation of training program of the diploma, graduate and postgraduate courses.
- Suspension of practice of the profession by its member.
- Granting recognition to the training institutes and periodical inspection, as the council is the governing authority of physical and clinical facilities in almost all the nursing courses conducted in the institution
- Prescribing syllabus and curriculum for various nursing courses conducting qualifying examination
- Registration and gratify certificate to qualified persons to practice their profession and to watch and take action against practice of profession by quacks and check malpractice as well as to take action.

Duties of Registrar

Registrar Administration and Finance

- All matters of administration and finance of the nursing council
- Convening nursing council meeting
- Registration renewal
- Recognition of nursing schools, licensing of nursing establishments
- Legal matters
- Conducting elections.

Nurse Registrar

- All matters connected with the examination, convening examination board meeting and declaration of results
- All matters connected with the examinations of GNM, ANM and health visitors
- Setting up of syllabus, conducting workshop and seniors and implementation of new syllabus
- Issuing examination certificates
- Admission approval
- To prepare the diploma certificates and registration certificates of nurses who have been qualified
- To arrange for inspections to ascertain that the institutions are carrying out the educational programs according to syllabus, rules and regulations laid down by state council.

Discussion

Limitations and constraints of INC.

Establishment, Incorporation and Constitution of the Council

1. **The state government may, by notification, establish a council to be called the Karnataka Nursing Council** for the purpose of carrying out the provisions of this Act. Such a council shall be a body corporate having perpetual succession and a common seal with power, subject to the provisions of this Act, to acquire, hold and dispose of property and to contract and may, by the same name, sue and be sued.
2. **The Council shall consist of the following members:**
   a. **As ex-officio members:**
      i. The Director of Health and Family Planning Services in Karnataka or such other officer as the state government may nominate
      ii. The Superintendent of Nursing Services, Government of Karnataka
   b. **As elected members:**
      i. **Eight persons** to be elected from amongst themselves by nurses, midwives, auxiliary nurse midwives and health visitors registered in the register, the number of persons to be elected from each category being so divided as to be in the proportion of the number of their members in the register:
         - Provided that in determining the said proportion, a fraction of one-half or less shall be neglected and a fraction of more than one-half shall be counted as one
         - Provided further that the number of members to be elected representing any particular category shall be at least one
      ii. **Two persons** to be elected from amongst themselves by the heads of the affiliated institutions
      iii. **Two persons** to be elected from amongst themselves by the matrons and nursing

superintendents of the affiliated institutions in the State of Karnataka

    iv. **One person** to be elected from amongst themselves by the sister tutors of the affiliated institutions

    v. **One person** to be elected by the Karnataka Medical Council

    vi. **One person** to be elected by the Karnataka State Branch by whatever name called of the Indian Medical Association

    vii. **One person** to be elected by the Karnataka State Branch of the Trained Nurses' Association of India.

  c. **As nominated members**, three persons to be nominated by the State Government of whom at least one person shall be a woman.

Provided that the members to be elected under clause (b) shall in respect of the first Council, be nominated by the State Government from persons who in the opinion of the state government are entitled to be included in the electorate or body concerned and shall hold office for a period of 2 years.

3. **The President and Vice-President of the Council shall be elected from among the members of the Council.**
4. **The election of the President and Vice-President shall, subject to the provisions of this Act, be held at such time and place and in such manner as may be prescribed.**

Registration Process

Maintenance of Register

The Council shall maintain a register of (a) nurses, (b) midwives, (c) auxiliary nurses and (d) health visitors, consisting of four sections, in such form, containing such particulars and divided into such parts as may be prescribed.

Persons Entitled to Registration

Persons who have undergone such courses of training have passed such examinations and who fulfil such other conditions as may be prescribed shall, on payment of the prescribed fee and on making an application in the prescribed form, be entitled to registration.

Refusal of registration and removal and re-entry of names:
- Subject to such conditions as may be prescribed, the Council may, after giving an opportunity to the person concerned to be heard in his defense and after holding an inquiry in the prescribed manner, refuse to enter in the register the name of any person or may order the removal of the name of such person from the register.
- The order passed under sub-section (1) shall be in writing and shall be served on the person concerned in the prescribed manner.
- The Council may direct that the name of any person against whom an order under sub-section (1) has been passed shall be entered or re-entered in the register, as the case may be.

Appeal from order under Section 14:
- Any person aggrieved by any order of the Council made under Section 14 may, within 90 days from the date on which such order is served, appeal against such order to the state government.
- The order of the state government on any such appeal shall be final.

Renewal fee:
- Notwithstanding anything contained in Section 13, the Council may, with the previous sanction of the state government, direct that for every 3 years a renewal fee of 1[five rupees]1 shall be paid by each person registered under this Act for the continuance of his name on the register.
- If the renewal fee is not paid before the date fixed by the Council, the Council may after giving notice to the defaulter concerned remove the name of the defaulter from the register.

Provided that the name so removed may be re-entered in the register on payment of the renewal fee in such manner and subject to such conditions as the Council may, after giving notice to the defaulter concerned.

State Nursing Boards

History

More than 100 years ago, state governments established boards of nursing to protect the public's health and welfare by overseeing and ensuring the safe practice of nursing in India. Boards of Nursing are state governmental agencies that are responsible for the regulation of nursing practice.

Roles and Responsibilities

- To coordinate and bring a uniform standard of nursing education
- To verify the eligibility requirements of the students before each examination
- To arrange for conducting examination and issuing certificates to successful candidates
- To prepare the calendar of events at the beginning of each academic year
- To appoint the examiners before each examination

Nursing Registration Board

Roles and responsibilities

- Enforcing the Nurse Practice Act and nurse licensure
- Accrediting or approving nurse education programs in schools and universities
- Responsible to maintain the register in prescribed manner for nurses, midwives and health visitors is called Indian Nurses Register
- Developing policies, practice standards and administrative regulations.

University

A University is an institution of higher education and research which grants academic degrees in a variety of subjects and provides both undergraduate education and postgraduate education.

Roles and Responsibilities

- Regulation of its own colleges and affiliated institutions
- Conducting inspection and granting permission for admission
- Conducting examination and announcing the results
- Conducting the graduation, postgraduation and doctoral programs
- Ensuring faculty welfare and development
- Ensuring student welfare and development
- Organizing various programs such as book exhibition, job fair, seminars, conferences, inter-college competitions, sport meets, etc.

Recent Strategies of University

- Internationalization strategies
- Quality and competitiveness strategies
- Web-based learning strategies.

CONCLUSION

The provincial regulatory bodies have responsibility for monitoring and approving nursing education. All nursing education programs must prove that their nursing curriculum prepares graduates to practice professionally and meet the required standards and competencies. The government sets out the legislation for the protection of the public. It is the nurses themselves who carry out this legislation under the specific mandate and structure required by the law.

CHAPTER 6: Professional Organizations

CHAPTER OUTLINE

- Definition and Meaning of Professional Organizations
- Major National Professional Organizations
  - Indian Nursing Council
  - State Registration Council
  - Trained Nurses Association of India
  - National Students Nurses Association
  - International Council of Nurses
  - National League of Nursing
  - Health Visitors League
  - Midwives and Auxiliary Nurse Midwives Association
  - Nursing Research Society of India
  - State Nurses Associations
- International Professional Organizations
  - American Nursing Association
  - Royal British Nurses Association
  - Canadian Nurses Association
  - Sigma Theta Tau International Honor Society of Nursing
- Other Associations
  - Commonwealth Nurses Federation
  - The Christian Nurses League
  - The Catholic Nurses Guild of India
  - The Indian Red Cross Society

INTRODUCTION

It is time for governance of nursing practice, education and functioning of health care system under law. Effective contribution of nursing care is possible by organized effort through organization and association of nursing as well as regulatory body, e.g. Nursing Council of India.

DEFINITION OF ORGANIZATION

Organization is the form of every human association for the attainment of common purpose and the process of relating specific duties or function in a whole. **—JD Mooney**

Organization is a system of co-operative activities of two or more persons. **—Chester/Bernard**

Professional organizations are the organizations that sets standard for practice and education. **—Carol Taylor**

MEANING OF PROFESSIONAL ORGANIZATION

Professional organization provides a means through which your own professional development can be channeled with authority of their representative character. It provides you an opportunity to express your viewpoints, develop your leadership qualities and abilities, and keep you well informed of professional trends and current issues.

All qualified nurses must participate in their professional State and National Organizations informed of new developments and upgrading the profession.

MAJOR NATIONAL PROFESSIONAL ORGANIZATIONS (TABLE 6.1)

Some of the Organizations are discussed below:
1. Indian Nursing Council (discussed in Chapter 5)
2. State Registration Council (discussed in Chapter 5)
3. Trained Nurses Association of India

Table 6.1: Major nursing professional organizations.

National organizations:	International organizations:
- Indian Nursing Council - State Registration Council - Trained Nurses Association of India - National Student Nurses Association - National League for Nursing - Health Visitors League - Midwives and Auxiliary Nurse Midwives Association - Nursing Research Society of India - State Nurses Associations	- American Nurses Association - Royal British Nurses Association - Canadian Nurses Association - International Council of Nurses - Sigma Theta Tau International Honor Society of Nursing **Other associations:** - Commonwealth Nurses Federation - The Christian Nurses League - The Catholic Nurses Guild of India - The Indian Red Cross Society

TRAINED NURSES ASSOCIATION OF INDIA

History of TNAI

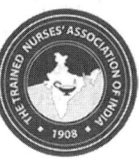

Before 1946, trained birth attendants used to gather in a forum, which never made any group activities. When Delhi and Vellore started graduation, nursing care took a different direction to establish themselves as an organized group.

By 1952, we could see an organized effort of grouping among trained nurses, but without any registered body. Various specialized courses are being made available, such as community health nursing, midwifery, operating assistant and rehabilitation nursing.

By 1960, an organized group called TNAI has formed with an objective of involvement into community welfare activities such as:
- Nursing care of children
- Nursing care of elderly
- Blood donation campaign and campus
- First aid facility
- Vocational rehabilitation
- Relief work with Red Cross, Indian Medical Association (IMA) and general practitioners
- The TNAI is the national body of nurses at various levels.

Definition of TNAI

TNAI is a non-sectarian, non-political, professional organization whose membership is opened to all registered nurses who hold certificates of full training in nursing and are recognized by INC and State Nursing Registration Councils.

Basic Objectives of the Association Set up in 1908

- To uphold the dignity and honor of the nursing profession
- To promote team spirit, high standards of health care and nursing practice
- Apart from enabling the members to represent their grievances and express their point of view to the concerned quarter in problematic situations
- It strives to update the knowledge of nurses and improve their skills.

Aims

- To standardize, upgrade, develop nursing education and to elevate nursing education
- To improve the living and working conditions of the nurses and also develop the educational standards for nursing
- To provide registration for qualified nurses and reciprocity of registration within different states in the country and within different countries

Membership

The membership consists of:
- **Full members:** Fully qualified registered nurses
- **Associate Members:** Health visitors, midwives and junior health assistants
- **Affiliate Members:** Student nurses and members of the affiliated organizations. Example: Christian Nurses League (CNL).
- Membership of TNAI is obtained by application and submission of the copy of one's State Registration Certificate. One can apply for life membership.
- Membership can also be transferred from SNA by transferring a certificate from the institution within six months of completion of the course.
- **Institutional membership:** Any organization with similar objectives and philosophy as that of TNAI
- **Honorary fellowship:** The council shall select members of the association who have rendered service of a very high order to the cause of nursing and confer with them, the honorary fellowship of TNAI
- **All have voting rights except institutional members and honorary fellowship members**

Functions

- The association works towards the professional enlistment and development of nurses
- It organizes workshops, conferences, educational, cultural and social programs for overall development of nurses
- It makes the society understand the role of nurses and their commitment to the society
- The association helps the nurses to specialize, to practice independently and practice evidence-based nursing management
- Research programs and continuing education programs are periodically arranged
- The association wants the nurse to be qualified and registered to practice and to uphold professionalism
- It is supporting the implementation of nursing homes
- It is looking at lack of basic equipment in many institutions that are constraints for providing quality care.

The Head Quarters

The Head Quarters of TNAI was transferred from Madras and established in Delhi in 1942. In 1946, the association purchased half an acre plot for building site in Green Park, New Delhi. The foundation stone was laid by Dr. Radhakrishnan, Vice President of India on October 17, 1960. The office moved to L-16 and L-17, Green Park, New Delhi, on July 31, 1961. The opening ceremony was performed by Mrs Indira Gandhi on September 30, 1961.

Management (Flowchart 6.1)

The management of association constituents:
- President
- First Vice President
- Second Vice President
- Third Vice President
- Honorary Treasurer
- Secretary General
- Assistant Secretary cum SNA Advisor
- Assistant Secretaries
- Editor
- President or Vice President, one from each State or Union Territory
- Branch or joint secretaries
- Co-opted members
- Chairpersons of standing committees and interest sections
- Ex-officio members.

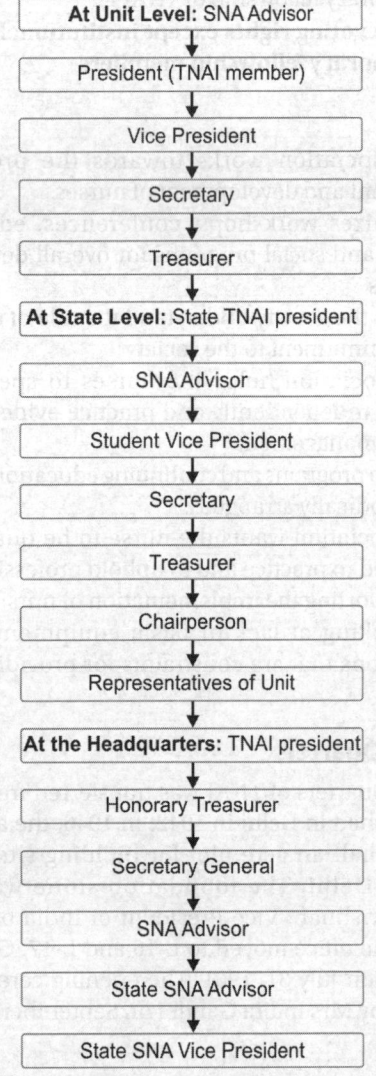

Flowchart 6.1: Organizational structure of TNAI.

Meetings

- *General meetings*: The general meetings of the members of the association shall be held biannually at which time and place as council may decide.
- *Special meetings*: The President of the TNAI may call a special meeting of the council/executive/house of delegates at any time necessary.

Elections

1. **Office bearers of the Council** of TNAI are the President, Vice President and Honorary Treasurer elected by the house of delegates.
2. **Executive Committee:** The nine members of the executive committee shall be elected by the Council from amongst its elected members at its meeting by ballet. The term shall be for 4 years.
3. **House of delegates:** There shall be one representative for every 200 members from states. For each fraction above 100, there shall be one representative. They shall be elected during general body meetings of the branch.

Activities Performed by TNAI

- Conducting conferences
- Organizing continuing education programs for the nurses of India at all levels
- Publishing journals and celebration of WHO day, International Nurses Day and International Women's Day and other related activities are carried out with the initiatives of TNAI in all states of the country
- Planning and implementation of socioeconomic welfare programs
- Participating with nursing regulation projects
- Coordinating the activities of student nurses associations and organizing extra-curricular activities at state and national levels.

Benefits of TNAI

- Representing various professional issues like Central Pay Commission
- Publishing journals and issuing publications with low cost for members and students
- Scholarship for TNAI members and student nurses
- Annual grant to state branches to hold activities
- One-fourth railway concession for TNAI members
- The guest room facilities at the Head Quarters and also in some states
- To establish functions, standards and qualifications for nursing practice
- Implementation of nursing standards through appropriate channel
- To establish a code of ethical conduct for practitioners
- To provide professional counseling and placement services for nurses
- To promote legislation

- To promote and protect socioeconomic welfare programs for destitute and elderly members
- To promote the general health and welfare of the public through all association programs, relationships and activities.

Publications of TNAI

The official organ of the TNAI is "The Nursing Journal of India" which is published monthly and impressive publication is "Indian Nursing Yearbook". Other publications include:
- Community Health Nursing Manual
- Nursing Administration and Management
- A Procedure Manual of Fundamentals of Nursing
- Simplified Micro Biology
- History and Trends of Nursing in India – 2006
- TNAI Handbook

The TNAI has Established the Following Organizations

1. Health Visitors League (1922)
2. Midwives and auxiliary Nurse Midwives Association (1925).
3. Student Nurses Association (1929–30).

NATIONAL STUDENTS NURSES ASSOCIATION

History

The National Student Nurses Association (NSNA) is official pre-professional organization for nursing students, formed in 1953; it was established in 1929 at the time of annual conference of the TNAI, and in 1954, SNA celebrated the Silver Jubilee and number of units was 117. Now SNA have more than 506 units. SNA having separate biannual conference, there is a separate secretary for national level and was incorporated in 1959. The NSNA originally functioned under the agencies of the American Nurses Association (ANA) and National League for Nursing (NLN); however in 1968, the NSNA became an autonomous body, although it communicates with the NLN and ANA. In 1975, it was agreed by the TNAI Council that one student representative be included in the State Branch Executive Committee on trial basis before the students are included in the TNAI Council as representatives of SNA. To qualify for membership in the NSNA, a student must be enrolled in a state-approved nursing education program.

Objectives of SNA

- To help students to uphold the dignity and the ideals of profession for which they are qualifying.
- To promote a corporate spirit among students for common good.
- To furnish nurses in training with advise in their courses of study leading to professional qualification.
- To develop leadership ability, skills and help students to gain a wide range of knowledge of the nursing profession in all of its different branches.
- To encourage both professional and recreational meetings, games and sports.
- To help the students to increase their social contacts and general knowledge in order to help in the world where they have furnished their training.
- To provide a special section in the Nursing Journal of India for the benefits of the students.
- To encourage students to compete for prizes in the student nursing competitions.

Management of SNA

The Governing body of association shall be the Council of TNAI which will receive the recommendations of the general committee of the SNA for considerations. The general committee of SNA shall consist of:
- President of TNAI or one of the Vice Presidents if the President wishes to delegate this responsibility
- Vice Presidents of SNA State branches
- Honorary Treasurer of TNAI
- National SNA Advisor who must be full member of TNAI
- State branches SNA Advisors
- Secretary of the SNA State branches
- Secretary General of TNAI.

SNA General Body

At national level, comprises of:
- Members of SNA general committee.
- Three representatives from each unit, i.e. SNA Vice President, SNA Secretary and SNA Advisor.
- All SNA delegates attending the conference.

SNA General Body at State Level

It consists of State SNA Executive committee members (State branch President, Vice President, Advisor, Secretary, Treasurer and Program Chairperson) and SNA Unit representatives (Vice President, Secretary and SNA Advisor).

SNA Units

Each unit should elect its own members of Executive Committee in its general body meeting, and these members are SNA Unit Advisor, Vice President, Secretary and Program Chairperson. The SNA general body meetings should be held at regular intervals. The agenda for these meetings will be according to the needs of unit members and objectives of SNA. SNA Unit Advisor is responsible to see that, as soon as a nurse has graduated, she is given an SNA to TNAI form for membership in TNAI. This form must be signed by the

Nursing Head of the institution and sent to the Secretary General of TNAI.

Membership

Student nurses of GNM, Basic BSc Nursing, multipurpose health worker (female)/auxiliary nurse—midwives, lady health visitors from the training institutions recognized by INC, in which a student nurses unit has been established.

Activities of SNA

A wide variety of activities are encouraged for SNA. Keeping in view the objectives of association and to strengthen curricular and co-curricular components as follows:

- **Organization of meetings and conferences:** At the TNAI conference, two representatives of SNA from each state are invited as observer and these student representatives are Vice President and Secretary of the state branches. They are invited to attend business meetings as observer.

    Three to four days' conference is held for SNA members biennially. Members discuss and provide final solution for various problems faced by the students. These conferences are held biennially at state level. At the units usually the meeting is held monthly or bi-monthly.

- **Maintenance of diary:** This is a biennial record book drawn up for the use of unit secretaries. The diaries are assessed annually by the state and SNA Advisors, and two best diaries are sent by state to the national SNA Advisor for biennial evaluation and awards.

    These diaries are assessed for professional, educational, extra-curricular, social, cultural and recreational aspects.

- **Exhibition:** Exhibition is a very useful and very popular activity of the association. All categories are eligible to participate either individually or in groups. They can prepare models, charts and posters on the subjects taught in their course of studies. Now, their activity is completed at the state level and one best entry under each category and section is entertained at national level.

- **Public speaking and writing:** Public speaking and writing are encouraged to increase self-confidence and help them gain skill in communication through debates, panel discussions and seminar on the theme of conference. Students are also encouraged to write for nursing general of India on a professional topic.

- **Project undertaking:** At the time of celebration of International Nurses Day, students are given project work on health-related topics. Regular project work is also given by institution to students.

- **Propagation of nursing profession:** Other professional and general public should be invited to celebration of professional and non-professional activities such as nurse's week and WHO day. The other activities such as a variety of entertainment programs, game, sports days, etc. are organized by nurses to acquaint general public with nursing profession.

- **Fund raising:** To meet the expenses at head quarter and SNA state level unit, it is necessary to raise the fund through voluntary donation.

- **Sociocultural and recreation activities:** To channelize your student energy, fine arts activities such as drama, dance, music and painting are arranged and competitions are also held at state and national level. Sports and games competitions are also held.

HEALTH VISITORS LEAGUE

This is an associate organization of TNAI called Health Visitors League.

Objectives

- To uphold in every way, the dignity and honor of health visitors
- To promote, among all health visitors, esprit corps
- To enable members to take council together on matters affecting their profession
- To raise the standards of education and practice of health visitor

President

The President of TNAI will be the President of Health Visitors League.

Membership

Health visitors holding a certificate from any health visitors training school recognized by INC, or in case of foreign qualifications recognized by the government of the country concerned, shall be eligible for membership.

Management

The governing body of the League shall be the Council of TNAI. The committee consists of:

- Honorary Secretary of Health Visitors League–Convener
- Representatives of the Health Visitors League on state branch committee
- Secretary-General of the TNAI, Ex-officio
- Honorary Treasurer of TNAI, Ex-officio

    The committee shall deal with all matters affecting the League, but no change shall be made in the policy of TNAI, or the subscription or privilege of membership, without the approval of TNAI Council.

- **Meetings:** A meeting of the committee and of members of the League shall be held at the time of the general meetings of TNAI and as desired.

MIDWIVES AND AUXILIARY NURSE MIDWIVES ASSOCIATION

One of the associate organizations of TNAI shall be the Midwives and Auxiliary Midwives Association.

Objectives

- To uphold in every way, the dignity and honor of the midwives and auxiliary midwives
- To promote, among all the midwives and auxiliary midwives, esprit corps
- To enable members to take council together on matters affecting their profession
- To raise the standards of education and practice of the midwives and auxiliary midwives.

President

The President of TNAI will be the President of Midwives and Auxiliary Midwives Association.

Membership

Midwives and auxiliary midwives holding a certificate from any midwifery and auxiliary midwifery training school recognized by INC, or in case of foreign qualifications recognized by the government of the country concerned, shall be eligible for membership.

Management

The governing body of the League shall be the Council of TNAI. The committee consists of:

- Honorary Secretary of Midwives and Auxiliary Midwives Association–Convener
- Representatives of the Midwives and Auxiliary Midwives Association on state branch committee
- Secretary-General of the TNAI, Ex-officio
- Honorary Treasurer of TNAI, Ex-officio

The committee shall deal with all matters affecting the Association, but no change shall be made in the policy of TNAI, or the subscription or privilege of membership, without the approval of TNAI Council.

- **Meetings:** A meeting of the committee and of members of the Association shall be held at the time of the general meetings of TNAI and as desired.
- **Election:** Election of the Honorary Secretary shall be held at a meeting of Midwives and Auxiliary Nurse Midwives Association at the time of general meeting and procedure is same as that of TNAI. The term of office shall be 4 years.

NURSING RESEARCH SOCIETY OF INDIA

Introduction

The Nursing Research Society of India (NRSI) was established in May, 1986 to promote research within and around nursing environment. It is registered under the society's Act XXI of 1960 with Registrar of Societies, Delhi administration (certificate no. S/18421 dated 2nd December, 1987).

Names and Objectives

- Supports the development of nursing research activities, the universities and nursing health care institutions
- Provides a platform to nurse-scientists to exchange views on nursing research
- Promotes and sponsors specific meets, seminars and conferences to advanced nursing research
- Creates public interest in the contribution of promotive, preventive and restorative activities
- Establishes a nursing research journal of India and brings out other documents attaining to innovations in nursing

Governing Body of NRSI

Governing/Managing/Executive Committee

- Governing body consists of members who shall take care of day-to-day functions of the society to achieve its aims and objects
- Governing body would consist of President, Vice President, Secretary, Joint Secretary, Treasurer, Editor, elected regional representatives (President), immediate Past President and the Secretary
- Minimum and maximum strength of governing body would be 7 and 15, respectively.
- Election would be held every four years in the general body meeting
- Term of office of the governing body shall be of 4 years.

Power/Duties/Functions of the General Body

- Shall meet at least once in a year
- Shall be able to spend two third of the money in hand of various activities of the society but must get it approved during the general body meeting
- Quorum and notice of the meeting: one fifth of the members will make a Quorum
- *Filling up of the casual vacancies:* Vacancies occurring by resigning or otherwise during middle of the term or before general body meeting shall be filled ad-hoc basis by the governing body.

Power and Duties of the Office Bearers

President

- The president shall precede over at the general body and executive committee meetings
- President shall see to it that constitution of the society is adhered to
- Has right to attend any community meeting of the society
- Can spend ₹ 500/- a month on her/his discretion (subject to revision from time to time)
- Sign cheques and other negotiable instruments, jointly with treasurer or secretary.

President or Vice President

Performs all duties of the president in his/her absence.

Secretary

- Is the principle executive officer of the society
- Calls meetings (general body and executives)

- Spends money within limits laid down by its general body members and executive members
- Shall be in constant touch with the president and act in accordance with his/her advice and instructions
- Can spend ₹ 500/- per month on his/her discretion (subject to revision from time to time)
- Sign cheques, jointly with either President or Treasurer.

Joint Secretary Shall
- Assist the secretary in all activities
- Perform all duties of the secretary in his/her absence.

Treasurer
- Keeps accounts of the society
- Presents annual audited accounts for the previous year to the members of the society during meetings
- Presents budgets for the next year
- His/her work maybe deputed to any other member of the society by president in his/her absence due to illness/visit abroad/resignation
- Signs cheques and other negotiable instruments jointly with Secretary in the absence of president.

Editor

Helps publish periodicals for the society.

Executive Committee Members
- **President:** Dr Usha U Ukkande, Principal and Professor, Choithriam College of Nursing, Manik Bagh Road, Indore
- **Vice President:** Mrs Selva Titus Chacko, Professor in Nursing, Deputy Dean, College of Nursing, CMC Vellore, Tamil Nadu
- **Secretary:** Prof (Dr) Pity Koul, Professor in Nursing, School of Health Sciences, IGNOU, Maidan Garhi, New Delhi
- **Treasurer:** Mrs Santosh Yadav, Assistant Superintendent, Lady Reading Health School, New Delhi
- **Editor:** Prof HC Rowat, Principal University College of Nursing, Faridkot, Punjab
- **Jr editor:** Mrs Shantha Dey, Professor, Bharathi Vidyapeet, Pune, Maharashtra.

INTERNATIONAL PROFESSIONAL ORGANIZATIONS

American Nurses Association

The ANA is the national professional organization for nursing in the United States. It was founded in 1896 as the nurses associated Alumnae of the United States and Canada. In 1911, the name was changed to the American Nurses Association. It was a character member of the International Council of Nurses (ICN), along with organizations in Great Britain and Germany in 1899:
- In 1982, the organizations became a Federation of State Nurses Associations. Individuals participate in the ANA by joining their state nurses' associations.
- The official journal of the ANA is the American Journal of Nursing, and American Nurse is the official newspaper.
- A nurse in her nursing profession recognizes and understands the fundamental needs of a healthy person, a sick person and who knows how these needs can best be met. She possesses a body of scientific nursing knowledge, which is based on science and technology. She will apply this knowledge to an individual and the community. She discerns her area of work with the work of other health professionals.
- The term professional nurse is given to those who are graduates as per nursing council of India guidelines and affiliated to university of health sciences.
- A constituent of ANA South Dakota nurses' association has in one voice supported professional nursing through advocacy and communication, networking and collaboration across nursing specialties; the registered nurse as a patient advocates working to increase access to quality, upholding standards of excellence for the profession and implementing exemplary care in a highly visible fashion.

Purpose of the ANA:
- To foster high standards of nursing practice and to promote the educational and professional advancement of nurses so that all people have better nursing care.
- It is committed to meet societal needs through contemporary nursing practice. This association brings together a community of peers strengthening a mutual effort to attain high standards of nursing practice.

As early as 1937, ANA defined professional nursing as a blend of intellectual attainment, attitudes and mental skills based on the principles of scientific medicine acquired by means of prescribed course in a school of nursing affiliated to hospital recognized by the state and practiced in conjunction with curative and preventive medicine by an individual licensed to do so by the state.

Priority issues of ANA:
- A restructured health care system that delivers primary health care in community-based settings
- An expanded role for registered nurses and advanced practice nurses in the delivery of basic and primary health care
- Obtaining federal funding for nurse education and training
- Helping to change and improve the health care work place to enhance the health and safety of the patient and nurse.

Royal British Nurses Association

The first organized body of trained nurses was British Nurses Association in the year 1887. It was called Royal British Nurses Association (RBNA) by Bedyord Fenwick and his wife with HRH princess Christian, daughter of Queen Victoria as its first president. In 1897, Fenwick and Isu Steward founded the Matron's council of Great Britain and Ireland. The

Passing of the Midwives Act 1902 encouraged the campaign for registration of nurses. The Association helped to set up the Central Committee for the State Registration of Nurses in 1908. The RBNA drafted three parliamentary bills on nurse registration. The central committee for the state registration of nurses was formed in 1909, which introduced annual parliamentary bills on the nurse registration. The College of Nursing was established in 1916 and an effort was made to merge with RBNA. The general nursing council chaired by Fenwick was established in 1920. In the year 1995, the association decided to make the archives fully available to the public.

Canadian Nurses Association

The Canadian Nurses Association (CNA) is the national nurses' association in Canada. Nurses do not join the CNA independently, but obtain membership by paying a fee to the provincial chapters.

The CNA has developed standards and code of ethics, and it offers support to all provincial associations. The CNA prepares licensure examinations and offers research grants fellowship and scholarship to Canadian nurses.

The official journal of CNA is The Canadian Nurse, which is published monthly.

International Council of Nurses (ICN)

Introduction

- The ICN was established in 1899. Nurses from Great Britain, the United States, and Canada were among the founding members. The council is a federation of national nurses' associations, such as the ANA and CNA.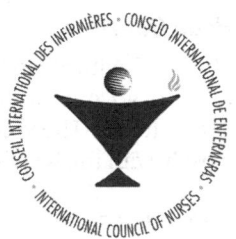
- The ICN provides an organization through which member national associations can work together for the mission of representing nursing worldwide, advancing the profession and influencing health policy. The five core values of the ICN are visionary leadership, inclusiveness, flexibility, partnership and achievement (ICN 2005).
- The official journal of ICN is "International Nursing Review."

Mission

To represent nursing worldwide, advancing the profession and influencing the health policy.

Purpose and Scope

ICN is a federation of nurses' association around the world which have bonded together to develop nursing contributions to the promotion of health and care of the sick. It was one of the health care organizations to adapt the strict policy of non-discrimination on matters regarding nationality, race, creed, color, politics, sex or social status. ICN accepts into membership of one association of nurses for each country.

Goals and Objectives

ICN's objectives are four-fold:
- To promote the development of strong national nurses' association
- To assist, national nurses' association to improve the standards of nursing and the competency of nurses. To assist national nurses' association to improve the status of nurses within their countries
- To serve as the authoritative voice for nurses and nursing internationally.

In short, there are three main goals:
- To bring nursing together worldwide
- To advance nurses and nursing worldwide
- To influence health policy.

Core Values

- Visionary leadership
- Inclusiveness
- Flexibility
- Partnership
- Achievement.

Head Quarters

The Head Quarters of ICN are placed at Geneva, Switzerland.

Membership

Membership is limited to one nursing organization per nation. In most cases, this is the national nurses' association such as the ANA. In 2001, the ICN permitted its members to adapt collaborative structures to be more inclusive of other domestic nursing groups. However, few member organizations have adapted the new structures (Fig. 6.1).

ICN is actively working for

1. **Professional nursing practice:**
   - Advance nursing practice
   - HIV/AIDS, TB and malaria
   - Women's health
   - Primary health care

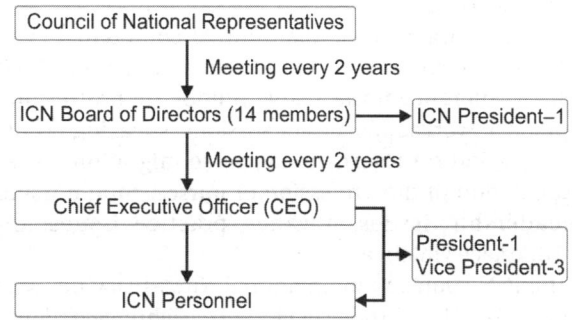

Fig. 6.1: ICN organization chart.

- Family health
- Safe water

2. **Nursing regulations:**
   - The ICN code for nurses is the foundation for the ethical nursing practices throughout the world
   - ICN standards, guidelines and policies for nursing practices, education and management are globally accepted as per the basis of nurses' policy
   - ICN advances nursing, nurses and health through its policies, partnership, advocacy and leadership development

3. **Socioeconomic welfare for nurses:**
   - Occupational health and safety
   - Human resources planning and policies
   - Career development
   - International trade in professional services.

Functions of ICN

- To provide policy directions to fulfill the objectives of ICN
- To establish categories of membership and determine their rights and obligations
- To act upon recommendations of the board of directors relating to admission and re-admission of member associations into ICN
- To receive and consider information from the board regarding activities
- To receive nominees for the board and to elect the board
- To act upon proposed amendments to ICN constitution
- To act upon recommendation of the board of directors for the amount of dues of national nurses' associations
- To act through mail or any written communication on ICN business that requires immediate attention.

Activities of ICN

- Focusing on the wide range of interests and needs of international membership, nursing education, economic and general welfare of nurses, nursing practice and service, nursing legislation, nursing research and cooperation with other health professions
- An important aspect of ICN's role is the coordination of activities with other international organizations in the health care field and acting as a spokesman of nurses at international level
- The ICN organizes a quadrennial conference every 4 years in conjunction with the meeting of the CNR. The conference hosts a large number of professional practice workshops, poster sessions, speaking events, discussion on international nurse migration issues, regulation of the profession of nurses, rural nursing, leadership issues, advance practice issues and workplace violence
- The ICN sponsors International Nurses Day on every May 12th, the birthday of Florence Nightingale's and it is supporting organization of health care information for all by 2015.

National League for Nursing

The NLN formed in 1952 is an organization of both individuals and agencies. Its objective is to foster the development and improvement of all nursing services and nursing education. People who are not nurses, but have an interest in nursing services, for example, hospital administration, can be members of the league.

- This feature of NLN involves non-nurse members, consumers and nurses from all levels of practice is unique.
- The NLN presents continuing education workshops for the remainder of its members. For school of nursing, the NLN offers testing services including preadmission testing for potential student and achievement testing through the program. The NLN also conducts yearly surveys of nursing schools, newly registered nurses and post-basic graduates. These surveys serve as primary sources of research data about nursing education in the United States. The National League for Nursing Accrediting Commission, an independent body within the NLN, provides voluntary accreditation for educational programs in nursing.
- The official journal of the NLN is Nursing and Healthcare Perspectives.

Head Quarters

The NLN, with Head Quarters in New York City, is led by a board of governors elected at large by the membership for 3-year terms. The volunteer president of the board works closely with the NLN's chief executive officer.

Core Values

The NLN implements its mission guided by four dynamic and integrated core values that permeate the organization and are reflected in its work:

- **Caring:** Promoting health, healing and hope and response to the human condition
- **Integrity:** Respecting the dignity and moral wholeness of every person without conditions or limitations
- **Diversity:** Affirming the uniqueness of and differences among persons, ideas, values and ethnicities
- **Excellence:** Creating and implementing transformative strategies with daring ingenuity.

Mission

The NLN promotes excellence in nursing education to build a strong and diverse nursing workforce.

Goals and objectives:

I. **Goal: Leader Nursing Education**—Enhance the NLN's national and international impact as the recognized leader in nursing education.

Objectives:
The NLN will:
- Be a key player in initiatives to build diversity in the nurse educator workforce
- Promote the education of the nursing workforce that contributes to health care quality and safety
- Be acknowledged as the leader in advancing excellence and innovation in nursing education.

II. **Goal: Commitment to members—Build a diverse, sustainable, member-led organization.**
Objectives:
- Continually seek out, engage and be responsive to full-time and part-time nurse faculty, individuals preparing for the faculty role, nursing education researchers and other health care and academic professionals
- Be the leading provider of products and services for the continuous professional development of nursing faculty.

III. **Goal: Champion for educators—Be the voice of nurse educators.**
Objectives:
- Promoting nursing education as an advanced practice role
- Shape and inform public policy on nursing education
- Expand and sustain alliances with other influential organizations.

IV. **Goal: Advancement of the science of nursing education—Promote evidence-based nursing education and the scholarship of teaching.**
Objectives:
- Promote the continuous development of faculty as educator-scholars
- Advocate for resources to support nursing education research.

Publications

The NLN's publications provide a broad spectrum of resources to our constituents and serve our mission to advance excellence in nursing education. Cutting-edge journal articles are published in the peer-reviewed, bi-monthly *Nursing Education Perspectives*.

NLN's print and electronic newsletters include *The NLN Report, NLN Member Update, Professional Development Bulletin* and *Nursing Education Policy*. Timely new releases keep you up-to-date on important events and activities at the NLN and around the world of nursing education.

Sigma Theta Tau International Honor Society of Nursing

Sigma Theta Tau, the international honor society of nursing was founded in 1922 and is headquartered in Indianapolis, Indiana. The Greek letters stand for the Greek words Storga, Tharos and Tima, meaning "love, courage and honor." The society is a member of the association of college honor societies. The society's purpose is professional rather than social. Membership is attained through academic achievement.

Students in baccalaureate programs in nursing and nurses in masters, doctoral and postdoctoral programs are eligible to be selected for membership, and potential members, who hold a minimum of bachelor's degree and have demonstrated achievement in nursing, can apply for membership as a nurse leader in the community.

The official journal of Sigma Theta Tau, **Journal of Nursing Scholarship** is published quarterly. The journal publishes scholarly articles of interest to nurses. The society also publishes **Reflections**, a quarterly newsletter that provides information about the organization and its various chapters.

OTHER ASSOCIATIONS

Commonwealth Nurses Federation

Introduction

The Commonwealth Nurses Federation is one of the 17 commonwealth-wide professional foundations receiving grant from commonwealth foundations.

The secretariat of the federation was established in 1973 at Royal Commonwealth Society, London. On that date, the member of associates was 25 and this number has increased now.

Aims and Objectives

The purposes for which the federation was established are as follows:
- To further the development of nursing for the benefit of the communities for countries within the commonwealth
- To promote the advances of nurses as profession
- To affect closer links between national nurses' association within the commonwealth as a means of providing mutual help and support
- To make available expert advice and assistance
- To disseminate professional information for the benefit of nurses
- To encourage the establishment of scholarship
- To organize commonwealth nurses' conferences from time to time
- To encourage establishment of national nurses' association in those commonwealth countries where none exists
- To cooperate with other commonwealth professional associations.

A regular CNF newsletter in the form of a federation supplement is made available to member associates.

The Christian Nurses League

Introduction
The Christian Nurses Association was formally organized in the year 1930, though it was actually born with the Christian Medical Association of India (CMAI), in the year 1926. Despite the great strides taken by nursing in India, the problems of nursing (education and service) remain the same though in a different nature. A very large number of nurses in the country are Christians.

Aim
The extension of the kingdom of Christ in India through the ministry of health and healing.

Objectives
- To encourage and promote spiritual fellowship
- To secure the highest standards in Christian nursing through the Christian nurses schools
- To promote highest efficiency in Christian nursing services
- To encourage the highest quality candidates to choose nursing as a desirable nurses vocation
- To help Christian nurses and institutions in solving their problems.

Membership
All Christian nurses from government, railways, industrial and military hospitals and overseas hospitals members are welcome to join the league and are encouraged to strengthen the bounds of fellowship. Students membership is also encouraged. The ANMs are accepted as associate members. Efforts are made to keep in touch with the nurses of other countries.

Activities
- **Christian nurses fellowship** is promoted through area conferences, retreats, rallies, prayer meetings and social gatherings. Christian medical conferences afford opportunity to develop good quality leadership and active participation in the programs.
- **Publications:** "The Christian Nurse," a bimonthly publication of the league, serves to promote fellowship and communication with one another in the country and abroad. Regional languages publication of nursing news is encouraged.

Professional Advancements
- As a liaison with the directorate general, health services and TNAI, the CNL recommends candidates for refresher courses and scholarships.
- **Conferences and contents:** CNL tries to keep in touch with all the members directly and through area secretaries to:
  - Answer question
  - Help solve problems
  - Provide prayer support
- **Projects:** A scholarship loan fund was built up:
  - To help needy student
  - Contributes to the various relief measures
  - Workshops and refresher courses—By the two nursing boards and the CMAI.

Other Projects
The CMAI shares the national concern of health and population problems and has been actively involved in the community of health and family planning program for more than a decade with Head Quarters at Bangalore.

The regional terms led by a nurse member are situated throughout the country, giving guidance and leadership in planning and carrying out the program.

Workshops
In community health, hospital administration, pharmacy and laboratory are presently being carried on under the direction of CMAI.

Economic Welfare of Nurses
The league has interest in suitable remunerations; living and service conditions of nurses in Christian hospitals. From time to time, negotiations are carried out to improve these conditions.

Nursing Education
The schools under the two nursing education boards and those outside (the boards) maintain high standards of education. The examining boards have been pioneering in publications of various nursing textbooks. Besides continuing education, workshops, preparing public health teaching aids and high quality examinations have been evolved.

Aims
- To promote the highest nursing efficiency in Christian nursing service
- Keeping abreast the changes and advances in medical and nursing education and postgraduate programs.

A high power commission was instituted:
- To make a study and find out ways and means of ascertaining adequate clinical specialists
- To look after financial components pertaining to keeping out the nursing school attention to student status
- To establish the type of education in terms of the needs for health delivery system in India

CONCLUSION
As professional organizations are the organizations that set standard for practice and education, it provides protection for professional rights, and it will give a detailed job description for its members and provides job security.

7

CHAPTER

Unions, Individual and Collective Bargaining

CHAPTER OUTLINE

- Definition and Types of Unions
- Unions/Labor Organization
- Nurses Unions and Associations
- Meaning and Definition of Collective Bargaining
- Objectives of Collective Bargaining
- Characteristics of Collective Bargaining
- Principles of Collective Bargaining
- Types of Bargaining
- Preparation for Collective Bargaining
- Process of Collective Bargaining
- Steps of Collective Bargaining
- Types of Strikes
- Levels of Collective Bargaining
- Importance of Collective Bargaining
- Advantages and Disadvantages of Collective Bargaining
- Research Abstract

COLLECTIVE BARGAINING

Introduction

The idea of collective emerged as a result of industrial conflict and growth of the trade union movement. The first collective bargaining agreement in India was concluded in 1920 at the instance of Mahatma Gandhi to regulate labor management relations in the textile industry in Ahmedabad. Collective bargaining is the most controversial and divisive issue in nursing. Some believe that collective bargaining reduces the professionalism of nursing, others view it as a mechanism to prevent employees from exploiting nurses. It has been seen as a complex legal issue, but dealt with by attorney and other experts specifically trained to handle the problem it presents.

DEFINITION OF UNIONS

The action of joining together or the fact of being joined together, especially in a political context.

TYPES OF UNIONS

Economists Ronald G Ehrenberg and Robert Smith, authors of "Modern Labour Economics," identify some of the unions: craft unions and industrial unions, and also third type is public sector unions.

1. **Craft unions:** Craft unions represent workers in a specific occupation. Modern craft unions continue to represent works in specific occupations, especially skilled trades. **Example:** Blacksmiths, bakers, autoworkers, electrical workers, etc.
2. **Industrial unions:** Industrial unions represent workers in a particular industry, regardless of workers' specific occupations.
3. **Labor unions:** There is a third type, which is public employee unions, which represent government workers, regardless of their specifications. These are similar to industrial unions, which includes government agencies, such as public schools, national education association, municipal employees, etc.

LABOR UNIONS

A labor union is an organization intended to represent the collective interests in negotiations with employees over wages, hours, benefits and working conditions.

A labor union is an organization that represents the rights and interests of workers to their employers. For example, in order to improve working conditions or wages.

UNIONS/LABOR ORGANIZATION

An organization in which employees participate for the purpose of negotiating with the employers about grievances, labor disagreement, wages, hours of work and conditions of employment.

NURSES UNIONS AND ASSOCIATIONS

Since its inception, the American Nurses Association (ANA) has had an active interest in the economics, security of nurses.

- ❖ *In the early 1900s:* Working conditions and salaries for nurses were extremely poor.
- ❖ *In 1929:* Some nurses began to recognize that protest and collective action were necessary to improve the conditions.
- ❖ *In 1945:* Shirley Titus, the Executive Director of the California Nurses Association, chaired a committee to study the employment conditions of nurses, and as a result of findings, ANA adopted what was called economic security program.
- ❖ *In 1974:* The health care amendments referred to earlier made it possible for nurses to use legal sanctions to ensure bargaining related to conditions of employment. Since the passage of amendments in 1978, many State Nurses Associations (SNAs) have qualified as legal bargaining agents for nurses.
- ❖ *In 1976:* ANA was to promote the useful honor and financial interest of nursing profession. Flannigan supported to shape the role of the profession by collective bargaining for nurses officially. ANA did not adopt an economic security program that included collective bargaining for nurses through the economics and general welfare program which currently is called the department of labor relations and work place advocacy.
- ❖ *In 1978:* Karnataka State Government Nurses Association started.
- ❖ *In 1982:* ANA changed structure to become a Federation of State Association. This change has rendered the state associations more direct representation of their member nurses.
- ❖ *In 1983:* The nursing leaders established the first organization, the American Society of Superintendents of Training Schools for Nurses, one of whose purpose was a commitment to promote the general welfare of nurses.

The ANA is a registered labor organization, but it does not engage in direct collective bargaining. The actual certification of units, negotiation of contracts and administration of contracts are conducted by the SNA.

The SNA have the freedom to independently decide their own level participation regarding collective bargaining.

MEANING OF COLLECTIVE BARGAINING

Collective bargaining consists of two words. Collective, which implies group action through its representative, and bargaining that suggests negotiating. It is a process between employers and employees to reach an agreement regarding the rights and duties of people at work. It aims to reach a collective agreement, which usually sets out issues such as employees' pay, working hours, training, health and safety, and rights to participate in work place or company affairs.

Collective bargaining is the means by which professional nurses can influence hospital nursing care delivery systems and labor management relations through a united voice.

DEFINITION OF COLLECTIVE BARGAINING

Collective bargaining takes place when a number of work people enter into a negotiation as a bargaining unit an employee or group of employee with the object of reaching an agreement on conditions of the employment of the work people.
—**Richardson JH**

Collective bargaining is an agreement between a single employer or an association of employees on the one hand, and a labor union on the other, which regulates the terms and conditions of employment.
—**Ludwig Teller**

OBJECTIVES OF COLLECTIVE BARGAINING

Collective bargaining has benefits not only for the present but also for the future employees, which lay foundation to voice for their rights:
- ❖ To provide an opportunity to the employees to voice their problems on issues related to employment.
- ❖ To facilitate reaching a solution that is acceptable to all parties involved.
- ❖ To resolve all conflicts and disputes in a mutually agreeable manner.
- ❖ To prevent any conflicts or disputes in the future through mutually signed contracts.
- ❖ To develop a conducive atmosphere to foster good organization relations.
- ❖ To provide stable and peaceful organization (hospital) relations.
- ❖ To prevent organization being locked at by strikes.

CHARACTERISTICS OF COLLECTIVE BARGAINING

- ❖ It is a group process wherein one group represents the employers and the other represents the employees.
- ❖ Negotiations form an important aspect which leads to the process of collective bargaining that includes scope for discussions, compromise or mutual give and take.
- ❖ Collective bargaining is a formalized process by which employees and independent trade unions negotiate terms and conditions of employment, employment-related issues regulated at national organizational and workplace levels.
- ❖ Collective bargaining is a process leading to demands that end with reaching agreement, which serve as the basic law governing labor management relations over a period of time in an enterprise. It is a flexible process and not fixed or static.
- ❖ It is a bipartite process where always two parties involve in collective bargaining between employees and the management.
- ❖ It is a complementary process, i.e., each party needs something. Labor can increase productivity and management can pay better for their efforts.

- It tends to improve the relations between workers and the union on the one hand, and the employer on the other.
- It is a continuous process. It enables industrial democracy to be effective.
- It takes all activities into account, such as day-to-day changes in policies, potentialities, benefits and interests.
- It is a political activity frequently undertaken by professional negotiation.

PRINCIPLES OF COLLECTIVE BARGAINING

For the Management

- It must develop and continues to follow a realistic policy for the welfare of employees.
- It must grant recognition to the unions and associations.
- It should extend fair treatment to the nursing associations and unions.
- It should deal only with one association in the organization.

For the Association/Unions

- The association should eliminate under democratic practices.
- Association leaders should not only function further to secure higher wages, short working hands and better working conditions for their members.
- Associations should go to strike only when all other methods of settlement of a dispute have failed.

For Both the Union and the Management

- It should be made an education as well as bargaining process.
- It must be as a means of finding the best possible solutions.
- Both parties should command the respect of each other.
- There must be good faith and a desire to make collective bargaining effective in practice.

TYPES OF BARGAINING

A collective bargaining process generally consists of four types of activities, i.e. distributive bargaining, integrative bargaining, attitudinal restructuring and intra-organizational bargaining.

- **Distributive bargaining:** It involves haggling, bargaining over the distribution of surplus. Under it, the economic issues such as wages, salaries and bonus are discussed. In distributive bargaining, one party's gain is another party's loss. This is, most commonly, explained in terms of a pie. Disputants can work together to make the pie bigger, so there is enough for both of them to have as much as they want, or they can focus on cutting the pie up trying to get as much as they can for themselves. In general, distributive bargaining tends to be more competitive. It is also known as conjunctive bargaining.
- **Integrative bargaining:** This involves negotiation of an issue on which both the parties may gain or at least neither party loses. For example, representatives of employer and employee sides may bargain over the better training program or a better job evaluation method. Here both the parties are trying to make more of something. In general, it tends to be more cooperative than distributive bargaining. This type of bargaining is also known as cooperative bargaining.
- **Attitudinal restructuring:** This involves shaping and reshaping some attitudes such as trust or distrust, friendliness or hostility between labor and management. When there is a backlog of bitterness between both the parties, attitudinal restructuring is required to maintain smooth and harmonious industrial relations. It develops a bargaining environment and creates trust and cooperation among the parties.
- **Intra-organizational bargaining:** It generally aims at resolving internal conflicts. This is a type of maneuvering to achieve consensus with the workers and management. Even within the union, there may be differences between groups. For example, skilled workers may feel that they are neglected or women-workers may feel that their interests are not looked after properly. Within the management also, there may be differences. Trade unions maneuver to achieve consensus among the conflicting groups.

PREPARATION FOR COLLECTIVE BARGAINING

- Preparation for collective bargaining should begin months before the contract talks.
- Chairperson should establish and maintain a pleasant relationship with union representatives by treating them continuously in social situation grievance hearing.
- Obtain information from other nurse executives about union activities in neighboring health agencies.
- Review other labor contracts negotiating in other agencies to determine what type of demands were made by various worker categories.
- Keep ongoing recording agency employees' grievances and analyze these before negotiation begins.
- Research the wage salary structures of other health agencies in the community and compare against agencies' current wage package.
- Should read the act to identify limitations.

PROCESS OF COLLECTIVE BARGAINING (FIG. 7.1)

1. **Prepare:** It involves a negotiation team, which consists of representatives of both parties with adequate knowledge and skills for negotiation between employees, representatives and union and examine their own situation. A correct understanding of the

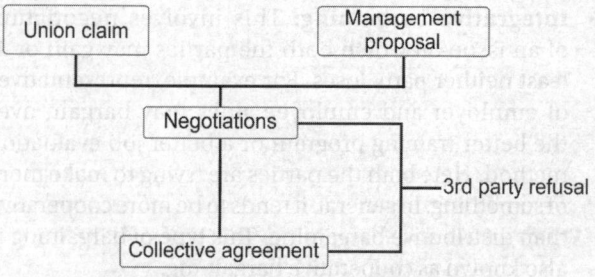

Fig. 7.1: Process of collective bargaining.

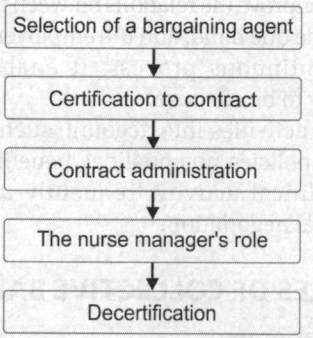

Fig. 7.2: Steps of collective bargaining.

main issues to be covered and intimate knowledge of operations, working conditions, production norms and other relevant conditions is required.

2. **Discuss:** The parties decide the ground rules that will guide the negotiations. A process well begun is half done and this is no less true in the case of collective bargaining. An environment of mutual trust and understanding is also created, which is leading to agreement.
3. **Propose:** This phase involves the initial opening statements and the possible options that exist to resolve them. This phase could be described as brain storming; the exchange of messages takes place and opinions of both the parties are sought.
4. **Bargain:** Negotiations are easy, if a problem-solving attitude is adopted. This stage comprises the time, and support is set forth, and the drafting of agreement takes place. Collective bargaining agreement may be in the form of procedural or substantive agreements. Procedural deals with the relationship between workers and management, and is adopted for resolving individual or group disputes. This normally includes procedures in respect of individual grievances, disputes and discipline. Frequently, procedural agreements provide information on the overall terms and conditions of employment, and codes of behavior. A substantive agreement deals with specific issues such as basic pay, overtime premiums, bonus agreements, holiday entitlements, hours of work, etc. In many companies, agreements have a fixed time scale and collective bargaining process will review the procedural agreement when negotiations take place on pay and conditions of employment.
5. **Settlement:** Once the parties are done with bargaining process, a consensual agreement is reached and both the parties agree to a common decision regarding the problem in issue. This stage is described as effective joint implementation of the agreement through shared vision, strategic planning and negotiated change.

STEPS OF COLLECTIVE BARGAINING (FIG. 7.2)

Selection of Bargaining Agent

This process is known as a representative election and is presided over by the National Labor Relationship Board (NLRB). For the election to occur, the union must demonstrate that 30% of the employees are affected by this action. The union can petition the national labor relations board to conduct an election. At the conclusion of this meeting, the board would have determined three things:

1. Who is eligible to participate in the union?
2. Whether the signatories are employees of the organizers?
3. A date for union election on election day, eligible employees are asked to choose representatives of the union.

Many unions represent registered nurses in collective bargaining. Therefore, the ballot may certain several choices for the bargaining agent. In addition to various SNAs, National Nurses Association and Trained Nurses' Association of India (TNAI), American Federation of Country and Municipal Employees (AFCME), Services Employees International Union (SEIU), selecting bargaining agent is important for the nurse, managers and staff nurses, and the rules of unfair labor practice apply.

Certification to Contract

Certification by the NLRB of a union to be the bargaining agent does mean that a group of people have the right to enter into a contract with an employee, a concept known as certification to contract. The actual contract and the provision must be written and voted on by the union membership. Issues considered as mandatory subjects of bargaining are rates of pay, wages, hours of employment and grievance procedure. Additionally, the contract may specify other areas provided that both parties agree that they can include:

- A union among security clause
- A management rights clause
- Seniority
- Fringe benefits
- Lay off and reduction in work language
- Floating procedure
- Insurance
- Retirement issues
- Professional issues.

The contract is considered to be in effect when both managements of the organizers and employees agree on its contract. Certification is obtained by a simple majority of eligible members who vote.

Contract Administration

The individual may be an employee of the union or a member of the nursing staff. It is the duty of the union representative to provide fair and equal representative to all members of the unit. The contract of union membership helps in the grievance process.

The Nurse Manager's Role

The nurse manager in a health care organization where nurses are organized into a collective bargaining unit participates in resolving grievances using the agreed upon grievance procedures.

Classification of Grievances

According to its cause, grievances agreement is classified as:
- Inadequate labor agreement
- Misunderstanding
- Lack of familiarity with the contract
- Intentional contract violations
- Ambiguous contract language or past practice
- Symptomatic problems outside.

The scope of the labor agreement frustration and labor relationship.

Grievance Process

- **Step 1:** The employee talks informally with her/his direct supervisor as soon as the incident has occurred, a written request for the next step is given to the immediate supervisor within 10 working days salary with representative of bargaining agent. The employee supervisor and agent will be present for any discussion.
- **Step 2:** If the response to step 1 is not satisfactory, a written appeal may be submitted within 10 work days to the director of nursing. The employee agent grievance chairperson and the top administrative or designs can be provided in 5 working days subsequent to these meetings.
- **Step 3:** The employee agent, grievance chairperson nursing administrative and director of human resources meet for discussions. The 10th and 5th day time limits for appeal and answer are again observed.
- **Step 4:** The final step is arbitration, which is involved when no solution suggested is acceptable. An arbitrator is a person who settles a dispute, and is a neutral third party who is selected and is present at these meetings. The submission of grievance may be required within 15 days after step 3 is completed.

Grievance Hearing

In the grievance hearing, remember this key behavior:
- Put the grievant at ease, do not interrupt or disagree
- Listen openly and carefully
- Discuss the problem calmly and with an open mind
- Get the story straight and get all the facts, and ask logical questions
- Consider the grievant view points
- Avoid snap judgment, do not jump to conclusion
- Make an equitable decision and then give it to the grievant promptly.

Decertification

Occasionally, members of a particular unit may decide that they want the union or that no union at all is needed. In such a case, the members of the bargaining unit have the right to either change their union affiliation or remove the union by using a process known as decertification. This process is essentially the same as that followed by the NLRB for a representation election.

TYPES OF STRIKES (FIG. 7.3)

Economic Strikes

Employees attempt to get their employer to meet their demands by their services. An employee cannot be fired for participating in an economic strike, and bill can be replaced.

Unfair Labor Strikes

Result from an unfair labor practice by an employer or a union.

Sympathy Strikes

Employees of one employer strike in support of another. Workers can refuse to cross to picket lines.

Jurisdictional Strikes

In jurisdictional strike, there is a work stoppage over the assignment of work to two or more unions. Employees may strike because the employer assigned a particular job to another union.

Recognition Strikes

It is a work stoppage to force an employer to bargain with a particular organization.

Illegal Strikes

The category of illegal strike comprises violent strikes, boycott or secondary strikes and wildcat or surprise strikes that are not authorized by the union.

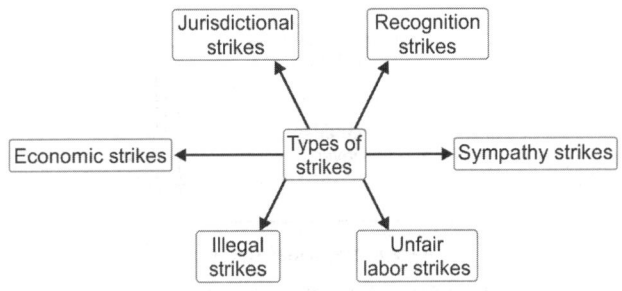

Fig. 7.3: Types of strikes.

LEVELS OF COLLECTIVE BARGAINING (FIG. 7.4)

- **National-level bargaining:** Economy-wide is a bipartite or tripartite form of negotiation between union confederations, central employer associations and government agencies. It aims at providing a floor for lower-level bargaining on the terms of employment, often taking into account macroeconomic goals.
- **Sectoral/industrial bargaining:** It aims at the standardization of the terms of employment in one industry, and includes a range of bargaining patterns. Bargaining may be either broadly or narrowly defined in terms of the industrial activities covered and may be either split up according to territorial subunits or conducted nationally.
- **Company/enterprise level:** This level involves the company and/or establishment. As a supplementary type of bargaining, it emphasizes the point that bargaining levels need not be mutually exclusive.

IMPORTANCE OF COLLECTIVE BARGAINING

Collective bargaining includes not only negotiations between the employers and unions but also includes the process of resolving labor management conflicts. Thus, collective bargaining is, essentially, a recognized way of creating a "system of" industrial jurisprudence. It acts as a method of introducing civil rights in the industry, that is, the management should be conducted by rules rather than arbitrary decision-making. It establishes rules, which define and restrict the traditional authority exercised by the management.

Importance to Employees

- It increases the strength of the workforce, thereby increasing their bargaining capacity group.
- Collective bargaining increases the morale and productivity of employees.
- It restricts management's freedom for arbitrary action against the employees. Moreover, unilateral actions by the employer are also discouraged.
- Effective collective bargaining machinery strengthens the trade unions movement.
- The workers feel motivated as they can approach the management on various matters and bargain for higher benefits.
- It helps in securing a prompt and fair settlement of grievances. It provides a flexible means for the adjustment of wages, and employment conditions to economic and technological changes in the industry, as a result of which the chances for conflicts are reduced.
- Collective bargaining develops a sense of self-respect and responsibility among the employees.

Importance to Employers

- It becomes easier for the management to resolve issues at the bargaining level rather than taking up complaints of individual workers.
- Collective bargaining tends to promote a sense of job security among employees, and thereby tends to reduce the cost of labor turnover to management.
- Collective bargaining opens up the channel of communication between the workers and the management, and increases worker participation in decision-making.
- Collective bargaining plays a vital role in settling and preventing industrial disputes.

Importance to Society

- Collective bargaining leads to industrial peace in the country.
- It results in establishment of a harmonious industrial climate, which supports and helps the pace of the nation's efforts towards economic and social development, since the obstacles to such a development can be considerable.
- The discrimination and exploitation of workers is constantly being checked. It provides a method or the regulation of the conditions of employment of those who are directly concerned about them.

ADVANTAGES OF COLLECTIVE BARGAINING

- Equalization of power
- Viable grievance procedure
- Equitable distribution of work
- Professionalism is promoted
- Nurses control practice.

DISADVANTAGES OF COLLECTIVE BARGAINING

- Adversary relationship
- Strikes may not be prevented
- Leadership may be difficult to obtain
- Unprofessional behavior

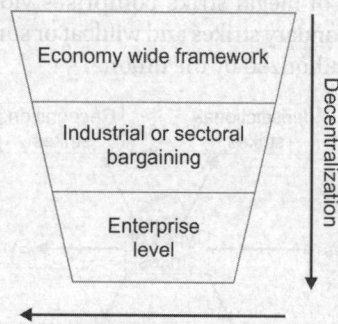

Fig. 7.4: Levels of collective bargaining.

- Interferes with management
- Decreased productivity of organization
- Must pay union dues
- Leads to dispute between employees and employer.

RESEARCH ABSTRACT

Collective bargaining has been recognized in almost all industrial settings as the most civilized way of resolving industrial conflicts and disagreements. The main objective of this paper is to determine the extent to which collective bargaining can effectively minimize industrial conflicts in Ghana with particular reference to the brewery industry in Ghana. It is a means of helping to foster cordial management-labor relationships towards industrial harmony. The study was carried out with a focus on Ghana Breweries Ltd. The results of the study show that collective bargaining is a powerful and effective tool that can be used to minimize industrial conflicts, and disagreements in industrial establishments. It is therefore recommended that employers should encourage the formation of trade unions to promote collective bargaining. It is further recommended that both management and labor should recognize collective bargaining as an effective tool for resolving conflicts and disagreements at the work place.

CONCLUSION

The collective bargaining has its own way between the labor and organization, but still the future of it is unknown for nursing community. Collective bargaining in labor relations procedure where an employer agrees to discuss the conditions of work by bargaining with representatives of the employees usually a labor union purpose may be either discussion of the terms and conditions of employment (wages, work hours, job safety or job security) or consideration of the collective relations between both sides, if a strike has occurred.

CHAPTER 8

Educational Preparations, Continuing Education and Career Opportunities—Professional Advancement, Role and Scope of Nursing Education

CHAPTER OUTLINE

- Meaning of Educational Preparation
- Need for Educational Preparation in Nursing
- Levels/Patterns of Educational Preparations in Nursing
- Concept of Nursing Education
  - Definition
  - Aims of Continuing Nursing Education
- Issues related to CNE
- Continuing Education Program
- Characteristics of Continuing Nursing Education
- Program Planning of CNE
- Evaluation of Continuing Professional Education
- Career Opportunities
  - Definition of Career Ladder
  - Model of Career Ladder
  - Preparation for Career Approach
- Preceptorship Model of Clinical Teaching
- Professional Advancement
- Role and Scope of Nursing Education

EDUCATIONAL PREPARATIONS

Introduction

The evolution of nursing education has been influenced by the conditions and changes in society over the past years. The rapidly changing health care system requires nurses to possess increasing knowledge, clinical competency, greater independence and autonomy in clinical judgments. Trends towards community-based nursing centers, private case management and complexity of home care are increasing. It's a sophisticated technology and society's orientation to health and self-care, and all are rapidly raising the educational needs of nurses.

Educational preparations for nurses are preparing the nurses at university level and state board level to develop career opportunities to work in hospitals, community or in educational institutions of nursing. For nursing to grow as a profession, knowledge is needed to predict with confidence the types of nursing interventions that will improve client outcomes.

There are different levels of nursing education in India. They are: The Indian Nursing Council (INC) at its meeting in 1950 came with some important decisions relating to future patterns of nursing training in India. One of the important decisions was that there should be two standards of training of nursing and midwifery.

MEANING OF EDUCATIONAL PREPARATION

Educational preparations for nurses means prepare the nurses at university level and state board level to develop career opportunities to work in hospitals or community educational institutions of nursing.

NEED FOR EDUCATIONAL PREPARATIONS IN NURSING

Nursing education is a professional education means to prepare professional nurses with the aims of harmonious development, correct attitude, knowledge and skill, aim, citizenship and many more in it, such as:

- ❖ *Nursing curriculum changes:* The curriculum focuses much on students' participation, competency-based learning, etc.
- ❖ *Latest technology:* Technology exerts greater influence on nursing education as a tool for teaching and learning
- ❖ *Opportunity for higher studies:* Nursing in India has reached its highest level of education, which includes MPhil and PhD, and a few short-term courses like nurse practitioners have been included in the curriculum
- ❖ *Preparation of global nurses:* Introduction of web-based nursing degrees, and student nurses have been trained for a global perspective to cater the public need not only in their own country but also in the other countries
- ❖ *Enhanced student status:* The horizon of nursing has widened so much that more and more students are joining this profession
- ❖ Expansion of employment opportunities
- ❖ Nursing shortage

- Evolution of nurses' roles due to professional advancement.

Levels/Patterns of Educational Preperation in Nursing in India (Table 8.1)

Multipurpose Health Assistants (MPHA), Multipurpose Health Supervisors (MPHS), Health Visitors.

The training grew out of the earlier auxiliary nursing and midwifery(ANM) course. The ANM training was for 2 years. Mainly covers maternal and childcare and family welfare. The Indian Nursing Council revised the ANMs syllabus in 1977 and reduced the duration to 18 months. At the end of the course candidates are eligible for working in health subcenters. There are nearly 500 schools offering this course in India at present.

It is 18 months training program, first started at St. Mary Hospital.

In Punjab in 1951 financial aid given by the Government of India under the scheme for preparing personnel to deliver the health care services to rural population within the community.

Female Health Supervisor Training (HV or MPHS-F)

This course was initially meant as a health visitor training course. It went to several modifications and finally became metamorphosed into the current six months promotional training. The female health supervisors or Multipurpose Health Assistant (F) course is being conducted in 21 centers in the country.

General Nursing and Midwifery (GNM)

The general nursing and midwifery course is conducted in 477 centers in the country.

The syllabus has undergone many revisions according to the change in the health plans and policies of the Government and changing trends and advancements in general education, nursing health sciences and medical technology. The latest revision of syllabus by INC in 2004 has increased the duration of the course from three year to three and half year, later it is reduced to 3 years. The basic entrance has become intermediate or class 12 instead of earlier class 10. Both science and arts students are eligible. The focus of general nursing education is the care of sick in the hospital. Schools of nursing are generally attached to teaching hospitals. Three Board examinations are conducted, one at the end of each year. On passing the candidates are registered as registered nurse and midwive by the respective state nursing councils.

Philosophy

The Indian Nursing Council believes that the basic course in nursing is a formal educational preparation which should be based on sound education principles. The council recognizes that the program as the foundation on which the practice of nursing is built and on which depends further professional education. It also recognizes its responsibility to the society for the continued development of student as individual nurse and citizens.

Purpose

The purpose of general nursing program is to prepare general nurse who will function as member of the health team beginning with competence for first level position in both hospital and community. The program is generated to the health needs of the society, the community and the individual and will assist nurses in their personal and professional development so that they may take their maximum contribution to the society as individual citizens and nurses.

Objectives

- Demonstrate awareness of and skills required in the nursing process in the provision of health care and nursing of patients.
- Apply relevant knowledge from the humanities biological and behavioral sciences in carrying out health care and nursing activities and functions.
- Show sensitivity and skill in human relationship and communication in his or her daily works.
- Demonstrate skill in the problem solving methods in nursing.
- Gain knowledge of health resources in the community and the country.
- Demonstrate skill in leadership.
- Demonstrate awareness of necessity of belonging to professional organizations.
- Promotion of health, precaution against illness, restoration of health and rehabilitation.

Students admission

- Age for the entrance shall be 17 years to 35 years, provided they meet the minimum educational requirement ie 12 years of schooling.
- Minimum education all students should pass 12 classes or its equivalent, preferably with science subjects.
- Admission of students shall be once a year.

Table 8.1: Levels of educational preparation in nursing.

Name of the course	Duration	Eligibility
ANM/MPHA	18 months	PUC with science/any other (arts; commerce)
GNM	3.5 years	+ 2 with science/any other (arts; commerce)
BSc Nursing	4 years	+ 2 with PCB
Post-basic BSc Nursing	2 years	Diploma in Nursing + 1 year experience
MSc Nursing	2 years	BSc Nursing + 1 year experience
PhD in Nursing	4 years—part time; 3 years—regular	After MSc Nursing and/or after MPhil Nursing

- Students should be medically fit. The selection committee should comprise tutors, nurse administrators, and educationalist/psychologist. The principal of the school shall be the chairperson.

Training program

The course in general nursing shall be of three years duration as follows, community health nursing and midwifery and which includes nursing administration and nursing research classes. There will be alternate course for male students in lieu of midwifery. The ANM who wishes to undertake general nursing course will not be given any concessions. The maximum hours per week per students shall be 36 hours, which includes instructions and clinical field experiences.

Bachelor of Nursing Course

Graduate nursing education started in India in the year 1946 in CMC, Vellore and in the RAK College of Nursing at Delhi University. At present several universities in India offer the course.

Eligibility for admission

A candidate seeking admission should have:
- pass the 2 year of preuniversity exam or equivalent as recognized by concerned university with science subjects, i.e. physics, biology and chemistry.
- student of vocational courses.
- obtained at least 45%of total marks in science subjects in the qualifying exam, if belongs to a scheduled caste or tribe, should have obtained not less than 40% of total marks in science subjects.
- completed 17 years of age at the time of admission or will complete this age on or before 31st December of the year of admission.
- is medically fit.

Objectives of study

The program is designed:
- To provide a balance of professional and general education
- To enable a student to become a professional nurse practitioner who has self direction and is a responsible citizen. Through planned guided experiences students are provided with opportunities to develop:
  - a broad concept of the fundamental principles of nursing care based on sound knowledge and satisfactory levels of skill in providing care to people of all ages in community or institutional setting
  - understanding of the application of principles from the physical biological and social sciences for assessing the health status
  - ability to investigate health care problems systematically
  - ability to work collaboratively with members of allied disciplines towards attaining optimum health for all members of the society
  - understanding of fundamental principles of administration and organization of nursing service
  - understanding of human behavior and appreciation of effective interpersonal relationship with individuals families and groups
  - ability to assume responsibility for continuing learning
  - appreciation of professional attitudes necessary for leadership roles in nursing appreciation of social and ethical obligations to society.

Course of study

The course of study leading to bachelor of nursing degree comprises 4 academic years.

Post Basic BSc Nursing (Post Certificate) for Qualified Nurses

The need for continuing education for higher was required for nurses who has completed diploma nursing and midwifery.

Philosophy and aims of the program

- The faculty believes that nursing is an integral part of the health care delivery system and shire responsibility in collaboration with other allied health professions for the attainment of optimal health for all members of the society. The faculty conceives education as a life long learning process. It seeks to render appropriate behavioral changes in students in order to facilitate their development, which assist them to live personally satisfied and socially useful lives.
- The goal of post certificate degree program leading to bachelor of science in nursing is the preparation of the trained nurse as a generalist who accept responsibility for enhancing the effectiveness of Nursing care.

Eligibility for admission

The candidate seeking admission must:
1. Hold a certificate in General nursing
2. Should be a registered nurse
3. Have minimum of two years of experience
4. Have passed preuniversity exam in the arts/science/commerce or its equivalent which is recognized the university
5. Should be medically fit
6. Have a good personal and professional record
7. Have working knowledge of English.

Program of study

Duration

The program of the study is two academic years from the date of commencement of program. Terms and vacations shall be as notified by the university from time to time.

Objectives

The goal of the postcertificate program leading to the bachelor of nursing is the preparation of the trained nurses as a generalist who accept responsibility for enhancing the effectiveness of nursing care.

- Administer high quality nursing care to all people of all ages in homes, hospitals and other community agencies in urban and rural areas
- Apply knowledge from the physical, social and behavioral sciences in assessing the health status of individuals and make critical judgment in assessing the health status of the individuals and make critical judgment in planning, directing and evaluating primary, acute and long term care given by themselves and others working with them
- Investigate health care problems systematically
- Work collaboratively with members of other health disciplines
- Teach and counsel individuals, families and other groups about health and illness
- Understand human behavior and establish effective interpersonal relationships
- Teach in clinical nursing situations
- Identify underlying principles from the social and natural sciences and utilize them in adapting to, or initiating changes in relation to those factors
- Acquire professional knowledge and attitude in adapting for leadership roles.

Degree of Master of Nursing

Philosophy

Nursing faculty presents the following beliefs about the master of nursing program:

1. The master of nursing program is offered by institution of higher education and is built up on a recognized bachelor's curriculum in nursing (in India by Indian Nursing Council)
2. The program prepares nurses for leadership position in nursing and other health fields who can function as specialists nurse practitioners, consultants, educators, administrators and investigators in a wide variety of professional setting in meeting the national priorities and the changing needs of the society
3. The program prepares nursing graduates who are professionally equipped, creative, self directed and socially motivated to effectively meet with the needs of the social changes. Further the program encourages accountability and commitment to lifelong learning which fosters improvement of quality care.

Objectives

Graduates of master of nursing program demonstrate:

- Increased cognitive, affective and psychomotor competencies and the ability to utilise the potentials for effective nursing performance
- Expertise in the utilization of concepts and theories for the assessment, planning and intervention in meeting the self care needs of an individual for the attainment of fullest potentials in the field of specialty
- Ability to practice independently as a nurse specialist
- Ability to function effectively as nurse educators and administrators
- Ability to interpret the health related research
- Ability to plan and initiate change in the health care system
- Leadership qualities for the advancement of practice of professional nursing
- Interest in lifelong learning for personal and professional learning advancement.

Eligibility

The candidate seeking admission must:

1. Have passed BSc Nursing/post certificate BSc, or nursing degree of any university.
2. Have a minimum of one year of experience after obtaining BSc, in hospitals or nursing educational institutions or community health setting.
3. For BSc, nursing post certificate, no such experience is needed after graduation the candidate shall be a registered nurse or registered midwife for admission to medical surgical nursing, community health nursing, pediatric nursing obstetric and gynecological nursing. A registered nurse for admission to psychiatric nursing.
4. The candidate shall be selected on merit judged on the basis of academic performances in BSc Nursing, post certificate BSc, or nursing and selection tests.

Specialties

Candidate will be examined in any of the following branches:

1. Branch 1-medical surgical nursing
2. Branch 2-community health nursing
3. Branch 3-paediatric nursing
4. Branch 4-obstetric and gynecological nursing
5. Branch 5-psychiatric nursing

Four common papers are there included in the syllabus. They are:

i. advanced concepts of health and nursing
ii. education and nursing education
iii. bio-statistics, research methodology and nursing research
iv. administration and nursing administration.

Master of Philosophy Program in Nursing (M Phil in Nursing)

In 1980 RAK College of Nursing started an MPhil program as a regular and part time course. Since then several universities started taking students for the MPhil course in nursing. Prominent among these are: MGR Medical University, Rajiv Gandhi University of Health Sciences, SNDT University and Delhi University and Manipal Academy of Higher Education.

Nurses who are interested in research and obtain higher degree of M Phil in nursing or M Phil in related disciplines of Master's degree specialized. It was first started in Raj

Kumari Amruth Kaur College of Nursing on October 15, 1986. This is the program for 1 ½ year for regular and 2 years for part-time candidates.

Philosophy

Nursing shares with the whole university a main focus of preparing its students for service and assisting them to achieve a meaningful philosophy of life. The student is encouraged to develop judgment and wisdom in handling knowledge and skills and achieve mastery of problem solving and creative skills. Commitment to life long learning is the mark of truly professional person. In order to maintain clinical competencies and enhance professional practice the student must stay abrupt of the new developments and contribute to the advancement of nursing knowledge.

Objectives

The objectives of MPhil degree course in nursing are:
- to strengthen the research foundations of nurses for encouraging research attitudes and problem solving capacities.
- to provide basic training required for research in undertaking doctoral work.

Duration

Duration of the full term MPhil course will be one year and part time course will be two year.

Course of study

At the time of admission each candidate will be required to indicate her priorities in regard to the optional courses. A candidate may offer one course from MPhil programme from the department of Anthropology, education, sociology and physiology or any suitable department. The MPhil studies will be into two distinct parts, part 1 and part 2.
- **Part 1:** It consists of 3 courses, i.e. research methods in nursing, major aspects of nursing, allied disciplines.
- **Part 2:** After passing the part 1 examination, a student shall be required to write a dissertation. The topic and the nature of the dissertation of each candidate will be determined by the advisory committee consists of 3 members. The dissertation may include results of original research, a fresh interpretation of existing facts, and date or a review article of critical nature of may take.

Doctorate of Philosophy in Nursing

Candidate for admission to the course for the degree of doctor of philosophy in the faculties of medical science must have obtained an MPhil degree of a university or have a good academic record with first or second class master's degree of an Indian or a foreign university in the concerned subject. The candidate shall apply to the university for the admission stating is qualification and the subjects he proposes to investigate enclosing a statement on any work he may have done in the subject. Every application for the admission of the course must be analyzed by the board of research studies.

Board of research studies (medical sciences)

Members:
- Dean and the head of the departments concerned
- Principals/head of institutions recognized for post graduate medical studies
- Two members nominated by the medical academic council
- Three persons nominated by the medical faculty for their special knowledge in the medical science.

Eligibility criteria

- The candidate should be postgraduate in nursing with more than 55% of aggregates of marks
- Should have research background
- May or may not published articles in journals
- The course duration is far regular PhD course is 3 years and for part time is 4 years
- **There are short term programmes to take up fellowship training, i.e. post basic nursing courses in a specialized areas.**

Registered nurse education

There are various educational routes for becoming a professional registered nurse (RN). As nursing increasingly defined its own body of knowledge, formalized educational process is developed to ensure a consistent level of education in institutions. Graduates in nursing or diploma in nursing holders are registered nurses.

PROBLEMS ASSOCIATED WITH CHANGING EDUCATIONAL REQUIREMENTS FOR LICENSURE

Several problems are associated with making any changes in educational requests for licensure.

Major Problems

- *Titling:* One of the most controversial problems associated with changing requirements for licensure involves titling or the use of titles
- *Scope of practice:* It may be limited to practice, lack of policies and inadequate professional autonomy.

CONCEPT OF NURSING EDUCATION

Jarvis (1984) differentiated continuing education and continuing learning, and assumes that the professional will endeavor to keep abreast of all new development through self-direction by reading and attending conferences. Continuing education suggests that education courses have to be supplied for the practitioner to attend. Learning in nursing is a continuous and never-ending process. Although many things are learned through experience, there are times when formal higher education is desired and necessary. Following international trends and recommendations made in the Bhore report, professional nursing authorities have aimed to develop general professional nursing education towards the collegiate level. It is believed that the combination of collegiate and semi-professional programs, with the large number on the level of the health worker will more adequately meet the minimum health needs of society as a whole.

National Staff Committee (1981) has argued that every nurse should be aware of the need to update and expand his/her knowledge and skills, and critically assess his/her own learning needs. It is important to understand how nurses view continuing professional education (CPE) and their perception of its relationships to nursing, clinical practice, professional development, job satisfaction, staff retention and career progress. Continuing education in nursing has frequently been identified as a necessary component of professional competence. Acquisition of new knowledge is critical, if nurses and other health care professionals are to continue to perform competently in the age of rapid change.

Definition

Continuing education is defined as, planned educational activities intended to build upon the education and experimental bases of the professional nurse for the enhancement of practice, education, administration, research theory development to the end of improving the health of the public.   **—ANA, 1974**

For continuing education to be meaningful, it must focus on the needs of the learners. It is important to note that regardless of age, marital status, parental status, level of nursing education or the number of years worked in nursing profession, nurses always demonstrated a great interest in continuing education by attending conferences and workshops.   **—Pennington, 1984**

Continuing professional education courses could positively affect clinical practice and thereby patient care. Effects upon the educational development were characterized by an increased knowledge base and an increased awareness of the need for further education.   **—Thurston, 1992**

On the evidence of scientific knowledge, it appears that the support of colleagues and superiors is the most important factor in determining the positive influence of education upon practice development. The influences upon nursing practice identified from the nurses having increased confidence improved knowledge increased self-awareness and increased awareness of professional issues in relation to the delivery of care, there is improved communication skills enhanced individualized care, research-centered practice.
  —Frank et al. 1995

Barber (1977) divided continuing education into two distinct categories:

1. Informal education, which includes activities such as reading, studying, watching TV and working on committees.
2. Formal education, i.e. seminars, conferences and planned education programs, changing and improving professional practice.

The educational process should provide practitioners with enhanced knowledge and skills to continue in their profession, and to develop an increased sense of critical awareness.   **—Jarvis, 1983**

Aims of Continuing Nursing Education

- Changing and improving professional practice
- Meeting the expressed needs/interests of nurses within a given practice area
- Providing competent and ultimately safe and effective patient care.

Issues Related to Continuing Nursing Education

During the present decade, there has been a wide range of changes in nursing education; predominantly in the preservice nursing area. There are many dimensions of increased pressure which professional nurses have to face today. One major pressure involves the demands placed on the nurse's role which flow from rapid technological improvements. With concomitant changes in medical practice, health (1980) offers a typical view of the problems arising in continuing nursing education (CNE):

- Inability to convince nursing managers that staff development is of vital importance for the service
- Failure to encourage qualified nurses to value their own continuing personal and professional development
- Failure to recognize that the training personnel also need help
- Lack of appropriate criteria for nurse managers to select staff for CNE program
- Ineffective methods for publishing program, activities and services or the in-service training department
- Little systematic attention to identify education and training needs
- Inadequate evaluation of effectiveness of staff development program
- Lack of coherent staff development plans
- Inadequate funding for staff development in the institutions.

Other Major Issues of CNE

- CNE curricula are determined by the needs of the employer health institution and not on the needs of the nurses. The program is often seen by the employer as a means to satisfy, reward and retain established nursing staff to cut down the expenses of termination and staff turnover.
- CNE curricula are mainly imposed on nurse either as mandatory CE requirements to renew registration or

by external (monetary) incentives to gain improved qualification.
- There are increased criticisms of the current techniques used in the delivery of CNE in that program often do not take the learning styles and career choices of the nurses into consideration.
- A persistent cause of failure of many CNE program is the absence of a coherent conceptual framework to guide the design of the nursing curricula. The planning of CNE curricula needs to be based on objective thinking and to be capable of meeting the health care requirements of modem society as well as professional interests and concerns of nurses themselves.
- CNE should maximize the nurse's own power and control needs to encourage nurses to be self-directed, and to choose for themselves what learning to pursue. Too often CNE activity focuses solely on the nurse as the responsible party for improving patient care without sufficient attention to other organizational and personal factors.

Need for Continuing Education
- Phenomenon of change basically arises as the need for continuing education arises from, change in what is known about man and how he functions in health and illness, changes in the way, in which people meet challenge to survive in a dynamic age, and change in the objectives, organization and financing health services.
- Altered professional roles: Due to the change in society and the technologies, knowledge emerges, and the professional roles get altered. The individual should not avoid the chance of acquiring new knowledge or his ability to adapt to changing demands.
- **Effective leadership and competent practitioners.** For the development of good leaders, continuing education must be there in nursing according to the demand of society and competent practitioners for the future.
- **To fulfill the needs of nurse practitioner.** Nursing profession itself and the larger society highlight the need for planned and programmed continuing education. These include changing functions of the nurse and increase towards advanced preparations or specializations.
- **Need to foster innovative and creative approaches to nursing care of patients.**
- **To achieve more effective behavior in nursing practice to improve the patient care.** To assume more responsibility in their respective jobs according to the levels at which they function.

CONTINUING EDUCATION PROGRAM

In-service Education
It is thought of as "on-the-job" training. It includes conferences, classes and demonstrations in the clinical area. It is aimed at helping to develop the skills needed, solve problems in everyday work and understanding broader health problems, to help continue learning new knowledge, principles and techniques, and to develop the ability to teach and supervise others who serve in the same area. It also serves to improve professional relationships within the institution with other professionals and members of the health team:
- Staff development program
- Journal presentation
- Special training
- Workshop
- Conferences
- Reference courses (refresher course; orientation course).

Characteristics of Continuing Nursing Education
Content may be developed on the basis of:
- Clinical areas, need like neonatal nursing, pediatric nursing, mental health nursing, neurological nursing, cardiopulmonary nursing, surgical nursing, etc.
- Level of group of nurses like graduates, under graduates, postgraduates, etc.
- Designation like staff nurses, junior health assistants, nursing tutors, etc.
- Experience like a new graduate or a nurse with 3 years' experience in a specific clinical area and so on.

Program Planning of Continuing Nursing Education
There are five components of the continuing education program that are planned and monitored, such as:
1. **Curriculum:** The program should be planned according to the content and outline of the lesson with objectives to be developed in terms of expected behavior. The program should be planned based on philosophy, adult education theory and importance of learners' participation.
2. **Teachers:** Teachers should have the expertise in teaching strategies to work effectively with adult learners. Experts from different areas can be invited as a resource person.
3. **Participants:** Participants should be well informed about the objectives, the topics being discussed, the arrangements and remuneration if any. Participants should be given adequate time to discuss the topic and give personal opinion. On completion of the program, a certificate should be provided.
4. **Resources:** When planning the staff education program, careful attention should be paid to assure that adequate resources are available for the comfort of the participants and for the achievement of the objectives; **for example**, what type of audio visual aids are needed, whether the participants are provided food, necessary equipment and stationary, etc. should all be given a proper thought.

5. **Administrative structure:** Finally, any continuing education program requires an adequate administrative structure to handle all of the tasks required.
   - Selecting the place
   - Inviting the participants
   - Arranging equipment
   - Ensuring the comfort of the participants
   - Handling the financial aspects

Program evaluation is done at the end of the CNE program to make a judgment about the success of the program in its attempt to meet the objectives. Using the systems model, three aspects are evaluated, i.e., input, output and process as given above.

Benefits of Continuing Education

According to Mitsunaga and Shores (1977), the benefits are divided into four main categories:
1. *Learner satisfaction:* While the overall purpose of continuing education in nursing may be increased quality of service through change in practice, it is learner satisfaction and knowledge acquisition that is most evaluated.
2. *Knowledge, skills and attitude change:* It is assumed that as knowledge, communication and assertiveness skills are increased, there is professional and educational development, and the nurse's ability to improve patient care is advanced.
3. Change in practice.
4. Ultimate quality of service framework to identify learning needs for CNE using information technology (Fig. 8.1).

Evaluation of Continuing Professional Education

Motivational factors may be multidimensional, but increased job competence and professionalization of nursing are major motivational factor.

—Kristganson and Scanlon, 1989

Ferguson (1994) has discovered four aspects of evaluation:
1. *Process evaluation:* Learner satisfaction with the course and how different processes within the course perform
2. *Content evaluation:* Acquisition of skills, knowledge and attitude change
3. *Outcome evaluation:* Change in practice by learner
4. *Impart evaluation:* Ultimate quality of the service.

Motivation and self-directedness are interlinked with the experience of CPE with the more motivated nurses being apparently more self-directed, and thus undertaking more CPE.

Nursing professional education: Thompson et al. (1987) identified the following advantages for a specific CPE:
- To make CPE available to nurses in a specific area
- To keep costs low
- To decrease staff shortages by offering the program in the clinical area. Therefore, students do not have to go away in order to attend CPE
- To reduce duplication
- To offer the program to as many nurses from the clinical area as possible
- To keep nurses up-to-date regarding new development in nursing
- To maintain/improve the standard of nursing care in that area.

Career Opportunities

Introduction

Education continues to be important after the nurse begins to practice, whether the practice setting focuses on the adult or child, the chronically or acutely ill or the home or hospital. Nursing encompasses an ever-widening range of roles. Multiple career paths and goals are open to new and experienced practitioners. Till the recent past, describing the role of nurse was simple, because there were few opportunities for variation. Today exploring job opportunities for nurses is more complicated as nurses are practicing in hundreds of diverse settings with a broad variety of clients.

The career opportunities for nurses are growing. Even though nursing roles have extended or expanded to different areas, the traditional functions of the nurse remain intact.

In the past, career mobility for nurses was somewhat limited. However, with expanding roles in nursing practice, this situation has changed. The clinical ladder approach to advancement has been discussed in many nursing journals and put into practice in various settings. The clinical ladder unifies clinical practice and nursing administration, fosters, collaboration between nursing education and service, and is a professional advancement system.

Definition of Career Ladder

The term career ladder is a metaphor or buzzword used to denote vertical job promotion. It contains structure,

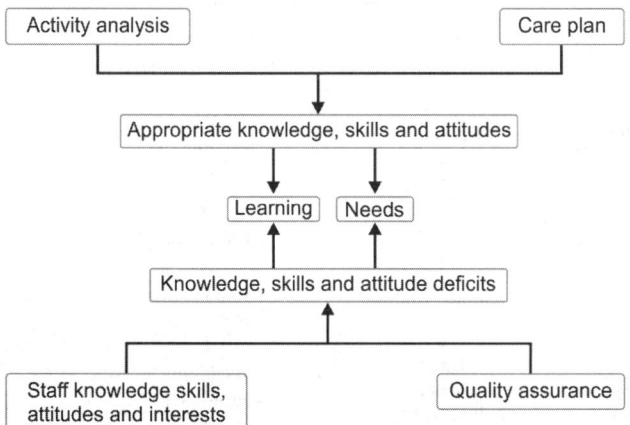

Fig. 8.1: Framework to identify learning needs for continuing nursing education using information technology.

criteria for claimed competencies, promotional procedures and incentives for advancement. The ladder describes progression from entry-level positions to higher levels of pay, skill, responsibility or authority. It is frequently used to denote upward mobility within a stratified promotion model. Because the ladder does not provide for lateral movement, it is assumed to be a singular trunk with the greatest benefits at the top.

Career ladder model (Fig. 8.2)

The structure is individualized for a specific institution and may include multiple levels on the clinical, administration, research and education pathways. There should be a measurable criterion for each level within the structure.

The clinical ladder is a method for career mobility by which one program can encourage and motivate nurses to remain in health care setting. Career counseling is another method of relation and promoting within the settings. Within a clinical ladder system, nurses are no longer promoted strictly on the basis of education and experience within the institution, but they are self-appraised and peer-appraised for career mobility within the system. The incentive for advancement may include increased autonomy of practice, raise in salary or promotion within the organizational structure itself, increased expertise and personal self-fulfillment.

Sources of career opportunities

- ❖ **Career day program:** In some colleges/schools, there would be annual learner day program during which recruiting officers or local health agencies inform senior students about employment opportunities.
- ❖ **Open house:** Opening of new service or educational program—invitation to individual nurses, group of special nurses, final-year student nurses to attend open house for recruitment.

Sources of career approaches:

Employee referral:
- ➢ From employees
- ➢ Ex-employees
- ➢ Political leaders
- ➢ Government officials
- ➢ Religious bodies

External sources:
- ➢ Door applicants
- ➢ Government employment exchange
- ➢ Private employment exchange
- ➢ Advertisement
- ➢ From other hospitals
- ➢ Teaching institution
- ➢ Internal circular for vacancies
- ➢ Friends or acquaintances
- ➢ Colleagues and co-workers
- ➢ Newspapers
- ➢ Job listings online.

Conceptual model for clinical specialization

This model evaluates the practice of the nurse on different levels.

Levels of competence

- ❖ **Novice:** It is the beginner; a student just learning about nursing is a novice, who is the nurse entering his or her first position.
- ❖ **Advance beginner:** Challenging patient care situations to have prior experience to apply to new situations. Without help from more experienced nurses.
- ❖ **Competent:** Nurses need 2–3 years of clinical role experience to achieve efficiency, organization skill and the ability to cope with complex needs of multiple clients.
- ❖ **Proficient:** Has learned from experience, and perceives the situation as whole. She demonstrates a new ability

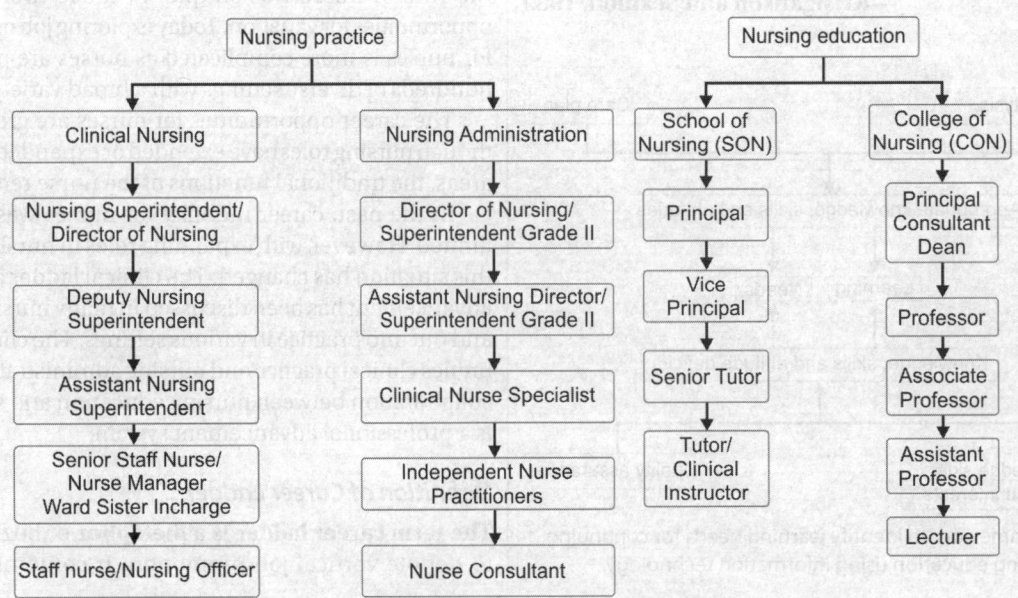

Fig. 8.2: Model of career ladder.

to identify the change in the situation and implement skilled responses to the situation. She is confident in her knowledge and practice.
- **Expert:** Has developed an extensive repertoire of skills, knowledge and clinic experience and an intuitive grasp of each situation. Accurately picture current and long-term implications, analytics skills and mentor for novice nurses.

It is important to recognize nurses' levels of competence while preparing for career responsibilities.

PRECEPTORSHIP MODEL OF CLINICAL TEACHING (BURNS AND PATERSON 2005)

Preceptorship has been used extensively with senior nursing students, graduate students for advanced practiced roles and for a new staff nurse.

Definition

Preceptorship is a time limited one-to-one relationship between learner and an orient-experienced nurse who is employed by the health care agency in which the learning activities take place.
- The preceptor provides intensive/individualized learning opportunities that improve the learner's clinical competence and confidence.
- Regardless of learners' level of education and experience, preceptorships provide opportunities for socialization into professional nursing roles. They also enhance personal and professional development of the preceptors.

Use of Preceptorship in Nursing Education

In academic programs that prepare nurses for initial entry to practice, preceptorships usually are used for students in their last semester; but providing perceptions for beginning students may have even greater benefits. Assignments that help to expand their basic skills develop independent self-confidence. Preceptorship is frequently used in graduate programs that prepare nurses for advanced clinical practice, administration and education roles. The student observes and participates in learning activities that demonstrate functional role components, allowing rehearsal of role behaviors before actually assuming an advanced practice administrative and teaching role.

In many health care organizations, preceptors participate in the orientation of newly hired staff nurses.

Advantages of Using Preceptors

- The presence of students in clinical environment tends to enhance the professional development, leadership and teaching skills of preceptors.
- Preceptors enjoy sharing their clinical knowledge and skill, which is appreciated.
- Students may assist preceptors with research or teaching projects.
- Preceptors model also produces opportunities to recruit potential staff members for the agency.
- The use of preceptors provides more clinical teachers for students and thus more intensive individualized guidance of students' learning activities.
- Helps faculty members to be updated/stay informed in current realities of practice, up-to-date clinical information benefits and ongoing curriculum development.

Disadvantages of Using Preceptors

- Use of preceptors may affect educational program.
- The preceptors program model requires considerable indirect teaching time for the development of relationships with agencies and preceptors.
- When preceptors are used as clinical teachers, faculty members may be responsible for more students in several clinical agencies.

Selecting Preceptors

The success of preceptorships largely depends on the selection of appropriate preceptors.

Qualities of Effective Preceptors

- Consider education preparation to be important
- Desire to teach and willingness to serve as a preceptor
- Clinical expertise or proficiency depending on the level of learner
- Psychomotor, problem-solving, critical thinking, reasoning and decision-making skills
- Leadership abilities
- Teaching skills
- Professional role behavior and attitudes.

Preparing Participants

Thorough preparation of preceptors and students for their role to success.
- The educational level and previous experience of the student
- Start with general orientation
- Continuing support of all participants
- Preparation can be formal or informal
- Learners also need to understand purposes and process of the preceptorship.

Content of Preceptorship Preparation Program

- Benefits and challenge of precepting
- Characteristics of a god preceptor
- Principles of adult learning
- Assessment of adult learning
- Clinical teaching methods—motivating, challenging, learners, dealing with difficult learning situations and when to use coaching techniques
- Evaluation of learning—effective feedback and use of clinical evaluation tools
- The preceptors' role in developing and implementing individualized learning contract

- The academic program curriculum structure, framework and goals
- The teacher, student and preceptor collaborate to plan and implement learning activities that will lead to the students' goal attainment.

Roles and Responsibilities of Participants' Preceptors

Role model behaviors important for preceptors to demonstrate can be classified into four categories:
- Technical skills
- Interpersonal skills
- Critical thinking
- Professional role behavior demonstrates enthusiasm/accountability and confidentiality.

Implementation

Successful implementation of preceptorships depends on students.
- Explanation of teacher and preceptor roles and review of unit policies specific to student practice
- Teacher may share samples of learning contracts or lists of activities
- Learning contract approvals, site visits/conference with faculty members
- Scheduling of clinical learning activities—according to work schedule, advising dates/examination/holidays, etc.
- Face-to-face interview
- Telephone conference with the teacher (written guidelines may be given to supplement the conference. Example: Graduate nursing students.

Teachers

- Pairing students with preceptors
- Preceptor and students.

Evaluating the Activities

- Monitoring the progress of learning
- Student performance.

Rewarding Preceptors

Preceptors make valuable contributions to nursing education programs and they should receive appropriate rewards and incentives for their participation. Other formal/informal ways of acknowledging are:
- Contributions—thank you note
- Preceptor badge
- Certificate of approval
- Annual receptor recognition event, including refreshments.

PROFESSIONAL ADVANCEMENT AND ROLE AND SCOPE OF NURSING EDUCATION

Advanced Practice Preparations

Specialized programs have been developed to help individual prepare for roles of used breadth and scope. Recent healthcare reform has resulted in a used emphasis in the role of advanced nursing practice in healthcare delivery and there demand for educational programs to prepare these practitioners clinical nurse specialists certified nurse midwives and certified registered nurse anesthetists.

Doctoral Preparation in Nursing

Nurses can earn a PhD in nursing having obtained the highest level of education in their field. PhD nursing programs will prepare nurse researchers and nurse scientists to better address the health care needs of individuals and their families, as well as the communities in which they live. Usually, this program will be affiliated to teaching hospitals, research facilities and universities. Other preparations include:
- Master's degree in his/her area of nursing expertise or with a doctorate in adult education
- Credentials with more publications
- Writing and organizing skills
- A continuing team
- Clinical expertise
- Depth of nursing knowledge and skills in its application
- Interest and enthusiasm in teaching
- Skills in working with adult learners
- Adequate knowledge about teaching skills and methods of teaching
- Diploma in nursing certificate to update their knowledge and obtain degree in nursing education.

Midwifery programs award standardized and rigorous cause of study lasting from 18 months to 2 years.

Advance Practice Nurse

Advance practice nurse is a graduate in nursing who chooses to further her education and obtain a master's degree by specializing in clinical nursing specialists. These nurses are certified by the national organizations as higher education in nursing with additional qualifications. MSc Nursing has specialists like community health nursing, obstetrical and gynecological nursing, pediatric nursing, psychiatric nursing and medical–surgical nursing. Advanced practice nurses are considered as expert clinicians to work as nurse anesthetists, nurse practitioners, nurse midwives and clinical nurse specialists.
- Nurses prepared at the graduate level function in a variety of roles as advanced practice nurses
- Role as a nurse educator
- Nursing educator provides leadership for the provision of health services
- A nurse educator helps in promoting health
- The nurse educator in a leadership role for health policies and programs
- The nurse educator serves as liaison between school personnel, family, community, health care providers, etc.
- A case manager participates as the health expert in an individualized education plan.

PROFESSIONAL ADVANCEMENT SYSTEM FOR NURSE CLINICIANS

This voluntary bonus program for direct care registered nurses represents a collaborative effort between nursing staff, nursing leadership and human resources to support nursing vision and philosophy, achieve organizational goals and enhance patient care. The criteria and processes of the professional advancement system are understood to be dynamic in order to promote professional development and balanced participation in evidence-based decision-making and practice changes.

Viewpoints of Nurses towards Professional Advancements

Victoria Hospital, BMCRI, Bengaluru, Karnataka State:

1. I'm a staff nurse, working as a skin bank In-charge. This is the only skin bank in Karnataka State since I have the advanced education of Masters degree in Nursing, I got the opportunity to have special training on skin banking at Bombay. My professional qualification played a good role in patient care, nursing administration and critical care to the patients and also to the institution.

   The well-educated nurse can do revolution in the field of nursing profession. Professional advanced education helping me to apply concepts of problem solving and evidence-based practice, and improving the healthcare organization and the quality of care. Career advancement system in nursing, also leads to increase performance in clinical skills, decrease turn-over and strengthen their motivation, and enhance the quality of nursing care.

   Mr Nagaraj BN (MSc N)
   Skin Bank In-charge
   Medical-Surgical Nursing

2. Nursing education programs provide specific challenges and strategies to improve advance practice in clinical field. Advanced education is helping me to work with all stake holders with a co-ordinated approach and to change some policies and bring innovations in specialized areas of practice. Some nurses are resistant to bring change, so advanced education is essential to meet many challenges of healthcare system. Ongoing update of knowledge is required to improve quality care management.

   Mrs Savitha R (MSc N)
   Psychiatric Nursing
   CSSD Department

3. In an increasingly complex healthcare industry advance practice, nurses are playing a vital role, they are becoming more skilled and evidence-based practitioners. As working in ICU the advance nursing education helping me to apply my abilities in a way that:

   - Obtaining health history and performing physical examination of the clients.
   - Interpreting the lab results and diagnostic studies related to disease conditions.
   - Evaluate patients response to plan of care and modifying as needed.
   - Maintaining patient's records and reporting appropriately.
   - Helping me Participate in research studies conducted in the organization.
   - Advancing our discipline and offering new solutions to enhance theoretical body of knowledge to our nursing profession.

   Mr Revanasiddappa (MSc N)
   Medical-Surgical Nursing
   Trauma ICU

4. Professional advancement in nursing career is one of the key factors that determine the patient care outcome. My Masters program has helped me that, in a fast paced society which is of technological advances in healthcare, it requires nurses with updated knowledge. Professional advancement helps nurses to stay current in their area of practice. It helps in effective communication, decision making, critical thinking and analysis thus, enabling nurses to provide skill-based nursing care. Professional advancement therefore helps nurses to establish themselves and demonstrate competency.

   Ms Beena (MSc N)
   Pediatric Nursing
   Trauma ICU

5. Today to meet the rapid changes in the nursing profession due to changes in the healthcare system all nurses must be motivated for achieving professional advancement. Advanced education is helping me to practice with advanced knowledge, skills, make more assertive, increase accountability and improve problem solving skills being working in ICU setting. So we can meet the criteria for standards of the profession.

   Ms Savitha (MSc N)
   Medical-Surgical Nursing
   Trauma ICU

Impact of Advanced Roles on Health Consumers

Social media provides consumers of health care with tools by which they can share with others their health concerns even as they arise and receive.

- Provide opportunities for online discussion with nurses
- Use of information and communication technology (ICT) and the Internet continues to grow in all regions of the world
- Social media is also finding a place in public health communication strategies
- Use of social media in nursing, i.e. gaining popularity among health care profession

- Caution is needed to use social media among individuals, health care institution and educational program ANA—Given resources of social networking principles—toolkit
- Examples of policy and guidance documents with a focus on social media and nursing include a statement of principles, a webinar, a feat sheet, a tip card and a tip section about the use of social media.

ROLE OF NURSING EDUCATOR IN TEACHING

Role towards Individual

A nurse educator promotes the:
- Education as growth of the individual dependence and adaptability
- Education as direction fixation of the activity
- Education as preparation of individual child for responsibilities and privileges of adult life.

Roles towards Society

- To encourage socialization, ancient social order and education, modern social order and education
- Education as continuous reorganization and integration of activities and experiences
- Experience as the basis of education.

Three permanent functions of education include:
1. **Conservative:** Preserve old traditions, values and ideals, and customs of students.
2. **Transmissive:** Transmitting the cultural heritage.
3. **Progressive:** Reconstruction of new experiences and new dimensions of knowledge.

Role towards Nation

Role of education in the national life inculcation of civic and social, national integration response, training for leaders.

Aims of Nursing Education

- To prepare nurses who will be expert at the bedside care
- To provide integration of health and social aspects
- To provide an adequate sound scientific foundation
- To provide opportunities to cooperatively manage through curricular and extra-curricular activities
- Ensure opportunities for initiative and resourcefulness
- To develop sense of responsibility towards the profession
- Provides the needed knowledge and skills required to practice the profession in a successful manner
- Promotes all round development of the physical, intellectual, emotional, social and spiritual abilities of the student
- To nurture leadership abilities among students
- Offers a variety of career opportunities.

Scope of Nursing Education

- Increase in health awareness among the people is demanding to provide quality health services. So, skilled and specialized nurses can get excellent employment opportunities in government or private hospitals. The roles have been extended to clinics, nursing homes, orphanages, old-age homes, industries, military services, schools and other places.
- Nurses can get jobs in specialized area like taking care of patients in pediatrics, orthopedics, psychiatry, obstetrics, geriatric, skin banks, etc.
- Nursing education provides the scope in teaching, supervision and higher level of administration.
- Nursing education has great scope for male nurses. They are valuable in activities of professional organizations.
- Nursing has great scope in abroad; they find jobs in specialized fields like ICU, CCU and emergency rooms.
- Nurses get high payment in abroad.
- Increased emphasis on collaboration between health care disciplines.
- Increased distance online learning.
- Schools of nursing providing ongoing professional development for competence requirements.
- Increased teaching of evidence-based practice.

CONCLUSION

Continuing education plays a very important role in all disciplines of education. In nursing profession also continuing education helps nurses to update, expand the knowledge and skills, and critically assess his/her own learning needs. CNE helps in changing and improving of professional practice, and nurse professionals provide quality care services that promote effective reach of organizational goals, which in turn leads to consumer satisfaction in the field of nursing practice and education as well. The need for evidence-based answers regarding the amount of clinical experience needed in an educational program and the amount of clinical practice needed before seeking an advanced degree have been identified. The authors have also highlighted the need for more research and dialog regarding the amount, type and measurement of clinical work needed for safe and effective patient care. Although the various stages of career ladders have indeed advanced the nursing profession, we need to continue seeking evidence to support the most promising career pathways in nursing.

CHAPTER 9

Role of Research, Leadership and Management

CHAPTER OUTLINE

- Role of Research in Nursing Profession
- Research Process
- Research Utilization
- Barriers Related to Research
- Strategies to Promote Research
- Nurse Researcher Roles
- Current and Future Strategies for Research Utilization
- Introduction to Leadership and Management
- Types of Leadership
- Styles of Leadership
- Roles of Leadership
- Techniques of Leadership
- Role of Management in Nursing Profession
- Common Management Functions
- Time Management Principles
- Five Rights of Delegation
- Responsibilities of Manager

ROLE OF RESEARCH IN NURSING PROFESSION

Introduction

Clinical nursing research is the research designed to generate knowledge to guide nursing practice and to improve the health and quality of life of a nurse's clients.

Because nursing is a practice profession, it is important that clinical practice be based on scientific knowledge. Nursing interventions should be proven to be of the highest quality and cost-effective. Nurses increasingly are expected to adopt an evidence-based practice (EBP), which is broadly defined as the use of the best clinical evidence in making patient care decisions. Nursing research is essential if nurses are to understand the varied dimensions of their profession.

Definitions of Nursing Research

Research is a systematic inquiry or study to validate and refine existing knowledge and develop new knowledge. The ultimate goal of research is the development of new knowledge. —**Burns and Grove, 1995**

Nursing research is systematic approach used to examine phenomena important to nursing profession including nursing practice, education, administration and informatics.

Research can create a strong scientific base for nursing practice and demonstrate accountability for the profession. —**Talbot, 1995**

Evolution of Nursing Research

Nursing research began with the work of Florence Nightingale during the Crimean War. After Florence Nightingale's work, the pattern that nursing research followed was closely related to the problems confronting nurses. For example, nursing education was the focus of most research studies between 1900 and 1940.

As more nurses received their education in a university setting, studies regarding student characteristics and satisfactions were conducted. As more nurses pursued a college education, staffing patterns in hospitals changed because students were not as readily available as when more students were enrolled in hospital-affiliated diploma programs. During this period, researchers became interested in studying nurses.

During the 1950s, more master's programs specific to nursing were developed and most of these programs included courses on research methods. Increased federal funding enabled more nurses to continue their studies at the master's level, and publications of nursing research became more common. The journal *Nursing Research* began publishing the results of studies by individuals and schools of nursing. At about the same time, a 5-year research project sponsored by the American Nurses Association (ANA) focused on nurses' activities and functions.

Federal funding for graduate study and research continued in the 1960s. The profession of nursing was strengthened with the development of conceptual frameworks (an early stage of theory development wherein interrelated concepts help shape the proposed research) and the use of scientific method in nursing practice. Nursing organizations established priorities for research investigations. Such research endeavors led to improvements in the quality and specificity of nursing care.

Rapid growth in nursing research continued during the 1970s and 1980s. Three more journals of nursing research were born in the 1970s:
1. Advances and Nursing Science
2. Research in Nursing and Health
3. Western Journal of Nursing Research

The ANA commission on nursing research in 1980 recommended further research in the areas of health promotion, illness prevention, cost-effective health care and nursing care for high-risk clients. Researchers examined the conceptual frameworks that arose in the 1960s and 1970s.

The Institute of Medicine, in a 1983 study, urged the federal government to increase the level of funding for nursing. As a result, the National Center for Nursing Research was established under the National Institutes of Health. The purpose of the center was to place nursing securely in the sphere of scientific investigation and to support research and training into client care, health promotion, disease prevention and the mitigation of effects of acute and chronic disabilities. This center has continued to fund and support nursing research.

Groups began to establish priorities in nursing research during the 1980s. In 1985, the ANA Cabinet on Nursing Research identified 11 priorities for nursing research, as listed in the accompanying display. In the late 1980s, *Applied Nursing Research*, a journal with studies related to the practice of nursing, began.

Scientific Process and Nursing Research

In general, research means the search for a valid answer to a question. The scientific method, the problem-solving method and the nursing process all use a method of research. Ways of seeking answers and acquiring knowledge in any field include classes, clinical experience, discussions with classmates, scientific problem-solving, continuing education and research studies relevant to the area of interest.

These methods of seeking knowledge have the following in common:
❖ Identifying what one needs to know
❖ Deciding how to approach the goal of answering the problem
❖ Devising a plan to do so
❖ Implementing the plan.

Differences between clinical nurse and researcher.

Clinical nurse	Researcher
Assessment of a problem	Recognize the general problem area
Make a nursing diagnosis	Defining the specific problem
Planning and intervention	Propose hypothesis and manage data
Evaluate the outcome	Analyze and disseminate the findings

Beginning nurses can use the nursing process framework to begin to formulate and answer questions. The outcome will be improved client care and services, and the advancement of nursing as a profession. Another way to become involved in research is to be a research subject or a data collector for another person's research project.

Importance of Research in Nursing

Nurses increasingly are expected to adopt an EBP, which is broadly defined as the use of the best clinical evidence in making patient care decisions. Nurses are accepting the need to base specific nursing actions and decisions on evidence, indicating that the actions are clinically appropriate, cost-effective and result in positive outcomes for clients. Nurses who incorporate high-quality research evidence into their clinical decisions and advice are being professionally accountable to their clients. They are also reinforcing the identity of nursing as a profession.

Another reason for nurses to engage in and use research involves the spiraling costs of health care and the cost-containment practices being instituted in health care facilities. Now, more than ever, nurses need to document the social relevance and effectiveness of their practice, not only to the profession but also to nursing care consumers, health care administrators, third-party payers (e.g. insurance companies) and government agencies. Some research findings will help eliminate nursing actions that do not achieve desired outcomes. Other findings will help nurses identify practices that improve health care outcomes and contain costs as well.

Nursing research is essential if nurses are:
❖ To understand the varied dimensions of their profession
❖ To describe the characteristics of a particular nursing situation about which little is known
❖ To explain phenomena that must be considered in planning nursing care
❖ To predict the probable outcomes of certain nursing decisions
❖ To control the occurrence of undesired outcomes
❖ To initiate activities to promote desired client behavior.

Characteristics of Nursing Research

Traditionally, nursing has been concerned with the whole person, not the individual parts. Likewise, nursing research differs from biomedical research in that it has a holistic perspective. When nurses do research, they focus on the physiologic, psychological, sociologic, cultural and economic factors that affect the person. They view events from different perspectives and ask questions about what they see (Mateo and Kirchhoff, 1991). Diers (1979) listed four properties of nursing research which maintain the holistic perspective:
❖ The focus of nursing research must be on a variance that makes a difference in improving client care.

- Nursing research has the potential for contributing to theory development and the body of scientific nursing knowledge.
- A research problem is a nursing research problem when nurses have access to and control over phenomena being studied.
- A nurse interested in research must have an inquisitive, curious and questioning mind.

Purposes of Nursing Research

The general purpose of nursing research is to answer questions or solve problems of relevance to the nursing profession, as traditionally defined.

Qualitative

Identification

Study of a phenomena about which a little is known or yet to be clearly identified/or has been inadequately defined or centralized conceptualized.

Quantitative

Begin with a phenomenon that has been previously studied or defined. Identification precedes the inquiry.

- *Description:* Research observe count, delineate and clarify quantitative description prevalence, incidence size and measurable attributes of phenomena. Qualitative uses in-depth methods to describe the dimension variation importance of phenomena.
- *Exploration:* Begins with a phenomenon of interest and investigates full nature of phenomena. Exploratory qualitative research is designed to shed light on the various ways in which a phenomenon is manifested on underlying processes.
- *Explanation:* Goals are to understand the underlying principles of a specific natural phenomenon and to explain systematic relationship among phenomena linked with theories.
- *Prediction and control:* Some phenomena explanation. Yet, it is possible to make prediction to control phenomena based on research findings even in the absence of complete understanding. For example, increasing age leading to Down syndrome for the child.

Basic research is under to extend the base of knowledge in a discipline or to formulate or refine a theory. For example, a researcher may perform an in-depth study to better understand normal grieving processes, without having explicit nursing applications in mind.

Applied research focuses on finding solutions to existing problems. For example, a study to determine the effectiveness of a nursing intervention to ease grieving would be applied to research.

Basic research is designed to indicate how these principles can be used to solve problems in nursing practice.

Need/Role of Research in Nursing

Nursing research is needed to discover, verify, structure and restructure the professional knowledge through systematic inquiry.

Research is the only way to:
- Build a body of nursing knowledge
- Validate improvement in nursing
- Make health care efficient as well as cost effective.

1. **To mould the attitudes and intellectual competence and technical skills:** Nursing is a service to individual, families, and therefore, society. It is based on arts and sciences which mold the attitude, intellectual competencies and technical skills of individual nurse into the desired and to help people, well or sick and cope with their health needs.
2. **Filling the gaps in knowledge and practice:** Most of the medical and nurses' leaders believe that a gap is existing between the knowledge, which is affecting nursing and its application. This gap exists in both nursing education and nursing service. To meet the new challenges, investigate unsolved problems and to scrutinize the changes in nursing, the individual nurse must actively seek to understand and apply the basic principles of research.
3. **Fostering a commitment, accountability to clientele:** The ultimate goal of a profession is to improve the practice of its member so that services provided to clientele should have the greatest impact. This can be done by continual development of scientific body of knowledge fundamental to its practice that can be instrumental in fostering commitment and accountability to profession and clientele.
4. **Providing basis for professionalism:** Nursing has established itself as a profession. The increasing awareness of nurses to include research as an integral part of professional nursing behavior is rapidly increasing. Nurses are extending base of knowledge as a part of professional responsibility and are endorsing scientific investigations to broaden the body of knowledge. Research provides abstract knowledge that is the foundation for establishing nurses as a profession.
5. **Providing basis for professional accountability:** The quality of nursing care can be improved only if science becomes part of tradition. Accountability is essential for nurse teacher in dealing with students, for nurse practitioner dealing with patients and for nurse administrator dealing with clients or professionals of health care delivery system. It also includes scientific literature for new knowledge so that application of this knowledge becomes part of nursing practice.
6. **Identifying the role in changing society:** Nowadays, consumers of health care are recognizing health care as a right rather than a privilege due to spiraling costs of health care, so there is a need to evaluate the efficiency of presently existing nursing practices in all areas to

modify or abandon the practices that have no effect on health status and provide nursing services accurately to needs of clients.
7. **Discovering new measures for nursing practice:** Practice-oriented research is the key to discover for improving nursing practice that will improve the quality of nursing care. Scientific studies are indeed to understand, explain the functions and forms of nursing care in meeting the needs of society and helping individuals regain their health.
8. **Helping to take prompt decisions by the administration to related problems:** Nursing administrators are more frequently looking to the findings for research in solving persistent problems in organizing nursing personnel in most efficacious manner.
9. **Helping to improve the standards in nursing education:** Nursing educators utilize the findings from research in structuring programs of study, in developing course contents and in designing methods of teaching.
10. **Defining the existing theories and discovering new theories:** The primary test of nursing research is to develop and refine nursing theories which serve as a guide to nursing practice and which can be organized into a body of scientific nurse knowledge.

So, the research nursing helps the nurse practitioners, administrators and educators to understand the phenomena with which they deal and to explain, predict and control the occurrences of phenomena. Research aids nurses to be accountable to patients. Scientific inquiries provide information that facilitates effective nursing decisions. Nursing research clarifies the forms and functions of profession in meeting the health needs of the society.

RESEARCH PROCESS

While conducting research, the researchers move from the beginning point of a study to the end point in fairly linear sequences of steps that are broadly similar across studies.

Phase 1: Conceptual Phase

The early steps in a quantitative research project typically involve activities with a strong conceptual or intellectual element. These activities include reading, conceptualizing, theorizing, re-conceptualizing and reviewing ideas with colleagues or advisers. During this phase, researchers call on such skills as creativity, deductive reasoning, insight and a firm grounding in previous research on the topic of interest.

Step 1: Formulating and Delimiting the Problem

One of the first things a researcher must do is develop a research problem and research questions. Good research depends to a great degree on good questions. Without a significant, interesting problem, the most carefully and skillfully designed research project is of little value.

Quantitative researchers usually proceed from the selection of a broad problem area to the development of specific questions that are amenable to empirical inquiry. In developing a research question to be studied, nurse researchers must pay close attention to substantive issues, clinical issues and methodologic issues. The identification of research questions must also take into consideration practical and ethical concerns.

Step 2: Reviewing the Related Literature

Quantitative research is typically conducted within the context of previous knowledge. To build on existing theory or research, quantitative researchers strive to understand what is already known about a research problem. A thorough literature review provides a foundation on which to base new knowledge and usually is conducted well before any data are collected in quantitative studies.

For clinical problems, it would likely also be necessary to learn as much as possible about the "status quo" of current procedures relating to the topic and to review existing practice guidelines or protocols. A familiarization with previous studies can also be useful in suggesting research topics or in identifying aspects of a problem about which more research is needed. Thus, a literature review sometimes precedes the delineation of the research problem.

Step 3: Undertaking Clinical Fieldwork

In addition to refreshing or updating clinical knowledge based on written work, researchers embarking on a clinical nursing study benefit from spending time in clinical settings, discussing the topic with clinicians and health care administrators, and observing current practices. Sterling (2001) notes that such clinical fieldwork can provide perspectives on recent clinical trends, current diagnostic procedures and relevant health care delivery models; it can also help researchers better understand affected clients and the settings in which care is provided. In addition to expanding the researchers' clinical and conceptual knowledge, such fieldwork can be valuable in developing methodologic tools for strengthening the study. For example, in the course of clinical fieldwork, researchers might learn what extraneous variables need to be controlled or might discover the need for Spanish-speaking research assistants.

As with literature reviews, clinical fieldwork may serve as a stimulus for developing research questions and may be the first step in the process for some researchers.

Step 4: Defining the Framework and Developing Conceptual Definitions

Theory is the ultimate aim of science in that it transcends the specifics of a particular time, place and group of people, and aims to identify regularities in the relationships among variables. When quantitative research is performed within the context of a theoretical framework, that is, when previous theory is used as a basis for generating predictions that can be tested through empirical research, the findings may have broader significance and utility.

Even when the research question is not embedded in a theory, researchers must have a clear sense of the concepts under study. Thus, an important task in the initial phase of a project is the development of conceptual definitions.

Step 5: Formulating Hypothesis

A hypothesis is a statement of the researcher's expectations about relationships between the variables under investigation. Hypotheses, in other words, are predictions of expected outcomes; they state the relationships researchers expect to find as a result of the study. The research question identifies the concepts under investigation and asks how the concepts might be related; a hypothesis is the predicted answer. For example, the initial research question might be phrased as, is preeclamptic toxemia in pregnant women associated with stress factors present during pregnancy?

This might be translated into the following hypothesis. Pregnant women with a higher incidence of stressful events during pregnancy will be more likely than women with a lower incidence of stress to experience preeclamptic toxemia. Most quantitative studies are designed to test hypotheses through statistical analysis.

Phase 2: Design and Planning Phase

In the second major phase of a quantitative research project, researchers make decisions about the methods and procedures to be used to address the research question and plan for the actual collection of data. Sometimes the nature of the question dictates the methods to be used, but more often than not, researchers have considerable flexibility to be creative and make many decisions. These methodologic decisions usually have crucial implications for the validity and reliability of the study findings. If the methods used to collect and analyze research data are seriously flawed, then the evidence from the study may be of little value.

Step 6: Selecting a Research Design

The research design is the overall plan for obtaining answers to the questions being studied and for handling some of the difficulties encountered during the research process. A wide variety of research designs is available for quantitative studies, including numerous experimental and non-experimental designs. In designing the study, researchers specify which specific design will be adopted and what controls will be used to minimize bias and enhance the interpretability of results.

In quantitative studies, research designs tend to be highly structured, with tight controls over extraneous variables. Research designs also indicate other aspects of the research. For example, how often subjects will be measured or observed, what types of comparisons will be made and where the study will take place. The research design is essentially the architectural backbone of the study.

Step 7: Developing Protocols for the Intervention

In experimental research, researchers actively intervene and create the independent variable, which means that people in the sample will be exposed to different treatments or conditions. For example, if we were interested in testing the effect of biofeedback in treating hypertension, the independent variable would be biofeedback compared with either an alternative treatment (e.g. relaxation therapy) or with no treatment.

The intervention protocol for the study would need to be developed, specifying exactly what the biofeedback treatment would entail (e.g. who would administer it, how frequently and over how long a period the treatment would last, what specific equipment would be used and so on) and what the alternative condition would be. The goal of well-articulated protocols is to have all subjects in each group treated in the same way.

In non-experimental research, of course, this step would not be necessary. Data collection plan is a complex and challenging process that permits a great deal of creativity and choice. Before finalizing the data collection plan, researchers must carefully evaluate whether the chosen methods capture key concepts accurately.

Step 8: Developing Methods for Safeguarding Human/Animal Rights

Most nursing research involves human subjects, although some studies involve animals. In either case, procedures need to be developed to ensure that the study adheres to ethical principles. For example, forms often need to be developed to document that the subject's participation in the study was voluntary. Each aspect of the study plan needs to be reviewed to determine whether the rights of subjects have been adequately protected. Often that review involves a formal presentation to an external committee.

Step 9: Finalizing and Reviewing the Research Plan

Before actually collecting research data, researchers often perform a number of "tests" to ensure that plans will work smoothly. For example, they may evaluate the readability of any written materials to determine if people with below-average reading skills can comprehend them, or they may need to test whether technical equipment is functioning properly.

If questionnaires are used, it is important to know whether respondents understand questions or find certain ones objectionable; this is usually referred to as pretesting the questionnaire. During final study preparations, researchers also have to determine the type of training to provide to those responsible for collecting data. If researchers have concerns about their study plans, they may undertake a pilot study, which is a small-scale version or trial run of the major study.

Normally, researchers have their research plan critiqued by peers, consultants or other reviewers to obtain substantive, clinical or methodologic feedback before implementing the plan. When researchers seek financial support for the study, a proposal typically is submitted to a funding source, and reviewers of the proposed plan usually suggest improvements.

Students conducting a study as part of a course or degree requirement have their plans reviewed by faculty advisers. Even under other circumstances, however, researchers are well advised to ask individuals to assess preliminary plans. Experienced researchers with fresh perspectives can often be invaluable in identifying pitfalls and shortcomings that otherwise might not have been recognized.

Phase 3: Empirical Phase

The empirical portion of quantitative studies involves collecting research data and preparing those data for analysis. In many studies, the empirical phase is one of the most time-consuming parts of the investigation; although the amount of time spent collecting data varies considerably from one study to the next. If data are collected by distributing a written questionnaire to intact groups, this task may be accomplished in a matter of days. More often, however, data collection requires several weeks or even months of work.

Step 10: Collecting the Data

The actual collection of data in a quantitative study often proceeds according to a pre-established plan. The researcher's plan typically specifies procedures for the actual collection of data (e.g. where and when the data will be gathered), for describing the study to participants and for recording information.

Technological advances in the past few decades have expanded possibilities for automating data collection. A considerable amount of both clerical and administrative work is required during data collection. Researchers typically must be sure, for example, that enough materials are available to complete the study, that participants are informed of the time and place that their presence may be required, that research personnel (such as interviewers) are conscientious in keeping their appointments, that schedules do not conflict and that a suitable system of maintaining confidentiality of information has been implemented.

Step 11: Preparing the Data for Analysis

After data are collected, a few preliminary activities must be performed before data analysis begins. For instance, it is normally necessary to look through questionnaires to determine if they are usable. Sometimes forms are left almost entirely blank or contain other indications of misinterpretation or noncompliance. Another step is to assign identification numbers to the responses or observations of different subjects, if this was not done previously.

Coding of the data is typically needed at this point. Coding involves the translation of verbal data into numeric form, according to a specified plan. This might mean assigning numeric codes to categorical variables such as gender (e.g. one for females and two for males). Coding might also be needed to categorize narrative responses to certain questions. For example, patients' verbatim responses to a question about the quality of nursing care they received during hospitalization might be coded into:

- ❖ Positive reactions—1
- ❖ Negative reactions—2
- ❖ Neutral reactions—3
- ❖ Mixed reactions—4

Another preliminary step involves transferring the data from written documents onto computer files for subsequent analysis.

Phase 4: Analytic Phase

Quantitative data gathered in the empirical phase are not reported in raw form.

They are subjected to analysis and interpretation, which occurs in the fourth major phase of a project.

Step 12: Analyzing the Data

The data themselves do not provide answers to research questions. Ordinarily, the amount of data collected in a study is rather extensive; research questions cannot be answered by a simple perusal of numeric information. Data need to be processed and analyzed in an orderly, coherent fashion.

Quantitative information is usually analyzed through statistical procedures. Statistical analyses cover a broad range of techniques, from simple procedures that we all use regularly (e.g. computing an average) to complex and sophisticated methods. Although some methods are computationally formidable, the underlying logic of statistical tests is relatively easy to grasp and computers have eliminated the need to get bogged down with detailed mathematical operations.

Step 13: Interpreting the Results

Before the results of a study can be communicated effectively, they must be systematically interpreted. Interpretation is the process of making sense of the results and of examining their implications. The process of interpretation begins with an attempt to explain the findings within the context of the theoretical framework, prior empirical knowledge and clinical experience.

If research hypotheses have been supported, an explanation of the results may be straightforward because the findings fit into a previously conceived argument. If hypotheses are not supported, researchers must explain why this might be so. Is the underlying conceptualization wrong or was it inappropriate for the research problem? Or do the findings reflect problems with the research methods rather than the framework (e.g. was the measuring tool inappropriate?). To provide sound explanations, researchers not only must be familiar with clinical issues, prior research and conceptual underpinnings, but also must be able to understand methodologic limitations of the study.

In other words, the interpretation of the findings must take into account all available evidence about the study's reliability and validity. Researchers need to evaluate critically the decisions they made in designing the study and to recommend alternatives to others interested in the same research problem.

Phase 5: Dissemination Phase

The analytic phase brings researchers full circle. It provides answers to the questions posed in the first phase of the project. However, researchers' responsibilities are not complete until the study results are disseminated.

Step 14: Communicating the Findings

A study cannot contribute evidence to nursing practice if the results are not communicated. The most compelling hypothesis, the most rigorous study and the most dramatic results are of no value to the nursing community, if they are unknown. Another and often final task of a research project, therefore, is the preparation of a research report that can be shared with others.

Research reports can take various forms such as term papers, dissertations, journal articles, presentations at professional conferences and so on. Journal article reports—appearing in such professional journals as *Nursing Research*—usually are the most useful because they are available to a broad, international audience. There is also a growing number of outlets for research dissemination on the Internet.

Step 15: Utilizing the Findings

In practice, many nurses have conducted interesting studies without having any effect on nursing practice or nursing education. Ideally, the concluding step of a high-quality study is to plan for its utilization in practice settings. Although nurse researchers may not themselves be in a position to implement a plan for utilizing research findings, they can contribute to the process by including in their research reports recommendations regarding how the evidence from the study could be incorporated into the practice of nursing and by vigorously pursuing opportunities to disseminate the findings to practicing nurses.

▌RESEARCH UTILIZATION

Research utilization is a process of systematically integrating the findings of completed nursing research studies into clinical nursing practice. Rather than collecting data to answer a specific clinical practice question, the nurse would apply research findings that already exist in the literature.

Steps in Research Utilization

Step 1: Pre-utilization

The first step in using nursing research in nursing practice is the recognition that some aspect of nursing practice could be done in a more efficient, a more beneficial or simply a different way. This begins an exploratory phase in which colleagues in the practice setting are consulted regarding their opinion about the need to find a new approach for some aspect of nursing practice.

Step 2: Assessing

The next step is the identification plus critical evaluation of published research that is related to the practice problem you have identified. Nursing literature is searched to those studies that deal with the practice problem. The task is to analyze the research reports critically to determine which findings are adaptable to the practice problem and context. Organizing and summarizing the adaptable findings into a table format will provide with a primary working document for the remainder of the utilization.

Step 3: Planning

Planning of research utilization is accomplished in three phases.
1. ***Innovation:*** Determining new approach that will be used based on the findings from the review of literature and determining the practice outcomes that are expected in the context of the practice settings.
2. ***Specific plan:*** Establishment of a systematic method for implementing the new approach and is followed and applied appropriately. This phase includes staff training for utilization of the new approach.
3. ***Method for evaluating:*** Establishment of a method for evaluating the practice outcomes or effects of the new approach. These are usually some specific improvements in patient care.

Step 4: Implementing

Implement or apply a new approach along with the collection of the evaluation data. It is important to begin collecting the evaluation data at the same time so that you can clearly determine the effect of the new approach.

Step 5: Evaluation

Evaluate the implementation to determine if the new approach improved practice outcomes. The use of new approach in the practice setting may also be based on new technology, economic considerations or changes in staffing. If there is no change in outcomes, it can return to the previous practice. The evaluation phase may lead to another research utilization project. Currently there is extensive concern that nurses have failed to realize the potential for using research findings as a basis for making decisions and for developing nursing interventions.

BARRIERS RELATED TO RESEARCH

Barriers related to research use include:
- Studies are not focused on clinical problems
- Studies are not replicated
- Findings are not stated in terms that are understood by most practicing nurses.

There is evidence that nurses are not always aware of research results and do not effectively incorporate these results into their practice (Polit and Hungler, 1997). Major barriers related to nurses include:
- Nurses do not value research
- Nurses are unaware or unwilling to read research reports
- Nurses lack the ability to access research findings
- Nurses do not know how to apply research findings in practice.

However, even when nurses have an appreciation for research and want to incorporate findings into their practice, they are unsure of where to find quality studies on a specific topic or practice issue.

Health professionals should be familiar with two major research utilization projects that were implemented to address the problem of nurses failing to review and use research findings. These formal projects were:
- Western Interstate Commission for Higher Education (WICHE) regional nursing research development project
- Conduct and Utilization of Research in Nursing (CURN) project.

WICHE Project

WICHE project was a 6-year project in the mid-1970s and the members were recruited from various clinical settings and educational institutions to participate in a workshop focused on improving their skills in critiquing research, and participants select research-based interventions that they were willing to implement in practice and developed detailed plans for using selected research findings in practice. One of the major findings of the WICHE project was that there were few well-designed clinical studies with clearly identified implications for nursing care (Burns and Grove, 1995).

CURN Project

CURN project was a 5-year project (1975-1980) with a major goal to increase the use of research findings in nursing practice by disseminating research findings. For this project, research utilization was considered an organizational process rather than a process that should be implemented by an individual nurse. An outcome of the CURN project was the development of clinical protocols to direct the use of selected research findings in practice.

The research utilization process included the following steps:
- Synthesizing multiple studies on a selected topic
- Organizing the research knowledge into a clinical protocol for practice
- Transforming the protocol into nursing actions
- Evaluating the protocol to determine if it produced the desired outcome.

During the CURN project, clinical studies were examined for scientific merit, clinical relevance, feasibility for changing practice in an agency and cost-benefit ratio.

STRATEGIES TO PROMOTE RESEARCH

Strategies for Administrators

Burns and Grove (1995) predict that in the future accrediting agencies will require health care agencies to have protocols that are documented with research. Therefore, procedure manuals, standards of care and nursing care plans will need to reflect current nursing research. Progressive nurse executives are fostering a positive environment for conducting research and for implementing findings into practice. To challenge traditional practice, an attitude of openness and intellectual curiosity must exist. Administrators should use the following strategies suggested by Polit and Hungler:
- Foster a climate of intellectual curiosity by making staff aware that their experiences and problems are important
- Offer support in the way of encouraging individual staff members
- Establish research utilization committees
- Establish journal clubs
- Allow research studies to be conducted in the agency
- Offer financial and resource support for research utilization
- Include research utilization as a criterion in performance evaluation
- Facilitate the establishment of research committees for the purposes of promotion and implementation, and the review of proposals from employees or others seeking access to subjects for research projects
- Inform researchers about the agency and potential research opportunities.

Individual nurses must be empowered to be self-directed and encouraged to initiate innovative care based on research findings from sound, well-designed studies. It is important to determine the overall cost benefit of implementing findings from research into practice as well as the effectiveness before incorporating new techniques.

Strategies for Practicing Nurses

Strategies suggested by Polit and Hungler (1997) for practicing nurses to promote research utilization are as follows:
- Read widely and critically
- Attend professional conferences
- Expect evidence that support research utilization

- Seek environments that support research utilization
- Become involved in a journal club
- Collaborate with nurse researchers
- Participate in institutional research utilization projects.

All nurses should participate in nursing research at some level, depending on the level of educational preparation. The researcher role expands with advanced educational preparation although nurses at all levels of preparation should at least be consumers of research.

NURSE RESEARCHER ROLES

There are two nursing roles that are specifically focused on research: the clinical nurse specialist (CNS) and the clinical nurse researcher (CNR).

Clinical Nurse Specialist

The CNS is a Master's degree prepared nurse who is an expert clinician with additional responsibility for education and research. A CNS is in an ideal position to link research to practice by assessing the agency's readiness for research utilization, working with staff to identify clinical problems and helping staff find, implement and evaluate findings that are relevant to current practice. All CNSs are educated in the research process and can conduct their own investigations and collaborate with doctorally prepared nurses.

Clinical Nurse Researcher

The CNR should be a doctorally prepared nurse with clinical and research experience. Clinical nurse researcher:
- Can either focus on the conduct or facilitation of research and should possess knowledge of statistics, grantsmanship, evaluation research and administration
- Should have interpersonal skills such as patience, flexibility and approachability, which are imperative
- Should develop relationships with the staff nurses to identify the research questions that the staff nurses see as most significant in a particular setting
- Should be responsible for designing studies and assisting staff nurses with understanding of the implications of the study
- Should provide guidance to the staff regarding their role in the research process
- Should be responsible for disseminating findings of the research to not only staff nurses but also to administrators of the agency so that findings would be incorporated into practice
- May need to communicate results to legislators if the results potentially affect health policy.

If agencies do not have a CNR, they should be encouraged to develop relationships with researchers in university settings or other agencies. Professors in academic settings are expected to conduct research and often are interested in collaborating with health care agencies that might serve as a site.

Researchers have an obligation to take steps to ensure use of findings. Polit and Hungler (1997) suggest the following steps:
- Conduct high-quality research
- Replicate studies
- Collaborate with practitioners
- Disseminate findings aggressively
- Communicate clearly, eliminating jargon and provide nursing implications as a standard section of research reports and articles.

CURRENT AND FUTURE STRATEGIES FOR RESEARCH UTILIZATION

Incorporation of research findings into practice is a difficult and challenging process.

Although we expect that nurses use research to guide practice, this is not always the case.

Experts in the field of research utilization note that, in many ways, utilization presents more challenges to overcome than does the conduct of research. Influencing the behavior of multiple caregivers to let go of ritual-based practices is not an easy task. Diffusion of an innovation, such as a set of research findings, is influenced by the nature of the innovation (the research findings) and the manner in which it is communicated to members (nurses) of a social system (institution, nursing profession).

This framework is helpful for understanding the barriers to and strategies for facilitating research utilization activities within the institution and in the profession of nursing.

The following discussion discusses each of those areas in relation to barriers as well as current and future strategies to promote research utilization.

Social System Barriers

Characteristics of the social system:
- Lack of authority to change practice
- Insufficient time on the job
- Little cooperation from physicians or administrators.

Past and Current Strategies of Organizations

- Organizational values for research incorporated into governance documents
- Value of research operationalized in job descriptions, merit programs and committee structures
- Hiring a doctorally prepared nurse researcher in practice
- Allocation of human and monetary resources.

Future Strategies

- Use of investigative teams
- Combining RU and QI activities into one committee
- Creating partnerships with organizations in the same geographic location
- Implementation across integrated delivery systems.

Professional Perspective Barriers
- Priorities of universities and practice differences
- Majority of federal research funds allocated to academic centers
- Historical perspective of research occurring in academic centers.

Past and Current Strategies
Articulation of importance of research utilization in practice standards by:
- Professional associations and external accrediting agencies (e.g. JCAHO)
- Development and use of research utilization models.

Future Strategies
- Increase funding for doctoral preparation
- Multisite research utilization projects
- Identification by specialty organizations of content areas ready for RU.

Members
Nurses comprise the members of the social system within which research findings are used. The knowledge, skills and attitudes of these nurses vary, in part, because of the varying educational credentials of nurses in the profession.

Barriers
- Lack of awareness of research
- Isolated from knowledgeable colleagues
- Difficulty evaluating the quality of the research
- Feeling that research is not valued
- Not feeling rewarded for participation in RU.

Past and Current Strategies
- Development and use of educational aids
- Federally funded research utilization projects (WICHEN, CURN, NCAST, OCRUN) RU conferences and pre-conferences
- Administrative support for RU
- Reward system
- Feedback of data to illustrate how RU improves quality of care.

Future Strategies
- Incorporating journal clubs as a touching strategy in undergraduate programs
- Integrating RU skills into baccalaureate and graduate programs
- Requiring participation and or leadership for RU projects as part of the educational experience
- Increase educational activities that socialize nurses into reading research
- Use of textbooks that have research-based interventions.

Nature of Innovation—Quality of Research
Barriers
Few replication studies.

Past and Current Strategies
Emphasis placed on scientists building a program of research increasing numbers of nurses prepared at the doctoral level in nursing publication of integrative reviews and meta-analysis. Meta-analysis is a rigorous statistical procedure that synthesizes results from multiple primary research studies on a common clinical problem or issue. Meta-analysis provides the power to detect differences and effects across studies using similar variables in order to answer questions that a single study could not.

Critical meta-analysis is the incorporation of all relevant primary studies (significant/not significant, published/not published). To enhance the quality and significance of their work, meta-analysis includes unpublished studies and doctoral dissertations to reduce the bias toward published studies, as well as contact researchers for required statistics not found in their manuscripts. Researchers can advance nursing science by comprehensively reporting results and/or retaining and providing analysis required.

Future Strategies
- More emphasis and value for replication studies
- More emphasis on development of midrange theories
- Devoted programs of research on the science of RU.

Communication
Dissemination of research findings to nurses in practice:
- Manner in which statistics are reported
- Relevant literature not compiled in one place
- Research reports written in research, with implications for practice being unclear.

INTRODUCTION TO LEADERSHIP AND MANAGEMENT

Introduction
Leadership in nursing will be the product of a visionary view of well-being and health. Nursing leadership, unlike leadership in other disciplines, is intrinsically different. Nurses display leadership every day at all levels in different healthcare settings. This leadership will be a key factor in the success of the health for all movements. It is based on certain attitudes, knowledge, skills and attributes. Nurses are effective reputed leaders, observing his/her behavior by attending leadership training programs and obtaining direct counseling and guidance from a specialist in the field. Development of leadership takes in various ways, which help one to create his/her leadership abilities. Leadership abilities are obtained by various ways, for

example, attending management seminars. Acquiring skills on how to generate, apply, analyze, synthesize and evaluate information is crucial for a nursing professional. The capacity for critical thinking and decision-making by its members is a prerequisite for a profession, which claims autonomy and independent practice.

Nurse as managers play a pivotal role in a practicing environment, not only in client care, but in organizational management activities as well. Healthcare settings follow a trend of fewer managers and form more self-directed work teams, and thus making the development of leadership and management skills of equal importance in developing clinical skills through theory, application and practice.

Leadership has been a topic of society's interest and subject of numerous studies particularly over the last half of the 20th century.

Definition of Leadership

Leadership can be defined as a process of influencing people to accomplish goals, i.e. it is the ability to influence the behavior of others towards the achievement of a mutually established goal. **—Potter and Perry**

Leadership is a process by which the willing support of the group members is ensured towards achievement of organizational goals. It thus has the connotation of "influencing and of motivation;" its components are decision-making, influencing, relating, facilitating and communicating.

Definition of Management

Management is distinct process consisting of planning, organizing, actuating, activating and controlling, performed to determine and accomplish the objectives by the use of people and resources. **—George, 1988**

Management is the process and agency, which directs and guides the operations of an organization in realizing established aims. **—O' Tead**

TYPES OF LEADERSHIP

Leadership approaches represent six types of contemporary theories, and these conceptionalizations have evolved to successful leadership.

1. **Transactional leadership:** Transactional leadership is based on the principles of social exchange theory in which social interaction between leaders and followers is essentially based on economics, and success is achieved when the needs are met and work performance is a transactional enhanced. Leader works within culture and competency, supervises and coordinates the day-to-day management of a work unit.
2. **Transformational leadership:** Transformational leadership occurs when one or more persons engage with others in such a way that the leader and follower raise one another to higher levels of motivation (Burns 1978). It is a process that can lead to a revolutionary change in organization through a commitment. Transformational leadership consists of systematic purposeful and organized searches for change. The transformational approach matches well with professional needs and for work requiring high levels of decision-making and autonomy. According to Bas (1985), transformation leadership includes four components:
    i. Idealized influence provides the followers with a vision and sense of mission and gains respect, trust and confidence from them
    ii. Inspirational leader engages in confidence building of their subordinates
    iii. Intellectual stimulation
    iv. Individualized consideration.
    According to the current concepts, the transformed leadership type is more effective to adopt in administration of nursing education working practice.
3. **Charismatic leadership:** Charismatic leadership is based on valued personal characteristics and beliefs.
4. **Connective leadership:** A leadership that values collaboration and team work, and interpersonal skills are used to promote collegiality in achieving organizational goals.
5. **Shared leadership:** An organizational structure is one in which several individuals share the responsibility for achieving organizational goals.
6. **Servant leadership:** Leadership originates from desire to serve a leader emerges when others needs take priority.

STYLES OF LEADERSHIP

1. **Authoritarian (autocratic) leadership:**
    - Concerns task accomplishment rather than relationships
    - Makes decision alone
    - Expects respect and obedience of staff
    - Lacks group support generally by participation
    - Exercises power with coercion
    - Proves useful in crisis situations.
2. **Democratic (participative) leadership:** Democratic (participative) leadership is a people-centered approach, which is detailed below:
    - It is primarily concerned with human relations and team work
    - Fosters communication that is open and usually two-way
    - Creates a spirit of collaboration and joint effort that results in staff satisfaction
    - According to the current trends, this type of leadership will lead to effective implementation of organizational goals that result in staff satisfaction.
3. **Permissive (Laissez-Faire) leadership:**
    - Tends to have few established policies, abstains from leading and avoids responsibilities delegating all decision-making to the work group

- It is not generally useful in highly structural organizations, e.g. healthcare institution.
4. **Bureaucratic leadership:**
    - Bureaucratic leadership lacks a sense of security and depends on established policies and rules
    - Exercises power by applying fixed relatively inflexible rules
    - Tends to relate impersonally to staff
    - Avoids decision-making without standards or norms for guidance.
5. **Situational leadership:** The leader may use any style at any time depending on the size of the work group, the maturity of the staff and the situations the work group encounters.

ROLES OF LEADERSHIP

Nurse Administrators as a Leader

The nurse administrator is nursing superintendent, supervisor or ward in-charge in a unique position to lead the staff in the desired direction, and ultimately help in achieving the goals of nursing department, i.e. quality nursing care.

It is absolutely essential for the nursing administration to possess the qualities of an effective leader.

To be an ideal and effective administrator, the following qualities are required (Fig. 9.1):

- ❖ **Clinical skills:** Experience in the different areas/fields of nursing.
- ❖ **Managerial abilities:** Managerial abilities in nursing are developed by participating actively in a nursing team, improving skills in ward management (clinical knowledge) skills and gains confidence to make right management decisions (in the unit) and last participating in planning process of staff selection, training and optimizing resources in a hospital equipment and supplies team coordinated functions in the ward.
- ❖ *Leadership qualities:*
    - Skills of personal behavior:
        ♦ Sense of humor
        ♦ A well-balanced personality
    - Effective communication skills
    - Good judgment and critical thinking skills
    - Insight and vision
    - Intelligence and ability to accept the responsibility
    - Skills of organization:
        ♦ Develop long- and short-range objections
        ♦ Break big problems into small ones
        ♦ Share responsibilities and opportunities
        ♦ Plan, act, follow-up and evaluate.

Nurse Educator as a Leader

Today's students are nurse practitioners and become nurse leaders of tomorrow, and teachers are the role models for their students.

Leadership in nursing education flows down from the top management of the institution or Dean through the Head of Department (HOD) of their faculty to the students.

Leadership Qualities of Nurse Educators

The top-level educationist shows the leadership qualities in the following manner:

- ❖ Emphasizes on participative leadership
- ❖ Transmits knowledge and experience
- ❖ Recognizes human values
- ❖ Creates a "we" feeling among her staffs and students
- ❖ Delegates responsibilities commensurate with appropriate authority to faculty
- ❖ Provides direction when needed
- ❖ Creates positive attitude among the faculty and students

Distinguish between leadership and management.

Leadership	Management
Leadership is the use of one's skills to direct and influence others to perform the best of their ability (Dosset, 1992)	Management involves handling the day-to-day operations of a work group to achieve a desired outcome
It is the interpersonal relationship between followers and the person who is leading	Management is more impersonal and passive, and the focus keeps evolving
Effective leaders must be able to make people want to accomplish something and to therefore get work done (Dosset, 1992)	Individuals on cause and directed toward organization goals to remain productive
A leader can be in any type of organizational position	Managers are not automatically leader, but effective managers often become leaders
Leader empowers others	Managers guide, direct and motivate (Manthey, 1990)

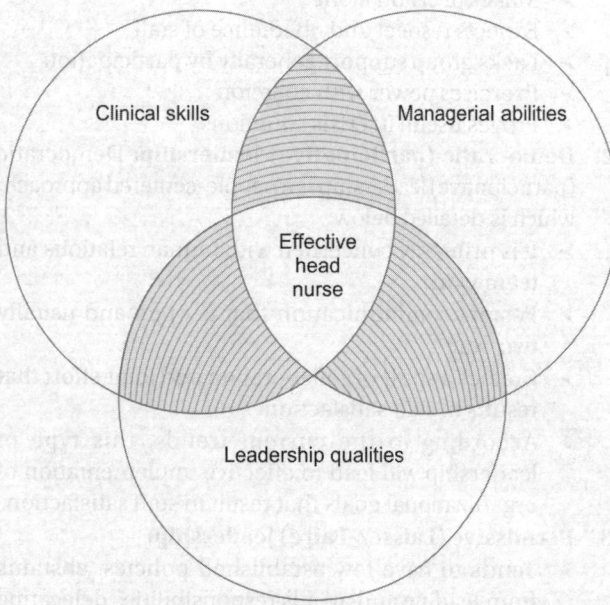

Fig. 9.1: Leadership qualities.

❖ Is a trend setter in teaching administration and professional participation

Leadership Qualities of a Public Health Nurse

The public health nurse must cultivate qualities such as:
❖ Alertness of mind to take a decision
❖ Cooperativeness and ability to coordinate
❖ Understanding of human nature
❖ Ability to mobilize and motivate people
❖ Empathy to mobilize and motivate people
❖ Empathy with social and traditional norms
❖ Ability to assess the situation correctly
❖ Competence at assessing the sociocultural and economic needs of the group
❖ Public speaking and communication skills
❖ A high frustration tolerance level
❖ Emotional maturity.

TECHNIQUES OF LEADERSHIP

❖ Planning and organizing the work schedule according to availability of personnel and materials
❖ Assigning work to subordinate which should be defined and recorded with clear cut directions
❖ Proper teaching and guidance to subordinates
❖ Cooperation and coordination between superior and subordinates
❖ Identifying talented subordinates and involving them in planning
❖ Democratic supervision
❖ Evaluation of performance of subordinates and self.

ROLE OF MANAGEMENT IN NURSING PROFESSION

With the vision of nursing established, it is the manager who directs and supports staff in the realization of the vision. The nurse executive supports managers by establishing a management structure that will help to achieve organizational goals and provide appropriate support to care delivery staff. The leader facilitates change in staff's attitudes and behavior, and gains their commitment.

Decentralized Management

Decentralized management has an advantage over others in creating an environment where managers and staff become more actively involved in shaping healthcare organizations, and is determined as success. Staff has more problem-solving abilities; choosing strategies and evaluating the outcomes of their work. Working in decentralized units creates more collaborative effort, increased competency of staff, and ultimately, a greater sense of professional accomplishment.

Centralized Management

A single administrator leads the organization with directors overseeing departmental responsibilities. Decisions are made from top to down with minimal input from staff. Managers tend to have minimal responsibility and accountability in the operation of nursing unit.

Matrix

Traditional hospital departments become organized into business units. Staff may report to more than one manager.

COMMON MANAGEMENT FUNCTIONS (FIG. 9.2)

❖ *Planning:* Determining long- and short-term objectives, e.g. nursing staff in oncology unit improve client's satisfaction with pain control. Actions are taken to assess client's pain more accurately and implementation of non-invasive pain control measures.
❖ *Staffing:* Includes selecting the personnel to carry out these actions and placing them in positions appropriate to their knowledge and skills. For example, the manager of the nursing unit selected a staff committee to interview applicants for a new clinical nurse specialist position.
❖ *Organizing:* Includes mobilizing human and material resources, so institutional objectives can be achieved, e.g. staff development program is conducted to plan new nurse specialist to attend teaching classes on pain assessment for the medical oncology unit staff.
❖ *Directing:* Includes motivating and leading personnel to carry out action needed to achieve the institution's or unit's objectives, e.g. the manager gave the new staff an objective to achieve by communicating the new standards of care for pain management on the unit. The committee met weekly for the first month to review pain management literature for oncology clients and share the objective by communicating the new standards of care for pain management on the unit. The nurse manager discusses ways in which new pain management interventions could be best incorporated into their practice.

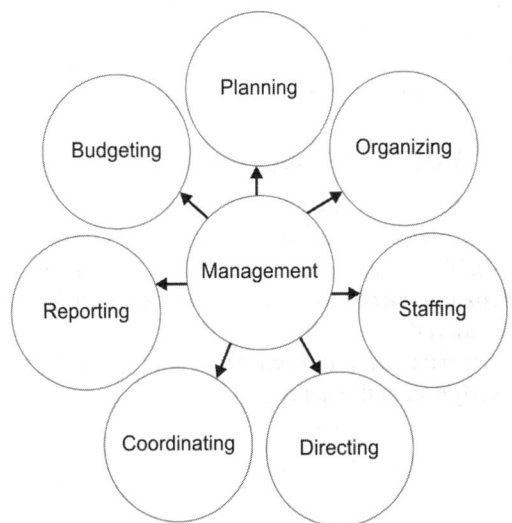

Fig. 9.2: Management functions.

❖ **Controlling:** Includes comparing results with predetermined standards of performance and taking corrective action when performance does not meet standards, e.g. the practice committee established two outcome measures. Client satisfaction with pain control and staff competency. The manager set the expectation that the staff would participate in additional training, if competency levels were not met. Satisfaction results from clients were reviewed weekly by the practice committee. If satisfaction results showed no improvement, the committee investigated causes and redesigned approaches.

❖ **Decision-making:** It includes identifying a problem, searching for solution and selecting the alternative that best achieves the decision-maker's objective, e.g. 3 months after the staff have been trained and new practice guidelines for pain must have been implemented, the manager reviewed client records and found documentation of pain assessment practice; committment the manager to identify the documentation out adding unnecessary charting requirements.

❖ **Coordinating:** It is inter-relating in various activities of functions performed by different individuals for achievement of objectives. Hence, a manager has to develop some means of coordinating the subordinates' efforts and blend all the activities into a unified action.

❖ **Reporting:** Reporting is a process of keeping a superior informed, to whom the subordinates are responsible and accountable, records, returns and checking. The progress can therefore be assessed through the reporting system.

TIME MANAGEMENT PRINCIPLES

❖ Goal setting
❖ Set priorities
❖ Time analysis
❖ Interruption control these activities, which interrupt client care to be controlled
❖ Evaluation at the end of the day, discuss with instructor or a more experienced staff member.

FIVE RIGHTS OF DELEGATION

1. **Right task:** Tasks for specific client.
2. **Right circumstances:** Appropriate client setting, available resources and other relevant sources.
3. **Right person:** Right tasks to right person factors are considered.
4. **Right direction/communication:** A concise, clear description of the tasks.
5. **Right supervision:** Appropriate monitoring and evaluation of interventions.

RESPONSIBILITIES OF MANAGER

❖ Assist staff in establishing annual goals for the unit and systems needed to accomplish goals
❖ Monitor professional nursing standards of practice in the unit
❖ Develop ongoing staff development plan including one for new employees
❖ Recruit new employees
❖ Conduct routine staff evaluation
❖ Establish self as a role model for positive customer service
❖ Submit staffing schedules for the unit
❖ Conduct regular client rounds and solve problems of the client or family complaints
❖ Establish and implement a unit quality improvement plan
❖ Renew and recommend new equipment for the unit
❖ Conduct regular staff meetings
❖ Establish and support staff, and interdisciplinary committees.

RESEARCH ABSTRACT

A study conducted by Morison and Fuller (1997) a regional medical center, "Alabama" to find out the relationship between leadership styles and its effects on job satisfaction among nursing staff concluded that transformational leadership appears to have a powerful influence on job satisfaction; both directly and indirectly through its influence on a person's intrinsic task motivation and empowerment.

CONCLUSION

Experimental research lacks in nursing. Current and future strategies are to be followed for research utilization. Research is essential in any profession except in the field of nursing. Nursing implications are applied to all fields including nursing administration, nursing education and nursing practice.

Leadership is to be effective in nursing. The nurse leader has to possess all leadership qualities and has to apply certain techniques to implement the activities. Effective leader and managerial functions lead to reach the goal of any organization. In health care organization and educational institution, leadership and management plays a very important role in improving quality services and harmonious maintenance of human resources.

10 CHAPTER
Quality Assurance in Nursing

CHAPTER OUTLINE

- Terminologies
- Meaning and Definition of Quality Assurance
- Historical Development of Quality Assurance in Nursing and Healthcare
- Concept of Quality Assurance in the Nursing Profession
- Quality Assurance of Nursing in India
- Goals of Quality Assurance
- Criteria in Quality Assurance System
- Definition of Standards
- Nursing Standards
- Techniques of Quality Assurance in Nursing
- Components of Quality Assurance Program
- Nursing Audit
- Factors Affecting Quality Nursing Care
- Measurable Initiatives for Continuous Quality Improvement in Nursing

INTRODUCTION

Quality assurance (QA) is now an essential part of healthcare and nursing service. In view of the increasing demand to maintain service excellence in patient care, managers and professionals are being asked to develop QA tools and to demonstrate concern for quality of services.

Growing awareness in the consumers for quality healthcare, standardized nursing education, advanced medical technology and various social, political and economic factors are pressurizing the profession to redefine the word "quality" in nursing.

TERMINOLOGIES

- **Quality:** A judgment of what constitutes good or bad
- **Audit:** A systematic and critical examination to examine or verify
- **Standard:** It is the desired quality, quantity or level of performance that is established as criterion against which workers' performance will be measured
- **Measurement:** It is the objective process of determining capacity, quantity or dimension of the object, phenomenon or outcome
- **Feedback:** It is the information about system performance that is reflected back into the system on a basis for monitoring system operation
- **Quality healthcare:** It is the appropriate application of medical science knowledge to patient care while balancing the hazards associated with each intervention with the benefits resulting from the intervention
- **Accountability:** It is the obligation to provide reasoning for one's actions to the persons who delegate authority for that action
- **Quality control:** It is a specific type of controlling that refers to activities that evaluate, monitor or regulate services rendered to consumers. Audit is a tool for quality control.

MEANING OF QUALITY ASSURANCE

Quality assurance is a systematic approach to achieving by monitoring the desired level of patient care. QA can also be interpreted as a formal guarantee of a degree of excellence in assuring patients an acceptable standard of care.
—Sale, 1990

DEFINITION OF QUALITY ASSURANCE

The World Health Organization (WHO) in 1992 defined QA as making sure that the services provided by the hospital are the best possible given the existing resources and current medical knowledge.

Quality assurance can be defined as the measurement of the actual level of the service provided, plus the efforts to modify when necessary, the provision of their services in the light of the results of the measurement.
—Willamson, 1982

Quality assurance is the promise or guarantee that certain standards of excellence are being met in care delivered.
—Lalonde, 1988

HISTORICAL DEVELOPMENT OF QUALITY ASSURANCE IN NURSING AND HEALTHCARE

Quality assurance approaches have been evident in nursing since the days of Florence Nightingale. In 1860, Nightingale called for the development of a uniform method to collect and present hospital statistics to improve hospital treatment. Nightingale was a pioneer in setting standards for nursing care. The impetus for establishing nursing schools in the United States came in the late 1800s from a desire to set standards that would upgrade nursing care. In the early 1900s, efforts were begun to set similar standards for all nursing schools.

From 1912 to 1939, the interest in quality nursing education laid to the development of nursing organizations involved in accrediting nursing programs. Licensure has been a major issue in nursing since 1892.

By 1923, all states had permissive or mandatory laws directing nursing practice.

After World War II: The attention of the emergency nursing focused on establishing a scientific method of practice. The nursing process was the chosen method and included evaluation of how the activities of nurses helped clients (Maibusch, 1984). QA involves the evaluative step in nursing process.

The 1950s brought the development of tools to measure QA. One of the first tools created was the Phaneuf Nursing Audit (1952, 1965). In 1966, the American Nurses Association (ANA) created the divisions on practice in its by-laws. As a result of this, in 1972, the congress for nursing practice was charged with developing standards to be used to institute QA programs.

In 1972, the Joint Commission on Accreditation of Hospitals Organization (JCAHO) clearly stated the responsibilities of nursing in its description of standards for nursing services; the JCAHO called on the nursing industry to clearly plan, document and evaluate nursing care provided. In the mid-1980s, JCAHO became the Joint Commission on Accreditation of Health Care Organizations (JCAHCO) and began developing quality control standards for home, health nursing and for hospital nursing.

Also in 1972, the Social Security Act (Public Law 92-603) was amended to establish the Professional Standards Review Organization (PSRO) and to mandate the review of the delivery of healthcare to the clients of Medicare, Medicaid and maternal and child health programs. The PSRO program was modified to become the Professional Review Organizations (PROs) by 1983 Social Security Amendments. The purpose of the PROs is to monitor implementation of the prospective reimbursement system for Medicare clients. PSRP and PRO have made QA a primary issue for all healthcare professionals.

CONCEPT OF QUALITY ASSURANCE IN THE NURSING PROFESSION

Quality assurance in healthcare is often taken to be an innovation of the late 12th century but its gestation has a much longer history. In the 19th century, the concept of quality in nursing was first introduced by Florence Nightingale. She prepared the cycle of standard settings—observation, review and improvement. The improvements that affected in the hospital at Scutari were only possible because her observations allowed her to demonstrate that hospitalization of wounded soldiers led to an increase rather than a decrease in mortality.

According to Ellis and Whittington (1993), Nightingale's "Notes on Nursing" were in fact standards for the nursing care and remained benchmarks for high, but achievable quality for many years; the same author described in brief the development of the process of QA programs in nursing. As early as in 1965, the Royal College of Nursing, United Kingdom (UK) set up a "standards of care" project. This has now developed into a major program of research development and education.

The ANA first disseminated generic standards in 1973 and followed up with standards for maternal child nursing, psychiatric/mental health nursing, community health nursing, medical-surgical nursing and gerontological nursing. Canada has also prepared standards in nursing care using Donabedian's model of QA (Nagpal, 1987). Thus, various developed countries that are involved in QA programs in India are still at a rudimentary stage where baseline studies are needed to know the status of nursing and its involvement in QA. Though awareness of quality among professionals is an essential prerequisite for quality, very little is done so far due to various hindrances.

QUALITY ASSURANCE OF NURSING IN INDIA

The concept of quality in nursing standards is not new in India. However, the amount of stress on these areas is negligible. Though standardization in nursing education is noteworthy, there is no significant initiation or progress in provision of standards in nursing care process. Various committees and commissions were set up to look into the healthcare delivery system. Though these committees have dealt with the issues of training shortage of man owe, creation of more posts, vacancies, improvement of service ions, none have listed or highlighted the importance of improving the standards of nursing (Fig. 10.1).

The licensing bodies, the Indian Nursing Council and the State Registration Councils, which are responsible for the preparation of minimum standards have limited their role to nursing education, examination and qualification. Today, while speaking of nursing care, almost all the senior professionals in India say that nursing standards are very

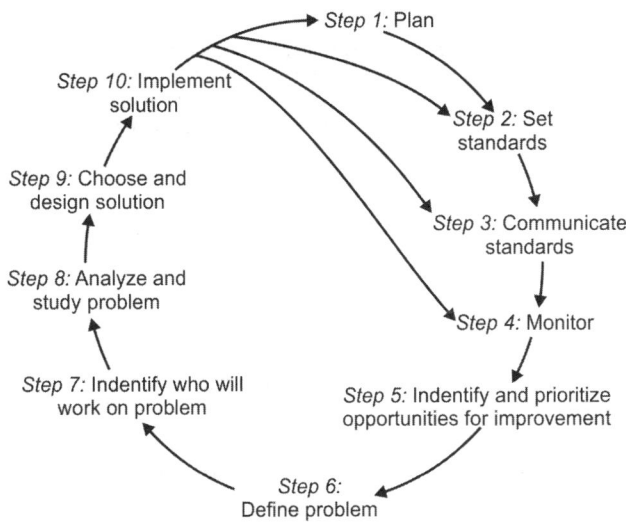

Fig. 10.1: Quality assurance cycle.

poor. Many of the consumers opine that nurses' role is mainly restricted to administration of drugs, treatment, bed making, recording, assisting the physician, etc. This is perhaps because consumers rarely come in contact with professional nursing.

Recent studies have explored healthcare utilization in general, which show that around 60–70% of healthcare contacts are made in the private health sector (George, Nandraj, et al, 1994). In Andhra Pradesh, except few hospitals, almost all the private nursing homes are manned mainly by unqualified persons who are designated as nurses. Any woman who gets elementary training by a doctor is called "nurse" in some private sector hospitals. Non-availability of qualified nurses and financial constraints in private hospitals are responsible for recruitment of unqualified and underqualified staff.

Analyzing today's situation where nursing profession occupies a distinct position in healthcare services, there is an indication that lack of proper standards in nursing care may cause a severe threat to the existence of the profession leading to the profession merging into other professions.

Hindrances to Standards of Nursing in India

- In India, there are various categories of nursing. Auxiliary nurse midwife (ANM) diploma, graduate, postgraduate, MPhil and doctorate nurses. The standard of education is different for each one. This could be one of the reasons why many of the procedures could not be standardized in a definite way as these standards are based on the knowledge of that particular group.
- The descriptions are not standard objectives and proper job for nurses in various sectors. Lack of proper job descriptions for each category of nurses is another obstacle to set uniform standards. For example, an ANM working in a hospital (especially private hospital) is supposed to carry out all the procedures similar to a qualified nurse, whereas her course curriculum is mostly based on community health. Hence, there is a need for setting minimum standards of nursing practice based on qualifications and job descriptions.
- Lack of adequate nurse administrators is one of the reasons for poor initiation of any innovative project in nursing profession.
- *Inter-professionality problem:* Many times, nurses do not have the right to do the procedures, which are said to be purely for nursing actions. Sophisticated procedures are always taken up by medical profession. Nurses are mostly restricted to giving physical care, medicine administration, record keeping and ward management (linen, equipment, drugs, etc.). Higher-level functions, critical judgments and decisions are not permitted by nurses in a healthcare system dominated by the medical profession.
- In India, there is no regulatory body to assess the standards of nursing services.

Indian publications on nursing are very few. Though, there are many resource persons, hardly few publications are available especially on local application of knowledge and utilization of available resources according to Indian situation.

GOALS OF QUALITY ASSURANCE

The goals of QA are:
- To ensure the delivery of quality client care
- To demonstrate the efforts of the health provider to provide the best possible results

The process of healthcare includes two major components:
1. Technical interventions.
2. Interpersonal relationships between practitioner and client.

CRITERIA IN QUALITY ASSURANCE SYSTEM

The QA system should know the following criteria; phonic "Rumba" can be used as criteria:

R: Relevant
U: Understandable
M: Measurable
B: Behaviorally stated
A: Achievable/Attainable

Models of Quality Assurance

To measure the quality of nursing care, we need some yardsticks, i.e. setting of standards in nursing practice.

The models of quality assurances (QA) in healthcare are detailed in Table 10.1.

Donabedian model:
Donabedian (1966, 1985) proposed a model for the structure, process and outcome of quality that is a widely

Table 10.1: Models of quality assurances in healthcare.

Donabedian's model 1960s	Wilson's model 1980s	Royal Marsden Hospital	Ellis and Whittington, 1993
• Structure • Process • Outcome	• Inputs: 　▪ People 　▪ Equipment; environment • Methods and procedures • Outcomes: 　▪ Productivity 　▪ Quality 　▪ Client satisfaction	• Resources • Professional practice • Outcomes	Operationalized Donabedian's model into a more practical form

used framework for assessing a method of measuring quality care. This model depicted as lineal model as in Figure 10.2.

FRAMES OF REFERENCES FOR EVALUATION OF NURSING CARE

Three frames of references can be used for setting standards and evaluating nursing care services; they are structure, process and outcome standards (Fig. 10.2).

Structure

Evaluation of structure is designed to find out whether facilities, equipment and manpower resources are conducive to effective delivery of nursing care. Structure evaluation focuses on characteristics of the nursing staff, the setting or the core environment. Structure deals with the care providing system and the resources, and relates to the framework that provides support for actual provision of care.

Structure standards or structure-based criteria are designed to identify necessary, but not sufficient conditions for quality of nursing care. Criteria based on structure give conditions under which it is likely that good nursing will take place, but such criteria do not assure good care. To evaluate structure information needed may be related to physical facilities, building, supplies and equipment, staff number, type of training, qualification, policies and organization, administrative setup, lines of communication, policies and objectives.

Process

Evaluation of process aims to find out whether nursing activities, techniques, processes and procedures are carried out properly. Process evaluation focuses on nursing performance. The actual activities in providing care are crucial in determining the quality of care.

Process standards help measure such factors as: the degree of skill with which techniques or procedures are carried out, the degree of client participation in care, the nature of interaction between nursing personnel and client, or at higher level, the evaluator could determine the accuracy with which the patients' needs are identified, the adequacy of nursing activities planned and the skill with which these are performed. Process standards are generally stated in terms of desired level of nursing performance,

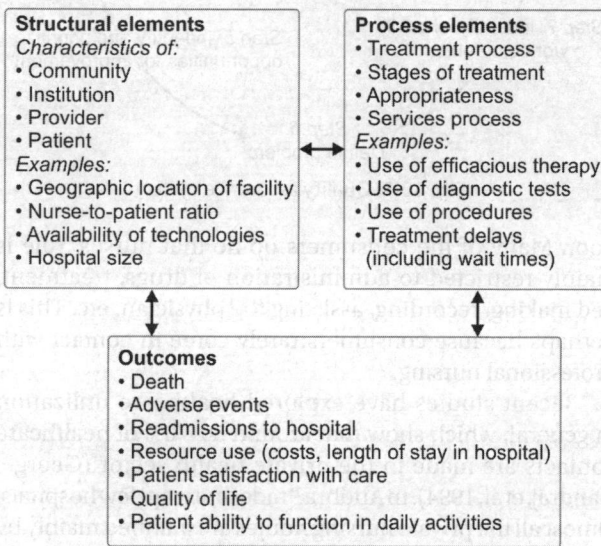

Fig. 10.2: Donabedian model of quality assurance.

i.e. quantity of care, adequacy of care, quality of care, appropriateness of care, etc. A critical difference between structure standards and process standards is that process standards require a professional judgment in determining whether the criteria are met.

Outcome

Evaluation of outcome is designed to find out the effect of nursing care on health status of patients. Outcome evaluation is focused on the effects of nursing care on clients or patients. Outcomes are considered by many experts to be the ideal frame of references if they could be based on the findings of sophisticated research that clearly identifies nursing contribution to the outcome.

DEFINITION OF STANDARDS

A statement can be defined as a professionally agreed level of performance for a particular population and which is achievable, observable, desirable and measurable.

Standards are one of the main building blocks in any QA activity. Standards setting provide a system, which all grades of staff can use easily. It provides direction. These provide a base line for evaluation quality of nursing care.

Types of Specification in Standards

Standards can establish a wide range of specifications for products, processes and services.

- **Prescriptive specifications** obligate product characteristics, e.g. device dimensions, biomaterials, list or calibration procedures, as well as definition of terms and terminologies.
- **Design specifications** set out the specific design or technical characteristics of a product, e.g. operating room facilities or medical gas systems.
- **Performance specifications** ensure that a product meets a prescribed test; e.g. strength requirements, measurement accuracy, battery capacity or maximum defibrillator energy.
- **Management specifications** set out requirements for the processes and procedures that companies put in place, e.g. quality systems for manufacturing or environmental management systems.

Purposes

- Provide reference criteria that a product, process or service must meet
- Provide information that enhances safety, reliability and performance of products, processes and services.

Conformity Assessment with Standards

- A product's conformity to standards is commonly assessed by direct testing.
- A process can be assessed by audit. Certification organizations or regulatory authorities attest that products or processes conform to a standard by authorizing the display of their certification mark.
- The conformity to management standard by an organization is known as management systems registration. Management system registration bodies issue registration certificates to companies that has management standards.
- Accreditation is used by an authoritative body to give formal recognition that an organization or a person is competent to carry out a specific task.

NURSING STANDARDS

Definition

A nursing care standard is a descriptive statement of desired quality against which to evaluate nursing care.

Purposes

- Standards give direction and provide guidelines for performance of nursing staff
- Standards provide a baseline for evaluating quality of nursing, ranging from excellent to unsafe care
- Standards may help to improve quality of nursing care, increase effectiveness of care and improve efficiency
- Standards may help to improve documentation of nursing care provided
- Standards may help to determine the degree to which standards of nursing care are maintained and take necessary corrective action in time
- Standards help supervisors to guide nursing staff to improve performance
- Standards may help to improve basis for decision-making and device alternative system for delivery of nursing care
- Standards may help justify demands for resources association
- Standards may help classify nurse's area of accountability
- Standards may help nursing to define clearly different levels of care.

Characteristics of Standard

- Statement must be broad enough to apply to a wide variety of settings
- It must be realistic, acceptable, flexible and attainable
- It should be phrased in positive terms and indicate acceptable performance
- Nursing care must express what is desirable at optional level
- It must be understandable and stated in unambiguous terms
- It must be based on current knowledge and scientific practice
- It must be reviewed and revised periodically.

Sources of Nursing Care Standards

- Professional organization, e.g. Trained Nurses' Association of India (TNAI), etc.
- Licensing bodies, e.g. statutory bodies, Indian Nursing Council (INC), etc.
- Institutions/healthcare agencies, e.g. university, hospitals, health centers
- Department of institutions, e.g. Department of Nursing
- Patient care units, e.g. specific patients unit
- Government units at national, state and local governments' limits.

Standards in Nursing

Standards formulation is of great advantage to a profession. Standards help in:

- Improving the quality of nursing care
- Evaluation of nursing care
- Provision of scientific and rationalized care with a definite direction
- Supervision and performance appraisals
- Attaining a district position by drawing a demarcating line (of standards) as to how nursing is different and unique from other professions
- Justifying demands in resource allocation

- Time conservation and time management
- Proper utilization of available resources
- Avoiding duplication of work (as healthcare involves multidisciplinary team).

TECHNIQUES OF QUALITY ASSURANCE IN NURSING

There are a few techniques used for preparation of standards in nursing profession. In the quality-specific techniques, the following are usually used (Fig. 10.3):
- Professional standards technique
- Comprehensive review systems
- Process appraisal techniques.

Professional Standards System

The professional standards category contains the various guidelines and standard documents, which healthcare professionals have published basis for QA.

American nurses have prepared a model of QA, which was meant for the nursing profession, but was used by various other professionals in healthcare. This is a cyclical model. All the QA systems involve appraisal of quality standards followed by action for quality improvement. The ANA cycle of QA is an elaboration of the sequence. At each stage in the cycle of observations, the events of the previous stage influence the decision to be made, and the action to be undertaken in the next. The cycle is known as "open" system. This openness is necessary to allow the idea of continuous quality improvements. Today's highest possible standards may not satisfy the consumers and professionals of tomorrow.

Comprehensive Review Systems

Many professional bodies have specified standards and guidelines for practice, which are taken and applied in all of the settings where the relevant professionals work. These standards are at a high level of generality, and several professional bodies suggest that their central standards should be used as a framework for more local exercises in specific standards setting.

The local and specific should thus grow out of the central and more general. But nursing profession has adopted the opposite strategy. It provides guidelines for a process for local standard setting on the assumption that at some later date, general standards may grow from the local and specific ones, e.g. Royal College of Nursing dynamic standard setting system established in 1965 (UK) is typically carried out at the ward level. Dynamic standard setting system (DySSSy) is designed based on comprehensive review systems. This system is designed to facilitate local standard setting as well as quality appraisal and improvement.

Process Appraisal Techniques

Process appraisal techniques contain methods, which focus particularly on appraisal of the quality of the processes of care. Process standards have been more extensively developed in nursing than in any other professional area and almost all instruments for measuring process quality are designed for use in nursing.

The process of care comprises all the procedures and activities through which the health professionals and support workers deploy their time, skills, knowledge and resources in pursuit of improving patient health and well-being. It has technical interpersonal and moral components and includes access, diagnosis, treatment, discharge aftercare, health education and promotion. Professions vary in the extent to which they have developed instruments for measurement of the process of care. Nursing is in the forefront of the other health professions in its work on instruments for measuring process quality.

COMPONENTS OF QUALITY ASSURANCE PROGRAM

There are five major components of a QA program. They are:
1. Setting standards
2. Comparing these standards to actual practice
3. Analyzing and interpreting these comparisons
4. Selecting and implementing action to change practice
5. Evaluating the effectiveness of these actions.

AUDIT

Introduction

To most people, the word "Audit" is familiar in relation to financial transactions justifying the use of financial resources and thereby establishing a guide for future financial operations. While standards provide the yardstick for the measurement of quality of care, audits are the tool. Hospitals or medical services are no exception to such audits, however, far more important aspects of activities and transactions in hospitals directly relate to patients. This aspect when viewed as a means of justifying the use of medical and nursing care resources and thereby establishing

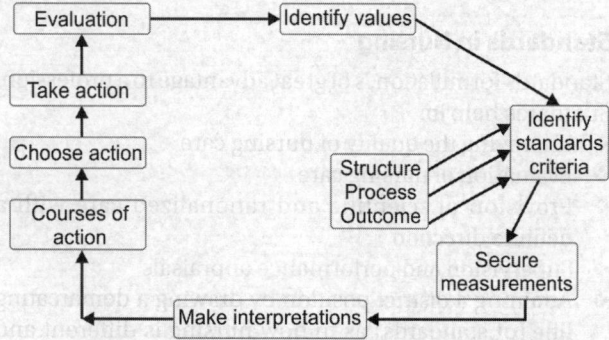

Fig. 10.3: American Nurses Association model of quality assurance.

Chapter 10: Quality Assurance in Nursing

a guide for future medical and nursing care operations has come to be known as the medical audit and nursing audit.

Definition

"Audit is an independent appraisal activity within an organization for the review of accounting, financial and other operations as a basis of services to the management. Audit seeks to investigate all the practices related to accounting of materials, labor or any activity that involves a cost".

"An audit is a systematic and official examination of a record, process or account to evaluate performance".

Audit refers to the monitoring of the budget process. Here, the budget reports are needed to monitor expenditure and keep the budget process focused on long-range objectives. The following are the most common budget monitoring tools.

Types of Audit

The audits most frequently used in quality control include outcome, process and structure audits.

- ❖ **Outcome audits:** Outcomes are the end results of care, the changes in the patient's health status and can be attributed to the delivery of healthcare services. Outcome audits determine what results if any occurred as a result of specific nursing invention for clients. These audits assume the outcome accurately and demonstrate the quality of care that was provided. Examples of outcome traditionally used to measure quality of health services include mortality, morbidity rates, etc.
- ❖ **Process audit:** Process audits are used to measure the process of care or how the care was carried out. Process audit is task-oriented and focus on whether or not practice standards are being fulfilled. These audits assume that a relationship exists between the quality of the nurse and the quality of care provided.
- ❖ **Structure audit:** Structure audit monitors the structure or setting in which patient care occurs, such as the finances, nursing service, medical records and environment. This audit assumes that a relationship exists between quality care and appropriate structure.

Audit Tools

A variety of audit tools can help achieve the best and most comprehensive data. These tools are record reviews, checklists, questionnaires and surveys.

Audit Process (Fig. 10.4)

The audit process consists of six steps:
1. Selection of a topic for study
2. Selection of explicit criteria for quality care
3. Review of records to determine whether the criteria are met
4. Peer review of all cases that do not meet the criteria

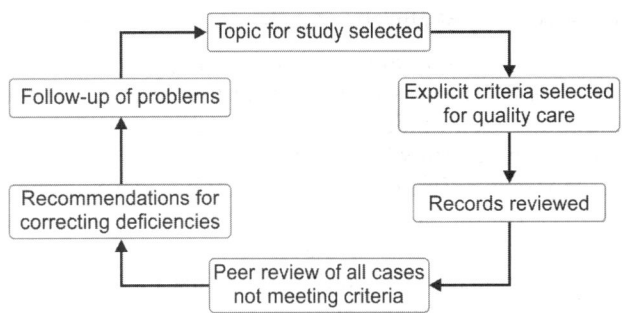

Fig. 10.4: Audit process.

5. Specific recommendations to correct problems
6. Follow up to determine whether problems have been eliminated.
   a. **Assessment:** Subjective and objective data are collected from various sources. It can be either primary or secondary sources.
   b. **Diagnosis:** Based on the data collected, diagnosis is made. The collected data will be related to demographic features, housing, environmental sanitation, vital statistics such as morbidity and mortality, maternal and child health (MCH) program, antenatal program, accessibility to some nutritional deficiencies, cases of complications, intranatal and postnatal services, etc.
   c. **Prioritizing the needs** on the basis of risk approach, like infants and neonates, mother and child, old-age people, etc.
   d. **Identify the resources** available to carry out the plans
   e. **Set the standards** according to the resources available
   f. **Committee reviews** the records and reports and identifying the strong and weak points.

Monthly audit committee meeting is held in community and report is submitted to the medical officer in primary health center. From primary health center, this will be sent to district health officer and from there to the Directorate of Family Welfare.

Involving the entire staff in the process is essential to increasing incentives for adhering to the standards. The information gathered can also support plans for revising and perhaps modifying the standards, as clients need changes. In some instances, the audit committee is empowered to implement those changes. Otherwise committee should revise follow-up reports on their recommendation from those who have taken the actions. In either cases, the results of recommended actions should be re-evaluated at a specified future date by the same group.

■ NURSING AUDIT

Meaning

Nursing audit (a) is the assessment of the quality of nursing care; (b) uses a record as an aid in evaluating the quality of patient care.

Brief History of Nursing Audit

Nursing audit is an evaluation of nursing service. Before 1955, very little was known about the concept. It was introduced by the industrial concern and the year 1918 was the beginning of medical audit.

First report of the nursing audit of the hospital published in 1955. For the next 15 years, nursing audit is reported from study or record from the last decade. The program is reviewed from record of nursing plan, nurses' notes, patient condition, nursing care, etc.

Nursing Care Audit

Audit is related to the planning, delivery and evaluation of patient care. It is an important component of nursing care.

Definition of Nursing Audit

According to Elison, "Nursing audit refers to assessment of the quality of clinical nursing."

According to Goster Walfer, "Nursing audit is an exercise to find out whether good nursing practices are followed."

"The audit is a means by which nurses themselves can define standards from their point of view and describe the actual practice of nursing."

"Nursing audit is the process of analyzing data about the nursing process of patient outcomes to evaluate the effectiveness of nursing interventions."

Purposes of Nursing Audit

- Evaluating nursing care given
- Achieves deserved and feasible quality of nursing care
- Stimulant to better records
- Focuses on care provided and not on care provider
- Contributes to research.

Methods of Nursing Audit

Retrospective View

This refers to an in-depth assessment of the quality after the patient has been discharged, and has the patient's chart to the source of data.

Retrospective audit is for evaluating the quality of nursing care by examining the nursing care as it is reflected in the patient care records for discharged patients. In this type of audit, specific behaviors are described, and then they are converted into questions and the examiner looks for answers in the record. For example, the examiner looks through the patient's record and asks:

- Was the problem solving process used in planning nursing care?
- Whether patient data were collected in a systematic manner?
- Was a description of patient's pre-hospital routines included?
- Whether laboratory test results were used in planning care?
- Did the nurse perform physical assessment? How was information used?
- Where nursing diagnoses stated?
- Did nurse write nursing orders? And so on.

The Concurrent Review

This refers to the evaluations conducted on behalf of patients who are still undergoing care. It includes assessing the patient at the bedside in relation to pre-determined criteria, interviewing the staff responsible for his care and reviewing the patients' records and care plan.

Method to Develop Criteria

- Define patient population
- Identify a time framework for measuring outcomes of care
- Identify commonly recurring nursing problems presented by the defined patient population
- State patient outcome criteria
- State acceptable degree of goal achievement
- Specify the source of information
- Design the type of tool
  - QA must be the priority
  - Those responsible must implement a program not only a tool
  - A coordinator should develop and evaluate QA activities
  - Roles and responsibilities must be delivered
  - Nurses must be informed about the process and the results of the program
  - Data must be reliable
  - Adequate orientation of data collection is essential
  - Quality data should be analyzed and used by nursing personnel at all levels.

Audit Cycle

Audit cycle involves following steps (Fig. 10.5).

Nursing Standards

Defines a standard as the desirable and achievable level of performance against which actual practice is compared. The standards must meet the needs of the patient.

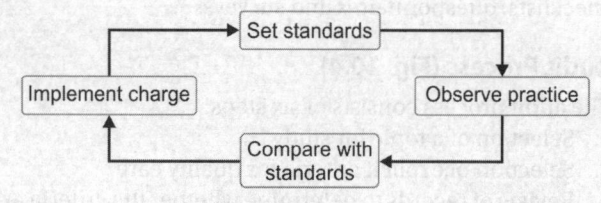

Fig. 10.5: Audit cycle.

Advantages of Nursing Audit

- Can be used as a method of measurement in all areas of nursing
- Seven functions are easily understood
- Scoring system is easily understood
- Results easily understood
- Assesses the work of all those involved in recording care
- May be useful tool as a part of a QA program in areas where accurate records of care are kept

Disadvantages of Nursing Audit

- Appraises the outcome of the nursing process, so it is not so useful in areas where the nursing process has not been implemented
- Many of the components overlap making the analysis difficult
- It is time consuming
- Requires a team of trained auditors
- Deals with a large amount of information
- Only evaluates record keeping. It only serves to improve documentation, not nursing care

Audit Committee

Before carrying out an audit, an audit committee should be formed, comprising a minimum of five members who are interested in QA, are clinically competent and able to work together in a group. It is recommended that each member should review not more than 10 patients each month and that the auditor should have the ability to carry out an audit in about 15 minutes. If there are less than 50 discharges per month, then all the records may be audited, if there are large number of records to be audited, then an auditor may select 10% of discharges.

Training for Auditors

It should include the following:
- A detailed discussion of the seven components
- A group discussion to see how the group rated the care received using the notes of a patient who has been discharged, these should be anonymous and should reflect a total period of care not exceeding 2 weeks in length
- Each individual auditor should then undertake the same exercise as above. This is followed by a meeting of the whole committee to compare and discuss their findings, and finally reach a consensus of opinion on each of the components.

FACTORS AFFECTING QUALITY NURSING CARE (FIG. 10.6)

Some quality management activities for community health nurses include daily prioritizing care for a caseload of

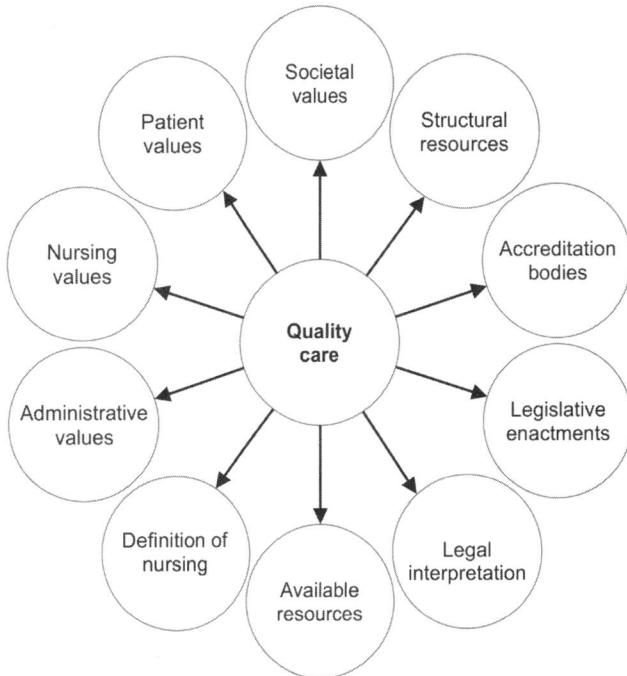

Fig. 10.6: Factors affecting quality nursing care.

students, seeking supervision or skills development for a difficult case, systematizing charting so that needed documentation is efficiently completed; proposing better ways to organize care of chronically ill clients or establishing new agency procedure.

Staff meetings, quality circle meetings and case conferences are common settings for nurses to bring the lessons of their practices to the larger group for examination and potential adoption.

MEASURABLE INITIATIVES FOR CONTINUOUS QUALITY IMPROVEMENT IN NURSING

- Error prevention and reporting
- Patient education
- Documentation improvement
- Billing efficiency
- Medical emergency preparedness
- Management of medication (MOM)
- Patient safety
- Discharge counseling
- Tissue viability
- Intensive care unit (ICU) care continuity
- Psychosocial approach to patient care
- Operation theater (OT) care continually/immediate post of care monitoring
- Surgical safety initiative and intraoperative safety
- Unit/ward specific patient feedback

- ❖ Theory application initiative for care quality, e.g. Kings, Orlando's theory
- ❖ Stay current and competent, and privileging competency.

CONCLUSION

Though the concept of QA is old, it is still in a rudimentary stage in India. There is no proper initiation of quality concepts in practice. Nurses are never involved in committees especially on local application of knowledge and utilization of available resources according to Indian situation. Nursing profession is badly in need of standards for various aspects of care especially in Indian context. The consumer organizations are demanding quality service. The challenge facing nursing profession is to demonstrate that nurses are cost-effective in delivering quality healthcare.

11 CHAPTER

Futuristic Nursing

CHAPTER OUTLINE

- Nursing Future Challenges
- Challenges in Nursing Practice
- Challenges in Nursing Education
- Trends of Nursing Education for Future
- Variation on Traditional Roles in Nursing
- New Millennium Nurses

INTRODUCTION

Nursing is a glorified noble profession. Nursing is rapidly growing day-to-day. Now nursing changed a lot than in the past, and in the future, it may have so many changes. The future promises existing and stimulating changes in the healthcare delivery system, and the nursing profession faces the challenge of taking an active part.

NURSING FUTURE CHALLENGES

Societal Challenges

There are five societal influences that are expected to have major impact on the future of the nursing profession:
1. Demographic challenges
2. Environmental deterioration
3. Unhealthy lifestyle and resulting illness
4. The need for cost control
5. Regulation of health care.

Demographic Challenges

Demography is the science that studies vital statistics and social trends. Demographers examine vital statistics such as birth rate, morbidity rate, death rate, marriage, the ages of various populations and migration patterns. From these health information, they will predict the future trends.

Four trends detected by demographers are particularly important to the future nursing:
1. Continuing increase in poverty
2. Rising numbers of elderly people
3. Increase in cultural diversity of population
4. Continuing trend towards urbanization.

Continuing poverty

When basic needs for food, clothing and shelter are unmet or uncertain, healthcare becomes a luxury. Children's immunization and prenatal care for women are neglected. Poor people tend to put off seeking care, until illness is advanced and harder to treat. Preventable conditions are often not prevented because of lack of education, lack of sanitations, crowded living conditions, etc. Poverty will continue to create increasing numbers of disenfranchised people, that is, people who have no power in political system with limited access to healthcare. Nursing as a profession values providing nursing care to all people, regardless of social and economic factors. The increasing number of medically disenfranchised people and the increase to limit healthcare expenditures will collide to create a conflict of values for nurses in the future.

Rising number of elderly people

The world future society predicts that by the end of the 21st century, average lifespan will approach 100 years.

Increase cultural diversity

Nurses need to take their beliefs into consideration when planning and implementing nursing care for individuals of diverse cultural background. Culturally sensitive care will be more important in the future than ever before.

Continuing urbanization

Urbanization is people moving from rural farming areas to cities. Decaying inner cities with large population of poor people create major social problems, such as homelessness, drugs-gangs, mental illness, violence and crime. Nurses of the future will be increasingly confronted with health problems created by the urbanization.

Environmental Deterioration

The related problems of environmental deterioration and over population are healthcare issues that future nurses will undoubtedly have to face the emergence of newer communicable and noncommunicable diseases.

Lifestyle Challenges
The twin epidemics of acquired immunodeficiency syndrome (AIDS) and drug abuse are two lifestyle issues that will profoundly affect the future of nursing. Nursing of the future will be called on to provide intensive nursing care to increase the number of substance abusers leading non communicable diseases such as, diabetes, hypertension and carcinomas, etc. and people with AIDS. Nurses will play an increasingly important role in educating people about wellness and self-care in the years ahead.

Cost Control
In future, nursing is high-quality, cost-effective and it may be an alternative to traditional medical care. One cost-effective method of providing basic healthcare to children is through school nurses and creating awareness on prevention of disease among people through mass media.

Regulation of Healthcare
Nurses will become active increasingly in developing health policies that improve access, quality and value in the delivery of health services.

CHALLENGES IN NURSING PRACTICE
Challenge of Technology
Technology will continue to advance at a dizzying pace in the 21st century. Nursing informatics, the organization and use of nursing date will change nursing practice dramatically.

Computerized health information network (CHIN) will allow immediate access to all patient data. This increased access to patient data will reinforce the need for patient confidentially. Voice-activated bedside computers will allow nurse to record patient information literally at the bedside. Advances in telecommunications will improve access to medical service for rural and elderly people. Nurses and physicians will examine and treat patients who are hundreds of miles away using two-way television system. They will evaluate and prescribe treatments via telephone. Telephone will become routine for those who live in remote areas.

Expanding Technology
Every person involved in healthcare delivery is well aware of the economic, political, professional, scientific and technological forces that exert pressure on the system.

For example, many nursing activities are already being done by technology. Vital signs will be monitored more accurately by machines than clinicians. Software has been devised, so that clients can perform much of their own psychotherapy without clinical assistance. Teaching machine will be available for clients to learn about their disease process and how to manage them. Sensors will monitor therapeutic drug levels and automatically replenish them without clinician interface. All the scientific and clinical information generated by worldwide research will be online and available to clinicians of all types.

Another very important area of current knowledge research is the genome-mapping project, which has the potential for introducing a very radical approach to both curing and preventing illness. Genetics may become the most studied field for the next few decades.

Computer Assistance
Computers become smallest and simpler to operate. They will be as common in homes as telephone presently are. Computer-assisted client care can reduce error, and helps in clinical planning process. It also can be used to evaluate client care. It will be possible to develop methods to assess the quality of the practitioners and the cumulative performance of the staff. Big computer companies, telecommunication firms and the government are trying to computerize two routine elements of hospital care diagnosis and prescription.

Electronic Mail
Electronic mail (e-mail) may be text or multimedia message sent from one computer to another via the Internet. Uses include communication and collaboration in clinically relevant ways. For example, nurses both at work and not at work can keep up-to-date with unit meetings, schedule changes, hospital or departmental news and announcements.

- ❖ Nursing administration can share news and views, policies and procedures, management practices, and stay in touch with local, national and international counterparts, and keep up-to-date with professional and union organizations
- ❖ Nursing research use mail to share research finding, database, program and information about research grants
- ❖ Community nurse use e-mail to stay in touch with their colleagues and with their administrative centers.

Web Browsers
Web browsers are of great significance for nurses and nursing, since more and more nurses and nursing organizations are publishing materials on worldwide web making them freely accessible to nurses globally. Now it is possible for nurses anywhere to obtain electronic access to text, abstracts, articles, policies, procedures and clinical guidelines. Using web technology, nurses may interact with colleagues, students or clients at a distance that is known as virtual nursing.

Robots

Robots are also being used in clinical settings. At the beginning of 1994, the University of Virginia Hospital was reported to have developed robots to conduct blood analysis. The use of robots in intensive care unit is not only time- and money-saving but also cut down human exposure to blood-borne infections. The blood analyzers have mechanical arms that handle blood specimens, so that healthcare workers have lower exposure. The robots also save time. They will have a 24 hours a day, 7 days a week availability.

Challenges of Practice in Expanded Settings

Community-based primary healthcare will continue to expand as cost-effectiveness remains a high priority.

Nurses-managed clinics will increasingly serve inner city and rural underserved populations.

Challenges of Technology and the Knowledge Explosion

Technological advances and the growth of nursing theories will create a knowledge explosion in nursing.

The traditional nursing lecture is now being augmented or replaced with computer-assisted instruction. Interactive programs will permit students to practice decision-making skills in a safe environment.

The use of videotaping and television in the classroom and in the practice laboratory has already proved to be an effective method to extend the ability of one instructor to assist many students. Videotaped demonstration eliminates the need for tedious repetition of basic procedure for a small group. Students can view videotapes at their own convenience and can use videotaped play back to assess their own skills.

CHALLENGES IN NURSING EDUCATION

As the profession of nursing matures, more nurses will recognize the value of bachelor's degree for beginning professional practice and master's degree for advanced practice.

Challenges of Outcome-Based Education

In the future, the quality of educational program will be judged by student competencies, that is, what student can actually do as a result of education. Nursing educational program will monitor their graduate's activity and achievements as professional nurse.

Future of nursing education: The millennium has become the metaphor for the extraordinary challenges and opportunities available to the nursing profession and to those academic institutions responsible for preparing the next generation of nurses.

Transformations taking place in nursing and nursing education have been driven by major socioeconomic factors, as well as by developments in healthcare delivery and professional issues unique to nursing.

TRENDS OF NURSING EDUCATION FOR FUTURE

- Changing demographics and increasing diversity
- The technological explosion
- Globalization of the world's economy and society
- The era of the educated consumer, alternative therapies and genomics and palliative care
- Shift to population-based care and the increasing complex of patient care
- Impact of health policy and regulation
- The growing need for interdisciplinary education for collaborative practice
- The current nursing shortage/opportunities for lifelong learning and work force development
- Significant advances in nursing science and research.

1. ***Changing demographics and increasing diversity:*** Population shifts in the United States have affected healthcare priorities as well as the practice of nursing. Due to advances in public health and clinical care, the average lifespan is increasing rapidly. By 2020, more than 20% of the population will be 65 and older, with those over 85 constituting the fastest growing age group greater life expectancy of individuals with chronic and acute conditions will challenge the healthcare system's ability to provide efficient and effective continuing care. Disparities in morbidity, mortality and other factors have led to increased violence and substance abuse. Nursing practice, education and research must focus on spiritual health, as well as the physical and psychosocial health of the population.

2. ***The technological explosion:*** The rapid growth in information technology has already had a radical impact on healthcare delivery and the education of nurses. Advances in processing capacity and speed, the development of interactive user interfaces, developments in image storage and transfer technology, changes in telecommunications technology and the increased affordability of personal computers have contributed to the explosion on information technology applications. Advances in digital technology have increased the applications of telehealth and telemedicine, bringing together patient and provider without physical proximity. Nanotechnology will introduce new forms of clinical diagnosis and treatment by means of inexpensive handheld biosensors capable of detecting a wide range of diseases from miniscule body specimen.

Dramatic improvements in the accessibility of clinical data across settings, and time have improved both outcomes and care management; the electronic medical record will replace traditional documentation systems. Through the Internet, consumers will be increasingly armed with information previously available only to clinicians.

3. ***Globalization of the world's economy and society:*** Globalization has been brought about by many factors, including advances in information technology and communications, international travel and commerce, the growth of multinational corporations, the fall of communism in Eastern Europe and the Soviet Union, and major political changes in Africa and Asia. With the "death of distance" in the spread of disease and the delivery of healthcare, there are both extraordinary risks and extraordinary benefits. Along with the potential for rapid disease transmission, there is potential for dramatic improvement in health due to knowledge transfer between cultures and healthcare systems.

4. ***The era of the educated consumer, alternative therapies and genomics, and palliative care:*** The educated consumer despite some information gaps, today's patient is a well-informed consumer who expects to participate in decisions affecting personal and family healthcare. With advances in information technology and quality measurement, previously unavailable information is now public information, and consumers are asked to play a more active role in healthcare decision-making and management. The media and the Internet have facilitated this trend.

   Technological advances in the treatment of disease have led the need for ethical, informed decision-making by patients and families. Consumers are thus becoming more interested and knowledgeable about health promotion as well as disease prevention, and there is increased acceptance and demand for alternative and complementary health options. The increased power of the consumer in the patient–provider relationship creates a heightened demand for more sophisticated health education techniques and greater levels of participation by patients. In clinical decisions, nurses must be prepared to understand this changed relationship and be skilled in helping patients and families maximize opportunities to manage their health.

   The impact of the human genome project and related genetic and cloning research is unparalleled. Gene mapping will drive rapid advances in the development of new drugs, and the treatment and prevention of disease. Nursing education and practices must expand to include the implications of the emerging therapies from both genetic research and alternative medicine, while managing ethical conflicts and questions.

   New settings for care, such as inpatient and home-based hospice, and new forms of care, including pain management, spiritual practices support groups and bereavement counseling are now likely to be part of well-developed healthcare systems. A significant gap in the body of scientific knowledge and clinical education with regard to palliative and end-of-life care remains, and nursing education must prepare graduates for a significant role in these areas.

5. ***Shift to population-based care and the increasing complexity of patient care:*** Rising costs and an aging population have led to new settings and systems of care across the healthcare continuum. The change of marriage age leading to fertility problems with rising cost requires nursing professionals to have an understanding of practice methods that improve quality, respond to clinical complexity and lower costs. Expanded life expectancy has led to increasing the complexity of the care provided and managing by clinicians. The community has largely become the setting for chronic disease management and prevention providing services for defined groups "covered" by managed care will demand skills and knowledge in clinical epidemiology, biostatistics, behavior science and their application to specific population. Nurses must demonstrate management skills at both the organizational and patient care levels. These concepts must be incorporated into the nursing curriculum.

6. ***Impact of health policy and regulation:*** Historically, nursing's influence on policy and regulation has been disproportionately low relative to the breadth of nursing practice and its importance within the healthcare delivery system. Nursing schools, scholars, executives and professional nursing organizations must more actively contribute to the development of health policy and regulations. Ethical issues involved in working in an integrated system constrained economic incentives are being defined more and more by government policy-makers, not healthcare professionals. Nursing leaders should contribute to the dialog that defines these issues, and students must be prepared for a meaningful role in the political arena.

7. ***Growing need for interdisciplinary education for collaborative practice:*** A wide range of knowledge and skills is required to effectively and efficiently manage the comprehensive needs of patients and population. The healthcare delivery system of the future will rely on teams of nurse practitioners, physicians, dentists, social workers, pharmacists and other providers to work together. While interdisciplinary and collaborative practice is still not the norm, there has been a heightened awareness of the need for coordinated care and a significant increase in the use of midlevel providers such as advanced practice nurses as part of the primary care team.

   With care management, a critical component in healthcare delivery, nursing must demonstrate leadership and competence in interdisciplinary and collaborative practice for continuous quality improvement. Team-based interdisciplinary approaches have been shown to be highly effective for improving clinical outcomes and reducing cost. Teaching methods that incorporate opportunities for interdisciplinary education and collaborative practice are required to prepare nurses for their unique professional role, and to understand the role of other disciplines in the care of patients.

8. ***Current nursing shortage/opportunity for lifelong learning and workforce development:*** Rapidly evolving technology, increasing clinical complexity in many patient care settings, advances in treatment and the emergency of new diseases are factors contributing to the increasing need for a strong emphasis on critical thinking and lifelong learning among professional nurses. Further, new clinical roles, the need for managerial and executing talent, the imperative to retain nurses in active practice over longer careers and the desire by practicing nurses to move up the economic ladder lead to the demand for continuing education and career mobility, and development schools of nursing have many of the core resources needed to deliver continuing professional education, and can provide appropriate courses efficiently and effectively. Affiliation with schools by nurses and active practice may lead to an increase in enrolment for advanced degrees. Healthcare and health-related organizations may serve as institutional partners in sponsoring such programs offering, which would contribute to their relevance and increase lower costs.

   In April 2001, the New York State Board of Regents named a Blue Ribbon Task Force on the Future of Nursing, chaired by Regent Diane O'Neill McGivern. The Regents Blue Ribbon Task Force has a critical role in addressing the current nursing shortage, solution to the problem and the long-term future of nursing. As a result of an ambitious agenda and a steadfast commitment to a story future for the nursing profession, the Task Force has released their findings and recommendation for resolving this looming healthcare crisis. In their report, Protecting the Public, the Task Force recommends the following solutions to the nursing shortage:

   > ***Recruitment:*** Expand the nursing workforce by recruiting additional numbers of men, non-practicing nurses and recent high school graduates.
   > ***Education:*** Provide additional academic and financial support systems to increase the pool of nursing school graduates and create career ladders.

   Technology: Increase the application of labor-saving technology to eliminate unnecessary, duplicative paper work and improve access to, and communication of, patient information, thereby improving workplace conditions.

   > ***Data collection:*** Develop a reliable central source of data on the future need for nurses in the workforce upon which employers, policy-makers, futurists, researchers and legislators may base public policy and resource allocations.
   > Clarify existing laws and regulation:
   >   ♦ ***Scope of practice for nurses:*** Issue practice guidelines to clarify the legal scope of practice of nursing, including those tasks, which do not require licensure. These guidelines will reaffirm the individual practitioner's responsibility for patient care, even within demanding workplace settings
   >   ♦ ***Patient abandonment:*** Familiarize field with existing regent regulations, which describe patient abandonment—clarifying that refusal to work a double shift or other mandatory overtime in ordinary circumstances does not necessarily constitute professional misconduct. This information will be provided to nurses, hospitals, nursing homes and home care agency administrators

9. ***Significant advances in nursing science and research:*** Nursing research is an integral part of the scientific enterprise of improving the nation's health. The growing body of nursing research provides a scientific basis for patient care and should be regularly used by the nation's 2.5 million nurses. Most studies concern health behaviors, symptom management, and the improvement of patients' and families' experience with illness, treatment and disease prevention. Research is conducted to improve patient outcomes and vulnerable population.

   An approach to examining future directions for nursing research is through the words of 60 major nurse researchers in the "Handbook of Clinical Nursing Research" by Hinshaw et al., 1999. For the major areas of evolving nursing science, **we could use the following directions for nursing research into the 21st century:**
   > Critical health needs of communities and vulnerable population
   > Practice strategies and outcomes
   > Family health and transition
   > Health promotion/risk reduction
   > Bio-behavioral manifestations of health and illness
   > Women's health
   > Health and illness of older population
   > Environments for optimizing client outcomes
   > Genetics research
   > End-of-life research.

   Many avenues for generating nursing knowledge provide opportunities for the future. A strong foundation has been built and the areas for future study are exciting. The effects are expected to be far reaching in the ability of nursing profession affecting the experience of health and illness of individuals, families and communities.

VARIATION ON TRADITIONAL ROLES IN NURSING

Advanced Roles

Advanced practice roles for nurse in tomorrow's healthcare system:

- ❖ **Case manager:** Accountable for planning, modifying and leading care to produce timely, cost-effective outcomes in accomplishing the overall plan of care for a particular client
- ❖ **Clinical educator:** Coordinates all educational activities for staff and patient's families within a defined clinical area
- ❖ **Clinical consultant:** Recognized for expertise as a resource to the clinical or management staff
- ❖ **Corporate nurse practitioner:** Responsible for developing group-specific health promotion and disease prevention programs, as well as diagnosis and management of acute and chronic illnesses
- ❖ **Patient care manager:** Operates one or more patient care areas in a cost-effective manner
- ❖ **Hospice nurse:** Hospice and palliative care nurses treat the symptoms of those with progressive terminal disease. These nurses work holistically with patients and families to maximize their quality of life rather than focus on quantity of life remaining
- ❖ **Informatics nurse specialist:** The American Nurses Association (ANA) defines informatics as the activities involved in identifying, naming, organizing, grouping, collecting, processing, analyzing, storing, retrieving or managing data and information. Healthcare systems face the inevitable need for data management for decision-making, and another nursing role has emerged—the informatics nurse specialist
- ❖ **Flight nurse:** Who need autonomous practice and opportunity to use advanced clinical skills. Critical care experience with certification in advanced cardiac life support is necessary
- ❖ **Telephone triage nurse:** In this practice, nurses interact with patients on the telephone to assess needs, intervene and evaluate. Telephone triage is used in a variety of setting including emergency rooms and physician practices.

Expanded Nursing Roles

An expanded nursing role is one that a nurse assumes by virtue of qualification and experience.
- ❖ **Nurse generalist:** An expert in any area of nursing care such as child health, school health, etc.
- ❖ **Nurse clinician:** First defined by Frances Reiter in 1966; provide bedside or direct care in a specialty area
- ❖ **Nurse practitioner:** Extension of the basic role (caregiver) with expertise in assessment, diagnosis and healthcare management
- ❖ **Nurse specialist:** Have advanced knowledge and skills in a particular area of nursing; with a master's degree in the particular area
- ❖ **Certified registered nurse anesthetist:** Nurse anesthetist is recognized as the first clinical nursing specialty. The most famous nurse anesthetist of the 19th century is Alice Macaw, and she is called the mother of anesthesia.

NEW MILLENNIUM NURSES

For the nursing profession to remain viable in the new millennium, nurses can and should:
- ❖ Become politically active with leadership strategies at the local, state and national levels lobbying for increased funding for nursing education
- ❖ Support professional nursing organization
- ❖ Become involved in recruitment and retention efforts for both nurses and students
- ❖ Write to newspapers and television station about the image and role of the professional nurse
- ❖ Educate potential students that nursing is a challenging and financially rewarding career
- ❖ Lobby for nursing salaries to rise in competition with other career salaries
- ❖ Capitalize on the latest technology by offering long distance continuing educations classes to nurses via the Internet
- ❖ Retain and recruit older workers who are drawn to nursing later in life.

CONCLUSION

At the dawn of the 21st century and the long awaited new millennium, nurse educators face a rapidly changing healthcare landscape, shifting student and patient demographics, an explosion of technology and the globalization of health care. In addition to a myriad of everyday challenges as we position ourselves.

SUGGESTED READING

1. Ann J Zwemer. Textbook of Professional Adjustments and Ethics for Nurses in India, 6th edition. Madras: BI Publications; 1995. pp. 139-47.
2. Ann Marriner Tomey. Nursing Theorists and their Work, 3rd edition. St Louis, Mosby Publication; 1994. pp 231-44.
3. Barbara Cherry, Susan R Jacob. Contemporary Nursing: Issues, Trends, and Management, 2nd edition. Mosby Publication; 2002. p. 419.
4. Barbara Kozier. Fundamentals of Nursing, 5th edition. California: Addison-Wesley Publishers; 1995. pp. 26-41.
5. Basavanthappa BT. Fundamentals of Nursing, 1st edition. New Delhi: Jaypee Brothers; 2002. pp. 1-11, 131.
6. Basavanthappa BT. Nursing Administration, 3rd edition. Jaypee Publishers; Bangalore; 2011. pp. 1-17, 114-7, 435-8f, 474-510, 516-7, 521-2, 543-56.
7. Basavanthappa BT. Nursing Research, 1st edition. Jaypee Brothers; 2005. pp. 1-38.
8. BT Basavanthappa, Management of Nursing Services and Education, 1st edition. Jaypee Publishers; 2011.
9. BT Basavanthappa. Fundamentals of Nursing. 1st edition, Jaypee Publishers; 2004.
10. Caroline Bunker Rosdahl. Textbook of Basic Nursing, 7th edition. Philadelphia, Lippincott; 1999. pp-7-9.
11. Cherry B, Jacob SR. Contemporary Nursing: Issues, Trends and Management. Missouri: Mosby Inc.; 1999;. pp. 3-28.
12. D Elakkuvana Bhaskara Raj, T Anbu, B Venkatesan. Management of Nursing Services and Education, 1st edition; 2010.
13. Ellis JR, Hartley CL. Nursing in Today's World: Challenges Issues and Trends, 5th edition. Philadelphia (PA): JB Lippincott Co.; 1995. pp. 22-8.
14. Gaberson KB, Oermann MH. Clinical Teaching Strategies in Nursing, 3rd edition. New York: Springer Publishing Company; 2010. pp. 285-301.
15. Gloria M Grippando, Paula R Mitchell. Nursing Perspective and Issues, 4th edition. Delmar publications, Canada; 1989. pp 17-37.
16. Grace L Deloughery. Issue and Trends in Nursing, 3rd edition. Mosby Company Publications; 2002. pp. 91-2.
17. Hamilton PM. Realities of Contemporary Nursing, 2nd edition. California: Addison-Wesley Publishers; 1996. pp. 1-26.
18. Indrani TK. History of Nursing (Ch 1). Jaypee Publishers; 2004. pp. 3-45.
19. Jean Barret. Ward management and teaching. Konark Publishers; 2003.
20. Joanne Come Mecloskey, Helan Kennedy. Current Issues in Nursing, 3rd edition. CV Mosby Company Publications; 2003. pp. 45, 116, 472-6.
21. Kamal S Joglekar. Hospital Ward Management Professional Adjustment and Trends in Nursing. Vora Publication; 1997. pp. 107-9.
22. Kay Kittrell Chitty. Professional Nursing Concepts and Challenges, 4th edition. Elsevier Sanders; 2005. pp. 2-27.
23. Laura Mae Douglass. The Effective Nurse: Leader and Manager, 4th edition; 1991. pp. 193-6.
24. Marcia Stanhope. Community Health Nursing: Process and Practice for Promoting Health. Mosby Publication; 1988. pp. 233, 347, 447-8.
25. Mary Lucita. Nursing Practise and Public Health Administration Current Concepts and Trends, 2nd edition. New Delhi: Elsevier Publications; 2001. p. 169.
26. Nancy Burns, Susan K Groove. Understanding Nursing, 1st edition. WB Saunders Company; 1995. pp. 1-9.
27. Navdeep Kaur Brar, HC Rawat. Textbook of Advanced Nursing Practice, 1st edition. Jaypee Publishers; 2015.
28. Neeraja KP. Textbook of Nursing Education, 1st edition. Noida: Jaypee Brothers Medical Publishers (P) Ltd; 2005. pp. 41-77.
29. Park K. Textbook of Preventive and Social Medicine, 20th edition. Jabalpur: Banarsidas Bhanot Publications; 2002. p. 640.
30. Patricia A. Potter, Anne Griffin Perry. Fundamentals of Nursing (Vol. I), 5th edition. India: Mosby Harcourt; 1997. pp. 367-80, 401-23.
31. Phipps WJ, Sands JK, Marek JF. Medical-Surgical Nursing: Concepts and Clinical Practice, 6th edition. Missouri: Mosby Inc.; 1999. pp. 3-5.
32. Potter A Patricia, Perry Griffin Anne. Basic Nursing Theory and Practice, 3rd edition. St. Louis (MO): Mosby; 1995. p. 8.
33. www.rakcon.com.
34. Rosdhal CB. Textbook of Basic Nursing, 7th edition. Philadelphia (PA): Lippincott Williams and Wilkins Inc.; 1999. pp. 3-5.
35. Rubenfeld GM, Scheffer BK. Critical Thinking in Nursing: An In-attractive Approach, 1st edition. Philadelphia (PA): JB Lippincott Co; 1995. pp. 28-9.
36. Rumhold G. Ethics in Nursing Practice, 2nd edition. Philadelphia (PA): WB Saunders Company; 1993. p. 163.
37. Sankara Narayana. Basics of Nursing Education, 1st edition; 2002. pp. 15-8.
38. Sorensen and Luckmann's Basic Nursing: A Psychophysiologic Approach, 3rd edition. WB Saunders; 1994. pp. 6-18.
39. Sr Nancy. Principles and practice of nursing, 6th edition. NR Publishing House. Indore; 2006.
40. Stevenes J. Nursing Management. New York: Mosby Publications; 1996.
41. Susan Kun Leddy, J Mae. Conceptual Basis of Professional Nursing, 2nd edition. JB Company Publication; 2005. p. 123.
42. Taylor Carol. Textbook of Fundamentals of Nursing: The Art and Science of Nursing Care (Vol. 1), 6th edition. Philadelphia (PA): Lippincott Williams and Wilkins Publication; 2008. p. 12.
43. The Board of Nursing Education Nurses League, CMAI. A New Textbook for Nurses in India; 1990. pp. 5-8.
44. Zerwekh Joann, Claborn JC. Nursing Today: Transition and Trends. Philadelphia (PA): WB Saunders Company; 1994. p. 40.

Journals

1. S Sridhar. Quality assurance in nursing Indian Journal of Nursing and Midwifery. 1998; Sept 2.
2. Indian Nursing Council. Teaching Material For Quality Assurance Model. Indian Nursing Council Publications. Nursing, 1st edition; 2006: 8,9.
3. T Dileep Kumar. "Independent Nurse practitioner, scope, settings and innovations". The Nursing Journal of India. 2001;December: 267.

4. Padma A. "The head nurse as a clinician, manager and leader: a personal experience". The Indian Journal of Nursing and Midwifery. 1999; September 2(3):27-31.
5. Barbara M Raudonis. "Thinking outside the Box" in Journal of Hospice and Palliative Nursing. 2003;5(3):120-121.
6. Nursing times. Nightingale. 2007;June (3):49-51.
7. TNAI. Nursing in India. Aravali Printers pvt. Limited. New Delhi: 145.
8. The Journal nursing outlook. 2008; July-August:152-156.
9. The Indian Journal of nursing and midwifery 1998. Vol-I, No. 2 Sept 1998.
10. The nursing journal of India health for all by 2004 chapter pp. 3-45.
11. Berger AM and Pattrin L. Advanced Practice Roles for Nurses in tomorrow's health care system. Clinical Nurse Specialist. 1996;10(5):250-2.
12. Ghai S and Ghai CM. History of Nursing in India. Nursing Journal of India. 1997; 28(6):131-132.
13. Hinshaw AS. Nursing Knowledge for the 21st Century; Opportunities and Challenges. Journal of Nursing Scholorship. 2000;(32):117-124.

Web Sources

1. education.portal.com4.currentnursing.com.
2. www.indiannursing council.ac.inl
3. www.karnatakacouncil.ac.in

REVIEW OF SECTION BASED QUESTIONS OF RGUHS

Long Essays

1. a. Explain why nursing is described as a profession.
   b. What is the perspective of nursing profession globally? (May 2011)
   c. Discuss the strategies that would enhance the image of nursing. (May 2011)
2. According to INC what are the strategies to maintain quality assurance.
3. Discuss the role of nurse in improving status and image of nursing. (May 2012)
4. Explain the image of nurses in our society. How can you improve the image of nursing profession. (2003)
5. Discuss the status of image of nursing. (2005, 2007 and May 2009, Nov 2012).
6. a. List the criteria necessary for the profession.
   b. What are the professional organisations of nursing present in India and explain their functions.
7. Explain in detail about ethical issues of ethical decision making process in nursing.
8. Discuss the role of regulatory bodies in nursing profession. (October 2016)

Short Essays

1. Nursing as a profession.
2. Criteria of the profession.
3. Role of regulatory bodies in nursing. (Nov 2012)
4. Collective bargaining.
5. Career opportunities.
6. Professional advancement.
7. Role and scope of nursing education.
8. Future of nursing. (April 2008)
9. Accountability. (2006)
10. Autonomy of nursing. (2003)
11. Assertiveness.
12. Quality of assurance in nursing. (2006, October 2016)
13. Role of INC with regard to nursing education in India.

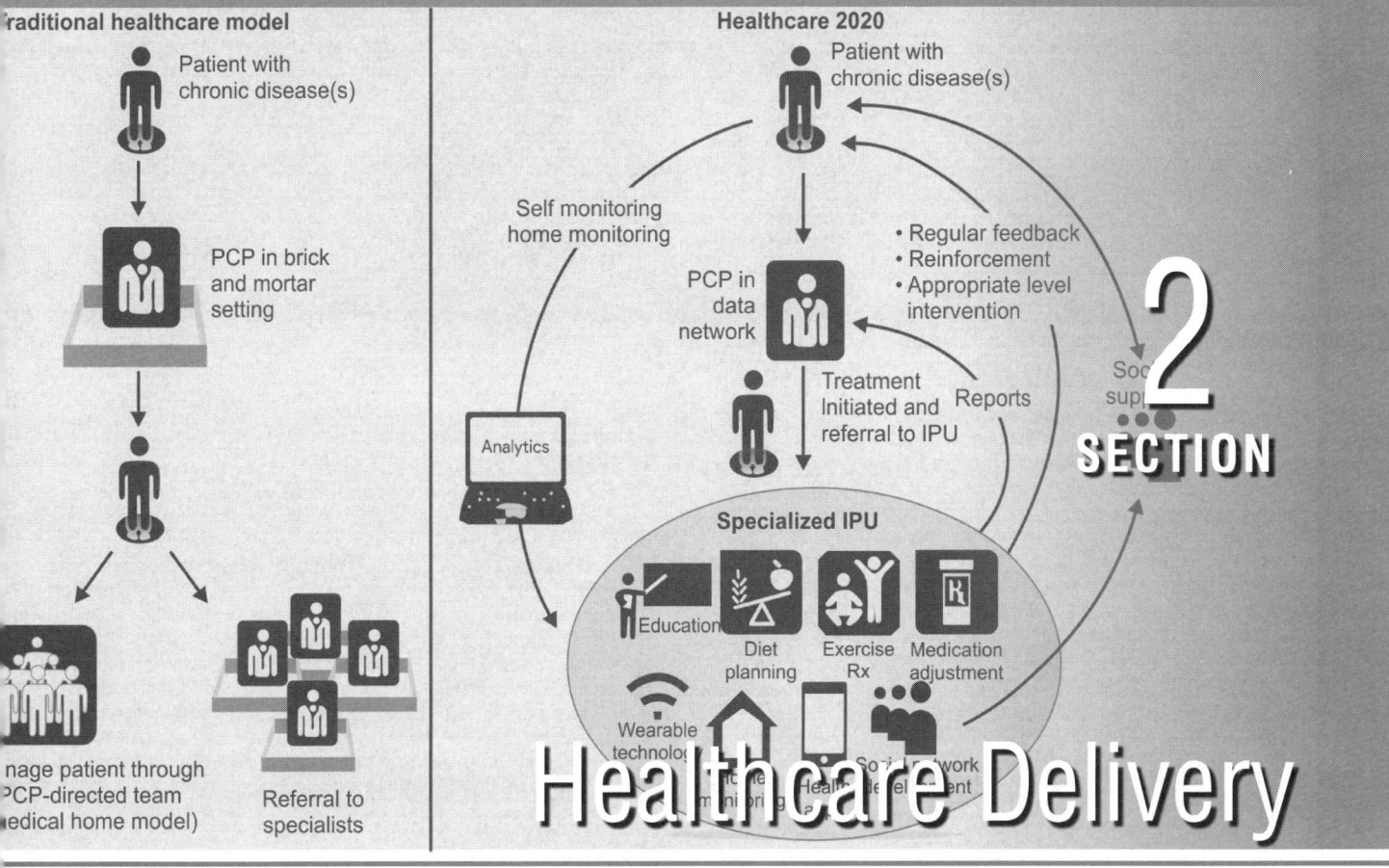

SECTION 2
Healthcare Delivery

Section Outline

12. Healthcare Environment, Economics, Constraints, Planning Process, Policies, Political Process Vis-à-Vis Nursing Profession
13. Healthcare Delivery System in National, State, District and Local Level
14. Major Stakeholders in the Healthcare System: Government, Nongovernment, Industry and Other Professionals
15. Patterns of Nursing Care Delivery in India
16. Healthcare Delivery Concerns, National Health and Family Welfare Programmes—Intersectoral Coordination, Role of Nongovernmental Agencies
17. Information, Education and Communication in Healthcare Delivery
18. Telemedicine/Telenursing

CHAPTER 12

Healthcare Environment, Economics, Constraints, Planning Process, Policies, Political Process Vis-à-Vis Nursing Profession

CHAPTER OUTLINE

- Health for All in the 21st Century
- Definition of Health
- Health Care Environment
  - Nightingale's Approach to Environment Theory
  - Environmental Health Hazards
  - Emerging Environmental Issues
- Environmental Protectional Agency
- Health Economics
  - Economic Indicators of Health Care
- Problems of Resources and Personnel in Health Care Services
- Health Planning Process
- Politics and Policy Making
- Role of Nurse in Politics

INTRODUCTION

Resources are needed to meet the vast health needs of a community. No nation, however, has enough resources to meet all the healthcare needs. Therefore, an assessment of available resources, their allocation and utilization are important considerations for providing efficient healthcare services.

In the democratic system of government, every citizen has political responsibilities because the government is of the people, for the people and by the people. So we shall discuss the various aspects of politics in nursing. Because several constituencies compete for the same resources in the policy arena, the political process is necessary to determine who gets what and how much. The political process is a means by which conflicting demands and desires for the allocation of resources are resolved. In the political system, decisions are made by voting.

HEALTH FOR ALL IN THE 21ST CENTURY

In 1977, the World Health Organization (WHO) had launched the universal goal of "Health for All." Since then Southeast Asian countries are expressing commitment to this goal, adapting primary health center (PHC) as the key approach to achieve "Health for All". The global priority is to maintain the highest attainment of health throughout their life.

DEFINITION OF HEALTH

According to WHO, health is a state of complete physical, mental and social well-being, and not merely an absence of disease or infirmity. The health of an individual is an integrated system within the context of the environment is termed as holistic health.

New Trends Influencing Health in the 21st Century

- ❖ Widespread absolute and relative poverty
- ❖ Epidemiological changes. Continuing high incidence of infectious diseases increased incidence of non-communicable diseases, injuries and violence
- ❖ Global environmental threats to human survival
- ❖ Globalization of trade, travel and the spread of values and ideas
- ❖ Advance in biotechnology
- ❖ New technologies, information and telemedicine services
- ❖ Demographic changes, aging and the growth of cities.

Health Outcomes

By 2005, the health equity indices will be used within and between countries as a basis for promoting and monitoring equity in health. In 2020, all countries through inter-sectoral action will have made major progress in making available safe drinking water, adequate sanitation, food and shelter in sufficient quantity and quality.

New Approaches to Development

In the eighth world conferences, WHO addressed some of the world's pressing problems and set priorities for a new future development agenda for the attainment of health for all as a priority:

- ❖ Development should be centered on human beings

- Central goals of development include the eradication of overt, the fulfillment of the basic needs of all people and the protection of human rights
- Investment in health education and training is critical to the development of human resources
- The improvement of the status of women, including their empowerment central to all efforts to reach sustainable development in all of its economic, social and environmental dimensions
- Diversion of resources away from social priorities should be avoided
- An open and equitable framework for trade investment for the promotion of sustained economy growth
- While the private sector is vital for economic development, government should take an active part in formulating, regulating and monitoring health social and environmental policies.

HEALTH CARE ENVIRONMENT

It refers to the environmental conditions, i.e. biological, chemical, physical and sociological forces in the environment that will affect the individual surroundings which influence on health and well-being of a person, family or community.

Importance of Health Care Environment

- Rising cost, suboptimal quality and a turbulent policy environment are increasing for those seeking high value care
- Maintaining a safe environment that reflects a level of compassion and vigilance for patient welfare is important as any aspect of competent health care. As a result, policy-makers and providers have intensified to understand and change organizational conditions, components and processes of healthcare systems. As they relate to patient safety
- Advise on preventable healthcare events related to patient's safety have major financial consequences to the patient, the provider, the insurer and often the family and caregivers
- Organizational climate.

Nightingale's Approach to Environmental Theory

Florence Nightingale was the first theorist who developed an environmental theory of nursing. Her main focus was the control of the environment of individuals and families, both, healthy or ill. She aimed to provide fresh air, light, warmth, cleanliness, quietness and a proper diet, and proved that manipulation of environment influences on rapid recovery of a client. Some of the individual's environment includes:

i. **Physical environment:** Nightingale viewed physical environment as a major component of nursing care. She identified ventilation and warmth, light, noise, bed and beddings, cleanliness of rooms, walls and nutrition as major areas of environment the nurse could control. When one or more aspects of the environment are out of balance, the client must increase the energy to counteract the environmental stress.

ii. **Psychological environment:** The effect of physical stress may influence the client's emotional climate. Therefore, emphasis is based on providing a variety of activities to keep his or her mind stimulated. Example: Manual work, appealing food and a pleasing physical environment.

iii. **Social environment:** It involves collecting the data relating to illness and disease prevention. It can be promoted by keeping the person's home, hospital room as well as the total community that affects the patient's specific environment.

So Florence Nightingale related the environmental concepts in promoting the maintenance of health care environment if the environment is well maintained which leads to optimal health and if the environment is not appropriately maintained, which delays the client's recovery in disease or illness.

Environmental Health Hazards

The environmental health hazards fall into four categories:

1. **Biological:** In which, disease-producing infectious agents that are capable of entering the human body as viruses, bacteria, etc.
2. **Chemical:** These include toxic agents such as polychlorinated biphenyls (PCBs), asbestos, lead, pesticides, insecticides, herbicides, rodents, industrial waste, emissions from motor vehicles, etc. Study results show that chemicals cause severe chronic health problems, thus leading to serious threat to human health.
3. **Physical:** Natural disasters such as earthquakes, volcanoes, accidents, noise, heat, vibration, radiation, insects, rodents and certain type of equipment fall into the category of physical hazards. Example: Air, temperature and humidity may be adversely affected in industries that use blast furnaces, laundry equipment, etc.
4. **Psychosocial:** Many of the stressors like violence, stress, substance abuse and dependence are known threat to health of individuals, families and communities.

Environmental Influences on Health

- **Air pollution:** The effect of air pollution on the health of individuals depend on the chemical properties of the pollutant and size of particle which, in turn, effects the side of deposition in the respiratory tract; adverse health effects from air pollution may range from mild to excessive. For example, mild irritation of respiratory tract can occur when larger particles are entrapped in the upper respiratory tree. On the other hand, severe respiratory problems and even asphyxiation may occur as a result of direct absorption of a pollutant such as carbon monoxide, from the alveoli into the blood. The risk of developing cancer or a chronic pulmonary disease increases with prolonged exposure to air pollutants.

- **Water pollution:** The most pressing health problems related to water quality involve contamination of waterways with the microbial pathogens found in human body wastes, a problem directly related to lack of faulty sewage disposal facilities. Swimming facilities such as swimming pools, hot tubs and natural bathing areas like lakes, rivers and ponds are sometimes dangerously polluted and disease increases with prolonged exposure to air pollution.
- **Noise pollution:** It can be defined as any unwanted or undesirable sound in the environment. Its effects can range from mildly annoying to psychologically and physically debilitating. The most severe health problem resulting from noise pollution is temporary or permanent hearing loss. It also affects an individual's psychological and physical health because it disrupts communication, sleep, leisure and work activities.
- **Accidents:** Unintentional injuries like those due to falls, drowning and fires kill more than 100,000 people each year and incapacitate millions of others with many lifelong disabilities. Of these, approximately 46,000 deaths are from motor vehicle related injuries.
- **Social hazardous wastes:** Wastes are being generated at an alarming rate. The amount of solid waste continues to soar, partly as a result of today's "Throwaway" attitude where many products are used once and then discarded. In addition to solid wastes, the disposal of hazardous waste is a critical issue.
- **Toxic agents:**
  - *Asbestos:* It has been linked to diseases such as lung and gastrointestinal cancer mesothelioma.
  - *Lead:* Lead biologically interferes with blood formation often resulting in anemia. It can also cause kidney damage, birth defects, injury to the central nervous system, poor memory, hair loss, hypertension, mental retardation, convulsions, coma and death.
  - *Pesticides:* Pesticide residues are contact poisons which tend to accumulate in fatty tissues of living organisms and remain in the body indefinitely.

Emerging Environmental Issues

Major Issues

Major environmental issues which will directly or indirectly affect health have been identified:

- **Population:** There was little change in population growth rates by the year 2000. The estimated world population by the end of century will be 6.3 billion.
- **Food production:** Worldwide food production was projected to increase by 90% between 1970 and 2000. However, the largest increase of food will occur in richer countries and the countries of Middle East. Africa and Southern Asia will continue to have inadequate amount of food for their people.
- **Natural resources:** Nonfuel resources appeared sufficient to meet demands through the year 2000, but discoveries and investments will be needed to maintain reserves.
- **Water:** Shortages will become more, over-pumping of ground water, poor land use practices and pollution of existing water supplies will reduce the availability of water at a time of rising need.
- **Forests:** Loss of forests will continue over the next 20 years.
- **Wild life:** Rates of extinction will increase sharply resulting in loss of hundreds of thousands of species, especially in the tropical forest regions.
- **Pollution:** Increased emissions of carbon dioxide and chlorofluorocarbons in the atmosphere are threatening to alter the world's climate and upper atmosphere significantly by 2050. Acid rain from the burning of fossil fuels is affecting increasingly wilder areas with damage to soil and crops.
- **Global warming:** As a result of increased burning of fossil fuels, deforestation and the production of certain synthetic chemicals, there is dramatic increase in heat trapping gases in the atmosphere. Carbon dioxide is the major offender, allowing energy from the sun to pass through, while absorbing radiation from the earth and creating a planetary hot house.

  NASA (National Aeronautics and Space Administration) has reported that the atmospheric ozone layer, which protects life from harmful ultraviolet radiations, has begun to thin globally. As ozone layer diminishes in the upper atmosphere, the earth receives more ultraviolet radiations, which promotes skin cancers and cataracts, and depresses the human immune system.
- **Acid rain:** Acid rain is caused by emission of sulfur-dioxide and nitrogen oxides. Nitrogen oxide, formed when fuel is burnt at high temperature, principally from motor vehicle exhaust, electric utilities and industrial boilers that burn coal or oil. Once released into the atmosphere, these compounds can be carried to long distances by prevailing winds until they return to the earth as acidic rain, snow, fog or dust. Fish and wildlife suffer harm, lakes are contaminated, buildings and status deteriorate and people experience health problems such as respiratory impairment.

ENVIRONMENTAL PROTECTIONAL AGENCY

Legislation establishing regulations and policy occurs at national level. The environmental protection agency (EPA) is an independent agency formed to coordinate environmental programs related to air and water pollution, solid and hazardous waste management, noise, public water supplies, pesticides and radiation. The agency also administers the municipal sewage treatment construction grant program authorized by congress in the 1972 Clean Water Act.

HEALTH ECONOMICS

Economics represents the study of allocating scarce resources among competing needs. Allocating resources refer to how each good produced is distributed to its consumers. Simply stated, economics becomes the intellectual liaison between nature and technology on the supply side, and the preferences and desires of consumers and overall society on the demand side.

The economics involved with health care is important on both the sides of the supply–demand equation. Economics provides a systematic mechanism to obtain information about the availability, potential and results of healthcare system. Also, economics can be used to trace relationships among the health of the population, the size and productivity of work force, and the demand for healthcare system. Also, economics can be used to trace relationships among the health of the population, the size and productivity of work force, and the demand for health care.

Economic Indicators of Health Care

- **Consumer price index (CPI):** CPI measures the average changes in prices of all types of consumer goods and services purchased by urban wage earners and clerical workers. This index is computed monthly by the Federal Government.
- **Hospital status:** Admissions, cost per inpatient day, length of stay, outpatient visits, occupation rates and staffed beds indicate consumption and cost of consumption for hospital care.
- **National health expenditure:** It includes both public and private expenditures for personal health care, medical research, the construction of medical facilities, program administration, insurance costs and government-sponsored public health programs.
- **Personal consumption expenditure (PCE):** PCE represents private payments for medical care.
- **Personal health care expenditure (PHCE):** It indicates expenditures for consumers whether insured or not. Included are expenses for non-prescribed drugs and medicines, household supplies and other items not covered by insurance.
- **Professional status:**
  Office visits: Indicate the number of office calls consumers make to a physician.
  Physician fee reflects charges for office and other physician visits.

Surgical charges indicate the fee for common surgical procedures and emergency medical procedures.

Economic Concepts in Health Care

The three basic concepts of *supply, demand and cost* are increasingly related in economics.

The **Supply** of health care refers to the amount of resources currently available for delivering health services. Resources include health care facilities, manpower and financing. Supply levels are constantly changing because of technological discoveries, costs for consumers, consumer demands and effect of government regulations.

The **Demand** for health care refers to the amount and type of health care the consumer requires and is willing to purchase (Feldstein, 1983). The demand level revolves around consumer needs and desires, costs of health care, treatment selections ordered by health care providers and general societal needs.

The **Cost** of health care refers to the amount a provider pays to produce health-related goods and services, as well as the amount a consumer pays to purchase these goods and services. Factors influencing the cost of health care are numerous, ranging from consumer demands to advancements in medical technology to the nation's economy.

PROBLEMS OF RESOURCES AND PERSONNEL IN HEALTH CARE SERVICES

Inadequate and Maldistribution of Resources for Health Services

Problems of resources are as follows:
- The developing world lacks human material and financial resources to meet the health needs; in some countries, there is absolute shortage under situation is often complicated by faculty utilization and distribution of resources that exist.
- Scarcity of money affects all parts of the health delivery systems. It first shows itself at the national level, both in rupee allocation of yearly budgets to the various sectors of economy and in the distribution of funds to the authorities responsible for National Development Plan (NDP). One useful index in financial resources per-capita. Health expenditure which is low in all developing countries, lowest in the neediest areas.

The shortage of financial resources affects the larger needier rural population more than the city dwellers. The health sector in India is hospital based, relies on sophisticated technologies and places emphasis on specialized medicine. As a result, it observes an unduly large share of health budget to serve the comparatively small, privileged clients. There is also shortage and maldistribution of human resources. The distribution of professional personnel within developing countries is almost inversely proportional to the distribution of

Table 12.1: Suggested norms for health personnel.

Category of personnel	Norms suggested
Doctors	1 per 3,500 population
Nurses	1 per 5,000 population
Health worker female and male	1 per 5,000 population in plain area, and 3,000 population in tribal and in hilly areas
Accredited Social Health Activist (ASHA)	One for each village (1 per 1,000 population)
Health assistant male and female	1 per 30,000 population in plain area, and 20,000 population in tribal and hilly areas
Health assistant male and female	Provides supportive supervision to six health workers male and female
Pharmacist	1 per 10,000 population
Laboratory technicians	1 per 10,000 population

the people. Outside the main cities and towns there are very few professional health personnel and they work in public, voluntary or mission services.
- Health personnel are also poorly distributed in most of the countries where a large number of professionals are trained. Most educational systems produce professional in accordance neither with countries' needs nor with the expectations of trainees (Table 12.1).

Non-utilization of Actual and Potential Resources
- Despite the shortage of all types of resources, there is underutilization of health services that are already available. The services are differing from culture to culture and situation to situation. In many cases, it reflects such factors as attitudes of health personnel, insufficient awareness of the need for community knowledge and involvement, physical and social inaccessibility, and poor transport.
- People who are often informed about available health services are not clearly aware of the type of health measures offered, and are the reasons for them; if people lack confidence in local health institution, they may ignore it. People who fell sick may go to private hospitals or traditional practitioners in rural and some urban areas, this leads to non utilization of available health facilities of the Government Studies indicate that the factors responsible for underutilization of studies are the consequences of inadequate services quality, failure to meet the communities, expectations, staff arrogance or discrimination, job dissatisfaction, exhausting workload and inappropriate use of staff time.
- Within the communities themselves resources lie and untapped, ignored by today's designers of health services; they include indigenous system for providing health care, traditional birth attendants, midwives, healers and others who are well established, but are unrecognized. The bypassing phenomenon may come into play.

Restricted Use of Primary Health Workers
- One of the major obstacles to the development of health services in rural areas has been the absence of clear thinking about the kind of health personnel needed to provide the necessary services at the village level.
- Offering alternative form of primary health care may rise a new set of problems related to primary health workers, selection and administration. For example, there is generally limited basic education and short period of preparation required, continuing on the spot training and full support of the whole health system.
- Existing health services have not provided training and support nor whole heartedly accepted the concept of utilization of primary health workers, because primary workers often work in remote areas without well-developed communication and transport; hence, it is difficult to ensure that they have the proper equipment and that patients can be easily referred to other levels of care. The remoteness of their posts also make more difficulty to supervise and evaluate their work. Other problems concerned with the use of primary health workers are social. Traditional healers and medicine men may be antagonistic to these workers because they are treating them as a threat to their power and livelihood. Customs and taboos often are against primary health workers' arid problem rising from the traditional division of activities which also complicate the establishment of a new system.
- Although basically they may be willing to stay in the villages, primary health workers may be discouraged by the problems they face and prefer to move to the cities and better paid jobs. If the primary health worker provides wrong treatment and do not refer patients when they should, the system will not function properly.

Rising Cost of Health Services
As the costs of basic commodities, fuel and agricultural products have increased, so did the costs in health care. The increasing cost of living and particularly food has aggravated the health problems of the vulnerable members of society and limited the ability of individuals and governments to pay for health services to few people. Low cost programmer should be promoted using less expensive primary health care personnel to reach large peoples of the community.

PROBLEMS OF THE GENERAL STRUCTURE OF HEALTH SERVICES

Lack of Effective Planning Machinery
The biggest weakness of many health planning endeavors is the lack of an overall health policy to guide them, lack of political will to provide resources necessary for implementation and lack of an effective executive

structure to complement the decisions; often planning is frequently focused on health services and not on meeting health needs. Many health administrations do not have competent planners or good planning systems, and the plans formulated are unrealistic and not cost-effective. The national planners and decision-makers concentrate their attention on economic development and health sector is neglected.

Weak Development of the "Total Systems" Concept

Health care delivery system, public and private, national and international, curative and preventive, peripheral, intermediate and central must be considered as a whole. In the health services, there is over centralization or authority and executive responsibility, which prevents effective and adequate delivery of health services at the periphery. It tends to lead to an over concentration of personnel, institutions and facilities, and so the maldistribution of resources. Central authorities became too far from the people and lost touch with community needs. Present system of reporting does not convey to the center the full picture of requirements. There is no proper integration of specialized programmers. The private health sector dominates.

Technical Weakness

Inadequate Health Education

High morbidity and high mortality, particularly among infants and children, are index not only of a community's low health level but also of inadequate health education. A great number of diseases could be prevented with little or no medical intervention. If people were adequately informed about them and if they were encouraged to take the necessary precautions in time:

- ❖ Health education is particularly needed where the network of services is weak, the people must learn to protect themselves from diseases and to seek help if they need it.
- ❖ Efforts in health education have often been limited to giving information dogmatically. The pattern of existing resources—economic, human and cultural—has been forgotten, and thus too has contributed to health educations' failure.
- ❖ A nucleus of health education specialist may be necessary to plan and guide health information activities in a country. Human resources, the teachers, agricultural extension workers, community development agents and depending on the culture, religious leaders, youth groups, traditional healers, can be used in education of the public, specially who are illiterates. Health education can make major contribution by giving people the self-repeat desired from the knowledge that they can prevent diseases, and thus change the course of their life by their own efforts.

Lack of Basic Sanitation

- ❖ The quality of basic sanitation in most developing countries is below the level considered necessity for the prevention and control of communicable diseases and the promotion and maintenance of physical, mental and social well-being, basic sanitation should aim at safe water a safe environment, uncontaminated food and a decent place to live.
- ❖ The development of sanitation measure should be linked with economic and social development and community action. A major problem is the lack of competent infrastructure to carry out a comprehensive range of functions effectively.
- ❖ As per WHO survey in 1970, more than 85% of the rural population had no safe drinking water available to them; furthermore, many of the piped urban supplies functioned only.
- ❖ The provision of basic sanitation for rural populations is a long-term undertaking on a vast scale. Quality standards and control are traditionally the responsibility of the Minister of Health. A multi-sectoral approach and close cooperation between government minister's department is also needed.

Deficiencies of Communication and Transport

Health service systems cannot operate adequately without proper communication among their various elements, including the primary health workers. In India, most of the problems in the delivery of health services to rural areas are the consequence of poor transport and communications. They include insufficient supervision or the staff, lack of consultation and referral facilities, inadequate supplies of drugs and other health requirement, feelings of isolation and neglect among the staff, and shortage information about needs.

Modern transport is not easily adopted to use in the developing world. Cost of operation is high in proportion to the country's limited resources, technical understanding is often lacking at central government level and the skills to operate complicated machinery may be in short supply.

Lack of Adequate Health Information

Statistical services fail to provide public health administrators with the information they need for sound decision in asking. If national system is to solve the real problems of communities, a reform of objectives and methods of data collection is required thoughtfully and intelligently planned, and periodic sample surveys or reporting may often be more useful information at lower cost. Information services should react according to the priorities of the health system and should be aimed strictly at problem solving.

Improper Utilization of Health Care Services by Community

- Government has provided the health services to all the sectors of the family, but the people are ignorant in utilization of health services because the negative replication on health team may be the inhibiting factor. This may be due to unwarranted behaviors from some of the non-professional people involved in the health care delivery system. For example, dais and other voluntary health workers though being untrained acting similar to quakes.
- The people may not have interest to go to hospital when they are sick because of wrong ideas about the health system
- The referral system by the health personnel may not be appropriate
- Lack of accessibility of health services at the needy homes of the people
- Community may not be satisfied with the services due to lack of some supplies and equipment, lack of health professional, etc.
- The lack of transport facility in the community
- Communication gap between the health personnel and the people of community
- Because of improper health education and counseling may lead to improper utilization of health services
- Attitudes of health professional may not be good towards the people
- Unawareness of the people about the health services, which are available
- Proper follow-up may not be there by the health personnel.

HEALTH PLANNING PROCESS

Planning is a process of analyzing and understanding a system, formulating its goals and objectives, assessing its capabilities, designing alternative courses of action or plans for the purposes of achieving these goals and objectives, evaluating the effectiveness of these plans, choosing the preferred plan, initiating the necessary action for its implementation and monitoring the system to ensure the implementation of the plan and its desired effect on the system.

Health planning: It is an orderly process of defining community health problems, identifying correct needs and surveying the resources to meet them, establishing priority goals that are realistic and feasible, and projecting administrative action to accomplish the purpose of the proposed program.

Characteristics of Planning

- Planning is essential for the entire job. Planning leads to more effective and rapid achievement because everyone involved is clear about what is to be done, how, when and why.
- Good planning should focus on the purpose, i.e. every program including health programs have their own purpose or objectives, e.g. reproductive and child health (RCH) programs.
- Although planning is a continuous process, there should be a provision for flexibility to some extent according to changes due to event or situation.
- Planning should not be based on high ideals and be blind to social and political conditions in the environment.
- Planning of health programmers must be precise in its objectives, scope and the nature.
- Planning should be documented because it serves as a blueprint for implementation.

Steps of Planning Process

- Analysis of the health situation
- Establishment of objectives and goals
- Assessment of resources
- Fixing priorities
- Write up the formulated plan
- Programming and implementation
- Monitoring
- Evaluation.

Planning process as follows (Fig. 12.1).

Analysis of Health Situation

It involves the collection, assessment and interpretation of information which provides a clear picture of health situation. The minimum requirements of data include:
- The population, its age and sex, statistics of mortality and morbidity
- The epidemiology and geographical distribution of different diseases

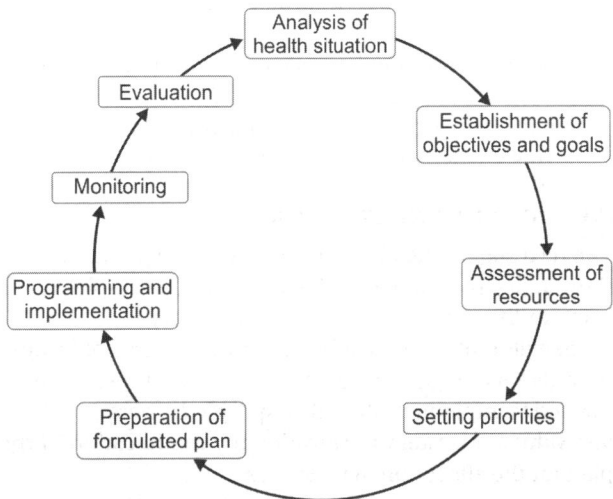

Fig. 12.1: Planning cycle.

- Medical care facilities such as hospitals, health centers, public and private agencies
- The man power of various categories
- Drawing facilities available
- Attitude and beliefs of populations towards disease, its cure and prevention.

The above data helps to analyze and interpret health problems, the health needs and health demands of the population.

Establishment of Objectives and Goals

For any program, planning the objectives are the key step to success. General objectives are established at top level. As it goes to lower level, specific objectives are set, and objectives or goals may be short-term or long-term. In setting objectives, time and resources are important factors to be considered. Objectives are not only a guide to action but also a yardstick to measure work after it is done. Modern management techniques are directed towards cost–benefit analysis and input–output study of health services.

Assessment of Resources

The resources imply the terms that include man power, money, materials skills, knowledge and techniques needed or available for the implementation of health programs. While planning resources, one should look into what is available and what is required.

Setting Priorities

Once the resources and objectives are determined, the next important step is to establish priorities and planning based on its importance. While setting priorities, attention is to be paid to financial constraints, mortality/morbidity rate, disease which can be prevented at low cost, saving the lives of younger people when there has been considerable social investment, and also political and community interests and pressures.

Example: Combined measles rubella vaccine program introduced in Karnataka in February 2017.

Once the priorities are done, alternate plans for achieving greater effectiveness are to be chosen.

Preparation of Formulated Plan

The next step in the planning process is the preparation of the detailed plan or plans. The plan must be complete in all ways for the execution of a program/project.

Skeleton of plan must be prepared in terms of inputs/outputs each stage of the plan is defined, and cost and time needed to implement should be specified. There should be an evaluation system to consider any modification of the plan for the allocation of resources.

Programming and Implementation

Once the plan has been selected and approved by the policy-making authorities, programming and implementation follow. Plan execution depends upon the effective organization of existence facilities organization must involve good organizational structure; specified procedures to delegate the authority with responsibility of different wishes for achieving the pre-determined objectives within the planned period.

Many consequences must be forecasted while implementation, including delays in critical supplies, inappropriate use of staff and similar factors. The implementation stage also makes important considerations, i.e.:
- Definition of roles and tasks
- The selection, training, motivation and supervision of the man power involved
- Organization and communication
- The deficiency of individual institutions such as hospitals and health centers.

Monitoring

Supervision and monitoring is the day-to-day follow-up activities during their implementation to ensure that they are proceeding as planned and according to schedule. Monitoring is a continuous process observing, recording and reporting on the activities of the project. Monitoring thus consists of keeping track of the course of activities and identifying deviations and taking corrective action if excessive deviations occur.

Evaluation

The purpose of evaluation is to assess the achievement of the stated objectives of a program, its adequacy and its acceptance by all people involved. While monitoring is day to day or ongoing operations evaluation is mostly concerned with the final outcome. Good planning will have well-built evaluation to measure the performance, output and cost effectiveness achieved.

POLITICS AND POLICY MAKING

Definitions

- Politics is the science or art of government.
- Politics is the business of conducting the affairs of the staff setting public policy and implementing laws that affect the lives of the citizens. **—Hamilton**
- Politics refers to the activities used by groups to exert control over their common affairs. **—Berger J Karen**
- A boycott is an organized refusal to deal with a person or organization to achieve certain goals. When consumers boycott a gasoline retailer because of price increases, their message is delivered clearly and effectively.

History of Politics

Historically, nurses' involvement in politics has been limited. Although individual nurses, e.g. Florence Nightingale used her contacts with powerful men in the government to obtain supplies and the personnel she needed to care

Health man-power in rural India as on March 2017.

Category	In position
1. Auxiliary nurse midwife at sub-center and primary health center	220,707
2. Multipurpose workers (male)	56,263
3. Health assistant (female)/lady health visitor	14,267
4. Health assistant (male)	12,288
5. Nursing staff at primary health center and community health center	70,738
6. Doctors in primary health centers	27,124
7. General duty of medical officers allopathic at community health center	14,350
8. Specialists:	
a. Surgeon	758
b. Gynecologist and obstetrician	1,463
c. Physician	864
d. Pediatrician	1,071
Total specialists at community health center	4,156
9. Radiographer	2,129
10. Pharmacist	25,193
11. Lab technician	18,952
12. Block extension educator (BEE)	3,517

Source: Park Textbook of Preventive and Social Medicine, 18th Ed.

for wounded soldiers in the Crimea (Woodham-Smith, 1983). Hannah Ropes was able to fight incompetence and obtain decent care for wounded Civil War soldiers because she understood who were the influential people in Washington and who would be receptive to her efforts, on behalf of the wounded soldiers. Also Lillian Wald and Margaret Sanger have influenced decision-making in areas such as sanitation, nutrition and birth control. Yet, nurses have accomplished less as a group. The recent women's movement, however, has inspired nurses to address health care issues. In addition, as more college-educated people enter the profession, they bring to nursing the activism and involvement of the university campuses.

In 1974, the American Nurses Association (ANA) formed the Nurses Coalition in Politics (N-CAP), which was the first Political Action Committee (PAC) for nurses. This organization, which was later renamed ANA-PAC, is a major PAC that is sought for support for candidates seeking federal offices (Mason 1990). Nurses' involvement in politics is receiving greater emphasis in nursing curricula, professional organizations and health care settings (Stanhope, Belcher, 1982). Professional nursing organizations have employed lobbyists to urge state legislatures and the United States (US) congress to improve the quality of health care.

Political Influence on Public Policy

Nursing agenda for health care reform is an example of public stand that demonstrates the professional values of health care for all. With active support, the role of profession and credibility increases. To gain respect of health care colleagues, legislators and the public, nurses must back their words with actions; this means communicating with legislators. Seeking positions in policy-making boards and managed care provider panels and engaging in informed dialog with consumers and other health care providers.

Political Favors

Political favors are given by individuals and groups when they contribute to campaign funds volunteer to work in campaigns or vote for candidates for public office. Requesting returns on favors previously given is a common and effective way of influencing policy-makers. Another highly visible and effective way of influencing policy-makers is through a boycott or the threat of a boycott.

Components of Political Action

Political action means getting involved in the process of change; such involvement is most effective when nurses use Vance (1985) calls the three **Cs** of political action.
- Communication that is assertive, dear and concise
- Collectivity a source of power and the foundation for networking, coalition-building and collaboration
- Collegiality, a sense of community, sisterhood and camaraderie, the foundation for building esteem and trust, and supporting and nurturing associates.

Nurses can use communication, collectivity and collegiality to take political action. To do so, they must become informed, vote, communicate with elected representatives and contribute time, money and effort.

Become Informed

Listen to daily news and in-depth reports of public radio and television stations—read news magazines and news sections of professional journals. Seek out special reports of such non-partisan groups as the League of Women Voters and common cause or partisan groups such as the Republican and Democratic Party. As a member of ANA, subscribe to capital update, a legislative newsletter published by the ANA. Learn the names and addresses of the elected representatives by calling a public, library or local newspaper. Learn how a bill becomes law. Obtain copies of proposed state laws by asking for them by number from state printing offices. Obtain proposed federal laws from US Senate Documents Office, Washington.

Vote

The most fundamental political action citizens can take is to vote. Nurses may feel they are too poor to contribute money, too busy to work for candidates or too involved to serve on boards and committees. However, nurses everywhere can be informed and vote.

Communicate with Representatives

Elected officials represent the people of their district or state. They seek input from, pay attention to and vote in accordance with the wishes of their constituents. The people who make their opinions known influence the outcome of issues and send long, rambling essays.

Contribute Time, Money and Effort

Political action takes time, money and effort. Besides telephoning, writing letters and sending telegrams, nurses can work on the campaigns of candidates and referendums, testify at public hearings, contribute money, serve on voluntary boards and commissions, seek appointment to positions of authority that will influence health policy and practice, and run for public office. By doing so, nurses provide pertinent facts that represent the viewpoint of nursing and increase its prestige and viability.

Political Focus

In the Community

Nurses can become politically active in their communities in countless ways from serving on school lunch committees to becoming mayors or cities. Because they are articulate, intelligent, highly motivated and energetic people, nurses are natural leaders. They can pursue their interest and make a difference in every areas of life in health care facilities, prisons, area of infant and aged care highway safety, and air quality in self-help groups and food, apply their knowledge of power and politics, and work for a more healthy society.

In Professional Organization

Professional nursing organizations are developed to advancing the profession and influencing health care. They exercise collective power by presenting a united voice for nursing. Individual nurses can participate in the activities of these groups in numerous ways at many levels. Professional advisory capacities to governmental agencies by supporting public and private initiatives. PACs are agencies devoted to advancing the interests of groups. Because not-for-profit organizations, such as the ANA, are prohibited by law from engaging in political action, they use PAC to carry out their agendas.

In the Work Place

Nursing is hard work. It requires enormous amounts of energy. Not much is left over for political action in the workplace. However, if nurses leave decisions about client care to others, others will make the decisions. If nurses are to exert power, they must become involved. By applying the interpersonal skills of political action (communication, collectivity, collegiality), nurses can affect change in the workplace. Here are some specific strategies:

- ❖ Volunteer to be a member of standing committees that make policy recommendations
- ❖ Use both the formal and informal information network of the agency to influence others. Many health care providers have an in-house newsletter or official communication system. All agencies have an informal communication network. Remember people who control information and hold power
- ❖ Use employee representatives if the agency has a collective-bargaining organization
- ❖ Pursue endeavors that earn respect and recognition, such as research and nursing excellence
- ❖ Seek position of authority. By serving in administrative positions, nurses gain the power to make decisions and to access others who hold power.

Political Strategies

While politics is the art or science of government, political strategies are tactics people use to influence governmental decisions. With energy and commitment, nurses can affect change by using the following strategies:

- ❖ Develop a sense of self and the ability to communicate effectively
- ❖ Seek position that gives you authority to grant rewards and mete out punishment
- ❖ Become expert in an area of interest, earn degrees and gain special skills
- ❖ Form coalitions with powerful persons of like mind
- ❖ Avoid people with sullied reputations
- ❖ Control information either by giving or withholding it
- ❖ Do your homework; learn all you can to out an issue you wish to change
- ❖ Be ready to move on issues; "Strike while the iron is hot"
- ❖ Compromise, if necessary; "Half a loaf is better than none"
- ❖ Display confidence; "Nothing ventured, nothing gained"
- ❖ Be prepared to give something in return; "qid pro quo"
- ❖ Be patient; "Rome was not built in a day"
- ❖ Watch for any change or weakening of position; "Get your foot in the door"
- ❖ Become sensitive to hidden agendas; "Read between the lines"
- ❖ Refrain from commitments that limit maneuverability of influence
- ❖ Try to understand another position; "Walk a mile in the other person's moccasins"
- ❖ Do not be discouraged by setbacks; "Look at the big picture"
- ❖ Gain collective power by joining the ANA and other nurse's groups.

Restriction on Political Activities

In an effort to prevent unfair political influence, the US Congress passed the Hatch Act in the 1930s. It prohibits employees of tax-supported agencies from engaging in activities on the behalf of a political party or in support of legislation that could be construed as support from a government agency. The act does not interfere with the right of private citizens to support parties, candidates or ballot measures. However, employees must be careful to speak and act only as private citizens, not as agency representatives. Because many have their own versions of the Hatch Act, nurses should learn about restrictions in their state.

Relationship Between Women, Power and Politics

In our culture, power and politics are associated with masculinity. Until recently, women have been socialized to be non-competitive, meek, compliant, passive and subservient and to shun power. In this view, authority and power are the birthright of men; compliance, the lot of women. In fact, in most world cultures today, men are the rulers and spiritual leaders. In general, women take over the reign of government only when family inheritance outweighs sexual bias and efforts to produce male heir fail. Small changes are being made, but women have a long way to go before they gain a significant share of the positions of power.

Because 88% of nurses in the United States are women (NLN Datasource, 1993), it is no surprise that nurses have difficulty assuming power or using power in the political arena. Many women nurses feel angry and sad, but powerless to change the system. Many nurses still think of power as anti-feminine, inappropriate and unprofessional. They view powerful nurses with suspicion and fear. This point of view is self-defeating and demeaning. Nurses have superior intellectual and organizational abilities. Moreover, they are nurturers and caregivers, committed to high ethical standards. What better group is there to lead the nation in areas of public policy and action? Nurses need not shun power, but embrace it. They need to apply their knowledge of power and politics to their personal, professional and public lives to bring about constructive change.

ROLE OF NURSE IN POLITICS

Nurses as Political Participants

Political involvement is an essential part of every nurse's professional role. Lobbying is an important way for a nurse to express professional values and identity.

Professional Organizations as Special Interest Groups

Nurses may belong to one or more professional organizations, each of which represents a specific constituency within the registered nurse community. The ANA in the Unites States and the Canadian Nurses Association (CAN) in Canada are the organizations with the largest membership. They are the "official" organizations or nursing practice. The ANA has a political action committee, ANA-PAC, which endorses candidates who have exhibited voting records and demonstrated leadership consistent with the ANA's political agenda.

Collaborating Through Nursing Coalitions

In an effort to resolve some of the intra-professional conflicts, leaders of the major nursing associations have formed the in-council composed of leaders from the ANA, the National League for Nursing (NLN), the Association of Nursing Executives (AONE) and the American Association of Colleges of Nursing (AACN); the Tri-Council meets regularly to discuss issues important to nursing practice.

In addition, representatives from various nursing specialty organizations such as the Association of Operating Room Nurses (AORN), the Association of Women's Health, Obstetric and Neonatal Nurses (AWHONN), and the American Association of Critical-Care Nurses (AACN) have likewise joined forces as the National Federation for Specialty Nursing Organizations so that they can better address issues relating to nurses who practice within a specialty area. It is clear that if nursing associations present a united front, their ideas will carry more weight.

Individual nurses have the responsibility to join those professional associations that are relevant to their particular area of practice. Any organization is only as strong as its membership. If nurses want their professional associations to have an impact on public policy, they must support them and participate in their activities.

Barriers of Collaboration

Coalitions are born out of political expedience and necessity because no two organizations or associations share similar views on political conflict and dispute.

Collaboration may be possible on some issues, but is probably impossible on all issues. It is critical that collaborators, either individual or associations identify which issues have potential for joint action.

If there are issues on which consensus cannot be reached, they may be acknowledged as areas in which individual errors may be more appropriate. Often, individuals or groups agree not to issue public policy statements on matters of concern to other coalition members during the time period the coalition is working toward a common policy direction on a more pressing issue.

Nurses and Electoral Process

Individual nurses may become involved directly in the electoral process in several ways. Many nurses begin active involvement by working for candidates who are seeking local state or national office. Involvement may be in the form of financial contribution to campaigns or more active grass roots involvement such as volunteering at campaign headquarters publicly supporting a candidate's position or sponsoring a political debate among candidates. Some elected officials attribute a substantial part of their campaign successes to nurses.

More and more nurses are seeking direct involvement in politics. The ultimate level of involvement for a nurse is to successfully seek election to local, state or federal office. Shirley Girouard, a nurse turned politician, credited much of the success of her campaign to a well-organized staff composed entirely of nurses. After winning a seat in the New Hampshire House 01 representative, she found that her expert knowledge as a nurse served her well and that she quickly became an effective and valued member of the legislature. Other nurses have had equally positive experiences as legislators at all levels of government.

Applying Power and Politics to Managing Nursing Care

The delivery of nursing services occurs at many levels in health care institutions/organizations. The effectiveness of care delivery is linked to the application of power and politics. For the staff nurse, the politics of bedside care involves influencing the allocation of scarce resources (e.g. equipment, supplies, time or personnel) for the delivery of nursing care. To maintain access to the resources needed for patient care, nurses must connect to the whole organization and beyond, not just their own unit. Staff nurses can use their power and the political skills of artful negotiation, collaboration and networking to obtain the necessary resources to provide care. Speaking on behalf of patient care, access and quality are what drives the politics of nursing care.

The politics of nursing care calls for an action plan, not just a care plan. Using power often means moving from being a passive observer to an active player. It means responding in politically shrewd ways by influencing and drafting policies rather than solely abiding by them.

To respond effectively to the limits placed on clinical nursing practice, nurses must speak out about the "things nurses do," physical assessment, patient education, primary care, home and hospice care, and other health-related activities. Besides being directly involved with policy-makers, nurses can hold grassroots organizational meetings to prepare new policy initiatives or changes. Another strategy is to identify a group of nurses to write letters to the editor of local newspaper or hospital paper explaining the impact the new policy will have on nursing. What happens in the workplace depends on the influences happening in the larger community, professional organizations and the government. The effective nurse manager understands the connections among these groups and uses them to the advantage of nursing patients and the health care organization.

CONCLUSION

Health care environment plays an important role in maintenance of safety, working environment in an organization and to promote health of the client, families and community. A good health economics will promote adequate planning of resources in health system. Nurses should have a political knowledge and policies for good administration of healthcare system.

CHAPTER 13

Healthcare Delivery System in National, State, District and Local Level

CHAPTER OUTLINE

- History of Healthcare System
- Healthcare Delivery System in India
- Organization and Administration of Health Services in India at Central Level
- State Level Ministry of Health and Family Welfare Services
- Organization of Health Service at District Level
- Organizational Chart of Primary Health Center

INTRODUCTION

Health is a fundamental right of every human being irrespective of race or creed. Health system is defined or intended to delivery of health services. The aim of a healthy system is health development of the population. Currently, the goal of the health system is to achieve "Health for All" by the year 2000 as per National Health Policy.

DEFINITIONS

Healthcare

Health care is defined as a multitude of services rendered to individuals and communities by the agents of the health services or profession for promoting, maintaining, monitoring or restoring health.

Healthcare Services

The purpose of health care services is to improve the health status of the population. Its goal is to reduce the mortality and morbidity rate, increase the expectation of life, decrease in population growth rate, improvements in nutritional status, provision of basic sanitation, health man power requirements and resources development, and contain other parameters such as food production, dietary note, reduced levels of poverty, etc.

Healthcare Delivery

Health care delivery is defined as activities designed to produce or restore the health of individual, families, groups and communities.

Healthcare Delivery System

It refers to the totality of resources that a population or society distributes in the organization and delivery of health population services. It also includes all personal and public services performed by individuals or institutions for the purpose of maintaining or restoring health (Stanhope, 2001).

HISTORY OF HEALTHCARE SYSTEM

Early History

The history of health in India goes back through the centuries to about 300 BC. The experiences and concern in health development date back to Vedic period between 300 and 1,400 BC. The excavations in the Indus Valley Civilization (e.g. Mohenjodaro and Harappa) planned cities with drainage, house and public baths built suggesting the practices of environment sanitation (300 BC). Actually this was followed by Dravidians, who lived at that time. After the invasion of Aryans, the Dravidian migrated to South. In 200 BC, Siddha system came into existence. The Manu Samhita prescribed rules and regulations for personal hygiene, food, spiritual and mental aspects of life. The system of hospital was developed during the Rahul Sankrityan period. The Arabic system of medicine known as Unani system was introduced in health services.

Pre-independence Era

- ❖ By the middle of the 18th century, the British had established their rule in India, which lasted till 1947
- ❖ A Royal Commission was appointed to investigate the causes of unsatisfactory condition of health in the British Army in 1859. In this period, they pointed out the need for the protection of water supply, construction of drainage and prevention of epidemics among British Army
- ❖ In 1864, sanitary commissioners were appointed in the three major provinces, i.e. Bombay, Madras and Bengal
- ❖ In 1880, the Vaccination Act was passed

- In 1896, a severe epidemic of plague occurred in India and Plague Commission was appointed
- In 1909, the Central Malaria Bureau was founded at Kasauli
- During 1920–1921, Municipality and Local Board Acts containing legal provisions for the advancement of public health were passed
- In 1930, the All India Institute of Hygiene and Public Health Calcutta was established with aids from Rockefeller Foundation. The Child Marriage Restraint Act (Sarda Act) came into effect
- In 1931, A Maternity and Child Welfare Bureau was established under the Indian Red Cross Society
- In 1939, the first Rural Health Training center was established at Singur, near Calcutta. In 1940, the Drug Act was passed and drugs were brought under the control for the first time
- In 1943, the Health Survey and Development Committee (Bhore Committee) was appointed by the Government of India to survey the existing position of health in India and to make recommendations for the future development. The committee recommended a short-term and a long-term program for the attainment of reasonable health services based on concept of modern health practice.

Components of Health System

- Concepts, e.g. health and disease
- Ideas, e.g. equity coverage, effectiveness, efficiency and impact
- Objects, e.g. hospitals, health centers and health programs
- Persons, e.g. providers and consumers.

Philosophy of Healthcare Delivery System

- Everyone from birth to death is part of the market potential for health care services
- The consumer of healthcare services is a client and not customer
- Consumers are less informed about health services than anything else they purchase
- Healthcare system is unique because it is not a competitive market
- Restricted entry into the health care system.

Goals/Objectives of Healthcare Delivery System

- To improve the health status of population and the clinical outcomes of care
- To improve the experience of care of patients' families and communities
- To reduce the total economic burden of care and illness
- To improve social justice equity in the health status of the population.

Principles of Healthcare Delivery System

- Supports a coordinated, cohesive health care delivery system
- Opposes the concept of fee-for-practice
- Supports the concept of prepaid group practice
- Supports the establishment of community-based, community-controlled health care system
- Urges an emphasis be placed on development of primary care
- Emphasizes on quality assurance of the care
- Supports health care as basic human right for all people
- Opposes the accrual of profits by health-care-related industries
- Supports individuals' unrestricted access to the provider, clinic or hospital
- Urges that in the establishment of priorities for health care funding, resource be allocated to maintain services for the economically deprived
- Supports efforts to eliminate unnecessary health care expenditures and voluntary efforts to limit increase in health care costs
- Endorses to provide old-age people with special health maintenance
- Supports public and private funding
- Condemns health care fraud
- Supports the establishment of a national health care budget
- Supports universal health insurance.

Functions of Healthcare Delivery System

- To provide health services
- To raise and pool the resources accessible to pay for health care
- To generate human and physical sources that make the delivery service possible
- To set and enforce rules of the game and provide strategic direction for all the different players involved.

Characters of Healthcare Delivery System

- Orientation toward health
- Population perspective
- Intensive use of information
- Focus on consumer
- Knowledge of treatment outcome
- Constrained resources
- Coordination of resources
- Reconsideration of human values
- Expectations of accountability
- Growing interdependence.

Financing

There are generally 5 primary methods of funding health care systems:
1. Direct or out-of-pocket payment
2. General taxation
3. Social health insurance
4. Voluntary aid and donation
5. Government funding.

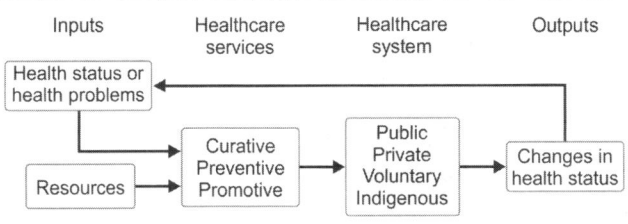

Fig. 13.1: Model of health care system.

Healthcare System Models (Fig. 13.1)

Many countries follow different healthcare models. As healthcare system is the organization of people, institutions and resources that deliver healthcare services to meet the health needs of population. There is a wide variety of health systems around the world. Implicitly, nations must design and develop health systems in accordance with their needs and resources, although common elements in virtually all health systems are primary healthcare and public health measures. The healthcare models helps to reduce the cost and effective utilization of services by the population, alternative models of healthcare delivery provide healthcare services that are reasonably inexpensive, and have the basic essentials required by rural population. The above Fig. 13.1 shows the organization of health care system or model of services catered in India.

HEALTHCARE DELIVERY SYSTEM IN INDIA (FIG. 13.1)

- Public health sector:
  - Primary health care:
    - Primary Health Centers (PHCs)
    - Sub-centers
  - Hospitals/health centers:
    - Community Health Centers (CHCs)
    - Rural hospitals
    - District hospital
    - Teaching hospital
  - Health insurance schemes:
    - Employees State Insurance (ESI)
    - Central government health scheme
  - Other agencies:
    - Defense services
    - Railways
- Private sector:
  - Private hospitals, polyclinics and nursing homes
  - General practitioners and clinics
- *Indigenous system of medicine:* Ayurveda, Siddha, Unani and Homeopathy
- Voluntary health agencies
- National health programs.

Organization and Administration of Health Services in India at Central Level (Fig. 13.2)

India is a union of 28 states and 9 union territories. Under the constitution of India, the states are largely independent in matters relating to the delivery of health care to the people. Each state, therefore, has developed its own system of health care delivery independent of the central government. The central responsibility consists mainly of policy-making, planning, guiding, assisting, evaluating and coordinating the work of the state health ministries, so that health services cover every part of the country and no state lags behind for want of these services.

The health system in India has three main links: central, state and local or peripheral.

The official organs of the health system at the national level consist of three units:
1. Union Ministry of Health and Family Welfare
2. The Directorate General of Health Services (DGHS)
3. The Central Council of Health and Family Welfare.

Union Ministry of Health and Family Welfare

Organization:

The Union Ministry of Health and Family Welfare is headed by a Cabinet Minister, a Minister of State and a Deputy Health Minister. These are political appointments and have dual role to serve political as well as administrative responsibilities for health.

Currently, the Union Health Ministry has the following departments:
- Department of Health
- Department of Family Welfare
- Department of Indian System of Medicine and Homoeopathy.

Department of Health

It is headed by a Secretary to the Government of India as its executive head, assisted by joint secretaries, deputy secretaries and a large administrative staff.

The Department of Health deals with planning, coordination, programming, evaluation of medical and public health matters, including drug control and prevention of food adulteration.

Functions

The functions of the Union Health Ministry are set out in the seventh schedule of the Article 246 of the Constitution of India under union list and concurrent list.

Union list:
- International health relations and administration of post-quarantine
- Administration of central institutes such as the All India Institute of Hygiene and Public Health
- Promotion of research through research centers and other bodies
- Regulation and development of medical, pharmaceuticals, dental and nursing professions
- Establishment and maintenance of drug standards
- Census, and collection and publication of other statistical data
- Immigration and emigration

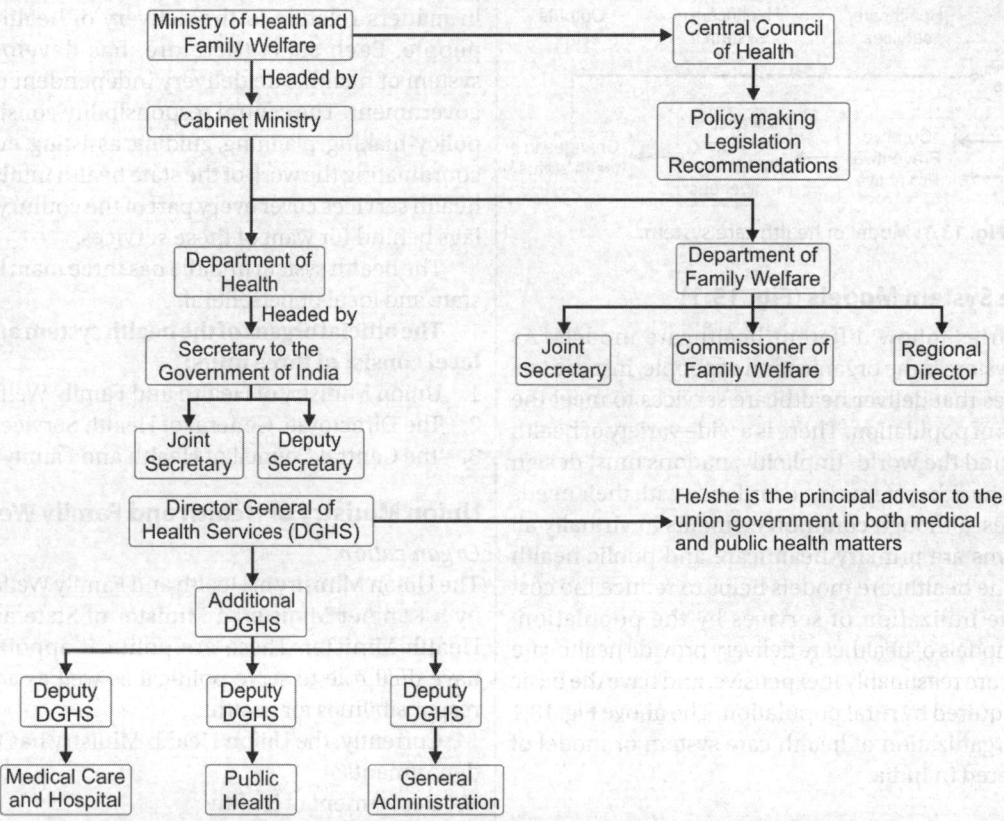

Fig. 13.2: Organization and administration of health services in India at central level.

- Regulation of labor in the working of mines and oil fields
- Coordination with states and other ministries for promotion of health.

Concurrent list: The concurrent list is the responsibility of both the union and state government. The concurrent list includes:

- Prevention of communicable disease from one unit to another
- Prevention of adulteration of foodstuffs
- Control of drugs and poisons
- Vital statistics
- Labor welfare
- Economic and social planning
- Population control and family planning.

Department of Family Welfare (Fig. 13.3)

It was created in 1966 within the Ministry of Health and Family Welfare. The Secretary to the Government of India in the Ministry of Health and Family Welfare is in overall charge of the Department of Family Welfare. He is assisted by an additional secretary and commissioner, and one joint secretary.

The following divisions are functioning in the Department of Family Welfare:

- Program appraisal and special scheme
- Technical operations: Looks after all components of the technical program, namely sterilization/intrauterine device (IUD)/nirodh, post-partum, maternal and child health (MCH), UPI, etc.
- Evaluation and intelligence: Helps in planning, monitoring and evaluating the program performance and coordinates demographic research
- Nirodh marketing supply/distribution
- Transport
- Universal immunization program
- Area project
- Mass education and media: Responsible for providing educational publicity and extent support to education.

Functions:

- To organize family welfare program through family welfare centers
- To create an atmosphere of social acceptance of the program and to support all voluntary organizations interested in the program
- To educate every individual to develop a conviction that a small family size is valuable and to popularize appropriate and acceptable method of family planning
- To disseminate the knowledge on the practice of family planning as widely as possible and to provide service agencies nearest to the community

Chapter 13: Healthcare Delivery System in National, State, District and Local Level

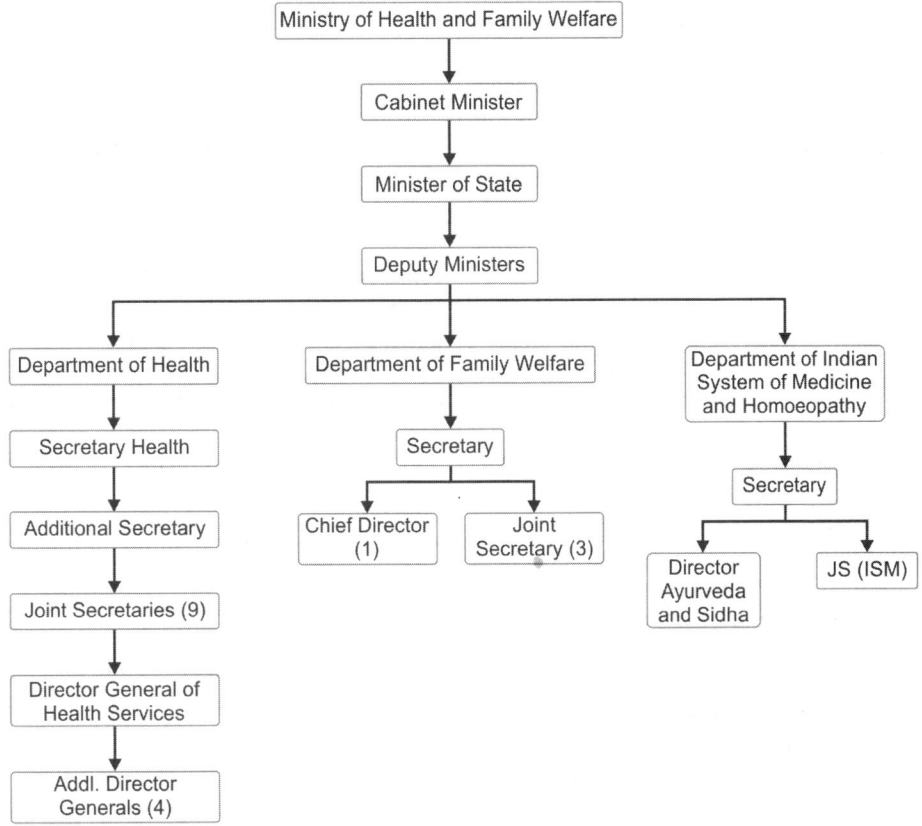

Fig. 13.3: Organization of Ministry of Health and Family welfare services.

- To organize basic research of human fertility, genetics and population dynamics, and the evolution of easy and reliable method of contraception
- To study the social factors that affect fertility and to take such steps that will reduce the number of children in a family
- To coordinate the family planning program with the child welfare and maternal health services throughout the country
- To organize production of contraceptive device in adequate quantities to maintain the supply at all levels at a minimum cost
- Indian system of medicine (ISM) and homeopathy helps to promote ISM in the country through training, research and use.

The Department of Indian System of Medicine and Homeopathy

- It was established in March 1995 and had continued to make steady progress. Emphasis was on implementation of the various schemes introduced such as education, standardization of drugs, enhancement of availability of raw materials, research and development, information, education and communication, and involvement of ISM and homeopathy in national health care.
- Most of the functions of this ministry are implemented through an autonomous organization called DGHS.

Directorate General of Health Services

Organization

The DGHS is the principal adviser to the Union Government in both medical and public health matters. He is assisted by a team of deputies and a large administrative staff. The Directorate comprises of three main units:

i. Medical care and hospitals
ii. Public health
iii. General administration.

Functions

- **General functions:** The general functions are surveys, planning, coordination, programming and appraisal of all health matters in the country.
- **Specific functions**
  - **International health relations and quarantine:** All the major ports in the country and international airports are directly controlled by the Director General of Health Services. All matters relating to the obtaining of assistance from international agencies and the coordination of their activities in the country are undertaken by the Director General of Health Services.
  - **Control of drug standards:** The drugs control organization is a part of the DGHS and is headed by the Drugs Controller. Its primary function is to

lay down and enforce standards and control the manufacture and distribution of drugs through both Central and State Government offices. The Drugs Act (1940) vests the central government with the powers to test quality of imported drugs.
- **Postgraduate training:** The DGHS is responsible for the administration of national institutions, which also provide postgraduate training to different categories of health personnel.
    - All India Institute of Hygiene and Public Health, Kolkata
    - All India Institute of Mental Health, Bengaluru
    - National Institute of Communicable Diseases, Delhi, etc.
- **Medical education:** The DGHS is directly in charge of the following medical colleges in India:
    - Lady Hardinge
    - Maulana Azad
    - Medical colleges at Puducherry and Goa

    Besides these, there are many medical colleges in the country which are guided and supported by the Center.
- **Medical research:** Medical research in the country is organized largely through the Indian Council of Medical Research (ICMR), founded in 1911 in New Delhi. The council plays a significant role in aiding, promoting and coordinating scientific research on human diseases, their causation, prevention and cure. The research work is done through the councils, and several permanent research institutes, e.g. Cancer Research Centre, TB Chemotherapy Centre at Chennai, etc. The funds of the council are wholly derived from the budget of the Union Ministry of Health.
- **National health programs:** The various national health programs for the eradication of malaria and for the control of tuberculosis, filaria, leprosy, AIDS and other communicable diseases involve expenditure of crores of rupees. The central directorate plays a very important part in planning, guiding and coordinating all the national health programs in the country.
- **Central health education bureau:** An outstanding activity of this Bureau is the preparation of education material for creating health awareness among the people. The bureau offers training courses in health education in different categories of health workers.
- **Health intelligence:** The Central Bureau of Health Intelligence was established in 1961 to centralize collection, compilation, analysis, evaluation and dissemination of all information on health statistics for the nation as a whole. It disseminates epidemic intelligence to states and international bodies.
- **National medical library:** The Central Medical Library of DGHS was declared the National Medical Library in 1966. The aim is to help in the advancement of medical, health and related sciences by collection, dissemination and exchange of information.

Central Council of Health

The Central Council of Health was set up by a Presidential Order on August 9, 1952, under Article 263 of the Constitution of India for promoting coordinated and concerted action between the center and the states in the implementation of all the programs and measures pertaining to the health of the nation. The Union Health Minister is the chairman and the state health ministers are the members.

Functions:
- To consider and recommend broad outlines of policy in regard to matters concerning health in all its aspects such as the provision of remedial and preventive care, environmental hygiene, nutrition, health education and the promotion of facilities for training and research.
- To make proposals for legislation in fields of activity related to medical and public health matters and to lay down the pattern of development for the country as a whole.
- To make recommendations to the Central Government regarding distribution of available grants-in-aid for health purposes to the states and to review periodically the work accomplished in different areas through the utilization of these grants-in-aid.
- To establish any organization or organizations invested with appropriate functions for promoting and maintaining cooperation between the central and state health administrations.

State Level Ministry of Health and Family Welfare Services

Historically, the first milestone in the state health administration was the year 1919, when the states (provinces) obtained autonomy, under the Montague-Chelmsford reforms, from the central government in matters of public health. By 1921–1922, all the states had created some form of public health organizations. The Government of India Act, 1935 gave further autonomy to the states. The state is the ultimate authority responsible for health services operating within its jurisdiction.

State Health Administration (Fig. 13.4)

At present, there are 28 states in India, with each state having its own health administration. In all the states, the management sector comprises the State Ministry of Health and a Directorate of Health.
- **State Ministry of Health:** The State Ministry of Health is headed by a Minister of Health and Family Welfare,

Chapter 13: Healthcare Delivery System in National, State, District and Local Level

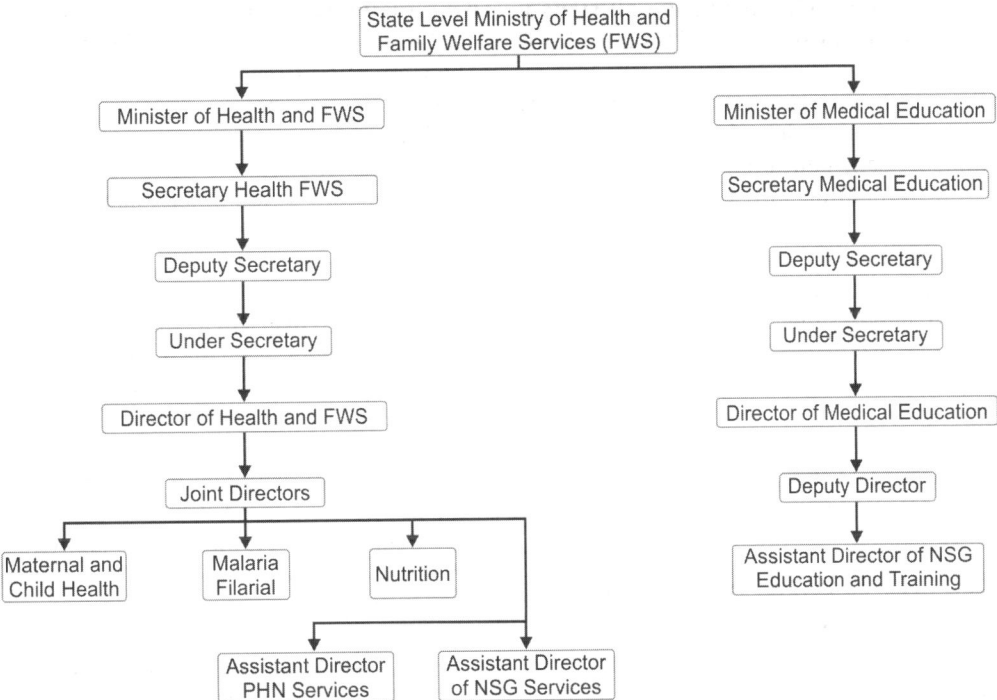

Fig. 13.4: Organization of State level Ministry of health and family welfare services.

and a Deputy Minister of Health and Family Welfare. In some states, the Health Minister is also in charge of other portfolios. The Health Secretariat is the official organ of the State Ministry of Health and is headed by a Secretary who is assisted by Deputy Secretaries and a large administrative staff.

Functions:
- Health services provided at the state level
- Rural Health Services through minimum needs program
- Medical development program
- MCH, family welfare and immunization program
- National Malaria Immunization Program (NMIP) and National Filaria Control Program (NFCP)
- National Leprosy Eradication Program (NLEP), National Tobacco Control Program (NTCP), National Program for Control of Blindness (NPCB), prevention and control of communicable diseases like diarrheal disease, Kyasanur Forest disease (KFD), Japanese encephalitis (JE), etc.
- Integrated Child Development Services, Anemia Control Programme, Iodine Deficiency Control Programme, etc.
- Laboratory services and vaccine production units
- Health education and training program, curative services, national AIDS control program.

❖ **State Health Directorate:** The Director of Health Services (DHS) is the chief technical adviser to the state government on all matters relating to medicine and public health. He is also responsible for the organization and direction of all health activities. With the advent of family planning as an important program, the designation of DHS has been changed in some states and is now known as Director of Health and Family Welfare. The Director of Health and Family Welfare is assisted by a suitable number of deputies and assistants. The Deputy and Assistant Directors of Health may be of two types:

i. The **regional directors** inspect all the branches of public health within their jurisdiction, irrespective of their specialty.
ii. The **functional directors** are usually specialists in a particular branch of public health such as mother and child health, family planning, nutrition, tuberculosis, leprosy, health education, etc.

Functions:
- Providing and planning curative and preventive services
- Promotion of health services
- Recruitment of health personnel
- Supervision of PHCs
- Prevention and outbreak of communicable diseases
- Planning and survey in relation to health.

Responsibilities:
The responsibilities of the state health directorate are as follows:
- It studies in depth the health problem needs in the state and plans schemes to solve them
- Providing curative and prevention services
- Provision for control of milk and food sanitation

- Takes total responsibility for taking all steps in the prevention of any outbreak of communicable diseases
- Establishment and maintenance of central laboratories for preparation of vaccines
- Promotion of health education
- Collection, tabulation and publication of vital statistics
- Promotion of health programs such as school health, family planning, occupational health, MCH
- Recruitment of personnel for all health services
- Supervision of PHCs
- Planning and carrying out surveys in relation to nutrition
- Establishment of training courses
- Coordination of all health services with other ministries of the state.

ORGANIZATION OF HEALTH SERVICE AT DISTRICT LEVEL (FIG. 13.5)

The district is the most crucial level in the administration and implementation of medical/health services. At the district level, there is a district medical and health officer or chief medical officer (CMO) who is overall responsible for the administration of medical/health services in the entire district.

Bhore Committee (1946) recommended integrated services at all levels and the setting up of a unified health authority in each district. The principal unit of administration in India is the district under a collector. There are 619 districts in India. Each district has six types of administration areas.
 i. Subdivisions
 ii. Tehsils (talukas)
 iii. Community development blocks
 iv. Municipalities and corporations
 v. Villages
 vi. Panchayats

Most of the districts in India are divided into two or more subdivisions, each in charge of an assistant collector or sub-collector. Each division is again divided into tehsils in charge of a Tehsildar. A tehsil usually comprises between 200 and 600 villages.

Since the launching of the community development program in India in 1952, the rural areas of the district have been organized into blocks known as **community development blocks**. The block is a unit of rural planning and development and comprises approximately 100 villages and about 80,000–120,000 population in charge of a block development officer (Fig. 13.6).

Finally, there are the village panchayats, which are institutions of rural local self-government.

The urban areas of the district are organized into the following local self-government:
- Town area committee: 5,000–10,000
- Municipal boards: 10,000–200,000
- Corporations: Population above 200,000

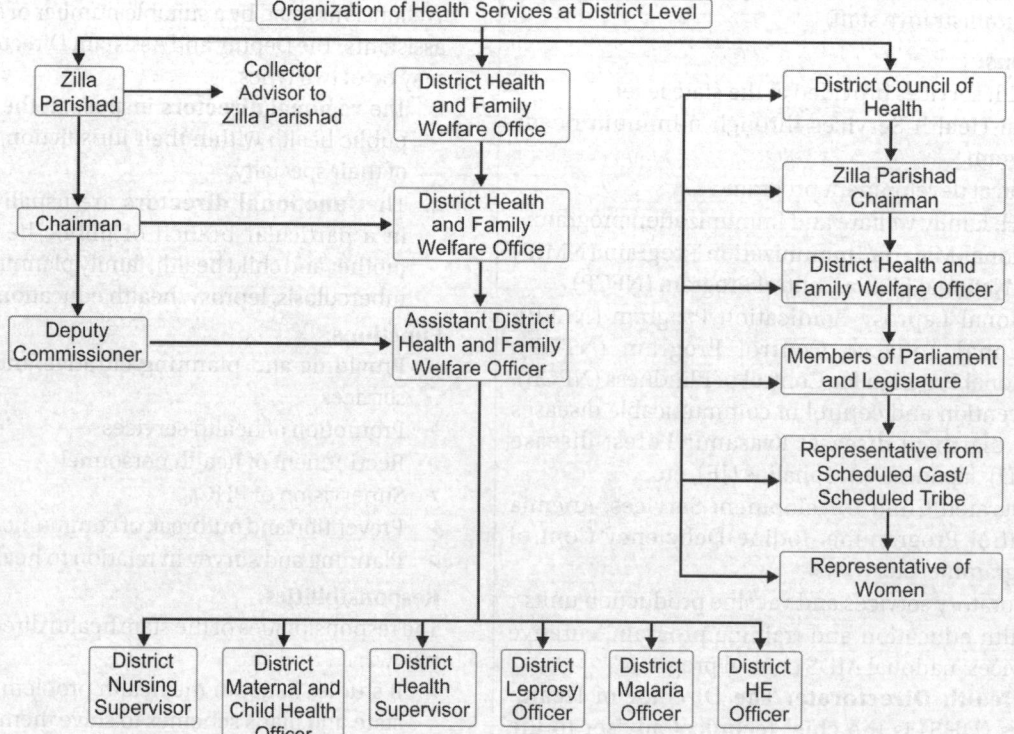

Fig. 13.5: Organization of health services at district level.

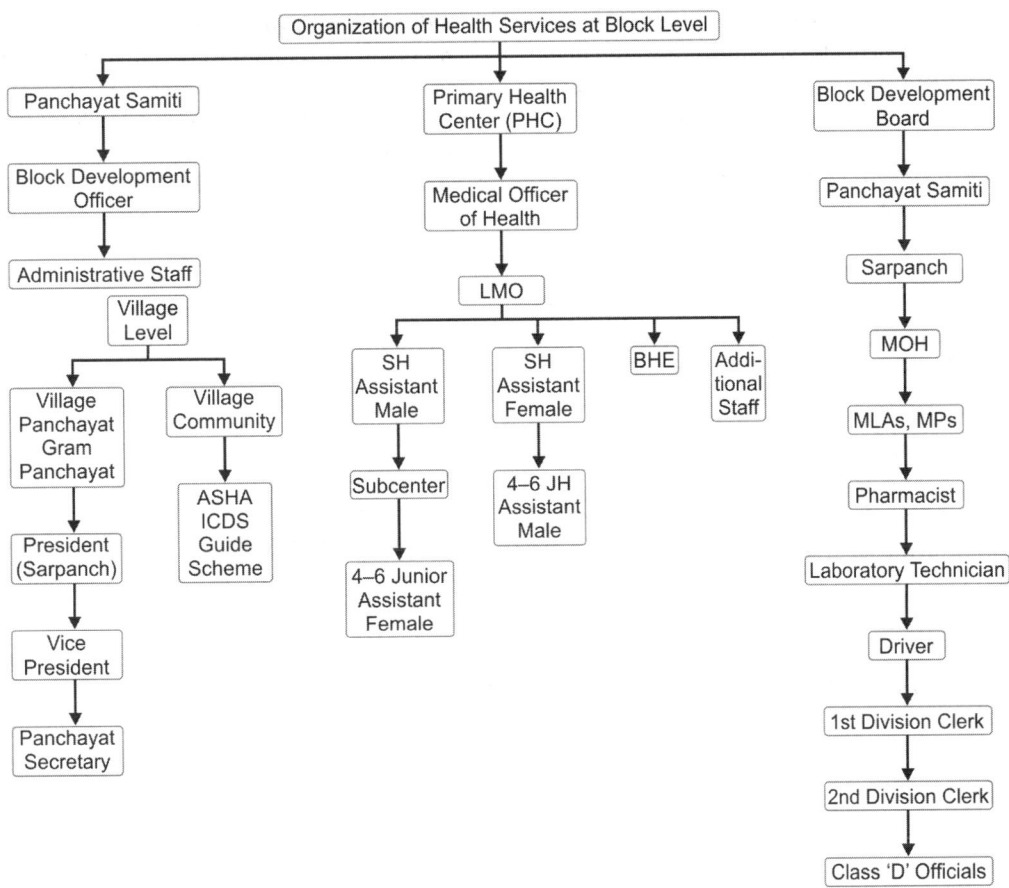

Fig. 13.6: Organization of health services at block level.
(LMO: Lady Medical Officer; MOH: Medical Officer of Health)

The **towns area committees** are like panchayats. They provide sanitary services.

The **municipal boards** are headed by a chairman/president, elected usually by the members. The term of a municipal board ranges between 3 and 5 years. The functions of a municipal board are construction and maintenance of roads, sanitation, drainage, street lighting, water supply, maintenance of hospitals and dispensaries, education, registration of births, deaths, etc.

Corporations are headed by Mayors. The councilors are elected from different wards of the city. The executive agency includes the commissioner, the secretary, the engineer and the health officer. The activities are similar to those of the municipalities but on a much wider scale.

District Level Organization

- District Medical Officer (DMO)
- Joint Director of Health Services (JDHS)
- District Health Officer (DHO)
- Joint Director of Rural Health Services (JDRHS)
- District Family Welfare Officer
- Joint Director of Family Welfare Services (JDFWS)

According to Alma Ata declaration (1978), "Health for All" can be achieved only through PHCs. The district level organization is as follows:

- Zilla Parishad (planning and policy-making)
- District Health and Family Welfare Office (implementation)
- District Council of Health (supervision, evaluation and monitoring)

Zilla Parishad

Zilla Parishad is the planning and policy-making body in district level. It has the following members:

- District heads of all departments and ex-officers in DHO
- All members of parliament and legislation in the district
- All chairman of block
- Representatives of scheduled caste, tribes and women
- The collector is designated as advisor to the Zilla Parishad

District Health and Family Welfare Offices

District Health and Family Welfare Department deals with the implementation of health programs at the district level.

Organization: The District Health and Family Welfare Offices are in charge of all health administration and health programs implemented in the district. He is assisted by Assistant District Health and Family Welfare Officer.

District Council of Health Organization

It is the monitoring, evaluating or supervisory body. Here, the members consist of:
- District Health and Family Welfare (DHFW) officer
- All members of parliament and legislature in the district
- All chairmen or block supports and representatives of scheduled caste (SC) and scheduled tribe (ST).

Rural Health Services

The government of India in 1977, launched a scheme known as Rural Health Service on the principle of planning people's health in people's hand. It is a three-tier system of health care delivery in rural areas:
1. Village level
2. PHC
3. Sub-center level.

Village level: The following schemes are available at village health scheme:

- *Village health guides scheme:* A village health guide is a person with an aptitude for society and service and is not a full-time government functionary. Their works are supervised by community health nurse (CHN) and health assistant.
- *Accredited Social Health Activist (ASHA)*: They play vital role in providing domiciliary, midwifery services in rural areas.
- *Anganwadi workers:* Under the Integrated Child Development Services (ICDS) scheme, one anganwadi worker for a population of 1,000. She will be selected from the community she lives. The services rendered by her are as follows:
  - Health education
  - Immunization
  - Supplementary nutrition
  - Health education
  - Non-formal preschool education and referral services.

Primary health center (PHC) (Fig. 13.7): PHC is the first contract point between village, community and the medical officer. PHC acts as a referral for six sub-centers.

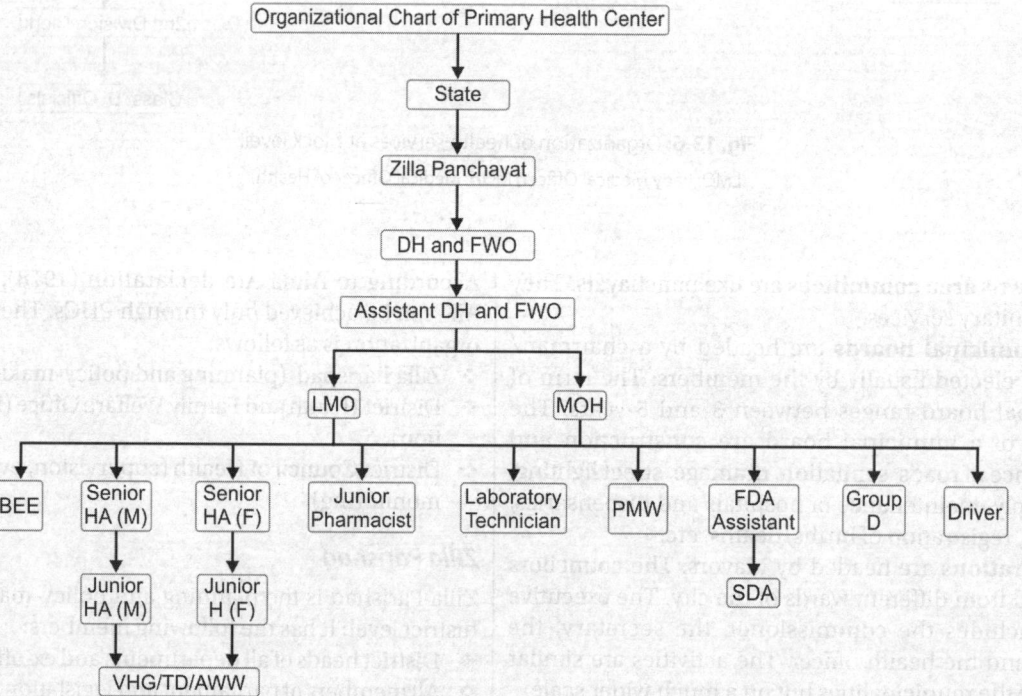

Fig. 13.7: Organizational chart of primary health center (PHC).

(AWW: anganwadi worker; Assistant DH and FWO: Assistant District Health and Family Welfare Officer; BEE: block extension educator; DH and FWO: District Health and Family Welfare Officer; HA: Health Assistant; LMO: Lady Medical Officer; TD: trained dai; MOH: Medical Officer of Health; VHG: Village Health Guide/Community Health Volunteer)

Organizational chart of primary health center:
- ❖ Functions of PHC
  - ➢ Medical care
  - ➢ MCH and family planning
  - ➢ Safe water supply and basic sanitation
  - ➢ Prevention and control of locally endemic disease
  - ➢ Collection and reporting of vital statistics
  - ➢ Health education
  - ➢ National health programs
  - ➢ Referral services
  - ➢ Education, training and research
  - ➢ Basic laboratory services.
- ❖ Staffing Pattern of PHC
  - ➢ Medical Officer—1
  - ➢ Pharmacist—1
  - ➢ Nurse midwife—1
  - ➢ Health worker (female)/auxiliary nurse midwife (ANM)—1
  - ➢ Health educator—1
  - ➢ Health assistant (male)—1
  - ➢ Health assistant (female)/lady health visitor (LHV)—1
  - ➢ Upper division clerk—1
  - ➢ Lower division clerk—1
  - ➢ Laboratory technician—1
  - ➢ Driver—1
  - ➢ Class IV workers—4

Sub-center Level (Fig. 13.8): The sub-center is the peripheral output of the existing health delivery system in rural areas, on the basis of one sub-center for every population. The work of the sub-center is supervised by male and female health assistants.

Staffing pattern of sub-centers are as follows:
- ❖ Health worker (female) ANM—1
- ❖ Health worker (male)—1
- ❖ Voluntary worker (pay 150 pm as honorarium)—1

Community Health Centers

CHCs were established by upgrading the PHCs. Each CHC corners a population of 80,000–1.20 lakhs. It serves as a referral center for four PHCs.

Staffing pattern of CHC level:
- ❖ Medical officer—4
- ❖ Nurse midwives—7
- ❖ Dresser—1
- ❖ Pharmacist—1
- ❖ Laboratory technician—1
- ❖ Radiographer—1

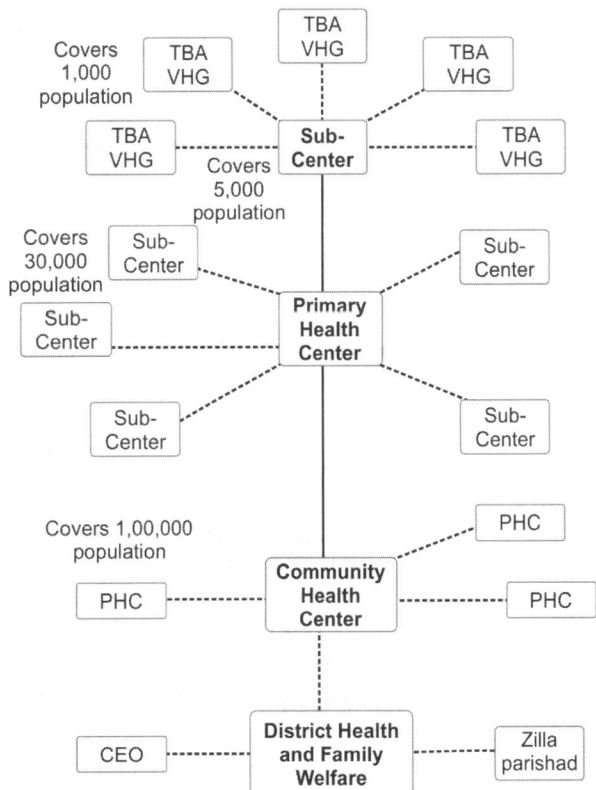

Fig. 13.8: Infrasructure of primary health care at district level.
(TBA: trained birth attendants; VHG: village health guides [Accredited Social Health Activist (ASHA) workers])

- ❖ Ward boys—2
- ❖ Dhobi—1
- ❖ Mali—1
- ❖ Sweepers—3
- ❖ Chowkidar—1
- ❖ Aya—1
- ❖ Peon—1

Hospital: Apart from the PHCs, the present organization of health services of the government sector consists of:
- ❖ Rural hospital
- ❖ District hospital
- ❖ Specialist hospital
- ❖ Teaching hospital.

The current opinion is that the hospital should not remain an Ivory Tower of Disease in the community, but should take an active part in providing health services to the community.

It is not to upgrade the rural dispensaries to PHCs and district hospital to district hospital center.

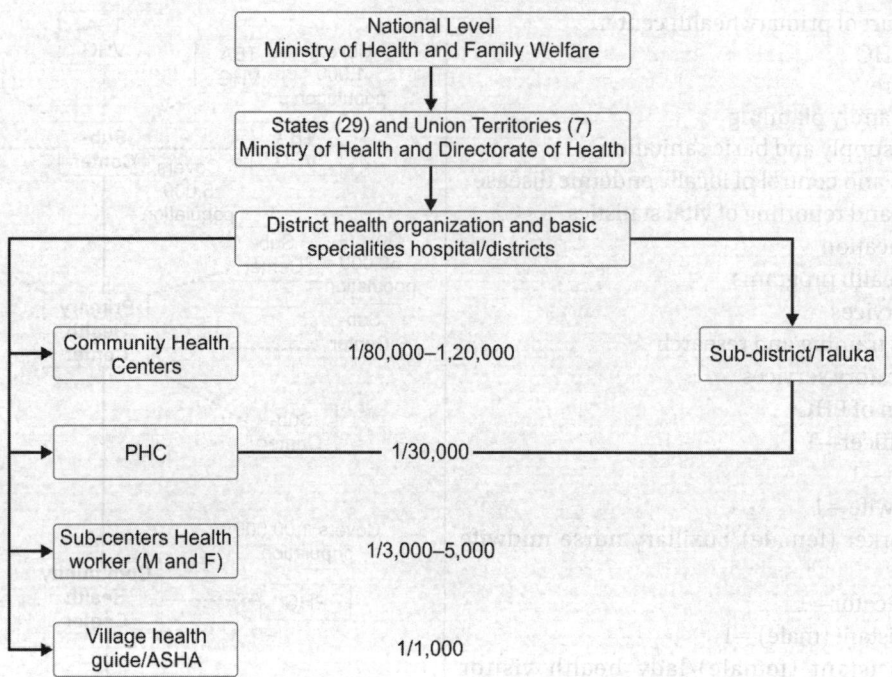

Fig. 13.9: Synoptic view of distribution of population with different healthcare services in India.

CONCLUSION

A health service system includes all formal and informal activities centered on the provision of health services for a given population and the utilization of such services by the population. Thus, health services can be described as permanent country wide system established institutions. The multipurpose objective of which is to cope with the various health needs and demands of population, and thereby provide health care to individuals and the community including preventive and curative activities and utilizing, to an extent, multipurpose health workers, resting traditionally on a three-tier hierarchy of central intermediate and peripheral levels.

14 Major Stakeholders in the Healthcare System: Government, Nongovernment, Industry and Other Professionals

CHAPTER

CHAPTER OUTLINE

- Stakeholders in Healthcare System
- Employee State Insurance Scheme
- Other Agencies
- Voluntary Health Agencies
- National Health Programs in India

INTRODUCTION

Stakeholder encompasses a wide sector of society; they include consumer or patients, community healthcare professionals, hospital healthcare professionals, pharmacists, nongovernmental organizations, suppliers, etc.

Stakeholder is a person, group, organization or system who affects and can be affected by an organizational action.

STAKEHOLDERS IN HEALTHCARE SYSTEM

- Government
- Public
- Providers
- Hospital administrator and governing boards
- Non-governmental organizations

Government

The role of government in the administration of healthcare cannot be overestimated. Many federal government healthcare efforts are headed by a cabinet-level officer, the secretary for health and human services, who runs the department of health and human services. The federal government makes budget and other planning related to expenditure in healthcare. As the major payer, the federal government has been active in regulating the healthcare industry.

Therefore, hospitals have great incentive to comply with regulations promulgated by the federal government, because they can be fined or decertified as a provider of care to medicare clients, if they do not. Noncompliance can result in the loss of lot of money and income for the hospital. Government regulation is frequently opposed by the healthcare industry because it often affects the healthcare practitioners' autonomy.

Public

The public has a stake in healthcare from several perspectives. As consumers of healthcare services or as patients, the public is concerned with quality, cost and access to care. Many people believe that healthcare is a right and should be universally available to all citizens, regardless of the cost. Paradoxically, however, most do not want to pay these costs. Patients want compassion as well as skill with clear communication.

They expect an employer to offer a wide variety of option for health coverage that can be customized to their specific needs. They also look for the employers to fund the majority of cost of health insurance. Overall, public values regarding healthcare are changing. People are interested in receiving quality care at a reasonable cost. In addition, the public has a more positive view of health promotion and illness prevention than in the past. Healthcare resources remain focused on illness, however, with only 1% of healthcare expenditures going to public health.

Providers

- Community healthcare professional
- Hospital healthcare professional.

Community Healthcare Professional

A community healthcare professional may be a public are highly skilled, in professions that usually require extensive knowledge including higher qualification in the field of community health care and acts as community health expert working for the common good of the society.

Hospital Healthcare Professional

i. **Physicians:** The role of physicians in the healthcare system is an important one. Physicians provide direct medical services to clients in a variety of settings, including offices, clinics, hospitals and freestanding centers. In addition, physicians control 60–70% of hospital costs through their decisions regarding the use of resources. Physicians decide which client to admit, where to admit, the length of stay, the ancillary services, whether to perform surgery, when to initiate and to discontinue treatment regimens and which medications to prescribe.

ii. **Nurses:** Nurse is an individual who provides care to clients. The extent of participation varies from simple patient care tasks to the most expert professional technique necessary in acute life-threatening situations. The ability of nurse to function independently and making self-directed judgment will depend on his/her professional development. Nurses provide a unique perspective on the healthcare system. The greatest impact and the most frequently discussed aspect of nursing has been the recurring shortage of nurses.

iii. **Pharmacists:** The roles of the pharmacist are changing. Some can now prescribe as well as dispense medicine. They are more interested in meeting the requirements of pharmaceutical industry.

Hospital Administrators and Governing Boards

The Chief Executive, Chief Financial Officer, Chief Nursing Officer and governing boards of hospitals strongly influence healthcare delivery in their institutions. In addition, most hospitals are members of some association, which represents the industries' efforts to influence legislation, regulation, judicial decisions and health policy (Table 14.1).

Table 14.1: Indicators of health.

Targets (2012–2017)	Achievements
Reduce IMR to 25/1000 live births	IMR reduced from 42 in 2012 to 39 in 2014
Reduce MMR to 1/1000 live births	IMR has reduced in 1.67 in 2011–2013
Reduce TFR to 2.0	TFR has reduced to 2.3 in 2014
Reduce annual incidence and mortality from tuberculosis by half	Tuberculosis incidence is at 167 per lakh population and mortality at 17 per lakh population in 2015
Reduce prevalence of leprosy to <1/10,000 population and incidence to 0 in all districts	Leprosy prevalence rate is <1/10,000 population
Annual malaria incidence to be <1/1,000	Annual malaria incidence is <1/1,000
Less than 1% microfilaria prevalence in all districts	Out of 225 endemic districts, 222 have reported microfilaria rate of less than 1%
Kala-azar elimination by 2015, <1 case per 10,000 population in all blocks	Out of 611 block PHCs, 454 have reported <1 case per 10,000

Source: Parks Textbook of Preventive and Social Medicine, 24th ed.

Nongovernmental Stakeholders

The voluntary agencies occupy an important place in community healthcare system. These organizations directly or indirectly act as stakeholder. These organizations are administered by autonomous boards, which hold meetings, collect funds from private sources and spend money for providing health services and health education to individual, family and community. There are many NGOs in India, which serves to society. Some of these organizations are given below.

❖ *Indian Red Cross Society:* Indian Red Cross Society was established in 1920 and has over 400 branches all over India. It has been executing programs for the prevention of diseases and promotion of health. Its activities are:
  ➢ Relief work
  ➢ Milk and medical supplies
  ➢ Armed forces
  ➢ Maternal and child welfare services
  ➢ Family planning
  ➢ Blood bank and first aid

❖ *Hind Kusht Nivaran Sangh:* It was founded in 1950 with its headquarters in New Delhi. Its precursor was the Indian Council of British Empire Leprosy Relief Association (BELRA), which was renamed as LEPRA in 1950. The programed work of the Sangh include rendering of financial assistance to various leprosy homes and clinics, health education, training of medical worker and physiotherapists conducting research and field investigation. The Sangh has branches all over India and works in close cooperation with the government and other voluntary agencies.

❖ *Indian Council for Child Welfare:* It was established in 1952. It is affiliated with international union for child welfare. The services of Indian Council for Child Welfare (ICCW) are devoted to secure for Indian children those opportunities and facilities, by law and other means, which are necessary to enable them to develop physically, mentally, morally, spiritually and socially in a healthy and normal manner and in conditions of freedom and dignity.

❖ *Tuberculosis Association of India:* Tuberculosis Association of India was formed in 1939. It has branches in all states of India. The activities of this association comprise of organizing tuberculosis (TB) campaign every year to raise funds, training of doctors, health visitors and social workers in anti-TB work, and promotion of health education conferences.

❖ *Bharat Sevak Samaj:* The Bharat Sevak Samaj (BSS), which is a non-political and non-official organization, was formed in 1952. One of the prime objectives of the Bharat Sevak is to help people achieve health by their own actions and efforts. The BSS has branches in all the states and nearly all the districts. Improvement of sanitation is one of the important activities of the BSS.

- *Kasturba Memorial Fund:* Created in commemoration of Kasturba Gandhi, after her death in 1994, the fund was raised with the main objective of improving the status of women, especially in the villages, through gram-savikas. The trust has nearly one crore of rupees and is actively engaged in various welfare projects in the country.
- *All India Women's Conference:* It is the only women's welfare organization in the country. Established in 1962, it has now branches all over the country. Most of the branches are running MCH clinics, Medical centers, adult education centers, milk centers and family planning clinics.
- *All India Blind Relief Society:* It was established in 1946 with a view to coordinate different institutions working for the blind. It organizes eye relief camps and other measures for the relief of the blind.
- *Professional bodies:* The professional bodies include the Indian Medical Association, All India Dental Association, the Trained Nurses Association of India for all men and women who are qualified in their respective specialties and possess registerable qualifications. These professional bodies conduct annual conferences, publish journals, arrange exhibitions, foster research, set up standards of professional education and organize relief camps during the periods of natural calamities.
- *Health insurance:* There is no universal health insurance in India; health insurance at present is limited to industrial workers and families. The central government employees are covered by Central Government Health Scheme.

EMPLOYEES STATE INSURANCE SCHEME

The Employees State Insurance (ESI) Scheme introduced by an Act of Parliament in 1948 is a unique piece of social legislation in India. ESI Act is an important measure of social security and health insurance in the country. The Act covers employees' drawing wages not exceeding 21,000 or less per month.

Act provides:
- Medical benefits
- Sickness benefits
- Maternity benefits
- Disablement benefits
- Dependent benefits
- Funeral benefit.

Central Government Health Scheme

The Central Government Health Scheme for the central government employees was first introduced in New Delhi in 1954 to provide comprehensive medical care to central government employees. The facilities under the scheme include:
- Supply of necessary drugs
- Outpatient care through a network of dispensaries
- Laboratory and X-ray investigations
- Domiciliary visits
- Hospitalization facilities
- Special consultation
- Emergency treatment
- Family welfare services.

OTHER AGENCIES

Defense Medical Services

Defense services have their own organization for medical care to defense personnel under the banner "Armed Forces Medical Services." The services provided are integrated and comprehensive, preventive, promotive and curative services.

Healthcare of Railway Employees

The railways provide comprehensive healthcare services through agency or railway hospitals, health units and clinics. Health checkup is provided at the time of entry into service, and there after every year.

Private Agencies

In a mixed economy, India's private practice of medicine provides a large share of health services available. The general practice constitutes 70% of medical professions and they concentrate in urban; they provide curative services for those who can pay.

Indigenous System of Medicine

The practitioners of indigenous system of medicine (Ayurveda, Siddha, Homeopathy, etc.) provide the bulk of medical care to the rural population. Studies indicate that nearly 90% of Ayurvedic physicians serve the rural areas. Most of them are local residents and remain close to the people socially and culturally. The Government of India is studying on how indigenous system of medicine could best be utilized for more effective and total health coverage.

VOLUNTARY HEALTH AGENCIES

Voluntary health agencies (VHA) may be defined as an organization that is administered by autonomous board, which holds meetings, collects funds for its support from private sources and expands money with or without paid worker for conducting programs for better public health.

VHA's main focus was on community health government that always looks up idea and new information from VHA. The main objective of VHA is planning for health of the people, and emphasizes more on preventive, curative health coverage.

Functions of VHA

- Supplementing the work of government agencies
- Pioneering

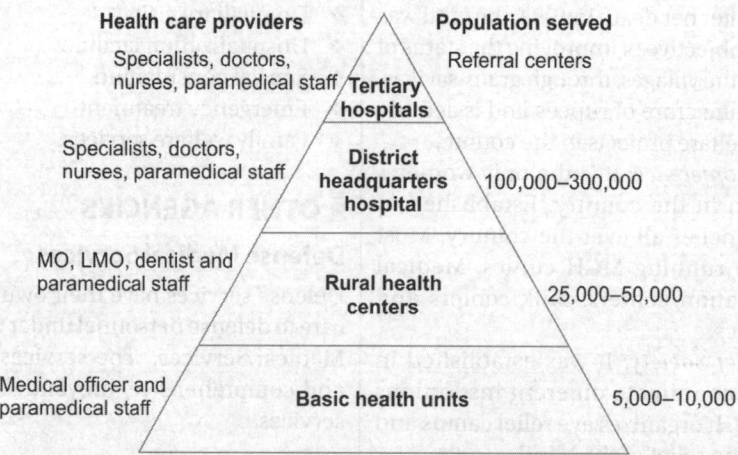

Fig. 14.1: Healthcare delivery system in India.

- Education
- Demonstration
- Guarding the work of government agencies
- Advancing health legislation.

VHA in India

- Indian Red Cross Society
- Hind Kusht Nivaran Sangh
- Indian Council for Child Welfare
- Tuberculosis Association of India
- Bharat Sevak Samaj
- Central Social Welfare Board
- The Kasturba Memorial Fund
- Family Planning Association of India
- All India Women's Conference
- The All India Blind Relief Society
- International Agencies.

NATIONAL HEALTH PROGRAMS IN INDIA

Measures had to be undertaken by the national government to improve the health of the people; prominent among these measures are the National Health Programs, which have been launched by the central government for the control/eradication of communicable disease, improvement of environmental sanitation, nutrition, control of population and rural health.

Various international agencies such as United Nations Children's Emergency Fund (UNICEF), United Nations Development Program (UNDP), Food and Agriculture Organization (FAO), Indian Labor Organization (ILO), United Nations Fund for Population Activities (UNFPA), World Bank and a number of foreign agencies have been providing technical and material assistance in the implementation of these programs. Some of the programs are:

Communicable Disease Programs

- National AIDS Control Program
- National Vector Borne Disease Control Program
- National Leprosy Eradication Program
- Revised National TB Control Program

Non-communicable Disease Programs

- National Program for Control of Blindness
- National Program for Prevention and Control of Deafness
- National Mental Health Program
- National Program for Prevention and Control of Cancer, Diabetes, Cardiovascular Diseases and Stroke
- National Iodine Deficiency Disorders
- National Tobacco Control Program
- National Program for Healthcare of Elderly
  - Expanded Program on Immunization
  - Diarrheal Disease Control Program
  - National Family Planning Program
  - National Water Supply and Sanitation Program.

CONCLUSION

Healthcare services can be implemented effectively with the supportive help of stakeholders. Nongovernment agencies, private, health insurance schemes and voluntary organization are indirectly supportive in delivery of services in health system and also intervenes the problems in healthcare system.

15 CHAPTER

Patterns of Nursing Care Delivery in India

CHAPTER OUTLINE

- Health
- Nursing
- Dimensions of Nursing Care
- Patterns of Nursing Care Delivery
- Comprehensive Nursing Care/Total Patient Care
- Progressive Patient Care Concept
- Team Nursing Concept
- Functional Method
- Case Method
- Primary Nursing Concept
- Self-care Concept
- Palliative Care Concepts
- Other Concepts of Nursing Care

INTRODUCTION

Nurse practice is ever-increasing in a variety of ways and settings. The focus of all nursing practice is the client, who may be an individual, a family, a group or a community. The practice of an individual nurse is determined largely by the setting and the needs of the clients served by the setting, e.g. in school children and their families. The nurse practicing in this setting must have special knowledge in pediatric growth and development, and health needs of school children. Other practice settings include hospitals, clinics, industry, extended care facilities and home health, and are regulated by the nurse practice acts of the area in which the nurse works. Nurses provide care for people in health and illness. The technologies of healthcare become more acceptable to human beings, if these are utilized with care and concern. The terminally ill require care and comfort. The central concern of nursing is care for people. All nursing practice is defined by the standards of the professional organization and regulated by the nurse practice acts of the area in which the nurse works.

HEALTH

The overall aim of nursing is to assist people to achieve their maximum health potential. Nursing is one of the health services which contribute to health and well-being of the individual, family and community. Health is a positive state of well-being in which harmonious development of mental and physical capacities of the individual lead to the enjoyment of a rich and full life. It implies adjustment of the individual to his/her total environment (physical and social).

NURSING

Nursing has been defined in various ways to explain the nature of nursing, the goals of nursing and the unique functions of the nurse. A wide definition of nursing by Virginia Henderson is that the unique function of the nurse is to assist the individual sick or well in the performance of those activities contributing to health or its recovery (or to peaceful death) that he would perform unaided if he had the necessary strength, will or knowledge. And to do this is such a way as to help him gain independence as rapidly as possible.

Study of this definition clearly indicates the following points:
❖ Nursing is viewed as a helping profession
❖ The nurse is a prime helper to the patient
❖ Scope of nursing is not limited to care of the sick
❖ Nursing encompasses help provided to healthy, sick or even dying persons
❖ Need for direct nursing assistance arose due to a person's specific inabilities
❖ Nurses promote independence to the patient as rapidly as possible.

Nursing has also been described as a humanistic science dedicated to concern for maintaining and promoting health, preventing illness, caring for and rehabilitating the sick and disabled. The goal of nursing is both to help people attain, maintain, retain and regain health, and to help them cope with crises, illness and death.

Nurse

A nurse is a person who has completed a program of basic nursing education, and is qualified and authorized in her country to supply the most responsible service of a nursing nature for the promotion of health, the prevention of illness and the care of the sick.

DIMENSIONS OF NURSING CARE

Nursing Practice

The recipients of nursing are sometimes called consumers, and sometimes patients. A consumer is called individual, a group of people or a community that use a service or commodity. A family that uses electricity in their home is a consumer of electricity. People who use healthcare product services are consumers of healthcare.

A patient is a person who is waiting for or undergoing medical treatment and care. The word patient came from a Latin word meaning to suffer or to bear. Traditionally, the person receiving healthcare has been called patient. Usually, people become patients when they seek assistance because of illness or for surgery. Some nurses believe that the word patient implies passive acceptance of the decisions and care of health professionals. Additionally, with the emphasis on the health promotion and prevention of illness, many recipients of nursing care are not ill. Moreover, nurses interact with family members and significant others in addition to the person actually receiving nursing care.

For these reasons, nurses are increasingly referring to the recipients of healthcare as clients. A client is a person who engages the advice of services of another who is qualified to provide these services. The term client presents the receivers of healthcare less as passive recipients and more as collaborators in the care, that is, as persons who are also responsible for their health professionals.

Focus of Nursing

Nursing involves an interrelationship of many people concerned with a client's response to potential or actual health problems. Today, nursing emphasizes the whole person; people are seen not merely as a physical being, but as biopsychological beings. Nursing practice involves a complex knowledge of skills applied to the whole. For this reason, a nurse must be aware of how the support person and community affect the client's well-being, and consider the well-being of this support person and the community. Nursing practice involves four areas related to health:

1. *Health promotion:* It means helping people develop resource to maintain or enhance their health and well-being. The focus of health promotion is "directed towards maintaining or improving the general health of individuals, families and communities." For example, explaining the benefits of good nutrition to all clients and encouraging a client to stop smoking.
2. *Health maintenance:* The nursing activities are those actions that help clients to maintain their health status. For example, an elderly person in a long-term care facility can be taught and encouraged to exercise to maintain muscle strength and mobility.
3. *Health restoration:* It means helping to improve health following health problems or illness. Examples of activities that help restore health are teaching a client to protect an incision and to change a surgical dressing, and assisting handicapped individuals to attain the highest level of physical strength of which they are capable of.
4. *Care of dying:* This area of nursing practice involves comforting and caring for people of all ages, while they are dying. Nurses carrying out these activities work in homes, hospitals and extended care facilities. Some agencies, called hospices, are specially designed for this purpose.

PATTERNS OF NURSING CARE DELIVERY (FIG. 15.1)

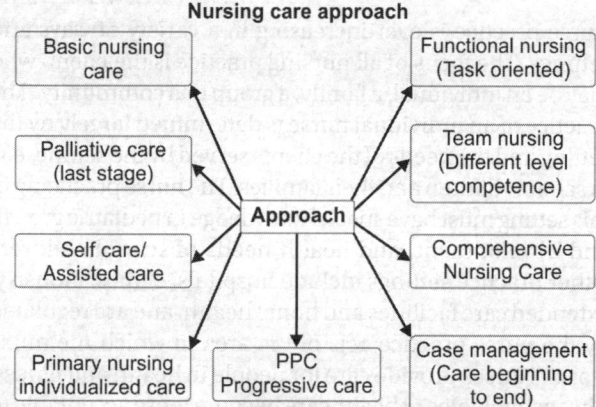

Fig. 15.1: Patterns of nursing care delivery.

COMPREHENSIVE NURSING CARE/ TOTAL PATIENT CARE (FIG. 15.2)

A concept was developed when the focus of nursing activities has to be changed from an excessively narrow

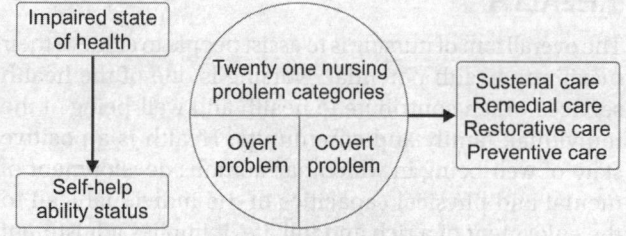

Fig. 15.2: Schematic diagram of comprehensive nursing care concept.

task-oriented functional one to a comprehensive personalized patient centered one. When nursing care is functionally organized, one nurse is responsible for hygienic care, a second nurse for medications, a third one for injections and a fourth one for other treatments. Nursing care becomes fragmented and tasks are performed in a depersonalized way.

Needs and problems of patients are not given the priority that it deserves. Nurses are more concerned about carrying out tasks, procedures and disease-related work.

The concept of comprehensive nursing care was proposed by a nursing theorist, Faye G. Abdellah, who stated that personalized nursing care should form the basis for professional nursing practice. Also each patient is a unique individual who has nursing problems, which can be derived from his health needs.

Definition

It has been defined as the care that is provided to the patient according to his/her needs in an appropriate, continuous and dynamic pattern. Nursing problem is a condition faced by the patient or his/her family that the nurse can assist him, her or them to meet through the performance of his/her professional functions.

- ❖ **Overt:** When it is an apparently obvious or observed condition, e.g. skin rash hyperpyrexia.
- ❖ **Covert:** When it is not obvious, hidden or concealed depression; these problems can be emotional, sociological or interpersonal in nature.

Nursing problems were identified according to the needs of the patient and categorized under 21 nursing problems:

1. To maintain good hygiene and physical comfort
2. To promote optimal activity, exercise, rest and sleep
3. To promote safety through prevention of accident or other trauma and through the prevention of the spread of infection
4. To maintain good body mechanics and prevent deformity
5. To facilitate the maintenance of oxygen supply to cells
6. To facilitate the maintenance of nutrition for all
7. To facilitate the maintenance of elimination
8. To facilitate the maintenance of fluid and electrolytes
9. To recognize the physiological responses of the body to disease condition—pathological, physiological and compensatory
10. To facilitate the maintenance of sensory functions
11. To facilitate the maintenance of regulatory mechanism and functions
12. To identify and accept positive and negative expressions, feelings and reactions
13. To identify and accept interrelatedness of emotions and organic illness
14. To facilitate the maintenance of effective verbal and non-verbal communication
15. To promote the development of productive interpersonal relationships
16. To facilitate progress toward achievement of personal and spiritual goals
17. To create and/or maintain therapeutic environment
18. To facilitate awareness of self as an individual with varying physical, emotional and development needs
19. To accept the optimum possible goal in the light of limitations, physical and emotional
20. To use community resources as aid for ill-resolving problems arising from illness
21. To understand the role of social problems as influencing factors in the cause of illness.

The 21 nursing problems focus on physical, biological, social and psychological needs of the patient. The problems are identified according to the condition of the patient and his self-help ability. The self-help ability of the patient refers to the ability of the patient to meet his healthcare needs. These abilities vary in accordance with the physical, mental and social capacities of the patient.

Comprehensive nursing care is based on the needs, requirements of the patient. These are classified in four broad categories:

1. *Sustenal care:* It is provided when self-help ability of the patient is reduced and he/she cannot meet his/her own personal needs.
2. *Remedial care:* Provided to correct and treat patients' impaired condition with a view to restore self-help ability of the patient.
3. *Restorative care:* It is provided to help patient develop new goals and teach him/her to live with his/her new self-help abilities.
4. *Preventive care:* It is provided to prevent an impaired state and to raise self-help ability of the patient.

Implementing the plan of care to the patient is the essence of comprehensive care, and helping the patient and his/her family to help themselves is an integral part of nursing. The present trend in nursing is to shift the emphasis from the disease-centered model to attend the total care of the patient.

PROGRESSIVE PATIENT CARE CONCEPT

The concept of progressive patient care (PPC) began to take shape in the 1950. The overall aim of this concept was to organize hospital services in such a way that the patient receives optimal care according to his/her medical and nursing needs.

Definition

Progressive patient care (PPC) is defined as the organization of hospital facility services and staff around, and segregated according to their diagnosis. For example, admitting patient to medical ward or a surgical ward. Under PPC system, the patient is classified and placed in different units of the hospital according to his/her needs. The patient may need intensive care or long-term care, and accordingly, he/she is admitted to the appropriate unit irrespective of his/her medical diagnosis. With the trend towards specialization, a variety of PPC elements have been established under a decentralized setup in major departments of large hospital.

Principal Elements of Progressive Care

- ❖ **Intensive care:** For critically ill patients who require intensive care round the clock, e.g. a patient with acute myocardial infarction. This unit is equipped with skilled personnel, life-saving equipment and supplies, and other resources required for revival, restoration and sustenance of the vital functions of the critically ill patients.
- ❖ **Intermediate care:** For moderately ill patients who may be ambulatory for a short period of time, e.g. a patient with appendicitis critically ill, he/she can be transferred to the intermediate care unit until condition improves and vital functions are stabilized. In many respects, the intermediate care units resemble the usual hospital wards, but facilities for convalescent care are better. Physical facilities in these units should include a dining room and a sitting room, so that a patient is not confined to a bed for the entire period of recovery.
- ❖ **Self-care:** For ambulatory patients, who are mostly self-sufficient in terms of daily care requirement, for example, an ambulatory patient who needs to undergo a series of diagnostic tests, which cannot be conveniently done on an outpatient basis. These patients require minimal normal care.
- ❖ **Long-term care:** For chronically ill patients or disabled patients who require nursing care for a prolonged period, e.g. a patient with cancer or a paraplegic patient. Rehabilitation care, occupational therapy and physical therapy may be needed for these patients. Patient teaching is emphasized with a view to help these patients learn how to adjust to their illness and disability.
- ❖ **Home care:** For patients who can be adequately cared for in the home through the extension of certain hospital services. A hospital-based home care program provides staff, equipment and supplies for care of the patient. For example, a patient with tuberculosis or a patient discharged after an operation who needs home care.
- ❖ **Outpatient care:** For ambulatory patients requiring simple diagnostic, curative, preventive and rehabilitative services, it is the more generally accepted activity of the average hospital.
- ❖ **Emergency care:** The hospital emergency service provides for the assessment of the ill or injured person, who is either treated or transferred to another institutional/department that offers the services needed by the patients.

Benefits of Progressive Patient Care

Patients:

- ❖ Receive specialized attention when they need it
- ❖ Get assistance in making adjustment to hospital and later to home and community
- ❖ Do not have to compete with critically ill patients for attention and assistance from nursing staff as they are segregated under this system of care
- ❖ Nursing personnel can make effective use of skills and capabilities
- ❖ Placement can be made according to skills and competencies of nursing staff
- ❖ Team can include semi-skilled to extend the nursing services to low-risk patients
- ❖ Can deliver increased quantitative improved quality of nursing services.

Hospital:

- ❖ Can make efficient use of high-qualified personnel and expensive high-tech equipment
- ❖ Can enhance the quality of patient care as a result of effective and efficient use of personnel beds, physical facilitating equipment supplies and funds can maintain continuity of case coordinate home care services.

Factors to be Considered in Progressive Patient Care

- ❖ Degree of illness
- ❖ Time required in meeting the needs
- ❖ Degree of activity permitted
- ❖ The teaching rehabilitation required by each patient
- ❖ The knowledge and experience of the professional and non-professional staff in the ward
- ❖ Proximity of the patient assigned to individual
- ❖ Orientation
- ❖ Job description
- ❖ Duration of patient care.

Advantages

- ❖ Installation of expensive equipment in your section of hospital
- ❖ More utilization of medical and nursing skills in intensive care unit (ICU)
- ❖ Individual patient cost could be less because of varying room rates
- ❖ Constant and continuous assessment of patient.

Disadvantages

- ❖ Fragmenting the care of the patient due to shifting from one unit to another several times during his/her stay in the hospital
- ❖ Reduced job satisfaction
- ❖ Same patient is seen by many nurses.

TEAM NURSING CONCEPT

Introduction

The team nursing concept is new and has developed as a way by which the patient can receive the quality care he/she needs from the individual competent person. This concept developed from a need to utilize the knowledge and skill of staff nurse to better advantage, and to ensure the supervision of the auxiliary nursing personnel. This concept has advantages over both the functional and patient methods of assign. Team nursing is based on levels of competencies and can make an effective contribution in nursing care.

Origin

In the early 1950s, in Columbia University, the concept was proposed which included professional and non-professional nursing to identify, plan, implement and evaluate comprehensive, client-centered care towards goal, and to reduce associated problems.

Overall Aim

The overall aim of team nursing is to provide nursing services to the individual patient in an efficient and effective manner.

Definition

Team nursing is a group of people led by a qualified nurse, provides for the health needs of an individual or a group of people though collaborative or cooperative effort.

—**Katherina V, 1980**

Composition of Team Nursing

A nursing team is made up of professional nurses, nursing auxiliaries and nursing aids who can work together cooperatively under a well-qualified team leader to provide a range of nursing services, which may vary from the very simple to the most complex nursing functions. A typical nursing team in a ward may include:
- Head nurses
- Staff nurses
- Nursing auxiliaries
- Nursing assistants
- Nursing students.

Spectrum of Nursing Functions

Team nursing recognizes that within the scope of nursing, there is a differentiation of functions. The spectrum of nursing functions includes:
- Simple nursing functions
- Technical nursing function
- Professional functions.

Simple nursing functions: Which require little knowledge skills. Judgment can be done by nursing aids who receive on-the-job training, e.g. giving a cold compress.

Intermediate nursing functions: Intermediate nursing function of a technical routine repetitive type can be earned out by technically trained nursing personnel, e.g. surgical dressing.

Complex nursing functions: Complex nursing functions, which require expert knowledge skills and judgments, can be performed by a nurse with professional nursing education background, e.g. organizing an infection control program in a surgical block of hospital.

Effective Teamwork

Effective teamwork has the following essential characteristics:
- Commonly agreed goals
- Clear division of labor
- Adequate resources, human and material
- Supportive and cooperative interpersonal relationships
- Open, honest communication
- Provision for evaluation and improvement.

Benefits of Team Nursing

- Provides a range of nursing services in an economical way
- More cost efficient as professional nursing staff are utilized for the performance of complex functions and nurses with a shorter duration of training are utilized for carrying out simple functions
- Work can be organized according to competencies of professional and non-professional nursing personnel
- Team nursing recognizes and respects valuable contribution of all categories of nursing personnel and patient care
- Members of the team are treated as equals
- Increase of job satisfaction in each member is deemed to be important
- Team members perform those functions that fall within the scope of their education and training
- There is appropriate utilization of staff
- Provides scope for developing nursing leadership skills
- Well-qualified, competent members can be given the opportunity to serve as team leaders.

Obstacles to Effective Team Work

Obstacles to effective team work in nursing may be due to:
- Poor leadership
- Ineffective communication
- Interpersonal conflicts
- Unfair division of labor
- Shortage of staff
- Insufficient time for planning team conference.

The chief disadvantage of team nursing is fragmentation of nursing care due to division of work.

A nursing team leader is expected to perform the following duties:
- Plan and evaluate work related to care of patient
- Assign work to team members

- Participate in direct care of patients and perform complex nursing functions
- Supervise and guide team members
- Conduct team conference.

Team conference is necessary for the following reasons:
- To share report of patient's progress
- To evaluate and modify nursing actions
- To discuss problems and alternative solutions
- To guide staff.

In team nursing, a synthesis of case method and functional method may be used for the assignment of work. Case method refers to the allocation of patients, and functional method refers to the assignment of specific functions and activities to be carried out by the member. A team member, for example, can be made responsible for the care of patients. And she can be given the specific assignment of requisitioning sterile supplies and dressing wound. The advantage of combining case methods and functional methods is that there is provision for individualizing patient care to get efficiency of functional method. All members of the nursing team need to develop a helping attitude towards each other for best results.

FUNCTIONAL METHOD

The functional method of delivering nursing care evolved as a result of World War II. Because nurses were in great demand in overseas to provide service at home. Many ancillary personnel were used to assist in patient care. These relatively unskilled workers were trained to do some simple tasks and gain proficiency by repetition. Persons were assigned to complete certain tasks rather than care of specific patients, for example, checking blood pressure, administering medication, changing linens and bathing patients. All the responsibilities are assigned to selected people in accordance with their expertise. The only person who has complete responsibility of the client is the head nurse or nurse acting in that role.

Merits
- The person can become particularly skilled in performing assigned tasks, and it can be efficient and economical
- Less equipment is needed, and what is available is better cared for when used only by a few personnel
- The potential for development of technical skill
- There is a sense of productivity for the task orient
- It is to organize the work of the unit and staff.

Demerits
- Client care may become impersonal compartment and fragmented. There is a tremendous risk for diminishing continuity of care
- Staff may become bored and have little motivational development, and self and others' work may become monotonous
- The staff members are accountable for the tasks; the nurse-in-charge of the unit has accountability for the individual care
- There is little avenue for staff development except that relating to tasks
- It is difficult to establish client priorities and operate the care plan reflecting it.

CASE METHOD

It is based on the concept of providing care on a continuum for persons with episodic or chronic illness. It uses a systematic approach to identify specific patients and to manage patient care of the optimum. The professional nurse is responsible for assessment of patient and family, establishment of the nursing diagnosis, development of the nursing care plan, delegation of nursing care to associates, activation of interventions, coordination and collaboration with the interdisciplinary team, and evaluation of outcomes. In this setting, the professional nurse case manager carries an active case load of approximately 40 patients, 10 in the acute care setting and 30 follow-up patients in the community. The case manager may have another 40–50 patients who have stabilized and require only a monthly telephone call for ongoing outcome evaluation. Initially, the case manager spends time with the patient and family to establish an open, working relationship and to gather information about previous and current levels of physical, psychological and spiritual functioning, and coping abilities and availability of resources and social support.

Merits
- The nurse can see better and attend to the total needs of clients due to the time and proximity of interactions. Coordination of all aspects of care is the main responsibility of the nurse, which include physical, emotional, medical regimen, teaching and all other aspects related to it
- Continuity of care can be facilitated
- Client may feel more secure knowing that one person is thoroughly familiar with the needs and the course of treatment for his/her disease.

PRIMARY NURSING CONCEPT

Under traditional system of nursing, in a typical hospital ward, the patient is not assigned to a nurse for the care that is provided to him/her during his/her hospitalization. Nursing functions are carried out by different nurses and no nurse is specifically assigned to assume responsibility for care of patient on a 24-hour basis during hospitalization. Under this system, it was difficult to promote accountability for nursing care provided to a patient. Primary nursing concept was developed as a solution to this problem. It was envisaged to promote individualized nursing care and to make qualified registered nurses assume responsibilities for nursing care provided to patients.

Chief Characteristics of Primary Nursing

- One nurse assumes total responsibility for the care of patient on a 24-hour basis
- The primary nurse is responsible for planning, carrying out and reviewing the nursing care provided to the patient
- The nursing care of the patient assigned to a primary nurse may be carried out by other members of the nursing team in the morning, evening or night shift, but responsibility is assumed by the primary nurse who is off-duty.

Basic Characteristics

- The primary nurse is said to be a triple "A" nurse having three basic characteristics:
  1. Autonomy
  2. Authority
  3. Accountability
- The primary nurse has autonomy to plan, control, review and revise the plan of care
- She has authority to determine what care is to be given, who will give it and how it is to be carried out
- The primary nurse is accountable for all decisions regarding particular patients assigned to her care. When one nurse is accounted responsibility for good or bad, nursing care is funneled back to the primary nurse
- Primary nursing promotes individualized patient-centered care; it provides for continuity of care. Since one nurse is made responsible for care of patient, it facilitates the coordination of care
- Patients know whom to approach, if plan needs to be modified or new problems develop. Patient cooperation and participation in planning care is encouraged under the primary nursing system.

Clinical Responsibilities of the Primary Nurse

- Assess conditions of patient and family on admission
- Identify problems and nursing care needs of the patient
- Prescribe nursing actions to be carried out in a plan of care
- Implement care and arrange for implementation of care in accordance with plan when primary nurse is off-duty
- Review and evaluate nursing actions carried out
- Revise plan based on the ongoing assessment of current problems and needs of the patient
- Collaborate with other members of the patient care team.

SELF-CARE CONCEPT

This concept is developed by the theorist Orem in 1971, which focuses on the individual and his/her self-care needs. Self-care is the practice of activities that individuals personally initiate and perform themselves in order to maintain health to prevent disease and promote health and restore function.

In nursing practice, nurses foster self-care inpatients by providing information about nutrition, sleep, exercise, stress management, psychological well-being, personal safety and environmental management.

The goal of Orem self-care deficit theory is helping client to achieve self-care. Nursing care is necessary when the client is unable to fulfill biological, psychological, developmental or social needs. In other instances, nurses help persons to maintain required self-care by performing some, but not all, care measures by supervising others who assist patients, and by instructing and guiding individuals as they gradually move towards self-care. There are basic types of nursing systems of Orem theory.

PALLIATIVE CARE CONCEPTS

Palliative care concept is one of the current concepts/modes of care adopted mainly for patients who are suffering from cancer. It is the care of patients whose disease is not responsive to curative treatment. Control of pain or other symptoms and of psychological, social and spiritual problems. The goal of palliative care is achievement of best quality of life for patients and their families. Palliative care affirms life and dying as a normal process, neither hastens nor postpones death, provide relief from pain and other distressing symptoms, integrates the psychological and spiritual aspects of care, offers a support system to help family cope up with the situation during the patient's illness and in their own bereavement.

OTHER CONCEPTS OF NURSING CARE

Extended Care

Hospitals are rapidly becoming healthcare facilities that deal almost exclusively with cases of acute injury or illness. Clients often receive care from other facilities for chronic conditions or after an initial crisis period ends. A broad continuum of care and assistance is available. Some facilities are referred to as extended care because they "extend" or continue care started in the hospital. Extended care facilities include sub-acute care facilities, medically complex at home receive home-based community services.

Expanded Role of Nurses

The expanded role of nurses can be described as a role which goes beyond the traditional nursing role to encourage or include additional responsibilities, and a wide range of functions in the community and clinical care settings. In an expanded role, trained nurses are urged to move out to the community and extend their services to the people. In institutional settings (e.g. a hospital), the new role will enable trained nurses with clinical expertise to retain the clinical role for direct nursing care in general units and expand their functions to meet the needs for specialized nursing care and skills in specialty units. This implies continued education and advanced nursing education of nurses in various fields of nursing. Nursing functions are being expanded in both developing and developed countries. Two major directions are indicated for expansion of nursing role:

- ❖ *Outward:* In order to extend nursing services to the community in support of primary healthcare
- ❖ *Upward:* To enable nursing experts to utilize their expertise for direct care of client; the client may be an individual, the family, a group or a community seeking healthcare
- ❖ The first outward direction indicated for the expanded role is meant to encourage trained nurses to move out from the curative sector into the community in support of primary healthcare
- ❖ The second upward direction indicated for expansion of nursing role is to enable nursing experts fulfill their potential in the hospital and in the community.

Nurse Practitioner

The nurse practitioner is a primary healthcare provider who assumes responsibilities of the expanded role to meet the healthcare needs of a group in the community. She is meant to provide first contact primary care to clients or case load of patients:

- ❖ All registered nurses can be called nurse practitioners, but currently the term, "nurse practitioner" is used for those assuming responsibilities of the expanded role whose work reflects the kind of nursing practice where encompassed additional functions and activities go beyond the scope of traditional nursing practice.
- ❖ Under expanded role, the nurse practitioners become delegated to medical responsibilities such as diagnosis and treatment of minor through standing orders in addition to traditional nursing responsibilities. She presents package of preventive, curative and rehabilitative services for promotion, maintenance and restoration of health of clients. Her clients are generally in the ambulatory category.

Nurse Clinician

The term nurse clinician was first coined by Reiter in the 1960s. She described the nurse clinician as a master practice who was competent in care and knowledgeable about cure.

The nurse clinician role was proposed when there was a need for senior nurse with experience and expertise. To retain their clinical expertise, they moved up the career ladder into supervisory and administrative positions. The clinician is expected to be clinically competent in carrying out care functions and counseling functions.

- ❖ *Care functions:* Include basic and technical nursing care based on the needs of the patient. These functions would encompass palliative care, physical care and protective care.
- ❖ *Cure functions:* Include those activities directly related to medical care, therapeutic regimen and overall clinical nursing management of patients.
- ❖ *Counseling functions:* Include psychological care, teaching patients and families, providing guidance in matters related to health and working with families for restoration, and maintenance of health.

Nurse Specialist

The nurse specialist is an expert practitioner in a specific branch of nursing with advance knowledge, high degree of skill and extensive experience in the care of clients or patients in the specialty concerned.

The nurse specialist's role evolved in response to the need for nursing experts, with appropriate educational preparation and experience, who could deliver high-quality nursing care in a defined area of specialization. In clinical nursing practice, the nurse specialist is a master clinician with high level of knowledge, skills and competence in a specialized area of nursing like cardiac nursing, cancer nursing, etc.

The nurse specialist has a multifaceted role, which encompasses the following:

- ❖ *Practitioner:* The nurse specialist is an expert practitioner who maintains direct contact with client, the client may be an individual, a family, a group or a community with specific health-illness problems.
- ❖ *Change agent:* The nurse specialist initiates change necessary for improvement of nursing care. She plays a key role in affecting change by linking findings of nursing research to improve nursing practice.
- ❖ *Consultant:* The nurse specialist serves as a consultant nurse, and other health workers utilize her expertise by making referrals for problems, which need to be handled by an expert in that particular field.
- ❖ *Coordinator:* The nurse specialist coordinates patient or client care to avoid fragmentation of care. She maintains links with other health professionals in the health team and collaborates with them for proper articulation of nursing services with other services for the patients and client.

CONCLUSION

The patterns of the nursing care was evolved from the theorist Faye G Abdelah compressive care concept and is more acceptable, providing holistic care to clients, families and community. The nurse administrators should be oriented to these concepts of care for effective implementation and it needs research. Nurses are working in all areas as expansion of technology, education and professional advancement brought changes in roles and functions.

16 CHAPTER

Healthcare Delivery Concerns, National Health and Family Welfare Programmes—Intersectoral Coordination, Role of Nongovernmental Agencies

CHAPTER OUTLINE

- National Health and Family Welfare Programmes
  - Reproductive and Child Health Programme
  - Child Survival and Safe Motherhood Programme
  - National Rural Health Mission
  - Family Welfare Programme under NRHM
  - Child Health Welfare Programmes
- Organization for Family Welfare Services
  - Family Welfare Services in Urban Areas
  - Family Welfare Service in Rural Areas
- Intersectoral Coordination
  - Nongovernmental Agencies

INTRODUCTION

India is a developing country, yet to be developed various ill effects making this country lag ill effects such as health problems, population explosion and unemployment. When we speak about health problems, it is understood that it comprises all the stages of individuals such as pediatrics, antenatal and postnatal mothers, geriatrics, etc. Nearly half of the population constituted mother and under-fives. So as to improve the health status of these groups, the Government of India has launched various maternal and child health (MCH) programmes with its effective delivery to the beneficiaries by health workers at village level, district level, state and union level.

NATIONAL HEALTH AND FAMILY WELFARE PROGRAMMES

Since maternal group and under-fives are the risk group, various programs are launched by central and state government. They include:
1. Reproductive and Child Health (RCH) Programme
2. Child Survival and Safe Motherhood (CSSM) Programme
3. National Rural Health Mission (NRHM)
4. Vande Mataram Scheme
5. Bhagyalakshmi Scheme
6. 24 × 7 primary health centre (PHC)/community health centre (CHC) services.

Components of NRHM Programs

It has following program components:

Maternal Health/Thayi Bhagya
- Janani Suraksha Yojana
- Prasooti Araike
- Madilu Yojane
- Public private partnership (PPP) scheme
- Family welfare under NRHM.

Child Health
- Integrated management of neonatal and childhood illness (IMNCI)
- Immunization
- Suvarna Arogya Chaitanya School Programs.

Other Programs
- Special nutrition program
- Integrated Child Development Services (ICDS) Programme
- Prophylaxis against national anemia
- Mid-day meal program
- Vitamin A prophylaxis to prevent blindness
- Prevention of vector borne diseases

Reproductive and Child Health Programme

Definition

The RCH is defined as people where the ability to reproduce and regulate their fertility. Women are able to go through pregnancy and childbirth safely. The outcome of pregnancy is successful in terms of maternal and infant survival and well-being, and couples are able to have sexual relations free of fear of pregnancy and of contracting disease.

RCH Programme—Phase I

The RCH phase I programme incorporated the components relating to CSSM and included two additional components, one relating to sexually transmitted disease (STD) and other relating to reproductive tract infection (RTI).

The program was started in August 1997. Financially, this program was supported by the World Bank and European Union.

RCH Package Services

Package services for mothers

- ❖ ***Essential obstetric care (EOC):***
  - ➢ The EOC includes early registration of pregnancy (within 12–16 weeks)
  - ➢ Provision of minimum three antenatal checkups
  - ➢ Promotion of institutional delivery provision of safe delivery at home
  - ➢ Provision of postnatal care and referral services.
- ❖ ***Emergency obstetric care (EmOC):*** The EmOC by identifying and strengthening first referral units (FRUs) under the RCH programme.
- ❖ ***At PHCs/CHCs 24-hour delivery services.***
- ❖ ***Referral transport:*** Provision has been made for the transport facility with the panchayat through district family welfare officers to be utilized by the families at the time of obstetric emergencies.
- ❖ ***Medical termination of pregnancy (MTP):***
  - ➢ Provision of MTP equipment to district hospital CHCs and PHCs wherever required
  - ➢ Assisting states/union territories (UTs) for engaging doctors trained in MTP to give their services once a week/fortnight in PHCs/CHCs and sub-district hospitals to overcome shortage of trained manpower
  - ➢ Provision of MTP equipment and free training in MTP techniques to nongovernment organizations (NGOs).
- ❖ ***Prevention, management and control of RTI and STDs:***
  - ➢ Various activities include setting up of RTI/STD clinics in FRUs
  - ➢ Collaboration with national AIDS control organization (NACO) for planning and implementation of services on RTI clinics
  - ➢ Training and counseling information education and communication (IEC) social marketing of condoms supply of RTI/STD drugs, and monitoring and evacuation.
- ❖ ***Training of accredited social health activists (ASHAs):*** Training is continuing under RCH programme. NGOs are involved in training of village workers to make it more local specific.
- ❖ ***RCH camps:*** Have been initiated in the remote areas where the existing services at the PHC level are under-utilized.

Package services for child

- ❖ ***Universal immunization programs:*** Under the program, the children are immunized as per schedule against six killer diseases of childhood, namely tuberculosis, diphtheria, pertussis poliomyelitis, measles, neonatal tetanus and hepatitis B:
  - ➢ Since 1998 a special campaign with the assistance of United Nations Children's Emergency Fund (UNICEF) has been taken up to protect children under 3 years of age. In slums, against measles, which occurs more in overcrowded area.
- ❖ ***Control of acute respiratory infections (ARIs):*** Health workers through training program are able to provide ARI management:
  - ➢ Cotrimoxazole is being supplied as the CSSM drug kit to health workers
  - ➢ Emphasis is given on IEC activities to educate mothers on recognition of symptoms, referral care of the child, etc.
- ❖ ***Essential newborn care:***
  - ➢ Essential newborn care is included as an intervention under the RCH program to decline infant mortality rate (IMR)
  - ➢ The related intervention include supply of equipment for newborn care to all the districts
  - ➢ Training of doctors and all other health workers on newborn care and use of compartments.
- ❖ ***Oral rehydration therapy for diarrhea control among children:***
  - ➢ Government supplies oral rehydration solution (ORS) packets to all the states to be made available at sub-centers to prevent mortality in children
  - ➢ Each sub-center is provided with two drug kits in a year each containing 150 ORS packets along with other drugs.
- ❖ ***Prevention and control of vitamin A deficiency among children:*** Under this program, vitamin A drops are administered to all the children under 5 years of age.
- ❖ ***Borders district cluster project (BDCP):*** The BDCP is launched in 47 identified districts of 16 states with the assistance of UNICEF. This project included additional input for implementation of RCH program to reduce infant mortality rate (IMR) and maternal mortality rate (MMR) by 50% over 4 years' period.
- ❖ ***National technical committee on child health:*** A national technical committee on child health has been set up to review critically existing program intervention, implementation achievements against indication related to prenatal. Infant and child mortality and suggest new additional cost effective feasible interventions, which helps decline infant and child mortality.

Initiatives taken after adoption of national population policy (2000):

- ❖ The RCH camps
- ❖ The RCH outreach scheme
- ❖ Operationalization of district newborn care
- ❖ Home-based neonatal care
- ❖ Border district cluster strategy (BDCS)

- Introduction of hepatitis and vaccination project
- Training of ASHAs.

RCH Phase II Programme

RCH phase II began from 1st April 2005. The focus of the program is to reduce maternal and child morbidity and mortality with emphasis on rural health care. The major strategies under the second phase of RCH are given below.

- **Essential obstetric care:**
  - *Institutional delivery:*
    - To promote institutional delivery in RCH phase II, it is envisaged that 50% of the PHCs and all the CHCs would be made operational as 24-hour delivery centers in a phased manner by the year 2010
    - These centers would be responsible for providing basic EmOC, essential newborn care and basic newborn resuscitation services round the clock.
  - *Skilled attendance at delivery:*
    - It is now recognized globally that the countries which have been successful in bringing down MMR are the ones where the provision of skilled attendance at every birth and linkage with appropriate referral services have been ensured
    - Guidelines for normal delivery and management of obstetric complications at PHCs/CHCs for medical officers and for antenatal care (ANC) and skilled attendance at birth for auxiliary nurse midwife (ANM)/lady health visitor (LHV) have been formulated and disseminated to the states.
  - *The policy decisions:*
    - ANMs, LHVs and staff nurses (SNs) have now been permitted to use drugs in specific emergency situation to reduce maternal mortality
    - They have also been permitted to carry out certain emergency intervention when the life of the mother is at stake.
- **Emergency obstetric care:**
  - Operationalization of FRUs and skilled attendance at birth are the two activities, which go hand in hand
  - Simultaneous steps have been taken to ensure tackling obstetric emergencies
  - It has been decided that all the FRUs be made operational for providing emergency and EOC during the second phase of RCH.

The minimum services to be provided by a fully functional FRU are:
- 24-hour delivery services including normal and assisted deliveries
- The EmOC including surgical interventions such as cesarean section
- Newborn care
- Emergency care of sick children
- A full range of family planning services including laparoscopic services
- Safe abortion services
- Treatment of sexually transmitted infections (STIs)/RTI
- Blood storage facility
- Essential laboratory services
- Referral services.

There are three critical determinations of a facility being declared as a FRU, which are:
- Availability of surgical intervention
- Newborn care
- Blood storage facility on 24-hour basis.

- **Strengthening referral system:**
  - Since there was no effective use of fluids by panchayats in running the scheme during RCH phase I, based on these experiences, different states have proposed different modes of referral linkage in RCH phase II.
  - Some of them indicated to involve local self-help groups, NGOs and women groups, whereas few others indicated to outsource it.

New initiatives

- **Training of MBBS doctors in life-saving anesthetic skills for EmOC:**
  - Provision of adequate and timely EmOCs has been recognized as the most important intervention for saving lives of pregnant women, who may develop complications during pregnancy and childbirth
  - The operationalization of FRU at sub-district/CHC level for providing EmOC to pregnant women is a crucial strategy of RCH II, which needs focused attention
  - The training of MBBS doctors will be undertaken for only such numbers who are required for the functioning of FRUs and CHCs, and shall be limited to the requirement of tackling emergency obstetrics situations only
  - Setting up of blood storage center at FRUs according to Government of India guidelines.

Vande Mataram Scheme

This is a voluntary scheme wherein any obstetrics and gynecology specialist in maternity home, nursing home, lady doctor/MBBS doctor can volunteer themselves for providing safe motherhood services

- The enrolled doctors will display "Vande Mataram Logo" at their clinic
- Iron and folic acid (IFA) tablets, oral pills, tetanus toxoid (TT) injection, etc. will be provided by the respective district medical officers to the "Vande Mataram doctors/clinics" for free distribution to beneficiaries
- It is a nation-wide program aimed at improving acute and postnatal care, which was launched on February 9, 2004.
- The scheme envisages free acute and postnatal checkup tips to avoid nutritional problems and anemia, and

counseling a small family norm, and is a major initiative in public-private partnership (PPP) during emergency
- "Vande Mataram Day" is considered on 9th of every month, and on this day, safe motherhood services are rendered.

Child Survival and Safe Motherhood Programme

It was launched on August 20, 1992; this program includes:
- Essential newborn care
- Immunization
- Oral rehydration therapy for prevention of death due to diarrheal dehydration
- Early treatment for lower respiratory tract infections
- Recognition of high-risk pregnancies and appropriate treatment complication of childbirth and pregnancy-related events.
- Availability of IFA tablets in adequate doses for all pregnant women to improve their general health and to reduce the number of premature and low birth weight infants
- Availability of vitamin A for all children under 3 years of age
- Promotion of breastfeeding and advice on healthy nutrition
- Training of traditional birth attendance (TBAs)
- In this program, 5Cs were envisaged clean surface, clean hand, clean cord tie, clean cord cutting and ligature as well as clean blade.

Later, since this program was ineffective, it was integrated with current RCH program in the year 1997. Major interventions are:
- EOC
- A 24-hour delivery services at PHCs/CHCs
- EmOC MTP
- Prevention of RTI and STDs
- District surveys/strengthening of PHCs.

National Rural Health Mission (NRHM)

Government of India launched "NRHM" on April 5, 2005 for a period of 7 years (2005–2012):
- The mission seeks to improve rural health care delivery system
- It is operational in the whole country with special focus on 18 states (Bihar, Jharkhand, Madhya Pradesh, Chhattisgarh, Uttar Pradesh, Uttaranchal, Odisha and Rajasthan) and North East states (Assam, Arunachal Pradesh, Manipur, Meghalaya, Mizoram, Nagaland, Tripura, Himachal Pradesh and Jammu and Kashmir)
- The main aim of NRHM is to provide accessible, affordable, accountable, effective and reliable PHC and bridging the gap in rural health care through creation of a cadre of ASHA
- The programs to be integrated are existing programs of health and family welfare including RCH II and other national programs.

Plan of Action to Strengthen Infrastructure
- Creation of a cadre of ASHA
- Strengthening sub-centers
- Strengthening PHCs
- Strengthening CHCs for first referral care.

Goals to be Achieved by NRHM (Table 16.1)
National level
- The IMR reduced to 30/1,000 live birth
- Maternal mortality ratio reduced to 100/100,000
- Total fertility rate reduced to 2.1
- Upgrading CHCs to Indian public health standards
- Increase utilization of FRUs from less than 20–75%
- Engaging 250,000 female ASHAs in 10 states.

As a part of the planning process, many different programs have been brought together under the overarching umbrella of National Health Mission (NHM), with NRHM and National Urban Health Mission (NUHM) as its two sub-missions. The main programmatic components include health system, strengthening in rural and urban areas, reproductive, maternal, newborn, child and adolescent health (RMNCH+A) and control of communicable and non-communicable. The Government of India has introduced a series of programs past the decades to address newborn health. The major milestones include:

1990—CSSM
1997—RCH1
2005—RCH2
2005—NRHM
2013—RMNCH + A strategy

Table 16.1: Indicators of health.

Targets (2012–2017)	Achievements
Reduce IMR to 25/1000 live births	IMR reduced from 42 in 2012 to 39 in 2014
Reduce MMR to 1/1000 live births	IMR has reduced in 1.67 in 2011–2013
Reduce TFR to 2.0	TFR has reduced to 2.3 in 2014
Reduce annual incidence and mortality from tuberculosis by half	Tuberculosis incidence is at 167 per lakh population and mortality at 17 per lakh population in 2015
Reduce prevalence of leprosy to <1/10,000 population and incidence to 0 in all districts	Leprosy prevalence rate is <1/10,000 population
Annual malaria incidence to be <1/1,000	Annual malaria incidence is <1/1,000
Less than 1% microfilaria prevalence in all districts	Out of 225 endemic districts, 222 have reported microfilaria rate of less than 1%
Kala-azar elimination by 2015, <1 case per 10,000 population in all blocks	Out of 611 block PHCs, 454 have reported <1 case per 10,000

Source: Parks Textbook of Preventive and Social Medicine, 24th ed.

2013—NHM
2014—India Newborn Action Plan (INAP).

Community level

- Health day at anganwadi level is a fixed day/month for provision of immunization ante/postnatal checkups and services related to mother and child health care including nutrition
- Improved access to universal immunization through induction of auto disabled syringes, alternate vaccine delivery and improved mobilization services under the program
- Improved facilities for institutional delivery through provision of referral transport escort and improved hospital care subsidized under the Janani Suraksha Yojanas (JSY) for the below poverty line (BPL) families.

ASHA

Selection of ASHA

- ASHA must be the resident of the village
- A woman (married/widow/divorced) preferably in the age group of 25–45 years with formal education up to eighth class, having communication skills and leadership qualities
- The general norm of selection will be one ASHA for 1,000 population.

Role and responsibility of ASHA in relation to MCH

ASHA will be a health activist in the community who will create awareness in health. Her responsibilities will be as follows:

- She will counsel women on birth preparation importance of safe delivery breastfeeding and complementary feeding immunization, contraception and prevention of common infections including RTI/STI and care of the young child.
- ASHA will mobilize the community and facilitate them in accessing health and health-related services available at the anganwadi/sub-center/PHC such as immunization, acute natal checkup, postnatal checkup, supplementary nutrition sanitation and other services being provided by the government.
- She will arrange escort/company to pregnant women and children requiring treatment admission to the nearest pre-identified health facility, i.e. PHC/CHC/FRU.
- She will also act as a depot holder for essential provision being made available to every habitation, such as ORT, IFA tablet, chloroquine, disposable delivery kits, oral pills, condoms, etc.; a drug kit will be provided to each ASHA.

Role of ASHA and integration with anganwadi

The anganwadi workers (AWW) will guide ASHA in performing following activities:

- Organizing health day once/twice a month. On health day, the women, adolescent girls and children from the village will be mobilized for orientation as health-related issues such as importance of nutritious food, personal hygiene, care during pregnancy, importance of antenatal checkup and institutional delivery, home remedies for minor ailment and importance of immunization. AWWs will inform ANM to participate and guide in organizing the health days at anganwadi center.
- AWWs and ANMs will act as resource person for the training of ASHA.
- The IEC activity through display of posters, folk dance, etc. on these days can be undertaken to sensitize the beneficiaries on health-related issues.
- The AWW will update the list of eligible couple and also the children less than 1 year of age in the village with the help of ASHA.
- The ASHA will support the AWW in mobilizing pregnant and lactating women, and infants for nutrition supplement. She would also take initiative for bringing the beneficiaries from the village on specific days of immunization, health checkup/health days, etc. to anganwadi centers.

Role of Integration with ANM

- The ANMs take help of ASHA in updating eligible couple for coming to sub-center for initial checkups
- She utilizes ASHA in motivating the pregnant women for coming to sub-center for initial checkups
- She also helps ANMs in bringing married couple to sub-center for adopting family planning
- The ANM guides ASHA in motivating pregnant women for taking full course of IFA tablets and TT injection
- The ANMs will orient ASHA on the dose schedule and side effects of oral pills
- The ANMs will educate ASHA on danger signs of pregnancy and labor, so that she can timely identify and help beneficiary in getting further treatment.

Schemes of NRHM

The NRHM has comprehensive health program, i.e., "Thayi Bhagya" a comprehensive health program for maternal care and child care to make this program more effective. They have been integrated under this program. The program has four schemes:

1. Janani Suraksha Yojana (JSY)
2. Prasooti Araike
3. Madilu Yojane
4. Public-Private Partnership (PPP) scheme.

Objectives of "Thayi Bhagya" Program

- Reducing maternal and IMR
- To provide health care to all pregnant women to make health care accessible to pregnant women living in tribal mountain and inaccessible regions

- Encouraging pregnant women for regular antenatal checkups
- To encourage deliveries in the hospital
- Participation of private institution in health care
- Encouragement for small family norms.

1. Janani Suraksha Yojana (JSY)

The JSY is a safe motherhood intervention under the NRHM, being implemented with the objective of:
- Reducing maternal and neonatal mortality by promoting institutional delivery among the poor pregnant women.
  - The Yojana launched on April 12, 2005 by the honorable Prime Minister is being implemented in all states and with special focus on low-performing states (LPS).
  - The JSY is a 100% centrally sponsored scheme and it integrated each assistance with delivery and post-delivery care.
  - The Yojana has identified ASHA; the ASHA has an effective link between the government and the poor pregnant women in 10 LPS, namely the eight empowered action group (EAG) states, Assam, Jammu and Kashmir, and the remaining North East (NE) states.

Role of ASHA associated with JSY:
- Identify pregnant women as a beneficiary of the scheme and report at facilitate registration for ANC
- Assist the pregnant women to obtain necessary certification wherever necessary
- Help the women in receiving at least three ANC checkups that include TT injection and IFA tablets
- Identify a functional government health center at an accredited private health institution for referral and delivery
- Counsel for institutional delivery
- Escort the beneficiary woman in the predetermined health center and stay with her till the woman is discharged
- Arrange to immunize the newborn till the age of 14 weeks
- Inform about the birth or death of the child, or mother to the ANM/medical officer (MO)
- Postnatal visit within 7 days of delivery to track mothers' health after delivery and facilitate in obtaining care wherever necessary
- Counsel for initiation of breastfeeding to the newborn within 1 hour of delivery and in continuance till 3–6 months and promote family planning.

Important features of JSY (Tables 16.2 and 16.3):
The scheme focuses on the poor pregnant women with special dispensation for states having low institutional delivery rates, namely the states of EAG. While these states have been named as LPS, the remaining states have been named as high-performing states (HPS).

Tracking each pregnancy:
Each beneficiary registered under this Yojana should have a JSY card along with a MCH card.

ASHA, AWW or any other identified link worker under the overall supervision of the ANM, MO or PHC should mandatorily prepare this.

The eligibility of cash assistance is as follows:
- **LPS:** All women including those from scheduled caste (SC) and scheduled tribe (ST) families delivering in government health centers such as sub-center, PHC, CHC, FRU, general wards of district and state hospitals at accredited private institutions. All birth delivered in health center government at accredited private health institutional will get the benefit.
- **HPS:** The BPL women aged 19 years and above, and the SC and ST pregnant women. The benefit is only up to 2 live births.

Flow of fund to JSY:
- State/district authorities would advance ₹5,000 and ₹10,000 for each ANM in HPS and LPS, respectively, as a recoupable impressed money from the JSY fund.
- This money could be kept in the joint account of ANM and Gram Pradhan as in the case of united fund placed with sub-centers so that the ANM could roll the entire amount by advancing ₹1,500 to ₹2,500 to ASHA/AWW per delivery and later she could recoup it from the PHC/CHC.
- There should be a clear authority for ANM to withdraw cash from this account for advancing it to the ASHA at AWW/any other health link worker needed for ready use towards disbursement in the pregnant and also for arranging the referral transport for escorting the pregnant women to the institution.

Payment to ASHA:
ASHA should bring her to the center:
- First payment for the transactional cost at the health center on reaching the institution along with the expectant mother.
- The second payment should be paid after she has made postnatal visit and the child has been immunized for Bacillus Calmette-Guérin (BCG).
- All payments to ASHA would be done by the ANM only. In this case too, a voucher scheme is introduced in such a manner that for every pregnant women she registers under JSY, ANM would give two vouchers to ASHA, which she would be able to encash a certification by ANM.
- ASHA package is available in all LPS, NE states and in tribal districts of all states and UTs.

In rural areas, it includes the following components:
- Cash assistance for referral transport for pregnant women to go to the nearest health center for delivery
- Balance amount to be paid to ASHA in lieu of the services rendered by her

Table 16.2: Microbirth plan for Janani Suraksha Yojana beneficiaries.

Activity	To be undertaken by	Proposed time line
Identification and registration of beneficiary	ANM/ASHA/AWW at any link worker	At least 20–24 weeks before the suspected date of delivery
Filling up of MCH card	ANM/ASHA/AWW	Immediately on registration
Inform dates of three ANC and TT injection and identify the health center for all referral Identify the place of delivery Inform suspected date of delivery	ANM/ASHA/AWW at any equivalent link worker Provide the first ANC Immediately on registration	Immediately on registration
Collecting BPL at necessary proofs/certificate	ANM/ASHA/AWW at any link worker	Within 2–4 weeks from registration
Submission of the completed JSY card in the health center for verification by the authorized/medial officer. Take necessary steps towards arranging transport or making available cash to the beneficiary to come to the health center Ensure availability of fund to ANM/ASHA, etc.	MO/PHC ANM/ASHA/AWW at any link worker ANM/MO/PHC	At least 2–4 weeks before the suspected date of delivery
Payment of cash benefit/incentive to the mother and ASHA	ANM/MO/PHC	At the institution
For complicated cases or those requiring cesarean section, etc.		
Action-1: Predetermine a referral health center and ultimate the pregnant women	By ANM/ASHA/Link worker	
Action-2: Familiarize the women with the referral center if necessary carry a letter of referral from MO, PHC	ANM/ASHA/Link workers	
Action-3: Preorganize the transport facility in consultation with family members/community leader	ANM/ASHA/Community	
Action-4: Arrange for the medical superior, if the same is not available in referred health center	MO/PHC	

(ANM: auxiliary nurse midwife; ASHA: accredited social health activist; AWW: anganwadi workers; MCH: maternal and child health; ANC: antenatal care; TT: tetanus toxoid; BPL: below poverty line; MO: medical officer; PHC: primary health center; JSY: Janani Suraksha Yojana)

Table 16.3: Scale of assistance under the scheme.

Category	Rural area			Urban area		
	Mother's package	ASHA's package	Total ₹	Mother's package	ASHA's package	Total ₹
LPS	1,400	600	2,000	1,000	200	1,200
HPS	700	–	700	600	–	600

(LPS: low-performing states; HPS: high-performing states; ASHA: accredited social health activist)

- The year 2006–2007 was declared as the year for institutional deliveries. During the year, scope of the scheme was extended to the urban areas of HPS, and restrictions of age and birth order were removed in the LPS
- The benefits of the scheme were also extended to all women belonging to ST/SC families for institutional deliveries
- During the year 2006–2008, about 28.11 lakhs pregnant women were benefited from the scheme out of which 18.72 lakhs had institutional deliveries.

2. Prasooti Araike

Launched on January 6, 2008:
- Government of Karnataka launched "Prasooti Araike," a scheme to boost the health of pregnant Dalit women living BPL in Karnataka. This program flagged off an immunization drive to fight hepatitis B.
- Implemented by Department of Health and Family Welfare, it is said that the Araike scheme had been launched as a pilot project in services backward districts of Karnataka to help SC and ST women get adequate nutrition and medical care.
- Women who are eligible for the scheme in the districts receive a sum of ₹2,000 in two instalments during the pregnancy and two sarees after the birth of the child.
- Women avail benefits of this scheme only for two pregnancies.
- Districts to be covered under the scheme are Bidar, Gulbarga, Bijapur, Bagalkot, Raichur, Koppal and Chamarajnagar.

❖ Government of Karnataka Health and Family Welfare (HFW) says it would soon be extended to other parts of the state.

3. Madilu Yojane

Madilu Yojane was launched on September 15, 2007 to encourage pregnant women to admit themselves in government hospitals for delivery.

❖ Scheme was aimed at protecting the health of the mother and the newborn bringing down the maternal and IMR, compulsory registration of births and encouraging poor women to admit themselves to government hospitals for delivery.
❖ Under this scheme, a kit will be distributed after the delivery at hospital.
❖ Each kit contains 19 items including a blanket, a towel, a napkin, a torch, a mosquito net and some emergency medicines.
❖ The benefit is limited to first two deliveries.

4. Public–Private Partnership (PPP) Scheme

PPP is a collaboration between the public and the private sector that enables fulfillment of certain common goals related to maternal care services.

The NRHM of India advocates PPPs to meet its EmOC provision. This is applicable to women either living BPL or from the SC/ST and above 19 years of age at the time of first two births. Under this, JSY has made a provision for women to give choice and preferring private facilities for her delivery. The scheme subsidizes the cost in such cases by providing ₹1,500 for contracting obstetric specialist when he/she produces the discharge. The district administration is to empanel the specialists for this scheme.

Family Welfare Programme under NRHM

Program Objectives

❖ Improve management performance by statewide implementation of policy change referred to as the participatory planning approach and institutional strengthening for timely coordinated utilization of project resources.
❖ Improve quality coverage by fixed day static approach and effectiveness of existing family welfare (FW) services.
❖ Progressively expand the scope and content of existing FW services to include more elements of a defined package of essential RCH services.
❖ In selected disadvantaged districts and cities, increase access by strengthening FW infrastructure, while improving in quality.

Suvarna Arogya Chaitanya School Health Programme

Provides health checkup for all students studying in 1–10th standard.

Detected cases of diseases to be treated free of cost in PHCs, Taluk hospital and district hospital.

Bhagyalakshmi Scheme

❖ It was launched on August 8, 2007.
❖ Bhagyalakshmi: the first ever insurance scheme for girl children of BPL families providing financial support for their education, health and marriage was launched by Government of Karnataka.
❖ In this scheme, the girl child gets health insurance cover up to a maximum of ₹25,000 a year. The girl would be given an annual scholarship of ₹300–1,000 up to 10th standard.
❖ Apart from these benefits, the parents would get ₹1 lakh in case of accident and ₹42,500 for natural death of the beneficiary.
❖ At the end of 18 years, the beneficiary would be paid ₹34,751.
❖ Under the scheme, the girl should be sent to an anganwadi till she attained the age of 6 years.
❖ Then she should study up to 8th standard to become eligible for receiving ₹34,751; such an arrangement would ensure that the girl got minimum education and was not married off early.

A 24 × 7 PHC Service

❖ Currently, the Government of Karnataka is providing round-the-clock services to obstetric care casualty services.
❖ Emergency comprehensive effective obstetric care is given by professionals with midwifery skills.
❖ No turning of subject away from hospital for any reasons.
❖ Casualty should be located close to the labor room and theater.
❖ Casualty should have obstetrician, life-saving drugs, emergency protocols, facility for examining the patient, transport system, etc.

Procedure performed

Vacuum extraction, forceps delivery, lower segment cesarean section (LSCS), emergency hysterectomy, manual removal of placenta, dilation and curettage, laparotomy and blood transfusion.

Child Health Welfare Programmes

Integrated Management of Childhood Illness (Fig. 16.1)

❖ It was launched in 2003 by Ministry of Health and Family Welfare of Government of India.
❖ It had been launched in four selected districts each in Uttaranchal, Madhya Pradesh, Odisha, Rajasthan, Maharashtra, Gujarat, Delhi, Haryana and Tamil Nadu.
❖ Indian version of IMCs has been renamed as integrated management of neonatal and childhood illness (IMNCI).
❖ It is the central pillar of the child health interventions under the RCH II strategy.

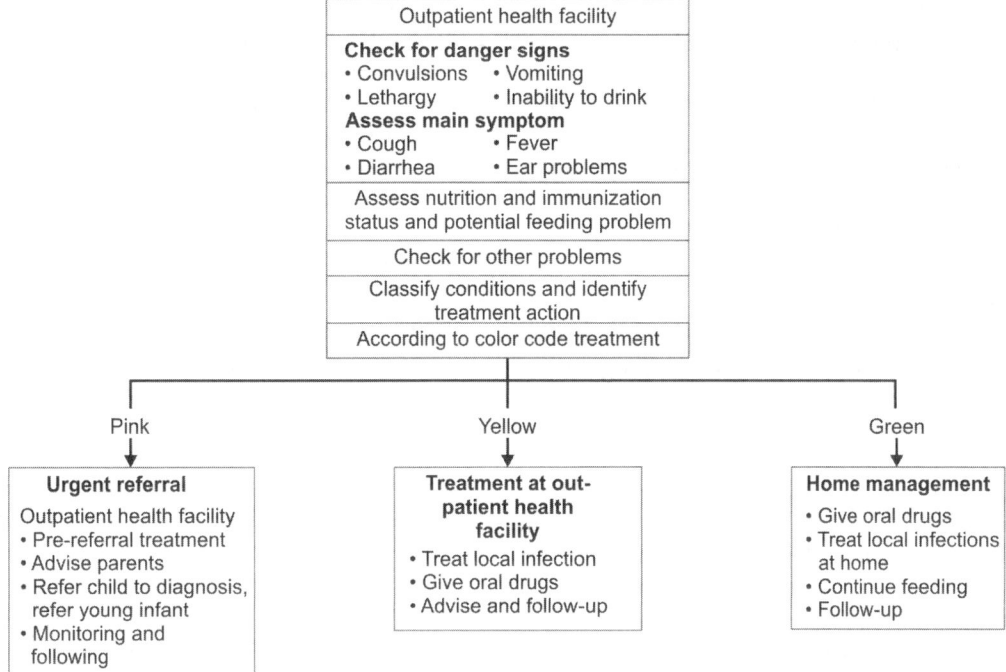

Fig. 16.1: Illustration of integrated management of neonatal and childhood illness management process.

The major highlights of the Indian adaptation are:
- Inclusion of 0–7 days' age in the program.
- Incorporating national guidelines on malaria, anemia, vitamin A supplementation and immunization schedule.
- Training of the health personnel begins with sick young infants up to 2 months.
- Proportion of training time developed to sick young infant and sick child is almost equal.
- It is skill based, and most sick children present with signs and symptoms of more than one of these conditions.

Hence, single diagnosis may not be possible or appropriate, and treatment may be complicated by the need to combine for several conditions. Hence, an integrated approach for managing sick children.

Other Programs

Special nutrition program
- This program was started in 1970 for the nutritional benefit of children below 6 years of age, and pregnant and nursing mothers, and is in operation in urban slums, tribal areas and backward rural areas.
- The supplementary food supplies about 300 kcal and 10–12 g of proteins per child per day.
- The beneficiary mothers receive daily 500 kcal and 25 g of proteins.
- This supplement is provided to them for about 300 days in a year.
- This program was originally launched as a central program and was transferred to the state sector in the five-year plan as part of the minimum needs program.
- The main aim of the special nutrition program is to improve the nutritional status of the target groups.
- Later it was gradually merged with the ICDS program.

1. ICDS program:
- The ICDS program was started in 1975.
- There is a strong nutrition component in this program in the form of supplementary nutrition vitamin A prophylaxis and IFA distribution.
- The beneficiaries are preschool children below 6 years and adolescent girls of 11–18 years, pregnant and lactating mothers.
- Workers at the village level who deliver the services are called AWW. Each anganwadi unit covers a population of about 1,000.
- A network of Mahila Mandal has been built up in ICDS project areas to help AWW in providing health and nutrition services.
- The work of anganwadi is supervised by Mukhya Sevikas, and field supervision is done by the child development project officer (CDPO).

2. Prophylaxis against nutritional anemia:
- In view of its public health importance, a national program for the prevention of nutritional anemia was launched by the Government of India during the fourth five-year plan.
- The program consists of distribution of IFA tablets to pregnant women and young children.
- The MCH centers in urban areas, PHCs in rural areas and ICDS projects are engaged in the implementation of this program.

3. Mid-day meal programme:
- The mid-day meal programme (MDMP) is also known as school lunch program.
- This program has been in operation since 1961 throughout the country.
- The major objective of the program is to attract more children for admission to schools and retain them, so that literacy improvement of children could be brought about.

4. Immunization programme:
- In May 1974, the World Health Organization (WHO) officially launched a global immunization programme known as expanded program on immunization to protect children against six vaccine-preventive diseases.
- The program now called universal immunization started from 1985.
- As per national immunization schedule, the first visit may be made when the infant is 6 weeks old.
- The second and third visits at intervals of 1–2 months.
- Oral polio vaccine may be given concurrently with diphtheria, pertussis and tetanus (DPT). BCG can be given with any of the three doses, but the site for the injection should be different.
- The schedule also covers immunization of women during pregnancy against tetanus.

These are the programs launched by central and state government so as to improve the family and child health services. The services are organized well at all the levels.

ORGANIZATION FOR FAMILY WELFARE SERVICES

The ministry of health and family welfare at the center and states play an important role in the government. The family welfare programme is fully funded by the central government and is implemented through the states. The administration and implementation of this program is done through an integrated structure of health care system. The primary responsibility for the delivery of services rests with the government through its health care system at the center and in the states.

At Center

- The family welfare programme is a centrally sponsored scheme and the states receive 100% assistance from the central government.
- The central government controls the planning financial management of the program (e.g. establishment of clinics' patterns of staffing expenditure).
- Training, research, the evaluation, and most important, the formulation of an overall policy.
- The current policy program is to promote family planning on the basis of voluntary and informed acceptance with full community participation.
- Emphasis is on a two-child family (small family).
- Recently, there have been two major changes in the approach to delivery of family planning services.
- First, a greater emphasis on spacing methods side-by-side with terminal methods, and second, to take the services to every door step and motivate families to adopt the small family norm.

Administrative Apparatus Consists of Three Departments

1. Department of Health
2. Department of Family Welfare
3. Department of Indigenous System of Medicine and Homeopathy

The department of family welfare deals with family welfare matters. The secondary to the Government of India in the ministry of health and family welfare is the overall in-charge of the department of family welfare.

There is an additional secretary and commissioner family welfare for this department. The additional secretary is assisted by a number of senior administrative and technical officers.

Additional secretary and commissioner (FW) supervise the implementation of the program in the state and coordinate the activities of and the functions of the technical division and the secretariat side of the Department of Family Welfare. On the technical side, the following divisions are functioning:

1. Program appraisal coordination and training and sterilization division
2. Technical operation division
3. MCH division
4. Evaluation and intelligence division
5. Mass education and media (including population education) division
6. Nirodh marketing division
7. Transport division
8. Project (area projects) division

On the secretariat side, the following divisions are functioning:

1. Policy division
2. Aided program division
3. An organized sector and voluntary organization division
4. A planned budget division

There are 17 regional offices of health and family welfare functioning under the ministry of health and family welfare located in the state capital, namely Hyderabad, Imphal, Bhubaneshwar, Patna, Chandigarh, Pune, Shimla, Jammu/Srinagar, Bengaluru, Thiruvananthapuram, Bhopal, Jaipur, Kolkata and Chennai covering all the states/UTs.

At State Level

The ministry of health and family welfare department, which has the responsibility of implementing family welfare programmes as planned and directed by the central government.

At present, there are 27 state family welfare bureaus functioning in the country.

- In 1979, the officer of the family welfare and national malaria eradication programmes were merged into one office and named as regional office for health and family welfare.
- These regional officers have been set up to maintain liaison with state governments and give technical assistance to them in connection with the implementation of the family welfare programme and other important health program.
- State level coordination of the family welfare activities between the state government and the central government are family welfare cell has been sanctioned for each state.

At District Level

The setup consists of a district family welfare bureau consisting of three divisions:

- An administrative division headed by the district family welfare officer
- Mass education and media division in-charge of district mass education and media officer
- Evaluation division in-charge of a statistical officer
- These are supported by 1,083 urban family welfare centers (UFWC) and 871 urban health posts.

Presently there are four types of urban health posts:
1. Type A for areas with population 5,000.
2. Type B for areas with population between 5,000 and 50,000.
3. Type C for population between 10,000 and 25,000.
4. Type D for areas with population between 25,000 and 50,000.

Type A, B and C health posts are attached to a hospital for providing referral and supervisory services.

Type D health post is attached to a hospital for sterilization MTP and refer only type D health post, and have a post of medical officer.

Presently, there are three types of UFWC:
1. Type I is for population between 10,000 and 25,000.
2. Type II is for population between 25,000 and 50,000.
3. Type III is for population above 50,000.

These are manned by two paramedical staff in type I and II centers and by six persons including medical officer in type III centers.

The UFWCs and health posts provide comprehensive integrated services of MCH and family planning. The staff pattern is different for different types of health posts and UFWCs.

At Community Health Center

The CHC is established and maintained by the state governments:

1. Presently, it is manned by four medical specialist supported by 21 paramedical and other staff.
2. Apart from the other EmOC, full range of family planning services including laparoscopic services and safe abortion services.

At Primary Health Center

- A rural family welfare center (RFWC) with a medical officer and supporting staff forms an integral part of the PHC
- A total of 5,435 RFWCs were established in the country at all block level PHCs sanctioned
- Medical officers are usually trained to provide MTP and sterilization services. The program of insertion of copper T or intrauterine devices (IUDs) has been intensified. It is intended that laparoscopic services, which have become very popular will be made more widely available at the PHC
- The sub-centers are to provide the main threat of the program. They are responsible for providing rudimentary health and MCH care
- Family planning motivation, supplies and services in spacing methods.

At Village Level

Two schemes are being implemented at the village level to improve the outreach of services and increase local participation.

- Village health guides: They are made responsible for spreading knowledge and information to the eligible couples and providing them with supplies of nirodh and oral pills
- About 3.23 lakh health guides are already in position
- ASHA: About 5.20 lakh have been provided with drug kits. At present, the village health guides, trained dais and ASHAs are the lynchpins of the family planning delivery system in India:
- The public sector provides a wide range of contraceptive services for limiting and spacing of births
- Government of India is promoting "fixed day static services" approach in sterilization services within the public health system with the aim of increasing access to sterilization services
- States are being provided technical and financial support for the development of human resources and upgradation of health facilities for the functioning of FDS
- In the states with high unmet need for limiting methods, sterilization camps will continue till the time FDS is implemented effectively
- Frequency of sterilization services at different health facilities at FDS is as follows:
  - District hospital—weekly
  - Sub-district hospital—weekly
  - CHC/block PHC—fortnightly
  - 24 × 7 PHC/sub-center—monthly.

Family Welfare Services in Urban Areas

Family welfare programme is implemented through the state government setup. The infrastructure division of the department of family welfare looks after the program in respect to urban services in India. It includes the following.

Postpartum Program

- This program was started during the year 1969 in 59 district level hospitals.
- The postpartum program is defined as a maternity-centered hospital-based approach to family welfare programme to motivate women. Within the reproductive age group (15–44 years), their husbands adopt small family norms through education and motivation particularly during prenatal and postnatal period.
- The postpartum centers also function as referral centers for providing MCH and family welfare services.
- At present, only 550 postpartum centers are functioning at the district level.
- Success of the program at the district level encouraged the Government of India to intend the postpartum program to sub-divisional taluka level hospitals as well.
- At present 1,012 sub-district level postpartum centers are functioning under the program.
- Under the postpartum program, a set pattern of inputs in the form of staff equipment construction of a ward and operation theater, etc. are provided.
- The program is 100% centrally assisted and is implemented through state governments. The contribution interns of performance of the postpartum program both at the district level and sub-district levels is quite encouraging.
- Under this program, 19% sterilization and 85% IUD insertion were performed during the year 1999–2000.

PAP Smear Test Facility Program

- For early detection of cervical cancer among women, this program has been approved by the Government of India in 105 medical colleges, which are equipped with a full-fledged department of pathology and services of a senior pathologist, i.e. professor of pathology.
- Under this program, a post of cytotechnician for preparation/examination of slides and contingent expenditure for purchase of glassware and chemicals, etc. have been provided by the Government of India.

Sterilization Bed Scheme

- This scheme was introduced during 1964 by reservation of sterilization beds in government voluntary organization and local body nutrition.
- The purpose of introducing this scheme was to provide facilities for tubectomy operation as the beds for such cases were not readily available in the hospitals.
- Under this scheme, a total of 3,217 beds are functioning at present (as on April 1, 2000).
- A recurring amount of ₹4,500/bed/annum is admissible for maintenance of the sterilization beds to local bodies/voluntary organization and achievement of 60 tubectomies per bed/annum.

Urban Revamping Scheme

- This scheme has been introduced with a view to provide improved service delivery outreach services of PHC, FW and maternity services in urban areas, particularly in slum areas.
- The state governments have established 871 health posts and 10 city family welfare bureaus.
- The city family bureaus are entrusted with the responsibility of coordination, monitoring supervision, etc. of the family welfare services provided by various institutions in the city.

Urban Family Welfare Centers

- The UFWCs have been functioning since 1950 to provide family welfare services in urban areas.
- There are three types of UFWCs based on the population covered by them.
- In all, there are 1,083 urban family centers functioning in the states/UTs as on April 1, 2000.
- These UFWCs will be reorganized into health posts gradually as and when these cities are considered for expansion under the urban revamping scheme.

Family Welfare Service in Rural Areas

The PHC infrastructure has been developed as a tier system and is based on the population norms given in Table 16.4.

Village Health Post

At the village level, village health posts are created, which are manned by village health guides to outreach services to people with their active participation.

- One village health post serves 1,000 people and is manned by one village health guide preferably a woman.
- She/he is responsible for giving information to and motivation of eligible couples, and supply them condom.
- Indigenous dais is another village-level workers, who are trained to conduct safe normal deliveries and motivate mothers for family planning.
- The target is to have one trained dais for 1,000 population. Both these local village-level workers are link between the community people and the village-level health functionaries.

Table 16.4: Infrastructure norms in rural areas.

Center	Population norms	
	Plain area	Hilly/tribal area
Village health post	1,000	1,000
Sub-centers	5,000	3,000
Primary health center	30,000	20,000
Community health center	120,000	80,000

Sub-centers

- Sub-centers are the most peripheral contact point between the PHC system and the community.
- These centers have mainly promotional and educational functions relating to maternal child health family welfare, nutrition, immunization, diarrheal control and control of communicable disease programs.
- The sub-centers are also provided with basic drugs for minor ailments purpose workers (male) and one multipurpose worker (female) ANM.
- Out of a total number of the functioning 137,271 sub-centers, 97,757 sub-centers are funded by the department of family welfare and the remaining are funded by the state government.
- It has been decided during 1997 that the state will have the choice of opening new sub-centers out of the funds provided to them. Under this scheme, there is provision for salary of female health worker/ANM. The salary of male health worker is provided by the state government.

Primary Health Centers

- The PHCs is the first contact point between the village community and the medical officer.
- These are established and maintained by the state government under the MNP/basic minimum services (BMS) program.
- A PHC is manned by a medical officer, health assistant (female and male), health worker (female), ANM, nurse and midwife, block extension educator, pharmacist, lab technician and is supported by 14 paramedical and other staff. It acts as a referral unit for six sub-centers and has 4–6 beds.
- The activities of PHCs involve curative, preventive, promotive and family welfare services. The number of PHCs functioning in the country is 22,975.

Community Health Centers

The CHCs are established and maintained by the state government under MNP/BMS program. It is manned by four medical specialists, i.e. surgeon, physician, gynecologist and pediatrician, seven nurse-midwives, each pharmacist/compound, dresser, lab technician, radiographer and other staff.

It has 30 indoor beds with X-ray, labor room, operation theater and laboratory facilities. It serves as a referral center for four PHCs and also provides facilities for obstetric care, specialized consultations. The number of CHCs functioning at present is 2,935.

Rural Family Welfare Centers

- There are 5,435 RFWCs functioning in the country at present.
- These were established at all the block level PHCs, sanctioned up to April 1, 1980.
- The states have integrated the RFWCs into their PHC system.
- Therefore, there is no separate identity for these RFWCs today. The Government of India, however, continues to provide financial support for maintaining these centers. One assistant surgeon supported by 11 paramedical and other staff operate on RFWCs.

INTERSECTORAL COORDINATION (FIG. 16.2)

The health care system is intended to deliver health care services. It operates in the context of socioeconomic and political framework of the country. In India, it is represented by five major sectors, which differ from each other. These are:
- Public sector
- Private sector
- Indigenous system of medicine
- Voluntary health agencies
- National health programmes

Intersectoral coordination is the basis of PHC. Intersectoral coordination is a crucial component for promotion of intersect, oral linkages, which is required for the effective implementation of health services throughout the country. Intersectoral coordination ensures convergence of basic social services in order to bring all health sector service providers into closer and more responsive working relationships for the benefit of the society. This will enable better equity and wider coverage.

The pulse polio drives have demonstrated that effective mobilization of civil society can achieve remarkable results, hence forging of partnerships with the government departments, NGOs, the corporate sector, trade unions, human rights commission, police, legal bodies, political parties, media and academic institutions will be promoted aggressively.

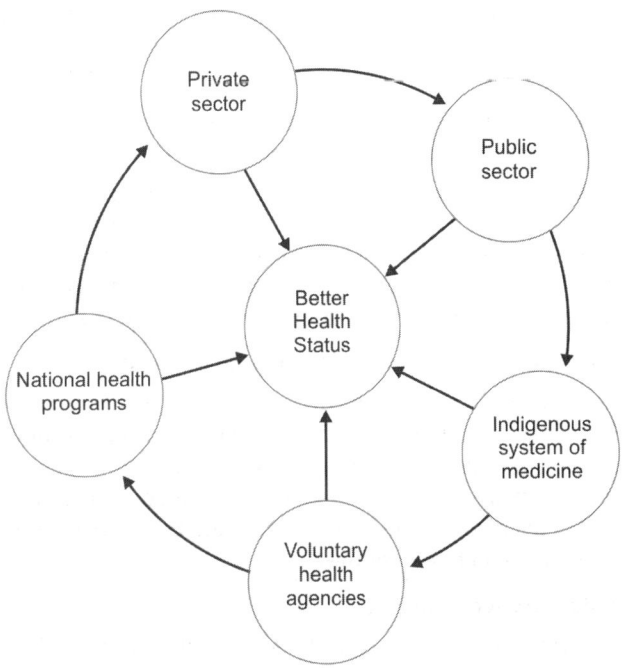

Fig. 16.2: Intersectoral coordination.

Health is not everything, but everything else is nothing without health

All the citizens of the country require enthusiastic and sustained participation in taking responsibility for their own health as well as that of their communities. An integrated multi-sectoral approach is appropriate to ensure coordination between ranges of activities.

Strategy for community participation and intersectoral coordination

The responsibility of seeking community participation and ensuring intersectoral coordination, which have been identified as key factors for the success of any program, can be integrated together. This responsibility can be shouldered by a single committee, which will be headed by the project officer. The community mobilization, coordination units and neighborhood councils will be important components of this committee.

Health care as a priority sector

To encourage increased participation by the private sector in providing secondary and tertiary health care, the government should announce health care as a priority sector and accord it all the benefits that accrue from being accorded a priority sector such as cheaper sources of funding.

Develop intersectoral linkages, especially in primitive and preventive services

There are several factors, which impact on the health of a community such as water, sanitation and sewage disposal. There are several agencies operating at different levels from the central government to the panchayat, operating individually on addressing these issues. There should be a massive effort in health education in the entire country, through school teachers, panchayat members, youth clubs, Mahila Mandals and health workers to help people inculcate a more rational and scientific understanding of health.

Develop intersectoral linkages in meeting finance and manpower requirements

India, considering its diversity, cannot have a single solution across the country. Our country would need a host of financing mechanisms to improve our health infrastructure. They have initiated schemes to encourage private sources of finance to augment constrained government spending.

Multiple financing options to provide for health care

The current system of individual spending should migrate to collective spending on health care. The government should facilitate this migration though introducing multiple health care financing schemes targeted at different socioeconomic segments of the population. This should be through a mix of private and public sources.

Voluntary sector in PHC

The voluntary sector should be involved in providing primary health care in a more effective manner, particularly in the neediest areas. A special fund such as center for advancement of people's action and rural technology (CAPART) should be set aside for this purpose.

Enhanced private sector participation for increased coverage

The government should enlist private providers to deliver preventive care through local delivery channels for specific preventive and primitive services. This would enhance the reach of the health delivery system and also reduce the need for extensive infrastructure to be established by the government.

Separate purchase and delivery functions

The government plays the roles of financier, purchaser and provider. These functions should be separated and the government should allow private providers to cover these roles in conjunction with the government agencies in providing better health services to the people.

Advantages of intersectoral coordination

- To provide sustainable basic health services to the community and to integrate these services with other health services provided by other health sectors
- Early detection, treatment of patients within the community itself
- To promote cooperation and mutual understanding among various sectors
- To take pressure off the one sector alone
- For attaining the goal such as health for all
- To make the services available to people with early and easy access.

Nongovernmental Agencies

Nongovernmental agencies arose because there was an unmet health need. They are the organizations that are formed by groups of people because of their interest in a particular health concern, such as diabetes, child abuse or environmental pollution. Voluntary agencies are funded by donations. They are accountable to their supporters and their activities are determined by supporter's interest, rather than legal proceedings.

Nongovernmental health agencies are of five types:
1. Voluntary agencies
2. Professional agencies
3. Philanthropic agencies
4. Service, social and religious organizations
5. Corporate agencies.

Voluntary Agencies

Voluntary agencies play an important role in research and education, although they may provide a few direct health services. In the field of health, their role is in promotion of health, creation of awareness among people about various measures to prevent illness and provision of welfare services for victims of different types of diseases.

Since official efforts alone are not sufficient to meet the health needs of the country, it is essential to have voluntary agencies to support and guard the work of official agencies. Indian Red Cross Society, Hind Kusht Nivaran Sangh, Indian Council for Child Welfare, Tuberculosis Association of India, Bharat Sewak Samaj, Central Social Welfare Board, Kasturba Memorial Fund, Family Planning Association of India, All India Women's Conferences and The All India Blind Relief Society are all the examples of voluntary agencies.

Role of voluntary agencies: They perform eight basic functions within the scientific health care subsystem:

1. **Pioneering:** Voluntary agencies explore areas that are underserved by the other components of the healthcare system, e.g., research that culminated in the development of a vaccine was the early focus of the March of Dimes. And now, polio immunization is largely a function of official agencies.
2. **Demonstration of pilot projects:** In health care delivery.
3. **Education:** Educating public and health professionals is the function of voluntary agencies.
4. **Supplementation:** This service is provided by the official health agencies. For instance, some voluntary health agencies provide transportation to clinics, despite care, special equipment and other services.
5. **Advocacy for public interests:** They advocate for the public health, e.g. a voluntary health agency may campaign against reduction of health care services due to budget cuts.
6. **Legislation:** Promoting legislation related to health is a closely related function.
7. **Health planning and organization:** Voluntary agencies often assist official agencies in determining health care needs in the population and in planning programs to address those needs.
8. **Assisting official agencies:** Voluntary agencies assist official agencies in developing well-balanced community health programs, e.g. voluntary agencies often provide services that fill gaps in services available from official agencies.

Professional Health Organizations

Professional agencies are made of health professionals who have completed specialized education and have met the standards of registration, licensure for their respective fields, e.g. American Nurse Association, INC, PNRC, etc.

Role of professional agencies

- Promoting high standards of professional practice for their specific profession, thus improving health of society.
- Certification of continuing education programs for professional renewal.
- Lobbying, e.g. INC has a powerful lobby nationally. Their purpose is to affect legislation in such a way as to benefit their membership and their profession.

Philanthropic Foundations

These foundations support community health throughout the world by funding programs and research on the prevention, control and treatment of many diseases, e.g. Rockefeller foundation funds, the international health projects. The development of vaccine for yellow fever by a scientist funded by the Rockefeller foundation is an example of one such long-range project.

Other such foundations are:
- Commonwealth fund (contributes to community health in rural communities)
- Ford Foundation (contributes to family planning efforts throughout the world).

Service, Social and Religious Organizations

The religious organizations play an important role in community health, e.g. rotary clubs, lions club, etc.

- Members enjoy social interactions with people of similar interests in addition to fulfilling the needs of communities
- Though their specific mission is not health, they make important contributions in that direction by raising money and funding health-related problems
- Religious groups donate money for missions. It should be noted that some religious groups have hindered the work of community health workers
- Almost every community in the country can provide an example where a religious organization has protected the offering of a school sex education program.

Corporate Agencies

Corporate agencies support health-related programs both at and away from the worksite. Worksite programmers aimed at trimming employee medical bills. Away worksite, the activities go beyond traditional sponsorship of youth and may include community health fairs, screening programmers for specific health problems.

CONCLUSION

National family welfare programme is executing vital role in promotion of family planning methods, thereby promoting women's health and child care services are being rendered at central levels, state level and district level; highly specialized care is provided at the tertiary level; referral services are provided at the state level and basic health service are provided at district level. In this way national family welfare programme is organizing well with adequate health man power for effective implementation of services.

17 Information, Education and Communication in Healthcare Delivery

CHAPTER OUTLINE

- Objectives of Information, Education and Communication
- Principles to Follow in Planning Information, Education and Communication Initiative
- Advantages
- Information, Education and Communication Tools
- Importance of Information, Education and Communication
- Training
- Need of Information, Education and Communication Specific Areas
- Gender Considerations

INTRODUCTION

Information, education and communication (IEC) was commissioned by the Department of Reproductive Health and Research at the World Health Organization (WHO) to examine lessons learned from more than two decades of experience in applying IEC interventions in support of public health. It represents an attempt to gather and synthesize experiences in IEC for public health and to succinctly analyze and share these experiences so that IEC can be effectively integrated into and support improved reproductive health programs and service delivery. This effort is intended to serve as an orientation or a "tour d'horizon," to future IEC work as educators, practitioners, policy-makers and communication specialists in all aspects of public health strive to build upon past experience in enabling people to affect more healthy behaviors.

DEFINITION OF INFORMATION, EDUCATION AND COMMUNICATION

The IEC initiatives are grounded in the concepts of prevention and primary health care. Largely concerned with individual behavior change or reinforcement and/or changes in social or community norms, public health education and communication seek to empower people vis-à-vis their health actions and to garner social and political support for those actions.

IEC can be defined as an approach, which attempts to change or reinforce a set of behaviors in a "target audience" regarding a specific problem in a predefined period of time. It is multidisciplinary and client-centered in its approach, drawing from the fields of diffusion theory, social marketing, behavior analysis, anthropology and instructive design.

OBJECTIVES OF INFORMATION, EDUCATION AND COMMUNICATION

- ❖ Have a clear objective (the specific behavior to change or reinforce)
- ❖ Target a specific audience, e.g. mothers of children below 5 years old
- ❖ Address a specific problem (e.g. offering increased fluids and continuing feeding a child with diarrhea) rather than attempt to change many problems at the same time
- ❖ Set a time frame within which results change in behavior or expected to occur
- ❖ The problem must be well-defined in IEC intervention to address.

PRINCIPLES TO FOLLOW IN PLANNING INFORMATION, EDUCATION AND COMMUNICATION INITIATIVE

The development of a poster without the following elements would not be a structured IEC initiative:
- ❖ Audience analysis
- ❖ Testing
- ❖ Plan with objectives
- ❖ Indicators and targets
- ❖ Clear target audience
- ❖ Distribution plan with follow-up
- ❖ Regular feedback through monitoring a formal evaluation.

ADVANTAGES

- Outcome oriented
- Use resources more efficiently
- Learn important lessons for the future from this experience.

INFORMATION, EDUCATION AND COMMUNICATION TOOLS

Countries often develop posters, flyers, leaflets, brochures, booklets, messages for health education sessions, logos and symbols on specific topics, radio broadcast or television spots, stories of materials, video cassette players, other materials, etc. as a means of promoting desired, positive behaviors in the community.

IMPORTANCE OF INFORMATION, EDUCATION AND COMMUNICATION

- It creates awareness, increases knowledge, changes attitudes and moves people to change or continue their behavior or to adopt an innovation
- To make a lasting change in one individual, the key influential must be identified and encouraged to support these changes
- Mass media helps to create an agenda for public debate. It reaches many people and is not that expensive. However, to be effective, mass media must be supported by interpersonal and group communication
- Communication channels should ensure availability of feedback mechanisms. This is important for reinforcement and for clarifying questions and issues
- Personal testimonies of affected people are far more compelling than any other form of communication. Fear arousal is seldom effective
- A mass communication program dealing with sensitive issues socially validates open discussion of these issues, thus making them a part of the everyday agenda
- A communication campaign to be successful, the relevant social services infrastructure should be prepared to satisfy the increased demand for services created by the campaign
- An important element in a health communication campaign is an adequate blend of entertainment and social messages
- Resources need to be devoted to producing salient materials in sufficient quantity, in establishing a workable distribution and reordering system and to show service providers how to use materials.

The IEC strategies involve planning, implementation, monitoring and evaluation. When carefully carried out, health communication strategies help to foster positive health practices individually and institutionally and can contribute to sustainable change toward healthy behavior.

Planning a Strategy

- The IEC succeeds when it is planned with a comprehensive strategy. This means having clearly articulated objectives, keeping the client at the center of what is being designed, conducting appropriate research, undertaking audience segmentation, carefully crafting and testing messages, knowing and using appropriate channel choices and planning for monitoring and feedback.
- Particularly in the case of reproductive health initiatives, it is important to know and incorporate community traditions (e.g. disposal of placenta, respecting preferred birth position), and to "follow the community at its own rhythm." Communities will test and credibility takes time.
- Much can be achieved through a comprehensive IEC intervention, which emphasizes long-term capacity building at the grassroots level. In this respect, the community is vital; it is not simply a message channel or a passive recipient of services or information.
- The IEC issues overlap with related issues of service delivery, quality of services, community participation and so on. There must be a true dialogue around a wide range of issues relevant to public health during the planning stage.
- Changing behavior is not an easy or quick task. An ideal campaign is sustained over time to foster changes in social and behavioral norms.
- It is important to remember that everything cannot be changed at once. Also, it is important to focus on what is relevant or irrelevant, and consider not only information, but also the "knowledge–behavior gap."
- The IEC interventions are more cost-effective when there are clear links with health care service delivery programs rather than when they are conceived as stand-alone IEC projects. From a communication perspective, this makes vital the quality of client–provider contact. Provider behaviors require monitoring, reinforcement and updating. The lack of a supportive environment from the health care provider is also a factor that can hinder individual behavior change.
- People learn new behaviors best when they are learning something. They feel it is useful when they can put into practice what they are learning, and when they receive feedback and are rewarded for doing well. Modeling is often the best way to teach complex behaviors.
- More effective campaigns combine mass media with community, small group and individual activities, and are supported by an existing community structure.
- Campaigns for preventive behavior are more effective, if they emphasize positive behavior change rather than the negative consequences of current behavior. Fear arousal as a campaign strategy needs to be used with caution. It is rarely successful as a long-term campaign strategy.

- The timing of a campaign helps to determine its effectiveness. For example, in diarrheal disease campaigns, seasonality is an important consideration since diarrheal disease often occurs in the rainy season.
- If more than one set of messages is being delivered via an umbrella campaign (e.g. several issues are being covered under one unifying theme), phasing of messages might be important to avoid information overload.

Implementing a Strategy

- Support of community leaders, public opinion leaders and decision-makers can lead to stronger results. The use of such identifiable and credible sources of information can enhance the success of an IEC initiative.
- Actively involving the target audience in the design, implementation and monitoring of a project is critical. Listen to local language, custom and experience. Negotiate the relevance of an intervention with the audience. Make sure the intervention addresses reality "on the ground."
- Establish linkages and relationships with, and actively involve, traditional healers, local nongovernmental organizations (NGOs) and local support groups, and recognize the important role each plays. Share information with them.
- The interaction between health care providers (at all levels) and clients is important for successful IEC interventions. This is where one stage of decision-making takes place. Provider behavior is critical and the need for behavior and attitude change among health workers has been established (physician resistance to change, as well as punitive actions by all other levels of health worker, is well documented). Training in interpersonal communication and counseling skills is absolutely critical to successful programing.
- Multimedia campaigns are most effective when mass media and popular traditional channels are used in combination with person-to-person interactions. There is less power in stand-alone multimedia campaigns than in campaigns that link the power of media and the power of individual persuasion with service delivery.
- A media campaign should use diverse broadcast and distribution channels, combining television, radio, print and traditional media, in order to maximize penetration and impact. More attention needs to be focused on the mix of channels used in a given situation. Achieving "reach and frequency" in communications takes careful research and planning.
- Decisions about media channels and frequency and intensity of broadcast or distribution should be closely tied to initial and ongoing research with the target population.
- Take advantage of local holidays and festivals to disseminate messages or for inaugural events.
- The IEC interventions cost money to implement and to sustain over time. There is an imbalance between expectations about what IEC can do and the resources allocated to carry out those interventions. It is important to realize that change within 5% of a designated population represents good progress. Remember, even Coca-Cola never stops promoting its product.
- IEC materials are more widely distributed when their distribution system is combined with relevant health commodities (e.g. distribution of contraceptive commodities simultaneously with posters for family planning).
- Distribution of print materials may occur more effectively, if contracted out to the private sector. The failure to plan for implementation and maintaining distribution systems is often a major failure of IEC efforts.

Monitoring and Evaluating a Strategy

- Monitoring has been neglected as a tool for understanding operational dynamics and for detecting what works and what does not. Inexpensive methods for monitoring can be used and should be explored (e.g., observation).
- Documentation of program inputs and implementation experiences is important for understanding successes and failures. Methods for doing this should be institutionalized as part of management information systems.
- Evaluation of IEC efforts is a complex task and should be considered from the very beginning, when projects are being planned and not just after they are underway or completed. Involving specialists in research design and evaluation can ensure that process and impact evaluations are valid and reliable.
- There is a need for extreme specificity in questions asked in an evaluation, especially in countries where multiple interventions have been carried out. Carefully constructed questions are very important. In designing questions, messages must be carefully analyzed so that primary messages (e.g. breast is best) are distinguished from secondary messages (e.g. promotion of weaning practices).
- The research and evaluation team should be given an opportunity to fully understand the project. The stronger the understanding between program staff and researchers, the better the product.
- Evaluation should be considered a learning tool by program staff and should be embraced as a resource for program redesign.
- An evaluation framework should be responsive to program needs and should feed information and data back to program staff to allow for corrections

and adjustments to program components during implementation. Evaluation should not impede implementation. As one evaluation expert put it, "one will rarely have evidence that is incontrovertible; nonetheless, one still need to act sensibly on the best evidence ever had."

❖ Recognizing that research and evaluation designs may have limitations and factoring in those limitations when assessing the effectiveness of program strategies can contribute to more successful outcomes.

TRAINING

❖ Provided with relevant training, non-IEC professionals can coordinate the development of good quality IEC materials and approaches. In order for training to be relevant, it must take into account the role and job description of the people being trained. People should not be trained just for the sake of training. All training designs should be seriously deliberated and individualized in order to meet the needs of the program and of those being trained.

❖ People need training in materials use and distribution as well as materials development.
Phased training, focusing first on skill building and then on skill transfer, is a successful model. It allows trainees to practice their new techniques counseling before actually becoming trainers of others in the same skill area. This enhances overall program sustainability. A competency-based approach for training is most effective at building skills.

❖ Training should be curriculum-based and apply the principles of adult education.

❖ Similar to other program components, training should be evaluated and those who are being trained should be involved in developing the curriculum.

❖ Even when trained, people have difficulty in discussing personal matters (such as sex) with others. IEC training needs to address this problem and provide specific techniques for opening dialog and moving it forward. It must also address the need for health care workers to come to grips with their own behavioral and cultural biases. For example: Can a midwife act against female genital mutilation in a believable way, if it has been done to her and she has allowed it to be done to her daughters?

❖ There is a pressing need for training in IEC techniques that effectively motivate people to express their genuine desires relating to reproductive health. Similarly, training design needs to take into account the desires of trainees and/or providers as well.

❖ It is most effective if the number of levels of trainers is kept to a minimum. That is, instead of having different trainers for each level (i.e. province, county, township, village, etc.), have perhaps two levels of trainers responsible for all training activities. The fewer the number of levels, the less opportunity for important content to be lost during training of trainers' workshops.

❖ Ensure that appropriate training materials are available for community-level workers. This includes budget considerations to assure funding so that adequate materials reach all levels, not just those at the higher levels.

❖ Include leaders and managers in the program or establish a parallel program for them to ensure they understand the importance of interpersonal communication work and will support it in future.

❖ A client-centered approach to training can have dramatic results in terms of service delivery. A consumer perspective requires that health workers understand the clients' circumstances, that they seek solutions to problems in collaboration with the client and that they are systematic about follow-up.

❖ Well-designed and tested training modules can serve as reference points for national and local training programs. In designing materials for widespread use or for local adaptation, three strategies can help assure relevance and widespread use—involving a wide range of potential user organizations in identifying needs and issues involving them in pretesting the materials in their respective programs and involving them in the translation and publication of materials.

❖ Incorporate interpersonal communication principles and skill training in regular, pre- and in-service training programs.

❖ Include in any training curricula, sessions on how to conduct audience research and how to use the results to adapt training materials for use at different levels.

❖ Include as many posters, models and other teaching aids as possible in training programs to supplement curricula and training materials.

❖ Schedule follow-up or refresher training.

❖ Be sure that clearly articulated job descriptions with realistic expectations are reviewed regularly and that supervision is ongoing.

NEED OF INFORMATION, EDUCATION AND COMMUNICATION SPECIFIC AREAS

❖ Peer education, support groups, counseling and interpersonal communication are important components of a reproductive health program.

❖ Counseling is a client-centered interactive communication process in which one person (usually trained) helps others make free, informed decisions about their personal behavior.

❖ Interpersonal communication is a broad term for person-to-person interaction and mutual understanding. It implies trust, support and frequent negotiation, and it is an extremely important part of any communication strategy.

GENDER CONSIDERATIONS

- ❖ ***Women's concern:*** Across all sectors of development is the importance of incorporating a gender perspective in program planning and policy-making. This lesson is also profoundly important in the spheres of reproductive health and IEC. Listening to women, including them in planning, implementation and decision-making, and validating the reality of their daily lives are all facets of a successful intervention.
- ❖ ***Family planning counseling:*** Issues of human sexuality, family planning and child spacing, conception, abortion, childbirth practices, obstetric events and so on are sensitive, private matters. Women need to feel that their attitudes, values, experiences and beliefs are respected.
- ❖ ***Men as partners:*** Reproductive health programs have increasingly understood that men's support and participation are essential to the ultimate success of any reproductive health initiative. Men need to be addressed in three specific roles—as individuals/partners, as community leaders and as government leaders. Thus, the term "men as partners" seems more appropriate than "male involvement" or "male responsibility" when discussing the importance of including men in reproductive health initiatives.
- ❖ ***Youth as an audience:*** Reproductive health projects for youth can be controversial. Parents, policy-makers, religious groups and other influentials often fear that by openly discussing sexuality and family planning, and by providing services, such projects foster premarital sex.
- ❖ Changing adolescent behavior requires intensive, long-term program efforts that incorporate a mix of media along with interpersonal communication and counseling. Guidance and facilitation help to keep youth focused on critical issues.
- ❖ ***Negotiation/life skills:*** Development of life skills is an important concept in promoting healthy behavior generally, and specifically with respect to reproductive health.

CONCLUSION

Information, education and communication are important components of any health care system in delivery of health services to the individuals, community and society. IEC materials are very good means of dissemination of knowledge to the population. At central and state operational system is developing IEC activities for health care personnel to provide health education to the public. WHO and reproductive welfare department is taking major steps in formulation and distribution of IEC materials to the community.

18 CHAPTER

Telemedicine/Telenursing

CHAPTER OUTLINE

- History
- Electronic Health and Telehealth
- Applications in Different Forms
- Types of Telemedicine
- Benefits and Uses of Telemedicine
- First Interactive Telemedicine System
- Specialties
- Telemedicine in India
- Telenursing

INTRODUCTION

Telemedicine is a rapidly developing application of clinical medicine where medical information is transferred through the phone or the Internet and sometimes other networks for the purpose of consulting and sometimes remote medical procedures or examinations.

Telemedicine may be as simple as two health professionals discussing a case over the telephone or as complex as using satellite technology and videoconferencing equipment to conduct a real-time consultation between medical specialists in two different countries.

DEFINITION

The term "telemedicine" has been derived from the Greek word "tele" meaning "at a distance," and "medicine," which is from the Latin word "mederi" meaning "healing." Time magazine called Telemedicine—healing by wire. Though initially considered futuristic and experimental, telemedicine is today a reality and has come to stay. This phrase was first coined in the 1970s by Thomas Bird.

Telemedicine generally refers to the use of communications and information technologies for the delivery of clinical care.

Telemedicine can be defined as the use of modern information technology, especially two-way interactive audio/video telecommunications, computers and telemetry to deliver health services to remote patients and to facilitate information exchange between primary care physicians and specialists at some distance from each other (telemedicine—theory and practice).

HISTORY

Care at a distance (also called absentia care) is an old practice, which was often conducted via post; there has been a long and successful history of absentia health care, which, thanks to modern communication technology, has metamorphosed into what we know as modern telemedicine.

In its early manifestations, African villagers used smoke signals to warn people to stay away from the village in case of serious disease. In the early 1900s, people living in remote areas in Australia used two-way radios, powered by a dynamo-driven set of bicycle pedals, to communicate with the Royal Flying Doctor Service of Australia. The idea of performing medical examinations and evaluations through the telecommunication network is not new. Shortly after the invention of the telephone, attempts were made to transmit heart and lung sounds to a trained expert who could assess the state of the organs. However, poor transmission systems made the attempts a failure.

Electrocardiography (ECG) Transmission (1906)

Einthoven, the father of ECG, first investigated an ECG transmission over telephone lines in 1906. He wrote an article "Le tele cardiograms at the Archives International Physiologies 4:132;1906."

Help for Ships (1920)

Telemedicine dates back to the 1920s. During this time, radios were used to link physicians standing watch at shore stations to assist ships at sea that had medical emergencies.

Telecare (1924)

The first exposition of telecare perhaps was the cover showed below of "Radio News" magazine from April 1924. The article even includes a spoof electronic circuit diagram, which combined all the gadgets of the day into this latest marvel.

Telepsychiatry (1955)

The Nebraska Psychiatric Institute was one of the first facilities in the country to have closed-circuit television in 1955. In 1971, the Nebraska Medical Center was linked with the Omaha Veterans Administration Hospital and veterans administration (VA) facilities in two other towns.

Massachusetts General Hospital (1967)

This station was established in 1967 to provide occupational health services to airport employees and to deliver emergency care and medical attention to travelers.

Satellite Telemedicine (1970)

Satellite telemedicine via ATS-6 satellites. In these projects, paramedics in remote Alaskan and Canadian villages were linked with hospitals in distant towns or cities.

Japan (1971)

First time implemented in two areas—Nakatsu-mura and Kozagawa-cho, Wakayama—using telephone line for voice and fax transmission and community antenna television (CATV) system for image transmission.

Japan (1972) between Aomori Teishin Hospital and Tokyo Teishin

Hospital over 4 MHz television channel and several telephone lines. Other systems came up for teleradiology in several places in Japan, such as Nagasaki, Tokai, etc.

ELECTRONIC HEALTH AND TELEHEALTH

Electronic health (e-health) and telehealth are at times wrongly interchanged with telemedicine. Similar to the terms "medicine" and "health care," telemedicine often refers only to the provision of clinical services, while the term telehealth can refer to clinical and non-clinical services such as medical education, administration and research. The term e-health is often used particularly in the United Kingdom (UK) and Europe, used as an umbrella term that includes telehealth, electronic medical records and other components of health information technology.

APPLICATIONS IN DIFFERENT FORMS

- Information exchange between hospitals and physicians
- Networking of group of hospitals and research centers
- Linking rural health clinics to a central hospital
- Videoconferencing between a patient and doctor, and among members of healthcare teams
- Training of health care professionals in widely distributed or remote clinical settings
- Instant access to medical knowledge base, technical papers, etc.

TYPES OF TELEMEDICINE

Telemedicine can be broken into three main categories, i.e. store-and-forward, remote monitoring and interactive services.

Store-and-Forward Telemedicine (Asynchronous)

It involves acquiring medical data (e.g. medical images, bio-signals, etc.) and then transmitting these data to a doctor or medical specialist at a convenient time for offline assessment. It does not require the presence of both parties at the same time. Dermatology (teledermatology), radiology and pathology are common specialties that are conducive to asynchronous telemedicine. A properly structured medical record preferably in electronic form should be a component of this transfer. A key difference between traditional in-person patient meetings and telemedicine encounters is the omission of an actual physical examination and history. The store-and-forward process requires the clinician to rely on history report and audio/video information in lieu of a physical examination.

Remote Monitoring

Remote monitoring, also known as self-monitoring/testing, enables medical professionals to monitor a patient remotely using various technological devices. This method is primarily used for managing chronic diseases or specific conditions, such as heart disease, diabetes mellitus or asthma. These services can provide comparable health outcomes to traditional in-person patient encounters, supply greater satisfaction to patients and may be cost effective.

Interactive Telemedicine Services (Synchronous)

Interactive telemedicine services provide real-time interactions between patient and provider, to include phone conversations, online communication and home visits. Many activities such as history review, physical examination, psychiatric evaluations and ophthalmology assessments can be conducted comparably to those done in traditional face-to-face visits. In addition, "clinician-interactive" telemedicine services may be less costly than in-person clinical visits.

BENEFITS AND USES OF TELEMEDICINE

- Telemedicine is most beneficial for populations living in isolated communities and remote regions and is currently being applied in virtually all medical domains

- Telemedicine is also useful as a communication tool between a general practitioner and a specialist available at a remote location
- Video consultations from a rural clinic to a specialist can aggravate prohibitive travel and associated costs for patients
- Videoconferencing also opens up new possibilities for continuing education or training for isolated or rural health practitioners, who may not be able to leave a rural practice to take part in professional meetings or educational opportunities.

FIRST INTERACTIVE TELEMEDICINE SYSTEM

- Operating over standard telephone lines, for remotely diagnosing and treating patients requiring cardiac resuscitation (defibrillation) was developed and marketed by MedPhone Corporation in 1989 under the leadership of its president and founder, S Eric Wachtel. A year later, the company introduced a mobile cellular version, the MDphone. Nearly 12 hospitals in the United States (US) served as receiving and treatment.
- Monitoring a patient at home using known devices like blood pressure (BP) monitors.
- Transferring the information to a caregiver is a fast-growing emerging service. These remote monitoring solutions have a focus on current high morbidity chronic diseases and are mainly deployed for the First World.
- In developing countries, a new way of practicing telemedicine is emerging better known primary remote diagnostic visits whereby a doctor uses devices to remotely examine and treat a patient. This new technology and principle of practicing medicine holds big promises to solving major health care delivery problems, for instance Southern Africa, because of primary remote diagnostic consultations not only monitors an already diagnosed chronic disease, but has the promise to diagnosing and managing the disease telecardiology.

ECG can be transmitted using telephone and wireless. Einthoven, the inventor of the ECG, actually did tests with transmission of ECG through telephone lines. This was because the hospital did not allow him to move patients outside the hospital to his laboratory for testing of his new device. In 1906, Einthoven came up with a way to transmit the data from the hospital directly to his laboratory.

TELETRANSMISSION OF ECG USING INDIGENOUS METHODS

One of the oldest known telecardiology system (teletransmission of ECG) was established in Gwalior, India in 1975 at GR Medical College by Ajai Shanker, Makhija S, Mantri PK using indigenous technique for the first time in India:

- This system enabled wireless transmission of ECG from the moving intensive care unit (ICU) van or the patient's home to the central station in ICU of the Department of Medicine. Transmission using wireless was done using frequency modulation, which eliminated noise. Transmission was also done through telephone lines. The ECG output was connected to the telephone input using a modulator, which converted ECG into high-frequency sound. At the other end, a demodulator reconverted the sound into ECG with a good gain accuracy. The ECG was converted to sound waves with a frequency varying from 500 to 2,500 Hz with 1,500 Hz at baseline.
- This system was also used to monitor patients with pacemakers in remote areas. The central control unit at the ICU was able to correctly interpret arrhythmia. This technique helped medical aid reach in remote areas. In addition, electronic stethoscopes can be used as recording devices, which is helpful for the purposes of telecardiology.

TELERADIOLOGY

Teleradiology is the ability to send radiographic images (X-rays) from one location to another. For this process to be implemented, three essential components are required, an image sending station, a transmission network and a receiving/image review station. The most typical implementation are two computers connected via Internet. The computer at the receiving end will need to have a high-quality display screen that has been tested and cleared for clinical purposes. Sometimes, the receiving computer will have a printer so that images can be printed for convenience.

The teleradiology process begins at the image sending station. The radiographic image and a modem or other connection is required for this first step. The image is scanned and then sent via the network connection to the receiving computer.

SPECIALTIES

Telemedicine covers a growing number of medical specialties such as homecare, emergency care, surgery, dermatology, psychiatry, oncology, pathology, ophthalmology, hematology, ear, nose and throat (ENT), nephrology, prehospital care, etc.

Growth of Telemedicine Applications

- 2001: Teleradiology—still images
- 2002: Telecardiology—moving images
- 2003: Telepathology and Teleophthalmology
- 2004: Teleoncology and Telesurgery
- 2005: Mobile telehealth—augmentation
- 2006: Telemedicine for primary health care

TELEMEDICINE IN INDIA (FIGS. 18.1 AND 18.2)

1. **Existing system limited only to private hospital:**
   - Apollo Group of Hospitals
   - RN Tagore Cardiac Hospital, Kolkata (Asia Heart Foundation)
   - No Telemedicine system for public health care
2. **Corporate sectors offering telemedicine systems:**
   - Apollo Group
   - Online Telemedicine System, Ahmedabad
   - Wipro GE
   - Siemens.

Telemedicine technology evolution in India:
- Point-to-point
- Point-to-multipoint
- Multipoint-to-multipoint
- Tele-education.

Data:
- Data related to a patient's personal information
- Data related to a patient's medical information
- Data for patient management in telemedicine
- Data related to the doctors
- Data for system management.

Personnel involved:
- Referral end:
  - A group of specialist doctors
  - System administrator
  - Studio technician
- Nodal end:
  - A group of general physicians
  - System administrator
  - Data entry operator
  - Studio technician
  - Patients
- Patient's personal information:
  - Patient identification
  - Name
  - Age
  - Sex
- Patient's medical information:
  - Textual
  - Plain text
  - Structured document
  - Image
  - Graphics
  - Video
  - Vector
- Data related to the doctors:
  - Doctor's personal information
  - Unique identification key
- Data for system management:
  - Users list
  - Password file
  - Log files.

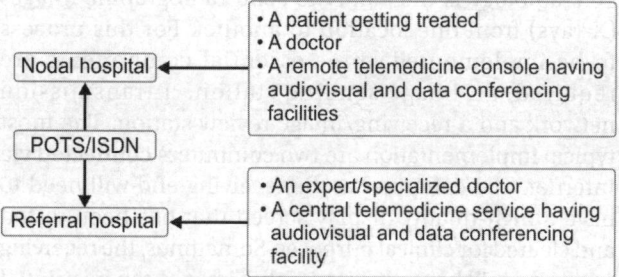

Fig. 18.1: Requirement specification.

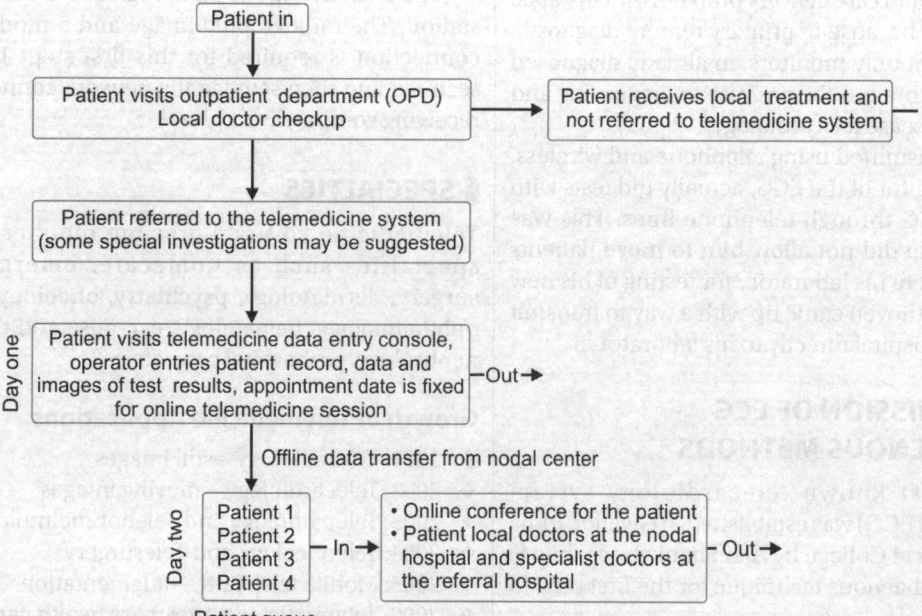

Fig. 18.2: Sequence of operation.

TELENURSING

Telenursing refers to the use of telecommunications and information technology for providing nursing services in health care whenever a large physical distance exists between patient and nurse or between any number of nurses. As a field, it is part of telehealth and has many points of contacts with other medical and non-medical applications, such as telediagnosis, teleconsultation, telemonitoring, etc.

Definition

- Telenursing means a telephonic communication between a patient and health care professionals, wherein the health care professionals' primary function is to provide the patient telephonic responses to patient's question regarding his/her or family members' medical care and treatment.
- Telenursing, the practice of nursing by telecommunication, is a new phenomenon. Nursing faculty is teaching via satellite to distant campuses. In some areas, nurses are practicing from their offices to patients' home through the use of camera and computer technologies.
- Telenursing is also being practiced across the state lines. The nurse on the hot line in one area may be advising client in another area or faculty members may be teaching students in any other area of the country. States require nurses to be licensed, where they are providing care. This model allows states to set and enforce standards to protect their citizens.
- Portable telemedicine units use a regular telephone line and are activated by the patient and nurse pushing one button simultaneously. The unit allows direct viewing of patients' measurement of BP and telephonic stethoscope for auscultation of heart and lung sounds.
- Telemedicine system consists of number of technologies such as audiovisual two-way interactive system, computer for storing and recording images, monitors to view and transmission over telephone lines. These systems are interfaced with the diagnostic tool depending on the purpose of the system. Such equipment has included ECGs, internally advanced scopes, cardiac monitors, BP and electronic stethoscopes.
- By watching the video screen at the central station, the nurse can assess the patient's mood and alertness and several neurologic functions. This more sophisticated unit can zoom close-up pictures of the patients and store these in medical records. When using this technology for chronic conditions, there is an increase in effective and efficient nurse–patient interactions, a reduction in unnecessary emergency department visits and a decrease in repeated hospitalization.

Advantages

- Increases accessibility to health care for patients in isolated areas or with transportation difficulties
- Decreased cost for the patient and health care system
- Decreases professional isolation
- Offers role expansion for advanced practice nurses (APNs) and home care nurses
- Provides an invaluable consultation resource, a monitoring device
- Means to provide an immediate feedback to anxious patients and their families.

CONCLUSION

Telemedicine will soon be just another way to see a health care professional, just as seeing friends and family, while talking to them on the phone is becoming commonplace. Technology manufacturers and telecommunication companies are already vying with each other to produce the low-cost equipment needed. Distance education is commonplace and most educational institutions and many companies allay travel costs for meetings by using video. Ten to fifteen years ago, we had no idea we would rely heavily on faxes, answering machines and e-mail, tools, which are now low-technology and taken for granted. Since the early 2000s, the ramifications of e-health—a general term encompassing health care delivery, administration and information dissemination and its relationship to telemedicine—are being analyzed.

SUGGESTED READING

1. Ann Marrinner-Tomey. Nursing Theorists and Their Work, 3rd edition. Toronto; Mosby Publications; 2009.
2. Basavantappa BT. Community Health Nursing (Vol. 2), 20th edition. New Delhi: Jaypee Brothers Publications; 2005. pp. 317, 333.
3. Decker Phillip J, Sullivan Eleanor J. Effective Leadership and Management in Nursing, 4th edition. California: Addison-Wesley; 1997. pp. 435-49.
4. Deloughery Grace. Issues and trends in nursing, 3rd edition. St Louis (MO): Mosby Company; 1998. pp. 448-60.
5. Gulani KK. Community Health Nursing Principles and Practices. 1st edition. New Delhi: Kumar Publishing House; 2005. pp. 33-5.
6. Hamilton Persis Mary. Realities of Contemporary Nursing, 2nd edition. California: Addison-Wesley; 1996. pp. 276-88.
7. Hickey JV, Ouimette RM, Vandral. Advanced Practice Nursing-Changing Roles and Clinical Applications, 1st edition. Philadelphia (PA): Lippincott; 1996. pp. 255-6.
8. HS2T1. Medical-Surgical Nursing. Block 1. New Delhi: IGNOU; 1999. p. 5.
9. Janice Rider Ellis, Celia Love Hartley. Nursing in Today's World: Challenges, Issues and Trends, 5th edition. Philadelphia (PA): JB Lippincott Company; 1995. pp. 342-69.
10. Kasturi Sundar Rao. An Introduction to Community Health Nursing, 1st edition. Madras: BI Publication Pvt. Ltd.; 1992. pp. 159-61.
11. Kennedy Grace Helen, McClosky Joanne Comi. Current issues in Nursing, 5th edition. St Louis (MO): Mosby; 1977. p. 13.
12. Kozier Barbara, et al. Fundamentals of Nursing Concepts, Process and Practice, 5th edition. Addison-Wesley Publishing Company; 1995. pp. 17-21.
13. Kozier Dugas. A Comprehensive Approach to Nursing, 4th edition. Harcourt Asia Pvt. Ltd.; WB Saunders Company; 1977. p. 13.
14. Lemone Priscilla, Taylor Carol, Lillis Carol. Fundamentals of Nursing –The Art and Science of Nursing Care, 4th edition. Philadelphia (PA): Lippincott; 2001. pp. 27, 28.
15. Park K. Textbook of Preventive and Social Medicine. 20th and 24th edition. India: M/s Banarsidas Bhanot; 2009 and 2017.
16. Patricia Potter, Anne Griffin Perry. Fundamentals of Nursing, 3rd edition. Philadelphia (PA): Mosby; 1992. pp. 24, 71.
17. Patricia Potter, Anne Griffin Perry. Fundamentals of Nursing, 5th edition. St. Louis (MO): Mosby; 2001. pp. 397-8.
18. Patricia S Yoder-Wise. Leading and Managing in Nursing, 1st edition. St Louis (MO): Mosby; 1995. pp. 476-94.
19. Phipps Wilma J, Long Barbara C, Woods Nancy Fugate. Shafer's Medical-Surgical Nursing, 7th edition. New Delhi: BI Publications Pvt. Ltd.; 1980. pp. 256-60.
20. Rinehart, Nancy Willis. Power and Related Concepts in Health Care, 1st edition. St Louis (MO): Ishiyaku Euro America, Inc. Publishers; 1991. pp. 1-9.
21. Rosdahl Caroline Bunker. Textbook of Basic Nursing, 7th edition. Philadelphia (PA): Lippincott; 1999. p. 1445.

Journals

1. Radha MS. Nursing yesterday, today and tomorrow. Health Action. 2003;16(10):14-5.
2. Atack L, Kenny R. Care co-ordination. An expanded role for nurses. Can Nurse. 1998;94(7):41-5.
3. Strengthening the performance of community health concerns in primary health care. Report of a WHO study group. Geneva: World Health Organ Tech Rep Ser. 1989;780:1-46.
4. Gonzalez RI. Assessing nursing's progress. Am J Nurs. 2002;102(4):24.
5. Trossman Susan. APRN's fight for their right to practice. Am J Nurs. 2002;102(1):63-5.

Internet References

1. www.gujhealth.gov.in/Medi – Servi/PPP
2. www.jstor.org/Stable/1965030
3. PSC refresh, blogspot.com/2009/07
4. www.deccanherald.com > Home
5. www.hindu.com/../2008/htm

REVIEW OF SECTION BASED QUESTIONS OF RGUHS

Long Essays

1. Illustrate the health care delivery system of India at the local level. (Oct 2010)
2. Explain current concept of primary health care. (May 2010)
3. Role of telemedicine in health care delivery system.
4. Health care environment versus nursing profession.
5. Discuss the various patterns of nursing care delivery in India. (Nov 2012, Oct 2016)
6. Explain in detail about the major stakeholders in health care system.
7. Discuss health care delivery system in India. (2007, May 2012)
8. Discuss on current health care delivery system in India. (May 2010)
9. Discuss current future roles of nurses within the health care delivery system. (May 2009, Oct 2010)
10. Discuss the appropriateness of the present heath care delivery system. (May 2009)

Short Essays

1. Information, education and communication.
2. Telemedicine and its uses in clinical practise. (May 2011)
3. National health and family welfare program.
4. Health care constraints.
5. People in the population.

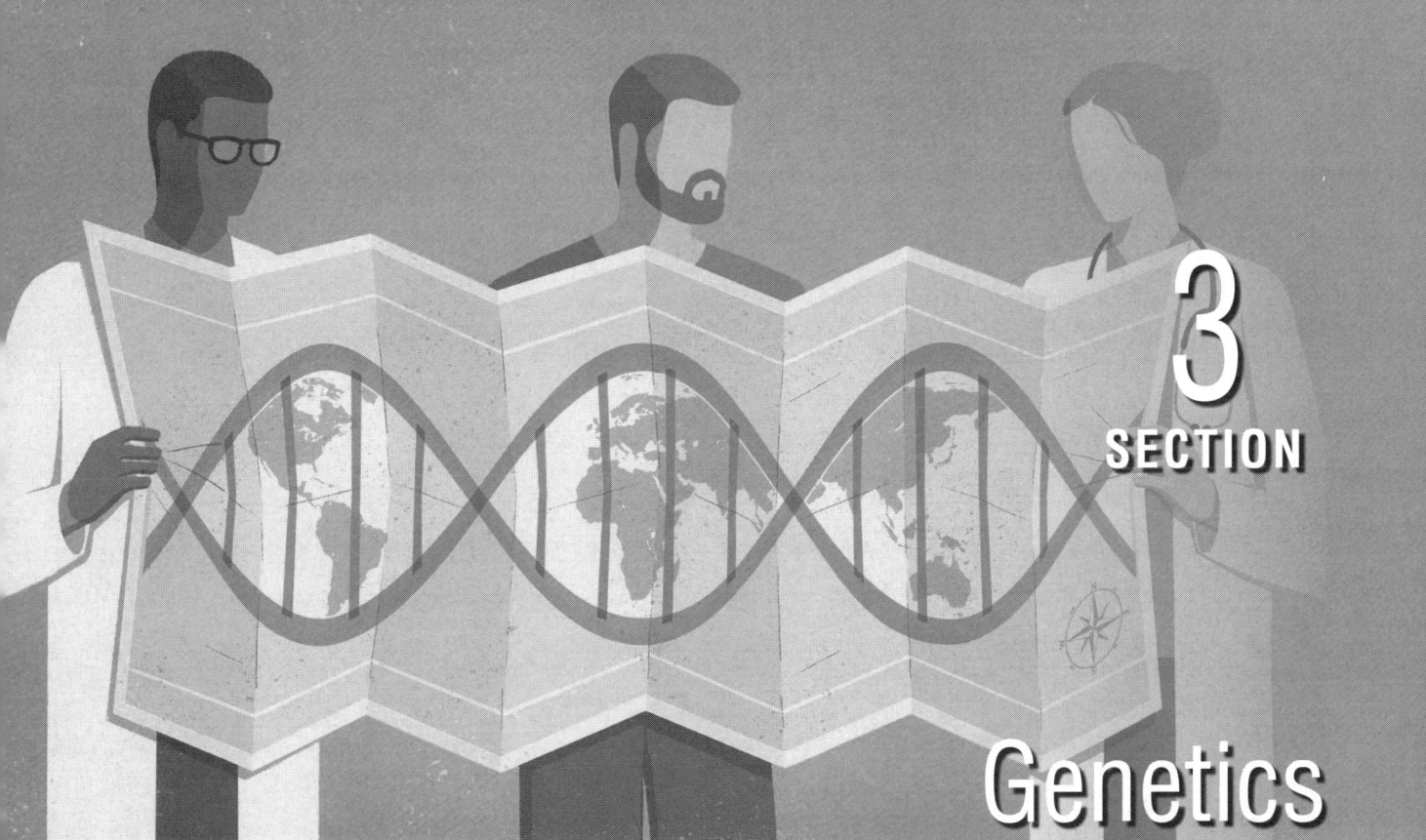

SECTION 3
Genetics

Section Outline

19. Review of Cellular Division, Mutation and Law of Inheritance, Human Genome Project, Genomic Era
20. Basic Concepts of Genes, Chromosomes and DNA
21. Approaches to Common Genetic Disorders
22. Genetic Testing: Basis of Genetic Diagnosis, Presymptomatic and Predisposition Testing, Prenatal Diagnosis and Screening
23. Genetic Counseling
24. Practical Application of Genetics in Nursing

19 CHAPTER
Review of Cellular Division, Mutation and Law of Inheritance, Human Genome Project, Genomic Era

CHAPTER OUTLINE

- Cell Structure
- Cell Membrane
- Cytoplasm
- Cell Organelles
- Cell Division
- Mitosis
- Meiosis
- Spermatogenesis
- Oogenesis
- Mutations
- Law of Inheritance
- Human Genome Project, Genomic Era
- Human Genome Project (HGP)
- Techniques and Analysis
- Ethical, Legal and Social Issues
- Genomic Era

INTRODUCTION

Human genetics deals with human variation—its variation, extent, origin and maintenance, its distribution in families and populations and its interaction with the environment. Unprecedented scientific and technologic advances have been made in human genetics during the past decade. Accompanying these advances are rapidly expanding service capabilities, the capacity to undertake mass screening to identify carriers of deleterious genes, the opportunities for prenatal diagnosis, the technology to sustain the lives of seriously ill and malformed newborns and the ability to increase the life expectancy of people affected by genetic disorders.

Johann Gregor Mendel (1822–1884) has laid the foundation for genetics, and our present knowledge base is given by his experiments on garden pea plants and followed by many others have contributed to the development of genetics worldwide.

CELL STRUCTURE (FIG. 19.1)

The cell is one of the most basic structural and functional units of life. The cell is the smallest unit of life in the bodies. It has outer membrane protecting from the outside environment called cell membrane. Cells usually increase in number by splitting, and the process is called cell division. In this, cells are divided into two cells. The cell which divides is called parent cell and the cell produced as a result of division are called daughter cells. Each cell grow old and die. These are replaced by new cells by cell division.

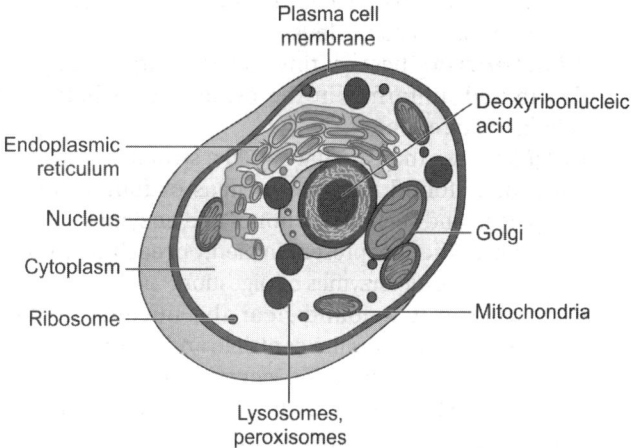

Fig. 19.1: Cell structure.

The cell is the basic living unit of the human body. The cell has a complete set of parts, neatly arranged in a mass of protoplasm surrounded by a membrane. The cell has a nucleus, cytoplasm and a cell membrane.

Centrally, there is a nucleus, which contain the cells deoxyribonuleic acid (DNA), the genetic code that coordinates protein synthesis and responsible for transmitting genetic information. It is composed of two pores that allow ribonucleic acid (RNA) molecules and proteins modulating DNA expression. DNA and protein associate to form a network of threads called chromatin, which forms rod-like chromosomes with the DNA. Nucleus has filamentous called nucleolus. It serves the RNA and protein components of ribosomes.

CELL MEMBRANE

Cell membrane is made up of two layers that contain large proteins and fatty substances, and forms a protective covering on the cell called plasma membrane. It can select substances entering and leaving a cell.

CYTOPLASM

Cytoplasm lies between the nucleus and the plasma membrane of the cell. The thick jelly-like material, which makes up most of each cell is called protoplasm. The cytoplasm forms the bulk and is made up of 85–95% of water, carbohydrates, protein, minerals and vitamins. It contains many living parts called organelles. The organic molecules are the nucleus, endoplasmic reticulum, mitochondria, Golgi apparatus, lysosomes and centrosome.

CELL ORGANELLES

In addition to the nucleus, there are many organelles inside the cell, which are given below:
1. *Endoplasmic reticulum:* It is a network of tubes that connect the plasma membrane with the nuclear membrane. There is rough and smooth endoplasmic reticulum. The rough forms fine granules called ribosomes. It participates in protein synthesis and transcription of cell nucleus.
2. *Mitochondria:* These are tiny bodies of varying shapes, distributed uniformly in the cytoplasm. It helps in cellular respiration.
3. *Golgi bodies:* They are flat sac-like structures, which are usually found near the nucleus or found in the cytoplasm, and secrete hormones and enzymes.
4. *Lysosomes:* They are present in plenty of each cell. They contain powerful enzymes of digestion.
5. *Centrosome:* It is found near the nucleus in the cytoplasm. It contains the centriole and is surrounded by some cytoplasm called centrosphere, with two centrioles, which together forms the centrosome. It plays a major role in cell division.

CELL DIVISION

Multiplication of cells takes place by cell division. Cells are reproduced by two different methods—mitosis and meiosis. Mitosis is the process by which body cells replicate to yield two cells with the same genetic make-up as the parent cell. First, the cell makes a copy of its DNA, then it divides and each daughter cell receives one copy of the genetic material. The purpose of mitotic division is for growth and development or cell replacement. Meiosis is the process by which gametes are produced.

MITOSIS

Beginning with the fertilized egg, or zygote, cell division is an ongoing process. Cell multiplication is equally necessary after the birth of the individual for growth and for replacement of dead cells. The chromosomes within the nuclei of cells carry genetic information that controls the development and functioning of various cells, tissues, and therefore, of the body as a whole. When a cell divides, it is essential that the entire genetic information within it is passed on to both the daughter cells resulting from the division. The life of individual cells is limited. They become worn out, die and are replaced by identical cells by mitosis. Mitosis can be divided into the following stages (Fig. 19.2):
1. *Interphase:* The period between two successive divisions is called interphase. During a specific period of the interphase, the DNA content of the chromosome is duplicated so that another chromatid identical to the original one is formed, the chromosome is now made up of two chromatids. DNA is the only type of molecule capable of independently forming a duplicate of itself.
2. *Prophase:* In this phase, two centrioles separate and move to opposite poles of the cell. They produce a number of microtubules that pass from one centriole to the other and form a spindle. Meanwhile, the nuclear membrane breaks down and nucleoli disappear.
3. *Metaphase:* With the formation of the spindle, chromosomes move to a position midway between the two centrioles (i.e. at the equator of cell); at this stage, chromosome looks shaped.
4. *Anaphase:* In this phase, the centromere of each chromosome splits longitudinally into two, so that the

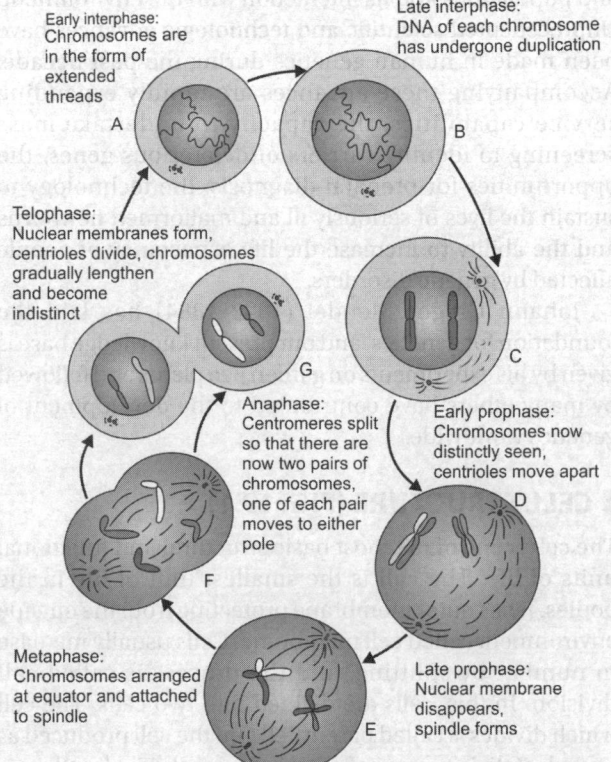

Fig. 19.2: Stages of mitosis.

Chapter 19: Review of Cellular Division, Mutation and Law of Inheritance, Human Genome Project, Genomic Era

chromatids now become independent chromosomes. Two chromatids, thus formed more apart to opposite ends of spindle than a single chromosome, are split into two new daughter chromosomes.

5. **Telophase:** In this phase, two daughter nuclei are formed by appearance of nuclear membranes. Chromosomes gradually lengthen and then become indistinct. Nucleoli reappear. The centriole is duplicated at this stage (or) in early interphase. The division of the nucleus is accompanied by the division of the cytoplasm. The cytoplasm divides equally into two daughter cells. Each daughter cell carries 46 chromosomes.

MEIOSIS (FIGS. 19.3A TO I)

A stage of reduction cell division when the chromosomes of a gamete are halved in number ready for union at fertilization. This consists of two successive divisions called first and second meiotic divisions. The cells resulting from these divisions differ from other cells of the body that is:
- The number of chromosomes is reduced to half the normal number
- The genetic information in the various gametes produced is not identical. This division occurs in the reproductive cells (gametes), i.e. the ova and spermatozoa

First Meiotic Division

Prophase

The prophase of the first meiotic division is prolonged and is usually divided into a number of stages as follows:
1. **Leptotene:** Chromosomes become visible. Although each chromosome consists of two chromatids, these cannot be distinguished at this stage.
2. **Zygotene:** Each cell consists of 23 pairs of chromosomes. The two chromosomes of each pair come to lie parallel to

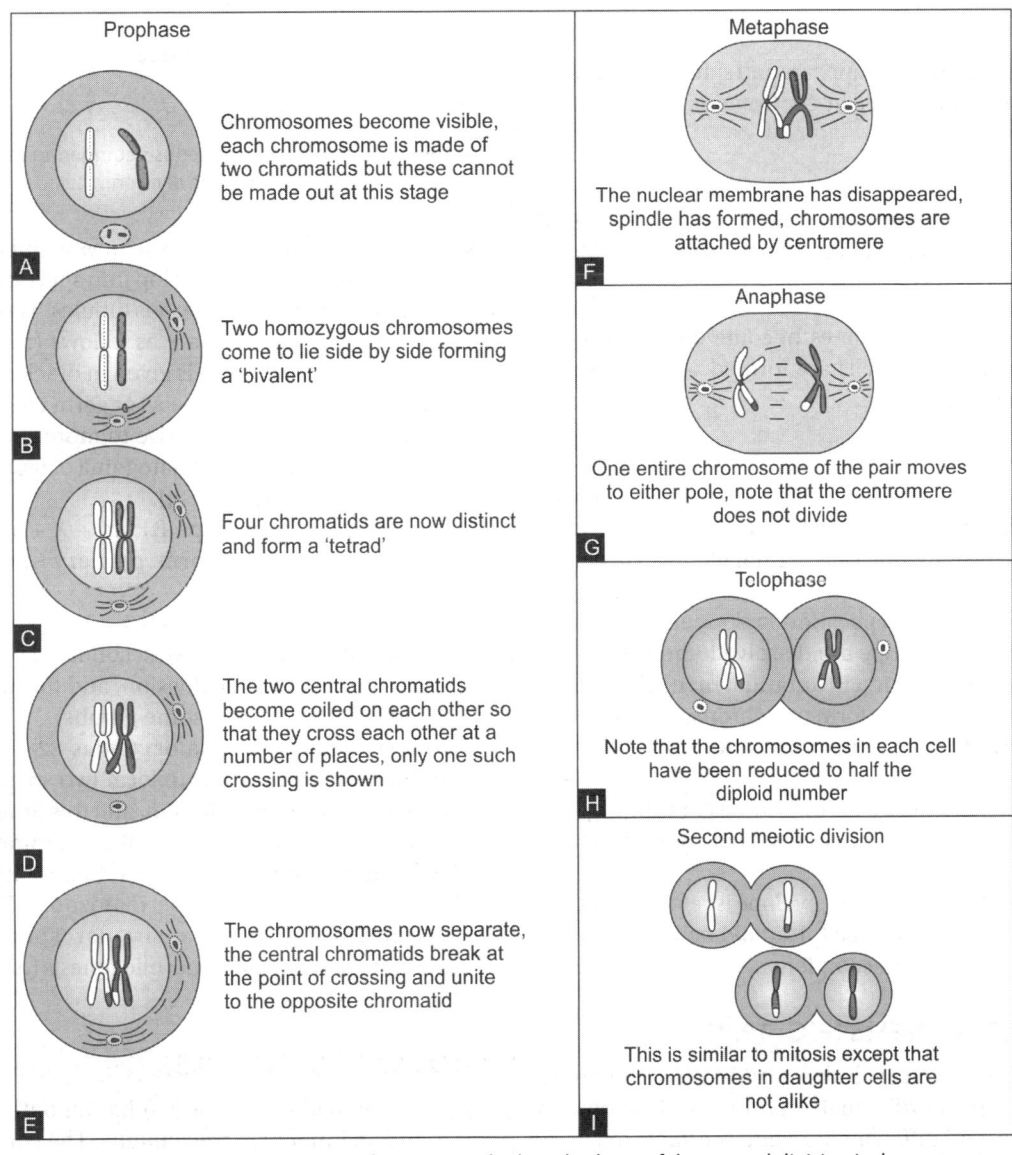

Figs. 19.3A to I: Main steps of meiosis. Only the telophase of the second division is shown.

each other and are closely apposed. Two chromosomes together constitute a bivalent.

3. **Pachytene:** The two chromatids of each chromosome become distinct. The bivalent now has four chromatids in it and is called tetrad. There are two central and two peripheral chromatids, which are from each chromosome. An important event now takes place. The two central chromatids become coiled over each other so that they cross at a number of points. This is called crossing over. At the site where the chromatids cross, they become adherent; the points of adherence are called chiasmata.

4. **Diplotene:** The two chromosomes of a bivalent now try to move apart. As they do so, the chromatids involved in crossing over "break" at the points of crossing and the loose pieces become attached to the opposite chromatid. This results in exchange of genetic material between these chromatids.

Metaphase

The nuclear membrane disappears and spindle has formed. Chromosomes are attached by centromere; the two tetrads line up in the center.

Anaphase

In this, there is no splitting of the centromeres. The tetrads split up into four chromosomes, which go to both poles.

Telophase

The two sets of chromosomes become enclosed by the nuclear envelope. Two cells are formed with two sets of chromosomes in each one.

Second Meiotic Division

The second meiotic division is similar to mitosis. However, because of the crossing over that has occurred during the first division, the daughter cells are not identical in genetic content.

- ❖ **Prophase II:** DNA replication is skipped and the two cells nuclear envelope are dissolved and the spindle reformed. The four chromatids in each cell are connected together to form two chromosomes.
- ❖ **Metaphase II:** The two chromosomes line up in the center.
- ❖ **Anaphase II:** The two chromosomes are split up into their daughter chromatids and moved towards opposite poles.
- ❖ **Telophase II:** The nuclear envelope is reformed around the two poles on each cell. Haploid cells remain as a result. Meiosis is now complete.

SPERMATOGENESIS (FIG. 19.4)

It is a process which includes a series of changes for conversion of primordial male germ cells, development of spermatids, and differentiation into spermatozoa in the seminiferous tubules of testis is called spermatogenesis.

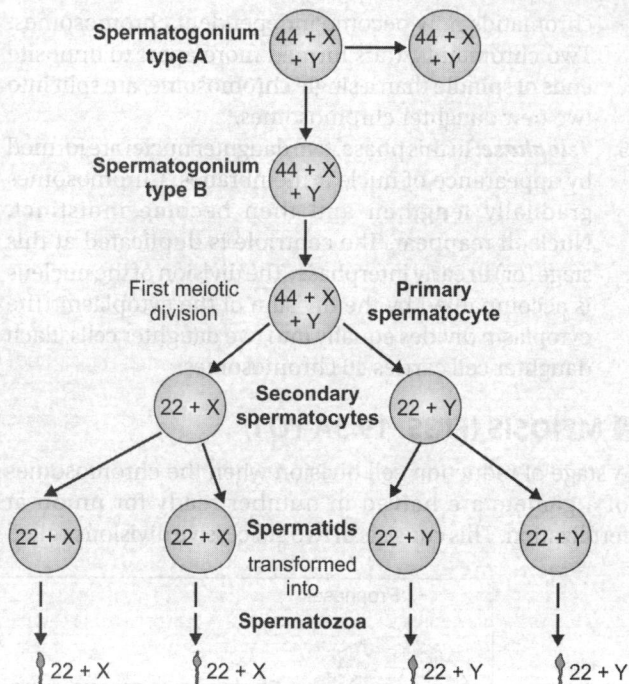

Fig. 19.4: Stages of spermatogenesis comparing each stage with meiotic division.

It starts at the age of 13–14 years in boys at puberty age and the primordial germ cells develop into spermatogonia and remain in the wall of seminiferous tubules. The various cell stages in spermatogenesis are as follows (the number of chromosomes at each stage is given in brackets):

1. The spermatogenesis (type A) or germ cells (44 + X + Y) divide mitotically, to give rise to more spermatogonia of type A and also to spermatogonia of type B (refer Fig. 19.4) (multiplication phase).
2. The spermatogonia (type B) (44 + X + Y) enlarge or undergo mitosis, to form primary spermatocytes (growth phase).
3. The primary spermatocytes (44 + X + Y) now divide so that each of them forms two secondary spermatocytes. This is the first meiotic division, and this time, there is no reduction in chromosome number.
4. Each secondary spermatocyte has 22 + X or 22 + Y chromosomes. It divides to form two spermatids. This is the second meiotic division, and this time, there is no reduction in chromosome number (maturation phase).
5. Each spermatid (22 + X or 22 + Y) gradually changes its shape to become a spermatozoon. This process of transformation or a circular spermatid to a spermatozoon is called spermiogenesis (differentiation phase).

OOGENESIS (FIG. 19.5)

The female gonad is the ovary. It has an outer part called cortex and an inner part, the medulla. The cortex contains many large round cells called oogonia. Around 2 million

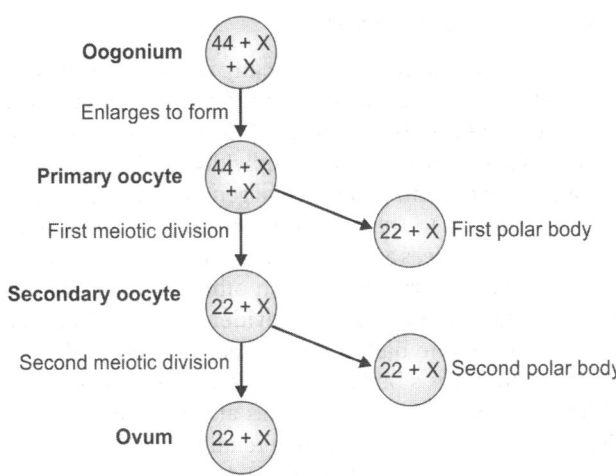

Fig. 19.5: Stages of oogenesis comparing each stage with meiotic division.

oogonia differentiate during fetal stage in ovary, during process of oogenesis. The oogonia are arrested in prophase I, each oogonium is called primary oocyte. All the oogonia to be used throughout the life of a woman are produced at a very early stage possibly before the birth and do not multiply thereafter. At puberty only 60,000–80,000 primary follicles are left in each ovary, out of which only 450 mature during the entire reproductive span in female.

Ova are derived from oogonia as shown in Figure 19.5, similar to the process of spermatogenesis. However, there are important differences:
1. One primary spermatocyte gives rise to four spermatozoa, one primary oocyte forms only one ovum.
2. When the primary spermatocyte divides, its cytoplasm is equally distributed between the two secondary spermatocytes formed. However, when the primary oocyte divides, almost all its cytoplasm goes to the daughter cell, which forms the secondary oocyte. The other daughter cell (first polar body) receives half the chromosomes of primary oocyte, but almost no cytoplasm. The first polar body is, therefore, formed to get rid of unwanted chromosomes.

MUTATIONS

Definition: Mutation is defined as a permanent change in the structure of DNA. Mutations of the germ cells are transmuted to the progeny and give rise to inherited diseases and that of the somatic cells can induce carcinogenesis and malformations.

Genetic Mutation

Each gene is made up of a series of bases, and those bases provide instructions for making a single protein. Any change in the sequence of bases and therefore in the protein instructions is a mutation. Similar to changing a letter in a sentence can change the sentence's meaning, a mutation can change the instruction contained in the gene. Some mutations have little or no effect on the protein, while others cause the protein not to function at all.

Sometimes normal genes also may be converted into abnormal ones; this change is also called mutation. It is a regular phenomenon in nature. The natural mutation rate is increased due to some absent reasons possibly environmental stress (spontaneous mutation), by exposure to mutagenes such as ultraviolet rays, radiation or chemical carcinogens (induced mutation) or some alteration in the possible generation in the genoma may express themselves by appearing a new creature.

Types of Mutations

- **Genome mutation:** Loss or gain of whole chromosome. Example: cystic fibrosis, phenyl ketonuria, color blindness, etc.
- **Chromosome mutations:** Rearrangement of genetic material with structural change in the chromosome.
- **Sub-microscopic gene mutation:** It may result in partial or complete deletion of a gene or often a single base.

These new features appearing may be life-threatening. When mutation does not affect the health of the individual, it is called genetic polymorphism:
- Mutation may occur due to the change in base sequence or due to altered protein with different aminoprotein
- Mutation may be due to change in RNA.

Problems of Mutations

Some mutations result in proteins that do not function normally, and may end up causing disease. There are several ways that gene mutation can change the way a protein function, including:

- *Altered function:* Some mutations result in a protein that cannot carry out its normal function in the cell or cannot carry out that function very well. One example of this type of mutation is sickle cell anemia. In this disorder, an altered protein in red blood cells (RBCs) alters the shape of the RBC, which causes the cell to become stuck in blood vessels. This prevents cells from carrying sufficient oxygen to the rest of the body.
- *Lack of protein:* Some mutations prevent the protein from being made. One example of this type of mutation is hemophilia. In this condition, a mutation results in the absence of a protein that causes blood to clot. The result is uncontrolled bleeding in response to injury.
- *Change in how much protein is made:* Some mutations cause too much or too little of a normal protein to be made. Although, the protein itself functions properly, it is not present in quantities that are appropriate. One example of this is in the development of some cancers. In this case, a protein that prevents additional mutations from building up can become turned off. Without this protein, the cell accumulates mutations and becomes increasingly cancerous.

LAW OF INHERITANCE

Gregor Johann Mendel was a 19th century Austrian priest/monk conducting experiments on garden peas, tall and short. Mendel chose seven physical traits (phenotype) to study. Mendel's goal was to reveal the genetic make-up (genotype). Mendel's work revealed following fundamental truths:

1. The physical traits are determined by factors, genes passed on by both parents.
2. Their factors are passed in predictable pattern from one generation to the next:
   Mendel's first law: Factors that determined physical traits segregate into both egg and sperm cells. Both egg and sperm carry physical traits to the offspring—the principle of segregation.
   Mendel's second law: Mendel explained a notation system to follow the inheritance of each trait. Mendel determines that an organism inherits two copies of the genetic material that determines an individual's physical traits, one copy coming from each of the male and female parent—the principle of independent assortment.
3. Individual genes can have different alleles, some of which (dominant traits) exert their effects over other (recessive traits)—the principle of dominance. Mendel's own words, "those characters which are transmitted entire or almost unchanged in the hybridization and therefore in themselves constitute the characters of the hybrid, are termed the dominant and those which become latent in the process recessive."

Dominant Trait (Fig. 19.6)

Traits caused by dominant alleles are the easiest to identify. Usually every individual who carries dominant allele manifests the trait, making it possible to trace the transmission of the dominant allele through the pedigree. The dominant trait's frequency of mutations is very low and is less viable for fertility problems. Most people show traits that are heterozygous for the dominant allele.

Recessive Traits (Fig. 19.7)

Those conditions that are clinically manifested only in individuals homozygous for the mutant gene (i.e. carrying double dose of the abnormal gene). So they are not easy to identify because they occur in individuals whose parents are not affected. Sometimes several generations of pedigree data are needed to trace the transmission of a recessive allele. Rare recessives are more likely to appear in a pedigree when spouses are related to each other. For example: In the first cousins, the increased evidence occurs because relatives share one half of their alleles by virtue of their common ancestry, siblings share one half their alleles, half siblings one fourth of their alleles and first cousins one eighth of their alleles. Thus, such relatives mate, and have a greater chance of providing child who is homozygous for a particular recessive allele than unrelated parents.

HUMAN GENOME PROJECT, GENOMIC ERA (FIG. 19.8)

Deoxyribonucleic Acid (DNA) Technology

The DNA technology depends on a number of basic tools that have been gradually developed over the past 20 years or so. A wide range of enzymes involved in DNA and RNA synthesis and repair have been identified and became available for laboratory use; nucleotide bases are available as laboratory reagents and specific DNA sequences can be synthesized at will. DNA diagnostic methods have been greatly simplified over the past 10 years. DNA has many advantages for genetic diagnosis. It is easy to obtain, since every cell of an individual or fetus contains the full DNA complement of that individual. Genes can be studied whether they are actively producing their product or not. A definitive diagnosis can usually be made in all genetic conditions.

Gene Therapy

Gene therapy is the introduction of a gene sequence into a cell with the aim of modifying the cell's behavior in a

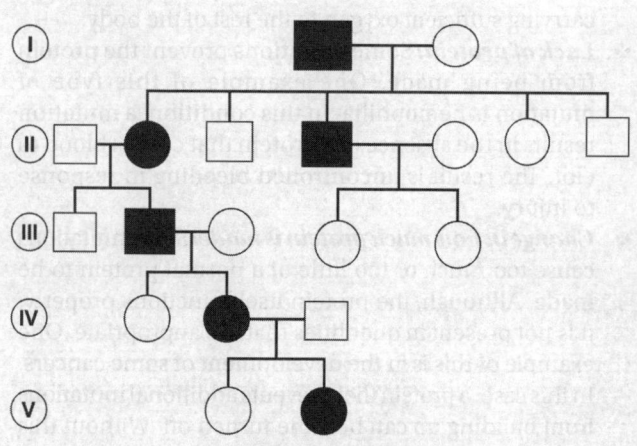

Fig. 19.6: Dominant trait.

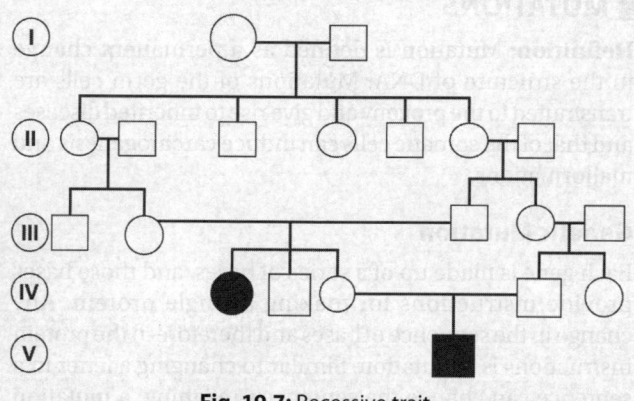

Fig. 19.7: Recessive trait.

Chapter 19: Review of Cellular Division, Mutation and Law of Inheritance, Human Genome Project, Genomic Era

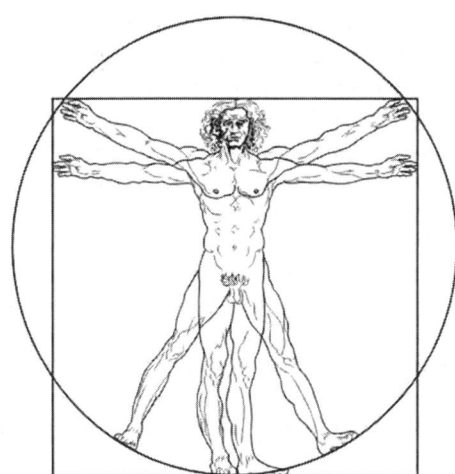

Fig. 19.8: Vitruvian Man (logo of Human Genome Project) is a drawing of Leonardo da Vinci around 1490.

clinically relevant fashion. It may be used in several ways, e.g. to correct a genetic mutation, to kill a cell or to modify susceptibility.

There are over 6000 inherited human diseases cataloged to-date, only a few are currently treatable.

Definition: It can be defined as replacement of deficient gene product or correction of an abnormal gene.

It can be done either in vitro or in vivo by treatment of cells/tissue by an affected individual in culture, with the reintroduction to the affected individual or in vivo if cells cannot be cultured or be replaced in the affected individual.

Function of Gene Therapy

Gene therapy involves adding a normal (wild type) copy of a gene to the genome of an individual carrying defective copies of the gene. A gene that has been introduced into a cell or an organism is called a trans-gene (transferred gene). To distinguish from endogenous genes and the organism carrying, the introduced gene is set to be transgenic. If gene therapy is successful, the trans-gene will synthesize the missing gene product and restore the normal phenotype.

Types of Gene Therapy

1. **Somatic cell or non-heritable gene therapy:** To perform somatic cell gene therapy, wild type genes must be introduced and expressed in cells homozygous for a mutant allele of the gene. In the wild type, gene could be delivered to the mutant cells by any of several different procedures; most commonly, viruses are used to carry the wild-type gene into cells. In case of retroviral vectors, the wild type of trans-gene is integrated along with the retroviral DNA into the DNA of the host-cell. Thus, retroviral vectors are used.
2. **Germ line or heritable gene therapy:** In higher animals such as humans, the reproductive or germ line cells are produced by a cell lineage separate from all somatic cell lineages. Thus, somatic gene cell therapy will treat the disease symptoms of the individual, but will not cure the disease. The defective gene will still be present in the germ line cells of a patient after somatic cell gene therapy and may be transmitted to his or her children. This is being performed on mice and other animals but not on humans.

Human gene therapy performed under strict guidelines was developed by the National Institute of Health (NIH) and it is scrutinized by review committees at both the local and national levels. Several requirements should be fulfilled before a gene therapy procedure will be approved.

- ❖ The gene must be cloned and well-characterized; it must be available in pure form
- ❖ An effective method must be available for delivering the gene into the desired tissues or cells
- ❖ The risks of gene therapy to the patient must have been carefully evaluated
- ❖ The disease must not be treatable by other strategies, data must be available from preliminary experiments with animal models or human cells and must indicate that the proposed gene therapy should be effective.

Recent Advances of Gene Therapy

Two recent applications of gene therapy have provided encouraging results:
1. Treatment of children with a rare form of congenital blindness—Laber's congenital amaurosis. Type II: This is caused by autosomal recessive mutations in any of at least 12 different genes, expressed in retinal pigment epithelium leading to blindness.
2. Treatment of Canavan Disease lacks an enzyme that breaks down the N-acetylaspartate produced in neurons. When the gene encoding the enzyme was introduced into brain cells, the missing enzyme was synthesized and neurological functions were improved.

So far, both of these gene therapy treatments have been successful.

Gene addition procedures: All past and current somatic cell gene therapy protocols simply add functional copies of the gene, i.e. defective in the patient to the genomes of recipient cells. As a result, more efficient targeted gene replacements are possible, and cells with the desired gene replacement can be identified more easily. In the future, targeted gene replacement will probably become the method of choice for somatic cell gene therapy of human diseases.

■ HUMAN GENOME PROJECT (HGP)

History of Human Genome Project

- ❖ The concept of a map of human genome was proposed as long ago as 1969 by Victor McKusik, one of the founder fathers of medical genetics
- ❖ Workshops regularly from 1973 to collate the mapping data

- A subsequent report on the technologies involved in detecting mutations in DNA and a further international meeting organized by US Department of Energy
- In the subsequent year, the US Congress approved a 15 years US Human Genome Projects (HGP) which started in 1991 with the estimated cost of $200,000 per annum
- This project HGP is run jointly under the auspices of the National Institute of Health and National Centre for Human Genome Research, headed by James Watson succeeded by Francis Collins and through National Laboratories.

The HGP was the international, collaborative scientific research project with the goal of determining the sequence of chemical base pairs, which make up human DNA and of identifying and mapping all of the genes of the human genome from both a physical and functional standpoint. It remains the world's largest collaborative biological project. The project was proposed and funded by the United States (US) government; planning started in 1984, got underway in 1990 and was declared complete in 2003. A parallel project was conducted outside of government by Celera Genomics, which was formally launched in 1998. Most of the government-sponsored sequencing was performed in 20 universities and research centers in the US, the United Kingdom (UK), Japan, France, Germany and China.

The HGP originally aimed to map the nucleotides contained in a human haploid reference genome (more than 3 billion). The "genome" of any given individual is unique; mapping "the human genome" involves sequencing multiple variations of each gene.

Objectives of HGP

- To map all human genes.
- To construct a detailed physical map of the entire genome.
- To determine the nucleotide sequences of all 24 human chromosomes by the year 2005.
- Development of informatics.
- Model organism genome projects.

Deoxyribonucleic Acid Replication

In May 1985, Robert Sinsheimer organized a workshop to discuss sequencing of the human genome, but for a number of reasons the NIH was uninterested in pursuing the proposal. The following March, the Santa Fe Workshop was organized by Charles DeLisi and David Smith of the Department of Energy's Office of Health and Environmental Research (OHER).

In 1990, the two major funding agencies, Department of Energy and NIH, developed a memorandum of understanding in order to coordinate plans and set the clock for the initiation of the project to 1990, assuming the role of overall Project Head as Director of the US NIH, National Center for Human Genome Research (which would later become the National Human Genome Research Institute).

A working draft of the genome was announced in 2000 and the papers describing it were published in February 2001. A more complete draft was published in 2003 and genome "finishing" work continued for more than a decade. Due to widespread international cooperation and advances in the field of genomics (especially in sequence analysis), as well as major advances in computing technology, a "rough draft" of the genome was finished in 2000 (announced jointly by US President Bill Clinton and the British Prime Minister Tony Blair on June 26, 2000). This first available rough draft assembly of the genome was completed by the Genome Bioinformatics Group at the University of California, Santa Cruz, primarily led by then graduate student Jim Kent. Ongoing sequencing led to the announcement of the essentially complete genome on April 14, 2003, 2 years earlier planned. In May 2006, another milestone was passed on the way to completion of the project, when the sequence of the last chromosome was published in Nature.

Mapping the Human Genome

Rapid progress was made in mapping the human genome from the launching of the HGP. Complete physical maps of chromosomes Y and 21 and detailed RFLP (restriction fragment-length polymorphism) maps of the X chromosome and all 22 autosomes were published in 1992. By 1995, genetic map contained markers separated by, on average, 200 kb. A detailed STR (short tandem repeat) map of the human genome was published in 1996, and a comprehensive map of 16,354 distinct loci was released in 1997. All of these maps have proven invaluable to researchers cloning genes based on their locations in the genome.

Unfortunately, the resolution of genetic mapping in humans is quite low—in the range of 1–10 mb. The resolution of fluorescent *in situ* hybridization (FISH) is also approximately 1 mb. Higher resolution mapping (down to 50 kb) can be achieved by radiation hybrid mapping, a modification of the somatic-cell hybridization mapping procedure. Standard somatic-cell hybridization involves the fusion of human cells and rodent cells growing in culture and the correlation of human gene products with human chromosomes retained in the hybrid cells. The polymerase chain reaction (PCR) is then used to screen a large panel of the selected hybrid cells for the presence of human genetic markers.

Sequencing the Human Genome (Figs. 19.9A to C)

While the gene-mapping work advanced quickly, progress toward sequencing the human genome initially lagged behind schedule. However, all that changed rapidly in 1998. During May 1998, J Craig Venter announced that he had formed a private company, Celera Genomics, with the goal of sequencing the human genome in just three years. Shortly thereafter, the leaders of the public HGP's sequencing laboratories announced that they had revised

Chapter 19: Review of Cellular Division, Mutation and Law of Inheritance, Human Genome Project, Genomic Era

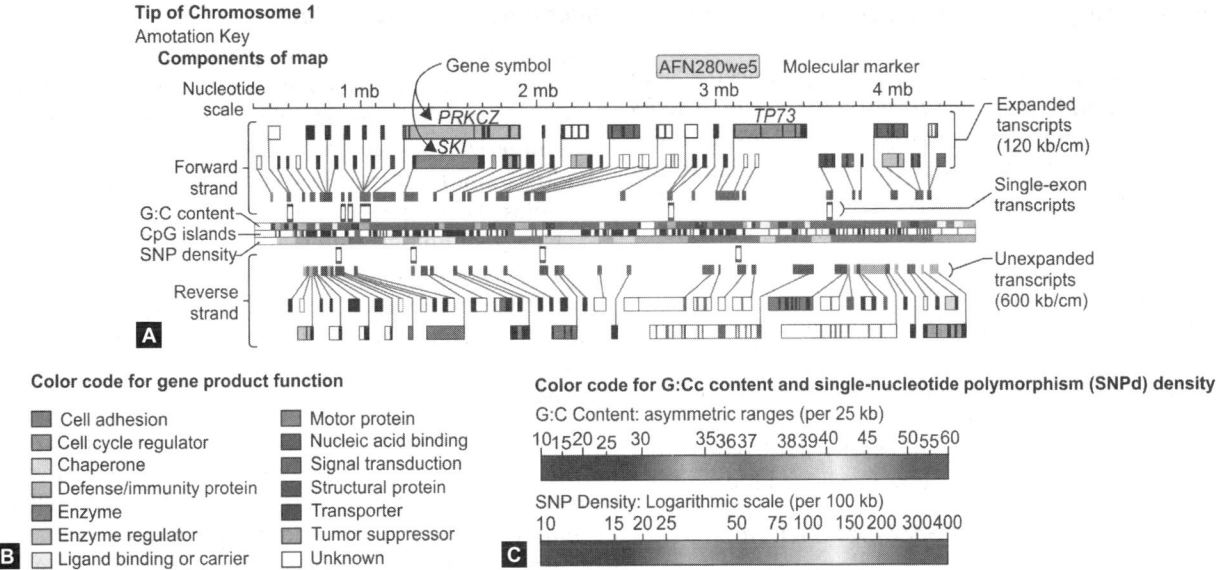

Figs. 19.9A to C: Annotated, sequence-based map of a 4-mb segment of DNA at the tip of human chromosome 1, assembled by researchers at Celera Genomics: (A) The top line gives distances in mb. The next three panels show predicated transcripts from one strand of DNA (the "forward strand"), whereas the bottom three panels show transcripts specified by the other strand of DNA (the "reverse strand"). The middle three panels give the G:C content, the positions of CpG islands, which occur upstream of genes, and the density of single-nucleotide polymorphisms (SNPs), respectively; (B) The color code for gene-product functions; (C) the color codes for G:C content and SNP density.

their schedule and planned to complete the sequence of the human genome by 2003, 2 years earlier than originally proposed. From that point in time, everything accelerated.

The complete sequence of the first human chromosome of the first human chromosome—small chromosome 22 was published in December 1999. The complete sequence of the human chromosome 21 followed in May 2000. Then, with intervention of the White House, Venter of Celera Genomics and Francis Collins, Director of the Public HGP, agreed to publish first drafts of the sequence of the human genome at the same time. The Celera and public sequences were both published in February 2001. The sequence provided 25,000–30,000 genes rather than the estimated 50,000–120,000 genes suggested by earlier studies.

On average, there is one gene per 145 kb in the human genome, some clustering of highly expressed genes with specific chromosomes. The average human gene is about 27,000 bp in length and contains nine exons. Exons make up only 1.1% of the genome, whereas introns account for 24% with 75% of the genome being intergenic DNA. Of the intergenic DNA, at least 44% is derived from transposable genetic elements.

The two first drafts of the sequence of the human genome were incomplete containing over 100,000 gaps. By October 2004, they had reduced the number of gaps to 341 and had completed the sequence of 99% of the euchromatic DNA in the human genome.

The Human Hapmap Project (Fig. 19.10)

Human genomes contain a large amount of generic variation. Small changes, insertions or deletions of one or a few nucleotide pairs are more frequent. The most common

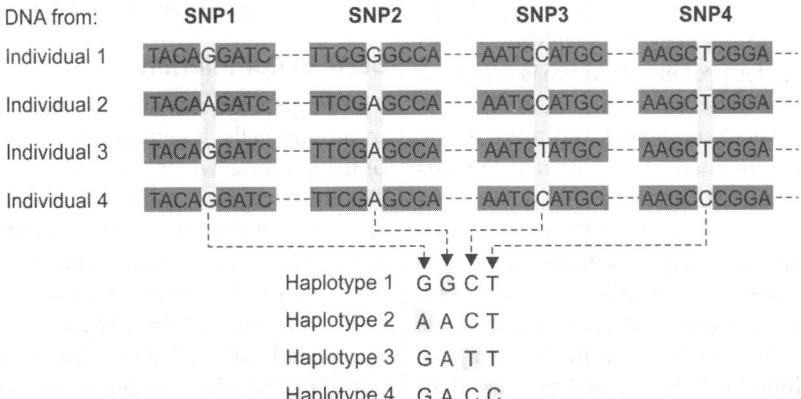

Fig. 19.10: Haplotypes are sets of linked SNPs and other genetic markers that tend to be inherited as a unit.

changes in human genomes are single nucleotide-pair substitutions, for example, A:T to G:C to A:T substitutions. Base-pair substitutions of this type have produced a large number of *single-nucleotide polymorphisms* (**SNPs** pronounced "snips") in human genomes. Most of these SNPs are not located in the coding regions of genes and do not result in mutant phenotypes. When the nucleotide sequences of the same chromosomes of two individuals are compared, an SNP is present, on average, in every 1,200 nucleotide pairs.

SNPs can be detected in human genomes by the microarray hybridization or "gene-chip" technology. In brief, hybridization probes can be synthesized that can detect single-nucleotide differences in DNA molecules. If a DNA molecule matches a probe exactly, it will bind to that probe; if it does not match exactly, it will not bind.

RNA and Protein Assays of Genome Function

Knowing the complete sequence of the human genome will help identify genes responsible for human diseases and should lead to successful gene therapies for some of the diseases. However, it will not tell us what these genes do or how they control biological processes. Indeed, by itself, the nucleotide sequence of a gene, a chromosome or an entire genome is uninformative. Only when supplemented with information about their functions, sequences become truly meaningful. Thus information about the functions of nucleotide sequences must still be obtained by traditional genetic studies and by molecular analysis. If geneticists want to understand the genetic control of the growth and development of a mature human from a single fertilized egg, they will need to know much more than the sequence of the human genome. But the availability of the ultimate map of the human genome, its nucleotide sequence, will certainly accelerate progress toward understanding the programs of gene expression that control morphogenesis. The new technologies such as "gene-chip" hybridizations are designed to take advantage of availability of the sequences of complete genomes.

Expressed Sequences

In large eukaryotic genomes, only a small portion of the DNA encodes proteins. In the yeast *S. cerevisiae*, almost 70% of the genome encodes protein and there is one gene for every 2 kb of sequence. In humans, only about 1% of the genome encodes amino acid sequences and there is one gene for every 130 kb of sequences. Thus, in order to focus on the protein-coding content of genomes, many scientists have identified cDNA clones (DNAs complimentary to RNA molecules) or ESTs (expressed sequence tags) rather than genomic clones. Multiple cDNAs can be obtained from different segments of a single gene transcript or alternative splicing of a gene transcript. For example, the human gene that encodes serum albumin is represented by more than 1,300 estimated sequences in public data bases.

Microarrays and Gene Chips

The sequence of an entire genome, geneticists can immediately begin to study the expression of every gene in the organism. Oligo nucleotide hybridization probes can be synthesized to segments of the transcripts of each open reading frame (ORF) and PCR can be used to make millions of copies of each gene in a genome.

New technologies now allow scientists to produce microarrays that contain thousands of hybridization probes on a single membrane. In case of gene chips, thousands of probes are synthesized on silicon wafers, 1–2 sq.cm in size. This can be used to study the expression of thousands of genes.

The green fluorescent protein as a reporter for protein synthesis: The discovery of a naturally occurring fluorescent protein, the green fluorescent protein (GFP) of the jellyfish *Aequorea victoria* has provided a powerful tool that can be used to study gene expression at the protein level in a wide variety of living cells. This fluorescence is introduced in the fusion protein in transgenic cells exposed to blue or UV light.

Bioinformatics

Knowledge of the nucleotide sequences of entire genomes has provided a wealth of information and a new challenge. This challenge has spawned a new scientific disciple called bioinformatics. It is the science of gathering, manipulating, storing, retrieving and classifying recorded information. It involves all biological information, most notably, DNA and protein sequences. Some of the more popular programs were developed by the genetics computer group (GCG) at University of Wisconsin. Earlier GENBANK, to search for DNA sequences similar to a query sequence by using BLAST software and the other programs, i.e. used for rapidly searching huge databases is called FASTA. The most elementary step in trying to identify genes within nucleotide sequences is to look for ORFs. GCG program is used to translate double-stranded DNA in all six reading frames. The standard three-letter amino acid abbreviations are quite common when dealing with large protein databases; therefore, single letter code is used in bioinformatic analyses.

State of Completion

The project did not aim to sequence all the DNA found in human cells. It sequenced only "euchromatic" regions of the genome, which make up about 90% of the genome. The other regions, called "heterochromatic," are found in centromeres and telomeres, and were not sequenced under the project. The HGP was declared complete in April 2003. An initial rough draft of the human genome was available in June 2000, and by February 2001, a working draft had been completed and published followed by the final sequencing mapping of the human genome on April 14, 2003. Although this was reported to be 99% of the euchromatic human

Chapter 19: Review of Cellular Division, Mutation and Law of Inheritance, Human Genome Project, Genomic Era

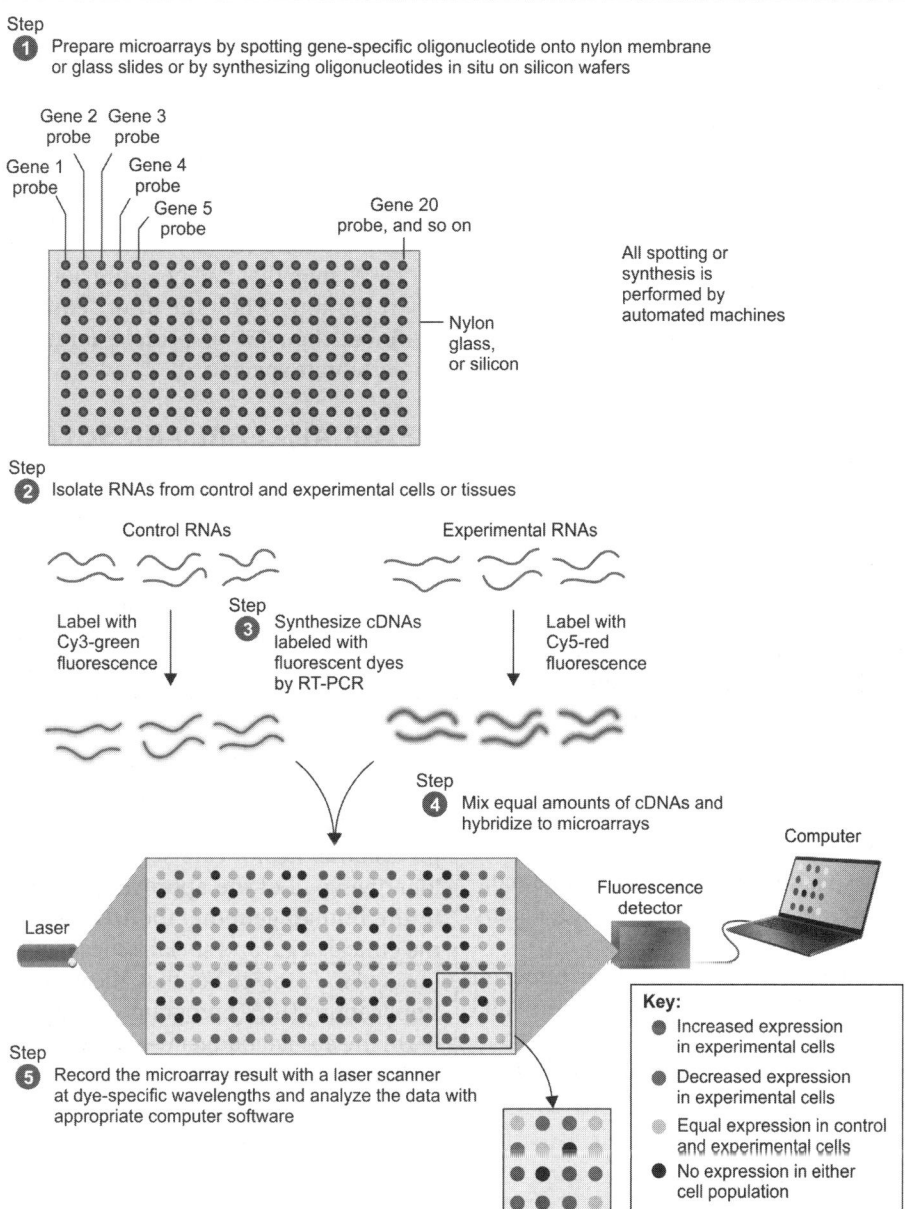

Fig. 19.11: Preparation and use of microarrays to study gene expression. RNAs are isolated from control and experimental tissues, for example, normal cells and cancer cells, and used to prepare cDNAs labeled with different fluorescent dyes. Equal amounts of the cDNA samples are mixed and hybridized; microarrays containing probes complementary to the cDNAs of the genes of interest. After hybridization, the microarrays are analyzed using sophisticated laser scanners and computer software that remove background noise and quantify the signals from the two fluorescent cDNA populations.

genome with 99.99% accuracy, a major quality assessment of the human genome sequence was published on May 27, 2004 indicating over 92% of sampling exceeded 99.99% accuracy, which was within the intended goal. Further analyses and papers on the HGP continue to occur.

Benefits of HGP

The sequencing of the human genome holds benefits for many fields, from molecular medicine to human evolution:

- ❖ The HGP, through its sequencing of the DNA, can help us understand diseases including genotyping of specific viruses to direct appropriate treatment.
    - ➢ Maintain major benefits to human kind, improving one's understanding and development of new strategies for the prevention and treatment of inherited diseases
    - ➢ Progress of HGP were planned and predicted. Projects likely to accelerate development of new

technologies and the convergence of findings from various component parts of the project
> It is importance to those individuals and families with or at risk of inherited diseases.
- Identification of mutations linked to different forms of cancer
- The design of medication and more accurate prediction of their effects
- Advancement in forensic applied sciences
- Biofuels and other energy applications are agriculture, animal husbandry and bioprocessing
- Risk assessment
- Bioarcheology, anthropology and evolution
- Another proposed benefit is the commercial development of genomics research related to DNA-based products, a multibillion-dollar industry
- The sequence of the DNA is stored in databases available to anyone on the Internet. The US National Center for Biotechnology Information (and sister organizations in Europe and Japan) house the gene sequence in a database known as GenBank, along with sequences of known and hypothetical genes and proteins
- Computer programs have been developed to analyze the data, because the data itself is difficult to interpret without such programs

Limitations of HGP
- Cost is more and expenditures is likely to be planned.
- Mindless sequencing project with devoid of any intrinsic biological interest.
- Misunderstanding of normal interaction between genetic makeup/evolution factors with developmental characteristic in order.
- Potential danger of misuse of information in the form of positive and negative energies.

TECHNIQUES AND ANALYSIS

The process of identifying the boundaries between genes and other features in a raw DNA sequence is called genome annotation and is the domain of bioinformatics. While expert biologists make the best annotators, their work proceeds slowly and computer programs are increasingly used to meet the high throughput demands of genome sequencing projects. Beginning in 2008, a new technology known as RNA-sequencing (RNA-seq) was introduced that allowed scientists to directly sequence the messenger RNA in cells. This replaced previous methods of annotation, which relied on inherent properties of the DNA sequence, with direct measurement, which was much more accurate. Today, annotation of the human genome and other genomes relies primarily on deep sequencing of the transcripts in every human tissue using RNA-seq. These experiments have revealed that over 90% of human genes contain at least one and usually several alternative splice variants, in which the exons are combined in different ways to produce two or more gene products from the same locus.

Key findings of the draft (2001) and complete (2004) genome sequences include:
1. There are approximately 20,500 genes in human beings, the same range as in mice.
2. The human genome has significantly more segmental duplications (nearly identical, repeated sections of DNA) than that had been previously suspected.
3. At the time when the draft sequence was published, fewer than 7% of protein families appeared to be vertebrate specific.

ETHICAL, LEGAL AND SOCIAL ISSUES

At the onset of the HGP, several ethical, legal and social concerns were raised in regards to how increased knowledge of the human genome could be used to discriminate against people. One of the main concerns of most individuals was the fear that both employers and health insurance companies would refuse to hire individuals or refuse to provide insurance to people because of a health concern indicated by someone's genes. In 1996, the United States passed the Health Insurance Portability and Accountability Act (HIPAA), which protects against the unauthorized and non-consensual release of individually identifiable health information to any entity not actively engaged in the provision of health care services to a patient. Along with identifying all of the approximately 20,000–25,000 genes in the human genome, the HGP also sought to address the ethical, legal and social issues that were created by the onset of the project. For that, the Ethical, Legal, and Social Implications (ELSI) program was founded in 1990. About 5% of the annual budget was allocated to address the ELSI arising from the project.

GENOMIC ERA

When the results of research studies immediately find practical applications. This issue of the Journal includes the last instalment in a monthly series on genomic medicine that began in November 2002. The series has focused on the ways in which the rapidly appearing tools of genomics have already begun to change the practice of medicine.

The genomic era can be said to have a precise birth date, it was in the midst of the appearance of the series, on April 14, 2003. That was when the international effort known as the HGP put a close to the pre-genomic era with its announcement (available at http://www.genome.gov/11006929) that it had achieved the last of the project's original goals, the complete sequencing of the human genome. The extent and pace of progress in genomics are suggested by the fact that this achievement occurred 11 days before the 50th anniversary of the publication of Watson and Crick's seminal description of the DNA double helix:

- In recent months, we have seen not only the promise of the genomic era with respect to medicine, but also its pitfalls. An example of the latter has been the revelation that confusion and misinformation have occasionally accompanied the counseling of persons who undergo screening for mutations in the cystic fibrosis transmembrane conductance regulator gene (CFTR); the gene responsible for cystic fibrosis. Different mutations in CFTR have different effects, leading to a range of phenotypes. Proper interpretation of screening results demands an understanding of the clinical implications of specific genotypes. For example, the relatively common 5T variant leads to the phenotype of classic cystic fibrosis only when it is accompanied by the R117H mutation on the same chromosome arm.
- Genomics provides powerful means of discovering hereditary factors in disease. But even in the genomic era, it is not genes alone but the interplay of genetic and environmental factors that determines phenotype (i.e. health or disease).
- It remains difficult to alter genes in humans (for both technical and ethical reasons). For the next couple of decades, we will generally use personalized modifications of the environment, and not of genes, to translate genomics-based knowledge into improvements in health for most of the patients. Clinicians will much more frequently suggest to patients with hereditary hemochromatosis that they avoid iron supplementation than that they consider gene therapy. Women who carry mutations will profit more from taking tamoxifen than from manipulations of their genotype.
- With the end of the pre-genomic era in sight, more than 600 experts recently collaborated to produce a vision for the future of genomic research and its applications to biology, health and society.
- Another social issue, with particular relevance in the United States, is the understandable concern of many patients that obtaining genetic information important to their health care is not worth the risk of discrimination stemming from the use of such information by potential insurers or employers. Although, more than 40 states limit employers' and insurers' access to or use of genetic information, many people believe that only the passage of legislation mandating uniform national protection against the misuse of such information will lead to full use of genetic testing.
- Other social issues require our attention, if genomic medicine is to benefit the patients. The Internet has recently had a proliferation of genetic-testing sites that feature claims grounded in greed and pseudoscience, rather than in data or reality. How will health care providers and the public distinguish between these and responsible testing services, whether they are available through the Internet or in the hospital?

While recognizing such challenges, look forward with curiosity and real hope to the advances of the next 50 years of the genomic era. As evidenced by the Genomic Medicine series, today's researchers and clinicians have already started to use the power of genomics to improve health, and we anticipate that this is a hint of the progress to come.

CONCLUSION

The HGP was one of the great feats of exploration in history, an inward voyage of discovery and an international research effort to sequence and map all of the genes together known as the genome of members of our species, Homo sapiens. Completed in April 2003, the HGP gave us the ability, for the first time, to read nature's complete genetic blueprint for building a human being and this has moved rapidly in applying basic knowledge clinically.

20 CHAPTER
Basic Concepts of Genes, Chromosomes and DNA

CHAPTER OUTLINE

- Genes
- Concepts of Genetics
- Chemistry of a Gene
- Deoxyribonucleic Acid
- Chromosomes

INTRODUCTION

Genes are the units of hereditary. They contain the hereditary information ended in their chemical structure for transmission from generation to generation. They affect development and function both normal and abnormal. It is said that we inherit about 50,000 genes from the mother. Genes are contained in the chromosomes, they also occur in pairs and are usually stable. Chromosomes are rod-like condensations of chromatin. They become visible in the nucleus only during cell division. Biochemically, the chromosomes are made up of deoxyribonucleic acid (DNA). Genetically, they consist of genes arranged similar to the beads of a necklace. All individuals of the same species have the same number of chromosomes.

GENES

- A gene is a segment of DNA molecule, located in a particular position on a specific chromosome, whose base sequence contains the information necessary for protein synthesis. The position of gene on the chromosome is called locus. There are approximately 100,000 gene loci in human chromosomes.
- A gene is a specific sequence of nucleotide bases whose sequence carry the information required for constructing proteins, which provide the structural components of cells, tissues as well as enzymes, and hormones for essential biochemical reactions, e.g. enzymes help us digest food, etc.
- The transfer of information from nuclear DNA to the site where proteins are synthesized in the cytoplasm is the function of ribonucleic acid (RNA). The formation of RNA is controlled by genes in the DNA, i.e. genetic information passes from DNA to RNA promoting protein synthesis.
- Dominant gene is one that is capable of transmitting its characteristics irrespective of the genes from the other parent. Recessive gene is one that can pass on its characteristics only if it is present with a similar recessive gene from the other parent.

CONCEPTS OF GENETICS

- The pattern of inheritance is determined by genetic material in the nuclei of the cell (23 chromosomes)
- Two members of the 23 chromosomes are homologous in both sexes
- Each spermatocyte contains 22 pairs of autosomes and one pair of sex chromosomes. In female *XX* chromosome and in male *XY* chromosome
- The portion of the chromosome, which codes for character is called gene
- The position of the gene in the chromosome is called locus
- Character coded by the chromosome may be same or different. For example, a black iris and blue iris have an altered form of gene which is known as alleles
- Alleles code the same character in same tract and is called homozygous state. Alleles' code for the different character is called heterozygous state
- If an allele clinically manifest itself in a heterozygous state is called dominant gene
- If an allele does not manifest clinically when other parent is normal, it is called recessive gene
- Genetic makeup pairs are called genotype
- Clinically manifest character is called phenotype
- Sometimes gene may be modified without any genetic polymorphism
- Chemically, chromosome is made up of DNA and histone. Only 3% DNA symbolizes your genes about

Chapter 20: Basic Concepts of Genes, Chromosomes and DNA

97% DNA has no clear function then it is called 'Junko' DNA.

CHEMISTRY OF A GENE

- Genes are made up of DNA. Most DNA resides in nucleus, and some genes are present in mitochondria
- It forms a double-stranded twisted helical structure
- Basic unit of DNA consists of a nitrogen base, purine and pyrimidine, sugar and phosphate
- Base of the two linked by hydrogen bond between purine of one strand and pyrimidine of other strand.

DEOXYRIBONUCLEIC ACID (FIG. 20.1)

The nucleus contains the body's genetic material in the form of large double chains of molecules of DNA, in a spiral arrangement (helical). It forms a double-stranded twisted helical structure. A DNA molecule consists of two strands that wrap around each other to resemble a twisted ladder. The basic unit of DNA strand is:
1. Nitrogenous base
2. Sugar
3. Phosphate

Each DNA strand is made of sugar and phosphate molecules and are connected by rungs of nitrogenous bases. Each strand is a linear arrangement of repeating similar units called nucleotides, which are each composed of one sugar, one phosphate and a nitrogenous base. The nitrogenous base consists of purine base and pyrimidine base:
- *Purine base:* Adenine and guanine
- *Pyrimidine base:* Thymine and cytosine

The bases occur in a set pattern. The purine of A in one chain is paired with T in the other chain of pyrimidine and G with C. That is:
- A...................T
- G...................C

Two bases linked by hydrogen bonds form each rung. In this way, the nucleotides are arranged in a precisely ordered manner in which one chain is complementary to the other.

CHROMOSOMES (FIG. 20.2)

Structure

Chromosomes are visible as compact, well-defined structures only during cell division, i.e. metaphase. The chromosome is made up of two rod-shaped structures or chromatids placed more or less parallel to each other. The chromatids are united to each other at a light staining area called the centromere. Each chromatid has two arms, one on either side of the centromere. Each chromatid has p and q arms. Upper arm is p and lower arm is q. Biochemically, chromosomes are made up of DNA.

Autosomes and Sex Chromosomes

A normal healthy individual receives 23 (haploid) chromosomes from each of the parent and shall have 46 (diploid) or 23 pairs of homologous (identical) chromosomes.

Of these, 22 pairs are autosomes. The remaining pair is concerned with the sex of an individual and are known as sex chromosomes (*X* and *Y*). Sex is determined as female, when there are two *X* chromosomes, i.e. *XX* and *XY* determine male sex. All the 46 chromosomes or 23 pairs of homologous chromosomes have definite size and structure, and are distinguishable from one another. Any deviation in the structure or number of these chromosomes leads to an abnormality.

Classification

- The autosomes have been classified and divided on the basis of length and certain morphological similarities into seven groups as follows:
  1. Group A: 1–3 pairs
  2. Group B: 4–5 pairs

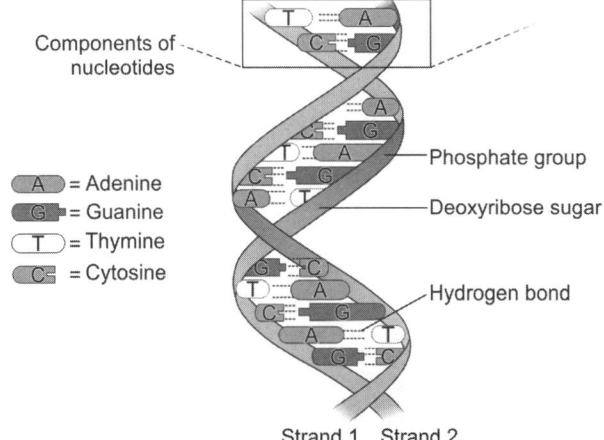

Fig. 20.1: Portion of a DNA molecule.

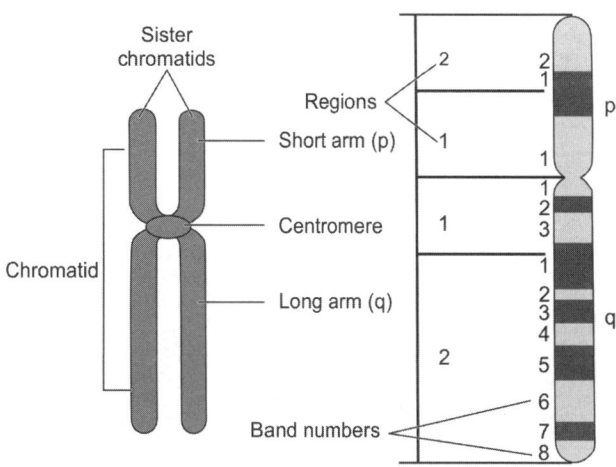

Fig. 20.2: Parts of a typical chromosome.

3. Group C: 6–12 pairs
4. Group D: 13–15 pairs
5. Group E: 16–18 pairs
6. Group F: 19–20 pairs
7. Group G: 21 and 22 pair.

- Classified as per the position of centromere, length and size:
  - **Telocentric:** Centromere is situated at the end having only one arm. Found in some animals, e.g. rats.
  - **Acrocentric:** Centromere is situated near the p arm having one very short and the other a long arm.
  - **Submetacentric:** Centromere is situated somewhere between the midpoint and the end of the chromosome.
  - **Metacentric:** Centromere is situated near the center chromosome making both arms almost equal.
  - **Satellite:** Small segments of chromatin distal to the secondary constriction on the short arms of acrocentric chromosomes.

Haploid and Diploid Chromosomes

During cell division, the chromatin network in the nucleus becomes condensed into a number of chromosomes. The number of chromosomes in each cell is 46. This is referred to as the diploid number. However, in spermatozoa and ova the number of chromosomes is only half the diploid number double, i.e. 23; this is called the haploid number (half):

- A typical cell contains 46 chromosomes (diploid number, i.e. 2n)
- A gamete contains 23 chromosomes (haploid number, i.e. n).

CONCLUSION

Chromosomes and genes play a very important role in genetic inheritance of an individual. Any change/abnormal compliment of chromosomes/genes leads genetic disorders.

21 CHAPTER
Approaches to Common Genetic Disorders

CHAPTER OUTLINE
- Definition of Genetics
- Incidence of Genetic Disorders
- Types of Genetic Disorders
- Management of Genetic Disorders

INTRODUCTION

Genetic disorders and congenital malformations have become major causes of morbidity and mortality in infants and children. Genetic and related disorders are also of increasing importance in the case of adults, particularly pregnant women and adults of reproductive age.

In recent years, the significance of genetics as an etiologic agent in disease and disability has assumed a more prominent place in the nursing care of infants and children. The expanded recognition of genetic diseases and defects as well as an increasingly well-informed public is creating a justified demand for genetic evaluation and diagnosis as well as information regarding risks to present and future generations. Unfortunately, however, persons who need expert genetic counseling often make uninformed on their own or are the victims of well meaning, but equally uninformed relatives and acquaintances or unknowledgeable paraprofessionals.

DEFINITION OF GENETICS

- Genetics is the science that deals with the transmission of characters from parents to offspring.
- Genetics deals with the study of underlying principles of heredity as well as its variations.
- Heredity is the transmission of both physical and mental characteristics to the offspring from the parents. The study of human genetics is becoming increasingly important to the childbearing process because genetic factors play a role in the etiology of many birth defects and a variety of human diseases.
- Genetics attempts to explore the secrets of the blueprints of life. It has been established that physical and biochemical characteristics are transmitted by the genes of the chromosome. Genetics today is doubtlessly the most significant and the youngest branch of medical science.

An elementary knowledge of the principles of genetics is essential for understanding the causation of several diseases.

INCIDENCE OF GENETIC DISORDERS

- Genetic diseases, also called hereditary diseases, are the most burdensome of all human afflictions. Genetic diseases are determined at conception, but can be expressed at any time in life span.
- Roughly 1 in 20 children admitted to hospital has a disorder, which is entirely genetic in origin and such disorders account for about 1 in 10 of childhood deaths in hospital. A number of surveys have indicated that at least 1 in 50 newborns has a major congenital abnormality.
- One in 200 has a major chromosomal abnormality. The incidence of autosomal dominant disorders is about 7 per 1,000 births. Autosomal recessive disorders are about 2.5 per 1,000 births. X-linked disorders are about 0.5 per 1,000 births.

TYPES OF GENETIC DISORDERS

Genetic diseases can be divided into following main categories:
- Chromosomal disorders
- Single gene disorders
- Multifactorial disorders.

Chromosomal Disorders

Live newborns are 0.5% and may have chromosomal anomaly types of chromosomal anomalies.

- These are due to abnormality in chromosome number or structure. The chromosome abnormality may involve autosomes or sex chromosomes. These chromosome abnormalities occur due to various genetic and environmental factors.

❖ Some of them are due to defective cell division during the formation of gametes in parents—advanced maternal age (more than 35 years), effect of drugs, chemicals, radiation and exposure to environment pollution.

These are:
❖ Changes in chromosome structure
❖ Changes in chromosome number
❖ Autosomal chromosome disorders of number
❖ Sex chromosome disorders of number.

Changes in Chromosome Structure (Fig. 21.1)

Chromosomal breakage with subsequent reunion in a different configuration resulting in a change or variation of genetic material is referred to as structural abnormality.

Causes: Ionizing radiation, chemicals, viral infections, etc.

Types of structural abnormalities

Deletion: In which a part of a chromosome has been deleted. A segment of chromosome may break off and may be lost, it can be detected by chromosomal staining called fluorescent in situ hybridization (FISH)

Duplication: It is just a duplication of a section of a chromosome

Inversion: In which a segment of a chromosome is reversed. Pericentric inversion is confined to a single arm of the chromosome, whereas pericentric inversion involves both arms and includes the centromere

Translocation: This is the transfer of a piece of one chromosome to a non-homologous chromosome. It is of two types:
1. Reciprocal: Chromosome material distal breaks into two and chromosomes are exchanged. Short/long arm involved
2. Robertsonian: Two breaks occur at or near the centromere of two acrocentric chromosomes, with subsequent fusion of their two long arms

Isochromosome: During mitotic cell division, chromosomes divide longitudinally, and rarely it may divide transverse across the centromere; that is, one may have a long arm or short arm

Chromosome ring: A ring chromosome happens in two ways. When there are deletions from both the ends of a chromosome, the ends may unite forming a ring chromosome.

Change in the Chromosome Number (Fig. 21.2)

Numerical changes in individual chromosomes represent loss or gain of chromosome sets. The term euploidy denotes the correct complete chromosome set that is present in humans. The diploid 2N = 46 and haploid N = 23 number of chromosomes.

Polyploidy: It refers to an exact multiple of the haploid set, e.g. 69(3N) chromosomes with three copies of each

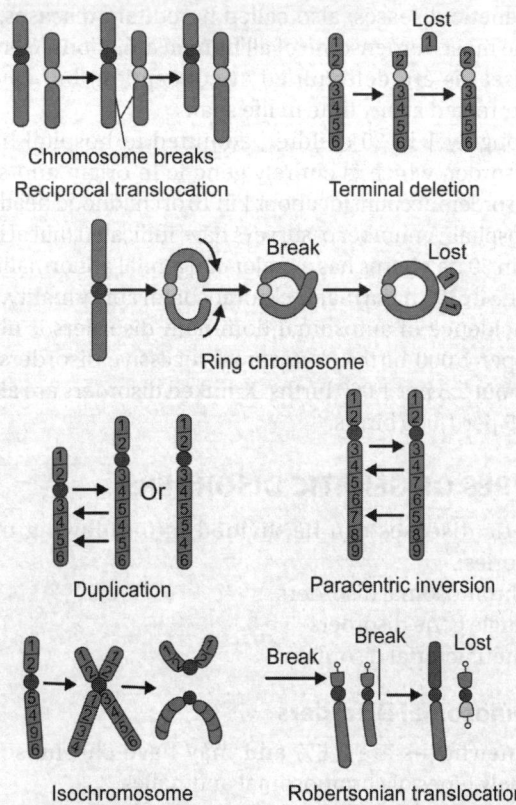

Fig. 21.1: Change in chromosomal structure.

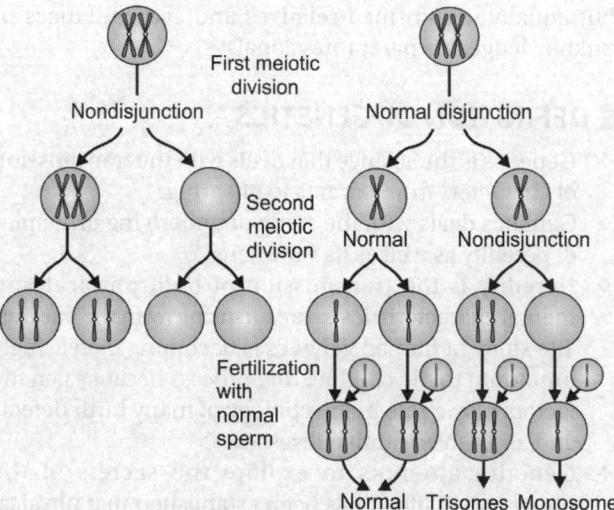

Fig. 21.2: Process of nondisjunction at the first and second meiotic divisions of the ovum and fertilization with normal sperm.

chromosome instead of two, i.e. more than four sets of chromosomes:
- Triploids: 3N or 3 sets of chromosomes
- Tetraploids: 4N or 4 sets of chromosomes

Aneuploidy:
- Depending upon the number of chromosome like loss of single chromosome is termed as monosomy and addition of one or more chromosomes are termed as trisomy, tetrasomy, etc. It is caused by nondisjunction (failure of the paired chromosome or sister chromatids to disjoin at anaphase) or anaphase lag (delayed movement of a chromosome of anaphase).
- Nondisjunction may occur either during meiosis or mitosis. Meiotic nondisjunction occurs at increased frequency with increased maternal age. The extra chromosome arising from nondisjunction at 15th meiotic division will contain both maternal and paternal homologous of the chromosome, and the chromosome arising from the second meiotic division will be either maternal or paternal.
- The occurrence of nondisjunction during mitosis results in another numerical change called mosaicism. An individual who is mosaic has two or more cell lines with different chromosome constitutions (e.g. 46 and 47 chromosome cell lines) originating from a single zygote.

Autosomal Chromosome Disorders of Number

There are several well-defined chromosome disorders in which a numerical abnormality of an autosome is present.

If three chromosomes are present instead of the usual pair, the abnormality is trisomy. Trisomies are the most common abnormalities of chromosome number. The usual cause of this numerical error is meiotic nondisjunction of chromosomes, resulting in a gamete with 24 instead of 23 chromosomes and subsequently in a zygote with 47 chromosomes. Trisomy of autosomes is associated with three main syndromes:
- Trisomy 21 or Down syndrome
- Trisomy 18 or Edwards syndrome
- Trisomy 13 or Patau syndrome

Infants with trisomy 13 and trisomy 18 are severely malformed and mentally retarded, and usually die early in infancy.
- **Trisomy 21:** One of the most common causes of mental retardation. The affected child has an extra chromosome 21 (with a total of 47 chromosomes). Incidence is 1 in 700 live births.
  Etiology: It arises from meiotic nondisjunction in either parents. The extra chromosome has been found to be of maternal origin in about 85% of cases and of paternal origin in 15%. Advanced maternal age is an important factor in the incidence of Down syndrome.
  Clinical features: Hypotonia, poor Moro reflex, flat facial profile, Brushfield spots, upward slanting palpebral fissures, epicanthal folds, small nose with low nasal bridge, low set ears, protruding tongue, incurving of the fifth finger (clinodactyly) excess skin folds on the back of the neck, short, broad hands with a single transverse retardation varies from mild to severe:
  1. Congenital heart defects occur in 40-60%
  2. Other complications are thyroid, gastrointestinal disorders, etc.
- **Trisomy 18 (Edward's syndrome):** Incidence is 1 per 3,500 live births.
  Etiology: Parental nondisjunction at either the first or second meiotic division. Translocation is rare.
  Clinical features: Low birth weight, failure to thrive, severe mental and growth retardation, congenital heart disease, prominent occiput, low set malformed ears, short sternum, clenched fists, rocker bottom feet. Anomalies of the kidneys and other organs may also be present. Thirty percent die within the first month, only 10% survive beyond the first year.
- **Trisomy 13 (Patau syndrome):** Patau syndrome is severe multiple malformation disorder with an incidence of about 1 per 5,000 live births.
  Etiology: Most affected infants have a regular trisomy due to meiotic nondisjunction in either parents.
  Clinical features: Severe mental and motor retardation, defects of forebrain, microphthalmos, cleft lip and palate, polydactyly, clenched fists, low-set malformed ears, microcephaly with sloping forehead, congenital heart disease and urogenital anomalies.

Sex Chromosome Disorders of Number

Numerical changes of the sex chromosomes similar to those of autosomes, arise chiefly through nondisjunction. Monosomy leads to Turner's syndrome (45, X) and trisomy leads to Klinefelter syndrome (47, XXY), (47, XYY) male and XXX female:
- Turner's syndrome 45, X
- Klinefelter syndrome XXY
- Triple X syndrome XXX
- XYY syndrome.

Turner's syndrome (45, X)

- *Incidence:* It is 1 in 2,000–2,500 live female births. This disorder is the only monosomy compatible with viability. The complete absence of the chromosome is present in about 50–60%.
- *Etiology:* Monosomy X may arise from parental nondisjunction. Since the maternal X-chromosome is present in many cases, it has been suggested that the error occurred in spermatogenesis or after fertilization.
- *Clinical features:* Short stature, low hairline, webbing of the neck, broad chest with widely spaced nipples, cubitus valgus (increased carrying angle of the arms),

hypoplastic nails and failure of secondary sexual development.

Klinefelter syndrome XXY (47, XXY)

- ❖ ***Incidence:*** It is 1 in 800 live male births.
- ❖ ***Etiology:*** The extra X-chromosome usually arises as a result of meiotic nondisjunction in either parents.
- ❖ ***Clinical features:*** Behavioral problems or dull mentality, long limbs, small penis or small testes, incomplete development of secondary sexual characteristics, inadequate testosterone production, gynecomastia, infertility, normal intelligence or varying degrees of mental retardation.

Triple X syndrome XXX

- ❖ ***Incidence:*** It is 1 per 1,000 female infants.
- ❖ ***Etiology:*** Meiotic nondisjunction in either parents is the cause of 47, XXX.
- ❖ ***Clinical features:*** Tallness with increased height velocity between 4 and 8 years of age. Menstrual irregularities, delay in speech and language development, mild mental retardation, problems in interpersonal relationships.

XYY syndrome

XYY syndrome occurs in approximately 1 in 1,000 male newborns.

Clinical features: May include tall stature, large teeth and severe acne at adolescence, behavioral problems with aggression and dull mentality. Intelligence tends to be about 10–15 points less than that of the normal siblings. The origin of 47, XYY is obviously paternal, arising from the production of a Y sperm during meiotic division or post-fertilization nondisjunction of the Y.

Single Gene Disorders

The transmission of traits or disorders according to specific patterns first described by the Austrian monk Gregor Mendel is known as Mendelian inheritance. Mendelian disorders are also called single gene disorders. Most disorders determined by single gene mutation follow the laws of inheritance described by Mendel. Two main laws were derived from his experiments:
1. Law of segregation (Mendel's first law)
2. Law of independent assortment (Mendel's second law).

In contrast to chromosome abnormalities, which involve an excess or deficiency of whole chromosomes or chromosome segments, single gene disorders are caused by a mutation of a gene at a single major error in the genetic information. If a particular trait disease or defect is controlled by a single gene, the pattern is called single gene disorders. There are four major patterns of Mendelian inheritance:
- ❖ Autosomal dominant
- ❖ Autosomal recessive
- ❖ X-linked dominant
- ❖ X-linked recessive.

Genes located on the autosomes are autosomal, whereas genes on the X-chromosomes are X-linked. Because chromosomes come in pairs, genes also exist in pairs. Genes at the same locus on a chromosome pair that govern a particular trait may occur in different or alternative forms called alleles. If the alleles of a gene pair are identical, they are referred to as homozygous. If the two alleles are different, they are referred to as heterozygous.

Genotype

It refers to the genetic constitution of an individual, with respect to either a specific gene pair, or less often, the total complement of genes. For example, a person who is heterozygous for one gene pair may be represented as Aa, whereas one who is homozygous might be AA or aa. It is relatively stable throughout the life of an individual.

Phenotype

It is the outward expression of the genetic constitution. The color, form, size and stature of individuals are all phenotypical expression of a particular genetic constitution. Certain phenotype characteristics of an individual may change from infancy to adulthood such as height, weight, body shape, etc.

Thus, there are two aspects of the genetic material—one fixed and other plastic. The fixed characters are the genotype and the plastic ones are the phenotype. These two types may best be compared to a given pellet of clay, which may be molded into any desired shape by an artist, but the weight, volume, density and chemical constitution of the pellet will remain the same.

Autosomal Dominant Inheritance (Fig. 21.3)

Autosomal dominant inheritance disorders are those in which the abnormal gene for the trait is expressed even when the other member of the pair is normal. The abnormal gene may appear as a result of a mutation, a spontaneous and permanent change in the normal gene structure, in which case the disorder occurs for the first time in the family. However, an affected individual usually comes from multiple generations having the disorder. An affected parent who is heterozygous for the trait has a 50% chance of passing the abnormal gene to each offspring. Males and females are equally affected.

Autosomal dominant disorders are not always expressed with the same severity of symptoms. The parent may have a minor abnormality that had not been diagnosed until the birth of a more severely affected child. There is no way offspring will have a minor or a severe abnormality. These are:
- ❖ Achondroplasia (dwarfism)
- ❖ Huntington's chorea
- ❖ Polydactyly (extra digits)

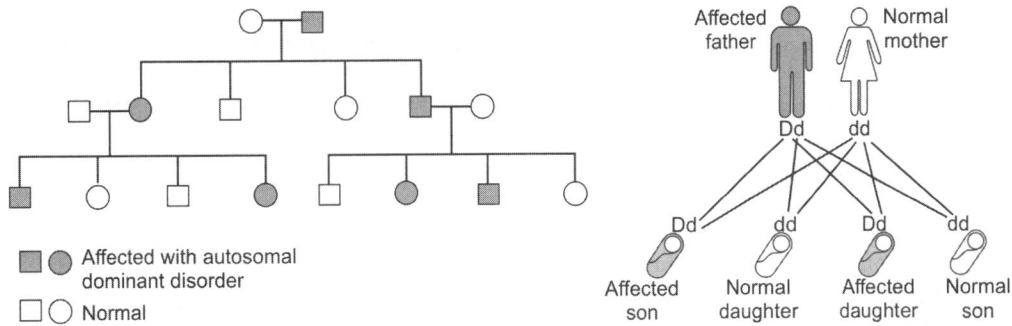

Fig. 21.3: Pedigree and the mechanism of transmission found in autosomal dominant inheritance.

- Marfan's syndrome
- Neurofibromatosis
- ABO blood group system.

Autosomal Recessive Inheritance (Fig. 21.4)

Autosomal recessive inheritance disorders are those in which both genes of a pair must be abnormal for the disorder to be expressed. Heterozygous individuals have only one abnormal gene and are unaffected clinically because their normal gene overshadows the abnormal gene. They are known as carriers of the recessive trait. Because these recessive traits are inherited by generations of the same family, an increased incidence of the disorder occurs in consanguineous mating (closely related parents). In order for the trait to be expressed, two carriers must each contribute the abnormal gene to the offspring may be a carrier of the gene. Males and females are equally affected.

Most recessive disorders tend to have severe clinical manifestations and affected offspring do not often reproduce. If they do, all of their offspring do not often reproduce. If they do, all of their offspring will be carriers for the disorder. They are:

- Phenylketonuria
- Galactosemia
- Sickle cell anemia
- Cystic fibrosis
- Tay-Sachs disease
- Hemoglobinopathies

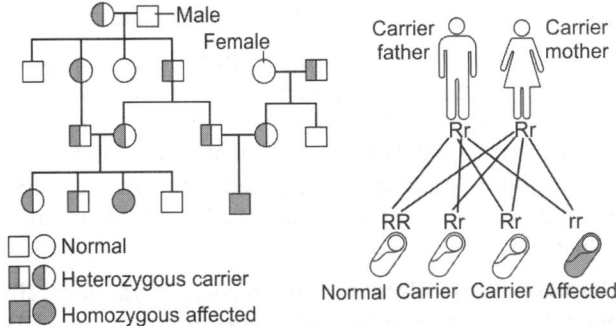

Fig. 21.4: Pedigree and the mechanism of transmission found in autosomal recessive inheritance.

X-linked Inheritance

Both recessive and dominant X-linked disorders are due to mutant genes located on the X-chromosome. A key characteristic of X-linked inheritance is that genes on the X-chromosome have no counterpart or corresponding locus on the Y-chromosome. Since males have only one X-chromosome, they are said to be hemizygous rather than heterozygous or homozygous, with respect to X-linked genes. A mutant gene on the X-chromosome will therefore always be expressed in the male. Females have two X-chromosomes and are either heterozygous or homozygous for X-linked mutant genes. Since no serious human diseases are known to be associated with the Y-chromosome, sex linkage is synonymous with X-linkage.

X-linked Recessive Inheritance (Fig. 21.5)

Abnormal genes for X-linked recessive inheritance disorders are carried on the X-chromosome. Females may be heterozygous or homozygous for traits carried on the X-chromosome because they have two. Males are hemizygous because they only have one X-chromosome genes with no alleles on the Y-chromosome. Therefore, X-linked recessive orders are most commonly manifested

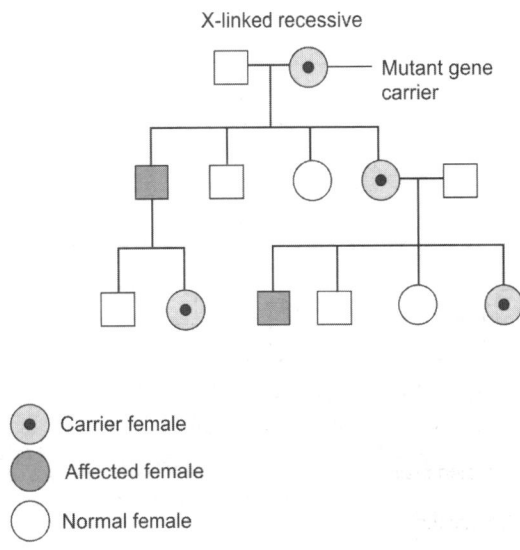

Fig. 21.5: X-linked recessive inheritance.

in the male with the abnormal gene on his single X-chromosome. The male receives the defective gene from his carrier mother on her affected X-chromosome. Female carriers have 50% probability of transmitting the abnormal gene to each offspring.

An affected male can pass the abnormal gene only to his daughters on the X-chromosome, but not to his sons. The daughters will be carriers of the trait if they receive a normal gene on the X-chromosome from their mother. They can be affected only if they receive an abnormal gene on the X-chromosome from their mother also. They are:
- Hemophilia
- Color blindness
- Hydrocephalus
- Retinitis pigmentosa
- A gamma globulinemia

X-linked Dominant Inheritance (Fig. 21.6)

X-linked dominant inheritance disorders occur both in males and heterozygous females. Because the females also have a normal gene and the effects are more severe in affected males. Affected males transmit the abnormal gene only to their daughters on the X-chromosome. Heterozygous females have a 50% chance of transmitting the abnormal gene to each offspring. An example of these extremely rare disorders is vitamin D-resistant rickets.

Multifactorial Inheritance and Disorders (Table 21.1)

- Most of the common congenital malformations result from multifactorial inheritance—a combination of genetic and environmental factors. The malformation may range from mild to severe, depending on the number of genes present for the defect or the amount of environmental influence.

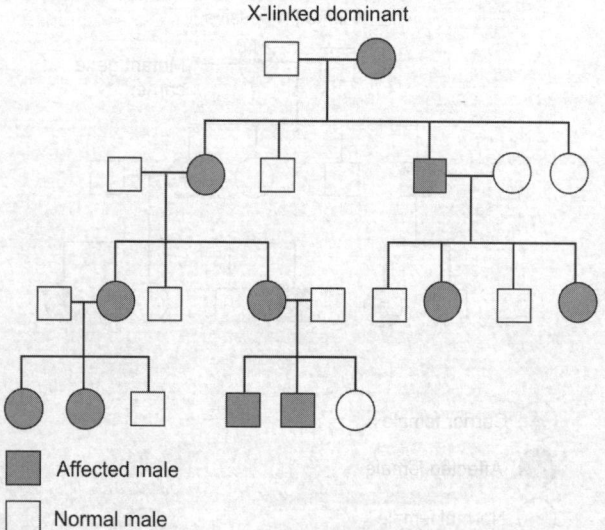

Fig. 21.6: X-linked dominant inheritance.

Table 21.1: Examples of multifactorial disorders.

Congenital malformations	Adult onset disease
Cleft lip	Hypertension
Cleft palate	Epilepsy
Congenital dislocation of hip	Obesity
Neural tube defects	Glaucoma, schizophrenia
Pyloric stenosis	Manic depression

- Some common congenital defects with a multifactorial basis are neural tube defects, cleft lip, cleft palate, congenital dislocation of the hip, congenital heart defects, clubfoot and pyloric stenosis.
- Most normal human traits such as height, intelligence, body build and blood pressure are also multifactorial. In addition, examples of common adult diseases that occur secondary to multifactorial causation include diabetes mellitus, schizophrenia, coronary artery disease, hypertension, peptic ulcer disease and some forms of cancer.
- The severity of the defect also influences recurrence risk estimation; that is, the more severe the defect, the higher will be the risk of recurrence.
- An important factor in multifactorial inheritance is the number of genes an individual shares in common with the affected person. The closer the relationship, the greater the number of genes shared in common. The risk to relatives is sharply lower for second degree than for first degree relatives and declines at a lower rate for third degree and more distant relatives. For example, for cleft lip with cleft palate, the empirical risks for first, second and third degree relatives are 40, 7 and 3 times that of general population incidence of 1 per 1,000 (Thompson et al, 1991).
- Some malformations occur more often in one sex or the other. For example, pyloric stenosis and cleft lip are more common in males and cleft palate is more common in females.

Role of Genetic Predisposition in Common Disorders

Genetic predisposition may lead to the premature onset of common diseases of adult life such as cancer, coronary heart disease (CHD), diabetes, hypertension and mental disorders.

Cancer: It is not yet certain whether most cancers are hereditary. But a genetic predisposition may be involved in as many as 10–25% of cases of cancer of the breast or colon. Numerous genes are being identified that may affect susceptibility to tumor development. This may lead to a general improvement in the diagnosis and treatment of cancer.

Coronary heart disease: Until recently, it was generally believed that environmental factors alone cause CHD. But investing family histories often uncover genetic predisposition to CHD are also genetically influenced. A combination of risk detection and lifestyle counseling with drug treatment, might cut the incidence of heart attacks to the low levels as two or three generations ago.

Diabetes: Evidence for a genetic element in insulin-dependent diabetes mellitus has emerged from studies showing a higher concordance in identical twins than in non-identical twins. About 85% of cases of diabetes in developed countries are of the non-insulin dependent form of the disease, which has a particularly string familial tendency. Diabetes of all types is an important candidate for future treatments such as gene therapy of pancreatic tissue transplantation.

Mental disorders: Evidence from family and twin studies demonstrate the existence of genetic predisposition to some common mental diseases. Alzheimer's disease, the most common form of senile dementia, has a strong familial tendency and is known to be caused by at least four different genes. Research may lead to the development of drugs useful in preventing or delaying the onset of the disease.

MANAGEMENT OF GENETIC DISORDERS

Currently, genetic disorders cannot be cured, although remedies can be implemented to preventive or reduce the harmful effects of a few disorders. Structural defects can sometimes be modified to produce normal or near normal function. Research is being conducted to devise methods to influence or change the genes directly by placing substitute DNA in the cells of those with a genetic mutation, thereby preventing or curing the disease process or relieving symptoms.

Researches continue to develop therapies for heritable diseases. Some possible methods of future management include replacement or stabilization by oral or parenteral medications or other methods, altering of intracellular DNA and other projected feats of genetic engineering.

CONCLUSION

Nurses involved in infant and child care continually encounter genetic disorder that needs expert evaluation. Early identification of a genetic disorder allows anticipation of associated conditions and implementation of available preventive measures and therapy to avoid potential complications and actualize or enhance the child's health potential. It may also prevent the unexpected birth of another affected child in the immediate or extended family.

CHAPTER 22

Genetic Testing: Basis of Genetic Diagnosis, Presymptomatic and Predisposition Testing, Prenatal Diagnosis and Screening

CHAPTER OUTLINE

- Types of Genetic Tests
- Indications for Prenatal Screening and Diagnostic Testing
- Goals of Genetic Screening
- Preventive and Social Measures
- Other Preventive Measures
- Reproductive Alternatives
- Ethical, Legal and Psychosocial Issues in Genetic Testing

INTRODUCTION

Genetic testing is essential for early diagnosis and treatment, and to identify the healthy carriers of genetic disorders. Antenatal and neonatal screening involves many risks of invasive procedures. There is need to discuss and make informed choices with couples when dealing with such issues.

Definition of Pedigree

The word pedigree came from "pied de grue" or crane's foot, a diagram of a family history indicating the family members, their relationships to the family tree is indicated by an arrow (pro-band) and their status with respect to a particular hereditary condition.

Pedigree Drawing (Fig. 22.1)

A Family Tree is a short-hand system of recording the pertinent information about a family and their relationships among the members of a family.

It is customary to represent males as squares and females as circles. A horizontal line connecting a circle and a square represents a mating. The offspring of the mating are shown beneath the mates starting with the first born at the left and proceeding through the birth order to the right. Individuals that have genetic condition are indicated by coloring or shading. The generations in a pedigree are usually denoted by Roman numerals, and particular individuals within a generation are referred by Arabic numerals following the Roman numeral.

It begins with careful assessment of the pattern of inheritance in the family. The process includes:

❖ **Family history:** A detailed family history is obtained to see if any disorders are presented in family members:
  ➢ The mother's age is important to obtain
  ➢ Previous obstetric history
  ➢ Menstrual history
  ➢ Any spontaneous abortions
  ➢ Any chromosomal abnormalities

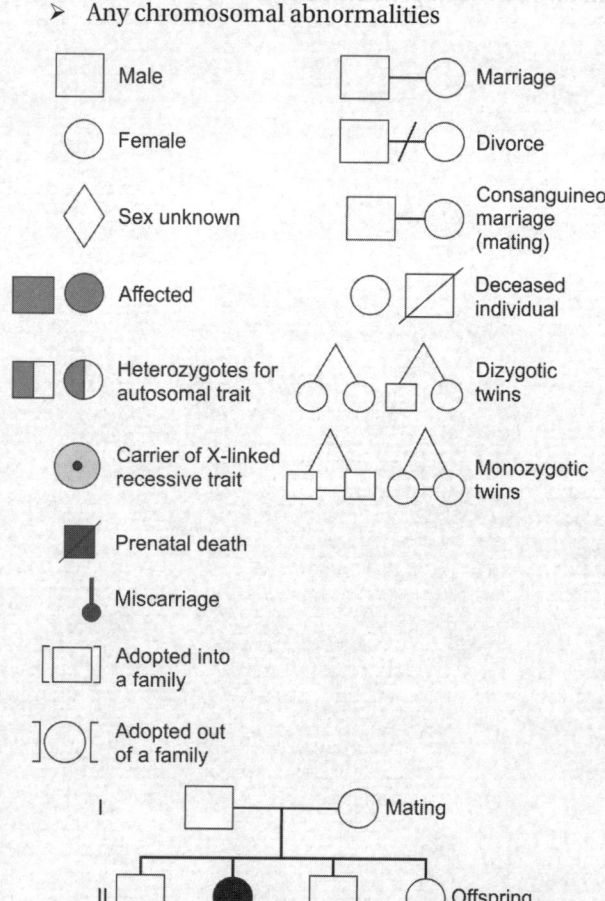

Fig. 22.1: Symbols used in construction of a pedigree.

- ➢ Related disease conditions
- ➢ Drawing a pedigree chart helps to know the mode of inheritance.
- ❖ **Physical assessment:** A careful physical assessment of all family members is important.
- ❖ **Laboratory analysis [biochemical, cytogenetic tests and deoxyribonucleic acid (DNA) studies]:** A genetic test is a laboratory analysis to detect DNA, ribonucleic acid (RNA) or chromosomal abnormalities that cause or likely to cause a specific disease or condition. Tests can also analyze proteins or metabolites that are the products of genes. There are many laboratory tests, which provide important clues of possible disorders.
- ❖ **Genetic tests:** They are used to predict risks of disease, screen newborns for disease, identify carriers of genetic disorders and establish prenatal or clinical diagnosis. Testing can be done using many different biological samples including blood, amniotic fluid, etc.
- ❖ **DNA studies:** The recombinant DNA technology (commonly called genetic engineering) is the latest investigation used for diagnosis of genetic diseases and research into molecular pathology of disease.

TYPES OF GENETIC TESTS

Some specific types of genetic tests are:

Carrier testing: It is performed to determine whether an individual carries one copy of an altered gene for a particular recessive disease. It is usually done in the context of reproductive planning and can be done before a pregnancy occurs.

Preimplantation diagnosis: It is used following in vitro fertilization to diagnose a genetic disease or condition in a preimplantation embryo.

Prenatal diagnosis: It is used to diagnose a genetic disease or condition in a developing fetus.

It is used to detect changes in the fetal genes or chromosomes before birth. This type of testing is done in couples with an increased risk of having fetus with genetic or chromosomal disorders.

Direct testing: It examines the DNA and RNA that make up a gene.

Biological testing: It assays certain enzymes or proteins, the products of genes.

Diagnostic testing: It is used to diagnose or rule out a specific genetic or chromosomal condition. Normally, genetic testing is used to conform a diagnosis when a particular condition is suspected based on physical mutations and symptoms. Diagnostic tests are not available for all genetic conditions, the result of a diagnostic test can influence a person's choices about health care and the management of the disease.

Predictive and presymptomatic testing: These tests are used to detect gene mutations associated with disorders that appear after birth, often later in life. These tests can be helpful in people who have family members with a genetic disorder, but have no manifestation of the disorder at the time of testing. Predictive testing can identify mutations that increase a person's chances of developing disorders with a genetic history, such as certain types of cancers. Presymptomatic testing can determine whether a person will develop a genetic disorder, before any signs or symptoms appear. This type of testing can provide information about a person's risk of developing a specific disorder, helping them to make decisions about their care.

Parental testing: This type of genetic test is used in special DNA markers to identify the similar inheritance patterns between related individuals.

Forensic testing: It uses DNA sequences to identify an individual for legal purposes. This testing is not used to detect gene mutations associated with diseases. This is used to identify crime or catastrophic victims, rule out or implicate a crime suspect or establish biological relationship between people.

Newborn screening: It is used just after birth to identify genetic disorders that can be treated early in life. The routing testing of infants for certain disorders is common and widespread in all the states, e.g. to rule out phenylketonuria and congenital hypothyroidism.

Research testing: These tests are used in special DNA markers to identify unknown genes, learning how genes work and advanced genetic conditions. The result of testing is done as a part of research study, and is usually not available to patients or their health care providers.

Pharmacogenomics: This is a type of genetic testing that determines the influence of genetic variations on drug response.

INDICATIONS FOR PRENATAL SCREENING AND DIAGNOSTIC TESTING

To detect abnormalities of the fetus, the prenatal diagnostic technique (Regulation and Prevention of Misuse Act) was passed on 20th September 1994. The main objectives were to regulate as well as prevent the use of prenatal diagnostic techniques for the purpose of prenatal sex determination leading to female feticide. This Act provides for regulation of genetic counseling centers, genetic laboratories and genetic clinics. According to the Act, the prenatal diagnostic techniques may be conducted for detecting the following abnormalities:

- ❖ Chromosomal abnormalities
- ❖ Advanced maternal age
- ❖ Genetic metabolic diseases

- Parental balanced translocation
- Affected parent with a micro deletion syndrome
- Abnormalities identified in pregnancy
- Family history of chromosomal abnormality, single gene disorder, neural tube defects, congenital abnormalities, etc.
- Two or more spontaneous abortions and exposure to certain teratogenic agents such as drugs, radiations, infections, etc.

GOALS OF GENETIC SCREENING

The principal goals of genetic screening are the early identification of potential risk and the determination of disease probability and etiology. These include karyotyping, Barr body determination, Alpha-fetoprotein (AFP) analysis, chorionic villi sampling (CVS), sonography and fetoscopy, etc.

Karyotyping

A karyotyping is a visual presentation of the chromosome pattern of an individual. For karyotyping, a sample of peripheral venous blood or a scraping of cells from the buccal membrane is taken. Cells are allowed to grow until they reach a stage of metaphase. Any additional lacking, abnormal chromosomes can be visualized by this method.

Fluorescence in situ Hybridization

Fluorescence in situ hybridization (FISH) is a rapid method for determining ploidy for a few specific chromosomes or confirming the presence or absence of a gene or large DNA sequence. It is not comparable to cytogenetic evaluation, because the chromosomes appear squat and the banding patterns are much less distinctive. Chromosome duplications, deletions and rearrangements often cannot be detected by FISH. Cells are fixed on a glass slide, and fluorescently labeled chromosome or gene probes are allowed to hybridize to the fixed chromosomes. Each probe is complementary to a unique area of the chromosome or gene, thus preventing cross reaction with other chromosomes. If the chromosome or gene of interest is present, hybridization is detected as a bright signal visible by microscopy. The number of signals indicate the number of chromosomes or genes of that type in the cell being analyzed. FISH is usually used when ploidy status would change clinical management and time constraints prevent waiting for cytogenetic analysis.

Barr Body Determination

If a child is born with ambiguous genitalia a Barr body determination, a quick test to evaluate whether the child has two X-chromosomes can be done. Only one X-chromosome is functional in females; the non-dominant one appears to be uninvolved in cell metabolism. For this procedure, the cells are scraped from the buccal membrane of the inner surface of the child's cheek, then stained and magnified. The presence of Barr body confirms that the child is chromosomally female.

Alpha-fetoprotein Analysis

AFP is a glycoprotein produced by the fetal liver. The level of AFP present in amniotic fluid or maternal serum will increase from normal if a chromosomal or a spinal cord disorder is present. Most pregnant women have a serum test done at the 15th week of pregnancy. It will be decreased in a chromosomal disorder such as trisomy 21.

AFP is shed by the fetus into the surrounding amniotic fluid; from there, it crosses the placental barrier and gains access to maternal serum. Therefore, AFP levels can measure maternal serum alpha feto protein (MSAFP) as well as in amniotic fluid alpha-fetoprotein (AFAFP).

Purpose: The evaluation of MSAFP is to determine whether the fetus has an open neural tube defects, which include anencephaly, spina bifida, etc.

Procedure: This test is done between 15 and 18 weeks of gestation; the physician offers the woman the option of having the blood drawn to evaluate the concentration of AFP in her serum. She is informed that MSAFP is only a screening test required to investigate abnormal concentrations. If Level 1 ultrasound fails to explain the abnormal levels of AFP, Level 2 ultrasound with amniocentesis should be the next step. Amniotic fluid is analyzed for elevated levels of AFP and for acetylcholinesterase (AChE) is noted in association with open neural tube defects.

Interpretation of the results:
- MSAFP level is elevated
- Wrong gestational age
- Open neural-tube defects
- Multiple pregnancy
- Intrauterine fetal death (IUFD)
- Anterior abnormal wall defects
- Renal anomalies.

Low levels are found in:
- Down's syndrome
- Gestational trophoblastic disease.

Advantages:
- It is a simple procedure that requires only a sample of maternal blood
- It is the least invasive and the most economical procedure to screen for open neural tube defects
- Prenatal diagnosis allows parents' time to examine their options.

Limitations:
- MSAFP screening test is only viewed as the first step in a series of diagnostic procedures that are necessary if abnormal concentrations are found

- Timing also imposes some limits, MSAFP evaluation is performed between the 15th and 18th weeks of pregnancy
- Because closed neural tube defects do not produce elevated levels of AFP, normal levels of AFP do not guarantee a perfect baby.

Triple Test

It is a combination of biochemical tests, which includes MSAFP, human chorionic gonadotropin (hCG) and unconjugated estriol (UE3). In which, maternal age in relation to gestational age is conformed. It is used for detection of Down's Syndrome. In an affected pregnancy level, MSAFP and UE3 tend to be low while that of hCG is high. It is performed at 15–18 weeks. It gives a risk ratio, and for conformation, amniocentesis has to done; the result is considered to be screen positive if the risk ratio is 1:250 or greater.

Acetylcholine Esterase (AChE)

Amniotic fluid AChE level is elevated in most cases of open neural tube defects. It has got better diagnostic value than AFP.

Chorionic Villi Sampling

It is retrieval and analysis of chorionic villi for chromosome analysis. Although this procedure may be done as early as the 5th week of pregnancy, it is more commonly done at 8–10 weeks. In this procedure, a thin catheter is inserted vaginally or a biopsy needle is inserted abdominally or intra-vaginally and a number of chorionic cells are removed for analysis.

Risk: It causes excessive bleeding, leading to pregnancy loss. Parents should be informed about this risk before the procedure. There are some instances of children being born with missing limbs after the procedure. Not all inherited diseases can be detected by CVS. The test does not reveal the level of spinal cord abnormalities.

Amniocentesis (Fig. 22.2)

Amniocentesis is the withdrawal of amniotic fluid through the abdominal wall for analysis at the 14th–16th week of pregnancy. Analysis may include the karyotyping of skin cells obtained or analysis of AFP or AChE. Detecting the enzyme AChE in the amniotic fluid helps support the diagnosis of an abnormality. In virtually all cases of anencephaly, spina bifida, the AFP level is high and AChE can be detected in the amniotic fluid. High level indicates an increased likelihood of spina bifida, anencephaly, etc. Women who have a high AFP level also are more likely to have complications during pregnancy such as retarded growth or death of the fetus and early detachment of placenta.

Percutaneous Umbilical Blood Sampling (Cordocentesis) (Fig. 22.3)

Percutaneous umbilical blood sampling (PUBS) is the removal of blood from the umbilical cord using an amniocentesis technique. This allows for more rapid karyotyping than is possible when only skin cells are removed.

Ultrasonography (Levels 1 and 2)

Sonography is a diagnostic tool that is helpful in assessing a fetus for general size and structural disorders of internal organs, spine and limbs. Because some genetic disorders are associated with congenital defects, sonography may be helpful. Sonography may be used concurrently with amniocentesis, because it causes no apparent risk to the fetus.

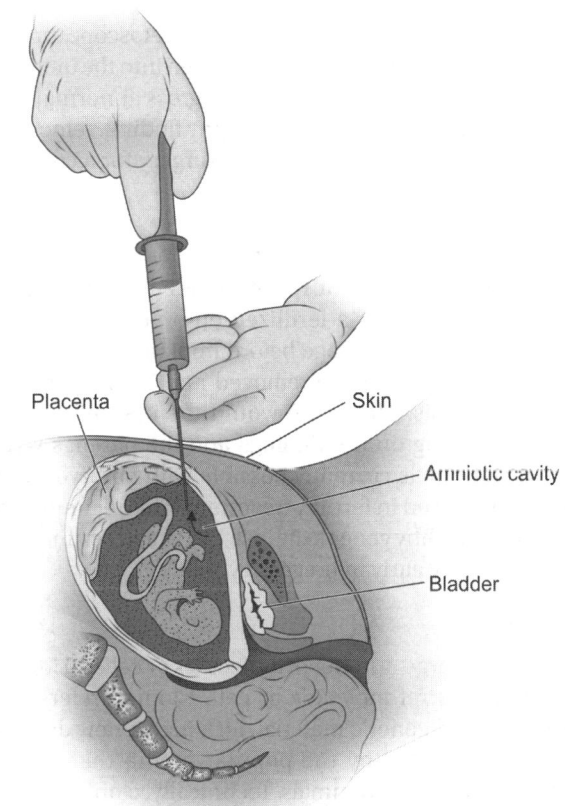

Fig. 22.2: Amniocentesis.

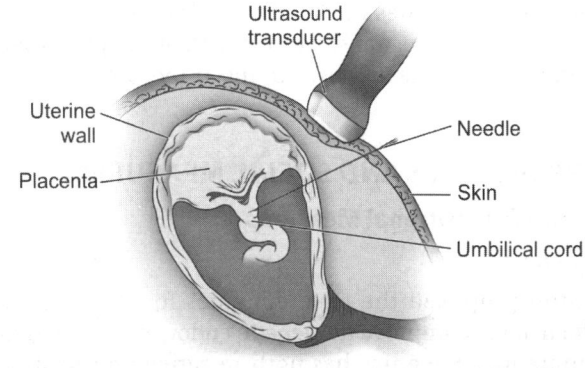

Fig. 22.3: Percutaneous umbilical blood sampling (PUBS) (cordocentesis).

Level 2 or targeted ultrasonography or anomaly scan is done to evaluate the systematic examination of fetal anatomy and physiology when there is increased risk for fetal abnormalities.

For example: The maternal history of giving birth to an infant with anomalies or a history of abnormal clinical findings such as hydramnios, oligohydramnios, neural tube defects, malformed kidneys, hydrocephalus, cleft lip and palate, cardiac defects can be detected with targeted ultrasound.

Fetoscopy

Fetoscopy is the insertion of a fiberoptic fetoscope through a small incision in the mother's abdomen into the uterus and membranes to inspect the fetus for gross abnormalities. It can be used to confirm a sonography finding, remove skin cells for DNA analysis or perform surgery for a congenital defect such as a stenosed urethra.

Preimplantation Diagnosis

Although currently not recommended, in the future it may be possible for a fertilized embryo to be removed from the uterus by lavage before implantation, with cells from the zona pellucida removed and biopsied for DNA or cell analysis. The ovum would then be reinserted or not, depending on the findings and the parent's wishes. The technique is currently possible with embryo transfer procedures used in fertility treatment. This technique may also allow healthy genes to be inserted to correct underlying disorders very early in pregnancy.

Cloning

A clone is a large number of molecules or cells all identical to one ancestral molecule or cell. Cloning refers to the replication of genetic material, although a new definition has been created by the popular media that includes replication of whole animals. Technically, cloning includes several laboratory techniques that enable pieces of DNA to be copied in large quantities by lower organisms. These techniques utilize various vectors, which are DNA molecules that replicate autonomously in its host cell. Restriction enzymes are used to cleave both the DNA sequence of interest and the vector DNA at appropriate sites, and DNA ligase is used to insert the DNA segment into the vector.

▮ PREVENTIVE AND SOCIAL MEASURES

Health Promotional Measures

Eugenics

Galton proposed the term eugenics for the science, which aims to improve the genetic endowment of human population. Eugenics has both negative and positive aspects.

Negative eugenics

Hitler sought to improve the German race by killing the weak and defective; this was negative eugenics. But nobody in the civilized world would approve of such a measure to improve the human race. The aim of negative eugenics is to reduce the frequency of hereditary disease and disability in the community to as low as possible. In spite of eugenic sterilization, new cases of hereditary diseases will continue to arise in the population partly because of fresh mutations, and partly because of marital alliances between hidden carriers of recessive defects; nevertheless, it may be hoped that should eugenic measures be applied, hereditary diseases would become less frequent.

Positive eugenics

It seeks to improve the genetic composition of the population by encouraging the carriers of desirable genotypes to assume the burden of parenthood. Its realization is difficult for two reasons.

The majority of socially valuable traits—let us say intelligence and positive character features, though partially determined biologically—are not inherited in such a simple way as say blood groups. These traits have a complex, multifactorial determination both genetical and environmental. It would be difficult to expect; therefore, positive eugenic measures will yield direct results. We cannot determine which gene we transmit to our children.

Euthenics

Mere improvement of the genotype is of no use unless the improved genotype is given access to a suitable environment, an environment which will enable the genes to express themselves readily. Studies with mentally retarded children indicate that exposure to environmental stimulation improve their IQ. Thus, the solution of improving the human race does not lie in contrasting hereditary and environment, but rather in the mutual interaction of heredity and environmental factors. This environmental manipulation is called euthenics and has considerable broader prospects for success.

Genetic Counseling

The most immediate and practical service that genetics can render in medicine and surgery is genetic counseling.

▮ OTHER PREVENTIVE MEASURES

Consanguineous Marriage

When blood relatives marry each other, there is an increased risk in the offspring of traits controlled by recessive genes, and those determined by polygenes. Therefore, a lowering of consanguineous marriages would be advantageous to the health of the community.

Late Marriage

The pendulum is swinging in favor of early marriages. The discovery of trisomy 21 in Mongols coupled with the knowledge that mongolism is more frequent in children born of elderly mothers tend to support from the view that early marriage of females is better than late marriage from the point of view of preventing mongolism. Its incidence in a mother at the age of 20 is only 1:3,000; by the age of 40, 60% of her eggs carries abnormal chromosomes.

Specific Protection

Increasing attention is now being paid to the protection of individuals and whole communities against mutagens such as X-rays and other ionizing radiations. Patients undergoing X-ray examination should be protected against unnecessary exposure of the gonads to radiation. X-ray examination of the pregnant uterus to determine the presence of twins or the lie of the fetus is to be strongly deprecated.

Early Diagnosis and Treatment

- *Detection of genetic carriers:* It is now possible to identify the healthy carriers of a number of genetic disorders, especially the inborn errors of metabolism. The female carriers of Duchenne type of muscular dystrophy, an X-linked disorder can now be detected by elevated levels of serum creatine kinase in 80% of carriers.
- *Prenatal diagnosis:* Amniocentesis in early pregnancy has now made it possible for prenatal diagnosis of conditions associated with chromosomal anomalies. The diagnosis of chromosomal anomalies is made by culture and karyotyping of fetal cells from the amniotic fluid, and of metabolic defects by biochemical analysis of the fluid. For the detection of neural tube defects, there is now the possibility of widespread screening by the determination of AFP levels in the maternal serum. If the test is positive, it can be confirmed by amniocentesis.
- *Screening of newborn infants:* We have today a long list of screening tests for the early diagnosis of genetic abnormalities—sex chromosome abnormalities, congenital dislocation of hip, sickle cell disease, etc.

Rehabilitation

Finally, rehabilitation with many genetic or partially genetic conditions causing physical or mental disability, much can be done for the patient and for his/her family in helping him/her to lead a better and more useful life.

REPRODUCTIVE ALTERNATIVES

Some couples are reluctant to seek genetic counseling, because they are afraid they will be told it would be unwise to have children:

- Artificial insemination by donor (AID) is an option for couples in whom the genetic disorder is one inherited by the male partner or is a recessively inherited disorder carried by both partners.
- If the inherited problem is one caused by the female partner, use of a surrogate mother (a woman who agrees to be artificially inseminated by the male partner's sperm and bear a child for the couple) is a possibility.
- Donor embryo transfer (an ovum is taken from a donor, fertilized in the laboratory by the husband's sperm, and then implanted in the wife's uterus) is a procedure performed in major centers.
- Pregnancy interruption or therapeutic abortion of any pregnancy that reveals a chromosomal or metabolic abnormality is yet another option.
- Diagnosis of a disorder during pregnancy and prompt treatment at birth to minimize the prognosis and outcome of the disorder is another possibility.
- Adoption is an alternative. Couples need support from health care personnel to decide on the alternative that is correct for them.

ETHICAL, LEGAL AND PSYCHOSOCIAL ISSUES IN GENETIC TESTING

Definition of ethical issues: Ethical issues can be defined as those which involve moral questions and dilemmas. Traditionally, they are approached by applying a set of moral principles, usually on a synthesis of the philosophical and religious views of well informed, respected, thinking members of the society. In this way, the code of practice evolves which is seen as reasonable and acceptable by a majority and which often forms the basis of professional guidelines or regulations.

Legal and Ethical Aspects of Genetic Screening and Counseling

When participating in genetic screening or counseling, there are a number of legal responsibilities to keep in mind. These include the following:

- Participation in genetic screening programs must be elective, not mandatory
- People desiring genetic screening should sign an informed consent form for the procedure
- Results may be interpreted carefully and relayed to individuals as promptly as possible
- The results must not be withheld from individuals
- The results must not be given to the persons other than those directly involved
- After genetic counseling, persons must not be coerced to undergo procedures such as abortion or sterilization. This should be a free individually dictated choice.

Genetic screening and counseling can raise serious ethical questions for a couple, particularly when they choose to abort a pregnancy based on CVS or amniocentesis. Some people argue that a decision to abort a child just because he or she will be mentally or physically handicapped is unethical. A woman who carries the gene for an X-linked disorder for which there is no prenatal screening test might choose to abort all male fetuses, even though each will have a 50% chance of not inheriting the disease. It is important to remember that the choice to be made is the couples not the counselors.

General Principles Related to Ethical Considerations

When undertaking any patient contact, there are a number of important general principles to keep in mind.
1. **Informed consent:** Patient is entitled to full explanation before any procedure or test is undertaken. Information should include details of the risks, limitations and implications of each procedure.
2. **Informed choice:** A patient is entitled to full information about all options available including the option of not participating. Potential consequences should be discussed. The doctor or nurse should not have a vested interest in the patients pursuing any particular course of action.
3. **Autonomy:** A patient is in charge. At any stage, he or she can decide to proceed no further.
4. **Confidentiality:** A patient has a right to complete confidentiality which can only on contract under extreme circumstances, such as, when patient behavior could convey a high risk of harm to himself or to others.

Common Legal Considerations in Clinical Genetics/Ethical Dilemmas

Potential areas of difficulty in clinical genetics include prenatal diagnosis, abortion, artificial insemination, population and family screening, predictive testing, genetic testing in children and genetic research (gene therapy).

- ❖ **Prenatal diagnosis:** Many methods are now widely available for diagnosing structural abnormalities and genetic disorders during the first and second trimester. The use of these techniques for monitoring pregnancies at risk generates little controversy. It is the ensuring possibility of termination of pregnancy on the grounds of fetal abnormality can be considered.

  Those who hold opposing views argue on religious, moral or ethical grounds that selective termination is little less than legalized infanticide. The cost–benefit ratio and social issues are to be considered.

  Indications for prenatal diagnosis:
  ➢ It is essential for genetic disorders for which there is unsatisfactory treatment
  ➢ When the risk of pregnancy is very high
  ➢ Disorder in which an accurate prenatal test is possible
  ➢ If the maternal age more than 35–40 years of age
  ➢ If one of the parents is a known carrier
  ➢ When the couple already have a child with genetic defects

- ❖ **Abortion choices:** The choice to abort any pregnancy is a moral problem wherever, duties to protect the interests of the women, the fetus and the society are to be held in conflict. One group argued that the destruction of certain fetuses was morally unacceptable, outweighing the possibility that given reassurance to some at-risk parents that their child would be unaffected. The other group contended that prenatal diagnosis was done largely with an intended abortion of an affected fetus for the purpose of medical indications which will harm the mother and the fetus. Elective abortion is the purposeful interruption of a viable pregnancy, the indication for elective abortion is by the request of the mother for reason of maternal or metal disease. It is called therapeutic abortion. MTP Act 1971, passed by parliament to provide some exception in provision of the penal code. According to this Act, abortion can be only done in case of pregnancy not exceeding 12 weeks and carried out at a licensed clinic or at a hospital by a licensed medical practitioner.

- ❖ **Artificial insemination:** It can be accomplished by two methods, i.e. artificial insemination from the husband (AIH). The second method, i.e. AID.

- ❖ **Population screening:**
  ➢ Programs that offered carrier detection for common autosomal recessive disorders have been in operation for many years.
  ➢ These have been well received for Thalassemia and Tay-Sachs disease, for which screening has been carefully planned with well-informed and highly motivated target populations.
  ➢ The differing receptions to these various screening programs illustrate the importance of informed consent and the difficulties of ensuring both autonomy and informed choice. **For example**, it has been suggested that screening for cystic fibrosis carrier status could be included in the neonatal screening program or to be introduced as an option for all school children at the age of 16 years.

- ❖ **Family screening:** It is widely agreed that the identification of a carrier of a condition could have incompletion for other family members should lead to the offer of tests for extended family. This applies particularly to carriers of balanced translocations and a series of X-linked recessive disorders. In case of translocations, sometimes referred to as autosomal recessive disorder such as cystic fibrosis, the cascade screening is applied and clinical geneticists would opt to respect their patients' confidentiality rather than break the trust which forms a cornerstone of the traditional doctor with relationship.

- ❖ **Predictive testing:** The development of molecular techniques of diagnosing single gene disorders either by direct mutational analysis or indirectly using linkages has made it possible to offer predictive presymptomatic testing for many adult onset disorders such as familial adenomatous, polyposis and Huntington's disease. This has raised several important ethical issues.

- **Fetal therapy:** Advances in technology have resulted in the ability to drain the spinal fluid from the brain of the fetus (cephalocentesis), catheterize the fetus in utero, remove its lower body from the uterus to repair a urinary tract obstruction, etc.; these are certainly milestones in the area of fetal therapy. Investigations are generally of experimental nature in many treatments. Ethical and legal questions and conflicts can emerge as these procedures and treatments are used more frequently. Risk-to-benefit ratio is favorable enough to cause this costly therapy to be a priority.
- **Genetic research:** All individuals who agree to undergo genetic testing in a service context are obviously entitled to a full and clear explanation of what the testing involves, how the results could have implementation for both themselves and other family members. The issues related to informed consent when participating in genetic research are just complex, and many people are perfectly willing to hold their arm for a blood testing which might help others, particularly if they have personal experience of a serious disorder in their own family who will be informed of the results and tests carried out, future techniques done. Informed consents are addressed when samples are collected for genetic research.

CONCLUSION

A wide variety of sophisticated methods has been made possible in early detection of physical abnormalities in fetus. Nurses play an important role in preventing risks and dealing with phase of detection, counseling to clients and their families.

It is clear that ethical considerations are of major importance in clinical genetics. Each new discovery has potential for good or bad and rises. New dilemmas for which there are often no easy answers. On a global scale, the computerized medical records completed with the widespread introduction of genetic screening make it essential that safeguards are introduced to ensure future population are not open to eugenic abuse.

CHAPTER 23

Genetic Counseling

CHAPTER OUTLINE

- Aims and Objectives
- Types of Genetic Counseling
- Purposes
- Clients Seeking Genetic Counseling
- Genetic Counseling Team
- Principles of Genetic Counseling
- Process of Genetic Counseling

INTRODUCTION

There is a need for nurses to play an active role in helping to identify and refer high-risk patients and their families for genetic services, and in meeting the special psychosocial needs of those dealing with genetic disorders and congenital anomalies. The most supportive nursing care can be given only when the nurse has a thorough understanding of the principles of medical genetics and the process of genetic counseling.

DEFINITION

Genetic counseling is a communication process that deals with the occurrence or risk of occurrence of a genetic disorder in a family (American Society of Human Genetics).

Genetic counseling is the process of communication between the parents of a child affected with a genetic condition and the counselor who conveys information regarding the prognosis and the available modes of therapy for the profaned as well as risks of recurrence, and methods of prevention.

The most immediate and practical service that genetics can render in medicine and surgery is genetic counseling.

AIMS AND OBJECTIVES

- Provide families with accurate information regarding recurrence risks when a member of the family has a disorder that might be genetically determined
- Reduce the numbers of children affected with a hereditary condition by prenatal detection of a disorder
- To reassure people who are concerned about their children inheriting a particular disorder that their fears are groundless
- To allow people who are affected by inherited disorders to make informed choices about future reproduction
- To educate people about inherited disorders and the process of inheritance
- To offer support by skilled health care professionals to people who are affected by genetic illness.

TYPES OF GENETIC COUNSELING

There are two types of genetic counseling:
1. Prospective genetic counseling
2. Retrospective genetic counseling.

Prospective Genetic Counseling

This allows for the true prevention of disease. This approach requires identifying heterozygous individuals for any particular defect by screening procedures and explaining to them the risk of them having affected children, if they marry another heterozygote for the same gene. If heterozygous marriage can be prevented or reduced, the prospects of giving birth to affected children will diminish, e.g. sickle cell anemia and thalassemia. It is possible that this kind of prevention may find wider application to cover a number of other recessive defects.

Retrospective Genetic Counseling

Most genetic counseling is at present retrospective and the hereditary disorder has already occurred with the family. The methods that could be suggested under retrospective genetic counseling are:
- Contraception
- Pregnancy termination
- Sterilization.

PURPOSES

- Advise couples before conception the probability of conception of an infant with a genetic disorder
- Advise couples after conception and fetal screening of whether or not the fetus has a genetic disorder
- Inform the couple of the options that are available to them including choosing not to become pregnant.

CLIENTS SEEKING GENETIC COUNSELING

- Persons who want to know if they have a genetic disease or if they are carriers of a genetic disease
- Persons who are concerned whether they are at risk for producing a child with a specific genetic disease
- Persons who are planning parenthood and who want to know the implications (prognosis and treatment) of a genetic disease affecting one or both parts
- Persons seeking help in making a decision about prenatal diagnosis, selective abortion and artificial insemination by donor or adaptation
- Persons seeking help for a child affected with a genetic disease
- Couples with consanguinity
- Persons with a family history of congenital abnormalities
- Recurrent abortions, still births, infant deaths, etc.

GENETIC COUNSELING TEAM

Genetic counseling requires teamwork. A general practitioner can provide genetic counseling in straightforward cases. Since an accurate diagnosis is important, a medical specialist is the ideal person for complex cases. A social worker is of great help in genetic counseling.

PRINCIPLES OF GENETIC COUNSELING

- Genetic counseling is a therapeutic measure
- It includes establishment of an accurate diagnosis, treatment of the affected individual as well as the prevention of the recurrence of genetic disorder
- A very important role that a genetic counselor can play is of allaying fears borne out of ignorance
- Genetic counseling requires a special aptitude in the art of communication
- Genetic counseling must be nondirective, while the information shall be complete, accurate and comprehensible to a layman
- The counselor shall exercise his/her judgment regarding the best possible manner in which the advice is to be given to the consultant
- The advice shall include information about the potential, medical, social, economical and psychological burdens on the one hand, and various reproductive options and alternatives available to the consultant on the other hand
- The final decision shall rest with the consultants
- Both parents should be counseled together as far as possible. Care must be taken to see that blame is not put on one of them
- Follow-up session is always desirable even in other cases to assess the accuracy and degree of understanding during genetic counseling
- One should not paint a very grim picture. It is best to be realistic, but not pessimistic.

Counseling Skills

The basic skills required to help the process of genetic counseling:

Attending: Attending is an active, rather than passive skill; it involves blocking out all distractions and giving total attention to the person speaking in which the midwife is using the skill of attending would be focused physically and psychologically on the client or the person in need.

Listening: The skill cannot be separated from the skill of attending. Listening involves using the mind and senses, and the midwife needs to be alert and free to concentrate on two levels of communication, i.e., Being Spoken and which is not.

Responding: The ways in which a midwife well respond to a person are varied and at many levels. Responses may be Spoken or Not Spoken.

A person in distress is more likely to express a non-verbal message of warmth and interest through ways of sitting or looking.

Questioning: It is the most obvious way of seeking information and useful way of enabling a person to hear herself tell about a situation. Asking a question influences how a question is heard. A question may be spoken in an authoritative way, responses are open and closed questions.

Allowing responses: Gives the person permission to express herself in a way true for herself. It is important that the midwife follows the cues of the person in difficulty and responds at her pace in an encouraging, open and supportive way.

Reflecting responses: These are to do with being like a mirror for the person in difficulty in order that they might see and hear what they are saying. The person will then pick up the message that she is hearing and take it on further in the way in which she wants to go in her own exploration of the difficulty.

Clarifying: When a person is in distress or difficulty, the emotional turmoil very often makes the situation unclear, so it is important for the midwife to make a clarifying response in this situation, rather than pretend that she has understood.

Supporting: The value of supporting responses is that they may give a person courage to go on working at her difficulty even when she is hurting inside. Particularly at the beginning of a counseling session, when the helping relationship is being formed on a basis of trust.

PROCESS OF GENETIC COUNSELING

The counseling process begins with an accurate diagnosis and a careful detailed family history. The diagnosis is frequently made on the basis of clinical manifestations, but may require special biochemical or cytological tests, especially in very rare or unusual cases. An accurate diagnosis is essential, a number of diseases have similar manifestations, but different modes of inheritance. The mode of inheritance determines the recurrence risks and sometimes the prognosis.

- **Estimation of risk:** The risks are determined by the mode of inheritance. The risk of recurrence for disorders caused by a factor that segregates during cell division can be estimated with a high degree of accuracy by application of Mendelian principles. In a dominant disorder, the risk is 50% that a subsequent offspring will be affected; an autosomal recessive disease carries one in four risk of recurrence and an X-linked inheritance. Translocation chromosomes present a high risk of recurrence.
- **Interpretation of risk:** Counselors explain the risk estimates to clients without making to recommendations or decisions (themselves whether risk, high or low) and avoid allowing their own biases to interfere. Counselor provide appropriate information about the nature of the disorder, the extent of the risks in the specific case, the consequences and alternative options available, but the final decision must be left to the family.

  The most important concept that must be emphasized to families is that each pregnancy is an independent event. For example, in monogenic disorders in which the risk factor is one in four that the child will be affected, the risk remains the same no matter how many affected children are already in the family. However, "chance has no memory" the risk is one in four for each pregnancy.
- **Discussion the options:** After the diagnosis and the risk estimation/recurrence, the counselor is obliged to ensure that consultants are provided with all the information necessary for them to come to their own informed decision. The information will include details that:
  - All ethical choices open to them involve lengthy discussion of reproductive option
  - Alternative approaches to conception such as artificial insemination by donor (AID)
  - Use of donor ova as well as review of the technique
  - Limitation and risk associated with methods available for prenatal diagnosis

These are the issues that should be discussed and whatever the views of the counselor/consultant are entitled of knowledge of those prenatal diagnostic procedure which are both technically feasible and legally permissible.

- **Communication and support:** Communication is a two-way process; not only does the counseling provide information but he/she also has to be receptive to the fears, aspirations, expressed or unexpressed, readiness to listen in a sympathetic and appropriate manner.

  Often individual or couple will be extremely upset when first made aware of genetic diagnosis, everyone involved in genetic counseling needs to remember that the delivery of the potential distressing information cannot be carried out in isolation. The setting should be agreeable, private and quite with ample time for discussion and questions. Questions should be answered openly and honestly. Convey every information and effective contact can be maintained.
- **Approach to genetic counseling:** Genetic counseling involves primarily the provision of information. The ultimate goal is to ensure that an individual or couple can reach their decision based on full information about risks and options.

  There is a universal agreement that genetic counseling should be non-coercive with no attempt being made to direct the consultant along a particular course of action. Non-directive and non-judgmental communication process, whereby factual knowledge is imparted to facilitate informed personal choice.

  Generally, they try to avoid being drawn to expressing an opinion preferring instead to suggest the consultant options. This approach sometimes referred to as scenario-based decision counseling. Counseling provides individuals with an opportunity for careful reflection, otherwise consultants/counselors will have to face the consequences of their decisions.

CONCLUSION

Genetic counseling plays an important role in prevention, diagnosis, screening and management of the genetic conditions in families and in the population. Genetic counseling should always be non-directive and non-judgmental, factual information should be given to make informed choices. Decision should be left to couples by explaining in terms of risk and benefits.

24 Practical Application of Genetics in Nursing

CHAPTER OUTLINE

- Nurses Role in Genetic Counseling
- Role of Nurse in Diagnostic Tests and Procedures
- Follow-up Care
- Role of the Administrator in Genetic Services

INTRODUCTION

Nurses are assuring an increasingly important role in counseling persons regarding genetically transmitted or genetically influenced conditions. Nurses who are actively involved in counseling require a minimum of a master's degree in genetics and related subjects. However, nurses without advanced preparation in genetics can be productive members of a counseling service. Nurses are usually the persons who provide follow-up care and maintain contact with the clients. Interviewing and counseling skills are an integral part of their professional practice.

NURSES ROLE IN GENETIC COUNSELING

Genetic disorders and variations are important in all phases of life cycle, and span all clinical practice divisions and sites, including the work place, schools, hospital, clinic, office and community health agency. It is time to integrate genetics into nursing education, practice and to encourage nursing personnel to think genomically (genetic testing). Her role as a genetic counselor is at two levels, i.e. preconception counseling and prenatal counseling.

Preconception Counseling

Ideally, couples who have the potential to transfer genetic disorders to their offspring should be counseled before pregnancy occurs. When preconception counseling is possible, the nurse should have a relaxed interview with the couple to discuss the issues related to risks. The most important requirement of preconception counseling is that it should be nonjudgmental and provided in an understanding atmosphere. The nurse should make an effort to avoid giving the couple an opinion about the advisability of getting pregnant. The decision to become pregnant despite significant risk is a very personal one for the couple. The role of the nurse is to provide factual medical information and to support the decision taken by the couple even if that decision does not agree with the nurse's personal opinion. Another aspect of preconception counseling is consideration of the financial burden, in terms of health care cost as well as working disability that the couple, specially the woman, will assume with high-risk factors. Many people are not aware of the high cost of the complex medical technology necessary for the care of their child born with a genetic disorder and many do not realize the limitations of the facilities available.

Preconceptional evaluation and some chromosomal and genetic testing will help the obstetrician to predict the risk if any, and help to counsel the client. The importance of preconceptional health, control of diabetics, hypertension to avoid smoking, alcohol, promote good health habits and risks associated with differing pregnancy to advanced age can be discussed so that the couple may go for planned pregnancy approach for early prenatal care.

Preconceptional counseling will also help all potential high-risk pregnancies with special importance to those rhesus (Rh) isoimmunization, history of repeated abortion or pre-termed labor. She may be referred to a genetic counselor or immunity against TORCH infections maybe evaluated.

Family history offers identification of genetic risks, client may be screened to identify more common autosomal recessive disorders like, thalassemia, sickle cell anemia, Tay Sach's Disease and cystic fibrosis. It allows the couple to make informed decision for next pregnancy, further needed investigations, if pregnancy occurs and subsequent decision regarding medical termination pregnancy (MTP) or continuation. The risk of Down's syndrome is more after 35 years, particularly in those having a family history; so marriage counseling and genetic counseling are essential today.

Prenatal Counseling

In prenatal counseling, the nurse has to identify women or couple who are at risk or having the potential for congenital disorders in their offspring. Would be parents with significant genetic risks are identified through clues provided in their history or physical examination. The task is made easy, since it is the responsibility of the health staff to register all pregnancies. The nurse working in the antenatal clinic should realize that genetic history taking is as important as obstetric and medical history taking.

In selected cases, invasive procedures like Chorion Biopsy and amniocentesis may be needed for cytogenetic study, and counseling of the client is needed as regards its value in identifying some autosomal disorders. The value of these tests, the risks associated and the cost involved should be discussed so that the client can form opinion whether to undergo these tests. Maternal alpha fetoprotein studies for neural tube defects and cytogenetic studies from cells obtained by amniocentesis are recommended in pregnancies over 30 years.

ROLE OF NURSE IN DIAGNOSTIC TESTS AND PROCEDURES

The family and persons directly involved with diagnostic procedures need to know the purpose of each test, what they can expect, and what they can do to facilitate the process. They may be concerned about whether or not the test will be painful, if they will be required to undress, and if they can be accompanied by a family member. Nurses can do a great deal to allay fears and to supply support and reassurance. The tests are not usually performed at the time of the initial interview, but at a subsequent visit or visits.

The pregnant woman who submits to chorionic villus sampling or amniocentesis for detection of genetic disease in a fetus is particularly anxious. Although the physical risk to fetus and mother is almost negligible, the procedure may be fraught with emotional issues and sequelae. When the fetus is found to be free of the disorder for which the test is carried out, the parents need only a thorough explanation of the procedure and support during the test.

FOLLOW-UP CARE

Maintaining contact with the family after genetic counseling testing or therapy is one of the most important nursing responsibilities. Most counseling services try to schedule at least one post-diagnostic or post-counseling visit to assess how well the family is beginning to incorporate this new information into their lives. Follow-up visits to the counseling services or visits to the home provide additional opportunities to re-explore all aspects of the situation and to answer any questions that may have occurred to the family, since the previous contacts. Clarifying information and misunderstanding of information are important nursing functions.

Besides providing genetic counseling, the public health nurse or midwife can also assess the following as a mediator, educator, service provider, risk taker and helper.

- Nurses have to act as a mediator between doctors and patients, husband and wife, couple and relatives or family members to explain the reality, causes, diagnostic procedures and preventive measures to be taken.
- Nurses have to educate the couple as well as general public regarding genetic disorders by means of health education and information.
- As primary health care providers, nurses have to help the couple prior to any investigation, during diagnostic procedure, total prenatal period, postnatal period and follow-up. Complete explanation regarding a procedure makes it easy for the person undergoing the test as well as the health team involved in conducting it.
- It is a challenge for nurse practitioners to inform the couple and significant others regarding genetic disorders, as it will affect the couple emotionally. Sometimes, it may lead to marital disturbance between husband and wife due to lack of accurate knowledge. The nurse takes a risk when she informs them and is responsible for tackling their psychological reactions and later in helping them to accept it and deal with it.

ROLE OF THE ADMINISTRATOR IN GENETIC SERVICES

As an administrator of hospital nursing services, the nurse can support the antenatal diagnosis of genetic disorders in the following ways:

- Promote refresher courses for nurses on genetics and genetic counseling. Special courses can be conducted on specialized genetic diagnostic procedures
- Provide special leave education programs to nurses to attend refresher courses and in-service
- Support research programs related to genetic disorders and encourage practicing nurses to participate in related research
- Fix a day in outpatient department to educate couples and other patients about genetic disorders

As an administrator of nursing education, the following functions can be performed to support diagnosis of genetic disorders and provide nursing care:

- More emphasis can be given on genetic counseling in community health and maternity nursing courses
- Practical sessions on genetic counseling should be arranged for students during clinical experience
- Short-term courses could be organized for faculty on genetic disorders and current diagnostic procedures
- Literature, for examination of booklets, pamphlets on genetic disorders can be published in leading newspapers to spread awareness
- Video films can be prepared on genetic counseling, in order to provide training nurses and students. These can

be telecast on the electronic media in local language for general public awareness.

Interest in genetics has resulted in the growth of a science called genetic engineering and many research studies are being conducted in this field. Nurses need to be aware of this research for use in counseling sessions in the clinical area. Nurses also need to undertake research regarding nursing care of patients with genetic disorders. The nurse can participate in development of this branch of science in the following ways:

- By supporting research related to nursing care aspects of genetic disorders and by selecting topics, which are directly related to nursing care
- By applying the positive findings of such research in her clinical work
- By publishing the findings of her own research related to nursing care
- By inviting suggestions from practicing nurses as well as experts in genetics regarding how to deal with problem cases.

CONCLUSION

Nurses are specially involved in care of mothers and children, and are in the best position to sustain a close relationship with clients, provide follow-up care, establish and support skilled care and thus improve the quality of life of clients affected with genetic disorders. Future of nursing, health care/genetics, involving the use of genomics in all of health care and nurses must be prepared to meet these.

SUGGESTED READING

1. Bobak IM, Jensen MD, Zalar MK. Maternity and Gynecologic Care: The Nurse and the Family, 5th edition. Toronto: Mosby; 2002.
2. Dutta DC. Textbook of Obstetrics including Perinatology and Contraception, 6th edition. Calcutta: New Central Book Agency; 2004. pp. 107-11.
3. Mueller RF, Young ID. Emery's Elements of Medical Genetics. Toronto: Churchill Livingstone; 1998. p. 44.
4. Park K. Textbook of Preventive and Social Medicine, 24th edition. India: Banarsidas Bhanot; 2017. pp. 857-67.
5. Pillitteri A. Maternal Child Health Nursing. Philadelphia (PA): JB Lippincott Company; 1995.
6. Rimoin D, Pyeritz R, Korf B. Principles and Practice of Medical Genetics (Vol. 1), 5th edition. Elsevier; Churchill Livingstone; 2007. pp. 53-60, 129-35, 767-85.
7. Singh IB, Paul GP. Human Embryology, 7th edition. Chennai: Macmillan India Ltd; 2002. pp. 1-25.
8. Snustad DP, Simmons MJ. Genetics, 6th edition. International Student Version. Singapore Pvt Ltd; Wiley Publications; 2012. pp. 46, 402-15, 450-5.
9. Swaminathan K. Pathology and Genetics for Nurses, 2nd edition. Tamil Nadu: Jaypee Brothers Medical Publishers (P) Ltd; 2012. pp. 421-81.

REVIEW OF SECTION BASED QUESTIONS OF RGUHS

Long Essay
1. Practical application of genetics in nursing.

Short Essays
1. Genetic counselling. (May 2011, May 2010)
2. Genetic testing. (May 2012)
3. Approaches to common genetic disorders.
4. Parental screening.
5. Legal and ethical issues in genetics.

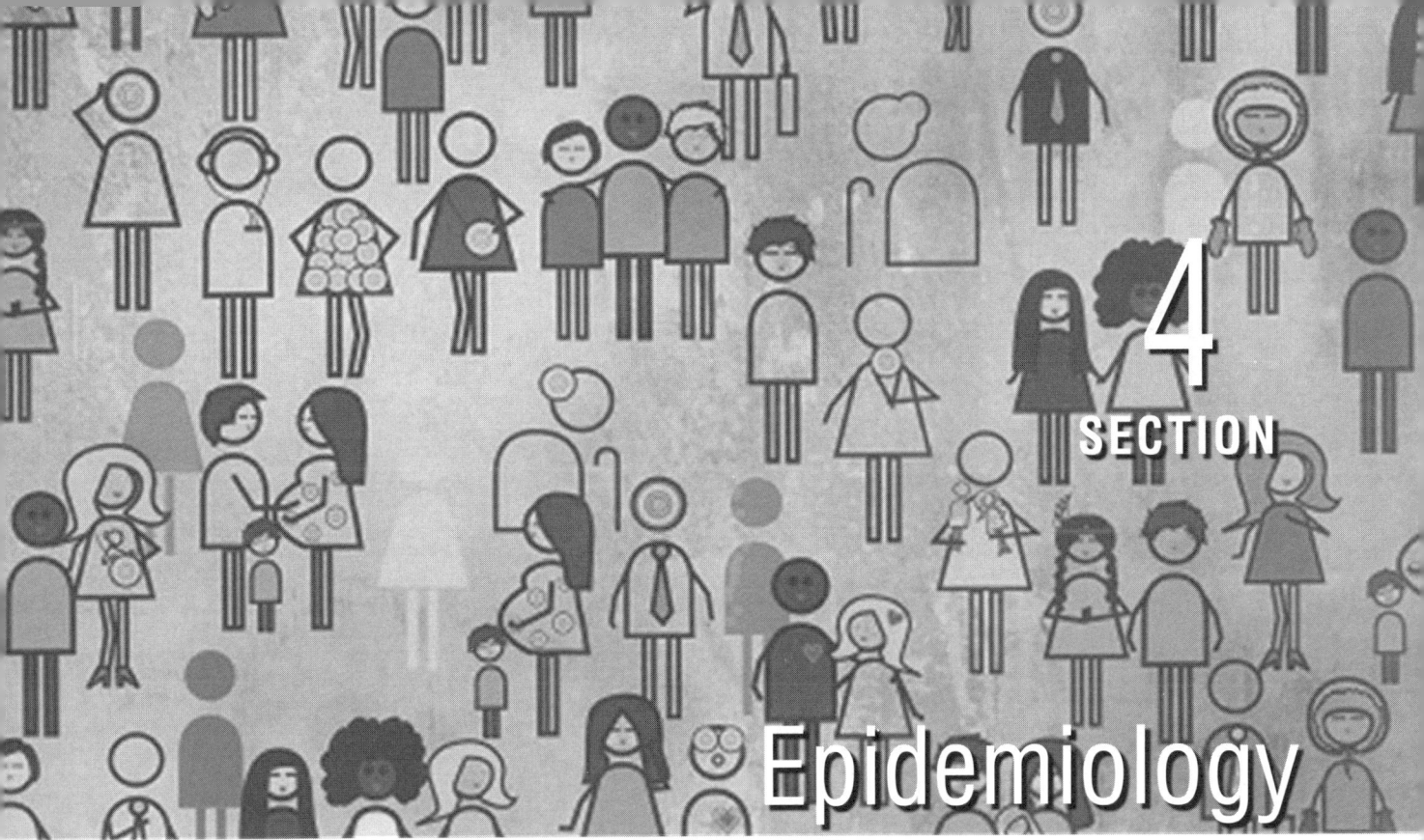

SECTION 4
Epidemiology

Section Outline

25. History, Scope, Aim, Epidemiological Approach and Methods
26. Mortality and Morbidity
27. Concepts of Causation of Diseases and their Screening
28. Application of Epidemiology in Healthcare Delivery, Health Surveillance and Health Informatics, Uses of Epidemiology
29. Role of Nurse in Epidemiology

25. History, Scope, Aim, Epidemiological Approach and Methods

CHAPTER OUTLINE

- History of Epidemiology
- Definitions and Modern Concepts of Epidemiology
- Scope of Epidemiology
- Aims of Epidemiology
- Epidemiological Approach
- Epidemiological Methods
- Case Control Study
- Cohort Study
- Experimental Epidemiology
- Association and Causation
- Epidemiological Investigation Process

INTRODUCTION

Epidemiology is the basic science of preventive and social medicine. It has evolved rapidly during past three decades. Modern epidemiology has entered the most exciting phase of its evolution. It has provided new opportunities for prevention, treatment, planning and improving the effectiveness efficiency of health services. This trend is bound to nurse in view of the increasing unimportance for epidemiological studies.

HISTORY OF EPIDEMIOLOGY

- The origin of epidemiology has been traced back to Hippocrates 460–441 BC who tried to explain the association of lifestyle and environmental factors with the occurrence of disease.
- In 19th century, foundation of epidemiology was laid a few classic studies made a major contribution to the saving of life. In 1850s Epidemiology Society of London, the society's main concern was the investigation of infectious diseases. The sudden growth of bacteriology had smothered the development of epidemiology in the universities.
- In 1920s, the United States, Winslow and Sedgwick both lectured on epidemiology although the subject was not given departmental.
- In 1927, WH Frost became the first professor of epidemiology in United States.
- Later major Greenwood became the first professor of Epidemiology and Medical Statistics in the University of London.
- Epidemiology has grown rapidly during the past three decades and it has now become firmly established in medical education.
- The application of epidemiology in nursing can be traced back to Florence Nightingale (1820–1910). Miss Florence Nightingale considered the issues related to hospital statistical and diseases classification and look suggestions from William Farr, the Chief Statistician, General Register office, England. She also contributed a lot towards bringing down morbidity and mortality among British soldiers during Crimean War in basis of systematic descriptive studies.

Meaning of Epidemiology

Epidemiology began with Adam and Eve, both trying to investigate the qualities of the "forbidden fruit." 3rd century BC, Meaning epidemiology given. Epi—"among," demos—"people," logos—"study."

DEFINITIONS AND MODERN CONCEPTS OF EPIDEMIOLOGY

Different definitions have been given by various epidemiologists based on their experience, background and changing trends. The difference is mainly about the extent of focus. In some definitions, the focus is on the investigation of disease, in others, disease is included as part of broader health disease spectrum, some of the definitions are reproduced below in chronological order:

- The epidemiology is that branch of medical science, which deals with epidemics. —**Parkin, 1873**

- Epidemiology is the science of mass phenomena of infectious diseases. —**Frost, 1927**
- Epidemiology is the study of disease, any disease, as a mass phenomenon. —**Greenwood, 1934**
- Epidemiology is the study of the distribution and determinants of disease prevalence in man. —**Mac Mohan, 1960**
- Epidemiology is the study of various factors and conditions that determine the occurrence and distribution of health, disease, defect, disability and death among groups of individuals. —**Clark, 1965**
- Epidemiology is concerned with the study of the processes, which determine or influence the physical, mental and social health of people. —**Cassel, 1965**
- Epidemiology is the study of the distribution of a disease or a physiological condition in human populations and of the factors that influence this distribution. —**Lilienfeld, 1980**
- Epidemiology is the study of the frequency, distributions and determinants of health-related states or events in specified population and the application of this study to control health problems. —**John M Last, 1988**

SCOPE OF EPIDEMIOLOGY

There are three components that are common to most of them:
1. Studies of disease frequency
2. Studies of the distribution
3. Studies of the determinant.

Each of these components confesses an important message.

Disease Frequency

Inherent definition of epidemiology is measured of frequency of disease. Disability or death and summarizing this information in the form of rates and ratios, e.g. prevalence rate, incidence rate and death rate, etc. These rates are essential for comparing disease frequency in different populations or subgroups of the same population in relation to suspected causal factors. Such important dues yield disease etiology. This is a vital step in the development of strategies for prevention or control of health problems.

Equally epidemiology is also concerned with the measurement of health-related events and states in the community. For example, health needs demands, activities, tasks, healthcare utilization and variables such as blood pressure (BP), serum cholesterol, height and weight, etc.

Distribution of Disease

The distribution of disease occurs in patterns in a community. An important function of epidemiology is to study these distribution patterns in the various subgroup of the population by time, place and person. That is the epidemiologist examines whether there has been an increase or decrease of disease overtime span, whether there is higher concentration of disease in one geographic area than in others. Whether disease occurs more often in men or particular age group and whether most characteristics behavior of those affected are different from those not affected. An important outcome of this study is formulation of etiological hypothesis.

Determinants of Disease

A unique feature of epidemiology is to test etiological hypothesis and identify the underlying causes (or risk factors) of disease. This requires the use of epidemiological principles and methods. This aspect of epidemiology is known as analytical epidemiology. This helps in developing scientifically sound health programs interventions and policies. In recent, this has contributed vastly to the understanding of the determinants of the diseases, e.g. lung cancer and cardiovascular (CV) diseases.

AIMS OF EPIDEMIOLOGY

According to International Epidemiological Association (IEA), epidemiology has four main aims:
1. To describe the distribution, and magnitude of health and disease problems in human population.
2. To identify etiological factors (risk factors) in the pathogenesis of disease.
3. To provide the data essential to the planning, implementation and evaluation of services for the prevention, control and treatment of disease, and to the setting up of priorities among those services.
4. The ultimate aim is to eliminate or reduce the health problem and to promote the health and well-being of society as a whole.

EPIDEMIOLOGICAL APPROACH

Epidemiological approach to problems of health and disease is based on two major foundations.

1. Asking Questions

- Examples, related to health events:
  - What is the event?
  - What is its magnitude?
  - Where did it happen?
  - When did it happen?
    - Who are affected?
    - Why did it happen?
- Examples, related to health actions:
  - What can be done to reduce the problem?
  - How can it be prevented?
  - What action should be taken by the community and by health services and activities carried out?
  - What resources are required and what activities organized/difficulties how to overcome?

This provides clues to disease etiology, and help epidemiology to guide planning and evaluation.

Making Comparisons

The basic approach in epidemiology is to make comparisons and draw inferences. This may be between two or more groups. One group having the disease or exposed to risk factor, or comparison between individuals. The epidemiology tries to find out the crucial differences between in the host and environmental factors between those affected, not affected. It requires standardization of definitions, classifications, criteria and nomenclature.

EPIDEMIOLOGICAL METHODS (FIG. 25.1)

Observational Studies

Observational studies allow nature to take its own course, the investigation measures, but do not intervene.

Descriptive Epidemiology

Descriptive studies are usually the first phase of an epidemiology investigation. These studies are concerned with observing the distribution of disease or health-related characteristics in human population and identifying the characteristics with which the disease in question seems to be associated.

Steps in descriptive studies:
- Defining the population to be studied population base, total number includes demographic characteristics such as age, sex, occupation, cultural characters, etc.
- Defining the disease under study—operational definition of disease, i.e. the criteria by which the disease can be measured.

Describing the disease by:
- *When:* Time, year, month, week, day, hour of onset and duration.
- *Where:* Place climatic zones, country region, urban or rural town cities, institutional.
- *Who:* Person's demographic characteristics—height, weight, BP, blood cholesterol and personal habits.

Time Distribution

Epidemiologists have identified three kinds of time trends or fluctuations in disease occurrence.

Short-term Fluctuations
- Common:
  - Single exposure or point source
  - Continuous or multiple exposure
- Propagated:
  - Person to person
  - Anthropod vector
  - Animal vector
- Slow (modern) epidemic.

Periodic Fluctuations

Seasonal trend

Noninfectious diseases: Sunstroke, hay fever, snake bite.

Cyclic trend
- Some diseases occur in cycles
- Spread over short periods of time
- Time, which may be day, weeks, months or years, e.g. outbreak of gastroenteritis, measles in prevaccination era appeared in cycles with major peaks every 2–3 years and rubella every 6–9 years, influenza pandemics 7–10 years due to antigenic variations.

Long-term or Secular Trends

Place distribution: Geographic patterns provide an important source of clues about the causes of the disease, the range of geographic studies concerned with local variations. At a broader level international comparisons may examine mortality and morbidity in relation to socioeconomic factors, dietary differences and the differences in culture and behavior. These variations may be classified as follows:
- International variations
- National variation
- Rural-urban differences
- Local distributions
- Migration studies.

Person distribution: In descriptive studies, the defining the persons who develop the disease by age, sex, occupation, marital status, habits, social class and of the host factors. These factors do not necessarily represent etiological factors, but they contribute to one understanding if the natural history of disease.

Measurement of disease: This information must be available in terms of mortality, morbidity, disability, etc. Measurement of mortality is direct and morbidity has

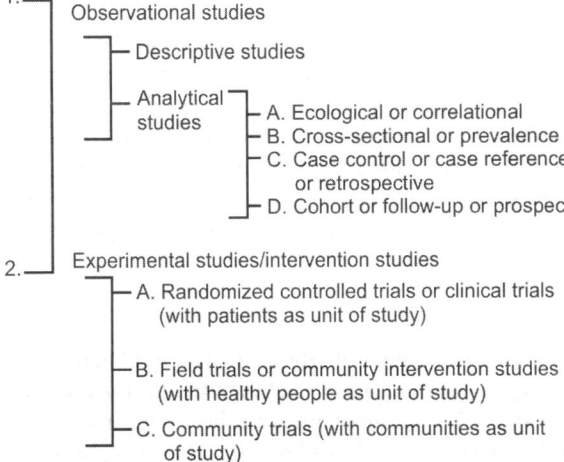

Fig. 25.1: Epidemiologic methods.

two aspects. Incidence and prevalence obtained from longitudinal studies.

Comparing with known indices: Compare between population and subgroups, increase risk of disease mortality, morbidity, incidence and prevalence can be assessed.

Formulation of hypothesis: It is often possible to formulate hypothesis arrived from observation as it can be accepted or rejected. Which includes hypothesis should specify the population characteristics applies, specific cause being studied, the expected outcome, cause response and time response relationship.

Analytical Epidemiology

Analytical epidemiology is second major type of epidemiological studies. Analytical studies comprise two distinct types of observational studies (Fig. 25.2):
- Case control study.
- Cohort study.

From each of these study designs one can determine:
- Whether or not a statistical association exists between a disease and a suspected factor.
- If one exists the strength of the association.

CASE CONTROL STUDY

Case control studies often called "retrospective studies" are a common first approach to last causal hypothesis. In recent years it has three distinct features:
- Both exposure and outcome (disease) have occurred before the start of the day.
- The study proceeds backwards from effect to cause.
- The use of a control or comparison group to support or refuse an inference.

Definition

A case control study involves two populations—cases and controls. In case control studies the unit is the individual rather than the group. The focus is on a disease or some other health problems that has already developed.

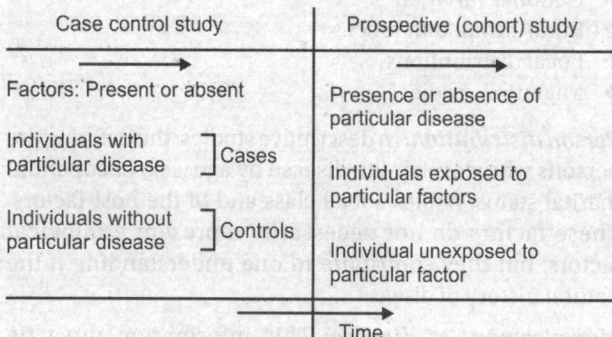

Fig. 25.2: Schematic diagram of the design of case control and cohort studies.

Basic Steps

There are four basic steps in conducting a case control study:
1. Selection of cases and controls
2. Matching
3. Measurement of exposure
4. Analysis and interpretation.

Selection of Cases

Definition of case

The prior definition of what constitutes a case is crucial to the case control study. It involves two specifications:
- *Diagnostic criteria:* The diagnostic criteria of the disease and the stage of disease if any, example breast cancer stage I to be included in the study must be specified before the study is undertaken.
- *Eligibility criteria:* A criteria customarily employed is the requirement that only newly diagnosed (incident) cases within a specified period of time are eligible than old cases or cases in advanced stages of the disease (prevalent cases).

Source of cases

The cases may be drawn from hospitals or general population:
- ***Selection of controls:*** The controls must be free from the disease under study. They must be similar to the cases as possible. As a rule a comparison group is identified before a study is done. Difficulties may arise in the selection of controls. If the disease under investigation occurs in subclinical forms whose diagnosis is difficult.
- ***Sources of controls:*** May be selected include hospitals. The controls may be selected from the same hospital as the cases, but with different illness other than the study disease.

For example, if we study cancer cervix, the control group cancer breast. Relatives, (spouses and siblings), neighbors and general population. Controls can be obtained from defined geographic areas, by taking a random sample of individuals free of the study disease.

To sum up, selection of proper cases and controls is crucial to the interpretation of the results of case control studies. Some investigations select cases from one source and controls from more than one source and controls from more than one source to avoid the influence of selection bias. It is also desired to conduct more than one case control study, preferably in different geographic areas.

Matching

The controls may differ from the cases in a number of factors such as age, sex, occupation, social status, etc. an important consideration is to ensure comparability between cases and controls. This involves what is known as matching. Matching is defined as the process by which we select controls in such a way that they are similar to cases with regard to certain pertinent selected variables are known to influence the outcome of disease if not adequately matched comparability could distort or confound the results. A "confounding factor" is defined as one, which is associated both with exposure and disease under investigation such association a risk factor for the disease.

Example to explain confounding: In the study of the role of alcohol in the etiology of esophageal cancer, smoking is a confounding factor because it is associated the consumption of alcohol and it is an independent risk factor for esophageal cancer. In these conditions the effects of alcohol consumption can be determined only if the influence of smoking is neutralized by matching. There are several kinds of matching procedures. One is group matching. This may be done by assigning cases to subcategories (strata) based on their characteristics (e.g. age, occupation, social class), and then establishing appropriate controls.

Measurement of Exposure

Definitions and criteria about exposure are just as important as those used to define cases and controls. Information about exposure should be obtained in precisely the same manner for cases and controls. This may be obtained by interviews, by questionnaires or by studying past records of cases such as hospital records, etc. It is important to recognize that when case control studies are being used to test associations the most important factor P values are obtained.

Analysis

The final step is analysis:
- Exposure rates among cases.
- Estimation of disease risk associated exposure.

Exposure rates (Table 25.1)
- Case = a/(a + c) = 33/35 = 94.2%
- Control = b/(b + d) = 55/82 = 67.0% P 0.001.

The frequency rate of lung cancer was definitely higher among smokers than among non-smokers. There is statistical association between exposure status and occurrence of lung cancer (P value is less than 0.001).

Estimation of risk: The second analytical step is estimation of disease risk associated exposure. It should be noted that if exposure rate was 94.2% in the study group, it does not mean that 94.2% of those smoked would develop lung cancer. The estimation of disease risk associated exposure is obtained by an index known as relative risk or risk ratio. It is given as:

$$\text{Relative risk} = \frac{\text{Incidence among exposed}}{\text{Incidence among nonexposed}}$$
$$= \frac{a+b}{s+c} \div \frac{b}{b+d}$$

A typical case control study does not provide incidence rates from which relative risk can be calculated directly, because there is no appropriate denominates or population at risk to calculate these rates. In general, the relative risk can be exactly determined only from a cohort study.

Odds ratio (cross product ratio): From a case control study, we can derive what is known as odds ratio (OR) is a measure of the strength of the association between risk factor and outcome). The odds ratio is the cross product of the entries in table, which is shown in Table 25.2.

Using the data in table the odds ratio would be estimated as follows (Table 25.3):

$$\text{odds ratio} = \frac{ad}{bc} = \frac{33 \times 27}{55 \times 2} = 8.1$$

In the above example, smokers of less than 5 cigarettes per day showed a risk of having lung cancer 8.1 times that of nonsmokers. Odds ratio is a key parameter in the analysis of case control studies.

Advantages and Disadvantages of Case Control Studies

Advantages
- Relatively easy to carry out.
- Rapid and inexpensive (compared with cohort studies).
- Require comparatively few subjects.
- Particularly suitable to investigate rare diseases or diseases about which little is known. But a disease, which is rare in the general population (e.g. leukemia in

Table 25.1: Age standardized death rates per 1,00,000 men per year by amount of current smoking.

Classification of exposure (cigarettes)	Number of deaths	Death rate
1/2 pack	24	95.2
1/2–1 pack	84	107.8
1–2 packs	90	229.2
2 packs +	97	264.2

Table 25.2: Diseases.

	Yes	No
Exposed	a	b
Not exposed	c	d

Table 25.3: A case control study of smoking and lung cancer.

	Cases of lung cancer	Control of lung cancer
Smokers less than 5 cigarettes/day	33 (a)	55 (b)
Nonsmokers	2 (c)	27 (d)
Total	35 (a + c)	82 (b + d)

adolescents) may not be rare in special exposure group (e.g. prenatal X-rays).
- No risk to subjects.
- Allows the study of several different etiological factors (e.g. smoking, physical activity and personality characteristics in myocardial infarction).
- Risk factors can be identified. Rational prevention and control programs can be established.
- No attrition problems, because case control studies do not require follow-up of individuals into the future.
- Ethical problems minimal.

Disadvantages

- Problems of bias rely on memory or past records, the accuracy of which may be uncertain; validation of information obtained is difficult or sometimes impossible.
- Selection of an appropriate control group may be difficult.
- We cannot measure incidence, and can only estimate the relative risk.
- Do not distinguish between causes and associated factors.
- Not suited to the evaluation of therapy or prophylaxis of disease.
- Another major concern is the representativeness of cases and controls.

COHORT STUDY

Cohort study is another type of analytical (observational) study, which is usually undertaken to obtain additional evidence to refute or support the existence of an association between suspected cause and disease. Cohort study is known by a variety of names—prospective study, longitudinal study, incidence study, and forward-looking study. The most widely used term, however, is "cohort study." The distinguishing features of cohort studies are:
- The cohorts are identified prior to the appearance of the disease under investigation.
- The study groups, so defined, are observed over a period of time to determine the frequency of disease among them.
- The study proceeds forward from cause to effect.

Indications for Cohort Studies

Cohort studies are indicated:
- When there is good evidence of an association between exposure and disease, as derived from clinical observations, and supported by descriptive and case control studies.
- When exposure is rare, but the incidence of disease high among exposed, e.g. special exposure groups such as those in industries, exposure to X-rays, etc.
- When attrition of study population can be minimized, e.g. follow-up is easy, cohort is stable, cooperative and easily accessible.
- When ample funds are available.

Types of Cohort Studies

Three types of cohort studies have been distinguished on the basis of the time of occurrence of disease in relation to the time at which the investigation is initiated and continued:
1. Prospective cohort studies.
2. Retrospective cohort studies.
3. A combination of retrospective and prospective cohort studies.

Prospective Cohort Studies

A prospective cohort study (or "current" cohort study) is one in which the outcome, (e.g. disease) has not yet occurred at the time the investigation begins. Most prospective studies begin in the present and continue into future. For example, the long-term effects of exposure to uranium was evaluated by identifying a group of uranium miners and a comparison group of individuals not exposed to uranium mining and by assessing subsequent development of lung cancer in both the groups.

Retrospective Cohort Studies

A retrospective cohort study (or "historical" cohort study) is one in which the outcomes have all occurred before the start of the investigation. The investigator goes back in time, sometimes 10–30 years, to select his study groups from existing records of past employment, medical or other records and traces them forward through time, from a past date fixed on the records, usually up to the present. This type of study is known by a variety of names—retrospective cohort study, "historical" cohort study, prospective study in retrospect and nonconcurrent prospective study.

Combination of Retrospective and Prospective Cohort Studies

In this type of study, both the retrospective and prospective elements are combined. The cohort is identified from past records and is assessed of date for the outcome. The same cohort is followed up prospectively into future for further assessment of outcome.

The outcome evaluated was death from leukemia or aplastic anemia between 1935 and 1954. They found that the death rate from leukemia or aplastic anemia was substantially higher in their cohort than that of the general population. A prospective component was added to the study and the cohort was followed, as established in 1955, to identify deaths occurring in subsequent years.

Elements of a Cohort Study

- Selection of study subjects
- Obtaining data on exposure
- Selection of comparison groups
- Follow-up
- Analysis.

Selection of Study Subjects

The subjects of a cohort study are usually assembled in one of two ways—either from general population or select groups of the population that can be readily studied (e.g. persons with different degrees of exposure to the suspected causal factor).

- ❖ **Special groups:** These may be special groups or exposure groups that can readily be studied.
- ❖ **Select groups:** These may be professional groups (e.g. doctors, nurses, lawyers, teachers and civil servants), insured persons, obstetric population, college alumni, government employees, volunteers, etc. These groups are usually a homogeneous population.
- ❖ **Exposure groups:** If the exposure is rare, a more economic procedure is to select a cohort of persons known to have experienced the exposure. In other words, cohorts may be selected because of special exposure to physical, chemical and other disease agents. A readily accessible source of these groups is workers in industries and those employed in high-risk situations (e.g. radiologists exposed to X-ray).

Obtaining Data on Exposure

Information about exposure may be obtained directly from the:

- ❖ **Cohort members:** Through personal interviews or mailed questionnaires. Since cohort studies involve large numbers of population, mailed questionnaires offer a simple and economic way of obtaining information. For example, Doll and Hill used mailed questionnaires to collect smoking histories from British doctors.
- ❖ **Review of records:** Certain kinds of information (e.g. dose of radiation, kinds of surgery or details of medical treatment) can be obtained only from medical records.
- ❖ **Medical examination or special tests:** Some types of information can be obtained only by medical examination or special tests, e.g. blood pressure, serum cholesterol, electrocardiogram (ECG).
- ❖ **Environmental surveys:** This is the best source for obtaining information on exposure levels of the suspected factor in the environment where the cohort lived or worked. In fact, information may be needed from more than one or all of the above sources. Information about exposure (or any other factor related to the development of the disease being investigated) should be collected in a manner that will allow classification of cohort members:
  - ➤ According to whether or not they have been exposed to the suspected factor.
  - ➤ According to the level or degree of exposure, at least in broad classes, in the case of special exposure groups.

In addition to the above, basic information about demographic variables, which might affect the frequency of disease under investigation, should also be collected. Such information will be required for subsequent analysis.

Selection of Comparison Groups

There are many ways of assembling comparison groups.

Internal comparisons: In some cohort studies, no outside comparison group is required. The comparison groups are in-built. That is, single cohort enters the study and its members may, on the basis of information obtained, be classified into several comparison groups according to the degrees or levels of exposure to risk, (e.g. smoking, blood pressure, serum cholesterol) before the development of the disease in question.

- ❖ **External comparisons:** When information on degree of exposure is not available, it is necessary to put up an external control to evaluate the experience of the expose group, e.g. smokers nonsmokers, a cohort of radiologists compared with a cohort of ophthalmologists, etc. The study and control cohorts should be similar in demographic and possibly important variables other than those under study.
- ❖ **Comparison with general population rates:** If none is available, the mortality experience of the exposed group is compared with the mortality experience of the general population in the same geographic area as the exposed people, e.g. comparison of frequency of lung cancer among uranium mine workers with lung cancer mortality in the general population where the miners resided; comparison of frequency of cancer among asbestos workers with the rate in general population in the same geographic area.

Follow-up

One of the problems in cohort studies is the regular follow-up of all the participants. Therefore, at the start of the study, methods should be devised depending upon the outcome to be determined (morbidity or death), to obtain data for assessing the outcome. The procedures required comprise:

- ❖ Periodic medical examination of each member of the cohort.
- ❖ Reviewing physician and hospital records.
- ❖ Routine surveillance of death records.
- ❖ Mailed questionnaires, telephone calls, periodic home visits preferably all three on an annual basis. Of the above, periodic examination of each member of the cohort yields the greatest amount of information on the individual examined, than would the use of any other procedure.

Analysis

The data are analyzed in terms of:

- ❖ Incidence rates of outcome among exposed and nonexposed.
- ❖ Estimation of risk.

Table 25.4: Applied to hypothetical cigarette smoking and lung cancer.

Cigarette smoking	Developed lung cancer	Did not develop lung cancer	Total
Yes	70 (a)	6,930 (b)	7,000 (a + b)
No	3 (c)	2,997 (d)	3,000 (c + d)

Incidence rates: In a cohort study, we can determine incidence rates directly in those exposed and those not exposed. A hypothetical example is given in Table 25.4 showing how incidence rates may be calculated:
- Among smokers = 70/7,000 = 10 per 1,000
- Among nonsmokers = 3/3,000 = 1 per 1,000
- Statistical significance = $P < 0.001$.

Estimation of risk: Having calculated the incidence rates, the next step is to estimate the risk of outcome, (e.g. disease or death) in the exposed and nonexposed cohorts. This is done in terms of two well-known indices (Table 25.6):
1. Relative risk.
2. Attributable risk.

1. ***Relative risk:*** Relative risk (RR) is the ratio of the incidence of the disease (or death) among exposed and the incidence among nonexposed. Some authors use the term "risk ratio" to refer to relative risk.

$$RR = \frac{\text{Incidence of disease (or death) among exposed}}{\text{Incidence of disease (or death) among nonexposed}}$$

In the hypothetical example.
RR of lung cancer = 10/1 = 10.

Estimation of relative risk (RR) is important in etiological enquiries. It is a direct measure (or index) of the "strength" of the association between suspected cause and effect. A relative risk of one indicates no association; relative risk greater than one suggests "positive" association between exposure and the disease under study. A relative risk of two indicates that the incidence rate of disease is two times higher in the exposed group as compared with the unexposed. Equivalently, this represents a 100% increase in risk. A relative risk of 0.25 indicates a 75% reduction in the incidence rate in exposed individuals as compared with the unexposed. It is often useful to consider the 95% confidence interval of a relative risk since it provides an indication of the likely and maximum levels of risk.

In the hypothetical example (Table 25.4), the relative risk is 10. It implies that smokers are 10 times at greater risk of developing lung cancer than nonsmokers. The larger the RR, the greater the "strength" of the association between the suspected factor and disease. It may be noted that risk does not necessarily imply causal association.

2. ***Attributable risk:*** Attributable risk (AR) is the difference in incidence rates of disease (or death) between an exposed group and nonexposed group. Attributable risk is often expressed as a percent. This is given by the formula:

$$= \frac{\text{Incidence of disease rate among exposed} - \text{Incidence of disease rate among nonexposed}}{\text{Incidence rate among exposed}} \times 100$$

Attributable risk in the example would be:

$$\frac{10-1}{10} \times 100 = 90\%$$

Attributable risk indicates to what extent the disease under study can be attributed to the exposure. The table is an example indicates that the association between smoking and lung cancer is causal, 90% of the lung cancer among smokers was due to their smoking. This suggests the amount of disease that might be eliminated if the factor under study could be controlled or eliminated.

3. ***Population-attributable risk:*** Another concept is "population-attributable risk." It is the incidence of the disease (or death) in the total population minus the incidence of disease (or death) among those who were not exposed to the suspected causal factor (Table 25.5). Deaths in total population = 74(c)

Individual RR = a/b = $\frac{224}{10}$ = 22.40

Populatin AR = (c – b)/c = 86%

The concept of population attributable risk is useful in that it provides an estimate of the amount by which the disease could be reduced in that population if the suspected factor was eliminated or modified. In the example (Table 25.5) one might expect that 86% of deaths from lung cancer could be avoided if the risk factor of cigarettes were eliminated.

Relative risk versus attributable risk: Relative risk is important in etiological enquiries. Its size is a better index than is attributable risk for assessing the etiological role of a factor in disease. The larger the relative risk, the stronger the association between cause and effect. But relative risk does not reflect the potential public health importance as does the attributable risk. That is, attributable risk gives a better idea than does relative risk of the impact of successful preventive or public health program might have in reducing the problem.

Two examples are cited (Tables 25.6 and 25.7) to show the practical importance of distinguishing relative and absolute risk. In the first example, the RR of a cardiovascular complication in users of oral contraceptives is independent

Table 25.5: Lung cancer death rates among smokers and nonsmokers.

UK physicians (deaths per 100,000 person/years)		
Heavy smokers	224	Exposed to suspected factor (a)
Nonsmokers	10	Nonexposed to suspected causal factor (b)

Table 25.6: The relative and attributable risks of cardiovascular complications in women taking oral contraceptives.

Cardiovascular risk (1,00,000 patients/ year)	Ages	
	30–39	40–44
Relative risk	2.8	2.8
Attributable risk	3.5	20.0

Table 25.7: Risk assessment, smokers versus nonsmokers.

Cause of death	Death rate/1,000 smokers	Nonsmokers AR (%)	RR
Lung cancer	0.90	0.07	12.86
Coronary heart disease	4.87	4.22	1.15

of age, whereas the AR is more than five times higher in the older age groups. This epidemiological observation has been the basis for not recommending oral contraceptive in those aged 35 years and over.

The second example (Table 25.7) shows that smoking is attributable to 92% of lung cancer and 13.3% of coronary heart disease (CHD). In CHD, both RR and AR are not very high suggesting not much of the disease could be prevented as compared to lung cancer.

Advantages and Disadvantages of Cohort Studies

Advantages

- Incidence can be calculated.
- Several possible outcomes related to exposure can be studied simultaneously that is we can study the association of the suspected factor with many other diseases in addition to the one under study. For example, cohort studies designed to study the association between smoking and lung cancer also showed association of smoking with coronary heart disease, peptic ulcer, cancer, esophagus and several others.
- Cohort studies provide a direct estimate of relative risk.
- Dose-response ratios can also be calculated and since comparison groups are formed before disease develops certain forms of bias can be minimized as misclassification of individuals into exposed and unexposed groups.

Disadvantages

- Cohort studies involve a large number of people. They are generally unsuitable for investigating uncommon diseases or diseases with low incidence in the population.
- It takes a long time to complete the study and obtain results (20–30 years or more in cancer studies) by which time the investigators may have died or the participants may have changed their classification. Even in very common chronic diseases, e.g. coronary heart disease, cohort studies are difficult to carry out. It is difficult to keep a large number of individuals under medical surveillance indefinitely.

Table 25.8: Main differences between case control and cohort studies.

Case control study	Cohort study
Proceeds from "effect to cause"	Proceeds from "cause to effect"
Starts with the disease	Starts with people exposed to risk factor or suspected cause
Tests whether the suspected cause occurs more frequently in those with the disease than among those without the disease	Tests whether disease occurs more frequently in those exposed, than in those not similarly exposed
Usually the first approach to the testing of a hypothesis, but also useful for exploratory studies	Reserved for testing of precisely formulated hypothesis
Involves fewer number of subjects	Involves larger number of subjects
Yields relatively quick results	Long follow-up period often needed, involving delayed results
Suitable for the study of rare diseases	Inappropriate when the disease or exposure under investigation is rare
Generally yields only estimate of RR (odds ratio)	Yields incidence rates, RR as well as AR
Cannot yield information about diseases other than that selected for study	Can yield information about more than one disease outcome
Relatively inexpensive	Expensive

- Certain administrative problems such as loss of experienced staff, loss of funding and extensive record keeping are inevitable.
- It is not unusual to lose a substantial proportion of the original cohort—they may migrate, lose interest in the study or simply refuse to provide any required information. Selection of comparison groups, which are representative of the exposed and unexposed segments of the population is a limiting factor. Those who volunteer for the study may not be representative of all individuals with the characteristic of interest.
- There may be changes in the standard methods or diagnostic criteria of the disease over prolonged follow-up. Once we have established the study protocol, it is difficult to introduce new knowledge or new tests later.
- Cohort studies are expensive.
- The study itself may alter people's behavior. If we are examining the role of smoking in lung cancer, an increased concern in the study cohort may be created. This may induce the study subjects to stop or decrease smoking.
- With any cohort study we are faced with ethical problems of varying importance. As evidence accumulates about the implicating factor in the etiology of disease, we are obliged to intervene and if possible reduce or eliminate this factor.

❖ Finally, in a cohort study, practical considerations dictate that we must concentrate on a limited number or factors possibly related to disease outcome.

EXPERIMENTAL EPIDEMIOLOGY

In the 1920s, "experimental epidemiology" meant the study of epidemics among colonies of experimental animals such as rats and mice. In modern usage, experimental epidemiology is often equated with randomized controlled trials.

Experimental or intervention studies are similar in approach to cohort studies excepting that the conditions in which study is carried out are under the direct control of the investigator. Thus experimental studies involve some action, intervention or manipulation such as deliberate application or withdrawal of the suspected cause or changing one variable in the causative chain in the experimental group, while making no change in the control group, and observing and comparing the outcome of the experiment in both the groups. This contrasts sharply with observational studies (e.g. descriptive, case control and cohort studies) where the epidemiologist takes no action, but only observes the natural course of events or outcome.

Aims of Experimental Studies

The aims of experimental studies may be stated as follows:
❖ To provide "scientific proof" of etiological (or risk) factors, which may permit the modification or control of those diseases.
❖ To provide a method of measuring the effectiveness and efficiency of health services for the prevention, control and treatment of disease, and improve the health of the community.

Advantages of Experimental Studies

❖ The experimental animals can be bred in laboratories and manipulated easily according to wishes of the investigator.
❖ They multiply rapidly and enable the investigators to carry out certain experiments, e.g. genetic experiments, which will take several years in human population.

Disadvantages

❖ Animal experiments are that not all human diseases can be reproduced in animals.
❖ All the conclusions derived from animal experiments may not be strictly applicable to human beings.

Types of Experimental Studies

Experimental studies are of two types:
1. Randomized controlled trials (i.e. those involving a process of random allocation).
2. Nonrandomized or "nonexperimental" trials (i.e. those departing from strict randomization for practical purposes, but in such a manner that nonrandomization does not seriously affect the theoretical basis of conclusions).

Randomized Controlled Trials (Fig. 25.3)

Too often physicians are guided in their daily work by clinical impressions of their own or their teachers. These impressions, particularly when they are incorporated in textbooks and repeatedly quoted by reputed teachers and their students acquire authority, just as if they were proved facts. Similarly many public health measures are introduced on the basis of assumed benefits without subjecting them to rigorous testing. The history of medicine amply illustrates this. For instance, it took centuries before therapeutic bloodletting and drastic purging were abandoned by the medical profession.

It is mainly in the last 35–40 years, determined efforts have been made to use scientific techniques to evaluate methods of treatment and prevention. An important advance in this field has been the development of an assessment method known as randomized controlled trial (RCT). It is really an epidemiologic experiment. Since its introduction, the RCT has questioned the validity of such widely used treatments as oral hypoglycemic agents, varicose vein stripping and tonsillectomy, hospitalization of all patients with myocardial infarction, multiphasic screening and toxicity, and applicability of many preventive and therapeutic procedures.

The design of a randomized controlled trial is given in Figure 25.3. For new programs or new therapies, the RCT is the number one method of evaluation. The basic steps in conducting a RCT include the following:
❖ Drawing up a protocol
❖ Selecting reference and experimental populations

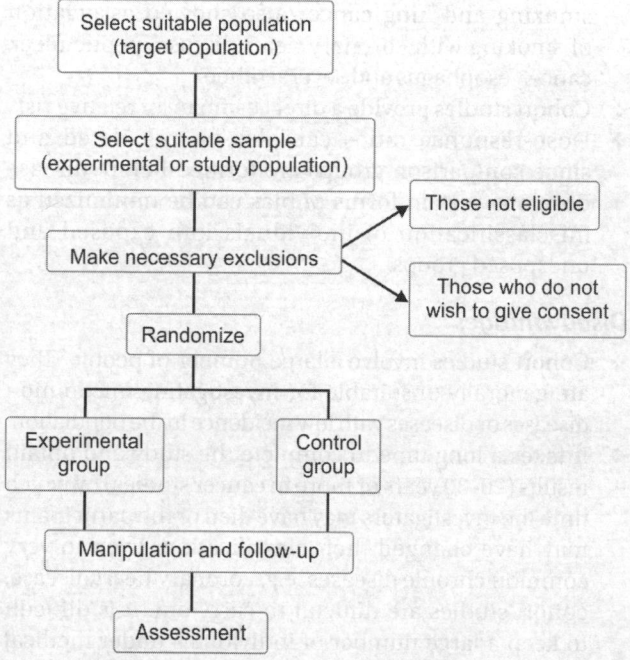

Fig. 25.3: Design of a randomized controlled trial.

- ❖ Randomization
- ❖ Manipulation or intervention
- ❖ Follow-up
- ❖ Assessment of outcome.

Protocol

One of the essential features of a randomized controlled trial is that the study is conducted under a strict protocol. The protocol specifies the aims and objectives of the study, questions to be answered, criteria for the selection of study and control groups, size of the sample, the procedures for allocation of subjects into study and control groups, treatments to be applied when and where, and how to what kind of patients, standardization of working procedures and schedules as well as responsibilities of the parties involved in the trial, up to the stage of evaluation of outcome of the study. A protocol is essential especially when a number of centers are participating in the trial. Once a protocol has been evolved, it should be strictly adhered to throughout the study.

Selecting reference and experimental populations

The reference population may comprise the population of a whole city or a population of school children, industrial workers; obstetric population and so on according to the nature of the study. The participants or volunteers must fulfill the following three criteria:

1. They must give "informed consent" that is they must agree to participate in the trial after having been fully informed about the purpose, procedures and possible dangers of the trial.
2. They should be representative of the population to which they belong, i.e. reference population.
3. They should be qualified or eligible for trial let us suppose, we are testing the effectiveness of a new drug for the treatment of anemia. If the volunteers are not anemic, we will then say, they are not eligible or qualified for the trial.

Randomization

Randomization is a statistical procedure by which the participants are allocated into groups usually called "study" and "control groups," to receive or not to receive an experimental preventive or therapeutic procedure maneuver or intervention. Randomization is an attempt made to eliminate bias allow for comparability.

The essential difference between a randomized controlled trial and an analytical study is that in the latter, there is no randomization because a differentiation into diseased and non-diseased (exposed or nonexposed) groups has already taken place. The only option left to ensure comparability in analytical studies is by matching.

Manipulation

Having formed the study and control groups, the next step is to intervene or manipulate the study (experimental) group by the deliberate application or withdrawal or reduction of the suspected causal factor (e.g. this may be a drug, vaccine, dietary component, a habit, etc.) as laid down in the protocol.

This manipulation creates an independent variable (e.g. drug, vaccine, a new procedure) whose effect is then determined by measurement of the final outcome, which constitutes the dependent variable (e.g. incidence of disease, survival time, recovery period).

Follow-up

This implies examination of the experimental and control group subjects at defined intervals of time, in a standard manner, with equal intensity, under the same given circumstances, in the same time frame till final assessment of outcome. The duration of the trial is usually based on the expectation that a significant difference (e.g. mortality) will be demonstrable at a given point in time after the start of the trial. Thus the follow-up may be short or may require many years depending upon the study undertaken.

Assessment

The final step is assessment of the outcome of the trial in terms of:

1. **Positive results:** That is benefits of the experimental measure such as reduced incidence or severity of the disease, cost to the health service or other appropriate outcome in the study and control groups.
2. **Negative results:** That is severity and frequency of side effects and complications, if any, including death. Adverse effects may be missed if they are not sought.

The incidence of positive or negative results is rigorously compared in both the groups, and the differences, if any, are tested for statistical significance. Techniques are available for the analysis of data as they are collected (sequential analysis), but it is more useful to analyze the results at the end of the trial.

Blinding

Blinding can be done in three ways:

1. **Single blind trial:** The trial is so planned that the participant is not aware whether he/she belongs to the study group or control group.
2. **Double blind trial:** The trial is so planned that neither the doctor nor the participant is aware of the group allocation and the treatment received.
3. **Triple blind trial:** This goes one step further. The participant, the investigator and the person analyzing the data are all blind. Ideally, of course, triple blinding should be used, but the double blinding is the most frequently used method when a blind trial is conducted. When an outcome such as death is being measured, blinding is not so essential.

Some Study Designs

It is useful to consider here some of the study designs of controlled trials.

Concurrent Parallel Study Designs

In this situation, comparisons are made between two randomly assigned groups, one group exposed to specific treatment and the other group not exposed. Patients remain in the study group or the control group for the duration of the investigation.

Crossover Type of Study Designs

This type of study design, each patient serves as his or her own control. As before, the patients are randomly assigned to a study group and control group. The study group receives the treatment under consideration. The control group receives some alternate form of active treatment or placebo. The two groups are observed over time. Then the patients in each group are taken off their medication or placebo to allow for the elimination of the medication from the body and for the possibility of any "carry over" effects, by the diagonal lines. After this period of medication (the length of this interval is determined by the pharmacologic properties of the drug being tested), the two groups are switched. Those who received the treatment under study are changed to the control group therapy or placebo and vice versa.

Advantages

- With such a design, all patients can be assured that sometime during the course of investigation, they will receive the new therapy.
- Studies generally economize on the total number of patients required at the expense of the time necessary to complete the study.
- This method of study is not suitable if the drug of interest cures the disease, if the drug is effective only during a certain stage of the disease or if the disease changes radically during the period of time required for the study.

Types of Randomized Controlled Trials

Clinical Trials

For the most part, "clinical trials" have been concerned with evaluating therapeutic agents, mainly drugs. The last three decades have been clearly the utility of clinical trials. Some of the recent, e.g., include evaluation of β-blockers in reducing cardiovascular mortality in patient surviving the acute phase of myocardial infarction; trials of folate treatment or supplementation before conception to prevent recurrence of neural tube defects; trials of aspirin on cardiovascular mortality and β-carotene on cancer incidence; efficacy of tonsillectomy for recurrent throat infection; randomized controlled trial of coronary bypass surgery for the prevention of myocardial infarction, etc. The list is endless.

Unfortunately not all clinical trials are susceptible to being blinded. For example, there is no way to perform a clinical trial of tonsillectomy and adenoidectomy without its being obvious who received surgery and who did not, a reason why the value of these procedures continues to be uncertain. Many ethical, administrative and technical problems are involved in the conduct of clinical trials. Nevertheless, they are a powerful tool and should be carried out before any new therapy, procedure or service is introduced.

Preventive Trials

In general usage, prevention is synonymous with primary prevention and the term "preventive trials" implies trials of primary preventive measures. These trials are purported to prevent or eliminate disease on an experimental basis. The most frequently occurring type of preventive trials is the trials of vaccines and chemoprophylactic drugs. The basic principles of experimental design are also applicable to these trials. It may be necessary to apply the trial to groups of subjects instead of to individual subjects. For example, extensive trial to test whooping cough vaccine from three manufacturers in ten separate field trials.

Risk Factor Trials

A type of preventive trial is the trial of risk factors in which the investigator intervenes to interrupt the usual sequence in the development of disease for those individuals who have "risk factor" for developing the disease; often this involves risk factor modification. The concept of "risk factor" gave a new dimension to epidemiological research. For example, the major risk factors of coronary heart disease are elevated blood cholesterol, smoking, hypertension and sedentary habits. Accordingly, the four main possibilities of intervention in coronary heart disease are reduction of blood cholesterol, the cessation of smoking, control of hypertension and promotion of regular physical activity. Risk factor trials can be "single-factor" or 'multi-factor' trials. Both the approaches are complementary and both are needed.

Cessation Experiments

Another type of preventive trial is the cessation experiment. In this type of study, an attempt is made to evaluate the termination of a habit (or removal of suspected agent), which is considered to be causally related to a disease. If such action is followed by a significant reduction in the disease, the hypothesis of cause is greatly strengthened. The familiar example is cigarette smoking and lung cancer. If in a randomized controlled trial, one group of cigarette smokers and the other group has given up, the demonstration of a decrease in the incidence of lung cancer in the study group greatly strengthens the hypothesis of a causal relationship. A large randomized controlled trial has been mounted to study the role of smoking cessation in the primary prevention of coronary heart disease.

Trial of Etiological Agents

One of the aims of experimental epidemiology is to confirm or refute an etiological hypothesis. The best known example of trial of an etiological agent relates to retrolental fibroplasia (RLF). Retrolental fibroplasia, as a cause of blindness, was nonexistent prior to 1938. It was originally observed and reported by TL Terry, a Boston ophthalmologist in 1942 and later in many other countries outside the USA.

Evaluation of Health Services

Randomized controlled trials have been extended to assess the effectiveness and efficiency of health services. Often, choices have to be made between alternative policies of healthcare delivery. The necessity of choice arises from the fact that resources are limited, and priorities must be set for the implementation of a large number of activities, which could contribute to the welfare of the society. An excellent example of such an evaluation is the controlled trials in the chemotherapy of tuberculosis in India, which demonstrated that "domiciliary treatment" of pulmonary tuberculosis was as effective as the more expensive in hospital or sanatorium treatment. The results of the study have gained international acceptance and ushered in a new era-the era of domiciliary treatment in the treatment of tuberculosis.

Nonrandomized Trials

Although the experimental method is almost always to be preferred, it is not always possible for ethical, administrative and other reasons to resort to a randomized controlled trial in human beings. For example, smoking and lung cancer, and induction of cancer by viruses have not lent themselves to direct experimentation in human beings. Secondly, some preventive measures can be applied only to groups or on a community-wide basis (e.g. community trials of water fluoridation). Thirdly, when disease frequency is low and the natural history long (e.g. cancer cervix) randomized controlled trials require follow-up of thousands of people for a decade or more. The cost and logistics are often prohibitive. These trials are rare. In such situations, we must depend upon other study designs these are referred to as nonrandomized (or nonexperimental) trials.

Uncontrolled Trials

There is room for uncontrolled trials, (i.e. trials with no comparison group). **For example**, there were no randomized controlled studies of the benefits of the Pap test (cervical cancer) when it was introduced in 1920s. Today, there is indirect epidemiological evidence from well over a dozen uncontrolled studies of cervical cancer screening that the Pap test is effective in reducing mortality from this disease. Initially uncontrolled trials may be useful in evaluating whether a specific therapy appears to have any value in a particular disease, to determine an appropriate dose, to investigate adverse reactions, etc. However, even in these uncontrolled trials, one is using implied "historical controls," i.e. the experience of earlier untreated patients affected by the same disease.

Since most therapeutic trials deal with drugs, which do not produce such remarkably beneficial results, it is becoming increasingly common to employ the procedures of a double-blind controlled clinical trial in which the effects of a new drug are compared to some concurrent experience (either placebo or a currently utilized therapy).

Natural Experiments

Where experimental studies are not possible in human populations, the epidemiologist seeks to identify "natural circumstances" that mimic an experiment. For example, in respect of cigarette smoking, people have separated themselves "naturally" into two groups, smokers and nonsmokers. Epidemiologists have taken advantage of this separation and tested hypothesis regarding lung cancer and cigarette smoking. Other populations involved in natural experiments comprise the following groups—migrants, religious or social groups, atomic bombing of Japan, famines and earthquakes, etc.

Before and After Comparison Studies

These are community trials, which fall into two distinct groups:
1. Before and after comparison studies without control.
2. Before and after comparison studies with control.

Before and after comparison studies without control

These studies center round comparing the incidence of disease before and after introduction of a preventive measure. The events, which took place prior to the use of the new treatment or preventive procedures are used as a standard for comparison. In other words, the experiment serves as its own control; this eliminates virtually all group differences. The classic examples of "before and after comparison studies" were the prevention of scurvy among sailors by James Lind in 1750 by providing fresh fruit; studies on the transmission of cholera by John Snow in 1854 and more recently, prevention of polio by Salk and Sabin vaccines.

Before and after comparison studies with control

In the absence of a control group, comparison between observations before and after the use of a new treatment or procedure may be misleading. In such situations, the epidemiologist tries to utilize a "natural" control group, i.e. the one provided by nature or natural circumstances. If the preventive program is to be applied to an entire community, he or she would select another community as similar as possible, particularly with respect to frequency and characteristics of the disease to be prevented. One of them is arbitrarily chosen to provide the study group and the other as a control group. In the example cited, (e.g. seat-belt legislation in Victoria, Australia), a natural "control" was sought by comparing the results in Victoria with other states in Australia where similar legislation was not introduced.

ASSOCIATION AND CAUSATION

The terms "association" and "relationship" are often used interchangeably. Association may be defined as the concurrence of two variables more often than would be expected by chance. In other words, events are said to be associated when they occur more frequently together than one would expect by chance. Association does not necessarily imply a causal relationship.

It will be useful to consider here the concept of correlation. Correlation indicates the degree of association between two characteristics. The correlation coefficients range from –1.0 to +1.0. A correlation coefficient of 1.0 means that the two variables exhibit a perfect linear relationship. However, correlation cannot be used to invoke causation, because the sequence of exposure preceding disease (temporal association) cannot be assumed to have occurred. Secondly, correlation does not measure risk. It may be said that causation implies correlation, but correlation does not imply causation.

Association can be broadly grouped under three headings:
1. Spurious association.
2. Indirect association.
3. Direct (causal) association:
   - One-to-one causal association.
   - Multifactorial causation.

Spurious Association

Sometimes an observed association between a disease and suspected factor may not be real. For example, a study in UK of 5,174 births at home and 11,156 births in hospitals showed perinatal mortality rates of 5.4 per 1,000 in the home births, and 27.8 per 1,000 in the hospital births. Apparently, the perinatal mortality was higher in hospital births than in the home births. It might be concluded that homes are a safer place for delivery of births than hospitals. Such a conclusion is spurious or artifactual, because in general, hospitals attract women at risk for delivery because of their special equipment and expertise, whereas this is not the case with home deliveries. The high perinatal mortality rate in hospitals might be due to this fact alone and not because the quality of care was inferior. There might be other factors also such as differences in age, parity, prenatal care, home circumstances, general health and disease state between the study and control groups. This type of bias where "like" is not compared with "like" (selection bias) is very important in epidemiological studies. It may lead to a spurious association or an association when none actually existed.

Indirect Association

The indirect association is a statistical association between a characteristic (or variable) of interest and a disease due to the presence of another factor, known or unknown, that is common to both the characteristic and the disease. This third factor, (i.e. the common factor) is also known as the "confounding" variable. Since it is related both to the disease and to the variable, it might explain the statistical association between disease and a characteristic wholly or in part. Such confounding variables (e.g. age, sex, social class) are potentially and probably present in all data and represent a formidable obstacle to overcome in trying to assess the causal nature of the relationship. Examples of an indirect association are given below.

Altitude and Endemic Goiter

Endemic goiter is generally found in high altitudes, showing thereby an association between altitude and endemic goiter (Fig. 25.4). According to current knowledge, we know, that endemic goiter is not due to altitude, but due to environmental deficiency of iodine. Figure 25.4 illustrates how a common factor, (i.e. iodine deficiency) can result in an apparent association between two variables, when no association exists. This amplifies the earlier statement that statistical association does not necessarily mean causation.

Direct (Causal) Association

One-to-one Causal Relationship

Two variables are stated to be causally related (AB) if a change in A is followed by a change in B.

If it does not, then their relationship cannot be causal. This is known as "one-to-one" causal relationship. This model suggests that when the factor A is present, the disease B must result. Conversely, when the disease is present, the factor must also be present. Measles may be one disease in which such a relation exists (Fig. 25.5).

Epidemiologists are interested in identifying the "cause." The most satisfactory procedure to demonstrate

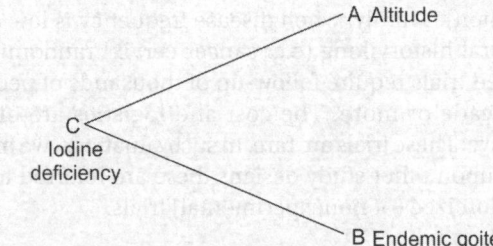

Fig. 25.4: Model of an indirect association.

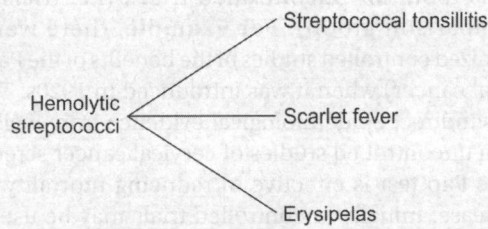

Fig. 25.5: Model in which one factor is shown to lead more than one disease.

this would be by direct experiment. But this procedure is scarcely available to the epidemiologist. And, in some cases, the "cause" is not amenable to manipulation.

The above concept of one-to-one causal relationship was the essence of Koch's postulates. The proponents of the germ theory of disease insisted that the cause must be necessary and sufficient for the occurrence of disease before it can qualify as cause of disease. In other words, whenever the disease occurs, the factor or cause must be present.

Although Koch's postulates are theoretically sound, the "necessary and sufficient" concept does not fit well for many diseases. For example, tuberculosis, tubercle bacilli cannot be found in all cases of the disease, but this does not rule out the statement that tubercle bacilli are the cause of tuberculosis. That the cause must be "sufficient" is also not always supported by evidence. In tuberculosis, it is well-known that besides tubercle bacilli, there are additional factors such as host susceptibility, which are required to produce the disease.

The concept of one-to-one causal relationship is further complicated by the fact that sometimes, a single cause or factor may lead to more than one outcome.

Multifactorial Causation

The causal thinking is different when we consider a noncommunicable disease or condition. For example, congenital heart disease. Where the etiology is multifactorial. There are alternative in lung cancer where disease causes more than one etiological factor. For example, smoking, air pollution, exposure, etc.

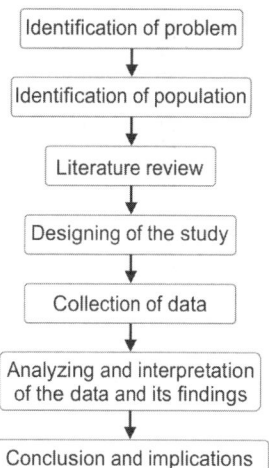

Fig. 25.6: Epidemiological investigation process.

EPIDEMIOLOGICAL INVESTIGATION PROCESS

There are seven steps of investigation process for doing any epidemiology study (Fig. 25.6).

CONCLUSION

Community health nurse should me knowledgeable and aware of epidemiological approaches, its scope to monitor the population by research application in the field. Study of epidemiology will help a nurse in the proper understanding and investigation of diagnosis and initiation of prompt treatment of a client, groups and families.

26 CHAPTER

Mortality and Morbidity

CHAPTER OUTLINE

- Basic Measurements of Epidemiology
- Tools of Measurement
- Mortality Rate (Death Rate)
- Morbidity Rates

BASIC MEASUREMENTS OF EPIDEMIOLOGY

Epidemiology focuses, among other things on measured of mortality and morbidity in human populations. The scope of measurements in epidemiology is very broad and unlimited, and includes the following:

- ❖ Measurement of mortality
- ❖ Measurement of morbidity
- ❖ Measurement of disability
- ❖ Measurement of natality
- ❖ Measurement of demographic variables
- ❖ Measurement of medical needs, healthcare facilities, utilization of health services and other health-related events
- ❖ Measurement of risk factors.

The basic requirements of measurements are validity, reliability, accuracy, sensitivity and specificity.

TOOLS OF MEASUREMENT (FLOWCHART 26.1)

The tools of measurement are rates, ratios and proportions.

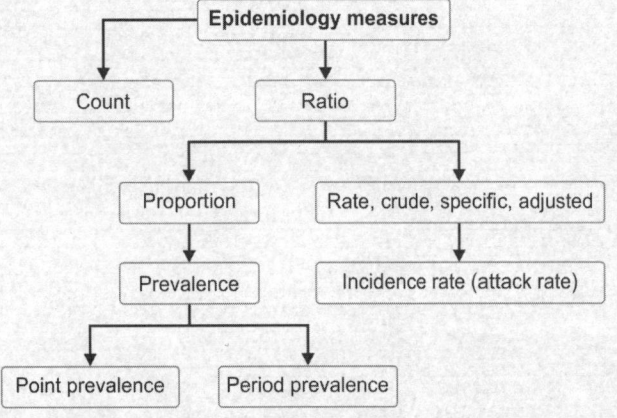

Flowchart 26.1: Epidemiological measurements.

Rate

A rate measures the occurrence of some particular event in a population during a given period of time. The event can be births, deaths, diseases, etc.

It is defined as a numerical statement of the frequency of an event obtained by dividing the number of individuals experiencing the event during a specified time period (the numerator) by the total midyear population who are capable of experiencing the event (the denominator or the population at risk) and multiply by a constant number, which is usually 1,000 but it can be some other round figure such as 10,000 and 100,000 (Table 26.1).

For example:

$$\text{Death rate} = \frac{\text{Number of deaths in 1 year}}{\text{Midyear population of the same year}} \times 1{,}000$$

The rates can be crude rates and specific rates.

Crude Rates

These are actual observed rates based on the entire population and are not reflective of any specific population group such as only females or any specific age group, etc. For example, crude birth rate, and crude death rate.

Specific Rates

These are actual observed rates based on specific population groups such as sex and age wise groups, disease wise groups, etc. or during specific time periods, e.g. annual rates, monthly rates, weekly rates, etc.

Ratio

Ratio is measure of events, which expresses a relation in size between two different factors occur in the population and it is obtained by dividing quantity of one factor with the other. For example, the number of males in the ratio of number of females, the number of children with malnutrition in the

Chapter 26: Mortality and Morbidity

Table 26.1: Commonly used rates and their formulae.

Sl. No.	Type of rate	Formula	Population factor (multiplied by)
1.	Crude death rate	Total number of deaths in an area during the year	1,000
2.	Cause specific death rate	Estimated midyear population in the same area during the same year. Number of deaths from specific cause in an area during the year	1,000
3.	Age specific death rate	Estimated midyear population in the same area during the same year. Number of deaths of a specified age group in an area during the year	1,000
4.	Sex specific death rate	Estimated midyear population of that age group in the same area during the same year. Number of deaths of males or females in an area during the year	1,000
5.	Case fatality rate	Estimated male or female population at midyear in the same area during the same year. Number of deaths from specified disease in an area during the year	100
6.	Proportionate mortality rate	Number of persons with the disease (old and new) in the same area during the same year. Total number of deaths from specific cause at a given time in a specified area	100
7.	Fetal death rate	Total number of deaths from all causes in the same area at that time. Number of fetal deaths at 20 weeks gestation or more in a community during the year. Number of live births plus fetal deaths of 20 weeks or more gestation in a community during the same year	1,000
8.	Perinatal mortality rate	Fetal deaths (7th month or more). Deaths under 1 week of birth in an area during the year	1,000
9.	Neonatal mortality rate	Total live births and late fetal deaths in the same area during the same year. Number of deaths under 28 days of age in an area during the year	1,000
10.	Postneonatal mortality rate	Number of live births in the same area during the same year. Number of deaths at 28 days of age to 1 year in an area during the year	1,000
11.	Infant mortality rate	Number of live births in the same area during the same year. Number of deaths under 1 year of age in defined populations in a year	1,000
12.	Maternal mortality rate diseases	Number of live births in the same population in the same year. Number of deaths from puerperal causes (pregnancy, postpartum) in a defined populations during the year	1,000
13.	Attack rate	Number of live births during that year. Number of new cases of specific occurring from time to time in a place during the specified period	100
14.	Incidence rate	Specific population at risk in the same place during the same period. All new cases of specific dieases occurring from time to time in a particular place during the year	1,000
15.	Prevalence (crude rate)	Estimated midyear population at the same place in the same year. All cases (old and new) existing in a particular place during a particular period. Estimated midyear population at the same place during the same period	1,000

ratio of normal children, etc. It is expressed in the ratio of X:Y or X/Y, i.e.

$$\text{Number of male:female} = \frac{\text{Number of males}}{\text{Number of females}}$$

$$\text{Doctor:population ratio} = \frac{\text{Number of Doctor}}{\text{Size of population}}$$

Proportion

A proportion is a ratio, which indicates the relation in magnitude of a part of the whole. The numerator is always included in the denominator. A proportion is usually expressed in percentage. For example,

$$\frac{\text{The number of children with malnutrition at a certain time in a community}}{\text{The number of total children at the same time in that community}} \times 100$$

Rates and ratios can help in making comparisons of one community with the other community and at different point in time. This facilitates in identification of trends, whether there is increase or decrease in morbidity and mortality, and accordingly one can evaluate the effectiveness of healthcare services. If the occurrence of a disease is in its usual frequency, it is then referred as endemic level and if it is more than endemic level, it is called epidemic level.

■ MORTALITY RATE (DEATH RATE)

The mortality rate can be crude mortality rate and specific mortality rate. The crude mortality rate is also called general mortality rate. In this, the numerator includes all the deaths occurring in a defined geographical area (community) in a particular year and the denominator includes the total population in the same area of the same year.

The specific mortality rate is cause, i.e. disease specific. For example, mortality rate due to measles. The numerator is the deaths due to measles in a particular area in a particular year and the denominator is midyear population of that area of the same year. This rate though is cause specific rate, but is an average rate and may not be useful for comparison for two different communities because measles deaths depend upon age group whereas denominator includes the whole population, i.e. all age groups. A community, which has more young children, will have higher mortality due to measles than another community that has significantly less young children and more elderly people. Thus, crude and average rates are not very useful for comparison of communities, which are different by composition.

For comparison of mortality rates, it is advisable to use specific rates for specific subgroups, e.g. age-specific mortality and sex-specific morality rates.

MORBIDITY RATES

The incidence and prevalence rates are the two most commonly used morbidity rates in community health.

Incidence Rate

It refers to the occurrence of new cases during a particular period usually 1 year in a population exposed to the risk in a particular area. It can be calculated as under:

$$\text{Incidence rate} = \frac{\text{Number of new cases of a specific disease occurring from time to time in a particular place during the year}}{\text{Midyear population of the same place during the same year}} \times 1{,}000$$

Incidence rate is helpful in monitoring the occurrence of new cases in a given population over time. For that reason, it is preferred to mortality rate. Any increase or decrease in incidence rates help in determining the causative or risk factors associated with disease, which can be further confirmed by case control or cohort studies. Similar to incidence rate is the attack rate, which represents the incidence of illness among the exposed population during the specified time period and can be calculated as:

$$\text{Attack rate} = \frac{\text{Number of new cases of a specified disease period occurring in a particular place during the specified period}}{\text{Specific population at risk during the same period}} \times 100$$

Prevalence Rate

Prevalence is of two types:
1. Point prevalence
2. Period prevalence

Point prevalence: Point prevalence of a disease is defined as the number of all current cases (old or new) of a disease at one point of time in relation to a defined population. The point in the point prevalence may for all practical purposes consist of a day, several days or a few weeks, depending upon the time, it takes to examine the population sample. Point Prevalence is given by the formula:

= Number of all current cases (old and new) specified disease existing at a given point in time estimated population at the same point in time × 100

The term prevalence rate is used without any further qualification it is taken to mean point prevalence. It can be made specific for age, sex and other relevant factors or attributes.

Period prevalence: It is less commonly used measure of prevalence is period prevalence. It measures the frequency of all current cases (old and new) existing during a defined period of time, (e.g. annual prevalence) in relation to a defined population. It includes cases arising before but extending into or through to the year to the year as well as those cases arising during the year.

Period Prevalence is given by the formula:

$$= \frac{\text{Number of existing cases (old and new) for a specified disease during a given period of time interval}}{\text{Estimated mid-interval population at risk}} \times 100$$

Relationship between Prevalence and Incidence

Prevalence depends upon two factors, the incidence and duration of illness. For example, assumption that the population is stable and incidence and duration unchanging. The relationship expressed as, $P = I \times D$
= Incidence × Mean Duration

Incidence 20 cases per 1,000 populations per year mean duration of diseases 5 years.

Prevalence = 20 × 5 = 100 per 1,000 population

Conversely it is possible to derive incidence and duration as follows:

Incidence = P/D
20 = P/5 years
P = 20 × 5 = 100
Duration = P/I = 100/20 = 5
Duration = 5 years

Example: In tuberculosis (TB), the higher prevalence rate is relative to incidence. This is because, new case TB keep cropping up through the year, while old one may persist for months or years so prevalence rate is relatively low than the incidence rate.

1. Morbidity indicators

Morbidity indicators are used to supplement mortality data to describe the health status of a population. Morbidity statistics have also their own drawback, they overlook a large no. of conditions which are subclinical or inapparent, i.e. hidden part of the iceberg of disease. The following

morbidity rates are used for assessing ill health in the community and
- ❖ Notification rates
- ❖ Attendance rates at out-patient departments, health centers, etc.
- ❖ Admission, readmission and discharge rates.
- ❖ Duration of stay in hospital
- ❖ Spells of sickness and absence from work or school.

2. Disability rates

The death rates have not markedly in recent years in spite of massive health expenditure, disability rates related to illness and injury have come into use to supplement mortality and morbidity indicators. It is based on the full range of daily activities. The commonly used disability rates fall into two groups.

- ❖ **Event Type Indicators**
  - ➢ Number of days of restricted activity
  - ➢ Bed disability days
  - ➢ Work-loss or school-loss days within specified period.
- ❖ **Person Type Indicators**
  - ➢ **Limitations of mobility**, e.g. confined to bed, confined to the house, special aid in getting around either inside or outside the house.
  - ➢ **Limitation of activity**, e.g. limitation to perform the basic activities of daily living, e.g. eating, washing, dressing, going to toilet, moving about, etc. Limitation of major activity, e.g. ability to work at a job, ability to house work, etc.
  - ➢ **Sullivan's Index**: This index is computed by subtracting from the life expectancy the probable duration of bed disability and inability to perform major activities.
  - ➢ **HALE (Health-adjusted Life Expectancy)**: The name of the indicator used to measure healthy life expectancy has been changed from Disability-adjusted Life Expectancy (DALE) to HALE. HALE is based on life expectancy at birth but includes an adjustment for time spent in poor health. It is most easily understood as the equivalent number of years in full health that a newborn can expect to live based on current rated of ill-health and mortality.
  - ➢ **DALY (Disability-adjusted Life Year)**: DALY is a measure of the burden of disease in a defined population and the effectiveness of the interventions. DALY express years of life lost premature death and years lived with disability adjusted for the severity of the disability. **One DALY is one lost year of healthy life.**

A "premature" death is defined as one that occurs before the age to which a dying person could have expected to survive if he or she was a member of a standardized model population with a life expectancy at birth equal to that of the world's longest—surviving population, Japan. However, their use as currently expressed and calculated may be limited because necessary data are not available or do not exist. Moreover, the concept postulated a continuum from disease to disability to death that is not universally accepted, particularly by the community of persons with disabilities.

3. National status indicators

National status is a positive heath indicator. Three nutritional status indicators are considered important as indicators of health status. They are:
- ❖ Anthropometric measurements of preschool children, e.g. weight and height, mid-arm circumference
- ❖ Heights (and sometimes weight) of children at school entry
- ❖ Prevalence of low birth weight (less than 2.5 kg).

4. Healthcare delivery indicators

The frequently used indicators of healthcare delivery are Doctor Population Ratio, Doctor Nurse Ratio, Population Bed Ratio and Population per Health center or subcentre, Population per Traditional Birth Attendant. These indicators reflect the equity of distribution of health resources in different parts of the country and of the provision of healthcare.

5. Utilization rates

In order to obtain additional information on health status, the extent of use of health services is often investigated. Utilization of services or actual coverage is expressed as the proportion of people in need of a service who actually receive it in a given period, usually a year. It is argued that utilization rates give some indications of the care needed via population and therefore the health status of the population. In other words, the relationship exists between utilization of healthcare services and health needs and status. Healthcare utilization is also affected by factors such as availability and accessibility of health services, attitude of an individual towards his health and the healthcare system.

Examples
- ❖ Proportion of infants who are fully immunized.
- ❖ Proportion of women who receive care or their deliveries supervised by the trained birth attendant.
- ❖ Percentage of the population using various methods of family planning.
- ❖ Bed occupancy rate (i.e. average daily inpatient census)
- ❖ Average length of stay (days of care rendered or discharges)
- ❖ Bed turnover ratio (Discharges or Average Beds).

6. Indicators of social and mental health

As long as valid positive indicators of social and mental health are less, it is necessary to use indirect measures, viz. indicators of social and mental pathology. These include suicide, homicide, other acts of violence and other crime; smoking; consumption of tranquilizers; obesity, etc. To these may be added family violence, battered-baby and battered-wife syndromes and neglected and abandoned youth in the neighborhood. These social indicators provide a guide to social action for improving the health of the people.

7. Environmental indicators

Environmental indicators reflect the quantity of physical and biological environment in which diseases occur and in which the people live. They include indicators relating the pollution of air and water, radiation, solid wastes, noise, exposure to toxic substances in food or drink. Among these, the most useful indicators are those measuring the proportion of population having access to safe water and sanitation facilities, e.g. percentage of households with safe water in the home or within 15 minutes walking distance from a water standpoint or protected well; adequate sanitary facilities in the home immediate vicinity.

8. Socioeconomic indicators

These indicators do not directly measure health but it is of great importance in the interpretation of indicators of healthcare. These include:

Increase in rate of population, per capita gross national product (GNP), level of unemployment, dependency ratio, literacy rates, especially female literacy rates, family size, housing—the number of persons per room, per capita calorie availability.

9. Health policy indicators

- The single most important indicators of political commitment are allocation of adequate resources. The relevant indicators are proportion of GNP health services, proportion of GNP spent on health related activities such as water supply and sanitation, nutrition and community development and proportion of total health resources devoted to primary healthcare. The degree of equity of distribution of health services:
- Community involvement
- Organizational framework and managerial process.

10. Indicators of quality of life

Increasingly, mortality and morbidity data have been questioned as to whether they fully reflect the health status of a population. The emphasis is based on increased life expectancy as an indicator of health is no longer considered adequate especially in developed countries. Quality of life is difficult to define and even more difficult to measure.

World Health Organization (WHO) defined the quality of life as a composite measure of physical, mental and social well-being as perceived by each individual or by group of individuals, i.e. happiness, satisfaction and gratification as it is experienced in life concerns as health, marriage, family work, financial situation, educational opportunities, self-esteem, creativity, belongingness and trust in others. People are now demanding a better quality of life. Therefore, governments all over the world are increasingly concerned about improving the quality of life of their people by reducing morbidity and mortality.

11. Other indicator series

Indicators selected for monitoring progress towards health for all.

Health status indicators:
- Low birth weight (%)
- Nutritional status and psychosocial developments of children
- Infant mortality rate
- Child mortality rate (1–4 years)
- Life expectancy at birth
- Maternal mortality rate
- Disease specific mortality
- Morbidity—incidence and prevalence
- Disability prevalence.

Millennium development goal indicators
- Prevalence of underweight children under 5 years of age.
- Proportion of population below minimum level of dietary energy consumption.
- Under five mortality rate.
- Proportion of 1 year old children immunized against measles.
- Maternal mortality ratio
- Proportion of births attained by skilled health personnel
- Human immunodeficiency virus (HIV) prevalence among young people aged 15–24 years.
- Condom use rate of the contraceptive prevalence rate.
- Number of children orphaned by HIV or acquired immune deficiency syndrome (AIDS).
- Prevalence and death rates associated with malaria.
- Proportion of malaria risk areas using effective malaria prevention and treatment measures.
- Prevalence and death rate associated with tuberculosis.
- Proportion of tuberculosis.
- Cases detected and curried under directly observed treatments, short-course (DOTS).
- Proportion of population using solid fuel.
- Proportion of population with sustainable access to an improved water source, urban and rural.
- Proportion of urban population with access to improved sanitation.
- Proportion of population with access to affordable essential drugs on a sustainable basis.

CONCLUSION

Mortality and morbidity indicators are important which helps to improve quality care services. Measurement of these indicators essential key to operate any programs.

27 CHAPTER

Concepts of Causation of Diseases and their Screening

CHAPTER OUTLINE

- Concept and Theories of Disease Causation
- Natural History of Disease

INTRODUCTION

Webster defines disease as a condition in which body health is impaired, a departure from the state of health, an alteration of the human body interrupting and the performance of vital functions.

The Oxford English Dictionary defines disease as a condition of the body or some part or organ of the body in which its functions are disrupted or deranged.

From an ecological point of view, disease is defined as maladjustment of the human organism to the environment.

From a sociological point of view, disease is considered a social phenomenon occurring in all societies, and defined and fought in terms of the particular cultural forces prevalent in the society.

The World Health Organization (WHO) has defined health, but not disease. This is because disease has many shades (spectrum of disease) ranging from in apparent (subclinical) cases to severe manifest illness. Some diseases commence acutely (e.g. food poisoning) and some insidiously (e.g. mental illness, rheumatoid arthritis). In some disease, a "carrier" state occurs in which the individual remains outwardly healthy and is able to infect others, e.g. typhoid fever. In some instances, e.g. diarrhea, the same organism may cause more than one clinical manifestations *(Streptococcus)*. Some diseases have a short course and some a prolonged course. It is easy to determine illness, when the signs and symptoms are manifest, but in many disease, the borderline between normal and abnormal is indistinct as in the case of diabetes, hypertension and mental illness. The end point or final outcome of disease is variable recovery, disability or death of the host.

Susser has suggested the following usages:
❖ Disease is a physiological or psychological dysfunction
❖ Illness in a subjective state of the person who feels aware of not being well
❖ Sickness is a state of social dysfunction.

CONCEPT AND THEORIES OF DISEASE CAUSATION

Before the discovery of microorganisms (bacteria by Louis Pasteur, 1822–1895), the French scientist in 1860, several theories explaining the causes of diseases were put forward from time to time.

Up to the time of Louis Pasteur (1895–1922) various concepts of disease causation were in vague. For example, the supernatural theory of disease, the theory of humors, the concept of contagious miasmatic theory of disease, the theory of spontaneous generation, etc. Discoveries in microbiology marked a turning point in our etiological concept. Some other theories of disease causation during the same period were theory of contagious, theory of humors by Greek and Ayurveda. With the discovery of microorganisms by Louis Pasteur mentioned above and Robert Koch (1843–1910), the bacteriologic era commenced in the late 1870, which was the turning point in disease causation. The earlier theories were discarded and germ theory was put forward by these scientists.

Germ Theory of Disease

According to this theory, microbes are the sole causes of disease. The concept of cause embodied in the germ theory of disease is generally referred to a one-to-one relationship between causal agent and disease. The disease model is: Disease Agent—Man—Disease.

The germ theory to disease, led many epidemiologists to take one sided, view of disease causation. It is now recognized that a disease is rarely caused by a single agent

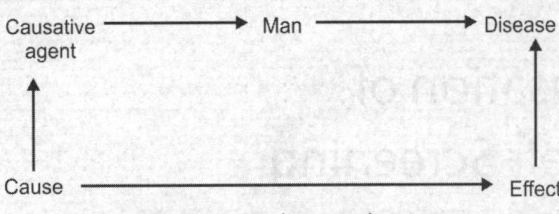

Fig. 27.1: Single cause theory.

alone, but rather depends upon a number of factors, which contribute to its occurrence. This is also called Single cause theory (Fig. 27.1). For example, diphtheria due to *Corynebacterium diptheriae*, cholera due to *Vibrio cholerae*.

Theory of Epidemiological Triad

The germ theory of disease has many limitations.

For example, not exposed to tuberculosis develops tuberculosis. The same exposure in an undernourished or susceptible person may result in clinical disease. Similarly, not everyone exposed to β-hemolytic streptococci develops acute rheumatic fever. This means it was not only the causative agent that was responsible for causing disease, but there were other factors related to man (host) and environment which contributed to the occurrence of a disease. There are other factors relating to the host and environment, which are equally important to determine whether or not disease will occur in the exposed host. This demanded a broader concept of disease causation that synthesized the basic factors of agent, host and environment.

This leads to the theory of epidemiological triad as shown in the epidemiological model given in Figure 27.2.

This model is also called ecological model and is evolved through the study of infectious diseases. According to this model, there are three elements or major factors, which are responsible for particular disease causation. These are agent, host and environment. The agent is considered to be the primary factor (e.g. bacteria, fungi, virus) without which a particular disease cannot occur. The host refers to human beings who come in contact with the agent. The host-related factors, which play an important role is genetic makeup, age, sex, race, immunity, health, behavior, etc.

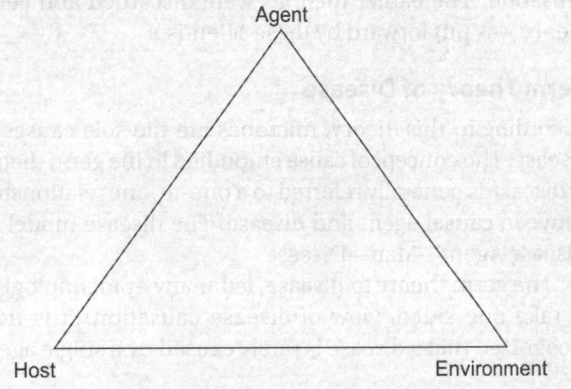

Fig. 27.2: Epidemiological triad.

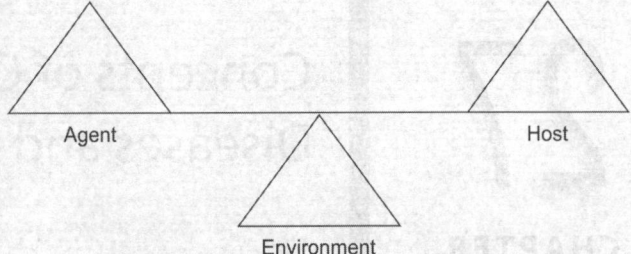

Fig. 27.3: Ecological model of health equilibrium.

The environment includes all that is external to the host and agent, but that may influence interaction between them. As long as they remain in equilibrium or in balance disease will not occur and is referred as state of health equilibrium (Fig. 27.3).

The disease will occur when equilibrium is disturbed due to change or disruption in any of these factors, e.g. poor environmental sanitation, open defecation, contamination of water, floods, etc. All these environmental conditions increase the possibility of people getting infected with disease producing organisms. Other examples of disruption that could increase the possibility of disease occurrence include conditions in the host such as severe malnutrition, disturbed immune system, poor specific resistance, etc. which increases his or her susceptibility to disease. The increased number and mutation of virus, which may increase their virulence and ability to infect the human host.

In fact there has to be optimal interaction of all the three factors to cause the disease in a man. It implies that disease will occur only when the agent is strong and enters the host through the right channel and in sufficient amount, the host is susceptible and when environmental conditions facilitate the interaction of host and agent. For example, the causation of pulmonary tuberculosis mentioned earlier, the live tuberculosis bacilli must enter through respiratory tract and in sufficient amount, the host must be susceptible, i.e. has no specific resistance and weak general body resistance and the environment must facilitate interaction of host and organisms, i.e. environment is crowded, dark and dingy (Fig. 27.4).

Multifactorial Causation Theory

The epidemiological triad model is applicable to infectious diseases only and has been in use for many years. It helps to understand different factors related to communicable diseases. However, it is not applicable to noninfectious and chronic diseases such as mental illness, coronary heart disease, rheumatoid arthritis, etc. It is because these diseases are not linked with specific causation agent and these cannot be prevented and controlled by immunization, isolation and quarantine techniques and by improvement of sanitation like infectious diseases.

According to this theory, diseases are due to multiple factors. For example, coronary heart disease is due to

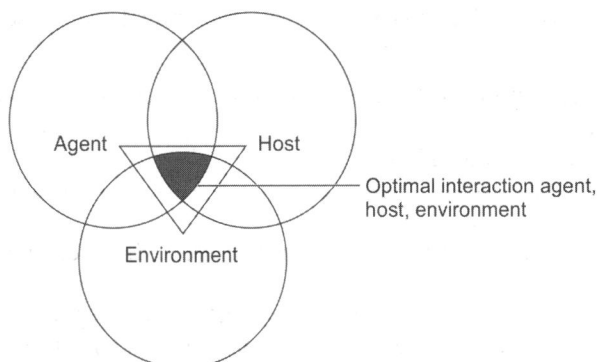

Fig. 27.4: Epidemiological concept of interaction of host, agent and environment.

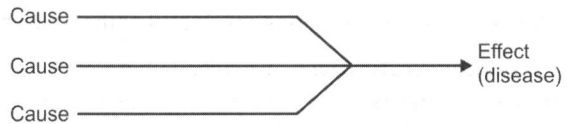

Fig. 27.5: Multiple cause or single effect model.

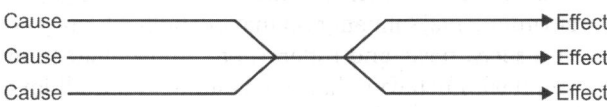

Fig. 27.6: Multiple causes or multiple effects models.

excess of fat intake, smoking, lack of physical exercise and obesity. Most of these factors are liked to lifestyle and human behavior (Fig. 27.5).

The multifactorial causation model helps epidemiologist to understand the various associated causative factors, prioritize these and plan preventive and control measures for a particular disease (Fig. 27.6).

It is also found that several causative factors produce many observed effects, e.g. air pollution, smoking, and specific form of radiation (causes) may produce lung cancer, emphysema and bronchitis (effects).

Web of Causation

This model of disease causation was suggested by MacMahon and Pugh in their book "Epidemiologic Principles and Methods."

The "web of causation" considers all the predisposing factors of any type and their complex interrelationship with each other.

The web of causation does not imply that the disease cannot be controlled unless all the multiple cause chains of causation or at least a number of them are appropriately controlled or removed. Sometimes removal of just one link or chain may be sufficient to control disease.

This epidemiological model suggests that there are cluster of causes and combinations of effects, which are related to each other and need to be studied to identify possible interventions to reduce the occurrence of a

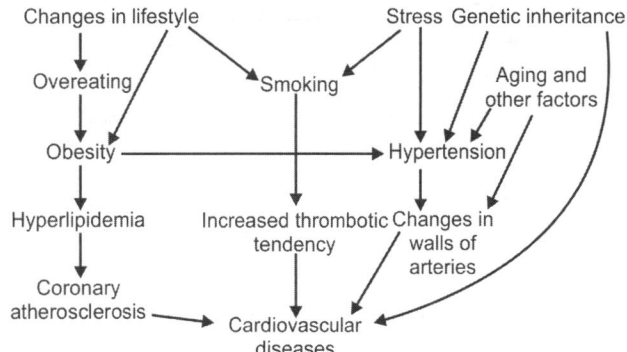

Fig. 27.7: Web of causation-cardiovascular diseases.

particular disease. For example, cardiovascular diseases may include avoidance of smoking, diet control, exercise, stress management, etc.

But fortunately, it is not necessary to understand the whole causal mechanism to effect prevention and control of a particular disease. It requires identification of the most important link(s) in the chains of causation of a disease. This model is particularly applicable to chronic diseases where the causative agent is unknown and which are due to interaction of multiple factors, e.g. cardiovascular diseases, cancer, etc. (Fig. 27.7).

Dever's Epidemiologic Model

This epidemiological model provides another approach to conceptualize interaction of various factors involved in the development of a particular condition. This model is based on Blum's model of health paradigms. The model is composed of four major categories of factors such as human biology, lifestyle, environment and healthcare system.

Iceberg of Disease

A concept closely related to the spectrum of disease is the concept of tile iceberg phenomenon of disease. According to this concept, disease in a community may be competed with an iceberg. The floting sea in the community, i.e. clinical cases. The vast submerged portion of the iceberg represents the hidden mass of disease, i.e. latent, inapparent, presymptomatic and undiagnosed cases and carriers in the community. The water line represents the demarcation between apparent and inapparent disease.

In some diseases (e.g. hypertension, diabetes, anemia, malnutrition, mental illness), the unknown morbidity, (i.e. the submerged portion of the iceberg) far exceeds the known morbidity. The hidden part of the iceberg thus constitutes an important undiagnosed reservoir of infection or disease in the community and its detection and control is a challenge to modem techniques in preventive medicine. One of the major determinants in the study of chronic disease of unknown etiology is the absence of methods to detect the subclinical state the bottom of the iceberg (Fig. 27.8).

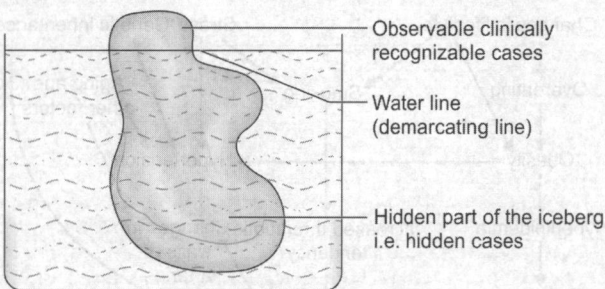

Fig. 27.8: Iceberg of disease.

NATURAL HISTORY OF DISEASE

A disease is the outcome of complex interaction of causative agent, host and environment. In the absence of any intervention, i.e. prevention or treatment, all diseases follow a natural course of events, which refers to "Natural History of Disease." The concept of natural history of disease was conceived by epidemiologists as early as 1860 in the United States as an argument for the clinical course of disease. But the concept was defined and associated with preventive and control strategies in 1953 by Leavell and Clark with the help of scheme of natural history of disease. The model was primarily used to explain infectious diseases, but it can be effectively used for chronic and noninfectious diseases and other health problems. Leavell and Clark have defined the natural history of disease model as "A narrative and schematic representation which portrays a chronological sequencing of departure from health. The sequence begins with the factors that promote health, but the model also addresses the very first force that inaugurates pathological departures. An innate function of this model is to describe various approaches to prevent and control pathological processes and this function is collectively known as the level of prevention."

The natural history of disease is depicted in Figure 27.9. It depicts its confrontation interaction of three essential elements, i.e. agent, host and environment to influence the onset of any disease, the continuum of pathogenesis.

This model is based on the following assumptions:

- **Health is a relative state:** It is assumed that everyone possesses some degree or level of health and it depends upon factors related to people (host) inherent or acquired characteristics, factors related to agents and factors related to environment in which people (host) live.
- **Disease is a process:** It is assumed that disease is not static. It is a process and begins before the individual is affected. It means that the conditions which stimulate illness are present in the environment and in the people (hosts) themselves. This process thus depends upon the nature and characteristics of agent, host and disease producing stimuli with in the environment and individual.
- **Disease is affected due to multiple causations:** As discussed in previous section, the occurrence of any disease depends on epidemiologic triangle composed of host, agent and environment.

There is no single force that can cause a disease. There must be:

- A susceptible host
- Causative agent or factor even if the exact nature of the agent is not known
- An environment which is conducive to the interaction of the host and agent.

There is multiplicity of interaction between the host and environment to cause various non-infectious and chronic diseases resulting in multifactorial causation and web of causation model. The precise mechanism of interaction to cause a disease is not known. The natural history of any disease as viewed by Leavell and Clark which has two stages or phases. These are prepathogenesis and pathogenesis.

1. **Prepathogenesis stage:** This stage is before the onset of disease and is also called as predisease stage. The causative agent has yet not entered the susceptible host (human being). But the factors that favor the interaction of agent and host exist in the environment, e.g. poor environmental sanitation, climatic conditions, presence of insects, pests and rodents, etc. unhygienic habits and health behavior, harmful cultural and traditional practices; and biological factors, i.e. age, sex, marital status, genetic and physiological status of people. This means people living in any particular environment are always predisposed to the risk of disease, i.e. they are in prepathogenesis stage of many infectious and noninfectious diseases. The disease will not occur in man unless these three factors, i.e. agent-host-environment, confront and interact to produce disease provoking stimuli as depicted in Figures 27.4 and 27.9. This stage thus happens in the environment where people live.

   This stage is described as stage of susceptibility by Mausner and Kramer because risk factors of various intensities related to host, agent and environment are present to contract the disease any time.

2. **Pathogenesis stage:**
   - **Prodromal period** (Phase of early pathogenesis): This phase begins with entry of causative agent in the susceptible human host as the agent enters the body through appropriate channel, e.g. in case of chickenpox, the agent varicella-zoster (VZ) virus, must enter through the respiratory tract; it induces tissues and physiological changes in the body. These changes are subclinical, i.e. clinical signs and symptoms of the disease are absent. The host remains apparently healthy and ambulant. After a lapse of some period, which is variable from disease to disease and ranges in a specific disease, the health equilibrium within the body is lost and the signs and symptoms of the disease begin to appear. This period, which lapses between the entry of causative agent and just before the appearance of clinical sign is called incubation

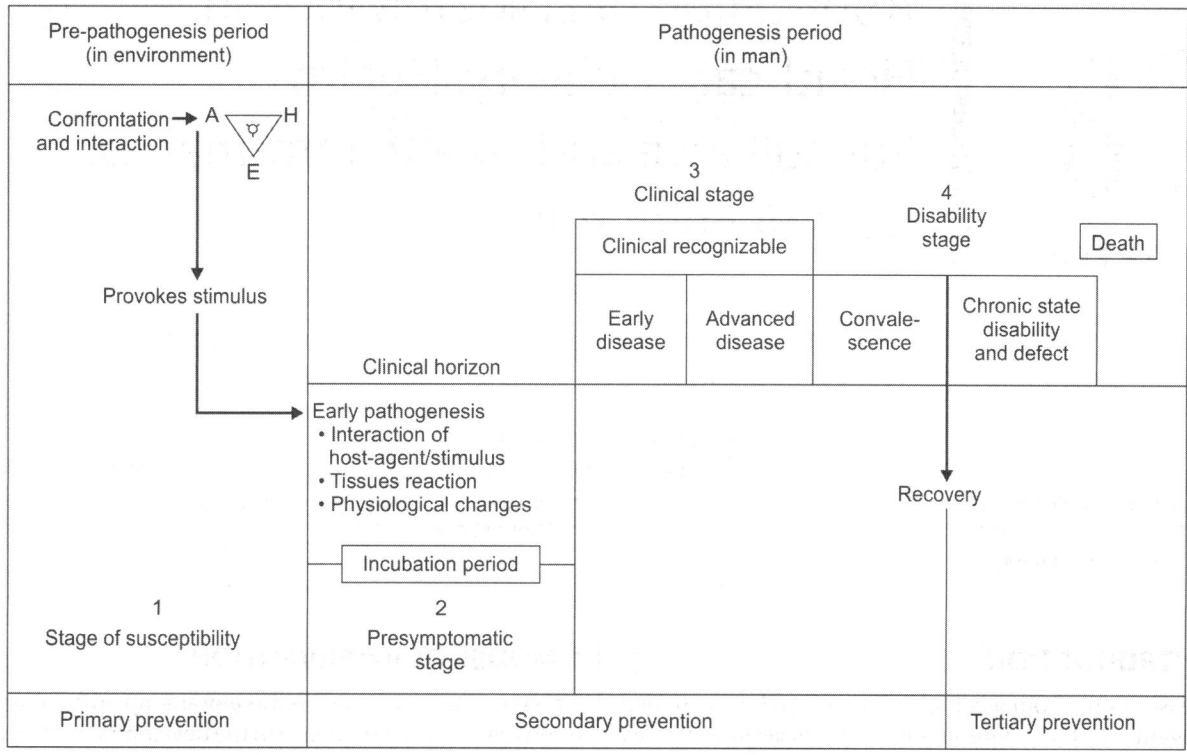

Fig. 27.9: Natural history of disease model based on Leavell-Clark and Mausner and Kramer.

period. In case of chickenpox, this period is usually 14–16 days. The signs and symptoms are sometimes vague during first few days of illness, e.g. in case of chickenpox running nose and watering of eyes, which are common to many other diseases.

- *Preclinical or subclinical phase:* This period is also called presymptomatic phase or stage by some epidemiologists (Mausner and Kramer) especially for chronic and noninfectious diseases. This presymptomatic stage corresponds to incubation period in communicable diseases. The length of presymptomatic phase or stage varies greatly ranging from instantaneous time to many years. For example, in case of accidental injuries it is instantaneous to few hours, and in case of diseases like cardiovascular and diabetes it can be many years.
- *Clinical phase or stage:* The pathological changes advance in the body system, the signs and symptoms become clear and clinical diagnosis can be done, e.g. appearance of skin rashes on different parts of the body in case of chickenpox and the diseases reaches its peak. But in many diseases especially chronic and noninfectious diseases, by the time recognizable signs and symptoms arise and clinical diagnosis is possible, the disease process or pathological changes are well in advance.
- *Disability phase or stage:* The end result of disease process may result in complete recovery. It takes time to recover and the period is called convalescence period or it may end into chronic

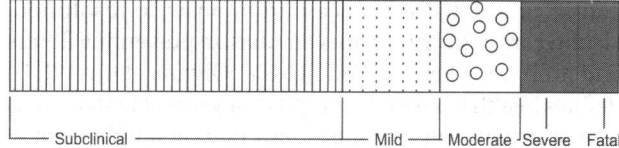

Fig. 27.10: Spectrum of disease.

state, varying level of disability defect or death. The reaction to infection and period of pathogenicity vary from disease to disease and from person to person for the same disease depending upon the virulence of causative agent and the susceptibility of the host and environmental factors. The infection may be clinical or subclinical, typical or atypical or the host may become carrier with or without having clinical disease, e.g. in case of typhoid fever and diphtheria. The period of pathogenesis can also be labeled as gradient of infection. The variation in the manifestation of the diseases in the pathogenesis phase ranges from subclinical to clinical cases. The clinical cases range in severity from mild-to-severe and fatal cases. These variations in the manifestation of a disease can be represented graphically and is called as spectrum of disease (Fig. 27.10).

CONCLUSION

Various expert views the causative agents are numerous and causes different diseases. Factual information can be demonstrated in diagnosing the cause for diseases. So, nurses should be knowledgeble about concept of disease and health.

28 CHAPTER

Application of Epidemiology in Healthcare Delivery, Health Surveillance and Health Informatics, Uses of Epidemiology

CHAPTER OUTLINE

- Concepts of Prevention
- Modes of Intervention
- Levels of Prevention
- Measures of Preventive Epidemiology
- Uses of Epidemiology

INTRODUCTION

Disease results from a complex interaction between men, an agent and the environment. Each disease has its own unique natural history, which is not necessarily the same in all individuals. The natural history of the disease is the course of the disease process from onset to resolution. Health care delivery services emphasize preventing illness and promoting health. World Health Organization (WHO) defines health is a state of complete physical, mental, social and spiritual well-being and not merely an absence of disease or infirmity. Study of epidemiology is useful to apply these concepts in prevention of disease and investigation of epidemics thereby treating the diseases.

CONCEPTS OF PREVENTION

The goals of medicine are to promote health, to preserve health, to restore health when it is impaired and to minimize suffering and distress. These goals are embodied in the work "prevention." Successful prevention depends upon a knowledge of causation, dynamics of transmission, identification of risk factors and risk groups, availability of prophylactic or early detection and treatment measures, an organization for applying these measures to appropriate persons or groups and continuous evaluation of and development of procedures applied.

It is not necessary to know everything about the natural history of a disease to initiate preventive measures. Often times, removal or elimination of a single known essential cause may be sufficient to prevent a disease. The objective of preventive medicine is to intercept or opposes the "cause" and they are by the disease process.

MODES OF INTERVENTION

"Intervention" can be defined as any attempt to intervene or interrupt the usual sequence in the development of disease in man. This may be by the provision of treatment, education, help or social support. There are five modes of intervention:

- ❖ Health promotion (primordial and primary prevention)
- ❖ Specific protection (primary prevention)
- ❖ Early diagnosis and treatment (secondary prevention)
- ❖ Disability limitation and rehabilitation (tertiary prevention).

LEVELS OF PREVENTION

In modern day, the concept of prevention has become broad-based. It has become customary to define prevention in terms of four levels. Each of these levels of prevention serves distinct purposes and involves specific intervention, which are applied to entire population considering its physical, mental, social and spiritual domains:

- ❖ Primordial prevention
- ❖ Primary prevention
- ❖ Secondary prevention
- ❖ Tertiary prevention.

Primordial Prevention

Primordial prevention, a new concept, is receiving special attention in the prevention of chronic diseases. This is primary prevention in its purest sense, i.e. prevention of the emergence or development of risk factors in countries or population groups in which they have not yet appeared. For example, many adult health problems, such as obesity, hypertension have their early origin in childhood because this is the time when lifestyles are formed those like smoking, eating patterns and physical exercises. In primordial prevention, efforts are directed towards discouraging children from adopting harmful lifestyles. The main intervention in primordial prevention is through individual.

Mode of Intervention

Health promotion (primordial prevention): Primordial prevention is defined of the action taken to develop a high level of wellness and is accomplished by influencing individual behavior and the environment in which people live. Health promotion is the process of enabling people to increase control over and to improve health. The well-known interventions in this area are:

- Health education.
- Environmental modifications.
- Nutritional interventions.
- Lifestyle and behavioral changes.
- ***Health education:*** This is one of the most cost effective interventions. A large number of diseases could be prevented with little or no medical intervention if people were adequately informed about them and if they were encouraged to take necessary precautions in time. The WHO constitution states that 'the extension to all people of the benefits of medical, psychological and related knowledge is essential to the fullest attainment of health'.
- ***Environmental modification:*** A comprehensive approaches to health promotion requires environmental modifications such as provision of safe water, installation of sanitary latrines, control of insects and rodents, improvement of housing, etc. Environmental interactions are nonclinical and do not involve the physician.
- ***Nutritional interventions:*** These comprise food distribution and nutrition improvement of vulnerable groups, child feeding programs, food fortification, nutrition education, etc.
- ***Lifestyle and behavioral changes:*** The action of prevention is one of the individual and community responsibilities for health, the physician and each health worker acting as an educator than a therapist. Health education is a basic element of all health activity. It is important in changing the views, behavior and habits of people.

Nurses Role in Health Promotion

Nurses have played key roles in prevention in areas such as prenatal care, immunization, occupational health and safety, cardiac rehabilitation and education, and public healthcare finding and early intervention:

- Meet health promotion needs of the patient whether practice is in the hospital, clinic, patient home, health maintenance organization, etc.
- Health promotion is primarily accomplished through patient education.
- Health promotion should occur through the life cycle with topics focused for infancy, childhood, adolescence, adulthood and old age:
  - For infancy, teach parents about the importance of prenatal care, basic care of infant's breastfeeding, nutrition and infant safety.
  - For childhood, teach about immunization, proper nutrition and safety practices.
  - For adolescence, motor vehicle safety, avoidance of drugs, alcohol and tobacco use, sexual decision making and contraception and prevention of suicide.
  - For adulthood, teach about nutrition, exercise and stress management to help them feel better. Also teach cancer-screening techniques such as breast and testicular self-examination and risk factor reduction for leading causes of death, heart disease, stroke and cancer.
  - For older age, stress on nutrition and exercise to help them live longer and stay fit.

Primary Prevention (Table 28.1)

Primary prevention can be defined as action taken prior to the onset of disease or the pre pathogenesis phase, which removes the possibility that a disease will ever occurs. It signifies intervention in the prepathogenesis phase of a disease or health problem [low birth weight (LBW)] or other departure from health. Primary prevention may be accomplished by measures designed to promote general health and well-being, and quality of life of people or by specific protective measures. Primary prevention precedes disease or dysfunction and is applied to clients considered physically and emotionally healthy. It is not therapeutic does not use therapeutic treatments and does not involve symptom identification.

Table 28.1: Primary prevention.

Health promotion	Specific protection
• Health education	• Use of specific immunizations l
• Good standard of nutrition adjusted to developmental phases of life	• Attention to personal hygiene
• Attention to personality development	• Use of environmental sanitation
• Provision of adequate housing and recreation and agreeable working conditions	• Protection against occupational hazards
• Marriage counseling and sex education	• Protection from accidents
• Genetic screening	• Use of specific nutrients
• Periodic selective examinations	• Protection from carcinogens
	• Avoidance of allergens

Primary prevention includes the concept of "positive health," a concept that encourages achievement and maintenance of an acceptable level of health that will enable every individual to lead a socially and economically productive life.

Information, Education and Communication (IEC) Activity

Provide educational programs, literature and posters of the food pyramid, in schools work sites, food stores and other public places to promote awareness. Encourage restaurants to offer healthy menu items.

Mode of Intervention

Specific protection (primary prevention): Primary prevention is a holistic approach. It relies on measures designed to promote health or to protect against specific disease agents and hazards in the environment. Primary prevention has become increasingly identified with "health education," and the concept of individual and community responsibility for health.

The following are some of the currently available interventions aimed at specific protection:
- Immunization
- Use of specific nutrients
- Chemoprophylaxis
- Protection against occupational hazards
- Protection against accidents
- Protection against carcinogens
- Avoidance of allergens
- The control of specific hazards in the general environment, e.g. air pollution, noise control, etc.
- Control of consumer product quality and safety of foods, drugs, cosmetics, etc. The concept of primary prevention is now being applied to the prevention of chronic disease such as coronary heart disease, hypertension and cancer based on elimination or modification of "risk factors" of disease.

Health Protection

Health protection is defined as the provision of conditions for normal mental and physical functioning of the human being individually and in the group. It includes the promotion of health, prevention of sickness and curative and restorative medicine in all its aspects.

The concept of primary prevention is now being applied to the prevention of chronic disease such as coronary heart disease, hypertension and cancer based on elimination or modification of "risk factors" of disease.

The WHO has recommended the following approaches for the primary prevention of chronic diseases. They are:
1. Population (mass) strategy.
2. High-risk strategy.

1. ***Population strategy:*** This is directed at the whole population irrespective of individual risk levels, e.g. studies have shown that even a small reduction in the average blood pressure or serum cholesterol of a population would produce a large reduction in the incidence of cardiovascular disease. The population approach is directed towards socioeconomic, behavioral and lifestyle changes.
2. ***High-risk strategy:*** The high-risk strategy aims to bring preventive care to individuals at special risk. Primary prevention is a desirable goal. It is worthwhile to recall the fact that the industrialized countries succeeded in eliminating a number of communicable diseases such as cholera, typhoid and dysentery, and controlling several others such as plague, leprosy and tuberculosis, not by medical interventions, but mainly by raising the standard of living. The application of primary prevention to the prevention of chronic disease is a recent development.

Primary prevention is a holistic approach. It relies on measures designed to promote health or to protect against specific disease agents and hazards in the environment. Primary prevention has become increasingly identified with "health education" and the concept of individual and community responsibility for health.

Secondary Prevention (Table 28.2)

Secondary prevention can be defined as action, which halts the progress of a disease at its incipient stage and prevents complications. The specific interventions are early diagnosis through screening tests, case finding programs and adequate treatment. By early diagnosis and adequate treatment, secondary prevention attempts to arrest the disease process, restore health by seeking out unrecognized disease and treating it before irreversible pathological changes have taken place, and reverse communicability infectious disease. It may also protect others in the community from acquiring the infection and thus provide at once secondary prevention for the infected individuals and primary prevention for their potential contacts.

Secondary prevention is largely the domain of clinical medicine. The health programs initiated by governments are usually at the level of secondary prevention. The drawback of secondary prevention is that the patient has

Table 28.2: Secondary prevention.

Early diagnosis and prompt treatment	*Disability limitations*
• Case finding measures; individual and mass screening surveys	• Adequate treatment to arrest disease process and prevent further complications
• Selective examinations	
• Care and prevention of disease process to prevent spread of communicable disease, prevent complications and shorten period of disability	• Provision of facilities to limit disability and prevent death

already been subject to mental anguish, physical pain and the community to loss of productivity.

IEC Activity

Conduct community screening programs for early detection of individuals with poor eating habits among groups such as adolescents, young female workers and the elderly. Initiate educational and incentive programs to improve dietary practices.

Mode of Intervention

Early diagnosis and treatment (secondary prevention): Early detection and treatment are the main interventions of disease control. The earlier disease is diagnosed and treated, the better in the prognosis and preventing the occurrence of further cases or any long-term disability.

Mass treatment: The rationale for a mass treatment program is the existence of at least 4–5 cases of latent infection for each clinical case of active disease in the community.

Tertiary Prevention

When the disease process has advanced beyond its early stages, it is still possible to accomplish prevention by what might be called "tertiary prevention." It signifies intervention in the late pathogenesis phase. Tertiary prevention can be defined as all measures available to reduce or limit impairments and disabilities, minimize suffering caused by existing departures from good health and to promote the patients adjustments to irremediable conditions. When defect and disability are more or less stabilized, rehabilitation may play a preventable role. Modern rehabilitation includes psychosocial, vocational and medical components based on teamwork from a variety of professions. Tertiary prevention extends the concept of prevention into fields of rehabilitation. Secondary prevention is an imperfect tool in the control of transmission of disease. It is often more expensive and less effective than primary prevention.

Restoration and Rehabilitation

- ❖ Provision of hospital and community facilities for retraining and education to maximize use of remaining capacities
- ❖ Education of the public and industries to use rehabilitated persons to the fullest possible extend
- ❖ Selective placement
- ❖ Work therapy in hospitals
- ❖ Else of sheltered colony.

IEC Activity

Case finding in school, work sites, etc. to determine people with eating disorders, addictions (such as alcoholism) or other lifestyle patterns that inhibit positive dietary practices and initiate treatment.

Mode of Intervention

Disability limitation and rehabilitation (tertiary prevention): When a patient reports late in the pathogenesis phase, the mode of intervention is disability limitation. The objective of this intervention is to prevent or halt the transition of the disease process from impairment to handicap.

Concept of disability: The sequence of events leading to disability and handicap have been stated as follows, disease—impairment—disability—handicap.

- ❖ **Impairment:** An impairment is defined as any loss or abnormality of psychological, physiological, anatomical structure or function, e.g. loss of foot, defective vision or mental retardation. Impairment may be visible or invisible, temporary or permanent, progressive or regressive. Further, impairment may lead to the development of "secondary impairment" as in the case of leprosy where damage to nerves (primary impairment) may lead to plantar ulcers (secondary impairment).
- ❖ **Disability:** Because of impairment, the affected person may be unable to carry out certain activities considered normal for his age, sex, etc. This inability to carry out certain activities is termed disability. A disability has been defined as any restriction or lack of ability to perform an activity in the manner or within the range considered normal for a human being.
- ❖ **Handicap:** As a result of disability, the person experiences certain disadvantages in life and is not able to discharge the obligations required of them and play the role expected of them in society. This is termed handicap. It is defined as a disadvantage for a given individual resulting from impairment or a disability that limits or prevents the fulfillment of a role that is normal for that individual. Taking accident as an example, the above terms can be explained further in Table 28.3.

Disability prevention: It refers to all the levels of prevention as follows:
1. Reducing the occurrence of impairment, viz. immunization against polio (primary prevention).
2. Disability limitation by appropriate treatment (secondary prevention).
3. Preventing the transition of disability into handicap (tertiary prevention).

Primary prevention is the most effective way of dealing with the disability problem in developing countries.

Table 28.3: Disease or disorder due to accidents.

Accident	Disease (disorder)
Loss of foot	Impairment
Cannot walk	Disability
Unemployed	Handicap

Selected Areas of Health Promotion

Counsel patients on the topics of proper nutrition, smoking cessation, exercise, relaxation and sexual health to promote health.

Nutrition or Diet

Diet is projected that 35% all cancers could be prevented with an improved diet recommended by national cancer institute. A low-fat and high-fiber diet is recommended. Fat should not account for more than 30% of calorie. More servings of fruits and vegetables should be included daily. If weight loss is desired, have the patient weigh in monthly and review the diet.

Smoking Prevention or Cessation

Smoking is a risk factor for hypertension, heart disease, peripheral vascular disease, cancer of lungs, colon, larynx, oral cavity, etc. Not smoking promotes health by increasing exercise tolerance, enhancing taste bud function and bad breath.

Smoking cessation can be accomplished through an individualized multidimensional program including information on the short and long-term health effects of smoking, practical behavior modification to help break the habit, use of medications designed to reduce physical dependence and minimize withdrawal symptoms.

Exercise/Fitness

Regular exercise as part of a fitness program helps achieve optimal weight, control blood pressure, lower-risk of coronary artery disease and improve the sense of well-being. Plan exercise according to individual tolerance, time allotment, interest and physical impairment.

Suggest walking, jogging, bicycling, swimming, water, aerobics, etc. Exercise program should include 5–10 minutes. Warm-up and cool down periods with stretching activity to prevent injuries. Advice patient to stop, if pair or shortness of breath, dizziness, palpitation or exercise sweating is experienced.

Relaxation or Stress Management

Stress is a change in the environment that is perceived as a threat, challenge or harm to the person's dynamic equilibrium. A limited amount of stress can be a time motivator to take action. Excessive or prolonged stress can cause emotional discomfort, anxiety and illness. In times of stress, sympathetic nervous system is activated and lead to high blood pressure, arteriosclerosis, cardiovascular disease, acute asthma attack, peptic ulcer, migraine, headache and other illnesses. Identify patient's physiological and psychological stress.

Steps of Relaxation Therapy

- ***Relaxation breathing:*** Breath slowly and deeply until relaxation therapy is achieved.
- Progressive muscle relaxation.
- ***Autogenic training:*** This can help relieve pain and induce sleep.
- ***Imagery:*** Uses imagination and concentration to take a mental vacation.
- ***Distraction:*** Uses patient's own interest and activities to divert attention from pain or anxiety and include listening music, watching TV, etc.

Assisting the patient with relaxation therapy: Encourage patient to combine techniques such as relaxation breathing, before and after imaginary or progressive muscle relaxation, along with autogenic training to achieve better result.

Sexual Health

Education, about sexual activity should begin during school age, heighten during adolescence and continue through adulthood. Teach about normal reproduction, unwanted pregnancy, contraception, sexually transmitted disease (STD) and mode of transmission, prevalence, signs and symptoms, and method of prevention.

Investigation of Epidemic

Investigation of epidemic is a systematic process and these steps help community health nurses to learn the process of investigation of epidemic.

Verification of Diagnosis of Disease

Verification of diagnosis of disease is done in the basis of clinical examination of sample of cases. Lab examination is done wherever necessary and applicable.

Confirmation of the Existence of an Epidemic

Confirmation of the existence of an epidemic is done on the basis of the frequency disease. If the frequency is more than normal expectancy in the community then it is considered epidemic. Often such comparison is not required because there is sudden increase in the number of cases within a short period, which happens with common source epidemic of cholera, hepatitis, food poisoning, etc.

Defining the Population at Risk

Defining the population at risk includes:
- Obtaining or preparing a map of the area. The map should show the natural boundaries landmarks, roads, sections and locations of all the dwelling units.
- Demographic study, which may include the study of total population or subgroups population at risk and their composition. This information is necessary for calculating various epidemiological measurements, e.g. morbidity and mortality rates and proportion, etc.

Identification of all Cases and their Characteristics

Identification of all cases and their characteristics can be done by organizing house to house search till the area is free of epidemic and medical examination of population at risk. An epidemiological sheet is prepared for every case. It includes basic information on age, sex, time of the onset of disease, signs and symptoms, information about contacts, movements, history of immunization, information on common source of infection according to the disease under investigation, e.g. parties attended, food eaten, source of water, etc. a properly designed epidemiological case interviewing guide must be developed and used the information.

Study of Ecological Factors

Study of ecological factors includes investigation of all those ecological factors, which might be responsible for epidemic. These include environmental factors, agent factors and host factors. This information will help in identification of source of infection, reservoir of infection and modes of transmission, and thereby planning of preventive and control measures. A proforma needs to be prepared to collect such relevant information correctly.

Data Analysis

The data analysis is the same as in descriptive epidemiology such as description of the cases in terms of person, place and time of distribution. A complete list of cases by chronological order is prepared to show the beginning of epidemic. Attempt is made to identify the first case and follow its movements to trace the source and spread of infection. Spot maps are prepared to find out the geographical distribution of cases. Concentration of cases (clustering) will indicate common source of infection.

Formulation of Hypothesis

Analysis of data will reveal the possible source, causes, agents, hosts and environmental risk factors of infection. These will help the investigator formulate the hypothesis, which may suggest further investigation and help in identification of interventions.

Recommendation for prevention and control: Based on the information revealed about the epidemic the epidemiologist health worker prepares a program of prevention and control of the epidemic not only for the present but also for its prevention in future.

Preparation of a Formal Report

A formal report should be prepared and communicated to health authority for information, evaluation and feedback for future actions.

MEASURES OF PREVENTIVE EPIDEMIOLOGY

Preventive epidemiology applied in identification of population at risk and environmental factors leading to ill health detects of persons with early, mild and asymptomatic diseases. These measures include:
- ❖ Health surveys
- ❖ Screening
- ❖ Surveillance
- ❖ Monitoring.

Health Surveys

Health surveys are investigations to identify the frequency, distribution and the determinants of health related events or states in the community. Health surveys help in knowing the community and making community diagnosis. The health surveys can be general health surveys and special or specific health surveys.

General Health Surveys

Provide comprehensive data about health and sickness status of the whole community. General health survey is not a regular practice in our country, it has been done twice in our country. Once in 1946 by Health Survey and Development Committee headed by Sir Joseph Bhore and again in 1962 by Health Survey and Development Committee headed by Dr Mudaliar.

Special or Specific Health Surveys

Deal with investigation of any aspect of health morbidity status, e.g. filaria, malaria or tuberculosis, etc. mortality and nutritional status. Whether general or specific, health surveys can be cross-sectional or longitudinal, descriptive or analytical or both. Cross-sectional surveys provide data about the prevalence and distribution of illness and the state of health of a community at one point in time. Longitudinal surveys provide valuable information about the natural history of diseases, incidence and prevalence of diseases and underlying causes, etc. By doing surveys on the same population over a longer period, but are difficult to organize and are time consuming, etc.

The data for health survey can be collected by using various methods. These are:
- ❖ Questioning
- ❖ Health examination and laboratory investigations
- ❖ Record review
- ❖ Observation.

  Each method has its own utility, advantages and disadvantages. A survey may require anyone or two or more methods depend upon the purposes of survey, sources of data available, the circumstances and feasibility, etc.
- ❖ ***Questioning:*** Questioning is an invaluable method to seek subjective information through interview and self-administered questionnaire. The interview is the most common method used especially for illiterate population. Self-administered questionnaire, which is usually sent by Mail is less expensive, but it is useful for literate and educated population. There is also high degree of nonresponse.
- ❖ ***Health examination and laboratory investigation:*** This method helps in getting more valid information than by questioning method about clinical cases. But this method is expensive and requires more time.

- ❖ **Record review:** Records are valuable source of health information and record review in a systematic way, which can help obtain health data. But this is a secondary source of information and reliability is in question. The informations may be incomplete because there are no set procedures and standards for record keeping.
- ❖ **Observation:** This is another very good method of obtaining objective information. But it requires lot of planning and systematic methods for data collection. This method is expensive and time consuming.

The most common sampling unit in community health surveys is the household. The sample should be randomized and the sample size could present the whole population. The data must be collected carefully as planned and recorded properly. The data collected are analyzed, i.e. these are compiled, computed, presented in tables, graphs, and charts, described, interpreted and concluded. The formal report is prepared. Such surveys provide baseline community health data and can help plan comprehensive health care programs to prevent diseases and promote health, etc.

Screening

Screening health point of view is defined as the method of search for unrecognized diseases by means of rapidly applied tests, examinations or procedures in apparently healthy population. Screening helps to detect persons with early, mild and asymptomatic diseases. The basic purpose of screening for disease protection is to identify from a large group of apparently well-population those who have a high probability of having the disease under study, so that they may undergo further investigations and if diseased brought to treatment. The screening tests are usually designed to be very simple, rapid and inexpensive because these are meant for large population. These are not diagnostic tests, e.g. mass chest screening by miniature X-rays for tuberculosis. This will help in detecting lesions in the chest, which major may not be tubercular and hence require further investigation. Similarly Pap smear for cancer cervix screening is advocated because it is believed that detection of diseases at its early stages will help in treatment, resulting in its cure, prevention and control of disability and mortality.

The important point, which is to be emphasize is that we must concentrate for early detection of those diseases for which early treatment is available and it is effective, e.g. tuberculosis, diabetes, cancer of cervix and breast. The screening should be part of health care program where treatment can be instituted. There are three types of screening namely:

1. **Mass screening:** In this screening of the whole population or the subgroups whether or not exposed to the risk of having the disease under study. It is not advisable under the present limited resources.
2. **Selective or high-risk screening:** In this screening of only those who are at high-risk to have a particular problem or disease, e.g. women above 35 years and lower social group have more chances of cancer cervix and if they are screened for that, then more chances of detecting the cases. Similarly people having family history of diabetes, breast cancer should be screened for such problems.
3. **Multiphasic screening:** In this screening number of tests for different diseases are grouped together to screen for number of conditions at the same time, e.g. test for lung diseases, cardiovascular diseases, diabetes, anemia, kidney diseases, cancer of the breast and uterus, visual and audio defects are grouped together. This refers to body scanning. But this is an expensive venture and its benefits are in question.

Criteria for Screening

The screening tests are generally directed to high prevalence (high-risk) groups, e.g. screening for HIV infection can be done for prostitutes, truckers, intravenous drug addicts. Some of the criteria, which are considered for screening, are as given below:
- ❖ The disease has high prevalence.
- ❖ The disease has early asymptomatic or latent stage and its natural history is clearly understood so that one knows at what stage it is irreversible.
- ❖ Simple, inexpensive and reliable tests are there to detect the disease prior to its onset.
- ❖ Facilities for further confirmation tests and treatment, etc. are available.
- ❖ Early detection and treatment will prevent and control morbidity, disability and mortality.
- ❖ Screening tests are reliable and valid.
- ❖ The tests acceptable to the people for whom it is done.

Health Surveillance

The dictionary meaning of surveillance is supervision or close watch especially on suspected person. Epidemiologically surveillance means close vigilance on occurrence and distribution of diseases and health-related problems, population dynamics, community behavior and environmental processes resulting in increased risk of ill health in the community. It involves identification of missed and suspected cases and contacts, their confirmation by laboratory investigations; identifying source of infection and channel of transmission. This information will help in planning and implementation of prevention and control programs for various diseases in the community. Thus, monitoring of the disease prevalence, its related risk factors and intervention of control program for the same are the important activities of surveillance. The epidemiological surveillance can be done at individual and family level, national and international level:

- ❖ **Individual or family surveillance:** It includes surveillance of an infected person in a family as long as the individual is source of infection to others, e.g. typhoid case and carriers.

- ❖ *Community or local population surveillance:* It includes active and passive surveillance of the whole community for early detection and prevention and control of a disease, e.g. malaria.
- ❖ *National surveillance:* It includes surveillance at the National level, e.g. surveillance of smallpox after its eradication.
- ❖ *International surveillance:* It includes surveillance of some of the diseases, which are listed by WHO, e.g. malaria, influenza, filaria, polio, etc. and are to be reported to WHO, which then provides information to the countries in the world to take timely actions.

Surveillance Process

Surveillance is a systematic process. The main steps involved are:
- ❖ Collection of relevant information about the disease under surveillance
- ❖ Analysis and interpretation of these information
- ❖ Reporting of the information to the concerned authority for decisions and actions leading to prevention and control of diseases.

Collection of relevant information about the disease under surveillance: Effectiveness of surveillance system depends upon identification of cases, collection of relevant information about the disease, their recording arid reporting. There are number of methods for collection of relevant information about the diseases under surveillance. It may be easier to identify some diseases, while it may be difficult to identify some others. Because of this difficulty no single method can be adopted for surveillance of all diseases. The various methods for surveillance are as under:

- ❖ *Routine reporting of cases* and deaths recorded at Health centers, dispensaries and hospitals: All these institutions are required to maintain record of cases reported in their outpatient department and clinics. A sample recording from which is usually practiced is given below:
  - ➢ From this record daily, weekly, monthly and yearly reports of disease occurred and reported at center are prepared.
  - ➢ This kind of routine reporting can help in making assessment of frequency and distribution of diseases by age, sex, area and time. Such reports are sent to the district and state health authorities. The practice of recording of cases under the routine reporting system is called passive surveillance.
- ❖ *Active surveillance:* It means actively looking for those types of cases who have not been recorded under the routine system. Active surveillance is done by health workers and community people, e.g. surveillance of malaria or tuberculosis cases.
- ❖ *Epidemiological investigations:* These are usually done, when there is occurrence of more than usual number of cases in a particular place during particular time period—when there is sudden outbreak of any disease and when a communicable disease, which has never occurred before, but it has occurred now. This will help in picking up cases and the associated causative factors. Thus epidemiological investigations provide important supplementary information, which are not obtained by other surveillance methods.
- ❖ *Sentinel centers:* These are those hospitals, health centers, laboratories, special disease hospitals, etc. that are identified for collecting information for selected diseases. The information are collected, compiled and forwarded to higher authority for use of immediate action and for making future plans and policies, etc. Sentinel surveillance can provide reliable information about selected diseases indicating the trend of disease prevalence in a particular area. Such information can call for immediate actions to control the disease and also timely remedial actions in future to prevent the occurrence of disease.
- ❖ *Special sample survey*: Special sample survey of disease is an active and efficient method of surveillance. There are different methods of sample surveys, but the survey by cluster sampling technique is recommended by the WHO. The target population, the sample size vary from disease to disease, e.g. the target population for poliomyelitis is 5–9 years, for diarrhea 0–4 years, preceding the date of survey.

Compilation and analysis of data: Once the surveillance data is collected for a reporting period by whatever method, it needs to be compiled and analyzed to assess the frequency and distribution by person, place and time. The reporting period can be a week, a month and a year. This information can be presented in tables, spot maps, charts and graphs. This kind of presentation helps in determining the pattern of occurrence of disease and whether there is decrease or increase in the number of cases.

Reporting of data and providing feedback: Feedback should be given to all the members of health learners and reported as and when desired by anyone.

Monitoring: Monitoring is day to day the assuring and analysis, i.e. making assessment of health status of people and their environment to determine any changes. It is also implementation of surveillance activities, which are planned.

Health Informatics

Health informatics plays very important role in identification and prevention of globally occurring current diseases in the world. Health information is an integral part of the national health system.

Definition

A mechanism for the collection processing, analysis and transmission of information required for organizing and operating health services, and also for research and training.

The primary objective of a health information system is to provide reliable, relevant, up to date, adequate, timely, and reasonably complete information for health manage at all levels. Sharing techniques and scientific information by all health personal participating in the health services of a country.

Requirements by Health Information System

According to WHO, expert committee identified the following requirements to be satisfied by the health information systems:
- The system should be population based.
- The system should avoid unnecessary agglomeration of data.
- The system should be problem oriented.
- The system should employ functional and operational terms, e.g. episodes of illness, treatment regimens and laboratory tests.
- The system should express information briefly and imaginatively, e.g. tables, charts, percentages, etc.
- The system should make provision for the feedback of data.

Components of a Health Information System

The comprehensive health information system requires information and indicates on the following aspects:
- Demography and vital events.
- Environmental health statistics.
- Health status—mortality, morbidity, disability and quality of life.
- Health resources—facilities, beds, manpower, etc.
- Utilization and nonutilization of health services attendance, admissions, waiting lists.
- Indices of outcome of medical care.
- Financial statistics (cost expenditure) related to the particular objective.

Uses of Health Information

Important uses of health information that may be applied are:
- To measure the health status of the people and to quantify their health problems and medical and healthcare needs.
- For local, national and international comparisons of health status. For such comparisons the data need to be subjected to rigorous standardization and quality control.
- For planning, administration and effective management of health services and programs.
- For assessing whether health services due accomplishing their objectives in terms of their effectiveness and efficiency.
- For assessing the attitudes and degree of satisfaction of the beneficiaries with the health system.
- For research into particular problems of health and disease.

Sources of Health Information

- **Census:** Census is important health information. It is taken in most countries of the world; first regular census in India was taken in 1881. The last census was held in March 2001. Without census data, it is not possible to obtain quantified health, demographic and socioeconomic indicators.
- **Registration of vital events**
  - Registration of births and deaths keeps a continuous check on demographic changes. If registration of vital events is complete and accurate, it serves reliable source of health information. The central births and deaths registration act 1969 promulgated by Government of India. The act provides for compulsory registration of births and deaths throughout the country and compilation of vital statistics in the states.
  - Some countries have attempted to employ first line health workers Village Health (VH) Guides record births or deaths in the community.
  - "Lay reporting of health information" a new approach has been developed in several countries. Transmission of information by health workers.
- **Sample registration system:** Since civil registration is deficient in India, a sample registration system was initiated in the mid-1960s to provide reliable estimates of birth and death rates at the national and state levels. The sample registration record system consisting of continuous enumeration of births and deaths an independent survey every 6 months in addition to serving as an independent check on the events recorded by the enumerator, produces the denominator required for computing rates.
- **Notification of diseases:** Reporting responsibility of notifiable diseases is now shifted from village chowkidar to the health workers. Legal provision is an essential prerequisite for any notification system, the enactment of a uniform act similar to the registration of births and deaths act 1969 is demined necessary for any improvement in the notification system in India. At the international level, the following diseases are notifiable to WHO in Geneva under the International Health Regulations (IHR), viz. cholera, plague, yellow fever and few others. This information is published by WHO on a worldwide basis. The expert committee on health statistics recommended that yearly data notification should be detailed by age and sex.
- **Community health risk assessment tools:** As the public has become more aware of harmful elements to the environment, risk assessment tools must be developed in future days, risk factor assessments complement vital statistics data systems and morbidity data systems by providing information on factors earlier in the casual chain leading to illness, injury or death.

- Risk factor systems are used throughout the country and may be local, regional, or national in scope, e.g. suicide prevention community assessment tool.
- National Health and Nutrition Examination Survey (NHANES).
- Youth risk factor surveillance system.
- Behavioral risk factor surveillance system (BRFSS).
- Determining the presence of risk factors in a community is a key part of a community risk assessment (CRA). The goal of a CRA is risk reduction and improved health and helps to set new properties for unmet needs and opportunities for action for local public health units. A CRA may also be used to monitor the impact prevention program.

❖ **Disease registers:** The term registration implies something more than notification. A register requires that a permanent record be established, that the cases be followed up and that basic statistical tabulations be prepared both on frequency and on survival.

Morbidity registers visit only in certain diseases and conditions such as stroke, myocardial infarction, cancer, blindness, congenital defects and congenital rubella. Tuberculosis and leprosy are also registers in many countries where they are common. If the reporting system is affective and the coverage is on a national basis, the register can provide useful data, treatment given and disease specific mortality can be determined.

Record linkage: The medical record linkage implies, the assembly and maintenance for each individual in a population. The events commonly recorded in a hospital admission and discharge. Record linkage is a particularly suitable method of studying associations may have etiological significance, therefore in practice record linkage has been applied only on a limited scale, e.g. twin studies, measurement of morbidity, diseases epidemiology and family and genetic studies.

❖ **Epidemiological surveillance:** In many countries, where particular diseases are endemic, special control or eradication program have been instituted, e.g. national disease control programs against malaria, tuberculosis, leprosy, filariasis, etc. These programs have yielded considerable morbidity and mortality data for the specific diseases.

❖ ***Agency support of epidemiology and monitoring of disease outbreaks:*** This is a need to define the role of federal, state and local primarily health agencies in the development of public health issues (PHI), and information technology applications. The availability of it today challenges all state hold in the health of the public to adopt new systems to provide adequate diseases surveillance and challenges us to improve outmoded process.

In the early 1990s, Centers for Disease Control and Prevention (CDC) launched a plan for an integrated surveillance system that moved from standalone systems to networked data exchange built with specific standards. Early initiatives were the National Electronic Telecommunications System for the Surveillance (NETSS) and Wide-ranging Online Data for Epidemiologic Research (WONDER).

Six current initiatives reflect the early vision is as follows:
1. Pulse Net USA: A surveillance.
2. The national electronic disease surveillance system facilities reporting on approximately 100 diseases with data feeding directly from limed lab creators allowing the early election.
3. Epidemic information exchange (EPIX): A secure communication system for practitioners to access and share preliminary health surveillance information.
4. Health alert network (HAN): A state and nationwide alert system.
5. Biosense provides improved real time biosurveillance and situational awareness in support of early detection.
6. Public health information network (PHIN) promotes standards and software solutions for the rapid flow of public health information.

❖ *Hospital records:* Developing country such as India Notification of Infections and Diseases is inadequate, hospital data constitute a basic and primary source of information about diseases prevalent in the community. The 8th report of the WHO expert committee on the statistics recommended that hospital statistics be regarded in all countries as an integral and basic part of the National Statistical Program.

Other health service records: A lot of information is also found in the records of hospital, input departments, primary health centers (PHCs) subcenters, polyclinics, private practitioners, mother and health centers, school health records, diabetic and hypertensive clinics, etc. For example, records of MCH centers provide information about birth weight, height, arm circumference, immunization, disease specific mortality, morbidity. Further the data generated by these records are mostly kept for administrative purposes rather than for monitoring.

❖ *Environmental health data:* Another area to which information is generally teaching is that relating to the environment. Health statistics are now sought to provide data on various aspects of air, water and noise pollution, harmful food additives, industrial toxicants, inadequate waste disposal and others aspects of the combination of population explosion with used production and construction of material good. This will be helped in the identification and qualifications of factors causative of disease.

- **Health manpower statistics:** Information in health manpower is by no means least in importance. Such informative relates to the number of physicians (age, sex, specialty and place of work), dentists, pharmacists, veterinarians, hospital nurses, medical technicians, etc. Their records are maintained by the State Medical Dental or Nursing Councils and the directorate of medical education. The institute of applied manpower research attempts estimates of manpower taking into accent different data, mortality and out turn of qualified persons from the different institutions. Planning commission publishes health information of India by the Government of India, in the Ministry of Health and Family Welfare.
- **Population surveys:** The health information system should be population based. The routine statistics collected from the above same. But they do not get the information about health and disease in the community. Surveys for evaluating of health status of a population, community diagnosis of health problems, surveys for investigation of factors affecting health and disease. Surveys relating to administration of health services, e.g. use of health services, expenditure on health and evaluation of population health needs and unmet needs, evaluation of medical care, etc.

Types of Survey Methods

- Health interview (face-to-face survey)
- Health examination survey
- Health records survey
- Mailed questionnaire survey.

a. ***Health disaster planning and preparation:*** Future public health information will offer real time surveillance data systems for planning, evaluation or implementation of public health interventions in management of any disasters.
b. ***Feedback to improve responses and promote readiness:*** Population health data must be considered an important infrastructure of all Regional Health Information Organizations (RHIOs), which are the building blocks for a National Health Information Network (NHIN). These effects call for collaboration of various organizations and agencies interested in clinical, public health and population health information to promote and protect the public's health.

Other Routine Statistics Related to Health

- **Demographic:** In addition to routine census data statistics on such other demographic phenomena as population density, movement and educational level.
- **Economic:** Consumption of consumer goods as tobacco, dietary facts and domestic coal, sales of drugs and remedies, information concerning per capital income employment and unemployment data.
- **Social security schemes:** Medical insurance schemes, make it possible study the occurrence of illness to the insured population other usable data comprise sickness, absence and disability benefit rates.

Non-quantifiable information: Health information mainly on quantifiable data. Health planners and decision makers require a lot of nonquantifiable information makers for instance information on health policies health legislation, public attitudes, program costs, procedures and technology, in other words, a health information system has multidisciplinary inputs. These should be proper storage, processing and dissemination of information.

USES OF EPIDEMIOLOGY

While study of disease distribution and cautions on remains centered to epidemiology. The techniques of epidemiology have a wide application covering many more important areas relating not only to disease but also health and health services. In this content Morris has identified seven distinct uses of epidemiology, extend epidemiology beyond search for causes of diseases and bring it close to day-to-day concerns of modern medicines. These are as follows:

- To study historically the rise and fall of diseases in the pollution
- Community diagnosis
- Planning and evaluation expanding health services to population
- Evaluation of individual's risks and chances
- Syndrome identification
- Completing the natural history of diseases
- Searching for causes and risk factors.

Other uses includes:

- Determine the usefulness and effectiveness of new innovative techniques, measure and programs, etc.
- Forecast the library occurrence of certain diseases on basis of epidemiological principles, e.g. changing trends in occurrence of malaria because of changes in climatic factors, e.g. rainfall.

CONCLUSION

Community health nurses working with vulnerable populations may fill numerous roles. They identify vulnerable individuals and families through outreach and case finding. They encourage vulnerable groups to obtain health services and develop programs that respond to their needs.

29 CHAPTER

Role of Nurse in Epidemiology

CHAPTER OUTLINE

- Role of Nurse in Epidemiology

1. **Epidemiology is one of the basic sciences applicable to nursing. Nurses working in the community deal with the people in various settings and help them to solve their health problems.** Nurses make use of nursing process, which is comparable to epidemiological process in solving the problems:
   - Identifies and investigates the problems.
   - Formulates and tests hypothesis regarding causes.
   - Formulates alternative interventions and implements to prevent and control problems.
   - Evaluates the effectiveness of interventions.
   - She may deal with independently, especially when these are nursing problems, minor ailments, or simple health conditions.
   - She may participate as one of the team members, especially when it is large-scale investigations, e.g. occurrence of any epidemic or community level general health survey, surveillance activities and screening.
   - She participates in data collection, data analysis, planning, implementation, and evaluation.

2. **Nurses in the community have an active role in prevention and control of communicable diseases, which include:**
   - Participation in early diagnosis and treatment, i.e. identification of all cases.
   - Notification of certain specific diseases like measles, diphtheria, tetanus, hepatitis, rabies, sexually transmitted diseases to the health authority.
   - Trace the contacts, keep them under surveillance.
   - Identify source of infection, methods of spread of infection.
   - Health education of people in general.

3. **Nurses in the community as a member of a health team participate in:**
   - Surveillance at all levels, which will depend upon existing situations, her preparation, the level at which she works.
   - At times, she may be the only one available at the community and find herself responsible for surveillance activities.
   - She can make interpretation and take decision to plan and implement, prevention and control measures.
   - She also participates in policy-making procedures and consults with other members of the team at the block and district level.
   - Community health nurse can teach and supervise other health workers surveillance activities.

4. **The nurses working in the community:**
   - Nurses working in the community are required to take notice of any unusual occurrence of any disease or in large number and report to the authority.
   - Participate in investigations regarding frequency and distribution and possible determinants, analysis of information collected, comparison with previous findings and with rates at the national level, and planning and implementation of prevention and control program.

5. **Nurses in the community have an important** role in prevention and control of chronic and noninfectious problems such as cardiovascular conditions, accidents, cancer, mental health problems, etc. through health education and helping people to change their lifestyle.

CONCLUSION

Therefore knowledge of basic concepts involved in epidemiological process is essential for any nurse, not only for those who are working in the community setting but also for those who are working in the hospitals. Nurses play a key role in prevention and control of diseases as well as in restoring and maintain optimum health. Wherever they practice, epidemiological concepts and methods must be included as an integral part of both theory and practical of nursing curricula. Students must be given an opportunity to apply epidemiological concepts during their clinical and field practice.

SUGGESTED READING

1. K Park. Textbook of Preventive and Social Medicine, 17th edition. M/s Banarsidas Bhanot Publishers; 2002. pp. 14, 27-37.
2. Marcia S, Jeanette L. Community Health Nursing, 4th edition. USA: Mosby and WB Saunders Co.; 1996. pp. 638-42, 214.
3. Patricia A Potter, Anne Griffin Perry. Fundamentals of Nursing, 3rd edition. USA: Mosby and WB Saunders Co.; 1992. pp. 47-50.
4. Sandra M Nettina. The Lippincott Manual of Nursing Practice, 6th edition. Philadelphia, USA: Lippincott Williams and Wilkins; 2010. pp. 10-17.
5. Susan Clemen-Stone, Diane Gerber Eigsti, Sandra L McGuire. Comprehensive Community Health Nursing, 5th edition. Maryland Heights, Missouri: Mosby; 1998. pp. 77-8, 100-1.
6. Janice SM, Mary A. Community Health Nursing. Philadelphia: WB Saunders Company; 1993. pp. 175-6, 116.
7. Bullough Bonnie, Bullough Vern. Nursing in the Community. Maryland Heights, Missouri: The CV Mosby Company; 1990. pp. 121-3, 25-6.
8. Carole Lium Edelman, Carol Lynn Mandle. Health Promotion throughout the Life Span, 3rd edition. Maryland Heights, Missouri: Mosby; 1994. pp. 13, 15-9.
9. Barbara Walton Spradley, Judith Ann Allender. Community Health Nursing: Concepts and Practice, 4th edition. New York, USA: Lippincott; 1996. p. 15.

REVIEW OF SECTION BASED QUESTIONS OF RGUHS

Long Essays

1. Concepts of causation of diseases and their screening.
2. Role of nurses in epidemiology.
3. Discuss in detail the scope, aim, approaches and methods of epidemiology.
4. Application of epidemiology in health care delivery.

Short Essays

1. Caution of diseases.
2. Uses of epidemiology. (May 2011)
3. Health surveillance and health informatics.
4. Morbidity and mortality.
5. Concepts of disease. (May 2012)
6. Importance of epidemiology in clinical practice. (Oct 2010)
7. Nursing informatics.

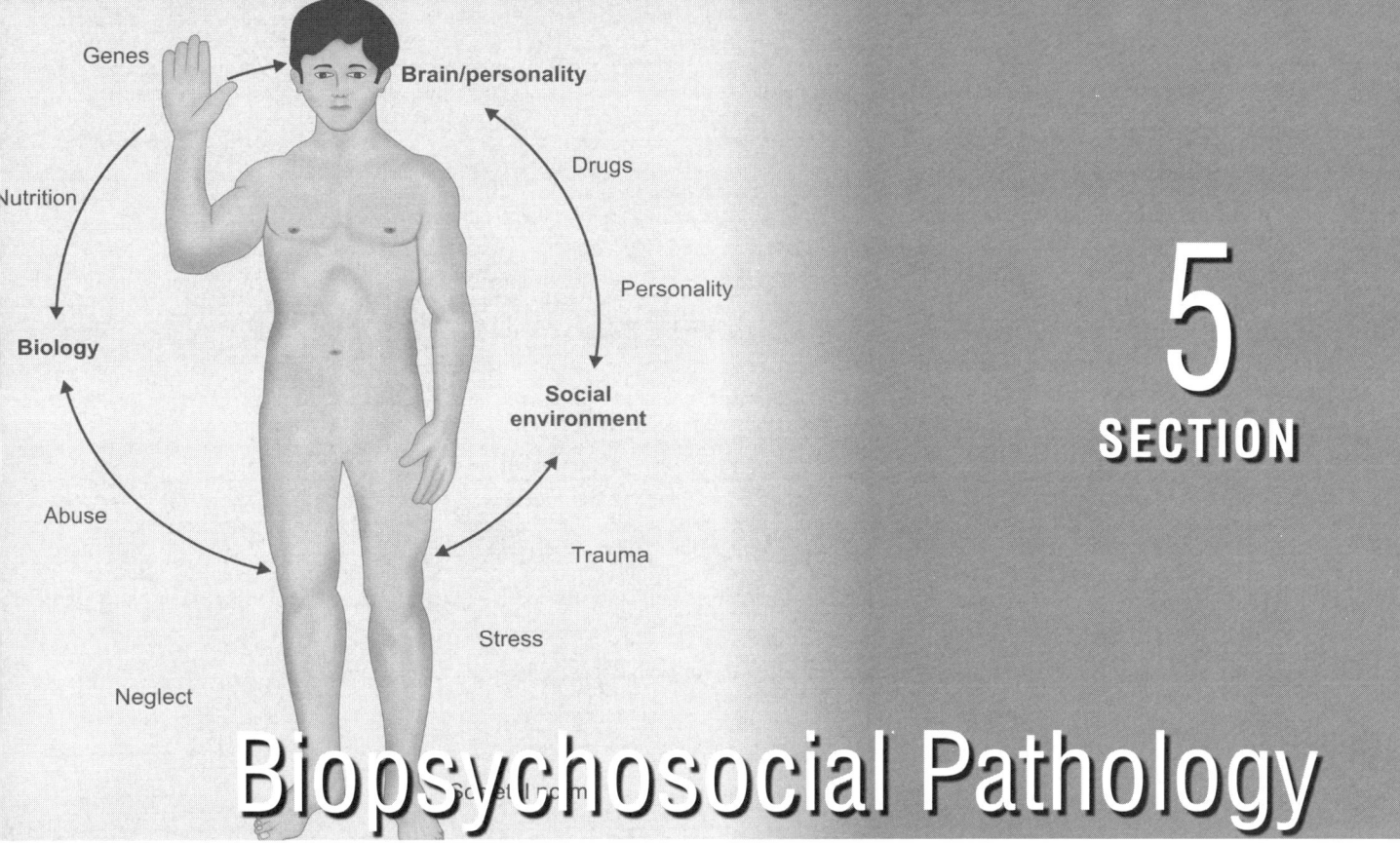

SECTION 5

Biopsychosocial Pathology

Section Outline

30. Pathophysiology and Psychodynamics of Disease Causation
31. Life Process, Homeostatic Mechanism, Biological and Psychosocial Dynamics in Causation of Disease and Lifestyle
32. Common Problems
33. Treatment Aspects: Pharmacological, Pre- and Postoperative Care Aspects
34. Cardiopulmonary Resuscitation
35. End-of-Life Care
36. Infection Prevention (Including HIV) and Standard Safety Measures
37. Biomedical Waste Management

30 CHAPTER
Pathophysiology and Psychodynamics of Disease Causation

CHAPTER OUTLINE

- Psychobiology
  - Definition of Psychobiology
  - Psychological Revolution
- Neuroanatomy
  - Neurons
  - Brain
  - Brainstem
  - Extrapyramid System
- Peripheral Nervous System
- Autonomic Nervous System
- Neuroregulation
  - Neurotransmitter Regulation and Psychiatric Illnesses
  - Neurotransmitters are Related to Psychiatric Symptomatology
- Diagnosis of Psychobiological Disorders
- Psychobiology and Nursing

PSYCHOBIOLOGY

Introduction

Man has the capacity for thought, and thought is the integrative activity of the brain. With great advances in technology, scientists have been able to objectively document the inner workings of the brain and its relation to behavior. Today practitioners, researchers, teachers, and students are faced with the challenge of integrating the rapidly expanding information about the brain and its behavior. At the transition of the 20th century, Adolph Meyer (1866-1950) introduced the concept of psychobiology, noting that psychology and biology are not mutually exclusive aspects of mental illness. Scientists continue to explore the relationship among physiological functions and anatomical structures and their association with mental processes, including consciousness, memory, and emotions.

Definition of Psychobiology

- Psychobiology is the study of the relationship between behavior and the brain.
- Psychobiology is the study of biochemical foundations of thought, mood, emotion, affect, and behavior.

—Wilson, 1994.

Psychobiological Revolution

Variations in biologic processes and hormonal imbalances have long been recognized as the cause of some psychiatric disturbances. Behavioral changes that manifest as brain lesions give further evidence of possible neurophysiologic determinants of some psychiatric disorders. Introduction of psychotropic agents in the early 1950s, notably reserpine and Thorazine®, restimulated research on the biochemistry of psychiatric disorders. Over the last 40 years, advances in biotechnology, immunology, genetics, endocrinology, and brain imaging have led to an explosion of investigations on the role of psychobiology in mental illness. It has been generally accepted that there is no real division between the mind and body, the mental and the physical health, and the brain and thought.

It has been observed that 'mind' is an integrative capacity developed by the brain. Thinking, decision-making, memory, intelligence, emotions, and control over one's behavior and talk, and awareness of surroundings are the different functions of the mind. Mind is the active part of ourselves and is the source of all our activities. The brain carries out all the functions of the mind. The brain is an organ of the body and is vulnerable to diseases as other body organs. Research on the functions of the brain including the role of neurotransmitters has led to reinterpretation of most functional psychiatric disorders (previously considered to have no organic basis) as brain diseases. The challenge is to find the loci of deficits in brain tissue, chemistry, physiology, and anatomy that cause manifestation or aberrant behaviors labeled as mental illness. Psychobiology is rapidly becoming the basis for mental health practice.

NEUROANATOMY

- The part of the nervous system, which occupies the central axis of the body, is called central nervous system (CNS). It consists of the brain, the spinal cord, and associated nerves.
- The basic unit of the nervous system and the brain is the neuron. The brain is made up of millions of neurons.

Neurons

Neurons are nerve cells having a cell body (soma) and extensions or protoplasm called neutrite. Neutrites that relay impulses toward the nerve soma are dendrites and those conducting impulses away from the soma are axons. Synapses are specialized areas of contact between neuron where impulses cross. Billions of neurons in the CNS are connected to one another electrochemically. Most are mediated by chemical substances known as neurotransmitters.

Brain

The brain has two hemispheres: left and right. The cerebral cortex is the gray matter at the surface of the two hemispheres of the brain. Fissures (sulci) and convolutions (gyri) of variable extent make up the cortex. Sulci serve to separate the cortex into areas of distinct function. Gyri are connected by short fibers that link different lobes of the brain. There are four major lobes of the brain on each hemisphere, i.e. the frontal, parietal, temporal and occipital lobes.

1. *The frontal lobes* influence the functions or learned motor activity and the planning and organizing of future expressive behavior. They allow versatile responses of the mind and are concerned with judgment, personality, and intellectual function.
2. *Parietal lobes* affect attention selectivity. They integrate somatic stimuli to recall form, texture, and weight. The parietal lobes also integrate these perceptions with other sensations to create self-awareness of both inner and outer worlds.
3. *Temporal lobes:* Structures of temporal lobes are critically involved with visual recognition, auditory perception, memory, and emotions.
4. *Occipital lobes* are primarily concerned with vision, including form recognition, color recognition, and integration of visual stimulation from partial objects into perceptions of a coherent whole.

Corpus Callosum

It interconnects matching areas of the two hemispheres. It contains 300 million fibers and is the largest fiber tract a superhighway of information exchange between the hemispheres that keep them working together. Embedded deep within the cerebrum are several large masses of gray matter called basal ganglia. The basal ganglia are extensively connected with association and limbic structures and are involved in complex behavior. Diseases of the basal ganglia, such as Huntington's and Parkinson's diseases, are usually associated with major changes in mental states. Gathering, processing, integrating, and storing information about internal and external conditions are done through a hierarchy of neural interconnections that form networks distributed throughout the cerebrum. The neurons of the CNS are concerned with the three major operations responsible for thoughts, feelings, and behaviors. These are as follows:

1. Input, receiving and registering sensory stimuli from outside and from within.
2. Output, planning and execution of complex motor acts.
3. Intermediary processing interposed between input and output. Manifestations of intermediary processes include functions of thought, language, memory, self-awareness, and many aspects of mood and affect.

Limbic System (Fig. 30.1)

The limbic system is the principal location for these intermediary processes and is primarily concerned with the integration of affective (emotional) aspects of behaviors, memory, and basic drives required for the individual. A basic principle of psychiatry is that thoughts, feelings, and behaviors are deviant from some norm and therefore induce distress in the individual and those close to him/her. The limbic system is believed to be the point of origin for these psychiatric disorders of mood and thought.

Limbus: Limbus means a border. The limbic system refers to a set of structures comprising a vertical limbus on each side or the brain surrounding the corpus callosum and a cerebral peduncle or stem-like connecting part, and a horizontal limbus surrounding the midbrain. The structures included in this system are the hippocampus, thalamus, hypothalamus, and amygdala. The components of the limbic system are interconnected through many neural circuits and may contain common immunological properties. One can conceptualize the limbic circuits as divided into hippocampal and amygdala spheres of influence with the hippocampus and its connections being more closely associated with memory functions, while the amygdala and its pathways are more closely related to affective components of events. The thalamus, besides being part of the limbic system, is integrated into the motor and sensory system, regulating activity, sensations, and

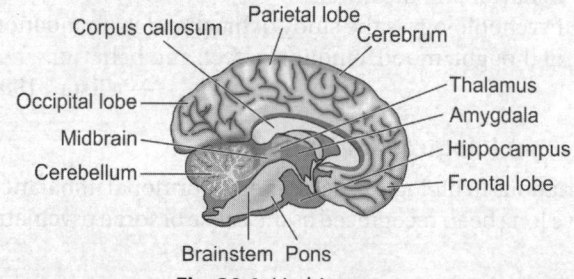

Fig. 30.1: Limbic system.

emotions. It relays impulses up to the hippocampus and to the wide areas of the cerebral cortex.

Hypothalamus

It is the gray matter below the thalamus. It is the chief coordinator of instincts and drives. The homeostatic and survival functions of the hypothalamus act to regulate body temperature, blood circulation, food, and water intake, the sleep cycle, defensive mechanisms, and sexual drives. Emotion is thought to be generated and coordinated chiefly by the hypothalamus through the integration of endocrine and motor responses including autonomic responses. The amygdala is thought to be associated with the generation of the emotion itself. It acts by directing the emotions to a proper object and proper mental content. The largest concentration of opiate receptors in the entire brain is found in the amygdala. Acute stressful situations activate the amygdala and releases endogenous opiates into the blood stream. The limbic system and higher brain structures link the hypothalamus to the outside world.

Cerebellum

It is the largest part of the hindbrain. It lies below the cerebrum and under the occipital lobes and is the center for motor coordination. It is responsible for the smooth contraction and relaxation of muscles and is essential for muscle tone and balance. Smoothing action is also crucial for both automatic and voluntary movements. However, the cerebellum does not initiate movement, nor does it have any role in intelligence and perceptions of conscious sensations. This process takes place on an entirely unconscious level. Staggering gait, clumsiness, and slurred speech observed in acute alcoholic states are symptoms of a generalized malfunction of the cerebellum.

Brainstem

The brainstem is involved in the transmission of all ascending and descending impulses. Structures of the brain stem are in descending order, the midbrain, pons, and medulla oblongata. They provide the many motor neurons, fibers, and tracts that relay information to and from the forebrain.

The midbrain merges into the thalamus and hypothalamus, thus interacting with the limbic system that was previously identified as the emotional center of the brain.

Pons and medulla structures are connecting pathways with the spinal cord. Norepinephrine cells in the pons called locus coeruleus and other norepinephrine systems are implicated in the production of anxiety. The medulla contains autonomic centers that are vital for the regulation of the heart and blood vessels, respiration, salivation, and swallowing.

Permeating the core of the brainstem is a network of neurons known as reticular formation (RF). The ascending limb of RF that extends into the thalamus and hypothalamus is the reticular activating system (RAS). RAS signals from internal and external environment meet and decide the level or arousal of the cerebral cortex. Level of consciousness and sleep-wake cycles are affected by the RAS. The hypothalamus with which the RAS is linked has anatomical connections to the optic nerve that respond to light within the hypothalamus are the basic mechanisms of the circadian clock that regulates the rhythm of many body functions, including sleep. Therefore, disturbances of the RAS have significance for sleep irregularities and seasonal affective disorders and may exacerbate other psychiatric disorders. Investigators have found that their clock can be reset through planned exposure to a light stimulus.

The pyramidal tracts take their name from the pyramid-like structure or the medulla. These are a collection of nerve fibers that originate in the motor cortex and travel through the pyramids of the medulla en route to the spinal cord. Within the pyramids at the pyramidal decussation, nerve fibers cross from one side of the brain to the opposite side of the spinal cord. The pyramidal tracts mediate voluntary movements especially those that are coordinated and purposeful and require skill.

Extrapyramid System

Extrapyramid system (EPS) consists of all the motor nerve tracts and pathways connecting the cerebral cortex, basal ganglia, thalamus, and cerebellum. RAS and spinal cord in complex circuits are not included in the pyramidal system. It is involved with the regulation or stereotyped reflex movement of muscles, maintenance of muscle tone, and control of body movements as in walking. Disturbances in EPS characteristically produce hypertonicity of the muscles. This is evident in dystonic reactions often seen with the use of antipsychotic medications.

Peripheral Nervous System

Peripheral nervous system (PNS) refers to all parts of the nervous systems that lie outside the CNS (brain and spinal cord). It includes the 12 pairs of cranial nerves and the 31 pairs of spinal nerves and their branches. Cranial nerves enter and exit the brain and primarily supply the head and neck. Spinal nerves enter and exit from the length of the spinal cord and enervate the rest of the body. Peripheral nerves carry messages from organs, glands, and muscles to the CNS and back. Afferent nerves relay impulses from the CNS to other areas of the body. Nerves of the PNS carry fibers that can functionally be divided into somatic and autonomic fibers. Somatic fibers innervate the skeletal voluntary muscles. Autonomic fibers innervate the smooth involuntary muscles and regulate bodily functions that are mostly out of conscious control such as the heart and intestinal movement.

Autonomic Nervous System

Autonomic nervous system (ANS) is of particular interest, as emotional states are related to specific patterns of autonomic responses. It is partly contained within the peripheral nerves and partly within the CNS, directly connecting with the hypothalamus. This association with the limbic system accounts for the powerful influence the amygdala and hypothalamus. The ANS is further subdivided into sympathetic and parasympathetic systems. The sympathetic system prepares the body for the "fight-or-flight" response by increasing the body alertness. It speeds the heart, dilates the pupils of the eye, causes the hair to stand on end, makes skin sweat, and releases norepinephrine as a neurotransmitter.

Parasympathetic system counteracts the responses induced by the sympathetic system and releases the neurotransmitter acetylcholine. Interplay of the two systems is important to the maintenance of equilibrium in the face of external and internal challenges to the organism. Sustained arousal or the sympathetic system related to stressors can result in physiologic changes. Physical conditions commonly cited as being affected by "psychologic factors" are hypertension, peptic ulcer, migraine, and colitis.

NEUROREGULATION

When a neuron is stimulated, an impulse is generated that causes the release of a neurotransmitter from the portion of the neuron closest to a neighboring neuron (dendrite) into a space between two neurons called synaptic cleft. The neurotransmitter crosses the synapse and binds to a receptor on the neighboring neuron, triggering an extracellular electrical signal that causes or inhibits a response. Neurotransmitters are derived from amino acids synthesized within neurons and stored at the nerve terminal in distinct vesicles. The ability of a neuron to generate an action potential depends on the presence of sodium (Na^+), chloride (Cl^-), potassium (K^+), and calcium (Ca^{++}) ions that affect the permeability of the cell membrane through electrical polarization and depolarization. A rise in concentration of Ca^{++} causes release of neurotransmitter molecules by fusing the wall of the vesicles to the nerve terminal, creating an opening through which the neurotransmitter is expelled into the synaptic cleft. The neuron releasing the neurotransmitter is the presynaptic neuron and the neuron receiving the neurotransmitter is the postsynaptic neuron. Transmission by a neurotransmitter can be increased or decreased in response to a given physiologic situation. When an individual thinks, talks, or does anything, many such neurotransmitters are actively involved. When changes occur in the neurotransmitters, the functioning of the mind gets disturbed. Major neurotransmitters are mentioned in Figure 30.2.

Release of acetylcholine stimulates cholinergic (parasympathetic) receptors that act on blood vessels, and most of the internal organs. Dopamine, norepinephrine, and serotonin are catecholamines that chemically contain a benzene ring with adjacent hydroxyl groups (catechol) and an amino group on a side chain. This is the reason

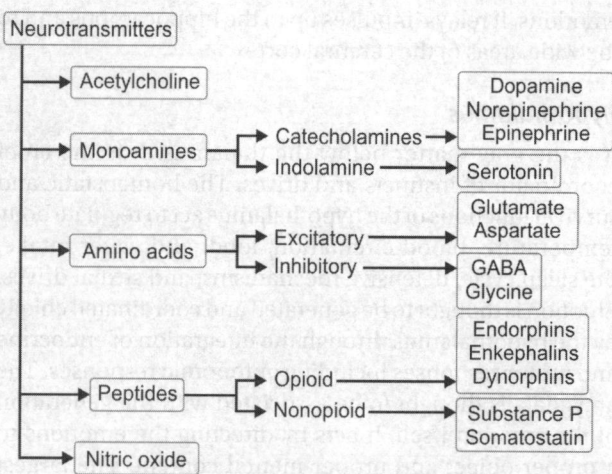

Fig. 30.2: Neurotransmitters.
(GABA: gamma-aminobutyric acid)

that these compounds are also known as monoamines. Under stressful conditions, including vigorous exercise, release of dopamine is greatly increased. The buildup of dopamine concentrations makes the body ready for action by increasing the heartbeat, raising blood pressure, and constricting key blood vessels. Dopamine plays an important role in controlling emotions, cognition, and movements and has side effects observed with the use of antipsychotic drugs. A number of neurologic and psychiatric disorders are linked to the dysfunction of dopamine. These include Parkinson's disease, schizophrenia, mood disorders.

Serotonergic pathways originate in the lower midbrain and the upper pons. Serotonin synthesis begins with tryptophan and is widely distributed in the tissues, particularly in the CNS and intestinal wall and in blood platelets. Serotonin is implicated in depression and sleep disturbances, but the exact mechanism is not well understood. Gamma aminobutyric acid is the major inhibitory neurotransmitter in the brain and is estimated to be present in 30% of all synapses. Gamma aminobutyric acid binds to receptors and decreases neuronal firing. It inhibits activation of neurons containing monoamines that mediate arousal and anxiety-related behaviors. When an individual is clinically anxious, it is thought that there is a change in balance between inhibitory neurotransmitters such us gamma aminobutyric acid and excitatory neurotransmitters such as acetylcholine. This imbalance results in a lack of inhibitory control over noradrenergic firing in the locus coeruleus and the manifestation of symptoms of anxiety. Endorphins play a role in opioid drug addiction.

A number of neurologic and psychiatric symptoms are caused by problems in the activity of neurotransmitters as they interact at critical sites in the brain. Drugs that affect the nervous system most often adjust the neurotransmission process. They can increase or decrease the synthesis, storage, release, metabolism, or receptor activity of neurotransmitters. Correction of neurotransmitter defects implicated in the disorder is the therapeutic purpose of these drugs. For instance, the antipsychotic drug Thorazine® affects receptor activity resulting in reduction of dopamine transmission.

Neurotransmitter Regulation and Psychiatric Illnesses

In contrast to neurological disorders, which are often associated with structural lesions in the CNS, psychiatric disorders are thought to be influenced by an abnormal pattern of interaction between neurochemical messenger systems in the brain. The role of the major neurotransmitter systems in behavior, emotion, and cognition is as follows:

- Neurotransmitters typically are synthesized, stored, and released by the neuron.
- The classification of neurotransmitters is based on their chemical structure.
- The stimulation or inhibition of neurotransmitters receptors results in biological and behavioral responses that include both desired and unwanted effects. For example, administration of a neuroleptic antipsychotic medication that blocks the dopamine D2 receptor may result not only in relief of psychotic symptoms but also in extrapyramidal symptoms (EPS), e.g. tremors, dystonia, akinesia, and dyskinesia.

Neurotransmitters are Related to Psychiatric Symptomatology

- *Schizophrenia:* Several lines of evidence are consistent with a dopamine hypothesis of schizophrenia, which proposes that psychotic symptoms associated with this illness result from excessive dopamine activity in area of a CNS associated with cognitive functioning. Self-administration of high doses of stimulant drugs, e.g. amphetamines, can result in psychotic symptoms. Research has shown that amphetamines can increase dopamine function by augmenting presynaptic dopamine release and blocking presynaptic reuptake of the neurotransmitter.
- *Mood disorders:* Major depression has been associated with norepinephrine hypothesis, which suggests reduced norepinephrine functioning in the CNS as a cause for depression. Monoamineoxidase inhibitors (MAOIs) prevent the breakdown of norepinephrine. This pharmacological effect increases norepinephrine concentrations available for interacting with receptors and appears to contribute to the therapeutic response to MAO in many patients with depression.
- *Anxiety disorders, eating disorders, and impulse-related disorders:* Anxiety disorders and mania have been linked to increased norepinephrine concentrations in the CNS. Behavioral symptoms of arousal sometimes noted in cocaine abusing patients may be related with cocaine interference with normal re-uptake of norepinephrine (as well as dopamine), which results in the presence of increased quantities of this neurotransmitters in the synaptic cleft.
- Serotonin is thought to play a role in regulating eating behavior, particularly satiety (how satiated or full one feels after a meal), e.g. bulimia nervosa (BN). Reduced levels of serotonin have been implicated in BN and also in impulsive and aggressive disorders. Current investigations are examining the relationship between serotonin and obsessive-compulsive disorder.
- *Other disorders:* Impaired memory may involve a number of neurotransmitters including acetylcholine, somatostatin, and nitric oxide. Alzheimer's disease has been associated with high concentrations or acetylcholine producing new neurons. Migraine headaches are thought to be associated with abnormalities in serotonic function.

DIAGNOSIS OF PSYCHOBIOLOGICAL DISORDERS

- *Brain imaging:*
  - Computed tomography (CT)
  - Magnetic resonance imaging (MRI)
  - Positron emission tomography (PET)
  - Single photon emission computed tomography (SPECT)
- *Neurophysiologic techniques:*
  - Electroencephalogram (EEG)
  - Polysomnography (sleep EEG)
  - Brain electroactivity mapping (BEAM)
  - Event-related potential (ERP)
- *Pharmacologic challenge:*
  - Dexamethasone suppression test (OST)
  - Thyrotropin-releasing hormone (TRH) challenge
- *Molecular genetics:*
  - Linkage map
  - Restriction fragment length polymorphisms (RFLPs)
  - Candidate genes.

PSYCHOBIOLOGY AND NURSING

Integrating psychobiologic principles into nursing practice will link the body, mind, brain, and behavior. Based on historical evolution nursing practice, it is recognized that our practice begins and ends with our clients, with their dysfunctions and disorders, their temptations and aspirations. What are the facts that count and why are behaviors the way they are? We must not cease to question. Understanding the client needs necessitates the full synthesis of communication, from molecular to verbal. An understanding or client's physical and social environment rounds out the mind–body connection.

Incorporating psychobiology will enable a nurse to fine-tune his/her assessments, diagnoses, interventions, and evaluations of human response patterns. The synthesis of this critical thinking will provide clients and families with quality care cost-effectively. Multifocal and multidisciplinary care incorporating psychobiologic dimensions will advance our ability to offer new, more effective assessments and less stigmatized interventions for our clients.

CONCLUSION

Anatomic systems within the brain such as the cortex and limbic system are associated with functions including memory, affect, and problem-solving. These may be dysfunctional in major psychiatric illnesses. From a psychobiologic perspective, the brain is the source of behavior, emotion, cognition, and "human-ness." Molecules make each of us unique. One aspect of mood or behavior may be linked to more than one neuromessenger and a single neuromessenger may be associated with more than one brain activity or behavior. Using the emerging data from psychobiology, such as the effect of biological rhythms on behavior, or negative symptom association with dopamine and serotonin, enables the psychiatric nurse to understand and advocate for the unique needs of the client.

31 CHAPTER

Life Process, Homeostatic Mechanism, Biological and Psychosocial Dynamics in Causation of Disease and Lifestyle

CHAPTER OUTLINE

- Life Processes
- Definition of Life Processes
- Homeostatic Mechanism
- Biological and Psychosocial Dynamics in Causation of Disease
- Terminologies
- Factors Influencing the Health Beliefs and Practices
- Variables Influencing Illness Behavior
- Psychological Stages of Illness
- Kinds of Emotions
- Health-illness States: Interaction Between the Mind and Body
- Role of Emotion in Health and Disease
- Illness with Negative Progresses
- Role of a Nurse
- Healthcare has Become Increasingly Focused on Health Promotion, Wellness and Illness Prevention

■ LIFE PROCESSES

Biology is the science that deals with living things. Sometimes it is necessary to make a difference between organisms that are alive and other things that are not alive.

Characteristics of Living Things

- Living things react to stimuli.
- Living things interact with their environment, which includes members of the same and other species.
- Living things have a metabolism—they take in food which they convert to the energy they need.
- Living things reproduce—they give birth to others of the same species. This is not true of all *individual* organisms. In eusocial organisms, some castes cannot reproduce. But, since the sterile workers are all the produce of a single queen, they are one collective.

■ DEFINITION OF LIFE PROCESSES

Various functions carried out by living beings which are necessary to maintain and continue life are called life process.

The following are the life processes in living beings:
- Nutrition
- Respiration
- Transportation of substances
- Excretion
- Movement
- Reproduction.

Nutrition

The process by which an organism takes food and utilizes it is called nutrition.

- **Need of nutrition**: Organisms need energy to perform various activities. The energy is supplied by the nutrients. Organisms need various raw materials for growth and repair. These raw materials are provided by nutrients.
- **Nutrients:** Materials which provide nutrition to organisms are called nutrients. Carbohydrates, proteins, and fats are the main nutrients and are called macronutrients. Minerals and vitamins are required in small amounts and hence are called micronutrients.

Types of Nutrition

- Autotrophic
- Heterotrophic

Autotrophic nutrition

The mode of nutrition in which an organism prepares its own food is called autotrophic nutrition. Green plants and blue-green algae follow the autotrophic mode of nutrition.

A process used by plants and other organisms to convert light energy, normally from the sun, into chemical energy that can be later released to fuel the organisms' activities.

- This chemical energy is stored in carbohydrate molecules, such as sugars, which are synthesized from carbon dioxide and water. In most cases, oxygen is also released as a waste product.

- ❖ Photosynthesis maintains atmospheric oxygen levels and supplies all of the organic compounds and most of the energy necessary for life on earth.
- ❖ Light energy is absorbed by chlorophyll, a green substance found in chloroplasts in some plant cells and algae.
- ❖ Absorbed light energy is used to convert carbon dioxide (from the air) and water (from the soil) into a sugar called glucose.
  - ➢ Oxygen is released as a by-product.

Heterotrophic nutrition

- ❖ The mode of nutrition in which an organism takes food from another organism is called heterotrophic nutrition.
- ❖ Organisms; other than green plants, and blue-green algae follow heterotrophic mode of nutrition.
- ❖ Heterotrophic nutrition can be further divided into three types, viz. saprophytic nutrition, holozoic nutrition, and parasitic nutrition.

Classification of Heterotrophs

Saprophytes

- ❖ In saprophytic nutrition, the digestion of food takes place before ingestion of food.
- ❖ This type of nutrition is usually seen in fungi and some other microorganisms.
- ❖ The organism secretes digestive enzymes on the food and then ingests the simple substances.
- ❖ Saprophytes feed on dead materials and thus help in decomposition dead remains of plants and animals.

Holozoic Nutrition

In holozoic nutrition, the digestion of food follows after the ingestion of food. Thus, digestion takes place inside the body of the organism.

Holozoic nutrition happens in five steps:
1. *Ingestion:* Taking in complex organic food through mouth opening.
2. *Digestion:* Change of complex food into simple form by action of enzymes.
3. *Absorption:* Passing of simple, soluble nutrients through blood or lymph.
4. *Assimilation:* Utilization of absorbed food for various metabolic processes.
5. *Egestion:* Expelling out the undigested food.

Nutrition in Amoeba

- ❖ Amoeba is a unicellular animal which follows holozoic mode of nutrition. The cell membrane of amoeba keeps on protruding into pseudopodia.
- ❖ Amoeba surrounds a food particle with pseudopodia and makes a food vacuole.
- ❖ The food vacuole contains the food particle and water.
- ❖ Digestive enzymes are secreted in the food vacuole and digestion takes place.
- ❖ After that, digested food is absorbed from the food vacuole.
- ❖ Finally, the food vacuole moves near the cell membrane and undigested food is expelled out.

Parasitic Nutrition

- ❖ Parasitic nutrition is a mode of heterotrophic nutrition where an organism lives on the body surface or inside the body of another type of organism (known as a host).
- ❖ The parasite obtains nutrition directly from the body of the host.
- ❖ Since these parasites derive their nourishment from their host, this symbiotic interaction is often described as harmful to the host.
- ❖ Parasites are dependent on their host for survival, since the host provides nutrition and protection.
- ❖ As a result of this dependence, parasites have considerable modifications to optimize parasitic nutrition and therefore their survival.

Nutrition in Humans

Human beings are complex animals and they have a complex digestive system. The human digestive system is composed of an alimentary canal and some accessory glands.

The alimentary canal is divided into several parts, viz. the esophagus, stomach, small intestine, large intestine, rectum, and anus. The salivary gland, liver, and pancreas are the accessory glands which lie outside the alimentary canal.

Structure of Human Digestive System

Mouth or buccal cavity: The mouth has teeth and tongue. Salivary glands are also present in the mouth. The tongue has gustatory receptors which perceive the sense of taste. Tongue helps in turning over the food, so that saliva can be properly mixed in it.

Teeth help in breaking down the food into smaller particles so that swallowing of food becomes easier. There are four types of teeth in human beings. The incisor teeth are used for cutting the food. The canine teeth are used for tearing the food and for cracking hard substances. The premolars are used for coarse grinding of food. The molars are used for fine grinding of food.

Salivary glands secrete saliva. Saliva makes the food slippery which makes it easy to swallow the food. Saliva also contains the enzyme salivary amylase or ptyalin. Salivary amylase digests starch and converts it into sucrose.

Stomach: Stomach is a bag-like organ. Highly muscular walls of the stomach help in churning the food. The walls of stomach secrete hydrochloric acid. Hydrochloric acid kills the germs which may be present in food. Moreover, it makes the medium inside stomach as acidic. The acidic medium is necessary for gastric enzymes to work. The enzyme pepsin, secreted in stomach, does partial digestion of protein.

The mucus, secreted by the walls of the stomach, saves the inner lining of stomach from getting damaged from hydrochloric acid.

Small intestine: It is a highly coiled tube-like structure. The small intestine is longer than the large intestine but its lumen is smaller than that of the large intestine. The small intestine is divided into three parts—(1) duodenum, (2) jejunum, and (3) ileum.

Liver: The liver is the largest organ in the human body. Liver manufactures bile, which gets stored in gall bladder. From the gall bladder, bile is released as and when required.

Pancreas: The pancreas is situated below the stomach. It secretes pancreatic juice which contains many digestive enzymes.

Large intestine: It is smaller than small intestine. Undigested food goes into the large intestine. Some water and salt are absorbed by the walls of the large intestine. After that, the undigested food goes to the rectum; from where it is expelled out through the anus.

Respiration

Aerobic Respiration

This type of respiration happens in the presence of oxygen. Pyruvic acid is converted into carbon dioxide. Energy is released and water molecules are also formed at the end of this process.

Anaerobic Respiration

- This type of respiration happens in the absence of oxygen. Pyruvic acid is either converted into ethyl alcohol or lactic acid.
- Ethyl alcohol is usually formed in case of anaerobic respiration in microbes; like yeast or bacteria.
- Lactic acid is formed in some microbes as well as in the muscle cells.
- When someone runs too fast, he may experience a throbbing pain the leg muscles. This happens because of anaerobic respiration taking place in the muscles. During running, the energy demand from the muscle cells increases. This is compensated by anaerobic respiration and lactic acid is formed in the process. The deposition of lactic acid causes the pain in calf muscles of the legs. The pain subsides after taking rest for some time.

Human Respiratory System (Fig. 31.1)

The human respiratory system is composed of a pair of lungs. These are attached to a system of tubes which open on the outside through the nostrils.

Nostrils: There two nostrils which converge to form a nasal passage. The inner lining of the nostrils is lined by hairs and remains wet due to mucus secretion. The mucus and the hairs help in filtering the dust particles out from inhaled air. Further, air is warmed up when it enters the nasal passage.

Pharynx: It is a tube-like structure which continues after the nasal passage.

Larynx: This part comes after the pharynx. This is also called the voice box.

Trachea: This is composed of rings of cartilage. Cartilaginous rings prevent the collapse of trachea in the absence of air.

Bronchi: A pair of bronchi comes out from the trachea, with one bronchus going to each lung.

Bronchioles: A bronchus divides into branches and sub-branches; inside the lung.

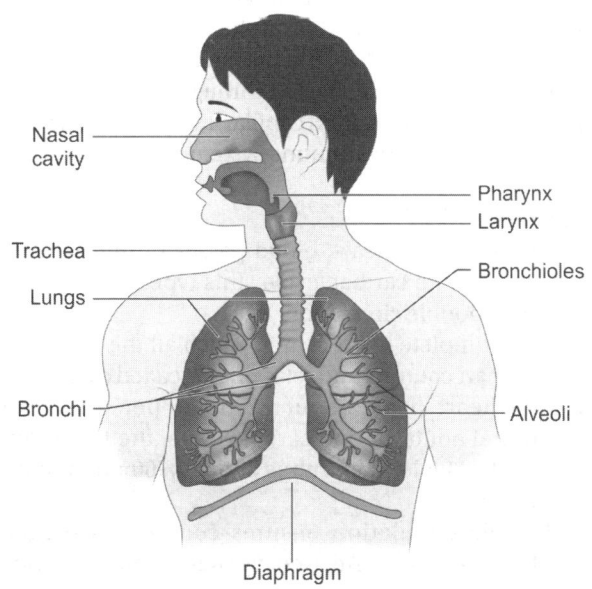
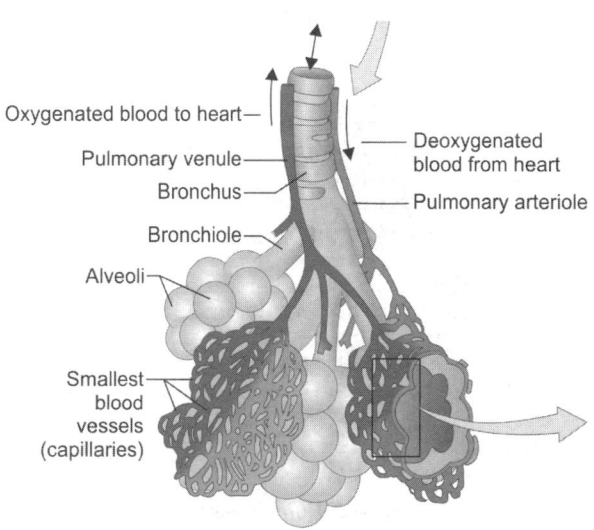

Fig. 31.1: Human respiratory system.

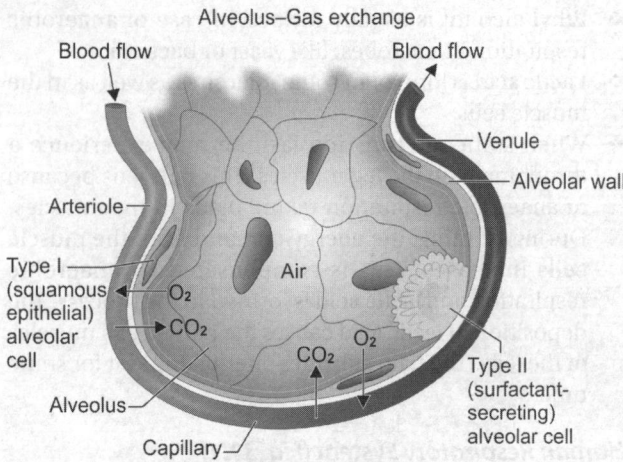

Fig. 31.2: Structure of alveoli.

Alveoli: These are air-sacs at the end of bronchioles. Alveolus is composed of a very thin membrane and is the place where blood capillaries open. This is alveolus, where oxygen mixes with the blood and carbon dioxide exits from the blood. The exchange of gases, in alveoli, takes place due to pressure differential. The structure of alveoli is shown in Figure 31.2.

Breathing mechanism: The breathing mechanism of lungs is controlled by the diaphragm and the intercostal muscles. Diaphragm is a membrane which separates the thoracic chamber from the abdominal cavity. When the diaphragm moves down, the lungs expand and air is inhaled. When the diaphragm moves up, the lungs contract and air is exhaled.

Transportation in Animals

Circulatory System

The circulatory system is responsible for transport of various substances in human beings. It is composed of the heart, arteries, veins, and blood capillaries. Blood plays the role of the carrier of substances (Fig. 31.3).

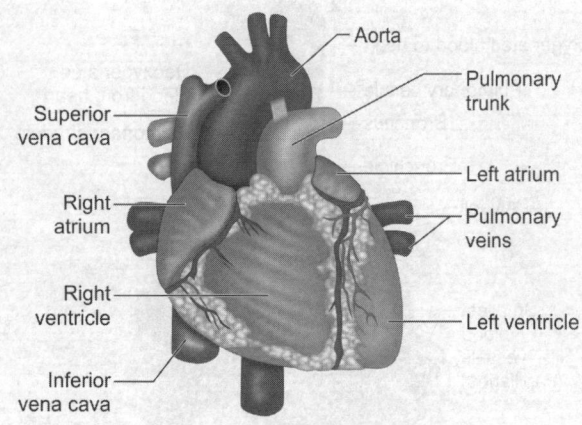

Fig. 31.3: Human heart.

Blood Vessels

Arteries: These are thick-walled blood vessels which carry oxygenated blood from the heart to different organs. Pulmonary arteries are exceptions because they carry deoxygenated blood from the heart to lungs, where oxygenation of blood takes place.

Veins: These are thin-walled blood vessels which carry deoxygenated blood from different organs to the heart. Pulmonary veins are exceptions because they carry oxygenated blood from lungs to the heart. Valves are present in veins to prevent backflow of blood.

Blood

Blood is a connective tissue which plays the role of the carrier for various substances in the body. Blood is composed of plasma, blood cells, and platelets.

Blood plasma: Blood plasma is a pale colored liquid which is mostly composed of water. Blood plasma forms the matrix of blood.

Blood cells: There are two types of blood cells—(1) red blood cells (RBCs) and (2) white blood cells (WBCs).

Red blood corpuscles (RBCs): These are of red color because of the presence of hemoglobin which is a pigment. Hemoglobin readily combines with oxygen and carbon dioxide. The transport of oxygen happens through hemoglobin. Some part of carbon dioxide is also transported through hemoglobin.

White blood corpuscles (WBCs): These are of pale white color. They play an important role in the immunity.

Platelets: Platelets are responsible for blood coagulation. Blood coagulation is a defense mechanism which prevents excess loss of blood, in case of an injury.

Lymph: Lymph is similar to blood but RBCs are absent in lymph. Lymph is formed from the fluid which leaks from blood capillaries and goes to the intercellular spaces in the tissues. This fluid is collected through lymph vessels and finally returns to the blood capillaries. Lymph also plays an important role in the immune system.

Double Circulation

- In the human heart, blood passes through the heart twice in one cardiac cycle. This type of circulation is called double circulation.
- One complete heart beat in which all the chambers of the heart contract and relax once is called cardiac cycle.
- The heart beats about 72 times per minute in a normal adult. In one cardiac cycle, the heart pumps out 70 mL blood and thus about 4,900 mL blood in a minute.
- Double circulation ensures complete segregation of oxygenated and deoxygenated blood which is

necessary for optimum energy production in warm-blooded animals.

Excretion

Removal of harmful waste from the body is called excretion. Many wastes are produced during various metabolic activities. These need to be removed in time because their accumulation in the body can be harmful and even lethal for an organism (Box 31.1).

Kidney: Kidney is a bean-shaped organ which lies near the vertebral column in the abdominal cavity. The kidney is composed of many filtering units called nephrons. Nephron is called the functional unit of kidney.

Nephron: It is composed of a tangled mess of tubes and a filtering part; called glomerulus. Glomerulus is a network of blood capillaries to which renal artery is attached. The artery which takes blood to the glomerulus is called afferent arteriole and the one receiving blood from the glomerulus is called efferent arteriole. Glomerulus is enclosed in a capsule like portion, called Bowman's capsule. The Bowman's capsule extends into a fine tube which is highly coiled. Tubes from various nephrons converge into collecting duct, which finally goes to the ureter.

Transportation in Plants

For transportation in plants, two things occur:
- Transport of water and minerals
- Transport of food and other substances
- Plants have tissues to transport water, nutrients, and minerals.
- Xylem transports water and mineral salts from the roots up to other parts of the plant, while phloem transports sucrose and amino acids between the leaves and other parts of the plant.

Excretion in Plants

Plants eliminate some waste through diffusion. During the day, excess oxygen gas produced by photosynthesis is released through the stomata. Carbon dioxide produced by respiration is normally used up during photosynthesis. At night, however, as photosynthesis slows, carbon dioxide is not used up as fast as it is produced, and it is released as a waste product.

Box 31.1: Some of the methods of excretion.

- Gums, resins, rubber and latex are exuded from various parts of the plant body.
- Crystals of certain chemical substances are stored in the plant body, e.g. calcium oxalate crystals in the leaf of colocasia, calcium carbonate crystals in the leaf of fig, etc.
- Some deciduous plants get rid of excretory matter when the leaves fall.
- In the bark and wood part of the trunk, tannin is stored. This makes the wood appear dark.

- Various functions carried out by living beings which are necessary to maintain and continue life are called life process.
- *Nutrition:* The process by which an organism takes food and utilizes it is called nutrition.
- *Respiration:* The process by which a living being utilizes the food to get energy is called respiration.
- *Transportation:* The action of transporting food materials or other substances.
- *Excretion:* Removal of harmful waste from the body is called excretion.

HOMEOSTATIC MECHANISM

Introduction

In human beings, the homeostatic regulation of body temperature as well as the generating heat through metabolic process. It is an organism's internal environment which stays the same. Human body includes mechanisms that help to regulate the body; this includes organs, glands, tissues, and cells. The adjusting of these enables the body to constantly be in a steady state. In practice, it comes down to providing stable environment for the cells of the body. The living process in the cells depends on the activity of enzymes. Any change in these conditions affects the function of the enzymes and may lead to death of the cells or, ultimately the whole organism. That is why the internal environment needs to be regulated and kept constant.

Definition

A condition in which maintenance of internal environment of the body, despite of changes in the external environment and various physiologic arrangements which serve to restore the normal state, for example, the maintenance of body temperature and the blood glucose levels.

Homeostasis is achieved through negative and positive feedback mechanism.

Negative feedback includes most homeostatic control mechanisms shuts off the original stimulus or reduces its intensity. Works like a household thermostat, for **example** control of blood pressure and temperature regulation.

Positive feedback increases the original stimulus to push the variables father, for **example** in blood clotting and during the birth of a baby.

Homeostatic mechanisms are designed to re-establish homeostasis when there is an imbalance.

The Home Heating System

- When the temperature of the room decrease below a set point, the thermostat electrically starts the furnace.
- As the temperature of the room rises to the set point, the thermostat shuts down the furnace.
- As the room cools, Step 1 is repeated.

- There are three components to this system:
  1. The censor which detects the stress
  2. The control center which receives information from the censor and sends a message to the effector
  3. The effector which receives the message from the control center and produces the response which re-establishes homeostasis

It should be noticed that the heat produce by the furnace shuts the furnace down through the thermostat. The original stress is reduced, i.e. the room warms up. Homeostatic mechanisms show that these two characteristics are operated by negative feedback.

Homeostasis using a neural pathway: Many homeostatic mechanisms use a nerve pathway in which to produce their effects. These pathways involve an afferent path which brings sensory messages into the brain and an efferent path which carries outgoing nerve messages to effectors.

Harmful effects of positive feedback: Positive feedback can be harmful. Specific examples of these harmful outcomes are:
1. Fever can cause a positive feedback within homeostasis that pushes the body temperature continually higher. If the temperature reaches 45°C, cellular proteins denature bringing metabolism to a stop and lead to death.
2. Chronic hypertension can favor the process of atherosclerosis which causes the opening of blood vessels to narrow; this will intensify the hypertension bring on more damage to the walls of the blood vessels.

Diagnostic evaluation for homeostasis: Homeostasis is a complex of various inter-related systems which function hand in hand to maintain the blood in a fluid state within the vessels and to form a clot whenever the circulation is interrupted. The most common presenting symptoms may be present when components systems are disturbed. The laboratory tests play a vital role in detecting the abnormalities. The following screening tests include:
- Complete hemogram with blood cell counts
- Examination of blood films
- Biochemical examination
- Clotting time
- Activated partial thromoplastin time (aPTT)
- Pro-thrombin time (PT)
- Differential tests for aPTT and PT
- Platelet
- Blood grouping and RH typing

These tests are carried out based on the symptoms and routinely.

BIOLOGICAL AND PSYCHOSOCIAL DYNAMICS IN CAUSATION OF DISEASE

Introduction

Nurses are in a unique position to assist clients in achieving and maintaining optimal level of health. Nurses understand the challenges of today's healthcare system and embrace the opportunity to use wellness activities to promote health and prevent illness. Nurses also identify actual and potential risk factors that predispose a person or a group to illness. When illness does occur, different attitudes about illness cause people to react in different ways to illness or that of a family member. Medical sociologists call the reaction to illness, illness behaviors. Nurses who understand how clients react to illness can minimize the effects of illness and assists the clients and their families in maintaining or returning to the highest level of functioning.

The two overacting goals for healthy people 2010 are:
1. To increase quality and years of healthy life.
2. To eliminate health disparities (USDHHS, 1998).

The document is divided into four areas:
1. Promoting healthy behaviors.
2. Promoting healthy and safe communities.
3. Improving systems for personal and public health.
4. Preventing and reducing diseases and disorders.

TERMINOLOGIES

- ***Health:*** WHO defines health as a state of complete physical, mental, and social well-being not merely the absence of disease or infirmity.
- ***Illness:*** Illness is a process in which the functioning of a person is diminished or impaired in one or more dimensions when compared with the person's previous condition.
- ***Acute illness:*** An acute illness usually has a short duration and is severe.
- ***Chronic illness:*** A chronic illness persists usually longer than 6 months and can also affect functioning in any dimension.
- ***Illness behavior:*** People who are ill generally act in a way that medical sociologists call illness behavior. It involves that how people monitor their bodies, define and interpret their symptoms, take remedial actions, and use the healthcare system (Mechanic, 1982).

FACTORS INFLUENCING THE HEALTH BELIEFS AND PRACTICES

There are internal variables and external variables which will affect the health of an individual. They are:

Internal Factors

Internal factors include biologic, psychological, intellectual, and spiritual dimensions.

Biological Factors

Genetic makeup influences biological characteristics, innate temperament, activity level, and intellectual potential. It has been related to susceptibility to specific diseases, such as diabetes and breast cancer.

Race is associated with predisposition to certain diseases. For example, Blacks have higher incidents of sickle cell anemia

Sex: Certain acquired and genetic diseases are common in one sex than the other. Disorders more common among females include osteoporosis and rheumatoid arthritis compared to males.

Age: It is also a significant factor that the distribution of the disease varies with age. For example, arteriosclerotic is common in middle aged males, but communicable diseases are common in children.

Developmental level has a major impact on health status. For example, toddlers who are learning to walk are more prone to falls and injuries. Declining physical, sensory and perceptual abilities limit the older adults to respond to environmental hazards and stress hours.

Psychological Factors

Psychological factors influencing health include mind–body interactions, self-concept, and job satisfaction. Emotional responses to stress affect body function. For example, a student who is extremely anxious before an examination may experience urinary frequency and diarrhea.

Intellectual Factors

Lifestyle choices include patterns of eating, exercise, use of tobacco, drugs, alcohol, and methods of coping with stress. Over eating, getting insufficient exercise, and being overweight are closely related to the incidents of heart disease, arteriosclerosis, diabetes, and hypertension.

Spiritual and Religious Factors

Spiritual and religious beliefs can significantly affect health behavior.

External Factors

External factors influencing health status beliefs and practices include:

Geography

Geography determines climate and climate affects health. For example, malaria and malaria-related conditions occur more frequently in tropical areas than temperature climates and natural disasters.

Environmental Conditions

People are becoming increasingly aware of their environment and how it affects their health. Pollution of water, air, and soil can affect the support of life. Poverty, slum neighborhoods, and crowded conditions lead to a state of deterioration.

Standards of Living

An individual's standard of living is related to health, morbidity, and mortality. Hygiene, food habits, and propensity to seek healthcare advice and follow health regimens vary among high-income and low-income groups. Low-income families often define health in terms of work, if people can work, they are healthy. They tend to be fatalistic and believe that illness is not preventable.

Family and Cultural Beliefs

In addition to transmitting genetic predispositions, the family passes on patterns of daily living and lifestyles to offspring, e.g. a woman who was abused as a child is also at high risk. Culture and social interactions also influence with health and illness. People of certain cultures may perceive home remedies.

VARIABLES INFLUENCING ILLNESS BEHAVIOR

People who are ill generally need a safety net in a way that medical sociologists call illness behavior. It involves how people monitor their bodies, define and interpret their symptoms, take remedial actions, and use the healthcare system. Personal history, social situations, social norms, and the opportunities can all affect illness behavior as affected by internal and external variables. Based on these variables, nurses can plan individualized care to assist clients coping with illness at various stages.

Internal Variables

Perception of Illness

If clients believe that symptoms of their illness disrupt their normal routine, they seek medical assistance; otherwise, they do not take it as serious.

Nature of Illness

Illness is a state of disequilibrium and imbalance, when you are ill, sick, or indisposed. The body is not working correctly, energy is sapped, and the spirits are low. Illness is the body's way of communicating its needs for attention. If the illness is of a physical nature, the body will attempt to restore, homeostasis, to being itself, back into balance until it exhausts its serves and falls over, unable to continue of the illness is psychological (dysfunction in the emotional, intellectual, social, or spiritual dimension of functioning), the body will adjust to the demands placed on it until it no longer capable of compensating.

A Client's Coping Skills

A client's coping skills, as well as, his or her locus of control or other external variables that affect the way the client behaves during illness.

External Variables

Visibility of Symptoms

A client with visible symptoms may be more likely to seek assistance than a client without such visible symptoms.

Social Groups

It helps in recognizing the threat of illness or supporting the denial of potential illness. Clients often react positively to social support while practicing positive health behavior.

Cultural Background

It teaches the person to be healthy, how to recognize illness.

Economic Variables

Because of economic constraints, a client may delay treatment and in many cases may continue to carry out daily activities.

Accessibility of the Healthcare System

It is closely related to economic factors. For many clients, entry into the healthcare system is complex or confusing.

PSYCHOLOGICAL STAGES OF ILLNESS

Whether an illness is acute or chronic, the sick individual experiences different stages of illness. The subjective experiences of the individual with illness or disability is highly personal. The illness experiences are roughly divided into five stages.

Stage I: Disbelief Anger

The illness experiences begin when a person becomes aware that something is not right. During this experience, an individual does the following:
- Becomes aware of one undesirable change.
- Analyzes and evaluates the change.
- Makes a decision that the change indicates an illness.
- Acts to remedy the situation based on the decision and the accompanying emotional responses. The patient usually undergoes a stage of disbelief and denial. He/she may be surprised as to how he/she got this disease; second, he/she may deny the fact that he/she is actually sick.

Stage II: Sick Role (Irritability Anger)

Once the person acknowledges the presence of an illness, he/she seeks to confirm it by talking with other people. This stage the person may usually have irritability anger. The irritability arises from a sense of that body mind it not acting as expected it is interfering with life to some degree.

Stage III: Attempting to Gain Control (Medical Care)

During the third stage of illness, an individual attempts to gain some control over the state of illness through self-diagnosis, applying what seems to be appropriate. If self-diagnosis interventions fail, the person usually seeks professional help.

Stage IV: Depression Despair (Dependency)

In this stage, the ill individual must be willing to accept the attentions of other people. He/she usually is depressed, feels hopeless. Depression induced by illness care varies in length intensity. The patient with lifelong chronic illness may plunge into a sudden deep depression on hearing the diagnosis. He/she may fight depression through his/her life, enjoying long periods of life where depression disappears with the help of family, friends, and caregivers who expect him/her to get well only. But the effect of disease and its interpretation vary according to cultural circumstances.

Stage V: Recovery Rehabilitation (Acceptance)

Movement in the recovery rehabilitation stage can occur suddenly (a response to drug therapy or the breaking of a fever) or more slowly (recovery from a stroke or mental disorder) if recovery is rapid complete, the individual gradually gives up the sick role resumes his/her normal obligations duties. For a person whose recovery is slow, usually tries to accept this stage by moving forward to whatever advice is given to recover or at least regain some of his/her abilities, and is depressed or elevated.

The internal changes that are brought about by emotions are psychological such as rapid pulse respiration, increased blood pressure, and tension pain. Usually, these changes are temporary subside when the individual returns to the normal.

KINDS OF EMOTIONS

Emotions in general can be categorized as positive emotions and negative emotions. Positive emotions are amusement, love, curiosity, joy and happiness that are helpful and essential to the normal development.

Negative emotions are fear, anger, jealousy, hate, moodiness, and sorrow which are harmful to the well-being development of an individual. Emotions with much intensity and frequency bring harmful effects.

Emotion

- The word emotion is derived from the Latin word "*emovere,*" which means to "stirrup" or to "excite."
- Emotion is an effective experience that accompanies generalized stirred up states in the individual that shows itself in his overt behavior.
  —**Crow and Crow, 1973**
- Emotion is an effective experience that one undergoes during an instinctive excitement.
  —**McDougall, 1949**
- Emotions as a complex affective experience that involves diffuse physiological changes can be expressed overly in characteristic behavior patterns.
  —**Charles G Morris, 1979**

Emotions motivate human behavior. An emotional experience is characterized by both external and internal changes in human beings. The external changes are those, which are apparent easily seen by others such as facial expression, changes in posture, e.g. angry or happy.

Characteristics of Emotions

Emotions have certain characteristics, which can be described as under:
- Emotions are universal—prevalent in every living organism at all stages of development from infancy to old age.
- Emotions are personal thus differ from individual to individual.
- The same emotion can be aroused by a number of different stimuli, object situations.
- Emotions rise abruptly, but subside slowly.
- Emotions have the quality of displacement. For example, an angry reaction caused by a rebuke by the boss can find expression in the beating of the children at home.
- An emotion can give birth to a number of other similar emotions.
- There is a negative correlation between the upsurge of emotions on the other hand. Emotional upsurge adversely affects the process of reasoning thinking powers.
- The emotional experiences are associated with one or the other instinct or biological drives.
- Every emotional experience involves many physical and physiological changes in the organism. Some of the changes which express themselves in our behavior are easily observable, for example, bulge of eyes, the flush of face, the flow of tears, the pulse rate, increased perspiration, the gooses flush, etc.
  In addition to these easily observable changes, these are internal physiological changes, example changes in circulation of blood, the impact on digestive system, the changes in the functioning of some glands such as adrenal glands, etc.

Emotional Reaction

The emotional reactions named anger, love, fear, etc. are some of the particular examples of the various emotional experiences reactions through which every individual passes at one or other occasion in the span of his life.

Anger

Anger represents one of the unpleasant or negative emotions that are learnt by the child during the course of his/her normal growth development. When an individual's need is wasted or his/her freedom is restrained or something happens against his/her wishes, he/she may get irritated or angry.

Sometimes when a person wants to protect himself/herself he/she expresses himself/herself through an emotional experience known as anger. This anger may provide a safety value or defense mechanism against damage done to one's personality on account of facing frustration.

Oral form of emotional reaction is verbal exchange of hot words, abusive words; however, if the intensity of anger increases, the individual becomes too violent, aggressive, biting or kicking even killing each other or damaging whatever comes in their way or is visible through their eyes.

In children, anger can be seen as kicking, thrashing out with arms, feet, throwing temper tantrums, etc. not talking for many days with the person they are angry.

Fear

Fear is also a negative emotion. Even though it is not bad to be fearful, as it helps us sometimes when we come across snakes, fire, so many other harmful things. Fear is always accompanied with the instinct of escape of feeling, the need to get rid of the threatened situation. But once the danger is passed, the fear also disappears. Fear responses are not inherited, but are learned in consequences of the experiences. These can also be unlearned as a result of reconditioning or pleasant experiences involving no fear.

Attempts should be made from the beginning to remove the fear feeling in the children. They should be provided stimulating environment full of encouragement incentives unnecessary fear, if any should be removed by applying the techniques of deconditioning behavior modification.

Love

Love as an emotional reaction that can be defined as affective experience that one organism exhibits for another. Writers have differentiated a variety of love such as, parental love, infant love, brotherly love, erotic love, paternal love.
- Parental love especially the maternal love is special kind of affectionate relationship involving care responsibility for the development or well-being of a child. The emotional attachment of the mother towards her child is totally unconditional. One exhibits this sort of love on account of performing one's duty or feeling a sort of satisfaction.
- Infant love is characterized by the infants close attachment to its mother. It is the outcome of the contact comfort that the mother provides than by her satisfaction of such basic needs as food warmth.
- Brotherly love is based on a belief in humanity a feeling that all people are one. It is in fact a love that is exhibited to all human beings is fundamental to any other form of living.
- Erotic love covers a wide concept. It is not limited to one or the other type of intimacy primarily sexual. It is based on complete fusion, for union with one other person:
  - Love is recognition.

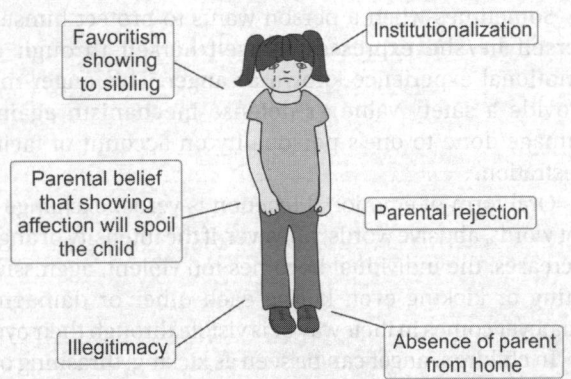

Fig. 31.4: Deprivation of love (common causes).

➢ Love is an understanding.
➢ Love is a response.

Deprivation of any emotion is harmful to the personality, but deprivation of love is especially damaging (Fig. 31.4). In early childhood, deprivation of an affectionate relationship is not very damaging. Deprivation of love can occur in a child due to institutionalization of the baby or child, owing to the economic or marital status of the parents the health of the baby or mother, the death of one or both parents, or some other causes.

Parents believe (in some cases) showing affection for the child will "spoil" him/her make feel too important under the roof alienation, seen mostly in us. Many adults also experience deprivation of love especially in old age after the death or divorce of a spouse. Deprivation can be almost as damaging to the self-concept in adulthood as in childhood.

Just as a child suffer under the root alienation, an adult may continue to love with a spouse but be "emotionally separated" from him/her. In many such cases, the individuals try to compensate for their deprivation of love by focusing their affection on a child or by having extramarital love affairs. Unmarried adults too experience deprivation of love whether their failure to marry is due to choice or inability to attract a member of opposite sex.

In old age as in childhood, the major source of affection is normally the family. But if these sources are fail to show affection either due to economic problems, rejected by the children or face deprivation of love. It is more damaging when their health is not good, loss of spouse or former friends.

Curiosity

Curiosity is a pleasant valuable emotion. It enables the person to discover new meanings thus to broaden his/her interests activity. It is valuable because it supplies the motivation for learning creativity. It prevents boredom stagnation by providing new avenues for thought action. Curiosity is harmful, while shifting takes place people who were once intelligence, bright creative who are likely to make the greatest contribution to the society can head to harmfulness to individual society. It is most damaging during early years.

Happiness

Happiness is a pleasant emotion, which results from when the individual get his/her wishes, needs fulfilled. Many people of all ages are deprived of experiencing the happiness, joy or elation. This again can be due to environmental obstacles or unrealistic levels of aspirations.

Pleasure

The emotion of pleasure manifests in smiling, laughing, hugging, kissing, or in contentment. It is evoked by situations, which give physical comfort to the infant or a young child. Absence of conditions, which causes non-satisfaction of normal wishes incongruous situations causes pleasure in adults, if a child or an adult feels that he/she is being loved, accepted, wanted, it gives him/her a feeling of great pleasure.

Jealousy

Jealousy is an unpleasant emotion, which stimulates from parents or adults showing more interest or gives more time to another child, the child feel jealous. This child may show his/her jealously, by attacking the child who is loved more by the parents.

Grief (Tears Sobbing)

Grief is the psychological process, which can happen when death of a loved one takes place or any other type of loss in life. For example, business loss, loss of position or breakup of a romantic affair, retirement separation from friend or a pet, or a loved toy (for children) can also cause grief to the individual.

Affection

Affection is a pleasant emotion anything that gives the child/individual pleasure, a person, a pet, a toy becomes the object of the person's affection. Wanting to the loved one, kissing, fondling or saying 'I Love You' shows this.

Envy

Envy is similar to jealousy. Here it is commonly seen in the children. The usual causes of envy are when the other child has a thing or can do something better than him/her.

Joy

Anything that makes a person feel satisfied or important such as doing something well or winning, it gives rise to feelings of happiness known as joy. Mild forms of joy is shown by smiling, laughing is stronger forms joy is shown as jumping up down, shouting with glee, hugging anything nearby him/her.

Hostility

Hostility is an abnormal emotion. Hostility is displayed as a subtitle expression in stubbornness or lack of cooperation. Hostility is often a response to hospitalization.

HEALTH-ILLNESS STATES: INTERACTION BETWEEN THE MIND AND BODY

In the recent past, physical illness with a major emotional component was referred to as psychophysiological disorder.

The specificity model; Alexander (1950) believed that prolonged psychological stress could sometimes lead to medical condition via activation of autonomic nervous system. He states that specific type of emotional conflict causes anxiety in the individual. In defending against this anxiety, the individual regresses to an earlier psychological physiologic stage of development. For example, a person may regress in the oral receptive stage in which there is unconscious wishes to be felt by the mother. This results in gastric hypersecretion. If the person has a vulnerable duodenal mucosa, peptic ulcer may result. Alexander hypothesized seven psychosomatic disorders:

1. Essential hypertension
2. Neurodermatitis
3. Bronchial asthma
4. Rheumatoid arthritis
5. Hyperthyroidism
6. Ulcerative colitis
7. Peptic ulcer.

He applied the specificity model to various cases examples. The researchers have developed a more useful model to find the relationship between emotions physical functioning. That is the multicausational concept of illness process (Fig. 31.5). Holmes and Rahe (1978), Multer and Schleifer (1966) and Rahe and Arthur (1978) have presented this concept in their research. These studies show that physical illness is commonly preceded by stressful life changes. It also suggests that physical disorders such as mental disorders are related to socioeconomic status. Individual with similar social situations define these situations differently, consequently bad different reaction.

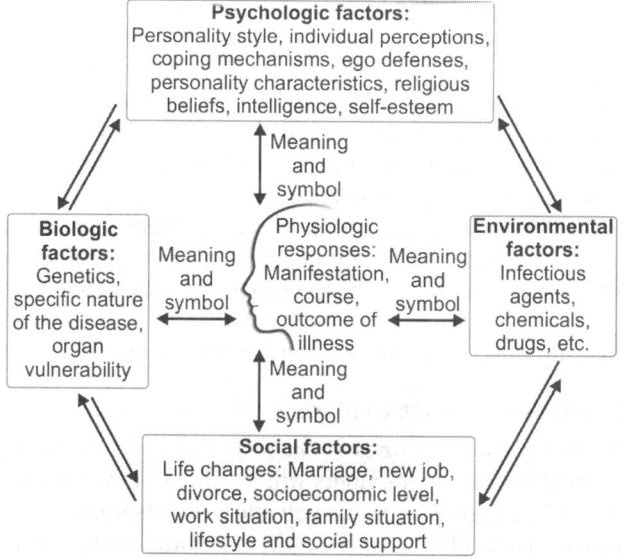

Fig. 31.5: Multicausational concept of illness.

The phrase meaning "symbol" refers to the fact that clients interpret all experiences in a highly individual manner.

ROLE OF EMOTION IN HEALTH AND DISEASE

Emotional states determine human behavior. Anger can cause a person to be rude sarcastic. Emotional disturbances can interfere with human efficiency such as lack of concentration, lack of appetite, increased risk of accidents, lack of sleep, palpitation, etc. In children, it appears in the form of temper tantrums, abdominal pain, spasms, tics, and antisocial behavior such as aggressiveness.

Psychosocial Illness

Group of diseases such as essential hypertension, peptic ulcer, asthma, and ulcerative colitis come under the psychosocial illness (mind acting on the body).

Control of Emotions

A well-adjusted mentally healthy person is one who is able to keep his/her emotion under control and is not carried away by one's emotions. Children should be shown love appreciation so that they may grow into emotional maturity. For adults, a happy family life is basic for emotional adjustment. Patients who are anxious need reassurance their fears must be allayed.

The following tips may be useful in controlling one's emotions:

- Cultivate hobbies, good habits of reading recreation
- Adopt a philosophy of life to enable you to avoid mental conflicts
- Try to understand your own limitations
- Develop a sense of humor.

Psychosomatic Illness

Psychosomatic illness is well known concept where the functions of the mind-body are inextricably related. Where the individual experience the emotions of fear, the body reaction is for fight or flight. A psychological reaction does not depend on the person's awareness of the emotions. In fact the existence of this response often serves to further observe the emotions. This process is termed as somatization.

In the past, stress-related illnesses were referred as psychosomatic illness. Unfortunately this term has been incorrectly incorporated into the languages meaning that the physical illness is not real, but rather a product of the person's imagination designed to elicit attraction sympathy.

Physiological Emotion Responses

Gastrointestinal System

Emotional factor plays a greater role in the development of duodenal ulcer, when tend to occur more in men than in women in younger age groups. Duodenal ulcer stem from sustained gastric hypersensitivity marked increase in gastric secretions, which eventually erode the lining of the subsequent exacerbations tend to be precipitated by stressful life events that bring the dependency-independent conflict disorder to the surface of consciousness.

Cardiovascular System

A major physiological emotional response affecting cardiovascular system is essential hypertension. It is a sustained elevation of systolic and diastolic arterial blood pressure in the absence of the demonstrable known causes of arterial hypertension. It is believed that tremendous amounts of repressed rage that have no acceptable outlet are the emotional dynamics underlying the development of essential hypertension.

Conversion Disorder

The major characteristics of the conversion disorder are a loss of physical functioning that suggest a physical disorder, but instead is an expression of a psychological need or conflict. The most common conversion symptoms suggest neurological disease such as paralysis, blindness, or seizures.

- ❖ *Primary gain:* It refers to the alleviation of anxiety in that conflict is kept out of awareness.
- ❖ *Secondary gain:* It refers to the gratification received as a result of how people in the patient's environment respond to illness. Current research suggests that genetic development learning personality sociocultural factors can predispose, precipitate and maintain these disorders. Stressful life events can also precipitate bodily concerns of somalizations.

Persistent "somatizers" are described as dependent, emotionally need, frustrated, chronically reserve persons who seek attention of or want to punish relative's physicians for not meeting their needs.

Emotional Disturbance or Reaction in Psychiatric Disorders

- ❖ *Mood disorder:* Extreme of emotion, soaring elation, or depression dominant the clinical picture.
- ❖ *Psychoneurosis:* Two essential features of psychoneurosis are that precipitate by emotional stressors, mental confusion and anxiety.
- ❖ *Mania:* The main characteristics of mania phase are general excitement and elation of mood.
- ❖ *Schizophrenia:* Schizophrenia is a group of psychotic disorders characterized by gross distortions of reality. Withdrawal from social interactions disorganization fragment of perception, thought emotion. Negative communication termed as expressed emotional over involvement that aggravates the schizophrenia.

ILLNESS WITH NEGATIVE PROGRESSES

To most people illness causes as an unwelcome intrusion, they have negative attitudes to illness. They also can affect normal roles within family social groups. The patient family may experience chronic emotional stress a decrease in the quantity of normal social functioning.

All patients do not cope equally well in a hospital setting experience because of increased physical stress. Certain unhealthy personality characteristics that were acquired during the patient's development may surface. These can undermine the patient's ability to adapt the hospital environment to the changes brought about by illness. These changes can undermine physical rehabilitation affect the patient's relationship with others.

Many nursing problems arise because sick people often behave not as adults, but as if they were much younger. Their attitudes to sickness are determined by childhood memories, by irrational fears, by unexpressed anger.

Stigma of Illness

In our modern age, attitudes to sickness are to a much less extent than firmly colored by disgust rejection. Some illness, however, still bears a stigma people suffering from mental disorder. From epilepsy, from tuberculosis or from venereal diseases are still occasionally treated as outcasts of society. Some people look upon the illness as a punishment they deserve other feel that they are unjustly treated wonder what they have done to deserve suffering.

Seeking Attention

Some children find that in illness they gain sympathy attention, which is denied then when they are well. In adulthood, there may still be the feeling that one is entitled to special consideration during illness. Adult patients are well-tried behavioral patterns quite unconsciously. Some mean, cry, complain display their suffering.

Roles in Illness Behavior

Parson's (1951) famous theory on the sick role behavior suggested that individual when suffering from an illness may behave in certain way in order to facilitate recovery. For instance, they may stay off work, avoid contacts and normal responsibilities. Repeated painful experience may lead to regression in behavior be manifested by regression to an earlier stage mobilizing, eating, bowel bladder habits. Some illness such as a light cold or a toothache usually mean that life goes as normal with only minor adjustment. It has been suggested that most symptoms do not result in any form of consultation this has been termed the "illness iceberg" (Last, 1963). Research has indicated that up to a one-third of symptoms will go unreported (Scrambler, 1981).

Family's Response to Illness

When a person becomes ill, the response of the patient to each of the family members will be different (McClowry, 1992). The response of one will affect the response of the others. If a child is ill, for example, the mother will respond to her child based on what the child's illness means to her, and how the child responds to the illness. The child's illness introduces a whole new dynamic in the father-mother relationship. The father in turn will respond based on his perception of the child's illness and by his/her own personality coping style.

ROLE OF A NURSE

Nurse as a Monitor

Nurses may be in a better position in a care giving team to monitor and evaluate the patient's family psychosocial progress during the patient's illness. Nurses spend more time with the patients than do any other member of the healthcare team.

Accordingly, they have the best opportunity to observe patients' progress to illness. They also observe how the patients interact with their family, friends, other members of the healthcare team. If psychological problems develop, the nurse most frequently observes them.

Nurses are usually viewed by patients as nurturing supportive people. Patients frequently are able to talk about their feelings with their nurses. The nurse should understand the emotions of the patients his/her own, so that he/she can help the patient to meet his/her needs. He/she can develop a care plan that will support more adaptive response better outcomes. The nurse has to give moral support is still in the patient's mind, a sense of belonging and a sense of attachment, which can bring about a profound change in the outlook of the patient. Consequently, the patient's speedy recovery is possible.

Nurse as an Advocate

Because nurses often have an intuitive awareness and sensitivity toward patients' needs, the patients' often choose to confide in them. Nurses may be in the best position in the healthcare team to be the patients' advocate. Accordingly, the nurse should be able to identify those patients who seem to ineffectively cope with their illness and mobilize the healthcare system resources to assist them in the adaptation process.

HEALTHCARE HAS BECOME INCREASINGLY FOCUSED ON HEALTH PROMOTION, WELLNESS AND ILLNESS PREVENTION

The rapid rise of healthcare has motivated people to seek ways to decrease the incidence and minimize illness or disability:

- ❖ Health promotion activities can be passive or active. With passive strategies of health promotion, individuals gain from the activities of others without acting themselves. By fluoridation of municipal drinking water with active strategies of health promotion, individuals are motivated to adopt specific health programs. Weight reduction and smoking cessation programs require clients to be actively involved to improve their further levels of wellness while decreasing the risk of disease. Motivating health promotion activities such as routine exercise and good nutrition, help clients maintain or enhance their present level of health.
- ❖ Wellness education teaches people, how to take care of themselves in a healthy way by including physical awareness, stress management and self-responsibility. Wellness is the ongoing and dynamic process of striving to achieve optimum health. Illness prevention activities such as immunization programs protect clients from actual or potential threats to health. The goal of a total health program is to improve the client's level of wellbeing in all dimensions, not just physical health.

Risk Factors Modification and Changing Health Behaviors

- ❖ Identifying the risk factors is the first step in health promotion, wellness education, and illness prevention activities.
- ❖ Health hazards should be discussed with the client following a comprehensive nurse assessment.
- ❖ In any program change, unhealthy lifestyle behaviors can be considered as a wellness strategy.
- ❖ Increase the quality of life and decrease the potential high costs of unmanaged health problems.
- ❖ Attempts to change are aimed to cease health damaging behavior. An understanding of the process of changing behaviors can cause behavioral change, followed by recycling. Nurses can assess the client with their adaptation to a changed and healthier lifestyle.

CONCLUSION

The concept of health and illness continuously change. It is dynamic state in which individual adapts to internal and external environment to maintain a mental wellbeing. To provide effective nursing care, a nurse must understand the biological and psychosocial dynamics that cause disease and lifestyle factors affecting health.

CHAPTER 32

Common Problems

CHAPTER OUTLINE

- Oxygen Insufficiency
- Oxygen Therapy
- Fluid and Electrolyte Balance
- Fluid Imbalance
- Nutritional Problems
- Client with Obesity
- Malnutrition
- Client with an Eating Disorder
- Hemorrhage and Shock
- Altered Body Temperature
- Unconsciousness
- Sleep Pattern and its Disturbances
- Physiology of Sleep and Arousal
- Stages of Sleep
- Pain
- Stress of Sensory Deprivation
- Stress of Immobility or Confinement
- Social Isolation

OXYGEN INSUFFICIENCY

Introduction

Oxygen is required to sustain life. Patients with respiratory dysfunction are treated with oxygen to relieve hypoxemia. The normal amount of oxygen in the arterial blood should be in the range of 80–100 mm Hg. If it falls below 60 mm Hg, irreversible physiological effects may occur. Thus, it requires immediate correction. Oxygenation is the process of treating a patient with oxygen.

Anatomy and Physiology of Respiratory System

The exchange of respiratory gases occurs between the environment and the blood. The lung transfers oxygen from the atmosphere to the alveoli, where oxygen is exchanged for carbon dioxide. The alveoli transfer oxygen and carbon dioxide to and from the blood through alveoli capillary membrane. There are three steps in the process of oxygenation—(1) ventilation, (2) diffusion, and (3) perfusion.

Structure and Function

Conditions or diseases that change the structure and function of the lung including the respiratory muscles, plural space, lungs, and alveoli essential for ventilation, perfusion, and exchange of respiratory gases alter respiration.

1. **Ventilation:** It is the process of moving gases into and out of the lungs. Ventilation requires coordination of the muscular and elastic properties of the lung and thorax. The major respiratory muscle of respiration is the diaphragm. It is innervated by the phrenic nerve.

2. **Diffusion:** It is the process of respiratory gas exchange between the alveoli and the capillaries of body tissues. Oxygen is transferred from the lungs to the blood; carbon dioxide is transferred from the blood to the alveoli and exhaled. Diffusion occurs at the alveolar capillary. The thickness of the membrane affects the rate of diffusion. Increased thickness of the membrane impedes diffusion because gases take longer time to transfer across the membrane.

3. **Perfusion:** The oxygen transport system consists of the lungs and cardiovascular system. Delivery depends on the amount of oxygen entering the lungs (ventilation), blood flow to the lungs and tissues (perfusion), rate of diffusion, and oxygen carrying capacity. Three things influence the capacity of the blood to carry oxygen—(1) the amount of dissolved oxygen in the plasma, (2) the amount of hemoglobin and (3) the tendency of hemoglobin to bind with oxygen. Regulation of respiration is necessary to ensure sufficient oxygen intake and carbon dioxide elimination to meet the body's demands, e.g. during exercise, infection, or pregnancy. Neural and chemical regulators control the process of respiration. Neural regulation includes the central nervous system (CNS) control of respiratory rate, depth, and rhythm. Chemical regulation involves the influence of chemicals such as carbon dioxide and hydrogen ions on the rate and depth of respiration.

Definition

Oxygen insufficiency or hypoxia is defined as a deficiency in the amount of oxygen reaching the tissues for which the person requires oxygen therapy.

Signs and Symptoms of Oxygen Insufficiency

- Tachypnea, dyspnea
- Anemia
- Pursed lip breathing
- Decreased skin turgor
- Dependent edema
- Lethargy
- Cyanosis, clubbing
- Pale conjunctiva
- Distension of neck veins
- Disorientation
- Decreased oxygen carrying capacity
- Low arterial oxygen tension.

Diagnosis of Oxygen Insufficiency

- Decreased respiratory rate, less than 16 breaths per minute
- Screening tests—blood specimens for complete blood count (CBC)
- X-ray chest, electrocardiogram (ECG)
- Peak expiratory flow rate (PEFR)—sputum of acid-fast bacilli and culture sensitivity
- Arterial oxygen tension should be checked
- Pulmonary function test
- Bronchoscopy, lung scan
- Thoracentesis
- Lipid profile, cardiac enzymes, ECG will be done.

OXYGEN THERAPY

Oxygen therapy is an intervention for administering more oxygen than is present in the atmosphere to prevent or relieve hypoxia.

Objectives

- To relieve hypoxemia
- To promote comfort
- To decrease work to the lungs/myocardium
- To relieve tissue hypoxia.

Indications

- Anemia and cyanosis—Hb% (decreased)
- Lung diseases that interfere with oxygen, which includes breathlessness due to asthma, emphysema, pulmonary embolism, coronary thrombosis, and cardiac insufficiencies.
- Patients with decreased respiratory capacity, atelectasis, pneumonectomy, thoracoplasty, etc.
- Poisoning—cyanide poisoning.

Cardiovascular Disorders

Shock and circulatory failure, congestive cardiac failure, left ventricular failure (LVF), myocardial infarction (MI), dysrhythmia, etc.

- Patients under anesthesia
- Patients who are critically ill
- Patients with psychologically induced breathlessness
- Asphyxia
- CNS conditions such as overdose of narcotics, anesthesia, head injury, and sleep apnea
- An environment low in oxygen content, e.g. high altitude.

Methods of Oxygen Therapy

Oxygen can be delivered to the client by nasal route in the following ways:

- ***Nasal cannula:*** It is simple comfortable device used for oxygen administration. Oxygen is supplied via cannula with a flow rate of 2–6 L/min. Usually, 4 L/min is used in order to prevent drying effect on the mucosa. Flow of oxygen meets 24–40%.
- ***Masks:***
  Simple facemask: It is used for short-term oxygen therapy. It fits loosely and delivers oxygen concentration from 35% to 50%. This is effective for mouth breathers/patients with nasal disorders. It is contraindicated in clients with carbon dioxide retention because retention can be worsened.
  Facemask with reservoir bag: It delivers higher concentration of oxygen from 35 to 60% (6 L/min) in partial breathers and 60–90% in non-rebreather and flow rate 10 L/min. Reservoir bag always remains inflated with oxygen.
  Venturi mask: It is used to deliver oxygen concentration of 25–55% with oxygen flow rate 4–8 L/min.
- ***Face tent:*** Provides comfortable fit and is useful for patient with facial trauma and burns facilitates humidification. Flow of oxygen 8–12 L/min and meets oxygen concentration 30–60%.
- ***Tracheostomy collar:*** Facilitates humidifying and warming oxygen flow rate 4–10 L/min and T piece supplies 24–100% of oxygen concentration.

Oxygen Hazards

- Oxygen support fire combustion
- Potential for oxygen toxicity
- Infection
- Dryness of the respiratory tract
- ***Atelectasis:*** Collapse of the alveoli
- ***Oxygen-induced apnea:*** Carbon dioxide washed off, when oxygen concentration is high
- ***Retrolental fibroplasia:*** Oxygen therapy affects retina and lens of the eyes in infants
- ***Asphyxia:*** Tent/Mask inhalation by not protected leads depletion.

General Instructions to be Followed While Giving Oxygen Therapy

- Oxygen is a drug. It must be prescribed in specific doses.
- When using oxygen cylinder, use a regulator and humidifier.
- Every part of the apparatus should be clean.
- Change nasal catheter every hour.
- Lubricate the nasal catheter, if it is used.
- Control the rate of flow/valve should not be handled on administration.
- Oxygen therapy should be discontinued gradually.
- There should be a calling signal near the patient.
- Pay attention for kinks in tubing, loose connections and faulty humidifying apparatus.
- Watch for any signs of oxygen hazards.
- Take precautions of fire by keeping "no smoking" board on clients room or over the bed.

Nurses' Responsibility in the Preparation of the Patient (Table 32.1)

Preliminary Assessment

- Keep equipment ready.
- Identify the patient with name/identification number, indication for oxygen therapy.
- Assess for the general condition/patient ability to cooperate during procedure.
- Explain to the patient and family members about safety of oxygen therapy.

Preparation of Environment

- Follow precautions of fire
- Provide privacy
- Provide a well-ventilated and lighted area
- If oxygen cylinder place it near head end of the bed.

Procedure

- Inspect the patient signs and symptoms associated with hypoxia and presence of airway secretions.
- Explain the procedure to the patient and family about the need for oxygenation.
- Wash hands.
- Fill the three-fourth humidifier with suitable sterile water/distill water.

Table 32.1: Equipment required for oxygen therapy.

Preparation of equipment	Others include
• Manual oxygen cylinder with regulator and humidifier • Oxygen mask, oxygen tubing • Oxygen source • Oxygen flowmeter	• Suction apparatus • Suction catheter • Water container • Sterile swabs • Sterile gloves • Paper bag/kidney tray

- Position the client in semi-Fowler's position. If not contraindicated.
- Clear the nostril, if required.
- Connect the tubing to the source of oxygen.
- Open the regulator.
- Check the flow of oxygen by placing the tip of the connecting tube in a bowl of water.
- Connect the oxygen regulator.
- Connect the tube to the oxygen administration device.
- Open the regulator and all the oxygen to flow at the rate prescribed.
- Secure the oxygen administration device.

After Care of the Client and Equipment

- Make the client comfortable
- Monitor the vital signs
- Clean, dry, and replace the equipment in a proper place.
- Wash hands.

Documentation

Record the time when the procedure was done, observation made and client's condition during and after the procedure.

FLUID AND ELECTROLYTE BALANCE

Introduction

Water is the most vital component of our body, so lack of fluids leads to illness or even death. The phrase fluid and electrolyte balance implies homeostasis or consistency of fluid, and electrolyte levels. It means that both the amount and distribution of fluids, and electrolyte levels are normal and constant. For homeostasis to be maintained, body input of water and electrolyte must balance the output. Cell function depends not only on a continuous supply of nutrients and removal of metabolic waste but also on the physical and chemical homeostasis of the surroundings fluids.

Terminologies

- *Homeostasis:* Relative stability or equilibrium of the internal environment between the kidney, liver, heart, thyroid, and adrenal gland
- *Extracellular:* Outside the cell
- *Intracellular:* Within the cell
- *Interstitial:* Between the cell and blood vessel
- *Intravascular:* Plasma portion of blood.

Definitions

- *Fluid:* It is a substance composed of molecules, which freely change their relative position without separation of mass.
- *Fluid balance:* A state in which the volume of body water and its solutes is within normal limits and there is normal distribution of fluids in the intracellular and extracellular.

- *Electrolyte:* A compound which, when dissolved in a solution will dissociate into ions. These ions are electrically charged particles and thus will conduct electricity.
- *Electrolyte balance:* The maintenance of the correct balance between the different elements in body tissues and fluids.

Distribution of Body Fluids

The body fluid is distributed into two distinct compartments, one consisting of the intracellular fluid and the other the extracellular fluid (ECF).
- *Intracellular:* It comprises all fluid within body cells. In adults, approximately 40% of body weight is intercellular fluid.
- *Extracellular:* It comprises all fluid outside a cell, which consist of interstitial fluid (fluid present between the cells and blood vessels) and intravascular fluid (blood plasma). In addition, the transcellular fluids such as cerebrospinal, pleural, peritoneal, and synovial fluids are also considered as extracellular fluid.

Composition of Body Fluids (Table 32.2)

The body fluid contains substances called electrolytes that are sometimes mineral or salts. An electrolyte is an element or compound which, when dissolved or melted in water or another solvent, separates into ions and is capable of carrying an electric current positively charged electrolytes are called cations (Na^+, K^+, Ca^{2+}, etc.) and negatively charged are called anions (Cl^-, HCO_3^-, SO_4^{2-}, etc.).

Movement of Body Fluids

Osmosis

Osmosis involves the movement of a pure solvent such as water through a semipermeable membrane from an area of lesser solute concentration to an area of greater solute concentration in an attempt to equalize concentration on both sides of the membrane. Osmotic pressure is the drawing power of water and depends on the number of molecules in solution.

Diffusion

Diffusion is the movement of a solute in a solution across a semipermeable membrane from an area of higher concentration to an area of lower concentration. The result is even distribution of solute in a solution, e.g., internal respiration.

Filtration

Filtration is the process by which water and diffusible substances move together in response to fluid pressure, moving from an area of higher pressure to one of lower pressure.

Active Transport

Unlike diffusion, osmosis, and filtration, active transport requires metabolic activity and expenditure of energy to move materials across cell membranes. This allows cells to admit larger molecules, e.g., Na^+, K^+ pump.

Capillary Dynamics

Fluid movement at the capillary level is dynamic and continuous in order to maintain homeostasis of vascular and intestinal fluid.

Arterial end fluid moves from capillary tissues to capillaries.

Venous end fluid moves to capillaries.

Homeostasis will maintain kidney, liver, thyroid gland, heart, and adrenal gland.

Regulation of Body Fluids

Fluid Intake (Fig. 32.1)

Fluid intake primarily is through the thirst mechanism. The thirst control center is located within the hypothalamus in the brain. Thirst is the conscious desire for water and is one of the major factors that determines fluid intake. A number of stimuli trigger this center, including the osmotic pressure of body fluids, vascular volume, and angiotensin. For example, a long distance runner loses significant amount of water through perspiration and breathing, increasing the concentration of solute and the osmotic pressure of fluids. This increase osmotic pressure stimulates the thirst center,

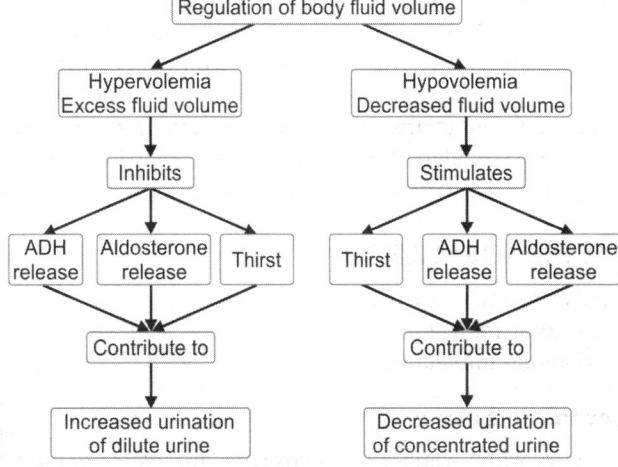

Fig. 32.1: Regulation of body fluids.
(ADH: antidiuretic hormone)

Table 32.2: Composition of normal ranges of electrolytes.

Electrolytes	Serum value (in mg/L)
Sodium (Na^+)	135–145
Potassium (K^+)	1.5–5.5
Calcium (Ca^{2+})	4.5–5.5
Bicarbonate (HCO_3^-)	22–26
Chloride (Cl^-)	90–110
Magnesium	1.5–2.5
Phosphate	1.7–4.6

causing the runner to experience the sensation of thirst and the desire to drink to replace lost fluids.

During periods of moderate activity at moderate temperature, the average adult drinks about 1,500 mL/day, but needs 2,500 mL/day, an additional 1,000 mL; this added volume is required from foods.

Fluid Output

The routes of fluid output or average fluid losses from the body:

Kidneys are major regulatory organs. They receive 70% of plasma and 1.5% of urine through filtration. Urine formed by the kidneys and excreted from the urinary bladder is the major avenue of fluid output. Normal urine output for an adult is 1,500 mL/24 h. Urine volume automatically increases as intake increases.

Skin activates sympathetic nerve system, losses occurs through sweat glands by physical exercise, elevated temperature, and increased metabolic rate. Insensible fluid loss occurs through the skin and lungs 400 mL during expansion and 200 mL gastrointestinal (GI) tract. Other types of insensible loss are in the exhaled air. In adults, this is normally 300–400 mL/day. Sensible loss occurs through (600–1000 mL) perspiration.

GI tract: An average adult loss only 100–200 mL of fluid through feces each day.

Hormonal Regulation

Antidiuretic hormone (ADH)

It regulates water excretion from the kidney and synthesized in the anterior portion of the hypothalamus and acts on the collecting ducts of the lobule. When serum osmolality rises, ADH is produced, causing the collecting ducts to become more permeable to water. This increase more water to be reabsorbed into the blood. As more water is reabsorbed, urine output falls and serum osmolality decreases.

Renin-angiotensin-aldosterone system

If blood flow or pressure to the kidney decrease, renin is realized. Renin causes the conversion of angiotensinogen to angiotensin-I, which is then converted to angiotensin-II, by angiotensin-converting enzyme. Angiotensin-II acts directly on the nephrons to promote sodium and water retention. In addition, it stimulates the release of aldosterone from renal cortex, which also promotes sodium retention.

FLUID IMBALANCE

Fluid imbalances are of two basic types:
1. Isotonic imbalance
2. Osmolar imbalance.

Isotonic Imbalance

It occurs when water and electrolytes are lost or gained in equal proportion, so that osmolality of fluid remains constant. There are two types of isotonic imbalance:

1. Fluid volume deficit
2. Fluid volume excess.

Fluid Volume Deficit

It occurs when the body losses both water and electrolyte from the ECF in equal proportion.

Etiology and risk factors
- Loses from the GI systems such as from diarrhea and vomiting
- Loss of plasma or whole blood such as with burns or hemorrhage
- Excessive perspiration
- Fever
- Decreased oral intake of fluids.

Clinical manifestations
- Thirst
- Oliguria
- Weak pulse
- Dry mucous membrane
- Poor skin turgor
- Lethargy
- Oliguria
- Postural hypertension
- Tachycardia.

Diagnosis
- Urine specific gravity greater than 1.030
- Increased blood urea nitrogen (BUN).

Management
- Monitor vital signs and check weight daily
- Assess breath sound and skin turgor
- Monitor fluid intake and output
- Administer oral and intravenous (IV) fluid as indicated
- Provide frequent mouth care
- Implement measures to prevent skin breakdown.

Fluid Volume Excess

Definition
Fluid volume excess occurs when the body retains both water and electrolyte in similar proportion to the ECF.

Etiology and risk factors
- Congestive heart failure
- Renal failure
- Cirrhosis of the liver
- Increased serum aldosterone and steroid level
- Excessive sodium intake or administration
- Inappropriate secretion of ADH.

Clinical manifestations
- Rapid weight gain
- Edema
- Hypertension
- Polyuria
- Neck vein distension
- Crackles in lungs on auscultation.

Diagnostic evaluation
- Serum osmolality: <2.75 mg/kg
- Serum sodium: <135 mEq/L, >145 mEq/L
- Decreased hematocrit: <45%
- Specific gravity: Below 1.010
- Decreased BUN: <8 mg/dL.

Management
- Pharmacologic treatment
- Diuretics
- Digitalis
- Dietary management: Low/high sodium diet.

Nursing management
- Monitor vital signs and check weight daily
- Assess breath sound
- Improve fluid balance
- Relieve dyspnea and dependent edema
- Clear chest sounds
- Absence of dependent edema
- Relief neck vein enlargement do not give semi-Fowler's position
- Decrease body weight
- Maintain urine output and intake
- Administer diuretics as ordered
- Restrict dietary sodium
- Restrict fluid intake.

Osmolar Imbalance

Osmolar imbalance involves the loss or gain of only water, so that osmolality of the serum is altered. Osmolar imbalance is of two types:
1. Dehydration
2. Overhydration

Dehydration

Dehydration occurs when water is lost from the body without significant loss electrolytes. Monitor risk of dehydration among infants, clients with neurological or psychological impairments, older adults, clients who are restrained unable to perceive or respond to thirst mechanism.

Etiology
- Patient receiving tube feeding who are not given adequate free water or who are feed hypertonic formulas are at risk
- Decreased thirst mechanism
- Unmonitored use of potent diuretics
- Vomiting
- Diarrhea
- Diaphoresis
- Diabetes
- Decreased secretion of ADH.

Clinical manifestations
- Thirst
- Decreased urine output
- Dry and cracked lips
- Coated tongue
- Sunken eyes
- Weak pulse
- Increased heart rate
- Postural hypotension
- Restlessness
- Headache
- Hallucinations
- Maniac behavior
- Confusion and coma.

Diagnostic findings
- Plasma sodium level >145 mEq/L
- BUN greater than 25 mg/dL
- Urine specific gravity >1.0.

Management
- If the fluids loss is mild, oral fluids can be given to restore the fluids loss.
- When the fluid loss is severe or life-threatening IV fluids are used for replacement.
- Urine output, body weight, and laboratory values of sodium.
- BUN and potassium are monitored closely.
- Antiemetic, antidiarrheal drugs may be prescribed to correct problems associated with vomiting and diarrhea.

Nursing management
- Assess the vital signs every 2–4 hours
- Check weight daily
- Monitor intake and output
- Provide frequent mouth care implement measures to prevent skin breakdown.

Overhydration

In overhydration, water is gained in excess of electrolytes.

Etiology
- Excess amount of saline IV fluid
- Ingestion of sodium high food
- Heart failure
- Lymphatic or venous obstruction
- Renal disorder
- Hyperaldosteronism
- Syndrome of inappropriate ADH.

Clinical manifestations
- *Respiratory manifestation:*
  - Coughing
  - Dyspnea
  - Crackles on auscultation
  - Pleural effusion.
- *Cardiovascular manifestations*
  - Bounding pulse
  - Elevated blood pressure (BP)
  - Jugular vein distension
  - An extra heart sound (S3) can be auscultated.

- *Others:*
  - Edema
  - Rapid weight gain.

Diagnosis
- Plasma osmolality <275 mEq/L
- Plasma sodium <135 mEq/L
- BUN <8 mg/dL
- Urine specific gravity <1.010.

Management
- Sodium intake is restricted in clients with cardiac and renal diseases.
- A mildly restricted sodium diet contains 4–5 mg of sodium, a moderately restricted diet contains 2 mg of sodium and severely restricted diet contains 0.5 mg of sodium.
- Administer diuretics to promote fluid loss.
- Treat the underlying cause.

Nursing management
- Monitor vital signs every 2–4 hours.
- Assess breath sound for crackles.
- Check weight daily; maintain intake and output chart.
- Palpate the sacrum and legs for pitting edema and observe for hand and bilateral neck engorgement.
- Provide meticulous skin care to prevent skin breakdown.

ELECTROLYTE IMBALANCE

An electrolyte imbalance is present whenever there is an excess or deficit in the plasma level of an employee. The types of electrolyte imbalance are detailed below.

Sodium Imbalance

There are two types of sodium imbalance—(1) hyponatrenia and (2) hypernatremia.

Hyponatremia

Hyponatremia is defined as serum sodium level of <1.35 mEq/L.

Etiology and risk factors
- Sodium loss from GI tract:
  - Vomiting
  - Diarrhea
  - GI drainage
- Profuse perspiration
- Diuretics
- Aldosterone deficiency
- Inadequate sodium intake
- Syndrome of inappropriate ADH (SIADH)
- Congestive heart failure.

Clinical manifestations
- *Neurological manifestation:*
  - Confusion
  - Hallucination
  - Behavioral changes
  - Brain herniation resulting in coma and death.
- *Cardiovascular hypotension:*
  - Decrease in BP
  - Orthostatic hypotension
  - Weak and thread pulse.
- *Respiratory manifestation:*
  - Tachypnea
  - Dyspnea
  - Orthopnea
  - Cheyne-Stokes respiration
  - Apneustic breathing.
- *GI manifestation:*
  - Nausea
  - Vomiting
  - Hyperactive bowel sound
  - Abdominal cramps
  - Diarrhea.

Diagnosis: Serum sodium level <135 mEq/L.

Management
- Provide a balanced diet with sodium level of 126–135 mEq/L.
- Diuretics such as furosemide are given to prevent pulmonary fluid overload.
- Fluid restriction to a range of 1,000–1,500 mL/day.
- For serum sodium level of 125 mEq/L or less IV therapy is the treatment of choice.
- For sodium level 125 mEq/L—0.9% normal saline (NS) or lactated ringer is used.
- For sodium level 115 mEq/L or less saline solution such as 3% NaCl is used.

Nursing management
- Monitor vital signs every 2–4 hours.
- Check weight daily.
- The nurse must monitor intake and output.
- The nurse encourages foods fluids rich in sodium content.
- If the patient is receiving nutrition only through tube feeding, it is sometimes necessary to add extra salt to the feeding.

Hypernatremia

Hypernatremia is defined as serum sodium level >145 mEq/L.

Etiology and risk factors
- Administration of concentrated saline solution
- Accidental or intentional salt ingestion
- Increased aldosterone production
- Osmotic diuresis
- Decreased thirst.

Clinical manifestations
- *Cardiovascular system:*
  - Orthostatic hypotension
  - Tachycardia

- ➤ Increased BP
- ➤ Jugular vein distension
- ➤ Weight gain and generalized edema.
- ❖ *Neurological manifestations:*
  - ➤ Restlessness
  - ➤ Agitation
  - ➤ Irritability.
- ❖ *Pulmonary manifestations:*
  - ➤ Crackles
  - ➤ Dyspnea
  - ➤ Pleural effusion.
- ❖ Skin and mucous membrane becomes dry.
- ❖ Elevated temperature.

Diagnosis: Serum sodium level > 145 mEq/L.

Management
- ❖ For minor manifestation, the focus is on correcting the underlying disorder and giving oral fluid replacement.
- ❖ Severe cases require hospitalization and treatment with IV saline.
- ❖ To decrease total body sodium and replace fluid loss hypo-osmolar electrolyte solution (0.2 or 0.45% NaCl) or dextrose in water.
- ❖ Rate of infusion must not exceed 2 mEq/L.
- ❖ In hypernatremia due to diabetes insipidus, demopressin in the form of nasal spray is administered 500–2,000 mg/day.

Nursing management
- ❖ Monitor vital signs every 4–8 hours
- ❖ Maintain intake and output chart
- ❖ Assess the skin and mucous membrane
- ❖ Monitor for changes in the mental status
- ❖ Provide mouth care every 2 hours
- ❖ If enteral feeding is used, sufficient water must be administered to keep serum sodium and BUN within normal limits.

Potassium Imbalance

Hypokalemia

Hypokalemia is defined as serum potassium level <3.5 mEq/L.

Etiology
- ❖ Inadequate potassium intake; increased potassium loss
- ❖ Vomiting
- ❖ Diarrhea
- ❖ Nasogastric (NG) suctioning
- ❖ Medications: Potassium wasting diuretics (thiazide loop and osmotic diuretics), steroids, aminoglycosides, amphotericin B
- ❖ Increase level of sodium intake
- ❖ Hyperaldosteronism
- ❖ Barter's syndrome.

Clinical manifestations
- ❖ *Neurological manifestation:*
  - ➤ Fatigue and irritability
  - ➤ Paresthesia
  - ➤ Hyporeflexia
  - ➤ Confusion
  - ➤ Convulsion
  - ➤ Coma.
- ❖ *Cardiovascular manifestation:*
  - ➤ Dysrhythmia
  - ➤ Hypotension
  - ➤ Slow, weakened pulse.
- ❖ *Pulmonary manifestation:*
  - ➤ Shallow respiration
  - ➤ Shortness of breath
  - ➤ Apnea.
- ❖ Respiratory arrest
- ❖ *Musculoskeletal manifestation:*
  - ➤ Muscle weakness
  - ➤ Leg cramps.

Diagnosis: ECG show depressed and prolonged ST segment, depressed and inverted "T" wave, and prominent "U" wave. Serum potassium level <3.5 mEq/L.

Management
- ❖ Maintenance dose for client not taking any source of potassium is 40–60 mEq/day in IV solution.
- ❖ For minor potassium deficits or those with potassium wasting conditions, administering food rich in potassium is adequate therapy. An adult recommended allowance is adequate therapy.
- ❖ Mild-to-moderate hypokalemia is treated by correcting or controlling the cause of the loss or by supplementing potassium intake throughout the diet or with the medication.
- ❖ Oral potassium replacement therapy is usually prescribed for mild hypokalemia (plasma potassium 3.3–3.5 mEq/L) or for potassium wasting condition.
- ❖ A client with a plasma potassium level between 3 and 3.4 mEq/L needs approximately 100–200 mEq/L of IV potassium.
- ❖ Potassium level of less than 3 mEq/L, it takes approximately 200–400 mEq/L of IV potassium.
- ❖ Potassium given IV must always be diluted in IV fluids. The usual concentration of IV potassium is 20–40 mEq/L.
- ❖ For severe hypokalemia, 10–20 mEq/L of potassium can be given in every hour, if diluted in IV (i.e., NS is recommended). Dextrose as a diluent is avoided because it increases intercellular potassium shifting.
- ❖ Potassium is irritating to the vein, therefore concentration >20–40 mEq/L increase the risk of phlebitis.
- ❖ Potassium is not given intramuscularly and is never given as bolus.

Nursing management
- ❖ The nurse encourages the patient to take potassium-rich food like fruits and fruit juices (banana, melon, citrus, and coconut water), fresh frozen vegetables, fresh meat, milk, and processed foods.

Table 32.3: Regulation of electrolytes.

Sl. No.	Electrolyte	Regulation
1.	Sodium (Na⁺)	• Renal reabsorption or excretion • Aldosterone increase Na⁺ reabsorption in collecting duct of nephrons
2.	Potassium (K⁺)	• Renal excretion and conservation • Aldosterone increase K⁺ excretion. Insulin decreases calcium level
3.	Calcium (Ca²⁺)	• Parathyroid hormone and calcitriol increases serum Ca²⁺ level
4.	Magnesium (Mg²⁺)	• Conservation and excretion by kidneys. • Intestinal absorption increased by vitamin D and parathyroid hormone
5.	Chloride (Cl⁻)	• Excrete and reabsorbed along with sodium in the kidney • Aldosterone increases chloride reabsorption with sodium.
6.	Phosphate	• Excretion and reabsorption by kidney. • Parathyroid decreases serum level by increasing renal excretion • Reciprocal relationship with calcium
7.	Bicarbonate	• Excretion and reabsorption by kidney

❖ Carefully monitoring of fluid intake and output, be administered only after adequate urine flow established.
❖ Potassium should be administered only after adequate urine flow established.
❖ A decreased in urine volume <20 mL/h for 2 conservative hours is an indication to stop potassium infusion unless the situation is evaluated (Table 32.3).

Hyperkalemia

Hyperkalemia is defined as serum potassium level of >5 mEq/L.

Etiology and risk factors
❖ *Decrease potassium loss:*
  ➤ Renal failure
  ➤ Decreases selection of aldosterone
  ➤ Potassium sparing diuretics.
❖ *Excessive release of potassium:*
  ➤ Burns, crush injuries, severe infection
  ➤ Tumor lysis syndrome (TLS).
❖ *Excess potassium intake:*
  ➤ Dietary excess
  ➤ Excessive IV administration.

Clinical manifestation
❖ *Cardiovascular manifestation:*
  ➤ Impaired cardiac conduction and ventricular contraction
  ➤ Hypotension
  ➤ Cardiac arrest.
❖ *Neurological manifestation:*
  ➤ Paresthesia
  ➤ Convulsion
  ➤ Severe neuromuscular weakness progressing to flaccid and respiratory muscle paralysis.
❖ *Urinary manifestation:* Oliguria and anuria.

Diagnosis
❖ ECG shows prolonged flat P wave PR interval peaked T wave depressed ST segment.
❖ Serum potassium level above 5 mEq/L.

Management
❖ For plasma potassium <5.5 mEq/L, dietary restriction of potassium is all that needed.
❖ Improving urine output by forcing fluids, giving IV saline or giving potassium-wasting diuretics usually corrects mild hyperkalemia.
❖ In severe hyperkalemia, temporary corrective measures are done such as:
  ➤ Infusion of IV calcium gluconate to decrease antagonistic effect of potassium excess on the myocardium.
  ➤ Infusion of insulin and glucose or sodium bicarbonate to promote potassium uptake into the cells.
  ➤ Use of beta-agonist albulerol (0.5 mg IV), which results in a decrease in plasma potassium level within 30 min lasting for 6 hours.
❖ A cation exchange resin such as sodium polysterene sulfonate may be given orally or rectally.
❖ In TLS prevention is the key; adequate hydration, i.e. 300 mL of IV fluid is given 24 hours before therapy, during therapy and 48 hours after therapy.

Nursing management
❖ The nurse observes for muscle weakness and dysrhythmias.
❖ Potassium rich food should be restricted.
❖ Encourage patient to take with minimal potassium-containing food.

Calcium Imbalance

Hypocalcemia

Hypocalcemia is defined as a plasma calcium level <4.5 mEq/L.

Etiology and risk factors
❖ Inadequate dietary intake
❖ Inadequate intake of vitamin D
❖ Parathyroid disease
❖ Certain medications such as magnesium sulfate, aspirin, steroids, loop diuretics, etc.
❖ Intestinal disease.

Clinical manifestations
❖ *Mild hypocalcemia:*
  ➤ Numbness and tingling of the hands, toes, and lips
  ➤ Emotional liability.
❖ *Severe hypocalcemia:*
  ➤ Hypotension
  ➤ Dysrhythmias

- Trousseau's sign
- Chvostek's sign
- Seizure
- Tetany
- Cardiac collapse and eventually death.

Diagnosis
- Plasma calcium level less than 4.5 mEq/L
- ECG shows prolonged interval.

Management
- Asymptomatic hypocalcemia is corrected with oral calcium gluconate, calcium lactate, or calcium chloride **supplementation**.
- Chronic or mild hypocalcemia can be treated in part by having the client consume a diet high in calcium.
- For tetany from acute hypocalcemia, IV calcium chloride or calcium gluconate must be given slowly to avoid hypotension and bradycardia.

Nursing management
- Check for Trousseau's sign and Chvostek's sign in high-risk patients
- Monitor vital signs
- Monitor for bleeding
- Monitor IV sites for infiltration or phlebitis when calcium is administered
- Provide calcium-rich diet to the patient.

Hypercalcemia: Hypercalcemia is defined as a plasma calcium level of >5.5 mEq/L.

Etiology and risk factors
- Metastatic malignancies
- Hyperparathyroidism
- Excessive intake of calcium supplements with vitamin D
- Calcium-containing antacid
- Prolonged immobilization
- Metabolic acidosis.

Clinical manifestation
- Mild hypercalcemia with calcium level slightly above 5.5 mEq/L is usually asymptomatic.
- Moderate hypercalcemia level above 6.2 mEq/L manifests as anorexia, nausea, vomiting, polyuria, muscle weakness, fatigue, lethargy, dehydration and constipation.
- Depressed sensorium, confusion and eventually coma.

Diagnosis
- Plasma calcium level >5.5 mEq/L
- ECG changes include shortened QT interval and widened T- wave.

Management
- IV NS, given rapidly with furosemide to prevent fluid overload, promote calcium excretion.
- Calcitonin is administered as it decreases plasma calcium level by the effect of parathyroid hormone (PTH) on the osteoclast and increasing urinary calcium excretion.
- Thiazide diuretics should be changed to furosemide or another diuretic that does not cause retention of calcium.

Conclusion: Electrolyte imbalance is found in all age groups. It is for an individual to have only one electrolyte imbalance; more commonly multiple electrolyte and fluid imbalance are present debilitating disease, etc. Nurses play an essential role in health promotion, health maintenance, and health restoration for clients at risk for or experiencing fluid and electrolyte imbalance.

NUTRITIONAL PROBLEMS

Introduction
Nutritional problems can occur in all age groups, cultures, ethnic groups, and socioeconomic classes. The nutritional status of a person or family may be influenced by many factors. The major nutritional disorders affect many systems and organs. They often cause serious health problems, such as hypertension, heart disease, fluid and electrolyte imbalances, disability, and even death.

Terminologies
- ***Nutrition:*** The process by which the body uses food for energy, growth, maintenance, and repair of body tissue.
- ***Anabolism:*** Building up of tissues.
- ***Catabolism:*** Breaking down of tissues.
- ***Facilitation:*** Catalyzes process through renal system, DM, vitamin B_{12}.
- ***Metabolic:*** The liver is largest organ of the body. Manufacture accumulate alter and excrete large number of substances involved in metabolism. Liver's role is important in regulation of glucose protein metabolism. Fats in GI tract excrete the waste products from bloodstream and secreting them into bile. Gallbladder empties bile to intestine.

Characteristics
- Effects are global for every individual.
- Effects manifest through organ/system.
- Biochemical markers specific goiter, diabetes mellitus (DM).
- Congenital, traumatic, infective/neoplastic.

These may or may not be reversible, primary and secondary to the diseases, e.g. cirrhosis of liver.
- ***Anabolic phase:*** Digestive and endocrine system enzyme production/utilization, e.g. fat absorption, protein malabsorption, nutritional deficiencies.
- ***Biochemical/cellular level,*** e.g. aplastic anemia/sickle cell anemia.
- ***Facilitation:*** Input/output secondary to life supporting needs of organism, e.g. carbon monoxide poisoning.

Classification
- ***Hepatic dysfunction:*** Jaundice, portal hypertension and ascites, nutritional deficiencies, hepatic coma.

- ❖ *Hepatic disorders:* Viral hepatitis, toxic/drug-induced hepatitis, hepatic cirrhosis, bleeding esophageal varices, hepatic tumors, liver abscesses.
- ❖ *Biliary condition:* Cholecystitis, cholelithiasis.
- ❖ *Others:* DM.

Treatment

- ❖ *Cellular level therapy:* Cannot detect, progressive
- ❖ *Substitution:* Replacement of insulin or administration of oral antidiabetic drugs
- ❖ *Alternative:* Lifestyle modification, diet control, and diuretics
- ❖ Transplant, e.g. transplantation of pancreas in DM.

Nutritional Conditions

Malnutrition may be over or under.

Classification

There are two major types.

1. *Macronutrient deficiencies:* Proteins-PEM, i.e. kwashiorkor and marasmus, carbohydrates, e.g. DM, fats, obesity, phrynoderma, coronary heart disease, cancer colon and breast, other skin lesions, lipidosis, obesity, etc.
2. *Micronutrients deficiencies*
   Vitamins: Fat-soluble A, D, E, K and water-soluble B complex, minerals Ca/Fe/I and trace elements zinc/copper.
   Vitamin A: Keratomalacia, night blindness, Bitot's spots, conjunctival xerosis, xerophthalmia (dry eye)
   Vitamin D: Rickets, osteomalacia
   Vitamin E: Cytotoxic effect
   Vitamin K: Decreases the prothrombin content of blood and prolongs clotting time
   Vitamin B (thiamine): Peripheral neuritis, beriberi
   Vitamin B_2 (riboflavin): Aribofavinosis, angular stomatitis, others—cheilosis, glossitis, nasolabial dyssebacia
   Vitamin B_3 (niacin): Pellagra
   Vitamin B_6 (pyridoxine): Megaloblastic anemia—pregnancy and lactation, glossitis, cheilosis, and GI disturbance
   Vitamin B_{12} (cyanocobalamine): Megaloblastic anemia, (pernicious anemia), neurological lesions in spinal cord, and infertility
   Vitamin C (ascorbic acid): Scurvy.

Minerals

- ❖ *Calcium:* Rickets and osteomalacia tetany
- ❖ *Iron:* Iron deficiency anemia
- ❖ *Iodine deficiency disorders (IDD):* Hypothyroidism, retorted physical development, and impaired environmental function, increased abortion, stillbirth, myxedema, and cretinism.

CLIENT WITH OBESITY

Introduction

Obesity is an abnormal increase in the portion of fat cells. Overweight and obesity result from a complex interaction between genes and the environment. An energy imbalance between energy expenditure and energy intake from a long-term sedentary lifestyle and/or excessive calorie intake causes an individual to become overweight or obese. It is most common in the United States.

Incidence and Prevalence

The incidence of overweight is higher in women, in blacks and in economically disadvantaged people of all races. In the US, more than 30% of the adult population is obese.

Risk Factors

- ❖ *Genetic/biologic:* There is a strong correlation between the weight of adopted children and their biologic parents. Identical twin tends to have similar body mass indexes (BMIs), whether raised together or apart, providing further evidence of a genetic link to obesity.
- ❖ *Physiologic:* Inactive people consume fewer calories than active people and continue to gain weight due to lack of energy expenditure.
- ❖ *Psychologic:* Low self-esteem may precipitate unhealthy eating behaviors and the resulting weight gain in turn may diminish self-image even further. A person may overeat as an anxiety, depression, guilt, or boredom or as a means of getting attention.
- ❖ *Environmental:* Such as abundant and readily available food supply, fast food restaurants, advertising and vending machines contribute to increase food intake.
- ❖ *Sociocultural:* Include overeating at family meals, rewarding behavior with food, religious, and family gathering that promote food intake and sedentary life-styles.

Diagnosis

BMI is used to identify excess adipose tissue.
$$BMI = weight\ (kg)/height^2\ (m^2)$$

- ❖ Anthropometry to estimate subcutaneous fat.
- ❖ *Hydrodensitometry (underwater weight):* This technique involves submerging the whole body and measuring the amount of displaced water.
- ❖ Bioelectrical impedance uses a low energy electrical impulse to determine the percentage of body fat by measuring the electrical resistance of the body.
- ❖ *Waist circumference:* To determine body fat distribution:
  ➢ Men: 40 inches (102 cm) or greater
  ➢ Women: 35 inches (88 cm) or greater.

Other diagnostic tests
- Thyroid profile to rule out thyroid disease
- Serum cholesterol to assess for elevated level
- Lipid profile
- ECG to detect effect of obesity on heart.

Management

- *Appetite suppressing drugs:* Appetite suppressants reduce food intake through nonadrenergic or serotonergic mechanism in the CNS. Nonadrenergic agents include phentermine (Adipex-p, Fastin, Ionamin), diethyl propion (Tenuate, Tepanil), phendimetrazin (Bontril, Plegine), and benzphetamine (Didrex). Serotononergic drugs acts to either increase the release of serotonin or decrease its uptake, thus reducing its metabolism.
- *Nutrient absorption blocking drug:* Orlistat (Xenical), a drug that was developed for weight loss and maintenance, works by blocking fat breakdown and absorption in the intestine. It inhibits the action of intestinal lipases. The undigested fat is excreted in the feces.
- *Exercise:* An aerobic exercise program of 30–40 minutes of exercise 5 or more days a week promotes weight loss, while reducing adipose tissue, increasing lean body mass, and promoting long-term weight control.
- *Nutrition:* Diet should be low in kilocalories and fat and contain adequate nutrients, minerals, and fiber.
- *Behavior modifications*
  - Keeping food record.
  - Eliminate cues that precipitate eating like keeping food out of view, eliminating snack foods.
  - Changing the act of eating.
  - Controlling the environment.
  - Purchase low calorie foods.
  - Keep all food in the kitchen.
  - Store all food in the refrigerator or in the cabinets in opaque containers.
  - Prepare exact portion of food to eliminate leftovers.
  - Eat all foods in the same place, avoid eating in the kitchen.
  - Avoid eating when watching TV or reading.
  - Reduce frequency of eating out at restaurants, parties, and picnics.
- *Controlling physiological responses to food*
  - Eat slowly by taking small bites, allowing 20 minutes for a meal.
  - Eat a salad or drink a hot beverage before a meal.
  - Chew each bite thoroughly and slowly.
  - Put eating utensils or food down between bites.
  - Concentrate on the eating process, savor the food.
  - Stop eating with the first feeling of fullness.
- *Controlling psychological responses to food*
  - Appreciate the aesthetic experience of eating.
  - Use attractive dinnerware and prepare a formal setting for eating.
  - Use small plates and cups to make servings of food look larger.
  - Concentrate on conversions and socialization during the meal.
  - Use nonfood rewards for meeting a goal.
  - Acknowledge small successes and improvements in all behavior.
- Substitute other activities of eating (e.g., reading, exercise, hobbies).

Surgery

Bariatric surgery is a surgical procedure that is used to treat morbid obesity. It is the only treatment that has been found to have a successful and lasting impact for sustained weight loss for severely obese individuals. It has three broad categories:

1. *Restrictive:* Reduces the size of the stomach to 30 mL or less, which causes the patient to feel full quicker. For example, vertical banded gastroplasty (portioning the stomach into a small pouch in the upper portion along the lesser curvature of the stomach).
   Adjustable gastric banding (the stomach size is limited by an inflatable band placed around the fundus of the stomach).
2. A combination of malabsorptive and restrictive. For example, Roux-en-Y surgical procedure is removing approximately three-fourth of the stomach to produce both restriction of food intake and reduction of acid output. The remaining portion of the stomach is connected to the lower portion of the small intestine.
3. Biliopancreatic diversion (BPD) with duodenal switch (variation of the BPD procedure by including a duodenal switch, i.e. leave a larger portion of the stomach intact and a small part of the duodenum). For example, Roux-en-Y surgical procedure (the stomach size is decreased with a gastric pouch anastomosis that empties directly into the jejunum).

Cosmetic surgeries to reduce fatty tissue and skin folds. For example, lipectomy/adipectomy (remove unslightly flabby folds of adipose tissue), liposuction (suction-assisted lipectomy).

High Risk Associated with Obesity

- *Cardiovascular Problems*
  - Hyperlipidemia
  - Deep venous thrombosis
  - Hypertension
  - Cardiomyopathy.

- ❖ *Respiratory Problems*
  - ➢ Obesity hypoventilation syndrome
  - ➢ Sleep apnea
  - ➢ Asthma
  - ➢ Pulmonary hypertension.
- ❖ *DM*
- ❖ *Musculoskeletal Problems*
  - ➢ Osteoarthritis
  - ➢ Impaired mobility and flexibility
  - ➢ Gout
  - ➢ Chronic low back pain.
- ❖ *GI and Liver Problems*
  - ➢ Nonalcoholic steatohepatitis (NASH)
  - ➢ Gallstones.
- ❖ *Cancer:*
  - ➢ In women:
    - ♦ Endometrial
    - ♦ Breast
    - ♦ Cervical
    - ♦ Ovarian
    - ♦ Uterine
    - ♦ Gallbladder
  - ➢ In men: Prostate cancer
  - ➢ In both men and women: Colorectal.

MALNUTRITION

Introduction

Malnutrition is a deficit, excess, or imbalances of the essential components of a balanced diet. It results from inadequate intake of nutrients.

Incidence

The prevalence of underweight is 42.5%; the stunted growth of under-five is 48%. A majority of children suffering from malnutrition is 80% globally. Malnutrition is a big public health problem for more than half of 54% of all under-five mortality rates in India.

Types

- ❖ *Protein calorie malnutrition:* It is due to ingestion of food deficient in protein. This results from either primary (nutritional needs are not met as a result of poor eating habits) or secondary factor (alteration or defect in ingestion, digestion, absorption or metabolism).
- ❖ *Marasmus:* It is the result of a concomitant deficiency of both calorie and protein intake leading to generalized loss of body fat and muscle.
- ❖ *Kwashiorkor:* It is caused by a deficiency of protein intake that is superimposed on a catabolic stress event such as GI obstruction, a surgical procedure, cancer, malabsorption syndrome, or an infectious disease.

Risk Factors

- ❖ *Age:* Older adults are at greater risk for malnutrition due to a variety of factors
- ❖ Poverty, homelessness, inadequate food storage, and preparation facilities
- ❖ Functional health problems that limit mobility or vision
- ❖ History of weight loss more than 20% of usual weight
- ❖ Oral or GI problem that affects food intake, digestion, and absorption
- ❖ Inability to eat for 5 or more days
- ❖ Chronic pain or chronic diseases such as pulmonary, cardiovascular, renal, or endocrine disorders or cancer.
- ❖ Dementia, mental health disorders
- ❖ Medications or treatments that affect appetite
- ❖ Alcohol or drug addiction
- ❖ Acute problems such as infection, surgery, or trauma.

Clinical Manifestations

- ❖ Weight loss
- ❖ Wasted appearance
- ❖ Dry and brittle hair
- ❖ Pale mucous membranes
- ❖ Peripheral or abdominal edema
- ❖ Dryness of conjunctiva and cornea
- ❖ Cheilosis
- ❖ Anemia
- ❖ Decreases BP and pulse
- ❖ Polydipsia
- ❖ Polyuria
- ❖ Increase number of infection
- ❖ Depression
- ❖ Confusion.

Diagnosis

- ❖ *History and physical examination:*
  - ➢ To know the dietary history of foods eaten over the past week, i.e. dietary recall for a day/week
  - ➢ To know the past health history
- ❖ *Laboratory studies:* To know hemoglobin, hematocrit level, serum electrolyte level, etc.
- ❖ *Anthropometric measurements:* Includes gross measures of fat and muscle content.

Management

Multivitamins and mineral supplements.

Nutrition

Fluids and nutrients are carefully reintroduced in severely malnourished hospitalized clients.
- ❖ Oral feeding
- ❖ Enteral nutrition
- ❖ Parenteral nutrition
- ❖ *Oral feeding:* High calorie oral supplements may be used whose nutritional intake is deficient. This may include milk shakes, puddings, or commercial available products. These supplements should not be used as meal substitutes, but between meal and snacks. In some long-term care facilities, these beverages are used

- *Enteral nutrition:* Enteral nutrition or tube feeding may be used to meet the calorie and protein requirements in clients unable to consume adequate food. Tube feeding is usually administered through a soft, small caliber NG or nasoduodenal tube with a weighted mercury tip. They can also be administering through a gastrostomy or jejunostomy tube. Small-bored feeding tubes are easily displaced; appropriate tube placement should be periodically checked by aspirating the tube and checking the pH of the aspirated contents.
- *Parenteral nutrition:* Total parenteral nutrition (TPN) also known as hyperalimentation is the IV administration of carbohydrate, protein, electrolyte, vitamins, minerals, and fat emulsions. These hypertonic solutions are usually administered through a central vein such as subclavian vein. A peripherally inserted central catheter line may be used for short-term TPN.

  Partial parenteral nutrition (PPN) is used to support the client who is able to consume some nutrients or in conjunction with enteral feeding. PPN may be given through a peripheral vein.
- **Low birth weight** is one of the nutritional major public health problems in many developing countries, about 16% of the babies are low birth weight, i.e. birth weight <2,500 g as compared to 4% in some developed countries. The causes for the low birth weight, maternal malnutrition, and anemia appear to be significant risk factors and multifactorial in its occurrence.

  The interventions include, mothers are protected against nutritional deficiencies particularly protein, vitamin and minerals especially vitamin A and iodine deficiency. Fresh milk, capsules of vitamin A and D are also supplied free of cost in some maternal and child health (MCH) centers.

  To prevent low birth weight, Government of India has introduced many nutritional programs to protect young population, expectant mothers, and postnatal mother's nutritional status.
- Information, Education and Communication (IEC) activities on nutritional awareness are organized globally to impart the education in all health facilities.
- **Nutritional anemia:** Nutritional anemia is caused by malnutrition. According to World Health Organization (WHO), it is a condition in which the hemoglobin content of blood is lower than normal as a result of a deficiency of one or more essential nutrients, regardless of the cause of such deficiency.

  About 50–60% of women belonging to low socioeconomic groups are anemic, interventions include:
- An estimation of hemoglobin should be done to assess the degree of anemia.
- The Government of India has initiated a program in which 100 mg of elemental iron and 500 µg of folic acid are distributed daily for 4 months to pregnant women through antenatal clinics, primary health centers, and sub-centers.
- If anemia is suspected in children up to 2 years of age, one tablet of iron and folic acid containing 20 mg of elemental iron and 0.1 mg of folic acid should be given daily for 100 days. For children 6–60 months, ferrous sulfate, folic acid is to be provided in a liquid formulation, should be dispensed in bottles so designed that only 1 mL can be dispensed each time. For children, 6–10 years of age are to be provided 30 mg elemental iron and 2.5 mg folic acid per day for 100 days. Adolescents are given the same dosage and duration as adults.
- Iron fortification of salt with iron has been introduced by the National Institute of Nutrition, Hyderabad, as a supplementation.
- Other strategies include changing dietary habits, control of parasites, and nutrition education.
- **Endemic fluorosis:** In many parts of the world where drinking water contains excessive amounts of flurorine (3–5 mg/L).

  Dental fluorosis occurs during the first 7 years of life, skeletal fluorosis is associated with lifetime daily intake of 3–6 mg per liter or more, this leads to crippling fluorosis leads to permanent disability. Genu valgum is a new form of fluorosis, characterized by osteoporosis of the lower limbs.

Interventions: Changing the water source is one of the solution with a lower fluoride content (0.5–0.8 mg per liter), if that is possible.
- If this is not possible, the water can be chemically defluoridated in a water treatment plant, such treatment is moderately expensive.
- Other measures include, fluoride supplement should not be prescribed for children and they should not recommend fluoride toothpaste up to 6 years of age.
- **Lathyrism:** This is one of the nutritional problems and a paralyzing disease of humans and animals. In the humans, it is referred to as neurolathyrism because it affects the nervous system. Lathyrus sativus is commonly known as "*khesari dhal*," these seeds have a characteristic triangular shape and gray color. When dehusked, the pulse similar to red gram dal or Bengal gram dal. This is a good source of protein, but for it toxin which affect the nerves. It is eaten mostly by the poor agricultural laborers because it is relatively cheap.

Interventions: The possible intervention for the prevention and control of lathyrism are:
- Vitamin C prophylaxis: Daily administration of 500–1,000 mg of ascorbic acid for a week or so.
- Banning the crop is not feasible but, prevention of food adulteration act in India has banned lathyrus in all forms.
- Removal of toxin is done by soaking the pulse in hot water that is called steeping method. A large quantity

of water is boiled and the pulse is soaked in hot water for 2 hour.
- ❖ Para boiling, an improved method of detoxicating the pulse is para boiling.
- ❖ The public must be educated and the dangers of consuming this pulse and the need for removing its toxin before consumption.

CLIENT WITH AN EATING DISORDER

Introduction

Eating disorder is complex condition that arises from a combination of long-standing behavioral, emotional, psychological, interpersonal, and social factors. Eating disorder characterized by severely disturbed eating behavior and weight management.

Common Eating Disorders

Anorexia nervosa: It is characterized by a self-imposed weight loss, endocrine dysfunction, and a distorted psychopathologic attitude toward weight and eating. It begins during adolescence.

Manifestation: Characterized by self-starvation and excessive weight loss.

Symptoms

- ❖ Refusal to maintain body weight at or above a minimally normal weight for height, body type, age, and actively level
- ❖ Intense fear of weight gain or being "fat"
- ❖ Feeling "fat" or overweight despite dramatic weight loss
- ❖ Loss of menstrual periods
- ❖ Extreme concern with body weight and shape.

Bulimia nervosa: It is a disorder characterized by frequent being eating and self-induced vomiting associated with loss of control related to eating and a persistent concern with body image. It develops in late adolescent or early adulthood, often following failed attempts to lose weight through dieting.

Manifestation: Characterized by a secretive cycle of binge eating followed by purging. Bulimia includes eating large amounts of food—more than most people would eat in one meal in short periods of time, then getting rid of the food and calories through vomiting, laxative abuse, or over exercising.

- ❖ Repeated episodes of excess eating and purging
- ❖ Feeling out of control during a binge and eating beyond the point of comfortable fullness
- ❖ Purging after a binge (typically by self-induced vomiting, abuse of laxatives, diet pills, and/or diuretics, excessive exercise or fasting)
- ❖ Frequent dieting
- ❖ Extreme concern with body weight and shape.

HEMORRHAGE AND SHOCK

Introduction

Shock is a life-threatening condition with a variety of underlying causes. Shock is a complex clinical syndrome that may occur at any time and in any place. Shock is an emergency after requiring team action by many healthcare providers, including nurses, physicians, laboratory technician, pharmacist, and respiratory therapist. Shock, causes thousands of deaths and unknown number of permanent injuries each year.

Terminologies

- ❖ *Perfusion:* The passage of fluid through a tissue especially the passage of blood through the lung to pick up oxygen and the alveoli and release of carbon dioxide.
- ❖ *Baroreceptors:* A collection of sensory nerve endings specialized to monitor changes in BP.
- ❖ *Stroke volume:* It is the volume of blood ejected out per ventricle/beat (70–80 mL).
- ❖ *Cardiac output:* It is the volume of blood ejected out from each ventricle 5–6 L/min.
- ❖ *Pulse pressure:* It is the difference between systolic and diastolic BP.
- ❖ *Colloids:* IV solution that contains molecules too large to pass through rapid membrane.
- ❖ *Crystalloid:* Electrolyte solution that move freely between the intravascular compartment and interstitial spaces.
- ❖ *Anaphylaxis:* An emergency condition resulting from an abnormal and immediate allergic response to which the body has become intensely sensitized.
- ❖ *Preload:* Ability of myocardial fiber to stretch in order to accommodate sufficient quantity of blood from atrium to ventricle.
- ❖ *Afterload:* Resistant offered by process of fibers either by pulmonic circuit for outflow of blood.

Definition

Shock is defined as a condition in which systemic BP is inadequate to deliver oxygen and nutrient to support vital organs and cellular function.

—Mikkhail, 1999

Shock is defined as failure of a circulatory system to maintain adequate perfusion of vital organs. Disorders leading to inadequate tissue perfusion result in decreased oxygenation at the circulatory level.

It is defined as a complex life-threatening condition (syndrome) characterized by inadequate blood flow to the tissues and cells of the body.

Incidence

An exact incidence of all types of shock is not known. But shock is manifestation of a pathologic condition rather than hypovolemic shock.

The incidence of occurrence among the various forms of shock differs widely.

Hypovolemic Shock

It occurs most commonly when severe blood and fluid loss make the heart unable to pump enough blood to the body due to decreased preload.

Cardiogenic Shock

Cardiogenic shock is a condition in which heart suddenly cannot pump enough blood to meet the body's needs.

It occurs in 10.1% in 2010 of all clients following myocardial infarction and has a range of 27–51% in 2019.

Neurogenic Shock

It is seen with all spinal cord injuries. The incidence of occurrence for both septic and anaphylactic shock is variable.

Shock occurs when one of the following two things happen. (1) CVS fails to deliver adequate amount of oxygen glucose to the cells. (2) The cells are unable to use the available amount of oxygen and nutrients.

External Fluid Loss

Hemorrhage, severe vomiting and diarrhea, excessive diuretics, inadequate fluid intake, temperature elevation, and severe dehydration.

Internal Fluid Loss

Interstitial obstruction, burns, peritonitis, ascites, pancreatitis.

Risk Factors

Traumatic surgery, alcoholism, severe dehydration, vomiting, etc.

Classification of Shock

- Hypovolemic shock
- Cardiogenic shock
- Distributive shock or vasogenic—maldistribution of blood, neurologic, anaphylactic, and septic shock
- Obstructive shock occurs from obstructive blood flow.

Hyovolemic Shock

It is the loss of fluid electrolytes, blood, and plasma.

It is due to inadequate circulating blood volume resulting from hemorrhage with actual blood cell. It is most common type of shock developed when the intravascular volume decreases to the part where compensatory mechanism is unable to maintain organ and tissue perfusion. For example, burns with a loss of plasma proteins and fluid shifts or dehydration with a loss of fluid volume.

Pathophysiology

- Decreased blood volume
- Decreased venous return
- Decreased stroke volume blood flow
- Decreased cardiac output supply
- Decreased tissues perfusion—anoxia shock.

Clinical manifestation

- Initial increase in urine osmolality and specific gravity
- Decrease as shock progresses
- Marked diaphoresis
- Decreased tissue perfusion to the skin making it cold and clammy, pallor
- Increased heart rate and respiratory rate
- Cyanosis
- Decreased urine output.

Diagnostic evaluation

- CBC
- Hematocrit values
- Hemoglobin
- Coagulation studies
- ECG
- Levels of PCO_2
- Assessment for fluid/blood loss/vital signs.

Management of hypovolemic shock

Medical management: Major goals in treating hypovolemic shock:
1. Restore intravascular volume to reverse the sequence of events lead into inadequate tissue perfusion.
2. Redistribute fluid volume.
3. List the underlying cause of the fluid loss.

Treatment of the underlying cause
- If the patient has hemorrhage, efforts are made to stop bleeding by applying pressure to the site.
- If the cause of hypovolemia is due to diarrhea or vomiting, administer medication to treat diarrhea and vomiting.

Fluid and blood replacement
- Fluid replacement is of primary concern. At least two large gauge IV lines are inserted to establish access for fluid administration.
- Fluid used for replacement are:
  Crystalloids
  - 0.9% sodium chloride (NS), Ringer's lactate, hypertonic saline.
  Colloids
  - Albumin (5%, 25%), dextron (40, 70)
  - Blood products are administered if cause for shock is hemorrhage. Packed red blood cells are administered to replenish the patient's oxygen carrying capacity
  - A modified Trendelenburg position is recommended in hypovolemic shock. Elevating the legs promote the venous return.

Pharmacological therapy

- **Dobutamine:** It enhances the strength of cardiac contraction, improves stroke volume.

- **Nitroglycerin:** Venous dilator reduces preload.
- **Dopamine:** Dose 0.5–3 mg/kg/min increases the renal and mesenteric blood flow, thereby preventing ischemia of organ.
- **Vasoactive medication:** Administration of norepinephrine, epinephrine causes increase in BP and vasoconstriction.

Nursing management

- Closely monitoring who are at risk for fluid deficit and assisting with fluid replacement.
- Administer prescribed fluids and medication.
- Monitor the signs of complication and reporting.
- Monitor vital signs.
- Maintain intake and output chart.
- Administer oxygen, blood transfusion safely as prescribed.
- Provide psychological support.

Cardiogenic Shock

It is due to inadequate pumping action of the heart because of primary cardiac muscle dysfunction or mechanical obstruction of blood flow caused by MI, vascular insufficiency caused by disease/trauma. Cardiac dysrhythmias or obstructive conditions include such as pericardial tamponade, or pulmonary embolism, arrhythmias.

Cardiogenic shock results from major LV dysfunction, leading to heart failure, ineffective pumping of blood, inadequate cardiac output, and decreased tissue perfusion.

Risk factors

- Cardiovascular stress with previous myocardial damage
- MI heart failure, cardiomyopathy
- Acute MI involving 40% of LVF
- Massive pulmonary embolism, myocarditis
- Dysrhythmia
- Aortic aneurysms
- Obstructed LV function.

Pathophysiology (Fig. 32.2)

The most common initiating events in cardiogenic shock are acute MI. Dead myocardium does not contract and cardiogenic cause may result. On a mechanical level, a marked decrease in contractility reduces the ejection, fraction and cardiac output. These lead to increased ventricular filling pressures, cardiac chamber dilatation, systemic hypotension, and/or pulmonary edema that lead to shock.

Diagnostic evaluation

CBC, serum electrolytes, cardiac enzymes, coagulation profile, arterial blood gas (ABG) analysis, imaging studies such as radiography of the heart, computed tomography (CT) scan, ECG, and a bed side Echo.

Clinical manifestation

- Decreased tissue perfusion to the skin—cold and clammy
- Distention of jugular veins
- Elevated central venous pressure (CVP)
- Kussmaul's sign
- Enlarged cardiac contour on chest failure
- Reduced cardiac output leading to hypotension, tachycardia, dyspnea, restlessness, anxiety.

Management

Medical management.

Goals

- Limit further myocardial damage and preserve the healthy myocardium.
- Improve the cardiac function by increasing cardiac contractility, decrease ventricular after-load.

Initiation of first line of treatment

- ***Supplying of oxygen:*** In early stages of shock, supplemental oxygen is administered by nasal cannula, 2 to 6 L/min to achieve 90% oxygen saturation.
- ***Controlling chest pain:*** Morphine sulfate is administered intravenously for pain relief. It also relieves patient's anxiety. Cardiac enzyme levels are measured. ECG is done to assess the degree of myocardial damage.
  - Providing selected fluid support.
  - Administer vasoactive medication.
  - Implantation of transthoracic and IV pacemaker to control heart rate.
  - Implementing mechanical cardiac support by intra-aortic balloon counterpulsation therapy, ventricular assist system or extracorporeal cardiopulmonary bypass.
- ***Pharmacological therapy:***
  - Administered as per Table 4

Nursing management:
  - Identifying the patient at risk.
  - Administer adequate oxygen.
  - Monitor hemodynamic status. Arterial lines and electrocardiographic monitoring equipment must be maintained and check for its functioning. Assess for breath sounds, changes in cardiac rhythm, physical assessment should be done.

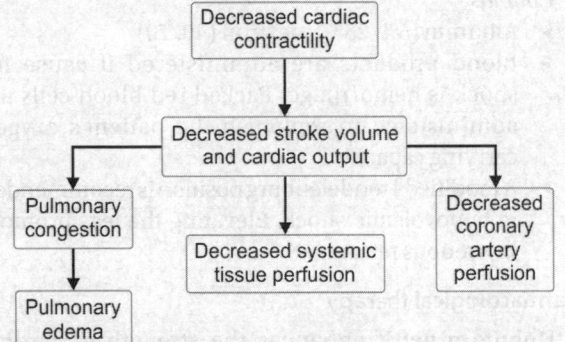

Fig. 32.2: Pathophysiology of cardiogenic shock.

- Administering medications and IV fluids
- Have active role in safeguarding the patient, enhancing comfort, reducing anxiety.
- Explanation of the treatment and disease condition to the patient and his family members.

❖ **Obstructive shock:** It is due to sudden obstruction of blood flow (cardiac tamponade, pneumothorax, pulmonary embolism).

❖ **Distributive shock (vasogenic shock) or circulatory shock:** It is due to changes in blood vessel tone that increase the size of the vascular space without increase in the circulating blood volume. It is further divided into three types.

1. Anaphylactic shock

It is a severe hypersensitivity reaction resulting in massive systemic vasodilation. It results from an antigen-antibody reaction that releases histamine or histamine-like substances.

Causes
- Adverse drug reactions
- Food intolerance
- Pollen hypersensitivity
- Hypersensitivity to insect stings
- Hypersensitivity to immune system (transfusion reaction).

Risk factors
- Unrecognized allergy
- Accidental exposure to known allergy.

Clinical manifestation
- Initially vague feeling of uneasiness
- Headache, severe anxiety, dizziness
- Disorientation, loss of consciousness, laryngeal edema, hoarseness, coughing, dyspnea, stridor, other includes pruritus, urticarial edema of eyelids, lips, and tongue.

2. Neurogenic shock

It results from generalized vasodilation and loss of vasomotor tone. It interferes with nervous system control of blood vessels such as with spinal cord injury, spinal anesthesia, or severe vasovagal reaction caused by pain or psychic trauma. The duration of neurogenic shock is usually 1–6 weeks as long as there is not irreparable cord injury.

Causes
- Spinal cord injuries
- Anesthetic paralysis
- Reflex vasodilation
- Head trauma
- Extensive pain.

Risk factors
- Traumatic injury
- Diseases of spinal cord
- Snake venom.

Clinical manifestation
- Bradycardia
- Hypotension
- Skin is dry to touch.

3. Septic shock (Fig. 32.3)

It is caused by a release of vasoactive substances. It is a syndrome marked by altered hemodynamics decreased tissue perfusion and loss of cellular energy it develops because of the body immune and inflammatory responses to endotoxin following bacteria.

Causes
- Gram-negative bacteria endotoxins most common
- Gram-positive bacteria—toxic shock.

Clinical manifestations
- Warm dry flushed skin (warm shock)
- Pale skin, cold and clammy skin, mottled skin
- Hypothemia
- Drowsiness
- Progressing to coma.

Stages of Shock

A convenient way to understand the physiologic responses and subsequent clinical signs and symptoms is divided into separate stages (Fig. 32.4):
- Compensatory stage

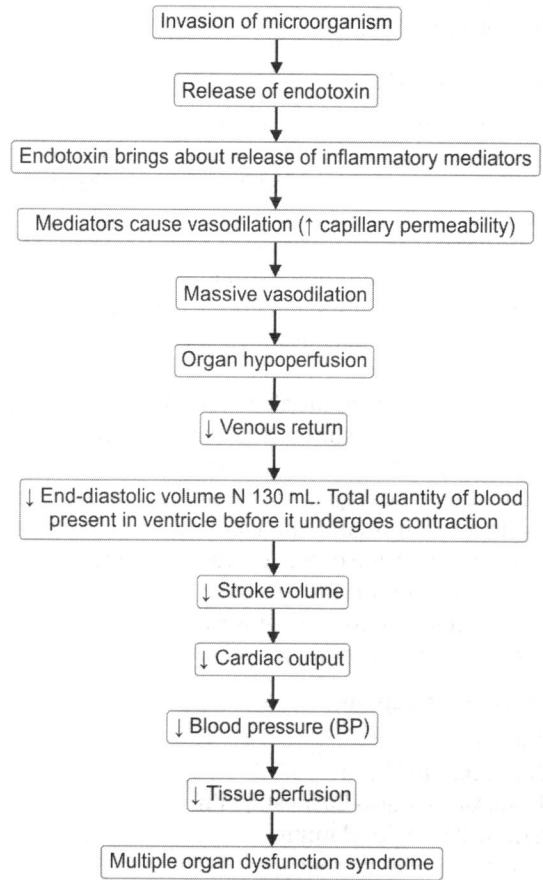

Fig. 32.3: Pathophysiology of septic shock.

Section 5: Biopsychosocial Pathology

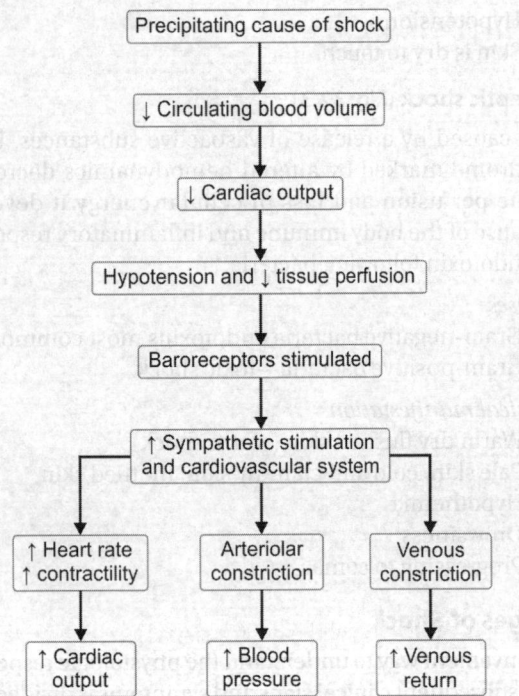

Fig. 32.4: Pathophysiology—compensatory mechanism for the restoration of circulatory blood volume in shock.

- Progressive stage
- Irreversible stage.

Compensatory Stage

When body sustains such as hemorrhage, extensive burns in heart failure a compensatory reaction occurs in the body. In compensatory stage of shock, the patient's BP remains within normal limits. Vasoconstriction, increased heart rate, and increased contractility of heart contribute to maintaining cardiac output. This results from stimulation of the sympathetic nervous system and subsequent release of catecholamines (epinephrine and norepinephrine).

The patient displays the often described "fight or flight" response. The body shunts blood from organs such as skin, kidneys, and GI tract to the brain and heart to ensure adequate blood supply to these vital organs. As a result, the patient's skin is cold and clammy, bowel sounds are hypoactive, and urine output decreases in response to the release of aldosterone and ADH.

Body attempts to compensate for decrease tissue perfusion in a variety of ways.

Clinical manifestations

- Normal BP
- Heart rate 100 bpm
- Respiratory status 20 breath/min
- Skin will be cold, clammy
- Urine output decreased
- Confusion state

- Respiratory alkalosis (hyperventilation).
  (If treatment begin in this stage, prognosis is good).

Management

Early intervention along with continuation of shock therapy is key improving patients prognosis.

- ***Monitoring tissue perfusion:*** In assessing tissue perfusion, the nurse observes for changes in level of consciousness, vital signs (including pulse pressure) urinary output, skin and laboratory values (serum sodium and blood glucose levels are elevated in response to the release of aldosterone and catecholamines).
- In-depth assessment of patient's hemodynamic status, administration of fluid, and medications.
- Relieve anxiety and promote safety.

Progressive Stage

In the progressive stage of shock, the mechanism that regulate BP can no longer compensate and mean arterial pressure (MAP) falls below normal limits with an average systolic BP of less than 90 mm Hg.

Pathophysiology (Fig. 32.5)

Although all organ systems suffer from hypoperfusion.

First, the over worked heart becomes dysfunctional, the body's inability to meet increased oxygen requirements

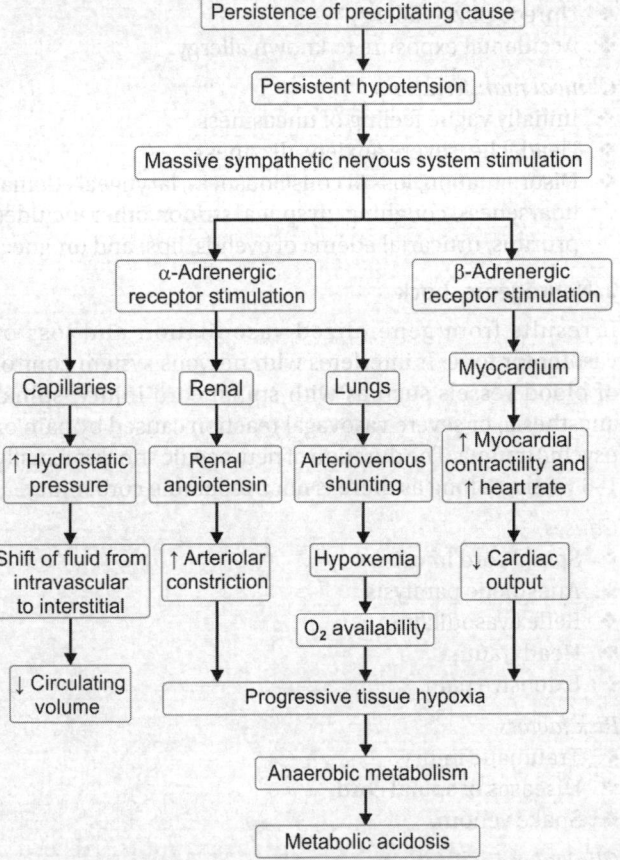

Fig. 32.5: Pathophysiology of progressive stage.

produces is chemical and biochemical mediators causes myocardial depression.

Failure of cardiac pump

Second, autoregulatory function of the microcirculation fails in response to numerous biochemical mediators released by cells.

Capillary permeability, with areas of arteriolar and venous constrictions, further compromise cellular perfusion. At this stage, patient's prognosis worsens.

The relaxation of precapillary sphincters causes fluid to leak from capillaries, creating interstitial edema, return less fluid to heart.

Clinical manifestation

- BP systolic less than 80–90 mm Hg
- Heart rate > 150 bpm
- Respiratory status: Rapid, shallow respiration, crackles
- Skin: Petechiae
- Urine output: 0.5 mL/kg/1 hour
- Mental status lethargic
- Metabolic acidosis.

Irreversible Stage/Refractory Stage

In this stage at which organ damage is so severe that the patient does not respond to treatment and cannot survive. BP remains low. Complete renal and liver failure.

It is compounded by the release of necrotic tissue toxins. Anaerobic metabolism contributes to worsening of lactic acidosis. The release ATP is completely depleted. Multiple organ dysfunction progresses to complete organ failure and death is imminent.

Clinical manifestation

- Requires intubation
- Asystole
- Skin: Jaundice
- Urinary output: Auric, requires dialysis
- Unconscious
- Profound acidosis.

Diagnosis

Noninvasive cardiology studies

- History and physical examination
- ECG, ECHO, multiacquisition scanning, radiographic studies
- Radiographs, CT scans, magnetic resonance imaging (MRI) scan
- Serial electronic BP monitoring
- Pulse oximetry
- Serial neurologic checks
- Core temperature measurement—probe ear.

Laboratory studies

- CBC and blood chemistry
- Serum electrolytes, ABG analysis
- Urine output
- Hemodynamic monitoring—CVP
- Peritoneal lavage
- Endoscopy
- Angiography.

Complications of shock

- Acute respiratory failure leading to death
- Metabolic acidosis
- Disseminated intravascular coagulation leading to death
- Sepsis due to tissue necrosis
- Cardiac temponade
- Multiple organ failure.

Management

Medical management

- Treatment shall be given when systolic BP 80 mm Hg or less
- Pulse pressure 20 mm Hg or less
- Pulse rate 120 or more
- Primary aim of treating shock is to increase tissue perfusion
- Prevent complications of shock through symptoms intervention.

Management for all phases of shock includes the following:

- Oxygen supply
- Fluid replacement to restore intravascular volume
- Vasoactive medications to restore vasomotor tone and improve cardiac function
- Nutritional support.

Respiratory support

- Airway
- Ensure ventilation by resuscitation
- Endotracheal intubation
- Oxygen supply can be increased by administration of oxygen
- Increase arterial oxygen saturation with supplemental oxygen and mechanical ventilation
- Maintain positive and expiratory pressure to prevent treatment of hypoxia
- Chest physical therapy of patients with acute respiratory distress syndrome (ARDS)
- Optimizing the cardiac output with drug therapy or fluid replacement.

Fluid replacement

The fluids are given to improve cardiac and tissue oxygenation. The fluids include crystalloids (electrolyte solutions that move freely between intravascular and interstitial spaces), colloids (large molecule IV solution), blood components. The large bore (14–16 gauge) IV catheter must be inserted. Common fluids are 0.9% sodium chloride, lactate Ringer's solution.

Medication therapy

Vasoactive medications are administered to improve the patient's hemodynamic stability. Vasoactive agents used in treating shock.

Nutritional support

- The patient in shock requires more than 3,000 calories daily.
- Parenteral or enteral nutritional support should be initiated as soon as possible.
- Glutamines can be administered through enteral nutrition.
- Enteral nutrition should be initiated within 24 hours.
- Weigh patient daily.

Emergency care in shock

- Call in all types of shock
- Assess for consciousness and open airway
- Ask the client for name, age and health history
- Keep the client warm in a supine position
- Feel the presence of carotid areas
- Reassure the client
- Stay client and have someone summon professional healthcare
- On arrival of trained emergency personnel—placement of IV line, oxygen therapy, and intimation of cardiac monitoring.

Care in hypovolemic shock

- Assess the client for evidence of bleeding
- Cover wounds with a clean cloth, if possible
- After IV line initiated recurrent laryngeal nerve stimulation (RLNS)
- Strict adherence to aseptic techniques
- Early detection of clinical manifestations
- Continuous monitoring
- After shock, assess and prevent complications and treatment.

Prevention

- Identify clients at risk and development of complications
- Clients with allergies to drugs—allergic person to wear identification card
- Fluid replacement in hypovolemia.

Nursing assessment: The initial assessment should be toward the ABC pattern. Further assessment focus on the assessment of tissue perfusion, level of consciousness, neurologic status, and capillary refill.

Nursing interventions

- Monitor vital signs frequently.
- Fluid replacement to restore intravascular volume.
- Close monitoring of the patient during fluid replacement.
- *Positioning:* Lower extremities elevated 45°, knee straight. Promotes increased venous return.
- Monitor nutritional need. Parental or enteral feeding should be initiated.
- Regular weight monitoring of patient.
- Apply elastic compression stocking and elevating the foot end of bed may minimize the pooling of blood in legs.
- Provide psychological support to relieve anxiety.

ALTERED BODY TEMPERATURE

Introduction

Changes in body temperature outside the usual range affect the hypothalamic set point. These changes can be related to excess heat production, excessive heat loss, minimal heat production, minimal heat loss, or any combination of these alterations. The nature of the change affects the type of clinical problems that a client experiences.

Terminologies

- *Febrile:* Client who has a fever
- *Afebrile:* Client who does not have fever
- *Fluctuation:* Variation in temperature.

Definition

There are two primary alterations in body temperature—(1) pyrexia and (2) hypothermia.

- *Pyrexia or fever:* A body temperature above the usual range is called pyrexia or fever.
- *Hypothermia:* It is a core body temperature below the lower limit of normal. The temperature falls below 95°F or 35°C.

Mechanism of Thermoregulation

Thermoregulation is one of the most fundamental physiological regulation in our body. Men are homeothermic, i.e. whatever may be the environmental condition, the temperature does not vary. This is the ability to keep the body temperature within a very narrow range. The temperature is operated by a thermoregulatory mechanism (Fig. 32.6).

Sources of Body Heat

- Metabolism
- External environment
- Channels of heat loss.

Channels of Heat Loss

- *Conduction:* It is the heat exchange between two materials that are in direct contact with each other, e.g. heat loss via lying in the floor, clothing, chair, etc.
- *Convection:* It is the transfer of heat by the movement of fluid (gases or a liquid) between areas of different temperature, e.g. by a breeze or a fan.
- *Radiation:* It is the transfer of heat in the form of rays between a warmer object and a cooler one without physical contact. The temperature of the body should

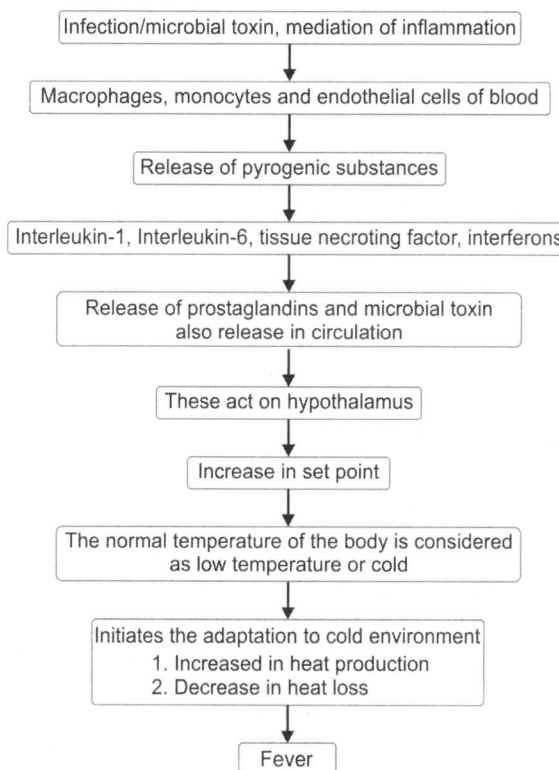

Fig. 32.6: Pathophysiology of fever.

be higher than the temperature of the environment otherwise the flow of the heat will be reversed and the body will gain heat.
- *Evaporation:* It is the conversion of a liquid to a vapor. Every milliliter of evaporation of water takes with it a great deal of heat 0.58 cal/mL.

Definition
Body temperature may be defined as the degree of heat maintained by the body or it is the balance between the heat produced and the heat lost in the body.

Types
- *Core temperature:* It is temperature of the deep tissues of the body, such as the cranium, thorax, abdominal cavity, and pelvic cavity. It remains relatively constant.
- *Surface temperature:* It is the temperature of the skin, the subcutaneous tissue, and fat. It by contrast rises and falls in response to the environment. The average body temperature of an adult is between 36.7°C (98°F) and 37°C (98.6°F).

Purpose
- To establish baseline data for subsequent evaluation.
- To identify whether the core temperature is within normal range.
- To determine changes in the core temperature is response to specific therapies (e.g. antipyretic medication, immunosuppressive therapy, and invasive procedure).
- To monitor clients at risk for alterations in temperature (e.g. clients at risk for infection or diagnosis of infection; those who have been exposed to temperature extremes; those with a leukocyte count below 5,000 or above 12,000).

Definition of Fever/Pyrexia
Fever/pyrexia results from an alteration in the hypothalamic set point. It occurs because heat loss mechanism is unable to keep pace with excess heat production, resulting in an abnormal rise in body temperature. The temperature is below 39°C (102.2°F).

Conditions of Increased Body Temperature
- *Hyperthermia:* An elevated body temperature related to the body's inability to promote heat loss or reduce heat production. There is no change in hypothalamic set point. The temperature is raised to 105°F.
- *Hyperpyrexia:* Fever due to any injury to CNS, hemorrhage or trauma. The temperature is above 105°F.
- *Hypothalamic fever:* In this, the hypothalamic function is increased, e.g. in case of tumor.
- *Neurogenic fever:* Fever occurs due to injury to hypothalamus.

Clinical Manifestations of Fever in Systemwise
- *Respiratory system:* Shallow and rapid breathing.
- *Circulatory system:* Increased pulse rate and palpitation.
- *Alimentary system:* Dry mouth, coated tongue, loss of appetite, indigestion, nausea, vomiting, constipation, or diarrhea.
- *Urinary system:* Diminished urinary output, burning micturition, high colored urine.
- *Nervous system:* Headache, restlessness, irritability, insomnia, convulsions delirium.
- *Musculoskeletal system:* Malaise, fatigue, body pain, and joint pain.
- *Integumentary system:* Heavy sweating, hot flushes—goose flush, shivering or rigors.

Types of Fever
- *Onset or invasion:* Body temperature is rising, it may be sudden or gradual process.
- *Crisis:* It is sudden return to normal temperature from a very high temperature within a few hours or days.
- *Lysis:* The temperature in zigzag manner for 2 or 3 days or week before reaching normal.
- *Continuous or constant fever:* In which the temperature varies not more than 2°C between morning and evening and does not reach normal for a period of days or weeks.

- ❖ **Intermittent fever:** The temperature rises from normal to high and back at regular intervals from few hours to days. Usually temperature higher in the evening than morning.
- ❖ **Remittent fever:** It is a fever characterized by variations of more than 2° between morning and evening but does not reach normal.
- ❖ **Inverse fever:** Highest range of temperature is recorded in the morning hours and the lowest in the evening, which is contrary to that found normal course of fever.
- ❖ **Hectic or swinging fever:** The difference between the high and low points is very great, i.e. hectic or swinging fever.
- ❖ **Relapsing fever:** There are brief febrile period followed by one or more days of normal temperature.
- ❖ **Irregular fever:** When fever is entirely irregular in its course. It cannot be classified under any one of the fever described above and it is called irregular fever.
- ❖ **Rigor:** It is a sudden severe attack of shivering in which the body temperature rises rapidly to a stage of hypopyrexia, e.g. malaria.
- ❖ **Low pyrexia:** Does not rise above 99–100°F.

Nursing Intervention for Fever (Table 32.4)

- ❖ Monitor vital signs
- ❖ Assess skin color and temperature
- ❖ Remove extra blankets when the clients feels warm, but provide extra warmth when the clients feels chilled
- ❖ Provide adequate nutrition and fluids
- ❖ Prevent dehydration
- ❖ Reduce physical activity
- ❖ Administer antipyretic drugs
- ❖ Provide oral hygiene
- ❖ Provide tepid sponge
- ❖ Provide dry clothing and bed linen.

Clinical Signs of Hypothermia

- ❖ Decreased body temperature, pulse, and respirations
- ❖ Severe shivering (initially)
- ❖ Feelings of cold and chills
- ❖ Pale, cool, waxy skin
- ❖ Hypotension
- ❖ Decreased urinary output
- ❖ Lack of muscle coordination
- ❖ Disorientation
- ❖ Drowsiness progressing to coma.

Nursing Intervention for Clients with Hypothermia

- ❖ Provide a warm environment
- ❖ Provide dry clothing
- ❖ Apply warm blankets
- ❖ Keep limbs close to body
- ❖ Cover the clients scalp with a cap
- ❖ Supply warm oral or IV fluid
- ❖ Apply warming pads.

UNCONSCIOUSNESS

Introduction

Unconsciousness or any other sudden change in mental status is a commonly occurring medical emergency. One of the nurse's most challenging tasks is to provide care to the unconscious patient. This task requires skill, sound judgment and the ability to make assessments and solve problems using only objective information. So, it is needed to explore the meaning of unconsciousness and to identify the causes of unconsciousness and how to provide care to the patients who are unconscious or are experiencing decreased level of consciousness.

Anatomy and Physiology of Central Nervous System

Central nervous system consists of higher levels of brain or cerebral cortex, lower levels of brain that include medulla, cerebellum, pans, basal ganglia, thalamus, hypothalamus, midbrain, and spinal cord.

Brain

It is a complex structure consisting of more than 100 billion neurons. It is a semisolid structure weights 1,400 g/3 pounds in an adult. Brain is divided into following areas.

Table 32.4: Example of nursing process for the management of pyrexia.

Assessment	Nursing diagnosis	Objective	Nursing intervention
Subjective data: Patient verbalized that he/she feels feverish **Objective data:** Patient temperature is 102°F	Hyperthermia related to disease condition	Fever will be reduced	• Assess the vital signs of temperature 102°F; pulse 80 beats/min; respiration 20 breaths/min, blood pressure (BP) 140/80 mm Hg • Provide cold sponge for 15 min • Provide increased fluid intake • Encourage to adequate rest • Provide antipyretic drug paracetamol as per doctor advice
Objective data: Patient is in unconscious state	Hypothermia related to trauma	Temperature will be maintained to normal	• Assess the vital signs temperature 95°F; pulse 85 beats per min; respiration 16 breaths per min; BP 100/60 mm Hg • Provide warm environment by giving blankets • Maintain the liquid and electrolyte balance as per the advice • Monitor the signs of consciousness • Proper management of trauma site

Cerebrum: The cerebrum is composed of two hemispheres joined by corpus callosum, the thalamus, hypothalamus, and basal ganglia. The cerebral hemispheres are divided into pairs of frontal, parietal, temporal, and occipital lobes.
- ❖ ***Frontal:*** The largest lobe functions are concentration abstract thought, memory, and motor function. It also contains Broca's area, which controls speech. It is also responsible for affect personality, judgment, and inhibitions.
- ❖ ***Parietal:*** Predominantly sensory lobe. The primary sensory cortex, which analyzes sensory information and relays this information to the thalamus and other cortical areas located in the parietal lobe. It is also essential to an individual awareness of the body in space as well as orientation in space and spatial relations.
- ❖ ***Temporal:*** Contains the auditory receptive areas also contains a vital area called the interpretive area that provides integration of somatization, visual and auditory areas and plays the most dominant role of any area of cortex in cerebration.
- ❖ ***Occipital:*** The posterior lobe of cerebral hemisphere is responsible for visual interpretation.

Hippocampus: It is the medical section of the temporal lobe, which plays an important function memory.

Basal ganglia: It consists of several structures of gray matter buried deep in cerebral hemispheres. It functions in the control of motor activity.

Brainstem: It is composed of midbrain, pons, and medulla. It consists of ascending pathways reticular formation, cranial nerves, and their nuclei and descending autonomic and motor pathways.

Diencephalon: Diencephalon consists of thalamus and hypothalamus. The thalamus channels all sensory information except smell to the cortical cells.

Hypothalamus controls the autonomic nervous system functions and also controls pituitary gland functions. It has also centers of hunger control, sleep-wake cycle, BP, aggressive behavior and emotional responses.

Limbic system: It is composed of hippocampus, diencephalon, and basal ganglia. It helps in olfactory sensations and emotional expressions.

Reticular formation: It is composed of complex network of gray matter (nuclei), ascending reticular, and descending reticular pathways. Its nuclei extend from superior part of spinal cord to diencephalon and communicate with basal ganglia, cerebrum, and cerebellum. Reticular formation assists in regulation of skeletal muscle movement and spinal reflexes. Also filters incoming sensory information to cerebral cortex.

Reticular activating system (RAS): RAS is a component of reticular formation, which controls sleep-wake cycle and consciousness.

Cerebellum: The cerebellum first separated from the cerebrum by a fold of dura mater. It is responsible for coordination of movement, fine movements, balance, position sense (awareness) of where each body part is an integration of sensory input.

Terminologies

- ❖ ***Coma:*** It is a state in which the person has no awareness or response except to painful stimuli.
- ❖ ***Syncope:*** A simple faint or temporary loss of consciousness due to cerebral ischemia, often caused by dilation of peripheral blood vessels and a sudden fall in BP.
- ❖ ***Toxin:*** Any poisonous compound, that is produced by bacteria.
- ❖ ***Hypoxia:*** A diminished amount of oxygen in the tissues.
- ❖ ***Ischemia:*** A deficiency of blood supply to a part of the body.
- ❖ ***Glasgow come scale:*** A standardized system for quickly evaluating the level of consciousness in a critically ill.
- ❖ ***Supratentorial lesions:*** These are lesions, which destroys compress reticular formation.
- ❖ ***CT scan:*** Computed tomographic scan.
- ❖ ***MRI:*** Magnetic resonance imaging.
- ❖ ***EEG:*** Electroencephalography.
- ❖ ***CSF:*** Cerebrospinal fluid.

Definition of Unconsciousness

Unconsciousness is a state in which a patient is totally unaware of both self and external surrounding, and unable to meaningfully to external stimuli.

Unconsciousness result from gross impairment of both hemispheres and/or ascending RAS or metabolically depress over all brain function.

Causes of Unconsciousness

- ❖ ***Structural brain lesions:*** It includes the abnormalities inside the brain, which increase the intracranial pressure (ICP). It is classified into two:
  1. ***Supratentorial lesions:*** These are which causes upper brainstem dysfunction that include:
     - ♦ Cerebral edema
     - ♦ Brain tumor
     - ♦ Brain abscess
     - ♦ Cerebral hemorrhage
     - ♦ Cerebral infarction (large)
     - ♦ Epidural hematoma
     - ♦ Aneurysm rupture.
  2. ***Infratentorial lesions:*** These are which compresses or destroy reticular formation that include:
     - ♦ Cerebella abscess
     - ♦ Brainstem or cerebella hemorrhage
     - ♦ Brainstem or cerebella infarction
     - ♦ Brainstem or cerebella tumor.

- **Metabolic disorders and diffuse disorders:** In this the causes outside brain which causes unconsciousness:
  - Diseases of other organs such as kidney, liver, heart, lungs, and endocrine glands
  - Poison intake, alcohol and drug abuse
  - Fluid electrolyte and acid–base imbalances
  - Seizures
  - Infections such as encephalitis and meningitis
  - Severe nutritional deficiencies
  - Hypoglycemia
  - Ischemia or anoxia
  - Syncope
  - Temperature regulation disorder
  - Electric shock
  - Sun stroke.
- Organic disease like mental illness.
- Emotional stress like psychogenic shock due to any unexpected events.

Pathophysiology

Consciousness is a complex function controlled by RAS and its integrated components. RAS begins in medulla and reticular formation connect to RAS and then to diencephalon. Integrated pathways connect the cerebral cortex to the limbic system via the thalamus and also connect to the brainstem. Reticular formation produces wakefulness whereas RAS and its higher connections are responsible for awareness of self and environment. Diffuse cortical connection allows maximum integration of all conscious-related activities/disorders that affect any part of RAS can cause unconsciousness.
- Direct compression or destruction of structures responsible for consciousness, e.g. tumor, hemorrhage.
- Decreased availability of oxygen or glucose, which are responsible for cerebral metabolism, e.g. hypoxia, ischemia.
- Toxic effect of substance on structures of RAS, e.g. toxic product from kidney, liver drug overdose, bacterial invasion.

Assessment of Unconsciousness

Assessment of unconsciousness includes various steps.

History Collection

A detailed history about the incident, any underlying diseases such as DM, renal diseases, respiratory or liver diseases, any psychological stress, etc., should be collected from the person who assisting the patient.

Physical Assessment

A thorough physical examination including head-to-toe examination and system wise examination should be done.

Neurologic Examination

Neurologic examination including checking of reflexes should be done, if possible. The pupillary movement also should be checked. Unequal pupils, fixed pupils indicate increased ICP.

Vital Sign Checking

Vital sign checking is an important past assessment after ABC has been established. It includes BP, temperature, pulse rate, and check of pupils.

A raising BP correlated with slowing pulse rate is indicative of increased ICP. Change in respiratory rate and temperature should also be reported to the physician.

Other Diagnostic Tests

Blood Investigation

Blood investigation includes total blood count, biochemistry investigations, and blood sugar level and paracetamol and aspirin levels.

MRI and CT Scans

These scans usually provide data that indicate whether the cause of coma is structural.

Lumbar Puncture

It is done to get CSF to check if any infection or bleeding is the cause of unconsciousness.

Electroencephalography

Electroencephalography can be used to determine whether the seizure activity causes unconsciousness.

Positron Emission Tomography

Positron emission tomography is used to assess any structural lesions in brain.

Glasgow Coma Scale

Glasgow coma scale is used to measure level of consciousness of patient based on scores (Table 32.5).

It has three components. Maximum score is 15 and minimum score is 3.

Clinical Manifestation

The person will be unresponsive to activity, touch, sounds, or other stimulation. The following symptoms may occur:
- Confusion
- Drowsiness
- Headache
- Inability to speak or move parts of body
- Light headedness
- Incontinence of both bowel and bladder
- Palpitations
- Pupillary response is slower.

Table 32.5: Assessment of Glasgow coma scale.

Components	Score
Eye opening	
Spontaneous	4
To speech	3
To pain	2
None	1
Verbal response	
Oriented	5
Confused	4
Inappropriate words	3
Incomprehensible	2
None	1
Best motor response	
Obeys commands	6
Localizes pain	5
Withdraws	4
Flexes	3
Extends	2
None	1

Management

First Aid

The goals of medical management are to preserve brain function and to prevent additional brain injury. The primary focus is on maintaining the supply of oxygen and glucose to brain:

- ❖ The patient's airway, breathing, and circulation must be maintained. A nasal or oral airway must be inserted. Ventilation and supplementary oxygen should be given, if necessary. Systolic BP is maintained between 100 and 160 mm Hg to maintain adequate cerebral perfusion.
- ❖ Raise leg approximately 20–30 cm to improve blood flow to brain.
- ❖ Loosen the tight cloth.
- ❖ If pregnant lady become unconscious, if possible place her left side.

Coma Cocktail

Although the treatment of coma depends on the cause, there are some general treatment rules. If the cause is unknown, what is often called "coma cocktail" is given to the patient it is a mixture of thiamine "a vitamin that helps in alcoholic or nutritionally starved patients." Glucose is used to correct hypoglycemia and naloxone (a substance that reverses the action of many narcotics and is used to treat overdoses).

- ❖ ***Correcting for electrolyte imbalance or toxic substance:*** Electrolytes are chemical like salts such as sodium and chlorine salt that are found in blood and throughout the body, and plays an important role in most physiological processes. IV fluids are administered to correct electrolyte imbalance.
  Renal dialysis, for example, is done to remove toxins and normal electrolyte balance of kidneys.
- ❖ ***Decreasing ICP:*** If coma is related to increased pressure in the brain, there are various things that can be done to reduce it, including hyperventilation, diuretics, and surgery.

Surgical Management

It is done to correct any structural deformities of brain, which lead to increase ICP, e.g. hemorrhage evacuation, meningioma excision, etc.

Urinary Catheterization

It is the treatment of urinary incontinence.

Antibiotic Management

It is done for any underlying infections and for prevention of diseases.

Nursing Management

Ineffective airway clearance related to altered level of consciousness.

Objective: Maintains effective airway clearance.
- ❖ ***Interventions:***
  - ➤ The unconscious should be placed in side-lying position to prevent tongue fall.
  - ➤ Suction the nose and throat to clear airway.
  - ➤ To prevent drying of mucous membrane of mouth and nose apply moistened swab or mineral oil. Humidification of air is also effective.
  - ➤ Endotracheal tube insertion.
  - ➤ Elective tracheotomy and mechanical ventilator, if necessary.

Deficient fluid volume is an inability to take in fluids by mouth.

Objective: Patient maintains adequate fluid volume.
- ❖ ***Interventions***
  - ➤ Administer IV fluids.
  - ➤ Insert an NG tube and provide feed 100–200 mL every 2–3 hours.
  - ➤ Gastrostomy feed can be given, if unconsciousness is prolonged.
  - ➤ Maintain I/O chart.

Impaired tissue integrity of cornea is related to diminished or absence of corneal reflex.

Objective: Maintains tissue integrity of cornea.
- ❖ ***Interventions***
  - ➤ Remove contact lenses to avoid injury to cornea.
  - ➤ Check cornea several times a day.

- If cornea reflex absent or any irritation or partially closed cover with an eye pad.
- Provide eye irrigation with physiologic solution of Nacil.
- Administer antibiotic eye ointments.

Ineffective thermoregulation related to damage to hypothalamic center.

Objective: Maintains effective thermoregulation.
- ❖ ***Interventions:***
  - Check rectal temperature every 4 hours.
  - Check for any underlying infections such as urinary tract infection (UTI) and pneumonia.
  - Ice bag can be applied to groin and axilla.
  - Administer aspirin and acetaminophen through NG tube.

Impaired urinary elimination (incontinence or retention related to impairment in neurologic sensing and control).

Objective: Maintains proper urinary elimination pattern.
- ❖ ***Interventions***
  - Provide more fluids through NG tube.
  - Insert a Foley catheter or condom catheter.
  - Check the output in volume.
  - Watch for any dysuria.
  - Clean the area of catheter daily.

Risk for injury related to decreased level of consciousness.

Objective: The patient remains free from injury.
- ❖ ***Interventions***
  - Observe the patient every 30 minutes.
  - Do not leave the patient alone for a long time.

Risk for complication, venous thrombosis related to decreased circulation secondary to immobility.

Objective: Patient maintains proper circulation.
- ❖ ***Interventions***
  - Patient must not left in position that restricts circulation to any part of the body.
  - Change positions every 1–2 hours will improve circulation.
  - Bony prominences should be protected from direct pressure.
  - Bed linen should be always dry and wrinkle free.
  - Administer antiembolism stockings.

Interrupted family processes related to health crisis.

Objective: Patient maintains good family environment.
- ❖ ***Interventions***
  - Listen to family members and to help to explore their thoughts.
  - Teach family to provide sensory stimulation (touch and speech), while staying at bedside.
  - Involve family members in giving care to the patient like positioning.
  - Put side rails of bed to prevent fall.
  - Care should be taken, while applying hot water bags or heating pads.
  - Care should be taken to prevent mouth injury, while suctioning and mouth case.

Risk for impaired skin integrity related to immobility.

Objective: Patients maintain skin integrity.
- ❖ ***Interventions***
  - Apply water bed or alphabed.
  - Bath with warm water daily.
  - Apply oil or moistening lotion to prevent drying of skin.
  - Avoid crumbles in bed and wet linen.
  - Comb hair and shampoo at least every 2 weeks.
  - Finger and toe nails cut every 2 weeks.
  - Change positions every 1–2 hours.
  - Provide back care and massaging over pressure points.

Complications

Many complications can be caused due to immobility and unconsciousness:
- ❖ Respiratory failure due to fall of tongue or due to secretions
- ❖ Pneumonia or infections
- ❖ Pressure or ulcers
- ❖ Aspiration
- ❖ Deep vein thrombosis
- ❖ Musculoskeletal deterioration
- ❖ Disturbed GI function.

Conclusion

Unconscious is a major problem, which requires complete observation and care. For easy recovery of the individual and prevent complications, nurses who are involved in the care of unconscious should provide physical and psychological care by focusing on touch and verbal communication, while ensuring that any clinical needs are met.

SLEEP PATTERN AND ITS DISTURBANCES

Introduction

A good night's sleep and a hearty laugh are the best for many illnesses. Moreover, if we want to be in good mood the whole day we need to sleep well and long enough. All sleep experts have the same opinion on this, unfortunately in this busy present day, fast paced world most of us feel that we cannot spend so much time for sleeping. Motivational orators encourage us to spend less time sleeping and more time working. But to be energetic and refreshed throughout the day, one must have enough good quality sleep.

Definition

Sleep

Sleep can be defined as a normal state of altered consciousness during which the body rests. It is characterized by decrease responsiveness to the environment, but a person can be aroused from sleep by external stimuli.

Sleep Pattern Disturbance

Sleep pattern disturbance is a nursing diagnosis that is defined as a disruption of sleep time that causes discomfort or interferes with a desired lifestyle.

PHYSIOLOGY OF SLEEP AND AROUSAL

A daily rhythmic activity cycle, based on 24-hour intervals, that is exhibited by many is called "circadian rhythm." The timing of sleep-wake cycle and other circadian rhythms such as body temperatures is controlled in part by the suprachiasmatic nucleus in the anterior hypothalamus located above the optic chiasm. This area receives input from the retina, which provides information about darkness and light. The suprachiasmatic nucleus controls the production of the hormone melatonin, which is believed to be a potent sleep inducer.

Arousal from sleep, wakefulness, and the ability to respond to stimuli rely on an intact RAS. The RAS is located in the brainstem and contains projections to the thalamus and cortex. The diffused network of neurons in the RAS is in a strategic position to monitor the ascending and descending stimuli through feedback loops. The neurotransmitters of the RAS serve as chemical messengers regulating the sleep–wake cycle and the stages of sleep. The onset of sleep and of each subsequent sleep stages is an active process involving delicate shifts in the balance of several of these neurotransmitters.

The transmission from the awaken state to a nonrapid eye movement (NREM) sleep is marked by decrease in concentrations of serotonin, norepinephrine, and acetylcholine and further decreases in serotonin and norepinephrine. As rapid eye movement (REM) sleep continues the concentrations of serotonin and norepinephrine increases eventually stopping REM sleep. The release of acetylcholine seems to reestablish REM sleep. The continuous interaction of these two systems produces the normal alterations between NREM and REM sleep. Other neuron transmitters such as gamma aminobutyric acid (GABA) and dopamine may be involved in the reciprocal process in shift sleep stage.

All these neurotransmitters are also actively involved in the waking process. For example, neurons that produce serotonin and norepinephrine play a role in the modulation of sensory input, mood, energy, and information processing including attention, laming, and memory. Imbalance in these neurotransmitters induces sleep pattern disturbance.

STAGES OF SLEEP

There are several different stages of sleep that people go through each night in which REM sleep and NREM sleep occurs. By EEG we can see the brain wave activities as person passes through delirious stages of sleep and to determine what type of sleep the person has entered.

A person who is wide awake and mentally active will show a brain wave pattern on the EEG called beta waves. Beta waves are very small and very fast. As the person relaxes, and gets drowsy slightly larger and slower alpha waves appear. The alpha waves are eventually replaced by even slower and larger waves.

Stage 1: NREM

- As theta wave activity increases an alpha wave activity fades always, people are said to be entering stage one sleep.
- This stage lightest level of sleep
- This stage lasts for few minutes
- Respiration begins to slow and muscles relaxes
- Person is easily aroused by sensory stimuli such as noise
- If awakened at this stage, person always claims that they were not asleep at all.

Stage 2: NREM

- Theta wave still predominates in this stage, but if people are awakened during this stage they will be aware of having been asleep.
- It is a period of sound sleep.
- The body temperature continues to drop, heart rate slows, and breathing becomes more shallow and irregular.
- Relaxation progresses.
- Arousal is still easy.
- This stage lasts for 10–20 minutes.

Stage 3: NREM

- The slowest and largest waves makes their appearance, these waves are called delta waves.
- In this stage, delta waves make up only 20–50% of the brain wave pattern.
- This is the initial stage of deep sleep.
- Sleeper is difficult to arouse and rarely moves.
- Muscles are completely relaxed.
- Vital signs decline, but remains regular.
- This stage lasts for 15–30 minutes.

Stage 4: NREM

- Once delta waves account for more than 50% of total brain activity. The person is said to have entered stage 4 sleep, the deepest stage of sleep.
- During this stage, growth hormones are released from the pituitary gland and reach their peak.
- It is the deepest stage of sleep.
- It is very difficult to arouse sleepers.
- Sleep lasts for approximately 15–30 minutes.
- Sleep walking and enuresis may occur.

REM Sleep

- After spending some time in stage 4, the sleeping person will go backup through stage 3, stage 2, and then into a stage in which the eyes move rapidly under the eyelids. The body is almost as aroused as in awakening state and the brain waves resemble beta waves.
- 90% of dreams actually take place in REM sleep.
- People have dreams in other NREM, but REM dreams tends to be more vivid, more detailed, longer and more bizarre than dreams in NREM sleep.

Factors Affecting Sleep

Factors that promote sleep in one person may hinder sleep in another. A single factor may not be the only course for a problem. Physiological, psychological, and environmental factors can alter the quality and quantity of sleep.

Physical Illness

Any illness that causes pain, physical discomfort such as difficulty in swallowing, anxiety, or depression can result in sleep problems. Person with such alterations may have trouble falling or staying asleep. Illness also forces clients to sleep in positions to reach they are unaccustomed. Assuming as awkward position while in traction, for example, can interfere with sleep.

Respiratory disease often interferes with sleep. Clients with chronic lungs disease such as emphysema are shortness of breath and frequently cannot sleep without two or three pillows to raise their head. A person with a common cold has nasal congestion, sinus drainage, and a sore throat, which impair breathing and the ability to relax.

Coronary heart disease is characterized by episodes of sudden chest pain and irregular heart rates. Clients with these diseases are often afraid to go to sleep because of the fear of heart attacks at night. Heart attacks occur more often during REM sleep. Death from heart disorder frequently occurs at night between 5 and 6 am, when REM sleep lasts longer.

Nocturia

Urination during night disrupts sleep and the sleep cycle. This condition is most common in older people with reduced bladder tone or person with cardiac disease, diabetes, urethritis, or prosthetic diseases. After a person awakens to urinate, returning to sleep may be difficult.

Older adults often experience "restless leg syndrome," which occurs during the presleep stage. People experience recurrent, rhythmical movement of the feet and legs. An itching sensation is felt deep in the muscle. Relief comes only from moving the leg, which prevents relaxation and subsequent sleep.

Drugs and Substances

Various types of drugs affect the pattern and quality of sleep such as diuretics cause nocturia, beta blockers cause insomnia, hypnotics interfering with reaching deeper sleep stage, etc.

Medications prescribed for sleep often causes more problems than benefit. Young and middle adults may rely on sleeping medications to deal with lifestyle stresses. Older adults often take a variety of drugs to control or treat chronic illness and the combine effects of several drugs can seriously disrupt sleep.

Lifestyle

A person's daily routine may influence sleep patterns. An individual working a rotating shift (e.g., 2 weeks of daytime work followed by a week of nighttime work) has difficulty adjusting to the altered sleep schedule. The body's internal clock might be set at 11 pm, but the work schedule forces sleep at 9 am instead. The individual often can sleep only 3 or 4 h because the body's clock perceives that it is time to be awake and active. Only after several weeks of working a night shift does a person's biological clock adjusts. Other alterations in routine that can disrupt sleep pattern include performing unaccustomed heavy work, engaging in late night social activities and changing evening meal time.

Sleep Pattern

The pattern and adequacy of sleep experienced each day affect a person's functioning. The most significant cause of daytime sleepiness is inadequate or abnormal sleep at night. Everyone has an increased sleep tendency from 2 to 7 am and to a lesser degree from 2 to 5 pm. For example, single vehicle accidents related to the driver falling asleep at the wheel occurs most often between midnight and 4 am. Sleep deprivation may result in difficulty in performing tasks and remaining active. Chronic lack of sleep is much more serious than temporary sleep deprivation and can cause serious alterations in the ability of daily functions.

Emotional Stress

Worry over personal problems of situations can disrupt sleep. Emotional stress causes a person to be tense and often leads to frustration when sleep does not come. Stress may also cause poor sleep habits.

Older clients frequently experience losses that lead to emotional stress. Retirement physical impairment, death of a loved one, and loss of economic security are examples of situations that predispose older adults to anxiety and depressions. With emotional stress older adults experience delay in falling asleep, earlier experience of REM sleep, frequent awakening, increase total bedtime, and early awakening.

Environment

The environment has a significant influence on the ability to fall and remain asleep. Good ventilation is essential for restful sleep. The size, firmness, and position of the bed can affect the quality of sleep. Sound also influences sleep. The level of noise needed to awaken people depends on the state of sleep. Low noises are more likely to arouse a person from stage one sleep whereas louder noises awaken people in stage 3 or 4 sleep. Some persons require silence to fall asleep whereas some prefer noise such as soft music.

Light level may affect the ability to fall asleep. Some clients may prefer a dark room whereas others such as children keep a soft light on at all times. Clients may also have trouble sleeping depending on the temperature of the room. A room that is too warm or too cold causes a client to become restless. Sleeping at temperature higher than 24°C causes poor quality sleep.

Exercise and Fatigue

A person who is moderately fatigued usually achieves restful sleep specially, if the fatigue is the result of enjoyable work or exercise. Exercising 2 hours before bedtime allows the body to cool down and maintain a state of fatigue that promotes relaxation. However, excess fatigue resulting from exhausting or stressful work can make falling asleep difficult.

Caloric Intake

Weight loss or gain influence sleep pattern. When a person gains weight sleep periods becomes longer with fewer interruptions. Weight loss can cause short and fragmented sleep. Certain sleep disorders may be the result of semistarvation diets popular in a weight conscious society.

Need for Sleep

Sleep is believed to have a restorative and protective function. During sleep sympathetic activities decreases while parasympathetic sleep may increase. Hormonal shifts facilitate anabolic process.

Rapid eye movement sleep may be especially important for maintaining mental activity such as learning, reasoning, and emotional adjustments. Sleep also appears to serve as energy conserving measure for most of the body except for the brain.

Normal Sleep Pattern

Sleep duration and quality vary widely among persons of all age groups (Table 32.6).

Table 32.6: Normal sleep pattern.

Age and condition	Average amount of sleep per day (hours)
Newborn	Up to 18
1–12 months	14–18
1–3 years	12–15
3–5 years	11–13
5–12 years	9–11
Adolescents	9–10
Adults	7–8 (+)

Neonates

A neonate's averages 16 hours of sleep a day with a range of up to 18 hours. For the first week, the neonate sleeps almost constantly to recover from birth. Approximately 50% of the sleep is REM sleep. This is essential for development because the neonate is not awake long enough for significant external stimulation.

Infants

Sleep patterns vary among infants. Active infants typically sleep less than less active infants. Infants usually develop a nighttime pattern of sleep during 3–4 months of age. The infants may take several naps during daytime, but usually sleeps an average of 8–10 hours during the night. Awakening commonly occurs early in the morning although it is not unusual for an infant to be awakened during the night. A large infant sleeps longer than a smaller one because of greater stomach capacity. An infant between 1 month and 1 year of age sleeps an average of 14 hours a day. REM sleep is predominant.

Toddlers

By the age of 2, children usually sleep through the night and take daily naps. Total sleep averages 12–15 hours/day. Naps may be eliminated at 3 years. It is common for toddlers to awaken during the night. The percentage of REM sleep begins to fall because toddlers have access to variety of meaningful external stimuli.

Preschoolers

An average preschooler sleeps about 11–13 hours a night and rarely takes naps. The preschoolers usually have difficulty relaxing after long active days. A preschooler also has problem with bedtime fears and nightmares. Parents are most successful in getting a preschooler to bed by establishing a consistent bedtime ritual. A child should not be allowed to become manipulated with by sleeping with parents or by staying up past a reasonable hour. When nightmares occur parents should comfort the child's own bed.

School-age children

The amount of sleep needed during the school years is highly individualized because of varying states of activity and level of health. The school age child usually does not require a nap. A 6-year-old requires an average of 11–12 hours of sleep a night whereas an 11-year-old child sleeps about 9–10 hours.

Adolescents

An adolescent's day is usually active and mentally and physically exhausting. Often the desire to spend time with peers prevents adolescent to sleep. An adolescent requires an average of 9–10 hours of sleep a night. Because of staying up late, an adolescent frequently sleeps late in the morning.

Young adults

Healthy young adults require rest and sleep to participate in the busy activities that fill their days. However, it is common for busy lifestyles to interrupt. Most young adults average 7-8 hours of sleep a night, but this can vary. It is unusual for young adults to take regular naps. Approximately 20% of sleep time is spent in REM sleep, which remains consistent throughout life.

Middle adults

During adulthood, the total time spent sleeping at night begins to decline. Also the amount of stage 4 sleep begins to fall continuing throughout older age. Sleep disturbances are common. Insomnia is particularly common because of the changes and stresses of middle age. Sleep disturbance can be caused by anxiety, depression, or certain physical ailments. Women experiencing menopausal symptoms may have insomnia. Members of this age group may rely on sleeping medication.

Older adults

The total amount of sleep does not change as age increases. However, quality of sleep deteriorates and REM sleep shortens. There an older adult has almost no stage 4 sleep. An older adult awakens more often during the night and total wake time increases. It may also take more time for an older adult to fall asleep. The changes in an older person's sleep pattern are due to changes in CNS that affect the regulation of sleep. Sensory impairment, common with aging, may reduce sensitivity to time cues that maintain circadian rhythms. An older adult's chronic illness may also impair the quality of sleep.

Sleep Disorders and Management

Dyssomnias

Dyssomnias include sleep disorders characterized by difficult initiating or maintaining sleep (insomnia) or by excessive sleepiness. The disorders may arise predominantly from within the body (intrinsic), from external sources (extrinsic) or from disruption of circadian rhythm.

Intrinsic sleep disorders

1. **Insomnia:** Insomnia is defined as difficulty with initiating or maintaining sleep. It is a symptom of clients who have chronic difficulty in falling asleep. The insomniac complains of insufficient quantity of sleep. Insomnia may signal and underlying physical or physiological disorders. This disorder is primary insomnia. To differentiate it from insomnia that is secondary to another sleep disorder, it specifies the symptoms must be of or at least 1 month duration and must cause significant impairment in social, occupational, or other important areas of functioning and must be to the direct effects of a substance, a general medical condition, or a mental disorder. Primary insomnia may be manifested by a combination of difficulty falling asleep and intermittent wakefulness during sleep. This disorder often becomes a vicious cycle when the individual becomes more and more distressed by the inability to achieve sleep and the additional stress in turn contributes to insomnia.

   Management of insomnia: It is complex. Clients often feel that they have already tried the usual intervention to promote sleep. Sleep habits can become increasingly erratic, client tries to sleep during the day to compensate for sleeplessness at night. Relaxation exercise can be helpful, but initially they should be practiced at times other than bedtime. In this way, by the time the exercises are introduced at bedtime, they are effective. Cognitive behavioral therapy has become an established approach for treating people with insomnia.

2. **Narcolepsy:** Narcolepsy is one of the disorders characterized by excessive daytime sleepiness. The client also experiences disturbed nocturnal sleep and repeated episodes of almost irresistible daytime drowsiness followed by brief periods of sleep especially when engaged in monotonous activities.

   Medical management: Medical management of narcolepsy usually consists of low doses of stimulants such as modafinil (Provigil) or methylphenidate (Ritalin). Emphasize on good sleep hygiene. They should maintain regular naps at times when clients are prone to increase sleepiness. Safety is a major issue for these clients.

3. **Sleep apnea syndrome:** Sleep apnea is characterized by association of breathing for 10 seconds or longer, occurring at least 5 times per hour. It can be classified as obstructive CNS apnea and mixed.

   a. *Obstructive sleep apnea syndrome:* In this case, respiratory efforts of the diaphragm and intercostal muscles are apparent, but infective against a collapsed or obstructed upper airway. Snoring indicates partial obstruction. Escalating snoring followed by a silent pause that ends with a gasp of snort probably indicates complete airway obstruction. As hypoxia ensures the person eventually awakens to breathe. The frequent awakening impair the normal sleep cycle.

   Management: The application of continuous positive airways pressure (CPAP) by means of a face mask covering the nose is the treatment of choice. The CPAP device provides room air under increased pressure, essentially providing a pressure splint to keep the upper airway open. It should be turned on whenever the client is ready to go to sleep and should be maintained throughout the sleep period. Additional humidification may be necessary especially in dry climate.

   b. *Central sleep apnea syndrome:* It is characterized by apneic periods during which no apparent respiratory effort occurs. Central apnea involves defects in the brains respiratory control center. The impulse to breathe temporarily fails and nasal airflow, and chest wall movement ceases. Cheyne-Strokes respiration is common with this symptoms (i.e. alternating periods shallow and deep respiration). The oxygen saturation of the blood falls slightly. The condition is seen in clients with brainstem injury, muscle dystrophy.

Management: Continuous positive airway pressure is the usual treatment. As with OSAS sedative and hypnotic drugs should be avoided. In severe cases with CNS involvement, the use of diaphragmatic pacemaker or mechanical ventilation may be required.

4. **Periodic limb movement disorder:** Periodic limb movement disorder may also contribute to daytime sleepiness and frequent nocturnal awakenings. It is characterized by period ice episodes of repetitive, stereotypic leg or arm movements during sleep causing partial arousal. It is more common in elderly population.

    Management: Clonazepam, a benzodiazepine or baclofen, a skeletal muscle relaxant, may be ordered to diminish the magnitude of the movement and the frequency of arousals. The antiparkinsonism drug carbidopa-levodopa (sinement) and the tricyclic antidepressant imipramine seem to act more directly and almost eliminate the movements.

5. **Restless leg syndrome:** Restless leg syndrome involves annoying, crawling, itching, or tingling sensation in the legs while at rest and causes an almost irresoluble urge to move. This syndrome is often most severe before sleep onsets.

    Treatment is similar to that for periodic limb movement.

Extrinsic sleep disorders

The extrinsic sleep disorders encompass a range of factors from environmentally to chemically induced disorders such as:

1. Inadequate sleep hygiene
2. Environmental sleep disorder.

Management: Extrinsic sleep disorder can be managed by:
1. Maintaining a consistent and a regular bedtime routine
2. Avoiding stimulants such as caffeine
3. Adequate sleep.

1. ***Circadian rhythm sleep disorders:*** In the general population, the circadian rhythm sleep disorders, such as time zone change syndrome and shifts, work sleep disorder are not uncommon. Older and clinically ill clients who live alone may be vulnerable to irregular sleep–wake pattern. In this disorder, prolonged ignoring or absence of external cues to time such as regular mealtimes, work periods, and daylight leads to erratic periods of sleeping and wakefulness. Internal circadian cues may also be damped as a result of aging or diffused brain disease.

2. ***Hospital-acquired sleep disturbance:*** Clients in the hospital may report difficulty getting to sleep, awakening frequently with difficulty getting back to sleep or early morning awakening. The etiologic mechanism and intervention range with the types of difficulty.

3. ***Sleep onset difficulty:*** Sleep onset difficulty is a common problem in hospitals because of the strange environment, noise, and the anxieties associated with illness and hospitalization.

    Management: Environmental controls, such as reduction of noise and interruptions, and conservative relaxation measures, such as back rub, should be given before restoring to a hypnotic agent. The rapid acting hypnotics, as Zolpidem are most effective with this type of insomnia.

4. ***Sleep maintenance disturbance:*** Sleep maintenance disturbance may be associated with sustained use or withdrawal from a variety of medication and related to substance. Alcohol hastens sleep onset, but leads to awakening later in the night. In acute intoxication, REM sleep is suppressed. Abrupt withdrawal, as occurs with hospitalization, may trigger massive REM rebound. Sustained use of or withdrawal from antidepressants, monoamine oxidase inhibitors, propranolol and phenytoin can also contribute to insomnia.

    Management: To reduce nocturnal stimuli by darkening the clients room, reduce as much noise as possible, etc. adjusting the temperature by providing bed covering according to the clients preference and by modifying room temperature such as by closing certain or adjusting ventilations.

5. ***Early morning awakening:*** Early morning awakening occurs frequently among older clients. Sensitivity to environmental disturbances increases toward morning in people of all ages, but even more so in older adults.

    Management: It can be treated by finding out the underlying cause for, such as delirium, depression, etc. Treating underlying cause will treat it.

6. ***Sleep deprivation:*** Sleep deprivation is a particular concern for clients in critical care units. The noise level, 24-h lighting, and frequency of caregiver interruptions create sensory overload and sleep deprivations. Clients who have had surgery are also at a risk of sleep pattern disturbance because of disruption of the circadian rhythms. The cause is unclear, but the disruptions may be related to the length and type of anesthesia, postoperative analgesia, or mechanism associated with the procedure itself.

Diagnostic Assessment

The primary diagnostic test for sleep disorders is polysomnography. Polisomnography is a comprehensive recording of the biophysiological changes that occurs during sleep. It is usually performed at night, when most people sleep, though some laboratories can accommodate, shifts

workers and people with circadian rhythm sleep disorders. The PSG monitors many body functions including brain (EEG), eye movement [electrooculography (EOG) and muscle activity electromyography (EMG)]. Clients may also have continuous recording of:
1. Arterial oxygen saturation by year or finger oximeter
2. Air flow as detected by monitoring expired carbon dioxide
3. Respiratory movement by means of transducers placed the chest and abdomen
4. ECG
5. Heart rate determination with standard limb leads.

A multiple sleep latency test (MSLT) may also be performed to assess impairment of daytime alertness. The MSLT is performed the day after a standard overnight polysomnogram. The time required for client to fall asleep when in a relaxed state is evaluated at 2-hour interval with each nap limited to 20 minutes. The type of sleep is also assessed making the test particularly useful in diagnosing narcolepsy.

Actigraphy, which is based on the fact that, in general, considerably fewer limb movements occur during sleep than during wakefulness. It consists of a movement detector and considerable memory storage.

PAIN

Introduction
Pain is a complex experience consisting of a physiologic response to a stimulus followed by psychologic response to that event. Pain is a multidimensional phenomenon and is difficult to define; pain is more than a system rather a problem. Pain is experienced by every person to some degree. It is unpleasant feeling of an individual and entirely subjective. Only person experiencing pain can describe or define. Pain accompanies many disorders. Pain is one of the major chronic problems in people with cancer. Relief of pain and discomfort is one of the goals of nursing intervention and, one that requires skill in both the art and science of nursing. It requires knowledge about concepts related to pain and useful therapies.

Meaning
Pain has different meanings for each person, which may differ for the same person at different times. In general, most persons view pain as a negative experience, but some may express pain as harm or damage, complication such as infection, new illness, loss of mobility, etc.

Definition
According to the International Association for the Study of Pain define that,
   "It is an unpleasant sensory and emotional experience associated with actual or potential tissue damage or described in terms of such damage."

Physiology
Pain is transmitted and perceived is still incompletely understood.

Pain Receptors and Stimuli
Pain receptors, called nociceptors, are free nerve endings of unmyelinated or lightly myelinated afferent neurons. Nociceptors are located extensively in the skin and mucosa and less frequently in selected deeper structures, such as viscera, joints, arterial walls, and bile ducts. Nociceptors respond to harmful stimuli that may be chemical, thermal, or mechanical. Chemical stimuli for pain include histamines, bradykinin, prostaglandins, and acids, some of which released by damaged tissues. The energy of these stimuli is converted to electrical energy. This energy conversion is known as transduction.

During this phase of stimuli (tissue injury), the release of biochemical mediators (e.g. prostglandins, serotonin, histamine, bradykinin) sensitize the nociceptors. Noxious or painful stimulation also causes movement of ions across cell membranes, which excite nociceptors. Pain medications can work during this phase of blocking the production of prostaglandin or by decreasing the movement of ions across the cell membrane.

Pain Transmission
Pain impulses are transmitted to the spinal cord by two types of fibers, i.e. thin myelinated faster-conducting A-delta fibers and slower-conducting unmyelinated *C fibers*. Pain that may be described as "sharp" or pricking and that can be easily localized results from impulse transmitted by the A-delta fibers. An example of this type of pain is that felt by a needle prick. *C fibers* transmit dull, aching pain. Lamina comprises an area called substantia gelatinosa (SG). Substance P is released at synapses in the SG and is thought to be a major neurotransmitter of the pain impulses. The pain impulse travels from the peripheral nerve fibers to the spinal cord through substance P of neurotransmitters enhancing the movement of impulses across the nerve synapse from primary afferent neuron to the second neuron. The most important ascending pathways for nociceptive impulses located in the ventral half the spinal cord are the spinothalamic tract (STT) and the spinoreticular tract (SRT). The STT is a discriminative system and conveys information about the nature and location of the stimulus to the thalamus, and then to the cortex for interpretation. Which go to the brainstem and part of thalamus activate the autonomic and limbic motivational-affective response.

Pain Perception
The third process is perception of pain when the client becomes conscious of the pain; it is believed that pain perception occurs in the cortical structures, which allows

for different cognitive behavioral strategies to be applied reducing the sensory and affective components of pain.

Pain Experience

The pain experience of every individual includes the perception of the pain sensation and the response to this perception. Tolerance to the noxious stimulus will influence both of these components:
- ❖ Stimulation of nociceptors:
  - ➢ Increased number of stimuli
  - ➢ Increased duration of the stimulus
- ❖ Alteration of transmission:
  - ➢ Damage to nerve endings
  - ➢ Inflammation, tumors or injuries to spinal cord
- ❖ Receptivity of cortex:
  - ➢ Inflammation, degenerative changes of brain
  - ➢ Depression of brain function
  - ➢ Anesthesia
- ❖ Interpretation in cerebral cortex:
  - ➢ Childhood training
  - ➢ Past experience with pain
  - ➢ Culture values
  - ➢ Religious beliefs
  - ➢ Physical and mental health
  - ➢ Knowledge and understanding
  - ➢ Attention and distraction
  - ➢ Fear, anxiety, tension
  - ➢ Fatigue
  - ➢ State of consciousness.

Pain perception therefore can be altered by usual activities, such as reading or socialization, as well as by abnormal conditions. Damaged nerve endings may not transmit pain sensation.

Pain Modulation

This fourth process occurs when neurons in the brainstem send signals back down to the dorsal horn of the spinal cord. Endorphins are thought to suppress pain by acting presynaptically to inhibit release of the neurotransmitter substance P or acting postsynaptically to inhibit conduction of pain impulses. These descending fibers such as endogenous opioids, serotonin and norepinephrine can inhibit ascending noxious impulses in the dorsal horn. These neurotransmitters are taken by the body, which limits the analgesic usefulness. The endogenous descending pain suppressive system is more effectively activated by nociceptive stimuli transmitted by A-delta fibers. Electrical stimulation by means of transcutaneous electrical nerve stimulation using low frequency and high intensity activates opiate analgesia. Acupuncture is also thought to use the opiate pathways.

Client with chronic pain may be prescribed tricyclic antidepressants, which inhibit reuptake of norepinephrine with serotonin. The action increases the modulation that helps to inhibit painful ascending stimuli.

Theories of Pain Transmission

Various theories of pain transmission have been proposed. The affect specificity and pattern theories that led to the development of the gate control theory. Although the gate control theory does not fully explain transmission, it serves as a base for understanding pain transmission.

Gate control theory: The gate control theory proposed by Melzack and Wall in 1965. The theory proposes that the SG in the spinal cord act as a gating mechanism to permit or inhibit passage of pain impulses, the gate can be closed (so that the contact is not made, thus interrupting the pain impulses) by nerve impulses from the large non-nociceptive A-beta and A-alpha fibers or from the descending pathways. Impulses conducted over large fibers not only close the gate but also are sent immediately to the cortex for rapid identification, evaluation, and modification of sensory inputs. Impulses sent to the brainstem, the center of motivational affective and sensory discriminative actions, can influence cognition or evaluation in the cortex. Impulses are then sent from the cortex back to the SG via corticospinal pathways to inhibit or permit passage of pain impulses.

Other Theories of Pain Transmission

- ❖ *Affect theory:* Pain is an emotion and its intensity depends on the meaning of the part involved does not include physiological aspects.
- ❖ *Specificity theory:* Specific pain receptors project impulses over neural pain pathways to the brain does not accounts for psychological aspects of pain preceptors and variability of response.
- ❖ *Pattern theory:* Pain results from combined effects of stimulus intensity and summation of impulses in the dorsal horn of spinal cord does not account for psychological aspects.
- ❖ *Gate control theory:* Pain impulses can be controlled by a gating mechanism in the dorsal horn of the spinal cord to permit or inhibit transmission. Gating factors include effect of impulse transmitted over fast or slow of descending impulses from the brainstem and cortex (Fig. 32.7 and Table 32.7).

Types of Pain

Pain is categorized according to characteristics include duration, location, intensity, and etiology (Fig. 32.8).

Pain Duration

Acute pain

It is very common daily occurrence and is usually defined as sudden onset, of relatively short duration, and of temporary mild-to-severe intensity. Pain in response to injury or another stimulus that resolves when the injury heals or the stimulus is removed. For example, a prick of the finger, appendicitis—pain is relieved after surgery.

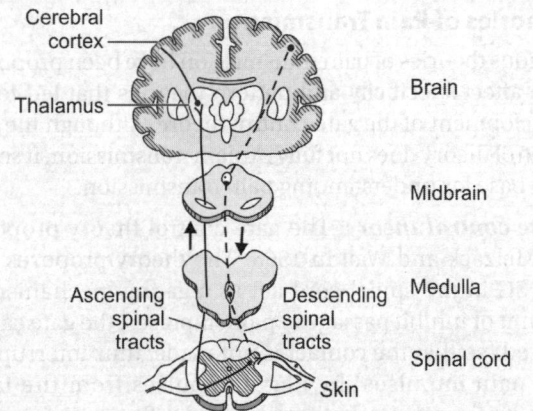

Fig. 32.7: Pathways of pain transmission to and from the cortex.

Table 32.7: Factors affecting pain transmission based on the gate control theory.

Site	Close gate (block transmission)	Open gate (permit transmission)
Fibers	Impulses transmitted by large fast myelinated	Impulses transmitted by slow small A-delta and C fibers. Stimulation of affected skin areas, e.g. sunburned skin
Brainstem (descending pathways)	Alpha and beta fibres. Stimulation of unaffected skin areas, e.g. massage, endorphin effect, sufficient or maximum sensory input, e.g. distraction	No endorphin effect, insufficient sensory input, e.g. monotony
Cortex	Past experiences, feeling of pain control	Past experiences, anxiety

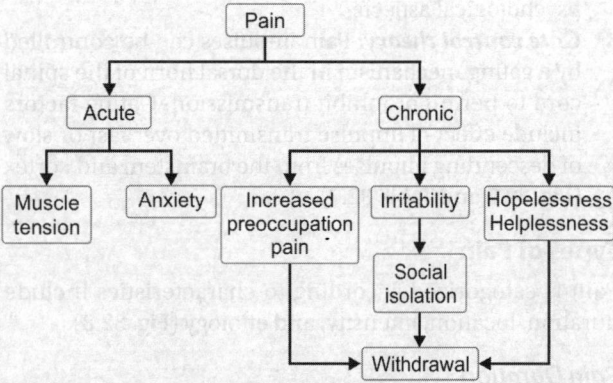

Fig. 32.8: Acute pain and chronic pain.

Chronic pain

Pain may be prolonged lasts for 6 months and interfere with normal functioning. It is long term; persistent type of pain which may remain primarily acute in nature.

Pain Location

Referred pain: It may appear when sensory fibers from the viscus enter the same segment of the spinal cord as somatic nerves, i.e. those from superficial tissues.

Pain appears from the originating areas

- ❖ *Visceral pain:* Normally the viscera all insensitive to cutting, burning, and crushing. The sensation of pain is dull, poorly located arises from hollow viscera.
- ❖ *Colicky pain:* Caused by muscle contractions of certain organs such as abdomen, uterus.

Pain Intensity

- ❖ Mild pain
- ❖ Moderate pain
- ❖ Severe pain.

Pain Etiology

- ❖ Physiologic pain
- ❖ Pathological pain.

Factors Influencing Pain

Pain is complex, involving physiological, social, spiritual, psychological, and cultural influences.

Physiological Factors

- ❖ *Age:* It is an important variable that influences pain; particularly infants are less sensitive to pain than older adults.
- ❖ *Ability:* Older clients with presence of multiple diseases express more symptoms of pain compared to adults.
- ❖ *Fatigue:* It increases the perception of pain.
- ❖ *Genes:* Recently research on animal models suggests that genetic information passed on by parents might increase or decrease the person sensitivity to pain.
- ❖ *Neurological function:* Awareness of a client on neurological function influence response to pain. For example, patient with spinal cord injury, peripheral neuropathy as in the case of DM.

Affective Factors

Clients with unrelieved pain often have concurrent emotional responses such as anger, fear, anxiety, sadness, or depression coping style that intensify pain perception.

Behavior Factors

When experiencing pain, express pain with many different behaviors. Patients may grimace, cry, rub the affected area, guard the affected area or immobilize it.

Others may moan, groan, grunt, or sigh. Not all clients exhibit the same behaviors and there may be different meanings associated with the same behavior.

Cognitive Factors

Exhaustion and lack of sleep contribute to a chronically fixed state, which may make it difficult to manage pain level of consciousness (sedation level), dementia, memory of past pain, source of motivation pain can dramatically influence the pain experienced.

Assessment of Pain Perception

The intensity and severity of pain can be measured by using different scales.

A Verbal Descriptive Scale

Verbal descriptive scale (VDS) consists of a line with three to six words descriptions equally and asks the client to choose the description that best represents the severity of pain.

A Numeric Rating Scale (Fig. 32.9)

The rate and scale of 0–10 represents no pain and 10 representing the worst pain. The scale worst best when assessing an individual client's pain intensity before and after therapeutic interventions to determine it is achieved.

A Visual Analog Scale (Fig. 32.10)

A visual analog scale (VAS) consists of a straight line without labeled subdivisions. The intensity of pain on a straight line of a scale has to be noted. A client indicates pain by marking the appropriate point on the VAS. This scale gives the client total freedom to identify pain severity.

Drawback

It cannot provide information on the emotional and sensory qualities of the client's pain.

Nursing Management

Assessment

1. Collect the health history and physical examinations and common signs and symptoms of pain.
2. History includes important nature of pain, onset, duration, location, intensity/severity, and record in pain scale.

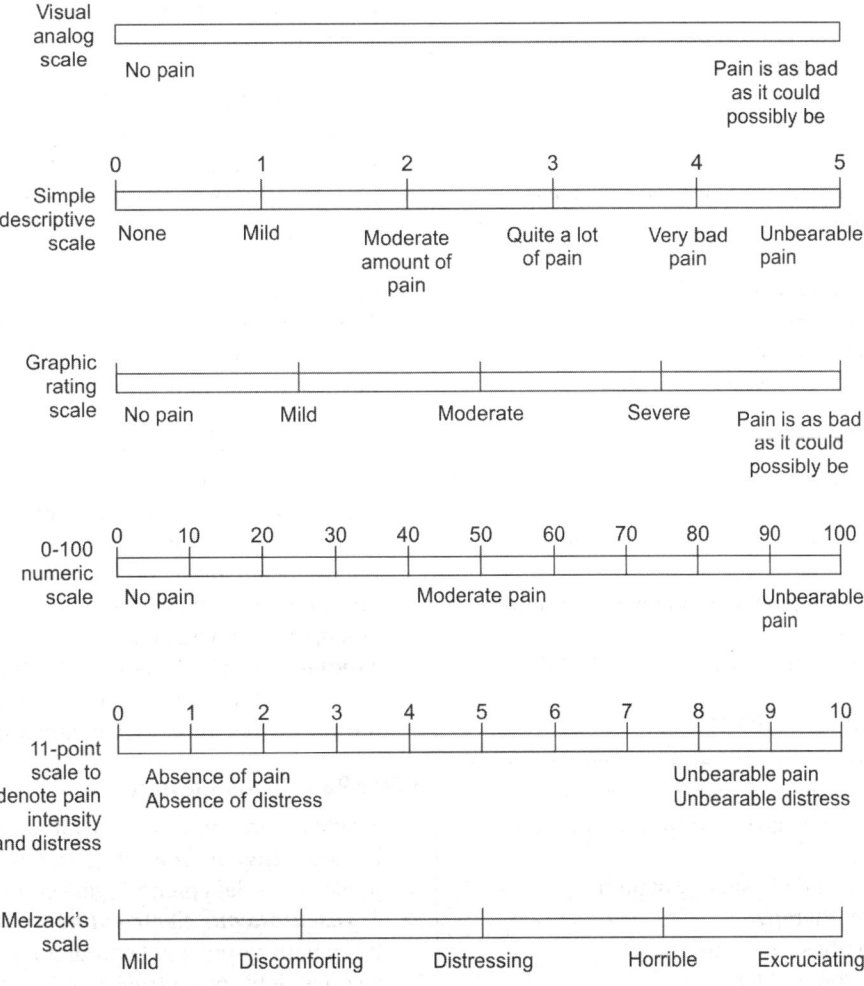

Fig. 32.9: Pain scale—visual analog scale (VAS), numerical rating scale.

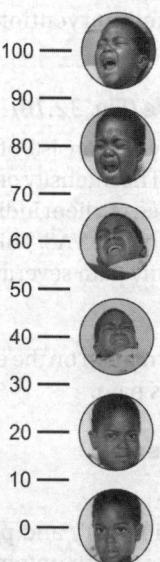

Fig. 32.10: Pain scale for children.

Physical Examination
- Assess vital signs.
- Inspect and observe. Note any behaviors of pain, painful area is assessed: warmth, edema, masses, enduration, tenderness, etc.

Nursing Diagnosis
- Anxiety related to increasing or threatened pain
- Ineffective breathing pattern related to pain in chest or abdominal
- Sexual dysfunction related to pain
- Self-care deficit related to pain
- Impaired physical mobility related to pain
- Sleep pattern disturbance related to pain.

Expected Patient Outcomes
- Patient states pain is relieved or reduced to a mild level.
- Pain-related behaviors or signs are decreased or absent.
- Patient with chronic pain state plans to participate in ongoing therapies.
- States plan for increasing independence in ADL.

Common Nursing Interventions
- All pain tends to be assessed as acute pain or chronic pain by using different parameters (pain scale).
- Analgesics need to be given around the clock, if pain levels are severe.
- Explain the cause and physiology of pain.
- Provide diversion therapy.
- Reduce external physical stimuli.
- Allow to express the problem.
- Reassure the client.

Pharmacologic Approaches to Pain Management

Analgesics
Two groups of analgesics as well as adjuvant medications are important components of effective pain management:
1. *Opioid analgesics:* Narcotics such as morphine acts mainly on the CNS to alter the perception of pain.
2. *Non-opioids:* Such as aspirin block impulses mainly in the periphery and decrease inflammatory related pain by inhibiting the synthesis of prostaglandins.

Patient controlled analgesia: This one method of providing more adequate pain control with opioids is the system of PCA. The system consists of a syringe type infusion pump that is filled with the prescribed opioid and is piggybacked into IV injection part. PCA is activated when the patient pushes a button to release a set amount of opioid by bolus.

Nonsteroidal anti-inflammatory drugs (NSAIDs): NSAIDs act primarily by inhibiting prostaglandin synthesis. In lower doses, these drugs have analgesics properties. In higher doses, there is anti-inflammatory action in addition to analgesia.

Aspirin: Acetylsalicylic acid is the most widely used analgesic for mild-to-moderate pain.

Other Drugs for Pain Relief
- *Smooth muscle relaxants* may be given for pain from muscle spasms and include Propantheline bromide and drugs of the belladonna group such as atropine. For example, belladonna and opium suppositories are effective in relieving bladder spasms after prostatectomy.
- *Sedatives and antianxiety agents* are sometimes prescribed for persons with pain. These drugs do not have analgesic effect, but may permit relaxation and decrease anxiety, and thus prevent potentiation of pain.
- *Trycyclic antidepressants* such as amitriptyline produce analgesia at doses lower than those of depression. These drugs are useful in nerve injury pain.
- *Counter irritants* are over the counter (OTC) drugs that relieve local pain by producing counter irritation, e.g., ointments containing methylsalicylate (oil of wintergreen, oil of cloves, etc.).
- *Nonpharmacologic approaches to pain management:* This type of intervention can alter pain transmission, modify the response to pain and modify pain stimulus.

After Pain Transmission
- *Electrical stimulators:* They modify the pain stimulus by blocking or changing the pain stimulus with perceived as less painful (gate control theory).
- *Transcutaneous electrical nerve stimulator (TENS):* It is a battery-powered stimulator worn externally. It is a convenient, nonintrusive, nonaddictive type of pain therapy that can be learned easily by the patient.

- ❖ **Spinal cord stimulators:** It is similar to the TENS except that they are intrusive procedures. Instead of electrode placement on the skin, the electrodes are placed on or near the spinal cord this is done either surgically over the ventral surface of the spinal cord or percutaneously through the back into the epidural space.
- ❖ *Neurosurgical procedures*
  - ➤ **Neurectomy:** It is the severing of nerve fibers from the cell body.
  - ➤ **Rhizotomy:** Resection posterior nerve root before it enters spinal cord interferes with the ability to perceive heat or cold.
  - ➤ **Cordotomy:** Severing of ascending anterolateral pain conducting pathways of spinal cords.
  - ➤ **Sympathectomy:** Excision or destruction of one or more synthetic ganglia or nerves.
  - ➤ **Nerve block:** A nerve block involves the injection of substances such as local anesthetics or neurolytic agents.
  - ➤ **Acupuncture:** It is an ancient form of diseases treatment that can be used for pain relief. The local stimulation of large diameter fibers by the needles "closes the gate" to pain. Nursing intervention includes careful client assessment and teaching.

Modify Pain Response

- ❖ **Behavior modification:** Consists of a planned change in the way a person behaves. For example, one protocol for patients with chronic low back pain is to set a limit 10 minutes for daily discussion of their pain experiences.
- ❖ **Biofeedback and autogenic training:** Some persons are able to alter their body functions through mental concentration. In biofeedback training, a machine that monitors brainwave activity is used. The nurse should encourage and price the person's effort. In autogenic training, the same type of self-regulation is used to alter various autonomic nerves system functions, e.g. meditation, methods of concentration, etc.
- ❖ **Hypnosis:** This may be used when conditions are aggravated by tension and stress. Individuals are helped to alter their perception of pain through the acceptance of positive suggestions made to the subconscious. Many persons are able to learn self-hypnoses.
- ❖ Explanation of the problems.
- ❖ Decreasing anxiety.
- ❖ Reducing additional physical stimuli.
- ❖ Cutaneous stimulation such as backrub, lightly rubbing the affected area, application of heat or cold, etc.
- ❖ Reducing auditory and visual stimuli.
- ❖ Reducing social isolation.
- ❖ **Therapeutic touch:** This may be helpful to patient whose pain is clearly understood. This is carried out when nurse undergoes brief period of medication before coming in contact with the patient. In which, the nurse quiets his/her internal energy levels and then touches the patient and transmits healing energies.
- ❖ Distraction and relaxation exercises.
- ❖ **Waking imagined analgesia:** Imagining a pleasant situation when a noxious stimulus is applied.
- ❖ **Relaxation:** Full relaxation decreases muscle tension and fatigue that usually accompanies pain.

Conclusion

Pain is a complex universal, yet individualized, experience. Opioids provide relief of severe pain many nursing interventions modify pain stimulus.

SENSORY DEPRIVATION

Introduction

Sensory deprivation occurs when there is an absence, blocking or alteration in reception perception that reduces sensory input below the level necessary for healthy functioning. Each person has an optimal level of sensory input that facilitates a sense of well-being and optimal cognitive and motor performance. Sensory input comes from environmental and internal sources. Sensory input is received through peripheral receptors transmitted via afferent neurons up the spinal cord, and channeled through the hypothalamus to the cortex, where it is interpreted in relation to previous patterns of experiences.

Definition

Sensory deprivation is a state in which the overall sensory input is decreased. With the overall reduction in stimuli, persons become more sensitive to the stimuli that are present in the environment and often supplement it with increasing internal stimuli, such as by day dreaming of reminiscing.

Conditions with Sensory Deprivation

- ❖ Strokes, head injury, Alzheimer's disease
- ❖ Eye disease, trauma, and surgery
- ❖ Hearing loss
- ❖ Loss of tasty or smell sensation
- ❖ Loss of tactile sensation (spinal cord injury)
- ❖ Language barriers, unfamiliar culture, isolation, and paralysis
- ❖ Monotonous surroundings
- ❖ Medication effects—sedatives, narcotics
- ❖ Individuals with old age, burns, leprosy, deafness, blindness, and fever.

Clinical Manifestation

- ❖ **Lack of sensory perception related to** hearing, vision, touch, smell and taste
- ❖ **Psychological and emotional:** Anxiety, fear, irritability, restlessness, boredom, depression, labile affect, mood swings

❖ *Cognitive:*
  ➢ Loss of sense of time
  ➢ Impaired problem solving
  ➢ Impaired concentration, inability to organize thought, memory problems
  ➢ Reduced motor coordination
  ➢ Vivid sensory images dreams
  ➢ Presence of illusions or hallucinations
  ➢ Confusion, disorientation
  ➢ Sleep disturbances, excess sleeping
  ➢ Varied somatic complaints
  ➢ Changes in thought processing.

Management

❖ The nurse's most important tool is sensitivity and awareness of the member; varieties of stimuli present in the practice environment and the potential these stimuli on the patient's mental status. The patient's family should be involved. The family can play important role in helping to structure an adequately stimulating environment. The family is an excellent source of information about the patient's likes and dislikes concerning music, reading material, television, or other strategies to inverse meaningful stimulation, which are effective in relieving sensory imbalance, meaningless stimuli increase the patient agitation.
❖ Human contact is one of the most meaningful forms of stimulation; nurse should use professional presence as well as visitation by family and friends to ensure meaningful human contact.
  ➢ It involves collaborative planning to ease routine constraints on visiting.
  ➢ The nurse will briefly explain all tests and procedures to the patient to help the patient established some sense of control over the environment.
❖ Provide pleasing environment.
  ➢ Nurse can place immobilized patients near windows when possible.
  ➢ Use room lighting to reinforce the natural daily patterns at light and dark color. Into the room linens, curtains, rugs, paint and wall paper is helpful.
  ➢ Pictures, calendars, and clock with large numerals can help keep and can be regularly incorporated into orientation activities.
❖ The patient should be encouraged and assisted to use any aid to sensory reception such as glasses, hearing aids, and dentures.
  ➢ The use of radio, tapes, or television can help increase sound stimulation, but their use and effectiveness needs to be carefully assessed. The wrong amount or wrong type of music or television can be disturbing to the patient and negate and positive effects.
❖ Patients are encouraged to participate in their own self-care to the degree possible.

❖ It is important to keep things simple and not to expect the patient to engage in a lot of decision making.
❖ Room objects should be kept in the same places and not rearranged, and the patient's attention is regularly drawn to their location and placement.
❖ Patient should be kept informed whenever circumstances require a break in the established routine.
❖ Reorientation is ongoing every 2–4 h.
  ➢ It provides the patient with the security of knowing where they are and why a calm quiet approach is reassuring reorientation is addressed directly, but constant of the patient should be avoided.

Stress of Change in Body Image

Introduction

Body image represents the picture that each of us has of ourselves. Serious illness and injury can abruptly interfere with that self-concept. Adapting to the changes imposed by illness and affects one's sense of identity. A major disability can be viewed a limitation to be challenged on the other hand it may lead to a feeling of being "crippled."

Definition

Body image describes an individual's perception on his/her body how the person thinks he/she looks, rather than an objective assessment of the person's characteristics. Body image is a factor in determining an individual's self-image, self-concept, and self-esteem.

It is made up of person's perceptions of the body, both internally and externally it includes feeling and attitudes toward the body.

Conditions with body image disturbance: After breast cancer surgery, renal transplant, vulvectomy, anorexia nervosa, atopic-dermatitis, bulimia, burns, cancer patients, colostomy client, plastic surgery, arthritis, obesity, multiple sclerosis, injury, psoriasis, systemic lupus erythematosus, and amputation.

Clinical Manifestations

Psychological

Feelings of shame, inadequacy and guilt, threat to self-esteem, anxiety, and embarrassment upsetting.

In healthcare setting, people deal with numerous situations that threaten their self-esteem violation of modesty and invasion of privacy cause anxiety and embarrassment.

Physical

❖ Treatments such as radiation or chemotherapy affect appearance changes in secondary characteristics and growth of facial hair.
❖ Exposure of the body during physical examinations and treatments like enemas and catheterizations may distress client.

- The need for using a bedpan or talking about bowel and bladder habits threat to self-esteem
- Changes brought by a colostomy or ileostomy procedure
- Treatments like radiation or chemotherapy affect appearance
- Changes in body image may result from side effects of medication like development of moon face from taking steroids
- Changes in secondary sex characteristics and growth of facial hair
- Changes in body structure and functioning due to injury or surgical intervention
- Subtle changes in progressive conditions such as arthritis, obesity, etc.
- Normal changes in body such as pregnancy and puberty
- Sexual disability.

Management

- The first step in understanding the concept of body image is to become more aware of one's own attitude toward health, illness, disfigurement, and changes in body functioning.
- Anxiety, revulsion, and pity are common responses to abnormal body appearance and functioning.
- To care for patients, who have these conditions, nurses must come to terms with their own feelings.
- A nurse reacting adversely to a patient's appearance can have a damaging effect on the person's ability to adjust in a positive manner.
- The nurse needs to learn what the body change means to the individual and what adjustment will be required.

  In formulating the nursing care plan, it is important to assess the ability of the family to help the patient cope with changes, to determine how realistic the person is about the body change and to identify specific problems in coping and methods of coping.
- Frequent reactions include grief, mourning, and anger. Yet hope is essential and must be supported and encouraged as must efforts at rehabilitation.
- The nurse needs to determine ways of supporting the family and the method of responding to the patient's reactions.
- *Social adjustments:* The person has to accept the change in body image and feels worth, and accepted by caregivers or she must adjust to dealing with the outside world many people respond negatively when they encounter someone who is disfigured or incapacitated stare or ask intrusive questions about the person conditions or treat the person as if he/she was completely helpless, patients may need help in learning how to handle such situations.

Nursing Intervention

- Provide privacy and assist the client to express feelings.
- Support the client in expressing feelings of grief or anger related to changes in body image.
- Provide reliable information about altered appearance and its effect on physical functioning.
- Provide information about appropriate supportive devices or prosthesis.
- Clarify any misunderstandings the client may have regarding appearance.
- Support the client in effects to view and touch changes in body appearance support the client or efforts to adapt to changes in physical functioning.
- Teach significant others necessary skills for assisting the client.
- Offer praise and encouragement to the client and significant others.
- Teach client new self-care necessary for adaptation.
- Reinforce instruction in occupational and vocational skill necessary for adaptation.
- Provide information on resources available for assistance.
- Encourage the client to participate in social activities
- Praise and encourage the client, and significant others.

STRESS OF IMMOBILITY OR CONFINEMENT

Definition of Immobility

Immobility can be defined as an inability to occupy space, the life space, from anywhere in the wide world to the confines of an upstairs bedroom. Its causes may be as diverse as inability to afford a car or an aeroplane ticket to agoraphobia, deafness, fear of falling, or the severe restrictions imposed by arthritis or a stroke; the effects of restricted mobility on an individual are equally diverse. Immobility is usually considered as a restriction in everyday activity.

Conditions with Immobility

Joint problems especially osteoarthritis in women, neurological deficit; impaired balance, stroke, Parkinson's previous falls, sensory deprivation; impaired vision, cardiovascular and respiratory diseases, mental barriers, accidents, fracture (injury), unconsciousness, paralysis.

Reactions or Manifestations

People who are unable to carry out the usual activities related to their roles (husband, mother) become aware of an increased dependence on others. These factors lower the person's self-esteem. Frustration and the decrease in self-esteem may in turn provoke exaggerated emotional reactions. Emotional reactions vary considerably some individuals become apathetic and withdrawn; some regress and some become angry and aggressive. Because the immobilized persons' participation in life becomes much narrower and the variety of stimuli decreases, the person's reception of time intervals deteriorates. Problem solving and decision-making abilities often deteriorate as a result of lack of intellectual stimulation, and the stress of the illness and immobility. In addition, the loss of control over events can cause anxiety. Immobility can impair the social and motor development of young children.

Management

- Assist the client to express feelings about role changes support the client in grieving over role loss.
- Help the client differentiate perceived from actual role requirements provide resources for role modeling or instruction regarding role change.
- Demonstrate role behaviors that the client needs to learn.
- Provide opportunities for practicing new role behavior.
- Praise and encourage the client when success in new role performance is demonstrated.
- Provide opportunities for discussing new role.

SOCIAL ISOLATION

Introduction

About 200 years ago, children were raised in extended families that consisted of several generations of family members who lived in closed proximity to one another. Large families were desired, members were interdependent, and socialization was accomplished by passing traditions from one generation to the next. Dynamic public policy and social changes, together with demographic trends, including expanded opportunities for higher education, diverse awareness of employment, have changed family life. At the beginning of the 21st century, family structures are more varied than in the past. The small, traditional family unit known as the nuclear family remains prominent; however, more than one-fourth of family units now consist of children who live with a single parent, blended families, extended families, cohabitated families, and communal families. In such conditions, the person may feel isolated. Social isolation may result when family members are separated, communication within families is poor, or others do not accept the family or its members. Isolation may be physical or psychological. Today many nuclear families, single adults, and older adults are separated from their extended families because the young have sought employment elsewhere, people may feel isolated in a new town without the usual family support.

Meaning

Social isolation is a sense of being alone as a result of having fewer meaningful relationships. It may occur because of declining health or income, transportation problem or ageism whatever the cause, prolonged social isolation has been associated with declining health and higher mortality rates.

Causes of Social Isolation

- Social isolation may result when family members are separated, communication within families is poor, or others do not accept a family or its members.
- Separation may result from hospitalization, job commitment or going away to college.
- Daily demands of a job, parenting, home maintenance, college studies, and illness may overburden the person involved.
- Geographic disturbance or desire to be independent may make family contact difficult, increasing isolation.
- Older adults are facing their final years away from their children and grandchildren, and may be living alone after their spouse die. They may feel isolated by a society that values youth, e.g. old age ashram.
- Poor communication within a family can isolate individual members.
- Discrimination of race, color, religion, ethnic group, or stigma associated with illness such as acquired immunodeficiency syndrome (AIDS), the person may also be isolated.
- Multiple social losses or fear of loss may lead to social isolation.
- Prolonged grief after the loss of a spouse, sibling, child or close friend may make the elder hesitant to become involved in other close relationships.
- Elderly patients experiencing organic cognitive impairment (such as Alzheimer's disease and related disorders) often withdraw from social contacts, daily routines.
- Sensory deficits such as hearing or vision impairment can also contribute to isolation for the elderly.

Social Isolation among Human Beings

Many researchers have found the social isolation in several species, including rodents, birds, and dogs. Among human beings, studies of hospitalization and orphans indicate an apparently need for affectionate stimulation. Infants receiving only-minimal adult attention are often retarded physically, intellectually, and emotionally, although their nutritional and cleanliness needs have been well met. Evidence comes partly from the Skeels and Dye (1939) study, in which a group of orphans received considerable attention from many older women, all whom were institutionalized. A small, busy nursing staff cared for a comparable group. A few years later, the children who had received considerable playful attention showed significantly greater intellectual development than did the control group. Furthermore, as adults they were significantly more often employed, more often involved with family or friends and more advanced in education. It is also proved that adults need companionship. The most common underlying theme in self-destruction among the rich, the poor; and other social classes is a loss of ties to the family, to friends and to the community at a large. The suicidal individual perceives himself/herself as a stranger in the world, no longer integrated into the society. People sometimes feel isolated even in a crowd. Reports of loneliness are common among college students, for whom there is a large group of potential friends. The sense of competition in and after college is partly responsible for this feeling. Among young adults, the suicide rate has risen dramatically, almost 250%, in recent years.

Patterns of Social Isolation

There are two forms of isolation. Isolation may be a choice, the result of a desire to interact with others. Isolation may also be a response to condition that inhibits the ability or the opportunity to interact with others. Many older adults experience social isolation, and the degree of isolation experienced may increase with age. Some older adults withdraw from social interaction because of feelings of rejection. Society's attitude about what is attractive and attitudes about aging as unattractive result in feelings of rejection for some older adults. Some of the patterns of social isolation are:

- ❖ **Type 1:** Lifelong extravert isolated by condition or situation:
  - ➢ Ameliorate the situation to the greatest extent possible
  - ➢ Seek to bring in contact with individuals and groups through internet, distance learning
  - ➢ Assist to identify like individuals who may enjoy frequent telephone contact
  - ➢ Establish pen-pal network.
- ❖ **Type 2:** Retiree whose contacts were mostly through work and who is now bereft of socialization opportunities:
  - ➢ Seek ready-made groups with some shared interests, often similar to work skills and expertise
  - ➢ Interest person in volunteer activities that will use particular skills
  - ➢ Provide opportunities to express particular skills in arenas where others will appreciate abilities.
- ❖ **Type 3:** Active extrovert who withdraws later in life because of events causing shame, e.g., divorce, alcoholism, poverty:
  - ➢ Assist with grief resolution, suggest counseling, and seek support, self-help group
  - ➢ Help find resources addressing specific alienating condition.
- ❖ **Type 4:** Lifelong isolate
  - ➢ Assist in finding resources to augments areas of interest, hobbies
  - ➢ Initiate dyadic interactions if individuals are willing.

Characteristics of Social Isolation

The social isolation is loneliness experienced by an individual and perceived as a negative or threatened state imposed by others. The defining characteristics of social isolation are as follows:

Major

- ❖ Expressed feelings of rejection or aloneness imposed by others
- ❖ Absence of supportive others (family and friends)
- ❖ Inability to meet expectations of others
- ❖ Incommunicable, withdrawn, lack of eye contact
- ❖ Inappropriate or immature interests/activities for developmental age/stage.

Minor

- ❖ Expressed anger, feelings of indifference from others, or feelings of insecurity in public
- ❖ Preoccupation with own thoughts
- ❖ Shows behavior unaccepted by dominant cultural group
- ❖ Repetitive, meaningless actions
- ❖ Projection of hostility in voice, behavior
- ❖ Desire to be alone, existence in subculture.

Related Factors

Absence of satisfying personal relationships; alterations in physical appearance, mental status, lifestyle, or state of wellness inadequate or community resources and/or unaccepted social values.

Social Isolation Among Different Age Groups

Among Children (Fig. 32.11)

Children who have abusive parents, drug-dependent parents, parents who commit suicide or any other problem that is not considered "normal" may hide their secrets from the outside world and the child may not interact with the society and also child may become socially isolated leading to social isolation. Hence, always the child should be assessed for signs of social isolation such as:

- ❖ Assess the child for evidence of isolation from others; sad appearance, lack of response to smiles, crying, loss of interest in toys and surroundings.

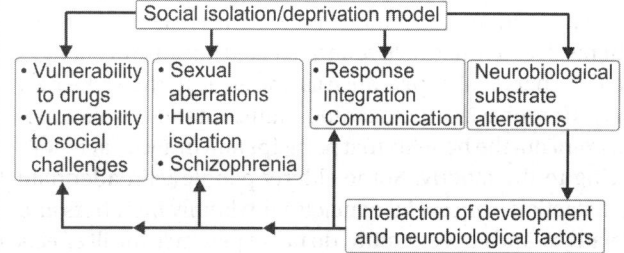

Fig. 32.11: Application of the social isolation-deprivation model of human psychopathology.

- ❖ Assess the child for child/parent relationship for bonding, eye contact, interaction, use of play materials, etc.
- ❖ Provide stimulation for child; colors, sounds, lights, toys, people, etc.
- ❖ Provide role model behavior showing "how to" stimulate and interact with the child.
- ❖ Utilize support person, e.g. "foster grandparent" to provide stimulation for child.
- ❖ Praise the child/parent when stimulation interaction occurs. Teach parents the need to provide stimulation for child. Based on growth and developmental needs.
- ❖ Initiate referral for family, if supportive care is needed.

Among Adults

Many young adults, having become accustomed throughout childhood and adolescence to depending on peers for companionship, experience loneliness from group of their peers. Those who were most popular during their school and college days, and who devoted much of their time to peer activities, find the adjustment to social isolation in adulthood especially difficult. Whether the loneliness comes from this isolation will be temporary or persistent depends on how quickly and how satisfactorily the young adults can establish new social contact to replace those of school and college days.

A competitive spirit and a strong desire to rise on the vocational ladder intensify isolation. To achieve success, they must compete with others thus replacing the friendliness of adolescence with the competitiveness of the successful adult and they must also devote most of their energies to their work, which leaves them little time for the socialization that leads to close relationships. As a result, they become self-centered, which contributes to loneliness.

Havighurst has explained that loneliness during the early adult years occurs because this is a relatively unorganized period in life, which marks the transition from an age graded to a social status graded society.

Among Older Adults

Many older adults experience social isolation, and the degree of isolation experienced may increase with age. Some older adults withdraw from social circles due to feelings of rejection. Society's attitude on attractiveness and generally considering aging as unattractive often results in feelings of rejection among some older adults. These older adults see themselves as unattractive and rejected because of changes in their personal appearance as one ages. Perhaps the best way to emphasize the hazardous nature of social isolation is to point out the benefits that participation in social activities bring to the elderly. Some elderly people gain adequate satisfaction from social contacts with family members and relatives, and consequently, do not experience the ill effects of social isolation. Studies on members in different types of voluntary association have revealed that active participation in social activities contribute greatly to psychological well-being and increase in life satisfaction.

Social Isolation Among Different Conditions

Among Clients Experiencing Grief and Loss

Social isolation occurs when the painful nature of grief causes those experiencing it to withdraw from their normal social support systems. These clients may have a sad, dull effect, be uncommunicative and withdrawn, express feelings of loneliness, and lack supportive others. Some people feel the need to display mastery of the situation or wish not to burden friends they may be afraid to test the strength of friendships. Social support is a major positive influence on the successful resolution of grief.

When external stimuli are decreased too much, the patient may lack distraction from the pain stimuli; thus pain perception is increased. Social isolation may occur for a variety of reasons; the serious nature of a patient's disease may necessitate being in a private room for an extended period, etc. each of the causes of isolation may have a different solution. In any event, careful assessment may indicate that social isolation is a problem for the patient.

Possible Nursing Intervention to Reduce Social Isolation (Table 32.8)

- ❖ Place the patient with a compatible roommate
- ❖ Plan frequent contact with health team members
- ❖ Facilitate visits by family and friends
- ❖ Help patient to be as comfortable as possible family and friends.

Among Clients with Burns

During the acute period of recovery from a major burn injury, the patient may experience a great deal of social isolation. Extensive bandaging and strict isolation procedures result in separation of the patient from the environment. Measures that bring the environment to the patient can reduce the social isolations. Visitors must be encouraged to look past the bandages and touch the patient. Tape recordings and videos of children or other family members that are unable to visit can be helpful. Other diversional activities such as music therapy and art therapy can be started as and when the patient's condition warrants.

Among Clients with AIDS

The psychological aspects of AIDS are devastating. The diagnosis of human immunodeficiency virus (HIV) infection, like a diagnosis of cancer, brings potential denial, fear, depression, and anger. The social stigma of AIDS, based on associations with homosexuality, IV drug abuse, and sexual transmission, cannot be minimized. One of the earliest issues that HIV-infected individuals face is sharing the information with significant others. Tremendous fear of family anger, rejection or abandonment is a real concern.

Table 32.8: Nursing process of a client with social isolation.

Outcome criteria	Nursing intervention	Rationale
• The client: Identifies factors/behaviors that produce social isolation • Formulates a plan to become more involved with others to reduce social isolation • Identifies community resources that will assist in decreasing social isolation	• Discuss with the client possible reasons for feelings of social isolation • Actively listen to the client • Encourage involvement in existing relationships reinforce efforts by the client and significant others to establish interaction • Suggest that the client form relationship with those who have common interest and goals • Encourage patients in developing relationships • Help the client become aware of strengths and limitations in communicating with others. • Encourage the sharing of common problems and honesty in presenting self to others • Give positive feedback when the client reaches out to others • Help the client to distinguish reality from perceptions • Schedule time to interact with the client • Discuss possibility of becoming involved in social and community activities. Provide information on community resources • Explore with the client the new interests and/or changing environment	• Identifying causes enables the nurse and client to focus on relevant interventions • Active listening facilitates expression of thoughts and feelings • Companionship is essential for physical and emotional well-being • Common interests and goals provide a basis on which to build a relationship • So that client does not become discouraged • This knowledge enables the client to make use of strengths and work on limitations if realistic • Failure to share self-honestly may be a barrier in forming relationships • The nurse should encourage the client to make the effort, especially if the clients perceived interventions as risky • Past isolation may have contributed to inability to interpret situations clearly • Interacting with the client provides support and stimulation • Becoming involved in these activities can offer a less person perhaps less threatening way to support system. These discussion may provide possibility of becoming involved stimulation and inventive to work on developing new relationships

Often families and friends who are struggling with their own anxieties and fears abandon the patient. When this happens, the nurse should try to assist the patient to find other sources of social support. HIV-infected individuals who have been exposed to contaminated blood or unknowingly through heterosexual relationship may feel unique and intense anger, and hostility. Their families and friends usually support these patients. Other persons who do not understand that HIV and AIDS are not spread by casual contact can isolate them.

Among Clients with Schizophrenia

Extreme anxiety about reality of others, often leads schizophrenic clients to withdraw from interaction and to isolate themselves. Some clients tolerate only a few moments of direct communication, whereas others can manage extended periods of contact. Assess the client's tolerance by briefly noting their contact with nurse and activities the client engages with others and when alone.

Nursing Diagnoses and Intervention of Social Isolation

Nursing Diagnoses

Aloneness experienced by an individual and perceived as a negative or threatened state imposed by others.

CONCLUSION

Social isolation is a sense of being alone and lonely as a result of having fewer meaningful relationships. Social isolation may result when family members are separated, communication within the family is poor, or others do not accept the family or its members. The social isolation can be reduced by encouraging the person to involved in existing relationships, reinforcing the efforts by the client and significant others to establish interactions. Perhaps the best way to emphasize the hazardous nature of social isolation is to point out the benefits that social belonging and participation in social activities bring to the person.

CHAPTER 33

Treatment Aspects: Pharmacological, Pre- and Postoperative Care Aspects

CHAPTER OUTLINE

- Concept of Perioperative Nursing
- History of Surgical Nursing
- Types of Surgery According to Urgency
- Purpose of Surgery
- Variables Affecting Surgical Problem Status
- Factors Influencing Surgical Outcomes
- Preoperative Nursing Care
- Preoperative Patient Admission
- Preparation of the Patient for Surgery
- Preoperative Phase
- Intraoperative Phase
- Postoperative Phase
- Anesthesia

■ DEFINITION

Perioperative nursing refers to the role of the operating room nurse provides preoperative and postoperative phases of surgery. It may take place in the hospital in a free-standing surgical center, in a surgical center attached to a hospital or in a physician office, or in ambulatory outpatient surgical units.

■ CONCEPT OF PERIOPERATIVE NURSING

- ❖ It is a fast-paced, changing, and challenging field to work.
- ❖ It is based on several characteristics including high quality teamwork.
- ❖ Effective and therapeutic concept common the client, client family, and the surgical team.
- ❖ Effective and efficient assessment in all phases.
- ❖ Advocacy for the client and family, cast containment.
- ❖ Nurse must practice good surgical asepsis.
- ❖ Thoroughly document care and emphasize client safety in all phases, e.g. atricarium muscle relaxant.
- ❖ Effective teaching and discharge planning are needed to prevent complications.
- ❖ It is based on the nursing process and the nurse is called upon to individualize strategies throughout perioperative period—admission and discharge.
- ❖ A client experiences a variety of stressors when facing surgery. The ability to establish an effective rapport with clients.

■ HISTORY OF SURGICAL NURSING

- ❖ Surgery became a medical specialty in the mid-19th century.
- ❖ Early surgeons had little knowledge of the principal aspects and anesthesia techniques were primitive and unsafe.
- ❖ 1840's anesthesia discovered and it made possible for surgeons to operate.

With the advent of antiseptic and later aseptic practices:
- ❖ Massachusetts General Hospital—first operating room edition for nurses in 1876.
- ❖ 1900s trend—operating room experience in each nurse's clinical instruction.
- ❖ 1956 association of operating room experience improvement nursing care of surgical clients.
- ❖ 1970s, change nursing education curriculum—eliminated operating room experience.
- ❖ However, today many schools experience, reinstituted clinical operating room experience.
- ❖ New development in the setting for operative procedures.
- ❖ Ambulatory surgery—outpatient or 1 day surgery is scheduled.
- ❖ 1995 cataract extractions, biopsies, cosmetic surgery.

Perioperative Care

Care that patients receive before, during, and after surgery.

—Barbaro

Surgery

Surgery is derived from the Greek words cheir and ergon, that is "hand and action" meaning work originating from hands. It is generally accepted that surgery is a branch of medicine to treat disease, injury, or congenital deformity by manual or instrumental operations.

Preoperative Phase

The preoperative period time that starts when patients are informed that surgery is necessary and ends when they are transported to the operating room:
- It may be short or long.
- One of the major factors affecting the length of preoperative period is the urgency with which surgery must be performed.
- The trend today is to keep the perioperative period as short as possible.

TYPES OF SURGERY ACCORDING TO URGENCY

- Optional surgery is performed at the request of patient—cosmetic purposes.
  - Elective—planned at the convenience of the patient, e.g. superficial cyst.
- Required surgery is necessary and should be done relatively, promptly, e.g. cataract.
  - Urgent surgery is required promptly within a day or two, e.g. malignant tumor if at all possible.
  - Emergency surgery is required immediately for survival, e.g. intestinal obstruction.

According to Stay in Hospital

Inpatient Surgery

Operative procedures performed on patient who overnight planned for who requires case more than 1 day and they receive instructions related to anesthesia and administers.

Outpatient Surgery

Operative procedure performed on patients who return home on the same day, ambulatory or same day of surgery.

Laser Surgery

- *Outpatient:* Advances in laser surgery.
- *Acronym:* Laser stands light amplification by the stimulated emission of radiation.
- Lasers convert a solid gas or liquid to light when focused the energy from light is converted to heat causing tissue to vaporize and bleeding vessels to coagulate. For example, carbon dioxide laser, argon laser, ruby laser.
- Laser surgery is used as alternative to many conventional surgical techniques attaching retina and revascularization ischemic heart muscle instead coronary artery bypass graft (CABG) surgery.

Advantages

- Cost effectiveness
- Reduced need for general anesthesia (GA)
- Smaller incisions
- Minimal blood loss
- Reduced swelling
- Less pain
- The decreased incidence of infections
- Reduced scarring
- Less time recuperating.

PURPOSE OF SURGERY

It is classified into:
- *Diagnostic:* Determine cause of symptoms biopsy.
- *Curative:* Remove a diseased body part or replace a body part to restore function—cholecystectomy.
- *Palliative:* Relieve symptoms without during disease—tumor resection associated with cancer.
- *Restorative:* Strengthen a weakened area—herniorrhaphy.
- *Cosmetic:* Improve appearance and change shape—mammoplasty face lift.
- *Preventive:* Removal of tissues before it causes problem.

VARIABLES AFFECTING SURGICAL PROBLEM STATUS

- Age: Old age
- Nutritional status: Malnutrition obesity
- Fluid and electrolyte status: Deficits or excess of
- Respiratory status: Acute respiratory infections
- History of chronic respiratory disease
- Cardiovascular status: History of pre-existing cardiac diseases
- Renal and hepatic status
- Neurological, musculoskeletal and integumentary status: Surgery position prolonged immobility
- Endocrine and immunological status diabetes immunosuppressive
- Medication: Chemical dependency.

Surgical Procedure Suffixes: Surgery Urgency Levels

- Ectomy: Removal by cutting
- Orrhaphy: Future or repair
- Oscopy: Looking into
- Ostomy: Formation of a permanent artificial opening
- Otomy: Incision or cutting into
- Plasty: Formation or repair.

Preoperative Phase

- Assist in data collection for developing the patient plan of care.
- Reinforce explanation and instructions given.
- Provide emotional support to patient and their family.

FACTORS INFLUENCING SURGICAL OUTCOMES

Emotional Responses

- Fears related to anesthesia
- *Age:* Older adult
- Hydration and nutrition
- Pain control
- Smoking and alcohol
- *Gerontological issues:* Mobility, respiratory functions, bowel function, urinary function, and delirium.

PREOPERATIVE NURSING CARE

Terminologies

- *Early ambulation:* Assisting the patient to get out of bed and to walk as soon after a surgical procedure as it is possible.
- *Embolus:* A dislodged blood clot that travels in the bloodstream.
- *Evisceration:* The separation of a wound with exposure of body organs.
- *Shock:* The reaction of the body to inadequate circulation or circulatory collapse.
- *Singultus:* Hiccups.
- *Thrombophlebitis:* Inflammation of a vein usually in the leg generally associated with the presence of a blood clot.
- *Thrombus:* A blood clot adhering to the wall of a blood vessel.
- *Trendelenburg position:* The position of the patient in bed with the feet elevated and the head lowered.

PREOPERATIVE PATIENT ADMISSION

Assessment

Subjective and objective data are collected:
- Data collection
- Personal and family history, physical assessment—fever, dentures, capped teeth, and any risk factors
- Problems with anesthesia
- Medication—allergies
- Diabetic patients on insulin
- Patient with oral steroid therapy
- During dependence
- Anxiety or fear related and potential change in body image
- Deficient knowledge related to lack of prior experience surgical routines and procedures.

Informed Consent

The clients are commonly fearful and anxious regardless of whether surgery is performed conventionally or using laser. The physician is responsible for providing information (criteria for informed consent). The client gives permission after an explanation of the risk, benefits and alternatives. A signed form witnessed by a nurse is evidence that consent has been obtained:

- If an adult client is confused or mentally incompetent, the client's spouse or nearest blood relative or someone of desirable power of attorney for the client's health care must sign the consent form.
- If patient under the influence of mind-altering drug or alcohol intoxication, the patient has delayed onset until drug is metabolized.
- Substituted judgment.

PREPARATION OF THE PATIENT FOR SURGERY

- Physiological preparation
- Physical preparation
- Psychological preparation.

Physiological Preparation

Nursing Assessment

- Admission procedure
- Surgical risk factors increase likelihood of complications are extremes of age, diabetes, cardiopulmonary disease, dehydration, malnutrition, drug and alcohol abuse, obesity, bleeding tendencies, smoking, low hemoglobin and red cells blood counts, anxiety, elevated temperatures, abnormal laboratory data, current infectious diseases, significant deviations in vital signs or pregnancy postpone/cancel the surgery
- Vital signs
- All laboratory investigations blood and radiological.

Preoperative teaching

- **Deep breathing:** It is a form of controlled ventilation that opens and fills small air passages in the lungs and reduces postoperative complications. This is especially good for patient who received GA/or breathe shallowly after surgery due to pain. For example, atelectasis, airless, collapsed lung, pneumonia (lung infection) and hypoxemia. Nurse should practice deep breathing patients before they undergo surgery by inhaling deeply using the abdominal muscles holding the breath for several seconds and exhaling slowly pursing the lips may extend the period of exhalation. Incentive spirometers are also used.
- **Coughing:** Impaired ventilation is accompanied by thickened respiratory secretions. Coughing is a natural method for clearing secretions from the airways:

- Deep breathing may produces coughing although forced coughing (purposely) may not be necessary for all patients who have thick sputum.
- All patients should receive instructions about the technique.

Performing forced coughing
- Sit up right
- Take a slow deep breath through the nose
  - Make the lower abdomen rise as much as possible
  - Lean slightly forward
  - Exhale slowly through the mouth
  - Pull the abdomen in ward
  - Repeat, but cough three times in arco, while exhaling
  - Teach the patient to splint, incision and cough.
- **Leg exercise:** It helps to promote circulation and reduce the risk of forming thrombus (stationary blood clot) in the veins and circulatory complications:
  - Surgical patients have reduced circulation because of postoperative restriction of food, fluid, and blood loss during surgery.
  - Blood tends to pool in the lower extremities because of the stationary position during surgery and patient reluctance to move.

Performing leg exercise
- Sit with the head slightly raised
- Bend on the knee, raise and hold the leg above the mattress few seconds
- Straighten the raised leg
- Lower the leg gradually back to the bed
- Do the same with the other leg
- Rest both legs on the bed
- Point the toes forward the mattress and toward the head
- Move feet in clockwise and then counter clockwise circles
- Repeat five times at least every 24 hours while awake.

- **Antiembolism stockings:** Elastic stockings are knee high or thigh high elastic stockings. These help to prevent the development of thrombi and emboli (mobile blood clots) by compressing superficial veins and capillaries redirecting more blood to larger and deeper veins. Where it flows more effectively toward the heart (intermitted pneumatic compression device), enhances good venous return.

Physical Preparation

Physical preparation depends on the time of admission to the hospital or surgical facility the number may perform some physical preparation includes:
- Skin preparation attention to elimination
- Restriction of food and fluids
- Care of valuables
- Disposition of prosthesis.

Skin Preparation

Skin preparation involves removing hair and cleansing the skin that decrease reservoirs of microorganism and prevent wound infections. For planned surgery—cleanse the particular area soap for several days before surgery.

Elimination

Indwelling urinary catheter preoperative for some surgeries—a distended bladder increased risk of bladder trauma and difficulty in performing procedure:
- Enemas or a laxative may be ordered to clean the lower bowel. A clean bowel allows for improving visualization of the surgical site and prevents trauma to the intestine or accidental contamination of the abdominal cavity with feces.
- If bowel surgery is scheduled—antibiotics may be prescribed to destroy intestinal microorganisms.

Food and fluids

Specific instructions—to restrict food and fluids preoperatively:
- Fasting from food and H_2O from midnight onward before surgery is common.
- It is used to prevent aspirating stomach contents, while client is anesthetized.
- Nowadays elective clear fluids may be taken 2 hours before surgery, light breakfast 6 hours before surgical procedure or have heavier meals 8 hours beforehand.
- Encourage clients to maintain good nutrition and hydration before the restricted time to promote nutrients.

Care of Valuables

- Any valuables should leave at home or with family member.
- *Healthcare agency:* Personnel itemize their place in an envelope and lock designated area, client sign a receipt and nurse notes items where about in clients medical records.
- If the client is reluctant to remove a wedding band, the nurse may slip gauze under the ring or then loop the gauze around the finger and wrist or apply adhesive tape around a plain wedding band.
- Removes eyeglasses, contact lenses places in safe surgical attire.
- Wear a hospital gown and surgical cap to operating room.
- Knee high or thigh high antiembolism stockings or legs are wrapped in elastic roller bandages before surgery.
- Hair ornaments are removed to avoid injury and equipment used to administer oxygen and inhalant anesthetic.
- Make up and nail polish are omitted to facilitate assessing oxygen.
- If a client has acrylic nails is removed to attach pulse oximeter.

Dentures and Prosthesis

- Depending on agency policy and the preferences of the anesthesiologist or surgeon, the client removes full or partial dentures. Doing so prevents the dentures causing airway obstruction.
- Well-fitting dentures remain—communicated and documented.
- When dentures are removed—they are placed in denture containers and stored at the clients bedside or with clients belongings. Other prosthesis, such as artificial limbs, are also removed unless ordered.

Preoperative medication

Common preoperative medication includes one or more of the following:

- Anticholinergics decrease respiratory secretion, dry mucous membranes and prevent vagal nerve stimulation.
- *Antianxiety drugs:* For example, lorazepam (Ativan) reduce preoperative anxiety cause slight sedation slow motor activity.
- Histamine-2 receptor antagonists decrease gastric acidity and volume.
- *Narcotics:* Decrease the amount of anesthesia needed and sedate the clients.
- *Sedatives:* Such as midazolam promote sleep or conscious sedation and decrease anxiety.
- Antibiotics destroy entire microorganisms before administering preoperative medication. The nurse checks the client's identification bracelet—asks about drug allergies, obtains vital signs, and asks the client to void and ensures that surgical consent form has been signed.

Preoperative checklist is a form that identifies the status of essential presurgical activities and is completed before surgery. The nurse verifies the following for completing and signing the checklist shift the client accompany till OT.

- Universal protocol for preventing wrong site
- Wrong procedure and wrong person surgery
- Preoperative verification process
- Marking operation site
- Time out immediately before starting the procedure to be followed.

Psychological Preparation

Preparing the client emotionally and spiritually is as doing so physically. It begins as soon as client is aware that surgery is necessary. Anxiety or fear if extreme can affect a client's condition during and after surgery. Careful listening and explaining what will happen and what to expect told by the nurse. Religious faith—source of strength. Clergy person or hospital chaplain may involve according to hospital policies.

PREOPERATIVE PHASE

- Assist in data collection for developing the patient's plan of care.
- Reinforce explanation and instruction given to the patient and family by the physician and registered nurse (RN).
- Provide emotional support for patients and their families.
- Reassure the patient and family.
- Pad bony prominences to protect against pressure ulcers and muscle, and bone discomfort.
- Teach what to expect before, after surgery diet changes, description and length of the surgical procedure activities in the recovery room, pain management, cough, and deep breathing exercises, procedures, and treatment (e.g. catheters, dressing).
- Ensure preoperative screening: Blood tests, radiographic studies, nutritional assessment, pulmonary function tests, and electrocardiogram (ECG).

Nursing diagnosis

Anxiety or fear related to potential change in body image, hospitalization, pain, loss of control, and uncertainties surrounding surgery.

- *Expected outcome:* Patient will state reduced anxiety or fear.
- *Deficient:* Knowledge related to lack of prior inter-inform patient about experience with signs.

INTRAOPERATIVE PHASE

- Begins with transfer to operating room and ends with admission to postanesthesia care unit (PACU).
- After transfer: Prepare patient in room and necessary equipment so it is ready for the patient return.
- When the patient is transferred to the operating table. Surgery may take place in a hospital operating room or force standing ambulatory.

The operation team members must perform a sterile surgical hand scrub with antimicrobial soap to reduce the amount of microorganism on their hands and arms:

- Keep surgical field sterile.
- The operation room is designed to enhance technique; clean and contaminated areas are separated.
- Before the patient undergoes surgery, a nursing plan of care is developed from preadmission assessment data.

Intraoperative nursing diagnosis/expected outcome

- Risk for perioperative-positioning injury related to positioning, chemical, electrical equipment, and effect of being anesthetized force from injury.
- Risk for impaired skin integrity related to chemicals, positioning, and immobility skin integrity.
- Risk for deficient fluid volume related to NPO status and blood loss.

- Risk for infection related to invasion and invasive procedures.
- Pain related to positioning incision and surgical procedure.

Receiving room is a place in the surgery department where clients are observed until the operating room and surgical team are ready:

- In some hospitals, preoperative medication is administered when clients receive in the receiving room. Skin preparation is also delayed.
- The nurse greets the patient, verifies the patient name, age, allergies, surgeon performing the surgery, informed consent.

Surgical procedures—site—right or left, medical history, answers questions, and alleviates anxiety:

- Patient is introduced to anesthesiologist who also verifies patient information, allergies rechecked.
- Intravenous fluids are started—prophylactic antibiotics.

POSTOPERATIVE PHASE

Postoperative patient hospital room preparation

- Bed linen should be clean and changed as needed.
- Place disposable, absorbent, waterproof pads on bottom sheet if drainage is expected.
- Apply lift sheet on bed of patient needing assistance with repositioning.
- Have extra blankets available.
- Fanfold top cover to end of bed or side of bed away from patient.
- Obtain extra pillows if needed for positioning, elevating extremities, splinting during coughing.
- Obtain intravenous (IV) pole.
- Have emesis basin at bedside.
- Have tissues and wash clothes in room.
- Have urinal or bedpan available in room.
- Prepare suction setup for tracheostomy, nasogastric tube or drains as needed.
- Have oxygen setup needed.
- Obtain special equipment as indicated by the surgical unit.
- Have vital sign equipment available.
- Obtain documentation.

ANESTHESIA

Various types of anesthesia cause partial or complete loss of sensation with or without loss of consciousness. They include general, regional, and local anesthesia.

General Anesthesia (GA)

General anesthetics are drugs act on the central nervous system (CNS) to produce loss of sensation, reflexes, and consciousness. General anesthesia are commonly administered via inhaled and intravenous (IV) routes. The patient closely monitored—effective breathing and oxygenation effective circulatory status including blood pressure (BP) and pulse within normal ranges, effective temperature regulation and adequate fluid balance.

Regional Anesthesia

Regional anesthesia interferes with the conduction of sensory and motor nerve impulses to a specific area of the body. The client experiences loss of sensation and decreased mobility to the specific anesthetized area. For example, local and spinal anesthesia, epidural and peripheral nerve blocks decreased risk of complication.

Monitors

For allergic reactions, changes in vital signs toxic reactions.

Conscious Sedation

Refers to a state in which clients are sedated a state of relaxation and emotional comfort, but not unconscious. They are free from pain, fear/anxiety. For example, diagnostic and short therapeutic surgical procedures:

- Monitor IV medications
- Ensure client's safety and comfort
- No equipment replaces a nurse's careful observation.

Reversal Drugs

Medications that counteract the effects of those used for conscious sedation must be readily available, e.g. naloxone antianxiety.

Surgical Waiting Area

It is where the family and friends await information about the client. It is staffed by volunteers who provide comfort support and news about how client surgery is progress.

Transfer from Surgery

When surgery is completed and anesthesia stopped, the patient is stabilized for transfer. After local anesthesia, the patient returns directly to a nursing unit. Patient goes to PACU or intensive care unit (ICU).

Patient Safety

Patient is never left alone:

- Ensuring a patient alone.
- Patient should be prevented from falls and injury from uncontrolled movements.
- Nurses transfer the patient until perianesthesia nurse is able to receive the report and assure care of the patient.
- This begins the final patient perioperative phase the postoperative period.

Postoperative Phase

It begins after the operation procedure is completed and the client is transported to an area to recover from the anesthesia and ends when the client is discharged.

PACU is also known as postanesthesia reacting (PAR) room or recovery room. It is an area in surgical department where clients are intensively monitored. Nurses ensure the safe recovery of surgical clients from anesthesia.

Postoperative nursing care after surgery is different during the immediate postoperative period than it is later, when clients are more stable:
- Initial or immediate postoperative care
- Admission to the postanesthesia care unit

Postanesthesia nurse's goal is to promote safe recovery from anesthesia. The nurse's role in the PACU begins by receiving a patient report from the nurse. An assessment by nurse systematically checks the following:
- Level of consciousness
- Vital signs
- Effectiveness of respirations
- Presence or need for supplemental/oxygen respiratory status and potency of airway
- Condition of the wound and dressing
- Location of drains and drainage characteristics
- Location type and rate of IV fluid
- Level of pain and need for analgesia
- Presence of airway catheter and urine volume.

Preparing the room

When the client is in the PACU the nursing team who will continue caring for the recovering client is alerted. They prepare the room for next stage of care.

Monitoring for complications

Postoperative clients are at risk for many complications some of which are more likely soon after surgery. Frequent focused assessment of the client and equipment facilitate a safe postoperative recovery:
- *Airway occlusion:* Obstruction of throat, tilt head and lift chin, and insert an artificial airway.
- *Hemorrhage:* Severe rapid blood loss.
- *Shock:* Inadequate blood flow.
- *Pulmonary embolus:* Obstruction of circulation through the lung as a result of a wedged blood clot that began as a thrombus.
- *Hypoxemia:* Inadequate oxygenation of blood.
- *A dynamic ileus:* Lack of bowel motility.
- *Urinary retention:* Inability to void.
- *Wound infection:* Proliferation of pathogens at or beneath the invasion.
- *Dehiscence:* Separation of incision.
- *Evisceration:* Protrusion of abdominal organs through separated wound.

Continuing postoperative care

After surgery, the client needs to resume eating and to demonstrate adequate elimination, circulation, and wound healing.

Food and oral fluids

- Food and oral fluids are withheld until surgical clients are awake and free of nausea and vomiting and bowel sounds are active.
- Postoperative clients usually progress from clear fluid diet to a surgical soft diet to normal solid diet.
- Nurses monitor fluid intake and output to ensure that clients are adequately hydrated.

Venous circulation

- Surgical clients ambulate assistance as soon as possible to reduce the potential for pulmonary and vascular complication. After some surgical procedures, antiembolism stocking, leg exercises ambulation, and elevation of lower extremities may not be enough to reduce swelling of the lower extremities, and the potential for thrombus formation.
- For clients who are potential for impaired circulation in one or both device (machine that promotes circulation of venous blood and relocation of excess fluid into lymphatic vessels).

Nursing Diagnosis

- Deficient knowledge
- Fear
- Acute pain
- Impaired skin integrity
- Risk for infection
- Risk for deficient fluid volume
- Ineffective breathing pattern
- Ineffective airway clearance
- Risk for impaired gas exchange
- Disturbed body image
- Risk for ineffective therapeutic regimens' management.

Wound Management

Nurses assess the condition of the wound and characteristics of drainage at least once each shift. The following are:
- Change dressing or reinforce if they become loose or saturated.
- Eventually sutures or staples are removed by sixth or seventh day.
- Most hospitalized clients are discharged within 3–5 days of surgery.

Discharge Instructions

The nurse provides discharge instructions, directions for managing self-care and medical follow-up before the client leaves.

Common areas to address when discharging clients who have undergone surgery:
- How to care for the incision site?

- Signs of complications to report
- What drugs to use to relieve pain?
- How to self-administer prescribed drugs?
- When presurgical activity can be resumed?
- If and how much weight can be lifted?
- Which foods to consume or avoid?
- When and where to return for a medical appointment?

The nurse should give information verbally and in written form.

CONCLUSION

Nurse plays an important role in treatment aspects of a client especially during pre- and postoperative care. This is the critical time the client approaches healthcare facility. The client is prepared physically, psychologically before the surgery starts with as soon as client approaches nurse and spends a lot of time in care of a client to support, assist, and educate the client throughout the phases of his/her recovery.

34 CHAPTER
Cardiopulmonary Resuscitation

CHAPTER OUTLINE

- Resuscitation
- Cardiopulmonary Resuscitation
- Aftercare
- Risks
- Neonatal Resuscitation

RESUSCITATION

Introduction
Establishing spontaneous breathing after birth is most crucial for the survival of a newborn baby. Most babies have a smooth transition from fetal to neonatal life and they are able to establish spontaneous breathing without any active assistance. Effective resuscitation demands availability of at least two persons.

Meaning
Resuscitation is restoration to life or consciousness of one apparently dead or whose respiration has ceased.

Definition
Cardiopulmonary resuscitation (CPR) is a procedure to support and maintain breathing, and circulation on a person who has stopped breathing (respiratory arrest) and/or whose heart has stopped (cardiac arrest).

CARDIOPULMONARY RESUSCITATION

It is an emergency technique used during cardiac arrest to reestablish the heart and lung function until more advanced life support is available.

Conditions Demanding Resuscitation
The CPR should be performed if a person is unconscious and not breathing. Respiratory and cardiac arrest can be caused by allergic reactions, an ineffective heartbeat, asphyxiation, breathing passages that are blocked, choking, drowning, drug reactions or overdoses, electric shock, exposure to cold, severe shock, or trauma. The existence of certain high risks during pregnancy and labor may alert the labor room staff to be fully prepared to meet the asphyxiated baby.

Purpose
The purpose is to restore and maintain breathing and circulation and to provide oxygen, and blood flow to the heart, brain, and other vital organs.

Precautions
The CPR should never be performed on a healthy person because it can cause serious injury to a beating heart by interfering with the normal heartbeat.

Description
The CPR is part of the emergency cardiac care system designed to save lives. Many deaths can be prevented by prompt recognition of the problem and notifying the emergency medical system (EMS), followed by early CPR, defibrillation (which delivers a brief electric shock to the heart in attempt to get the heart to beat normally), and advanced cardiac life support measures:

- ❖ The CPR must be performed within 4–6 min after cessation of breathing so as to prevent brain damage or death.
- ❖ It is a two-part procedure that involves rescue breathing and external chest compressions. To provide oxygen to a person's lungs, the rescuer administers mouth-to-mouth breaths and then helps circulate blood through the heart to vital organs by external chest compressions.
- ❖ Mouth-to-mouth breathing and external chest compression should be performed together, but if the rescuer is not strong enough to perform both, the external chest compression should be performed. This is more effective than no resuscitation attempt, as is CPR that is performed 'poorly'.
  - ➤ When performed by a bystander, CPR is designed to support and maintain breathing and circulation

Chapter 34: Cardiopulmonary Resuscitation

until emergency medical personnel arrive and take over. When performed by healthcare personnel, it is used in conjunction with other basic and advanced life support measures.

➤ According to the American Heart Association, early CPR and defibrillation combined with early advanced emergency care can increase the survival rates of people with a type of abnormal heart beat called ventricular fibrillation by as much as 40%. CPR by bystanders may prolong life during deadly ventricular fibrillation, giving emergency medical service personnel time to arrive.

➤ However, many CPR attempts are not ultimately successful in restoring a person to a good quality of life. Often, there is brain damage even if the heart starts beating again. CPR is therefore not generally recommended for the chronically or terminally ill or frail elderly. For these people, it represents a traumatic and not a peaceful end of life. Each year, CPR helps save thousands of lives in the United States. More than 5 million Americans annually receive training in CPR through the American Heart Association and the American Red Cross.

In addition to courses taught by instructors, the American Heart Association also has an interactive video learning system, which is available to more than 500 healthcare institutions. Both organizations teach CPR the same way, but use different terms. It is recommended that family members or other people who live with people who are at risk of respiratory or cardiac arrest be trained in CPR. A handheld device called CPR Prompt is available to walk people trained in CPR through the procedure, using the American Heart Association guidelines. CPR has been practiced for more than 40 years.

Performing Cardiopulmonary Resuscitation

The basic procedure for CPR is the same for all people, with a few modifications for infants and children to account for their smaller size.

Performing CPR on an Adult

The first step is to call the EMS for help and then to begin CPR, following these steps (Figs. 34.1 and 34.2):
- ❖ The rescuer opens a person's airway by placing the head face up with the forehead tilted back and the

- Check for danger
- Stay with the person
- Call for help and start resuscitation

1 Airway
- Quickly turn person on side
- Remove foreign material from mouth
- Place neck and jaw in correct positions
- Listen for breathing
- Watch for chest movement

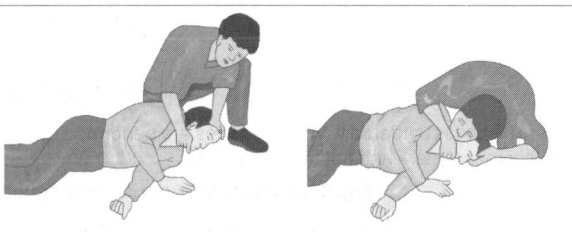

2 Breathing
If not breathing
- Quickly turn person on back
- Open airway
- Start mouth to mouth or mouth to nose
- 5 full ventilations in 10 seconds
- Check neck pulse
- If pulse is present, resuscitation at a rate of 15 per minute (one every 4 seconds) —check the circulation after 1 minute and then every 2 minutes
- If breathing returns: Place the person on side - keep the airway clear

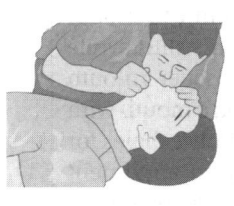 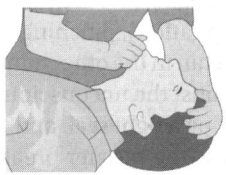

3 Compression
- Check neck pulse
If absent
- Begin external cardiac compression
- Place the heel of one hand on the lower half of the sternum
- Lock the other hand to the first by grasping wrist or interlocking fingers
- Keep fingers ot the chest
- Do 2 ventilations and 15 compressions every 15 seconds

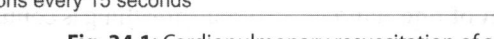

Fig. 34.1: Cardiopulmonary resuscitation of an adult.

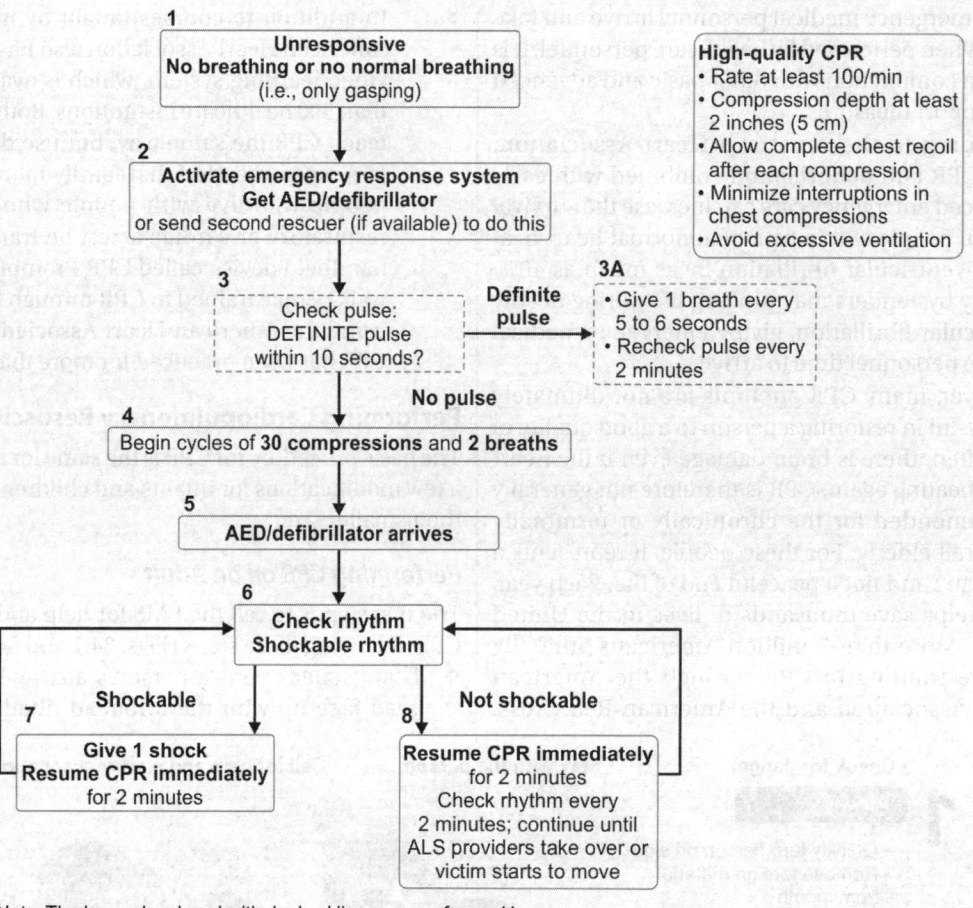

Fig. 34.2: Basic life support; cardiopulmonary resuscitation.
(AED: automated external defibrillator; BLS: basic life support; CPR: cardiopulmonary resuscitation)

chin lifted. The rescuer checks again for breathing (3–5 s), then begins rescue breathing (mouth-to-mouth artificial respiration), pinching the nostrils shut, while holding the chin in the other hand. The rescuer's mouth is placed against the unconscious person's mouth with the lips making a tight seal, and then gently exhales for about 1–1.5 s. The rescuer breaks away for a moment and then repeats. The person's head is repositioned after each mouth-to-mouth breath.

- After two breaths, the rescuer checks the unconscious person's pulse by moving the hand that was under the person's chin to the artery in the neck (carotid artery). If the unconscious person has a heartbeat, the rescuer continues rescue breathing until help arrives or the person begins breathing without assistance. If the unconscious person is breathing, the rescuer turns the person onto his/her side.
- If there is no heartbeat, the rescuer performs chest compressions. The rescuer kneels next to the unconscious person, placing the heel of one hand in the spot on the lower chest where the two halves of the rib cage come together. The rescuer puts one hand on top of the other on the person's chest and interlocks the fingers. The arms are straightened; the rescuer's shoulders are positioned directly above the hands on the unconscious person's chest. The hands are pressed down, using only the palms, so that the person's breastbone sinks in about 1 [frac12]–2 inches. The rescuer releases pressure without removing the hands, and then repeats about 15 times per 10–15 s intervals.
- The rescuer tilts the unconscious person's head and returns to rescue breathing for one or two quick breaths. Then breathing and chest compressions are alternated for 1 min before checking for a pulse. If the rescuer finds signs of a heartbeat and breathing, CPR is stopped. If the unconscious person is breathing, but has no pulse, the chest compressions are continued. If the unconscious person has a pulse, but is not breathing, rescue breathing is continued.

- ❖ For children over the age of 8, the rescuer performs CPR exactly as for an adult.

Performing CPR on an Infant or Child Under the Age of 8

- ❖ The procedures outlined above are followed with these differences.
- ❖ The rescuer administers CPR for 1 min and then calls for help. The rescuer makes a seal around the child's mouth or infant's nose and mouth to give gentle breaths. The rescuer delivers 20 rescue breaths per minute, taking 1 $\frac{1}{2}$–2 s for each breath.
- ❖ Chest compressions are given with only one hand for a child and with two or three fingers for an infant. The breastbone is depressed only 1–1 $\frac{1}{2}$ inch for a child and $\frac{1}{2}$–1 inch for an infant, the rescuer gives at least 100 chest compressions per minute.

AFTERCARE

Emergency medical care is always necessary after successful CPR. Once a person's breathing and heartbeat have been restored, the rescuer should make the person comfortable and stay there until emergency medical personnel arrive. The rescuer can continue to reassure the person that help is coming and talk positively until professionals arrive and take over.

RISKS

The CPR can cause injury to a person's ribs, liver, lungs and heart. However, these risks must be accepted if CPR is necessary to save the person's life.

Normal Results

In many cases, successful CPR results in restoration of consciousness and life. Barring other injuries, a revived person usually returns to normal functions within a few hours of being revived.

Abnormal Results

These include injuries incurred during CPR and lack of success with CPR. Possible sites for injuries include a person's ribs, liver, lungs, and heart. Partially successful CPR may result in brain damage. Unsuccessful CPR results in death.

Cardiac Arrest

Temporary or permanent cessation of the heartbeat.

Cardiopulmonary

Relating to the heart and the lungs.

Defibrillation

A procedure to stop the type of irregular heart beat called ventricular fibrillation, usually by using electric shock.

Resuscitation

Bringing a person back to life after an apparent death or in cases of impending death.

Ventricular Fibrillation

An irregular heartbeat where the heart beats very fast, but ineffectively. Ventricular fibrillation is fatal if not quickly corrected.

NEONATAL RESUSCITATION

Pathophysiology of Asphyxia

Birth asphyxia is associated with reduction in arterial oxygen tension, accumulation of carbon dioxide, and fall in oxygen and blood pH. These biochemical changes lead to right to left shunt with the perpetuating of birth asphyxia. Early phase of birth asphyxia—blood glucose (due to break on black board down of glycogen to glucose), but in severe hypoxia in preterm and growth retardation is associated with hypoglycemia. Hypothermia and hypoglycemia, accumulation of fatty acid and glycerol, anoxic damage to cells, release of potassium and phosphate in the extracellular fluid.

Assessment of Infant at Birth

Assessment of Apgar scoring system is conventionally used for assessing infant at birth, the condition of a newborn baby at 1 min after birth. The respiratory and heartbeat are crucial components in the Apgar scoring system because muscle tone, response to reflex stimulus, and color depends upon the gestational maturity and cardiorespiratory status (Table 34.1).

A normal infant in good condition at birth will achieve an Apgar score of 7–10. A score below seven indicates that baby requires some form of resuscitation.

Signs and Symptoms

The asphyxiated fetus initially behaves like a strangulated individual and makes violent efforts leading to exaggerated fetal movements, which is followed by reduced or absent fetal movements. Initially there is tachycardia follows by bradycardia and slow, and irregular heartbeats. And sphincter relaxes and the fetus may pass meconium.

Table 34.1: Apgar score.

Score/item	0	1	2
Breathing	Nil	Slow	Crying
Heartbeat	Nil up to 100	>100	
Tone	Flaccid	In between	Flexed
Reflex	Nil	Grimace	Sneezing
Color	Blue	Peripheral cyanoses	Pink

Gasping breathing movements triggered by hypoxia leads to aspiration of meconium stained liquor into the lungs.

Diagnosis

Diagnosis of asphyxia in intrauterine can be done by:
- Biophysical profile
- Oxytocin challenge test
- Nonstress test

Management of Birth Asphyxia

Clearing the Airway

The Apgar score is assessed in the normal manner at 1 min. The baby's airways should be cleared by gentle suction of the oro and nasopharynx and the presence of an apex beat verified. The baby should be placed in well-lit resuscitation area a flat and firm surface. The baby should be placed in a head low position to ensure drainage of oropharyngeal secretion. The mouth should be suctioned first followed by suctioning of the nose.
- The pressure of suction should be gentle and maintained at 100 mmHg.
- Sustaining should not be done for more than 5 s.

If the baby is not crying, he/she is gasping or having no breathing effort, must be given one or two flicks or slaps over the soles to stimulate breathing. If meconium is thick, then endotracheal suctioning should be done. The meconium stained baby should never be ventilated till the air passage is cleared.

Resuscitation Kit

The resuscitation kit/tray consists of a:
- Pencil handle laryngoscope with infant (0 and 1) blade
- Resuscitation bag and mask
- Endotracheal tubes (ETTs) with diameters of 2.5, 3, 3.5
- Suction catheters
- Syringes and needles
- Sodium bicarbonate
- Epinephrine in 10,000 solution
- Naloxone
- Oxygen cylinder should be working
- Sterile neonatal packs containing a bowl scissors, cotton swabs, and umbilical ties.

Bag and Mask Ventilation

If despite stimulation, the baby is still apneic (evidenced by heart rate less than 100). The baby should be given bag and mask ventilation. The mask should tightly fit on the face enclosing nose and mouth of the baby. The oxygen reservoir should be attached to the bag to increase the concentration of oxygen delivered to the baby. The infant should be ventilated at a rate of 40 breaths per minute. There should be a noticeable rise and fall of chest during each ventilation.

During bag and mask ventilation, heart rate should be closely monitored every 20-30 s. Record the heart rate for 6 seconds and then multiplied by 10.

If despite effective bag and mask ventilation heart rate is not coming up or it further slows down then chest compression is done.

Endotracheal Intubation

For endotracheal intubation, the size of the ETT to be selected according to weight and gestational age (Table 34.2).

Laryngoscope blade no. "0" for preterm and blade no. "1" for full term. The ETT should be prepared by shortening it to 13 cm and attaching connector. The ETT should be suctioned before starting positive pressure ventilation with a bag or machine. The ventilation can be stopped as soon as the baby establishes spontaneous breathing and heart rate is maintained above 100/min.

External Cardiac Massage and Medication

External cardiac massage is indicated in babies in whom heart rate drops below 60/min despite effective ventilation. The ventilation should be continued and simultaneously the heart should be massaged press the lower part of the sternum with rescuer's thumbs at the rate of 90 compressions and 30 ventilations in 1 min (3:1 ratio).

If heart rate is not picking up despite effective ventilation administer 0.5–1.0 mL of 1:10,000 solution of epinephrine through umbilical vein. The dose may be repeated after 10 min sodium bicarbonate 1–2 mL/kg of 7.5% solution administered IV.

Neonatal Resuscitation after Birth (Fig. 34.3)

After care of an asphyxiated baby

- Infant with birth asphyxia should be admitted to neonatal intensive care unit (NICU) for observation and management for 1–2 days. Neurological behaviors of the

Table 34.2: Selection of endotracheal tube according to weight and gestational age.

Weight	Gestational age	Size
1,000 g	28 weeks	2.5 mm
1,000–2,000 g	28–34 weeks	3.0 mm
2,000–3,000 g	34–38 weeks	3.5 mm
>3,000 g	>38 weeks	4.0 mm

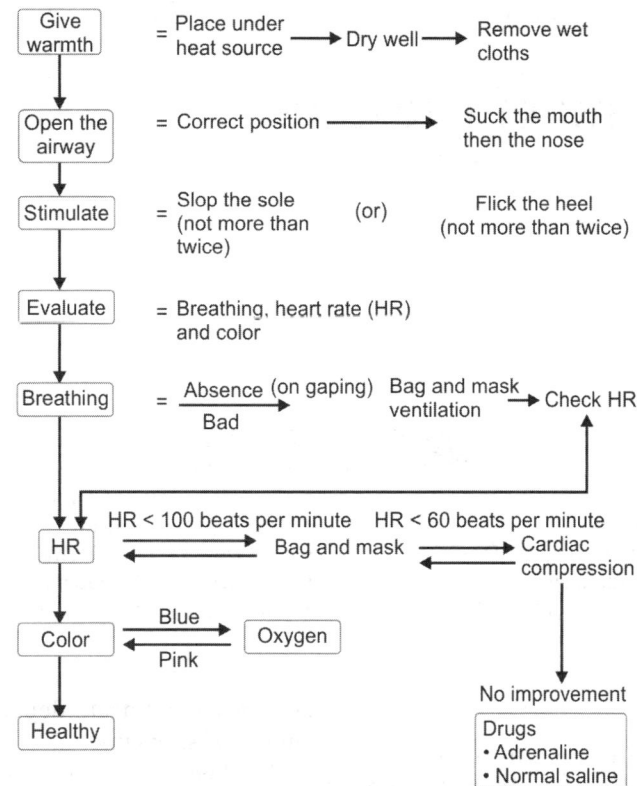

Fig. 34.3: Neonatal resuscitation.
(HR: heart rate)

infant should be closely watched until establishment of self-feeding.
* Provide opportunity to mother to see and hold her baby.
* Vitamin K 0.5–1.0 mg should be given 1 M.
* Provide opportunity for mother to see and hold her baby.

Complication of Resuscitative Technique
* Fractured ribs
* Injury to stomach
* Compression injury to the liver

CONCLUSION

Resuscitation is a life-saving emergency procedure. If done promptly, the patient's life can be saved. It is important as nurses to know the resuscitation technique to act during emergency.

35 CHAPTER

End-of-Life Care

CHAPTER OUTLINE

- Terminologies
- Concept of Death and Dying
- Changes in Healthcare Related to Dying and Death
- Standard for Healthcare in Providing End-of-life Care
- States of Awareness Manifested by Client and Family
- Common Fears and Concern of the Dying
- Journey toward Death
- 1–2 Weeks Prior to Death
- Journey's End: A Couple of Days to Hours Prior to Death
- Stages of Death and Dying

INTRODUCTION

Dying was once considered to be a normal part of the life cycle. Today, it is often considered to be a medical problem that should be handled by healthcare providers. Technological advances in medicine have led to depersonalized and mechanical care of those who are dying.

Our highly technological world calls for application of high-touch interventions with the dying. In other words, appropriate care of the dying should be administered by compassionate nurses who are both technically competent and able of impending death will prepare the nurse to render sensitive, effective care both to the client and family and to the client's body after death.

TERMINOLOGIES

- **Death:** The end of life of a person or organism.
- **Cessation:** Ending, termination, stopped breathing.
- **Hospice:** A home providing care for the sick, especially the terminally ill.
- **Palliative:** Relieving pain or alleviating a problem without dealing with the underlying cause.
- **Bereavement:** Deprived of a loved one through a profound absence, especially due to the loved one's death.
- **Burnout:** Physical or mental collapse caused by overwork or stress.

CONCEPT OF DEATH AND DYING

Dying is a part of living. It is the process of coming to an end. Death is inevitable conclusion of life. Death is the permanent cessation of all vital functions, the end of human life. The style of dying reflects a person's style of living and attitudes about death depend on a person's beliefs and emotional strengths.

In 1968, the world medical assembly adopted the following guidelines for physicians as indications of death:
- Total lack of response to external stimuli
- No muscular movement, especially breathing
- No reflexes
- Flat encephalogram
- In instances of artificial support, absence of brain waves.

Definition

End of life care is an important part of palliative care and usually refers to the care of a person during the last part of their life from the point at which it has become clear that person is in a progressive state of decline.

In medicine, end of life care refers to a medical care not only of patients in the final hours or days of their lives, but more broadly, medical care of all those with a terminal illness or condition that has become advanced, progressive, and incurable.

CHANGES IN HEALTHCARE RELATED TO DYING AND DEATH

- Before the 1950s, it was common for patients to die at home in their beds with assistance only from their family.
- From 1950s to 1980s, the healthcare system became highly mechanized and dying occurred mostly in institutions often with sophisticated equipment attached to the dying individual to prolong life.
- By the early 1980s, when diagnosis-related groups (DRGs) came into play, the trend again changed.

- Currently, only those patients who are considered medically at risk for complications or who need immediate hospital recovery time after surgery or special procedures are placed in hospital beds.
- The recuperating or terminally ill is often discharged to home, a convalescent center or a nursing home.

STANDARD FOR HEALTHCARE IN PROVIDING END-OF-LIFE CARE

- Providing appropriate treatment for any primary and secondary symptoms, according to the wishes of the patient and surrogate decision-maker
- Managing pain aggressively and effectively
- Sensitively addressing issues such as autopsy and organ donation
- Respecting the patient's values, religion and philosophy
- Involving the patient and the family in every aspect of care
- Responding to the psychological, social, emotional, spiritual, and cultural concerns of the patient and family.

Issues Related to Death and Dying
- Euthanasia
- Do not resuscitate (DNR)
- Advance directives
- Organ donations
- Rights of dying patients.

Euthanasia
Euthanasia in Greek stands for "easy death." Euthanasia may be:
- Active euthanasia
- Passive euthanasia

Active euthanasia is an action deliberately taken with the purpose of shortening life to end suffering or to carry out the wishes of a terminally ill patient.

Passive euthanasia is permitting the death of a patient that takes the form of withholding treatment that might extend life such as medication, life-support systems or feeding tubes.

The American Nurses Association (ANA) distinguishes relieving pain and euthanasia. Pain relief is central to nursing whereas euthanasia is viewed as unethical.

Do Not Resuscitate
- Patients and families should control any decisions relative to any conditions that withhold or withdraw treatment.
- A DNR decision should be a joint decision of the patient, family. All facts regarding the patient's condition should be explained to the patient and family as well as all treatment options.
- The DNR means is not only to resuscitate. It does not mean to withhold any other care such as hygiene, nutrition, fluids, or medications.
- In the event that the physician and patient has made a decision not to administer cardiopulmonary resuscitation, physician should write a "no code" or DNR order.
- Many times the decision regarding life-saving treatment is written in the patient's living will or durable power of attorney.

Advance Directives
Advance directives are signed and witnessed documents providing specific instructions for healthcare treatment in the event that a person is unable to make these decisions personally at the time they are needed. There are two basic advance directives:
1. Living wills
2. Durable power of attorney

The Patient Self-Determination Act (1991) requires hospitals, nursing homes, hospices, and home healthcare provider agencies to advise patients at admission of their right to refuse medical treatment and of their right to execute an advance directive. Under this act, it must be documented in the patient's record whether the patient has signed an advance directive.

- ***Living wills:*** Living wills are written documents that direct treatment in accordance with a patient's wishes in the event of a terminal illness or condition.
- ***Durable power of attorney:*** A durable power of attorney for healthcare designates an agent, surrogate, or proxy to make healthcare decisions on his/her own behalf. This agent is appointed to make healthcare treatment decisions based on the patient's wishes. Generally, two witnesses, neither of whom can be a relative or physician are needed when the patient signs the document.

Organ Donations
- Legally competent people are free to donate their organs for medical use.
- Consent forms are available for this purpose.
- In most states, required request laws stipulate that the time of a person's death a qualified healthcare provider must ask family members to consider organ or tissue donation.
- Vital organs are recovered after a patient is pronounced clinically dead or brain dead.

Rights of Dying Patients
I have right:
- To be treated as a living human being until I die
- To maintain a sense of hopefulness however changing its focus may be

- To express my feelings and emotions about my approaching death in my own way
- To participate in decisions concerning my care
- To expect continuing medical and nursing attention even though cure goals must be changed to comfort goals
- Not to die alone
- To be free from pain
- To have my questions answered honestly
- Not to be deceived
- To have help from and for my family in accepting my death
- To die in peace and with dignity
- To retain my individuality and not to be judged for my decisions, which may be contrary to the beliefs of others
- To be cared by caring, sensitive, knowledgeable people who will attempt to understand my needs and will be able to gain some satisfaction in helping me face my death

Dying Environment

- Acute care hospitals
- Long-term care
- Hospice
- Home care

Acute Care Hospitals

- Even though most deaths occur in healthcare institutions, the acute-care hospital or teaching hospital may be the least suitable place for the dying older adult or terminally ill patients.
- In the hospital setting, the disease process and diseased organ are the focus, with cure as the goal.
- Physicians and nurses often demonstrate discomfort and guilt when faced with those who are dying despite their efforts.

Long-term Care

- The atmosphere of the long-term care setting is less critical than that of the acute care setting.
- The client, family, and caregivers can express and carry out their wishes regarding death in a relaxed empathic setting.
- If previous decisions have been made regarding the dying process, death in a long-term care setting can occur in a calm, supportive atmosphere.

Hospice

- A hospice is a program or an institution designed to meet the needs of the dying.
- Emphasis is based on the relief of psychological and physical suffering, which includes pain relief.
- Programs vary, but include inpatient and outpatient services.
- Inpatient hospice facilities are provided in hospitals and outpatient and home care hospice services are often established through visiting nurse associations.

Home Care

- Another alternative may be to die at home. For this alternative, several factors must be considered because care of the dying at home imposes strain on the caregivers.
- Care at home depends heavily on the commitment and strength of several people to coordinate and provide care.

STATES OF AWARENESS MANIFESTED BY CLIENT AND FAMILY

Closed Awareness

In closed awareness, the client is not made aware of impending death. The family may choose this because:
- They do not completely understand why the client is ill.
- They believe the client will recover. Here the nurse is confronted with an ethical problem.

Mutual Pretense

In mutual pretense, everyone knows that the prognosis is terminal, but do not talk about it.

Mutual pretense permits the client degree of privacy and dignity, but places heavy burden on the dying person, who has no one in whom to confide.

Open Awareness

The client and others know it and feel free to discussing it. This awareness provides opportunity to finalize affairs and even planning for funeral arrangement.

COMMON FEARS AND CONCERN OF THE DYING

- Death itself
- Thought of a long and painful death
- Facing death alone
- Dying in the nursing home, hospital, or rest home
- Loss of body control, such as bladder or bowel incontinence
- Not being able to make decisions concerning care
- Loss of consciousness
- Financial costs and becoming burden on others
- Dying before having a chance to put personal affairs in order.

JOURNEY TOWARD DEATH

The dying process usually begins well before death actually occurs.

Death is a personal journey that each individual approaches in their own unique way. Nothing is concrete, nothing is set in stone. There are many paths one can take on this journey, but all lead to the same destination.

As one comes close to death, a process begins, a journey from the known life of this world to the unknown of what lies ahead. There are milestones along this journey. Because everyone experiences death in their own unique way, not everyone will stop at each milestone. Some may hit only a few, while another may stop at each one, taking their time along the way. Some may take months to reach their destination, others will take only days.

Journey Begins (1–3 Months Prior to Death)
- As one begins to accept their mortality and realizes that death is approaching, they may begin to withdraw from their surroundings. They are beginning the process of separating from the world and those in it.
- They may decline visits from friends, neighbors, and even family memories. They are beginning to contemplate their life and revisit old memories. They may be evaluating how they lived their life and sorting through any regrets.
- Food becomes less appealing as the body begins to slow down. The body does not need the energy from food that it once did. The dying person may be sleeping more now and not engaging in activities they once enjoyed.

1–2 WEEKS PRIOR TO DEATH

Mental Changes
- This is the time during the journey that one begins to sleep most of the time.
- Disorientation is common and altered senses of perception can be expected.
- He/she may also experience hallucinations, sometimes seeing or speaking to people that is not.

Physical Changes
The body is having a more difficult time maintaining itself. There are signs that the body may show during this time:
- The body temperature lowers by a degree or more.
- The blood pressure lowers.
- The pulse becomes irregular and may slow down or speed up.
- There is increased perspiration.
- Skin color changes as circulation becomes diminished. This is often more noticeable in the lips and nail beds as they become pale and bluish.
- Breathing changes occur, often becoming more rapid and labored. Congestion may also occur causing a rattling sound and cough.
- Speaking decreases and eventually stops altogether.

JOURNEY'S END: A COUPLE OF DAYS TO HOURS PRIOR TO DEATH
- The person is moving closer toward death. There may be a surge of energy as they he/she gets nearer. He/she may want to get out of bed and talk to loved ones. He/she may ask for food when he/she has not eaten in days. The surge of energy is usually short lived and then the previous signs become more pronounced as death approaches.
- Breathing becomes more irregular and often slower. Cheyne-Stokes breathing, rapid breathes followed by periods of no breathing at all, may occur.
- Congestion in the airway can increase causing loud, rattled breathing (death rattle).
- Hands and feet may become blotchy and purplish (mottled).
- Lips and nail beds are bluish or purple.
- The person usually become unresponsive and may have their eyes open or semiopen, but not seeing their surroundings.
- It is widely believed that hearing is the last sense to go so it is recommended that loved ones sit with and talk to the dying during this time.
- Eventually, breathing will cease altogether and the heart stops. Death has occurred.

STAGES OF DEATH AND DYING
Elizabeth Kubler-Ross identified five possible stages of dying that are experienced by clients and their families and not every client moves sequentially through each stage. These stages are experienced in varying degrees and for varying lengths of time. Understanding the stages of death helps increase sensitivity to the needs of the dying client.

Denial
In the first stage of dying, the initial shock can be overwhelming. Denial is a useful tool in coping and an essential and protective mechanism that may last for only a few minutes or may manifest for months. Denial may manifest as "doctor shopping," insisting that there must have been a mix-up or mistake in the diagnostic tests, avoiding the issue or going about their daily routines as though nothing in their lives has changed.

Anger
The initial stage of denial is followed by anger. The client's security is being threatened by the unknown and since the client has no control over the situation, he/she may become angry in response to this powerlessness.

Bargaining
The next stage is bargaining in which the client attempts to postpone or reverse the inevitable. The client's bargaining represents an attempt to postpone death and usually has self-imposed limitations. For example, the client will ask to live just long enough to see his/her first grandchild born in exchange for a promise to perform some service for the church.

Depression
When the realization occurs that the loss can no longer be delayed, the client moves to the stage of depression.

However, it may help the client detach from the life and thus be able to accept death.

Acceptance

The final stage acceptance may not be reached by every dying client. With acceptance comes growing peace and contentment. The feeling this all that could be done has been done is often expressed during.

CONCLUSION

The end of life care is very sensitive where nurse meets the family and being cared of a client with family after death. Legal and ethical considerations to be followed during end of life care and nurse should be able to convince the families in acceptance of a death of a person, explain causes and help them to adaptation in stages of grief.

36 CHAPTER
Infection Prevention (Including HIV) and Standard Safety Measures

CHAPTER OUTLINE

- Definition
- Hand Hygiene
- Key Points
- Infection Control and Standard Safety Measures
- Control Measures

DEFINITION

Standard Safety Measures

These are procedures and work practices used to reduce the risk of disease transmission, prevent and protect ourselves from infections.

Basic Principles of Infection Control (Fig. 36.1)

- All patients are potentially infectious
- Follow standard precautions for all patients
- Use of personal protective equipment (PPE) is based on risk of the procedure.

Prevention and Control of Infection

- Practice hand hygiene
- Use PPE when handling blood, body substances, excretions, and secretions
- Disinfection and sterilization
- Biomedical waste management.

HAND HYGIENE

Definition: Any action of performing hand hygiene with soap and water and other detergents containing an antiseptic agent for mechanically removing dirt, organic material, and micro-organisms.

Purpose: To prevent harmful germ transmission and/or infection.

Hand hygiene technique is used before doing any procedure, and the following procedures:
- Taking blood pressure
- Inserting a Ryle's tube
- Giving oral medication
- Conducting a delivery
- Cleaning a diabetic foot
- Before giving injection
- Giving feed to a neonate.

For all types of hand hygiene (Figs. 36.2 and 36.3):
- Keep nails short (1–2 mm)
- Do not wear nail polish
- Remove jewelry, bracelets, wrist watches (Figs. 36.2A and B)
- Do not dry hands on clothes/uniforms after hand washing.

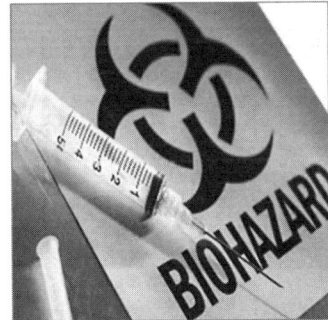

Fig. 36.1: Biohazard symbol with risk of transmission.

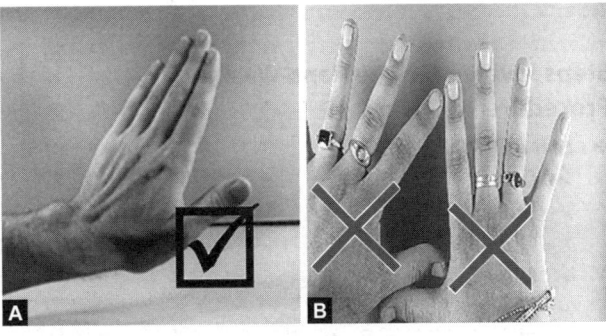

Figs. 36.2A and B: Do's and Dont's during hand washing.

Section 5: Biopsychosocial Pathology

How to handwash?
Wash hands when visibly soiled! otherwise, use handrub
- **Duration of the handwash (steps 2–7):** 15–20 seconds
- **Duration of the entire procedure:** 40–60 seconds

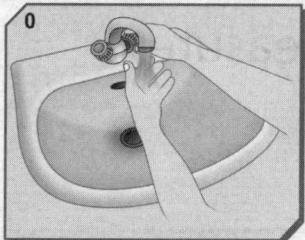
0. Wet hands with water

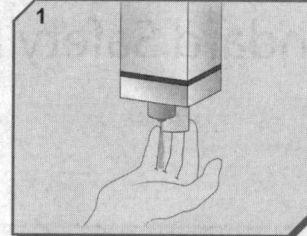
1. Apply enough soap to cover all hand surfaces

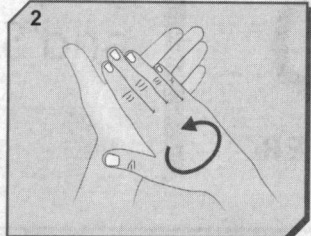
2. Rub hands palm to palm

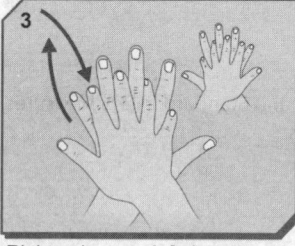
3. Right palm over left dorsum with interlaced fingers and vice versa

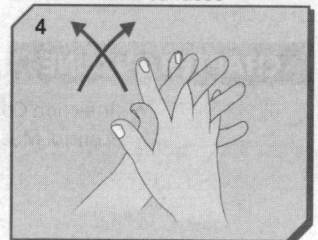
4. Palm to palm with fingers interlaced

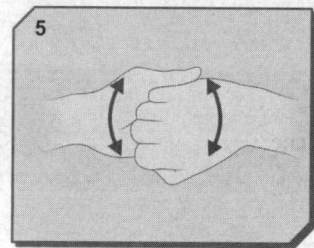
5. Backs of fingers to opposing palms with fingers interlocked

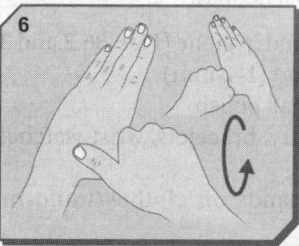
6. Rotational rubbing of left thumb clasped in right palm and vice versa

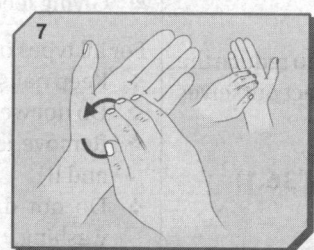
7. Rotational rubbing, backwards and forwards with clasped fingers of right hand in left palm and vice versa

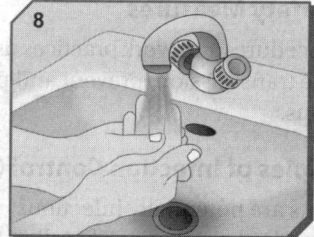
8. Rinse hands with water

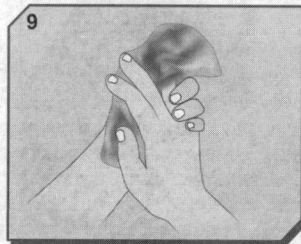
9. Dry thoroughly with a single use towel

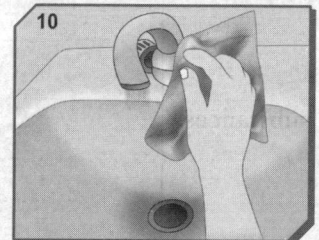
10. Use towel to turn off faucet

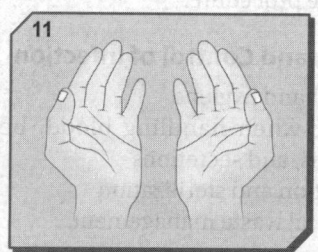
11. Your hands are now safe

Fig. 36.3: WHO steps of hand hygiene.

Steps Involved in the Hand Washing Procedure

- ❖ *List of PPE (Fig. 36.4):*
  - ➢ Cap
  - ➢ Mask
  - ➢ Goggles
  - ➢ Gloves
  - ➢ Gown
  - ➢ Shoe cover/leggings.

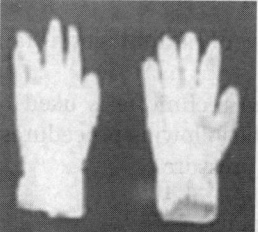

Fig. 36.4: Techniques of wearing sterile gloves (PPE).
(PPE: personal protective equipment)

Use of Personal Protective Equipment

Do's and Don'ts for Use of Personal Protective Equipment (Fig. 36.5)

Do's
- Use PPE based on risk of the procedure
- Change PPE completely after each procedure
- Discard the used PPE in appropriate disposal bags
- Dispose PPE as per the policy of the hospital
- Always wash hands after removing PPE
- Educate and train all junior and auxiliary staff in the use of PPE.

Don'ts
- Share PPE
- Use the same gloves between patients
- Reuse disposable gloves, eyewear, masks
- Use eyewear that restricts the vision
- Use masks when wet.

Safety of Instruments

- First choice, use disposable needles
- Never reuse a disposable needle or instrument
- Safely dispose all sharps (needles, lancets, scalpels) after use
- Disinfect reusable needles/syringes/instruments with hypochlorite first, then sterilize by autoclaving or boiling before reuse.

Agents Used in Disinfection (Effective against Human Immunodeficiency Virus)

- Household bleach/sodium hypochlorite
- Chlorhexidine (2–4%)
- Glutaraldehyde (2%)
- Ethanol (70%)
- Formalin (4%)
- Povidone iodine (2%).

Ineffective against human immunodeficiency virus (HIV)
- Savlon—poor effect
- Dettol solution—no effect
- Lysol—poor effect.

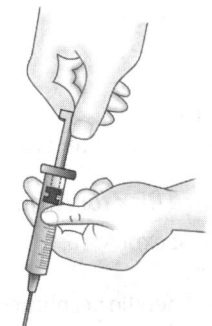

Fig. 36.5: Protect from PEP.
(PEP: post-exposure prophylaxis)

10% household bleach (as per WHO)
Contains 0.5% chlorine concentration, used to disinfect:
- Excreta
- Dead body
- Spills of blood/body fluids
- Vehicles and tires
- Also used to prepare 1:100 bleach solution.

1% household bleach (as per WHO)
Contains 0.05% chlorine concentration, used to disinfect:
- Surfaces
- Medical equipment
- Bedding
- Reusable protective clothing before it is laundered
- Rinsing gloves between contact with different patients (if new gloves are not available).

Preparation of Bleach Solution

10% bleach solution
- **Using bleach solution:** Add one volume of household bleach (e.g. 1 L) to nine volumes of clean water (e.g. 9 L).
- **For using 1% bleaching solution:** Mix 30 g or one ounce of bleaching powder to 1 L of water.
- For preparation of hypochlorite solution 1% or 10% follow the calculation according below formula as follows:
  Formula for dilution of stock solution of sodium hypochlorite to working concentration of sodium hypochlorite:
  Amount of required = (working conc. required/stock conc.)*(working solution volume required)

For example:
For preparation of 1% hypochlorite solution = (1%/5%) × 1000 mL

So, add 200 mL of hypochlorite solution to 800 mL of water.

Things to Remember

- Bleach solutions must be prepared daily as they lose their strength after 24 h.
- Any time the odor is not present, discard it.
- 1:10 bleach solution is caustic; avoid direct contact with the skin and eyes.
- Prepare the bleach solutions in a well-ventilated area.
- For all types of blood spills, it is recommended to use 10% bleach solution.
- Keep away from direct sunlight.

Nurse's Role in Disinfection and Sterilization

- Prepare bleach solution every day
- Keep a separate area for disinfection of patient care items
- Disinfect all patient care equipment contaminated with body fluids or secretions

- Maintain separate personal care items for patients, e.g. razors, toothbrushes
- Clean daily, surfaces in close proximity to patient (bed side rails, tables)
- Disinfect all reusable articles before sending for sterilization
- Clean all patient area and the unit thoroughly on discharge.

Standard Precautions Against Blood-borne Pathogens

- Hand hygiene
- Use PPE
- Disinfect and sterilize
- Proper waste management
- Prevent accidents
- Protect yourself from occupational exposure
- Disposal of needles:
  - Needle destroyer/burner/cutter
  - Disposal of sharps into the appropriate bin.

Nurse's Role: Reduce Risk of Sharp Injuries

- **Do's (Figs. 36.6A and B):**
  - Use needle cutter/destroyer.
  - Separate sharps from other waste.
  - Use rigid, puncture proof disposal bins.
  - Empty sharps containers when they are three-fourth full.
- **Don'ts (Figs. 36.7 and 36.8):**
  - Handle, empty, or transfer used sharps between containers.
  - Do not recap sharps before disposal.

Protect Yourself

- Take three doses of hepatitis B vaccine booster dose for every 5 years. It gives you lifelong protection.
- Take measures to prevent accidents.

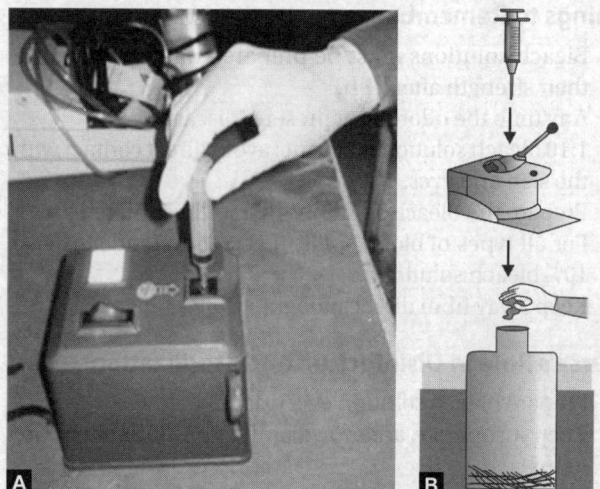

Figs. 36.6A and B: Disposal-needle destroyer/burner/cutter.

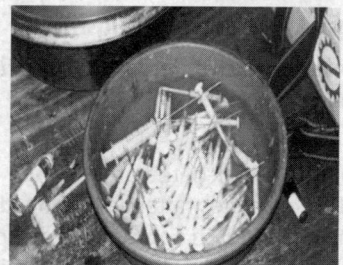

Fig. 36.7: Danger-incorrect disposal of sharps.

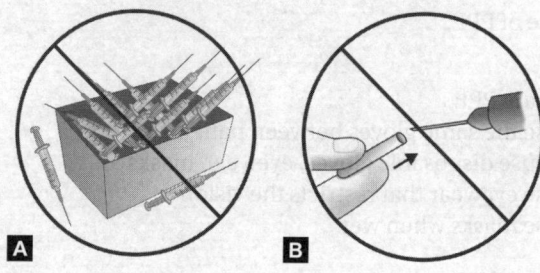

Figs. 36.8A and B: Dont's in handling sharps.

- Take post-exposure prophylaxis (PEP) in the event of any occupational exposure.
- Follow standard precautions at all times.

Types of Occupational Exposures

- Needle-stick or cut with sharp instrument infected with HIV, HBsAg, etc.
- Splash to eyes, nose, mouth
- Direct exposure involving non-intact skin.

Body Fluids that Have Risk of HIV Transmission

- Considered "at risk":
  - Blood
  - Semen
  - Breast milk
  - Vaginal secretions
  - Cerebrospinal fluid
  - Synovial, pleural, pericardial, peritoneal fluids
  - Amniotic fluid
  - Other body fluids visibly contaminated with blood.
- Considered "not at risk":
  - Tears
  - Sweat
  - Urine and feces
  - Saliva (unless they contain visible blood).

Factors That Influence Risk for Acquiring HIV

- Type and efficacy of exposure:
  - Depth of injury
  - Size and type of needle i.e. blunt or wide bore needle
  - Amount of blood
- HIV status of the source
- Amount of virus present in the contaminated fluid

- Types of procedures that carry a higher risk of transmission:
  - Procedures involving a needle placed in artery or vein
- Use of invasive devices visibly contaminated with blood.
- Whether PEP is taken within the specified time or not.
- Most exposures do not result in infection.

Steps Following Occupational Exposure
- Crisis management—remain calm.
- Dispose the sharp appropriately.
- First aid—wash and irrigate the site.
- Report to the appropriate authority.
- Get evaluated for PEP and baseline testing for HIV.
- The PEP should be started within 2 h of exposure, and not later than 72 h.
- The PEP must be taken for 4 weeks (28 days).
  A follow-up HIV testing (6 weeks, 3 months, 6 months). The National AIDS Control Organization (NACO) guidelines
- A follow-up counseling and care.

Management of Exposure: Immediate Measures
First Aid (Depending on Area of Exposure) (Box 36.1)
- **Wound or skin:** Wash with soap and water.
- **Mucous membrane:** Flush exposed membrane with water.
- **Open wound:** Irrigate with sterile saline or antiseptic solution.
- **Eyes:** Irrigate with clean water, saline, or sterile eye irrigants.
- **Mouth:** Do not swallow. Rinse out several times with cold water.

Post-exposure Prophylaxis
Post-exposure prophylaxis refers to the use of antiretrovirus prophylactically to prevent HIV infection following an occupational exposure.

General Guidelines for PEP
- Potential benefits weighed against potential risks and informed to the staff
- Adherence and adverse effects be monitored
- Baseline HIV test of staff with counseling

Box 36.1: Risk of occupational exposure.
- HBV: 30% (30 in 100)
- HCV: 3–5% (3–5 in 100)
- HIV: 0.3% (3 in 1,000)
- Occupational exposure to HIV very low risk

(HBV: hepatitis B virus; HCV: hepatitis C virus; HIV: human immunodeficiency virus)

- Follow-up:
  - Counseling and HIV testing
  - Monitor for drug toxicity.

Steps for PEP
- Assess nature of exposure
- Assess HIV status of source of exposure
- PEP evaluation
- PEP regimens—drugs and dosage for PEP
- Follow-up.

Follow-up
- Follow-up for drug toxicity monitoring: Complete blood count (CBC) and the liver function test (LFT) at baseline and at 2 weeks.
- Repeat HIV testing of exposed staff as per protocol (3 weeks, 3 months, 6 months).

KEY POINTS
- Standard precautions must be followed for all patients.
- Use of standard precautions could reduce the risk of blood-borne and airborne infections.
- Nurses have a key role in:
  - Following standard precaution protocols
  - Educating other healthcare personnel
  - Preventing occupational exposure
  - Protecting self and others from blood-borne pathogens including HIV
- PEP significantly reduces the risk of HIV transmission from occupational exposure.
- Existing PEP protocols should be followed.
- Ideally PEP should be given within 2 h and not later than 72 h after exposure.
- Exposed healthcare providers should be monitored for side effects and adherence.

INFECTION CONTROL AND STANDARD SAFETY MEASURES

Introduction
Infection control is the discipline, which is mainly concerned with preventing nosocomial infections. It is an essential part of the infrastructure of the health care. It mainly addresses the factors related to the spread of infections within the healthcare settings including prevention and control of the spread of the infections within the healthcare settings.

Definition
- An infection is the entry and multiplication of an infectious agent in the tissue of host and causing signs and symptoms.
- If the pathogens multiply and cause clinical signs and symptoms, then it is symptomatic.

❖ If the infectious agent fails to cause injury to cells and tissues, then the infections is asymptomatic.

Course of Infection by Stage

- ❖ *Incubation period:* Interval between entrance of pathogen into the body and appearance of first sign or symptom.
- ❖ *Prodromal stage:* Interval from the onset of nonspecific signs and symptoms (malaise, low-grade fever) to more specific signs and symptoms.
- ❖ *Illness stage:* Interval when client manifest signs and symptoms specific to the type of infection.
- ❖ *Convalescence:* Interval when the acute symptoms of infectious are after disappeared. Length of recovery depends on severity of infection and client's general state of health, Recovery may take place in several days to months.

Chain of Infection (Fig. 36.9)

The presence of pathogen does not mean that an infection will begin. Development of infection occurs in the cycle that depends on the presence of all the following elements:
- ❖ An infectious agent or pathogen
- ❖ A reservoir or source of pathogen growth
- ❖ A portal of exit from the reservoir
- ❖ A mode of transmission
- ❖ A portal of entry to host
- ❖ A susceptible host.

An infection will not develop if the chain remains intact. Nurses follow infection prevention and control practices to maintain the chain so that infection will not develop.

Infectious Agent

Microorganisms including bacteria, viruses, fungi, and protozoa are the infectious agents, which causes infections.

Reservoir

A reservoir is the place where the pathogen can survive, but may or may not multiply. For example, hepatitis A virus survives in shellfish, but does not multiply.

Human body, animals, food, water, insects, and innate objects can be reservoirs for infectious organisms.

Portal of Exit

After microorganisms find a place to grow and multiply, they must find a portal of exit, if they are ready to enter into another host and cause disease. Microorganisms can exit through a variety of sites such as skin, mucous membrane, respiratory tract, urinary tract, gastrointestinal (GI) tract, reproductive tract, and blood.

Modes of Transmission

There are many modes of transmission of microorganisms from the reservoir to the host. For example, droplet infection, waterborne, airborne, etc.

Entry Portal

Organisms can enter the body through the same routes they used for the exit.

Susceptible Host

Whether a person acquires an infection depends upon the susceptibility of an infectious agent. Susceptibility depends upon individual degree of resistance to pathogen. The more virulent an organism, greater is the likelihood of a person's susceptibility. A person's resistance to an infectious agent is enhanced by vaccines or by actually contracting the disease.

CONTROL MEASURES

The control measures include the following:
- ❖ Control or elimination of infectious agent
- ❖ Control or elimination of reservoir
- ❖ Control of portal of exit
- ❖ Control of transmission
- ❖ Protection of susceptible host.

Control or Elimination of Infectious Agent

Cleaning, disinfection, and sterilization of contaminated objects significantly reduce and often eliminate microorganisms.

Cleaning

It is the removal of all the soil from the object and surface. Cleaning involves use of water and mechanical action by hand washing.
- ❖ When cleaning the equipment that is soiled by organic materials such as blood, fecal matter, or pus, this need application of mask and protective eyewear and waterproof gloves.

The following steps ensure that an object is clean:
1. Rinse a contaminated object or article with cold running water to remove organic material. Hot water causes the protein in organic material to coagulate.
2. After rinsing clean the object with soap and warm water.
3. Use a brush to remove dirt or material in gloves. Friction dislodges the contaminated material and can be easily removed.
4. Rinse the object in warm water.
5. Dry the object and prepare it for disinfection.

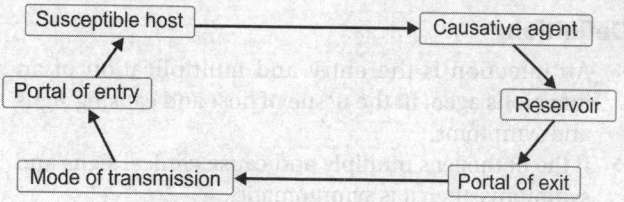

Fig. 36.9: Chain of infection.

Asepsis

- Asepsis is the absence of pathogenic microorganisms.
- The aseptic techniques refer to practices that keep a client as free from pathogens as much as possible.
- There are two types of aseptic techniques:
  - *Medical asepsis:* Includes the procedures to reduce and prevent the spread of microorganisms during medical procedures.
  - *Surgical asepsis:* Includes the procedures to reduce and prevent the spread of microorganisms including spores during surgical procedures.

Disinfection and sterilization

- Disinfection describes the process that eliminates many or all the pathogens with the exception of bacterial spores.
- It is the complete elimination or destruction of all the pathogens including spores steam under pressure, gas—hydrogen peroxide, etc.

Control or Elimination of Reservoir

To control or eliminate the reservoir site for infection the nurse eliminates or controls the sources of body fluids, drainage of solutions that might harbor microorganisms.

The nurse also carefully disinfects the articles that become contaminated with infectious material. The Occupational Safety and Health Act of 1991 set the standards for minimizing occupational exposure of blood borne pathogens or other potentially infectious materials.

Control of Portal of Exit

The nurse follows prevention and control practices to minimize or prevent infectious organisms from exit the body:

- To control organisms exiting via respiratory tract the nurse should avoid talking directly into the client's face, sneezing or coughing directly over incision wounds or sterile dressings.
- A nurse who has an upper respiratory tract infection and continues to work with clients should wear a mask when working closely with the clients. Another way of controlling the exit of pathogens is through the careful handling of the exudates, e.g. urine.
- Contaminated fluids can easily splash, while being discarding them.

Control of Transmission

- Effective control of infection requires a nurse to remain aware of the mode of transmission and ways to control them.
- In hospitals, home or extended care facility a client should have a personal set of care items. Sharing bed pans, urinals, basins, eating utensils can easily lead to transmission of infections.
- To prevent infections, the soiled items and equipment must be kept away from touching the nurses clothing. A common error is to carry dirty linen in the arms against the uniforms.
- Laundry hampers should be replaced before they are overflowing.
- Hand hygiene; the most important and basic technique in preventing and controlling infection is hand hygiene. It includes using an instant alcohol hand rub antiseptic before and after providing care, hand washing with soap and water when the hands are visibly soiled and performing a surgical scrub.

Control of Portal of Entry

- Many measures that control the exit microorganisms control the entrance of pathogen.
- Maintaining the integrity of the skin and mucous membrane reduces the chances of microorganisms reaching the host.
- The client's skin should be well lubricated by using lotion.
- After elimination the women should clean the anus and perineum by wiping from urinary meatus toward the anus.
- Frequent perineal care to the obstetric patients and older adult women who wear disposable continent pads.
- A final method of reducing the entrance of pathogens is the technique for cleaning wounds.

Protection of the Susceptible Host

- A client's resistance to infection improves as the nurse protects normal body defense against infection.
- The nurse also protects himself/herself and others through the use of isolation precautions:
  - Protective environment
  - Specimen collection
  - Surgical asepsis
  - Performing sterile procure
  - Gloving as goggles, N-95 mask, triple layer mask, gown, shoe covers, gloves.

Standard Safety Measures

Standard safety measures are those, which are used to prevent and to protect ourselves from infection. The standard safety measures are as follows:

- *Personal Protective Devices:* Following personal protective devices are useful in preventing the risk of hazardous infections:
  - Cap/scarf
  - Goggles/plain glasses
  - Mask
  - Apron/gowns
  - Gloves
  - Shoe covers and shoes.
- *General Protective Measures:*
  - All the nurses including staffs must be vaccinated against hepatitis B.

- Extreme care is needed while handling the needles and sharps, since most sharp injuries occur between the points of use and disposal.
- Sharps should be segregated at the site of generation and thereafter placed in a puncture proof container.
- All the disposable items must be dipped in 1% hydrochloride solution for at least half an hour to ensure that they are disinfected.
- Care during dealing with the HIV or Hepatitis B positive cases—keep these patients in isolation wards, always wear two pairs of gloves and use other protective devices.
- In operation theater glasses/goggles must be worn. Also the transfer of instruments should not be from hand between a nurse and surgeon or vice versa. Instead a bowl should be used to keep them.

❖ **Care of Injury Caused by Infected Sharps:**
- Special precautions need to be taken if the sharps are infected with HIV or hepatitis B cases.
- Clean the wound immediately, first with saline and then with spirit or Betadine
- An injection of tetanus toxoid (TT) is advisable.
- Dressing of the wound may be required.
- Consult the physician as early as possible.
- In case of infectious solution, spilled on the body:
  - Remove the soiled cloths and wash the part thoroughly with plenty of water.
  - Apply nonirritant antiseptic cream on that part.
- In case of spillage in eyes, wash it with water, avoid rubbing.
- Consult the physician.
  Post-exposure prophylaxis drug with antiretroviral drugs is advisable to nurses of healthcare workers within 2 h of exposure. Also follow the post-exposure guidelines of the National AIDS Control Organization.

❖ **Other Measures of Safety:**
- Nurses need to be well equipped with latest information, skills, and practices in managing and handling the contaminated things and patients with infectious diseases.
- The nurses should have thorough knowledge regarding biomedical waste management, which helps to prevent and control the spread of infections.

CONCLUSION

Infection is localized, proper care to control the spread and to minimize the infection. An infection that affects the entire body instead of just a single organ or part is systemic and can become fatal. The nurse is responsible for properly prevention and control of infections. Infection control is the discipline, which is mainly concerned with preventing nosocomial infections. So there is a need to follow strict and standard safety measures to prevent and control the infections.

37 Biomedical Waste Management

CHAPTER OUTLINE

- Types of Hospital Waste
- Treatment and Disposal
- Biomedical Waste Management and Handling Rules
- Nurse's Role

"Recycle and reuse our wastes for a cleaner and healthier environment."

INTRODUCTION

The World Health Organization (WHO) revealed that more than 50,000 people die every day from infectious diseases. One among the number of causes is the increase in improper waste management. India generates around 3 million tons of medical waste every year. The estimated waste generated in hospitals in India is 1–2 kg/bed/day.

Definition of Hospital Waste

Waste generated in healthcare establishment including hospitals, laboratories blood banks/camps, or similar establishments during healthcare research testing or related procedure on human beings or animals.

TYPES OF HOSPITAL WASTE (FIG. 37.1)

Waste is generated from healthcare units outpatient wards, labor wards, hospital staff, operation theaters, laboratories, etc. patients attenders, public, etc., staying and waiting places or biomedical waste (BMW) 15% general waste 85%.

Biomedical Waste (Fig. 37.2)

It means "any solid and/or liquid waste including its container and any intermediate product is generated during the diagnosis treatment or immunization of human beings and animals."

WHO Classification of BMW

- 85% of waste is non-hazardous.
- 10% of the BMW is infectious and 5% is non-infectious.
- Pathological
- Radioactive
- Others (general waste)

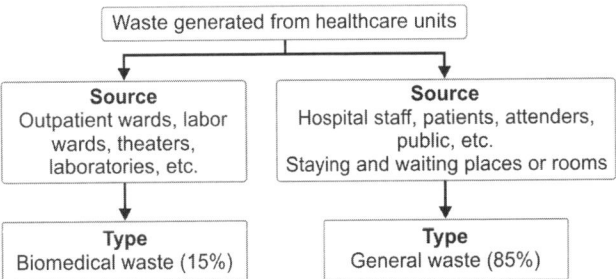

Fig. 37.1: Types of hospital wastes.

Health Hazards

- Infections
- Occupational health hazards
- Hazards to general public
- Hazards to animals and birds
- Hazards to environment

Objectives of Hospital Waste Management

- To prevent harm resulting from waste
- Minimize its volume
- Retrieve renewable materials
- Ensure safe of economical disposal.

Biohazard Symbol (Fig. 37.3)

The bins, bags, trolleys, transportation vehicles, storage rooms should carry the biohazard symbol, which should be non-washable and prominently visible.

Steps in Waste Management

- Waste survey
- Waste segregation
- Waste accumulation of storage
- Waster transportation
- Waste treatment and disposal
- Waste minimization

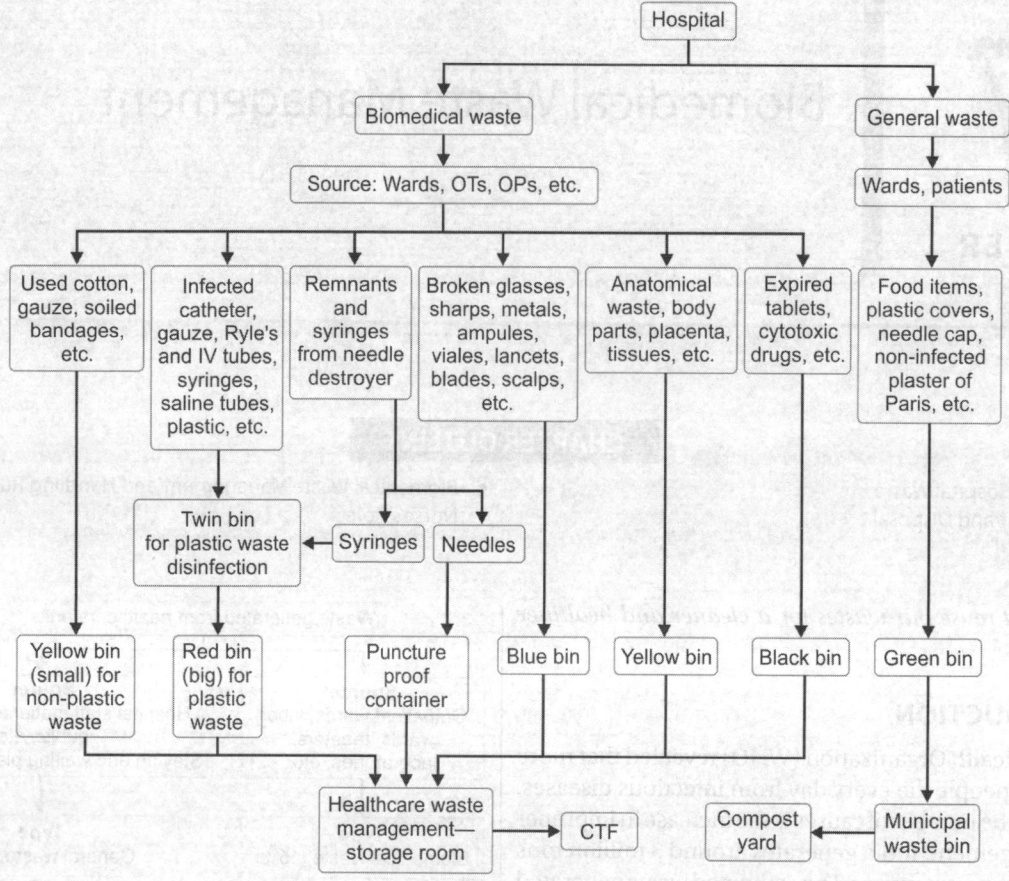

Fig. 37.2: Biomedical waste.
(CTF: centralized treatment facility; IV: intravenous; OP: outpatient; OT: operation theater)

Fig. 37.3: Handle with care.

Waste Survey

- Differentiate and quantify the waste
- Determine the method of disposal
- Determine the points of generation, type of waste level of generation, and the disinfection required

Waste Segregation

Segregation refers to the basic separation of different categories of waste generated at source and thereby reducing the risks as well as cost of handling and disposal.

This helps to:
- Prevent mixing of BMWs with general waste
- Prevent illegal reuse
- Provide opportunity for recycling
- Biodegradable waste can be composted and used for gardening.
- Recycling can help in revenue generation.

Twin bin (Fig. 37.4): Twin bin is closed double-basket system with perforated inner severe container.

Outer bin: Contains 1% sodium hypochlorite solution.

Inner sieve: Contains plastic wastes (syringes, intravenous (IV) tubes, Ryle's tubes, catheters, etc.).

The waste is soaked for 30 min and transferred to respective bag by lifting the inner sieve. The lid is to be closed to prevent chlorine escape. A fresh solution is to be prepared each time.

Waste Accumulation and Storage

- Accumulation refers to the temporary holding of small quantities of waste near the point of generation (wards, operation theaters, laboratories, kitchen, corridors, etc.).

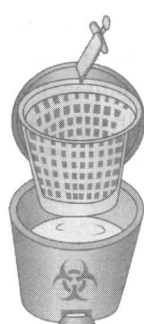

Fig. 37.4: Twin bin (for plastic waster disinfection) after 30 min of disinfection, put the plastic wastes in red bin (big).

❖ Storage is characterized by long-holding periods of large waste quantity offsite storage room.

Storage chambers

❖ This should be located from functional areas diesel generator sets, oil storage, gas storage, and other potential sources of fire.
❖ It should be fenced for netted to prevent access to animals and birds.
❖ Strict prohibition for unauthorized access of human beings.

Storage area: Floors and walls should be impervious to liquid and easy to clean:
❖ Should be disinfected regularly.
❖ Refrigeration may be required storage area should posted with "explicit" signs.

Waste Transportation
❖ The segregated BMWs after registering are transported in the trolleys to the storage chambers.
❖ The bags/containers containing BMWs should be tied/lidded.
❖ Offsite transportation vehicle should be market with name and address of the carrier.
❖ Biohazard symbol should be painted.

TREATMENT AND DISPOSAL

1. Incineration
2. Chemical disinfection
3. Wet and dry thermal treatment
4. Microwave irradiation
5. Inertization
6. Land disposal/deep burial

Incineration

❖ High temperature dry oxidation process that reduce organic and combustible waste into inorganic and combustible waste into inorganic incombustible matter. Resulting in significant reduction in waste volume and weight.
❖ Process is selected to treat waste that cannot be recycled, reused, or can be disposed in land.

Types of Incinerators
❖ Double chambered (for infectious waste)
❖ Single chambered (if double chamber not affordable)
❖ Rotatory kilns (for genotoxic waste)

Chemical Disinfection

❖ Commonly used for treatment of liquid infectious waste, e.g. blood, urine, stool, and hospital sewage
❖ Chemicals are added to waste to kill or inactive the pathogen it contains.

Wet and Dry Thermal Treatment

❖ Wet thermal treatment/steam disinfection is based on exposure if infectious waste to high temperature and high pressure steam similar to process of autoclaving, inappropriate for treating anatomical, chemical, and pharmaceutical waste.
❖ Screw feed technology: Dry thermal treatment in which waste is shredded and heated in rotating auger. 80% volume and 20–35 weight is reduced, suitable for infectious waste and sharps.

Microwave Irradiation

Microwave of frequency 2450 MHz and wavelength 12.24 cm used to destroy the microorganism. Water contained in the waste is rapidly heated by microwave and infectious components are destroyed by heat conduction.

Inertization

❖ Process of mixing waste with cement and other substances before disposal in order to minimize the risk of toxic substance migrating into surface water or ground water and to prevent scavenging.
❖ Proportion of 65% waste, 15% lime, 15% cement, and 5% water is used.

Waste Minimization

Waste minimization management step makes use of reducing, reusing, and recycling principles:
❖ General waste should never be mixed with BMW
❖ Designing eco-friendly biodegradable plastics
❖ Using electronic devices, etc.

Records to be Maintained
❖ Register for daily collection BMW
❖ Register of source wise collection of BMW
❖ The monthly consolidation register
❖ The register for needle-stick injuries

Section 5: Biopsychosocial Pathology

Managements of Needle Stick Injuries

- Follow standard precautions during post-exposure prophylaxis in the event of any occupational exposure.
- First aid: Wash and irrigate the sight.
- Report to the appropriate authority.
- Get evaluated for PEP and baseline testing for human immunodeficiency virus (HIV).
- PEP should be started within 2 h of exposure, and not later than 72 h.
- PEP must be taken for 4 weeks (28 days).
- Follow-up HIV testing should be done at 6 weeks, 3 months, and 6 months.
- Follow-up counselling and care.
- Inform doctor if pregnant or breastfeeding woman.

BIOMEDICAL WASTE MANAGEMENT AND HANDLING RULES

The Ministry of Environment and Forest, Government of India has issued a notification on BMW under the Environment (Protection) Act.

- The Environment Protection Act 1986 passed by environmental Law and Legislation.
- In 1998, the BMW management and handling rules were published by the Government of India.
- The BWM handling rules were revised in 2016 by the Central Government under Environment Protection Act.

Salient Features of the Rules

Waste Categories (Figs. 37.5 to 37.8)

- Waste categories schedules.
- Duty of the occupier: To ensure safe handling of BMW.
- *Segregation:* BMW are to be segregated properly according to the color codes and labeled.
- *Storage:* BMW storage to be maintained untreated BMWs shall not be stored for more than 48 hours.
- **Red bin:** It contains disinfected plastic waste recyclable placed in Red bag.
- **Yellow bin:** This is to dispose anatomical waste. (Placenta, tissues, body parts) Nonplastic waste (used

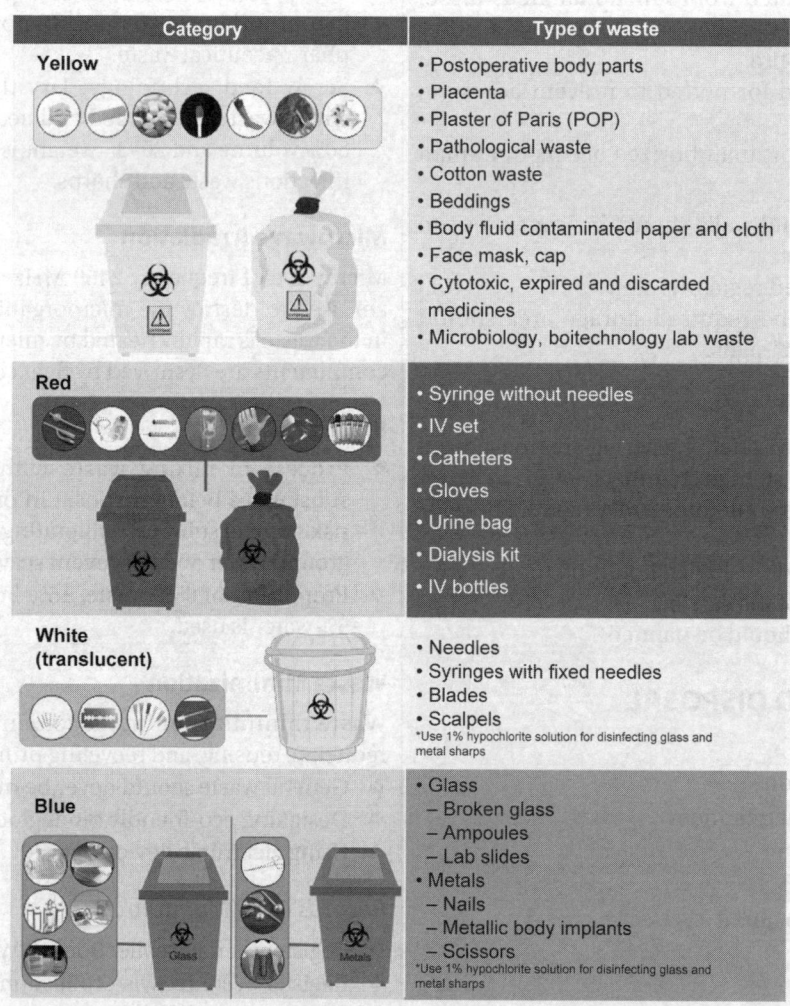

Category	Type of waste
Yellow	• Postoperative body parts • Placenta • Plaster of Paris (POP) • Pathological waste • Cotton waste • Beddings • Body fluid contaminated paper and cloth • Face mask, cap • Cytotoxic, expired and discarded medicines • Microbiology, boitechnology lab waste
Red	• Syringe without needles • IV set • Catheters • Gloves • Urine bag • Dialysis kit • IV bottles
White (translucent)	• Needles • Syringes with fixed needles • Blades • Scalpels *Use 1% hypochlorite solution for disinfecting glass and metal sharps

Blue	• Glass
	  – Broken glass
	  – Ampoules
	  – Lab slides
	• Metals
	  – Nails
	  – Metallic body implants
	  – Scissors
	*Use 1% hypochlorite solution for disinfecting glass and metal sharps

Fig. 37.5: Segregation of the waste. *(For color version, see color Plate 1)*

(IV: intravenous)

25 liters red bin (big) with
red bag for plastic wastes
A
B
C
D

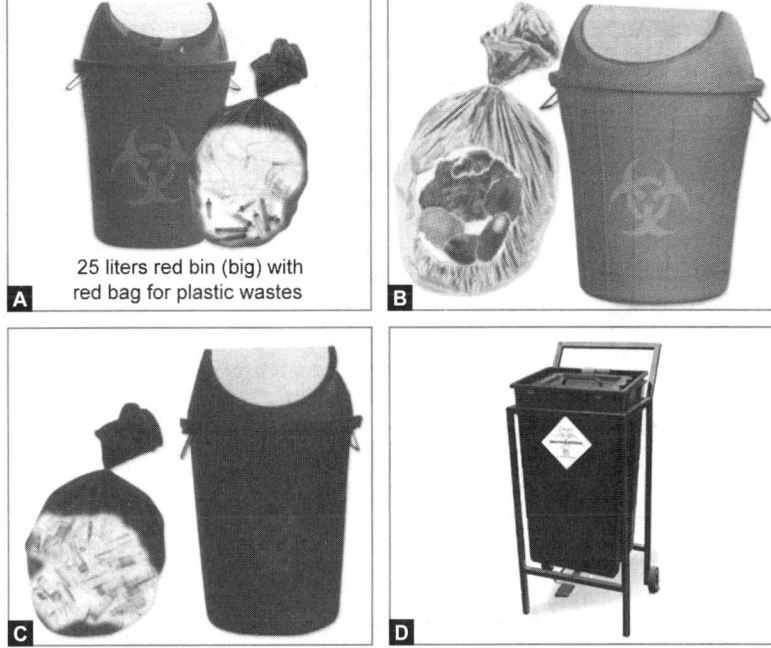

Figs. 37.6A to D: (A) Red; (B) Yellow; (C) Blue; (D) Black. *(For color version, see color Plate 2)*

cotton, gauze, soiled bandages, and expired drugs and cytotoxic drugs, etc.)

- **Blue bin:** BMW like sharps (ampoules, vials, broken glass, sutures, slides, etc.)
- **Black bin:** Black for wastes from disposables, i.e. general and covers, etc.
- ***Transportation:*** Use only vehicles authorized by competent authority.
- ***Authorization:*** The authorization authorities are state pollution control board, district environmental engineer, and municipal corporation.
- ***Records:*** Which are maintained and subject to verification.
- ***Noncompliance:*** Failure to act is punishable with 5 years imprisonment and a fine of 1 lakh Indian rupees.

NURSE'S ROLE

Waste Management

- Segregate at with site of waste generated.
- Daily prepare hypochlorite solutions.
- Keep with $NaHCO_3$, away from direct sunlight.
- Do not recap needles, if needed, use scooping technique.
- Adhere to the rules laid down by medical waste managements.
- Select the area to store with waste until it is disposed.
- Use trolleys to carry the waste.
- Provide Group D workers with all protective equipment, including utilizing gloves.
- Be up-to-date on infection control practices.
- Segregate hospital wastes appropriately.

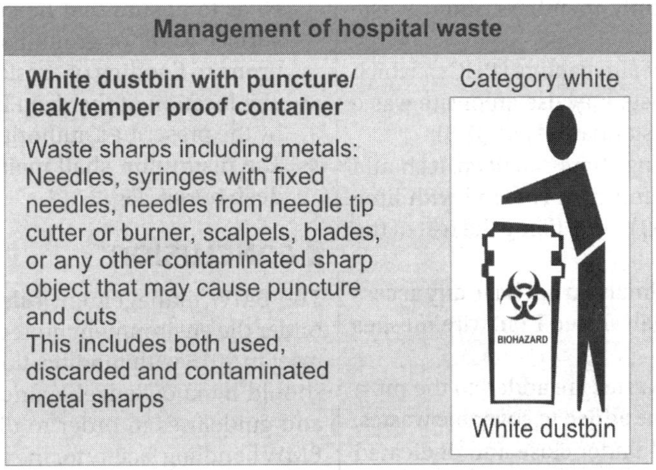

Management of hospital waste
White dustbin with puncture/
leak/temper proof container
Waste sharps including metals:
Needles, syringes with fixed
needles, needles from needle tip
cutter or burner, scalpels, blades,
or any other contaminated sharp
object that may cause puncture
and cuts
This includes both used,
discarded and contaminated
metal sharps
Category white
BIOHAZARD
White dustbin

Fig. 37.7: Disposal of sharps.

Categories of BMW

Color code	Type of bag/container	Type of waste	Treatment options
Red	Red colored non-chlorinated plastic bags or containers 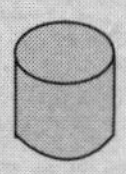	Contaminated waste (recyclable)	Autoclaving or micro-waving/hydroclaving followed by shredding or mutilation or combination of sterilization and shredding treated Waste to be sent to registered or authorized recyclers
White (Translucent)	Puncture proof, leak proof, tamer proof containers 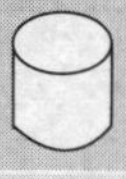	Waste sharps including metals	Autoclaving or Dry Heat sterilization folowed by shredding
Blue	Cardboard boxes with blue colored marking 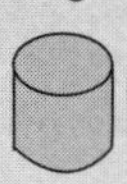	a. Glassware b. Metalic body implants	Disinfection and then sent for recycling.
Yellow	Yellow coloured non-chlorinated plastic bags 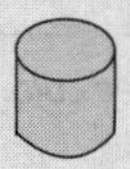	a. Human anatomical waste b. Animal anatomical waste c. Soiled waste	Incineration or plasma pyrolysis or deep burial
		d. Expired or discarded medicines	Returned back to the manufacturer or supplier for incineration
		e. Chemical waste	Disposed of by incineration or plasma mixing with other wastewater
	Separate collection system leading to effluent treatment system	f. Chemical liquid waste	Chemical liquid waste shall be pre-treated before mixing with other wastewater
	Non-chlorinated yellow plastic bags or suitable packing material	g. Discarded linen, mattresses, beddings contaminated with blood or body fluid	Non- chlorinated chemical disinfection followed by incineration or plazma Pyrolysis or for energy recovery
	Autoclave safe plastic bags or containers	h. Microbiology, biotechnology and other clinical laboratory waste	Pre-treat to sterilize with nonchlorinated chemicals on-site

Fig. 37.8: Categories of waste. *(For color version, see color Plate 3)*

- Teach, train, and supervise junior staff/students and cleaning, and other staff in the ward with regard to waste segregation and disposal.
- Educate patients and family members about waste management.

Small clinics or primary health centers (PHCs), which generate small volumes of waste may use an onsite waste burial pit as per the following standards (Fig. 37.8):

- A pit or trench should be dug about 2 m deep. It should be half filled with waste, and then covered with lime within 50 cm of the surface, before filling the rest of the pit with soil.
- It must be ensured that animals do not have any access to burial sites. Covers of galvanized iron/wire meshes may be used.
- On each occasion, when wastes are added to the pit, a layer of 10 cm of soil shall be added to cover the wastes.
- Burial must be performed under close and dedicated supervision.
- The deep burial site should be relatively impermeable and no shallow well should be close to the site.
- The pits should be distant from habitation, and sited so as to ensure that no contamination occurs of any surface water or groundwater. The area should not be prone to flooding or erosion.
- The location of the deep burial site will be authorized by the prescribed authority.
- The institution shall maintain a record of all pits for deep burial (Fig. 37.8).

CONCLUSION

The BMW management rules were established in 1998 under the environment protection act, the rules have been reset in 2016 with modification of set guidelines. So nurse should be knowledgeble and aware of the current rules and guidelines in order to dispose waste appropriately, BMW handling facility for the collection, reception, storage, transport, treatment, disposal or any other form of handling.

SUGGESTED READING

1. Atne PL, Szanne TE, Lackman. Medical Surgical Nursing, 4th edition. Philadelphia, PA: WB Saunder Company; 1996.
2. Barbara K. Fundamentals of Nursing Concepts, Process and Practice, 5th edition. California: Addison-Wesley Nursing Publishers; 1995. pp. 650, 861-2, 1280, 1283.
3. Barbara LC, Wilma PJ, Virginia CL. Medical Surgical Nursing, 3rd edition. Mosby Publishers; 1993. pp. 177, 254, 1524, 1581.
4. Benjamin SJ, Virginia SA. Comprehensive Textbook of Psychiatry, Vol 1, 7th Edition. Philadelphia, PA: Lippincott Publishers; 2000. pp. 555-6.
5. Boyle AJ, Wilson AM, Connelly K, et al. An evaluation during simulated cardiac arrest on a hospital bed. Resuscitation. 2002;54.
6. Chiang WC, Chen WJ. Better adherence to the guidelines during cardiopulmonary resuscitation through the provision of audio-prompts. Resuscitation. 2005;64(3):297-301.
7. Elizabeth HB. Development Psychology – A Lifespan Approach, 5th edition. New Delhi: AITBS Publishers; 1999. pp. 268-9, 416.
8. Fernald Dodge L, Fernald S. Peter Introduction to Psychology, 5th edition. New Delhi: AITBS Publishers; 1999. p. 304.
9. Kneisl W. Psychiatric Nursing, 5th edition. California: Addison-Wesley Nursing Publishers; 1996. pp. 310, 332, 336, 442-3, 486, 510-11.
10. Marlow DR. Textbook of Pediatrics for Nursing, 6th edition. WB Sarendees Co.; 2001. pp. 315-7.
11. Park K. Parks Textbook of Preventive an Social Medicine, 16th edition. Jabalpur; M.S Banarsidas; Bhanot Publications; 2001. pp. 16-18.
12. Parthasarathi A. Textbook of Pediatrics, 2nd edition. New Delhi: Jaypee Brothers Medical Publishers; 2000. pp. 47-52.
13. Patricia AP, Griffin PA. Fundamentals of Nursing, 5th edition. Noida: Elsevier Publishers; 2001. pp. 2218, 907, 940.
14. Pillitteri A. A Textbook of Maternal and Child Health Nursing, 4th edition. London: Lippincott Publications; 2003. Prevention of Infection. pp. 1299-301.
15. Potter PA, Perry AG. Fundamentals of Nursing, 4th edition; Mosby Publications; 1997; Infection Control. pp. 741-9.
16. Ruth CF, Hirnle J. Constance, Fundamentals of Nursing-Human Health & Function, 3rd edition. New-York: Lippincott Publishers; 2000. pp. 1216-62.
17. Stuart, Gail W, Laraira Michele J. Principles and Practice of Psychiatric Nursing, 7th edition. Philadelphia: Mosby Publication; 2001. pp. 299-312.
18. Suzzane SC, Brenda BG. Brunner and Suddarth's Textbook of Medical Surgical Nursing, 8th edition. Philadelphia, PA: Lippincot; 1995. pp. 106-16.
19. Townsend Mary C. Psychiatric Mental Health Nursing, 3rd edition. Philadelphia: FA Devis Company. pp. 632-49.
20. Tylor C, Lillis C. Fundamentals of Nursing, 6th edition. Lippincott Publication; 2008; Asepsis and Infection Control. pp. 699-704.

Journals

1. Delisle Isabelle, "La solitude", The Canadian Nurse Infirmer, November 1998;94(10):40-44.

REVIEW OF SECTION BASED QUESTIONS OF RGUHS

Long Essays

1. a. Discuss the various electrolyte imbalance and its management. (May 2010)
   b. Discuss the pathophysiology and immediate nursing care for hypovolemic shock?
2. a. What are the common nutritional problems prevalent among children in India?
   b. Describe the nutritional programs in our country to prevent nutritional problems. (May 2011)
3. As a nurse manager, how will you plan the bio-medical waste management for a hospital.
4. State the different causes of hemorrhage and shock? Explain in detail its pathophysiology?
5. What are the biopsychosocial pathology regarding sleep pattern disturbances?
6. a. What are various theories of pain?
   b. Write in detail the WHO strategies of pain management?
7. What are the biopsychosocial pathology regarding altered body temperature? How will you apply nursing process for a patient with altered body temperature?
8. What are the biopsychosocial pathologies of unconsciousness? Apply nursing process for a patient with unconsciousness?
9. How will you plan for care of patients undergoing abdominal surgery?
10. What are the postoperative complications and enumerate the steps to prevent it?
11. Discuss the role of nurse in preventing nosocomial infection. (Oct 2010)
12. Illustrate the pathophysiology of altered body temperature and discuss the management of hyperpyrexia. (Nov 2012)
13. Explain the role of nurse in biomedical waste management? (Nov 2012)
14. Explain the infection prevention and safety measures. (May 2012)
15. a. What are causes of anaphylactic shock?
    b. As a nurse how will you assess and manage the patient with anaphylactic shock?
16. List down the causes of unconsciousness and formulate a nursing care plan for an unconscious patient.

Short Essays

1. End of life care.
2. Oxygen insufficiency.
3. Cardiopulmonary resuscitation.
4. Standard safety measures.
5. Biomedical waste management.
6. Homeostatic mechanism.
7. Sleep problems and sleep hygiene. (Oct 2010)
8. Responsibility of a department supervision in infection control of the EMERGENCY UNIT. (May 2010)
9. Care of unconscious patient. (October 2016)

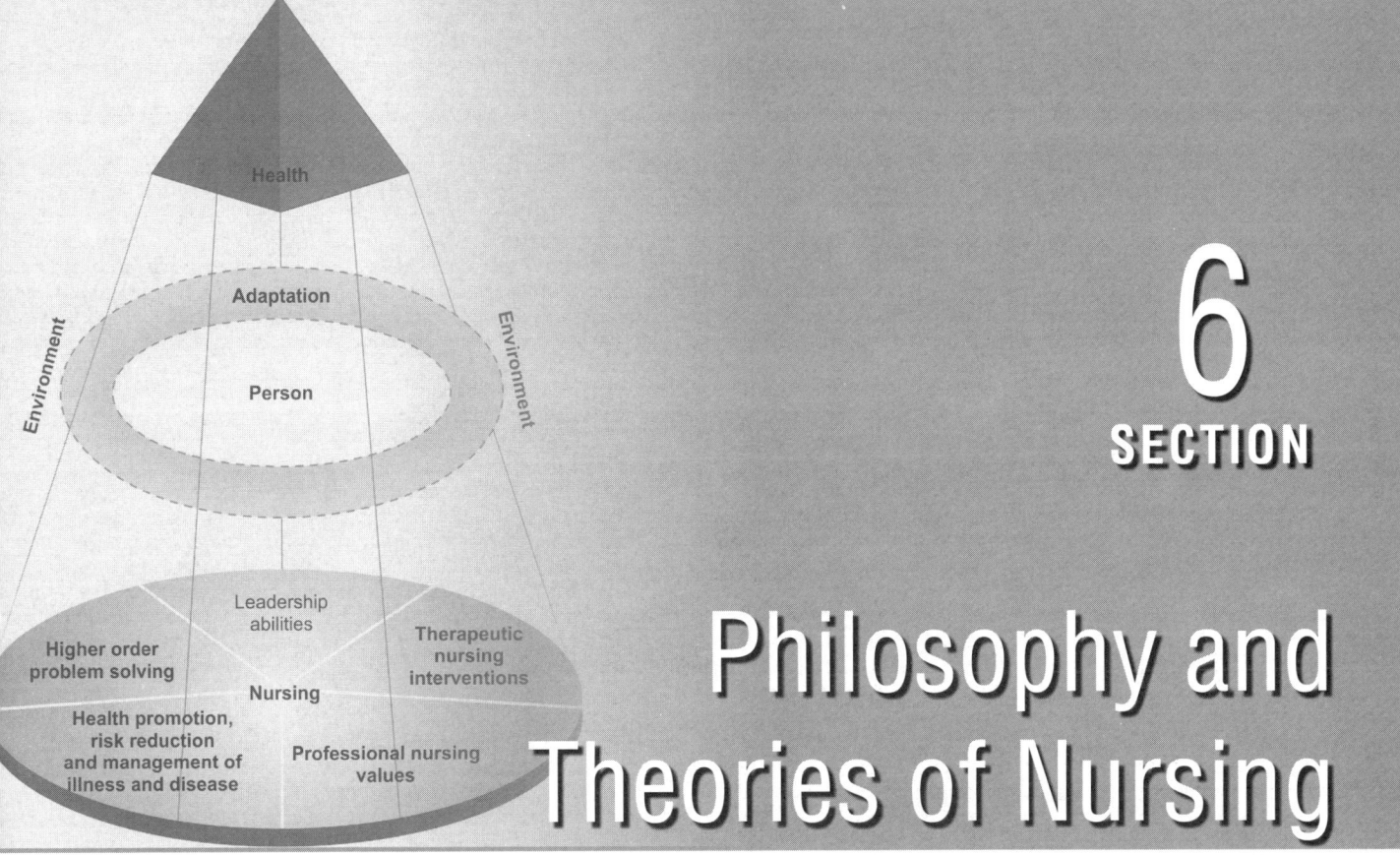

Section 6

Philosophy and Theories of Nursing

Section Outline

38. Values, Conceptual Models and Approaches
39. Nursing Theories
40. A Health Belief Model
41. Concept of Self-health
42. Evidence-based Practice Model

CHAPTER 38

Values, Conceptual Models and Approaches

CHAPTER OUTLINE

- Terminologies
- Introduction
- Model
  - Conceptual Model/Frameworks, Purposes, Significance, Uses of Conceptual Framework, Development of Conceptual Framework and Its Steps
- Theory
  - Definitions, Purposes, Significance, Components, Characteristics, Scope, and Classification of Theories

TERMINOLOGIES

- ***Phenomena:*** Occurrence of facts, i.e. directly perceptible by their senses (feel, hear, see), e.g. storm, rain, organization of meeting, etc.
- ***Concepts:*** Subject matter of the theory they are the symbolic representation of a thing or event. Concept is a systematic view of phenomenon; it is a complex mental function of object property or an event. It is derived from individual perceptual experience. It is an ideal mental image, which is generated and framed in the mind. It labels the phenomena.
- ***Abstract concept:*** It is completely independent of time and place, e.g. temperature.
- ***Concrete concept:*** It is specific to time and place, e.g. what is the room temperature.
- ***Facts:*** These are something, which is known with certainty, e.g. water flows, earth is round, fire burns.
- ***Assumptions:*** Statements supposed to be true without proof or demonstrations are beliefs about phenomena one must accept as true.
- ***Definitions:*** Statements are meaning of a word or phrase or statement, e.g. temperature means heat maintained by the body.
- ***Theoretical definition:*** Derived from theory exactly. It conveys the general meaning of the concept in manner that fits into the theory.
- ***Operational definitions:*** Specifies the activities or operations necessary to measure or construct or variable, e.g. perception, awareness.
- ***Theories:*** Theory is a set of concepts definitions or propositions of that project of systematic view of phenomena by designing a specific interrelationship among the concepts for the purpose of describing, explaining, and predicting.
- ***Propositions:*** Propositions are statements of theories, which are derived from axioms (generalizations). It means any ideas or hunch (inner feeling), i.e. present in the form of scientific statement.
- ***Axioms:*** Axioms state the most general relationship between concepts. So theories generate from axioms. Theory is composed of many axioms or propositions.
- ***Variables:*** These are dependent and independent:
  - ***Dependent variables:*** These are the behavior or characteristics of outcome researcher can understand, explain as the effect of independent variables, e.g. smoking (independent) leads to cancer (dependent).
  - ***Independent variable:*** This is the presumed cause is not affected by any variables, e.g. age, sex, etc. (in nonexperimental studies).
- ***Paradigm:*** A paradigm is a conceptual diagram. It can be a large structure used to organize theory.
- ***Meta paradigm:*** It is the most global conceptual or philosophical frame of a profession, which defines and describes relationships among major ideas and values. It guides the organization of theories and models for a profession.
- ***Person:*** It refers to the recipient of nursing care, including physical, spiritual, psychological, and sociocultural components of an individuals, family, or community.
- ***Health:*** It refers to the degree of wellness or illness experienced by the person.

- ❖ **Nursing:** It refers to the actions, characteristics, and attributes of the individual providing nursing care.
- ❖ **Environment:** It refers to all the internal and external conditions, circumstances, and influences, and affecting the persons.
- ❖ **Law:** A law is a statement that describes a relationship in which scientists have so much confidence they consider it an absolute truth.
- ❖ **Hypothesis:** Tentative prediction/explanation of the relationship between two or more variables to be tested.
- ❖ **Empirical generalizations:** These are patterns of events found in number of different empirical studies.
- ❖ **Causal:** One concept is believed to cause the occurrence of another concept, if they have a causal relationship, correlation is not causation.
- ❖ **Research:** It is application of systematic methods to obtain reliable and valid knowledge about empirical reality. Research may generate theory with an inductive approach or test it by deductive approach.
- ❖ **Theoretical statements:** It describes a relationship between two or more concepts.
- ❖ **Induction:** It is a form of reasoning the moves from the specific to the general. In inductive logic, a series of particulars is combined into a larger whole.
- ❖ **Deduction:** It is a form of logical reasoning that progress from general to specific. This process involves a sequence of theoretical statement derived from few general statements.

INTRODUCTION

Florence Nightingale taught us that nursing theories describe and explain what is nursing and what is not nursing. Today knowledge development in nursing is taking place on several levels with a variety of scholarly approaches contribute to advances in the disciplines' various paradigms and value systems that express the perspective held by several groups within the disciplines grant the knowledge and practice of nursing.

Theory helps provide knowledge to improve practice by describing, explaining, predicting, and controlling phenomena. Nurse's power is increased through theoretical knowledge because systematically developed methods are more likely to be successful. Theory provides professional autonomy by guiding the practice, education, and research functions of the profession.

The study of the theory helps to develop analytical skills, challenging thinking clarify values and assumptions and determine purpose of nursing practice, education and research. It is important to understand cyclical nature of theory, research and practice (Fig. 38.1).

The testing process for theory is clinical research. The more research conducted about specific theory, the more useful the theory is to practice. Practice is based on the theories of the discipline that are validated through research.

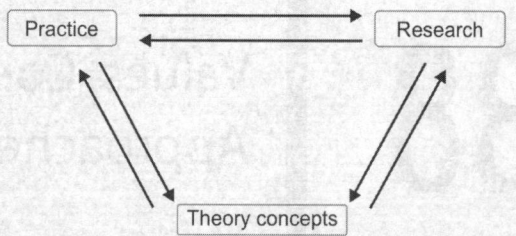

Fig. 38.1: Cyclical nature of theory, research, and practice.

MODEL

A model is any structure of events or systems, ideas, which purport to replicate, reproduce, or represent something else.

Conceptual Model

"It is the abstract, logical structure of meaning that guides the development of the study and enables the researcher to link findings to nursing body of knowledge."

—**Polit and Hungler**

"A conceptual model can be defined as a basic structure in which a complex of ideas are united to portray a large general idea."

Conceptual models are conceptual frameworks are made up of abstract and concepts (general ideas) and propositions that specify their relationships.

Conceptual Framework

- ❖ It is the brief explanation of theory or those portions of theory, which are to be tested.
- ❖ Theoretical and conceptual frameworks are commonly used in quantitative research studies.
- ❖ This helps to organize the study and provide a context for the interpretation of study results.

Purposes of Conceptual Framework

- ❖ To make research findings meaningful and generalized.
- ❖ For drawing together and summarizing accumulated facts.
- ❖ Framework may serve as a springboard for scientific advancement.

Uses of Conceptual Framework and Models

- ❖ Models are used for development of framework of the studies.
- ❖ It is the primary mechanism by which researchers organize findings into a broader context.
- ❖ Helps to stimulate research and extent of knowledge.
- ❖ Useful in clarifying concepts and their association.
- ❖ Helps in formulating research question and hypothesis.
- ❖ Models promote the association between research activities.
- ❖ Framework provides the structure for examining a problem.

❖ Framework serves as a guide to examine relationship between variables.
❖ Frameworks also can help to promote the association between research activities.

Developing Conceptual Framework and Models

It requires researcher's knowledge of theories, findings of previous similar research studies, and related field experience. It requires skills of creativity in identifying and relationship between two or more study concepts.

Facts about Framework Development

❖ Development of framework depends on the power of observation, understanding of a problem, imagination, and conceptualization about abstract ideas.
❖ Frameworks are usually developed through inductive reasoning.
❖ Concepts may be borrowed from personal real life experiences, findings of the previous research, and concepts of existing theories or theoretical models.
❖ A theoretical framework is developed on the basis of theoretical concepts, which are related to particular research study variables.
❖ Conceptual frameworks are constructed on the basis of researchers own experience in respective field and findings of the previous study or the concepts of the several existing theories.

Steps for Development of a Conceptual Framework (Fig. 38.2)

1. **Identification of general concepts:** Initially the researcher identifies the general concepts of the study; these concepts may be based on the study variables, previous research findings or existing theories and models.
2. **Gathering relevant information:** Gathering relevant information about concepts from the relevant existing theories, previous research findings, etc.
3. **Formulation of general scheme of relevant concepts (Fig. 38.3):** The researcher starts establishing the general relationship between the different related and relevant concepts.
4. **Development of logical construct (Fig. 38.4):**
   ➢ After establishing the logical relationship between two or more variables, the researcher develops final construct.
   ➢ Construct is highly abstract, complex description of a phenomenon (concept).
   ➢ It is denoted by a made-up or construed term.
5. **Evaluation and revision**
   ➢ **Concepts and constructs:** It acts as the building blocks for the framework, which are later evaluated for their relevance and their relationship to conclude or generalize the facts.

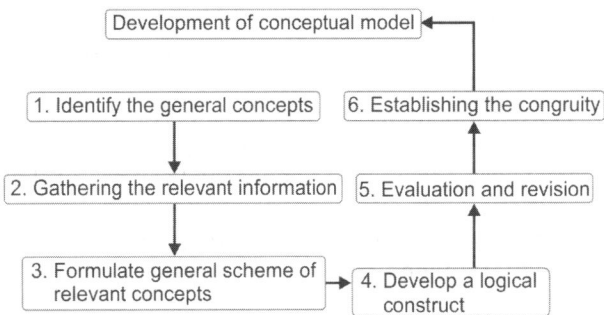

Fig. 38.2: Steps for development of a conceptual framework.

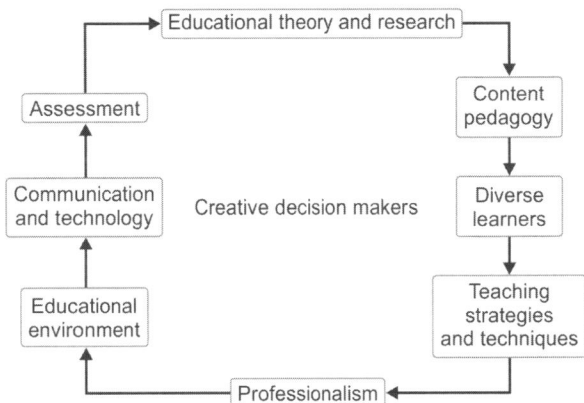

Fig. 38.3: Formulation of general scheme of relevant concepts.

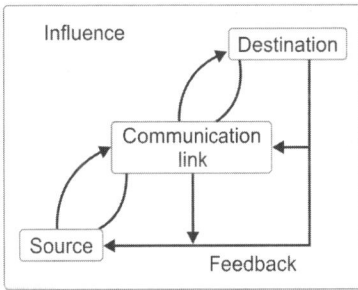

Fig. 38.4: Conceptual framework for implementation of defined practices and programs.

   ➢ After evaluation, revision may be made before development of a framework.
6. **Establishment of the congruity**
   ➢ Once the researcher develops a framework, it is important to establish the congruity between model and its components.
   ➢ The research problem.
   ➢ Hypothesis
   ➢ The description of operationalization of concepts
   ➢ The selection of research design.

Framework

A framework is the conceptual underpinnings of a study. Not every study is based on theory or conceptual model, but every study has a framework. The concepts in which a researcher is interested are by definitions abstractions of observable phenomena.

- ❖ *Conceptual models used in nursing research:* Nurse researchers have used both nursing and non-nursing frameworks to provide a conceptual context for their studies.
- ❖ *Conceptual models of the nursing process:* Nurses have formulated number of conceptual models of nursing practice. These models constitute formal explanations of what the nursing disciplines. As Fawcett (1989) has noted four concepts are central to models of nursing person, environment, health, and nursing.

The various conceptual models, however, define these concepts differently link them in diverse ways and give different emphases to the relationships among them. The grand theorists often included aspects of human beings, their environment, an health in the nursing conceptual models, e.g. Callista Roys adaptation model, Orem, Levine, Rogers, Johnson, Neuman, and King's theory.

THEORY

Meaning

Theory is Greek word "theoria" means speculation—expressing:

- ❖ It is a highly complex term with abstract meaning.
- ❖ It is a set of defined concepts and systematic logical network of relation statement or propositions.
- ❖ It varies in degree of abstract and concepts, and statements in the theory.

Definitions

Theory is a set of interrelated concepts, definitions, and propositions that provide an orderly way to view a phenomenon.

—**Kerlinger**

A theory is a set of concepts definitions and prepositions that project a systematic view of phenomena by designing specific interrelationships among concepts for purposes of describing, explaining, and predicting.

—**Chinn and Kramer M, 2004**

Nursing theory is a conceptualization of some aspect of reality (invented or discovered) that pertains to nursing. The conceptualization is articulated for the purpose of describing, explaining, and predicting or prescribing nursing care.

—**Meleis, 1997**

Purposes

- ❖ To build up the body of knowledge to provide foundations required for profession.
- ❖ To disseminate knowledge, facts and phenomena in nursing.
- ❖ Theories help to describe, explain, predict and control outcome of nursing activity.
- ❖ It increases understanding in knowledge of what and why nurses do certain things.
- ❖ Theory develops autonomy.
- ❖ It helps to develop analytical skills, thinking, and reasoning.
- ❖ It clarifies the values and assumptions.
- ❖ It helps to describe the goal for nursing practice, education, and research.
- ❖ It helps to identify goals in specific nursing practice.
- ❖ It serves as important use in nursing research.

Significance of Theories

- ❖ Theories and models provide sound philosophy and scientific knowledge, education, and practice and research.
- ❖ They reveal the nature of nursing as a distinct science.
- ❖ Establish a comprehensive and scientific is unique to nursing.
- ❖ It explains nature of phenomena, which is occurring in nursing.
- ❖ It helps to contribute toward explain attaining objectives.
- ❖ It provides direction of future development of nursing knowledge and practice.
- ❖ It helps in experimental research. It leads to verification of laws and in nursing research.
- ❖ Theory also helps in summarization of knowledge.
- ❖ It contributes toward professionalization.
- ❖ Theories helps to explain past events provides a sense of understanding current events and practices future events, and provides potentialities to control them.
- ❖ It helps to providing nurses a professional autonomy by serving a framework for nursing education and research.
- ❖ Many issues in nursing can be solved on the basis of theory. It forms the platform for continuous theoretical development.
- ❖ Theories help to determinate effect of hospitalization because of separation from family members and use rationale in understanding individual relationships and the hospital personnel.
- ❖ It provides platform for continually theoretical development. It is also source of internal control.
- ❖ It provides an ability to challenge healthcare activities of others.

Components of a Theory (Fig. 38.5)

Autonomy and Theories

There are number of issues critical to the topic of theory that will influence the direction and the level of autonomy that distinguishes advanced practiced nursing. These issues include:

- ❖ Reluctance of advanced practice nurses to recognize the significance of nursing theory

Chapter 38: Values, Conceptual Models and Approaches

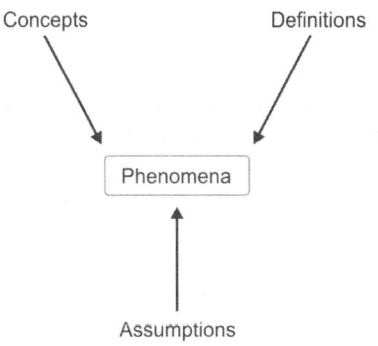

Fig. 38.5: Components of a theory.

- Lack of conceptual clarity as to what constitutes advanced nursing
- Negative consequences of nursing's history
- The interface between theory for nursing and theory for advanced nursing.

Role of Theory in a Practice Discipline

- A theory is general explanation used to explain, predict, control and understand commonly occurring events (Holder and Chitty, 1997) and is of unique interest to a discipline.
- Theory organizes and classifies events into a logical, conceptual whole that allows a practitioner to recognize, understand, and manage the phenomena at hand.

For example, a theory of pain would encompass notions of causation and response. Thus a well-defined theory of pain would enable nurse to recognize predictions and indication of pain. A theory of pain management would further facilitate a systemic approach to intervening to achieve goals relative to preventing or minimizing pain.

Characteristics of Theory

Torres (1990) provides the characteristics that enhance the utility of a theory:
- Theories relate concepts in such a way as to create new and more useful ways to look at a particular phenomenon.
- Theories must be logical in nature.
- Theories must be relatively simple yet generalized.
- Theories can be the basis for hypothesis that can be tested.
- Theories contribute to and assist in measuring the general body of knowledge within the discipline through the research implemented to validate them.
- Theories must be consistent with other validated theories, laws and principles, but they leave unanswered questions that need to be investigated.

Scope of Theories

Theories differ in their level of scope; the scope of theory relates:
- The range of phenomena to the theory relates.

- Theory is level of abstraction.

Theories may be very broad in their range of phenomena of interest and try to portray the larger picture or they may be very limited in their focus. While theories are classified according to their level of scope starting from broadest and moving to the most limited the different classification include the following.

Classification of Theories (Fig. 38.6)

Depending on Function

- ***Descriptive:*** To identify the properties and workings of a discipline.
- ***Explanatory:*** To examine how properties relate and thus affect the discipline.
- ***Predictive:*** To calculate relationships between properties and how they occur.
- ***Prescriptive:*** To identify under which conditions relationships occur.

Depending on the Generalization of their Principles

- ***Meta theory:*** Identifies specific phenomena through abstract concepts. This is oriented toward philosophical and methodological issues of theory development. This focuses on concerned related to the nature of theories. Meta theory asks questions about knowledge and about the broader issues within a discipline. It examines questions such as what are appropriate criteria for the analysis and evaluation and nature of theory.
- ***Grand theory or broad range theory:*** Provides a conceptual framework. Grand theories have the broadest scope and present general concepts and propositions. Theories at this level may both reflect and provide insights useful for practice, but are not designed for empirical testing. This limits the use of grand theories for directing explaining and predicting. Nursing in particular situations. Development of grand theories goal is to explain the totality of events related to discipline. Theoretical formulations within a grand theory are general. In nursing, a grand theory would attempt to explain the mission and goals of nursing care.

Examples of grand theories include Orem's self-care deficit theory, Roger's science of unitary human beings,

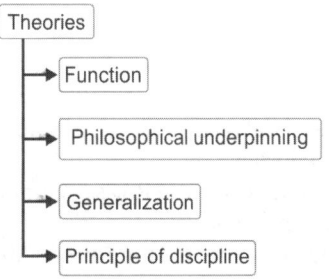

Fig. 38.6: Classification of theories.

King's theory of goal attainment, Myra Levine theory, Dorothea E Johnson, Sister Callista Roy theory, Betty Neuman's theory, etc.

Based on the Principles of the Discipline can be Identified Middle Range Theory

Middle range theory is more precise and only analyzes a particular situation with a limited number of variables. It has a narrow focus than grand theory and a broader focus that micro theory. However, the focus of midrange phenomena and concepts can be relevant to all nursing specialties and applicable to a number of nursing care situations. It seeks to provide answers to specific nursing questions. A midrange theory is based in specific practice concepts and is characteristically more concrete than a grand theory, but cannot be used to explain complex life situations and appropriate for empirical testing.

Example of midrange theories includes: Peplau's interpersonal relations theory, Leininger's cultural care theory, Rosemarie Rizzo Parse human becoming theory, Ida Jean Orlando, Joyce Travelbee, Joan Riehl-Sisca, Erickson, Ramona T Mercer, Kathryn E Barnard, Newman, Evelyn Adam, and Nola Pender.

Micro/practice theory: Explores one particular situation found in nursing. It identifies explicit goals and details how these goals will be achieved. It is also known as practice theory, empirical generalization, or partial theory. The range of micro theory is more limited and prescribed than that of midrange theory. Micro theories are the least complex and more specific. They are a set of theoretical statements usually hypothesis, that deal with narrowly defined phenomena.

The goal of micro theory is to provide a nurse with specific desired patient goals and precise practice directives.

Example of micro theory would be physiology of pain phenomena.

Based on the Philosophical Underpinnings of the Theories

- Needs theories
- Florence Nightingale theory
- Abdellah theory
- Henderson theory
- Dorothea Orem theory
- Lydia Hall theory
- Jean Watson theory
- Interaction theories
- Peplau theory, Orlando, King, Wiedenbach, Paterson and Zderad, Erickson, Tomlin and Swain, etc.
- Outcome theories
- Input output theories and Roy's, Neuman, etc.
- Humanistic theories
- Fl Nightingale, Virginea Henderson, Abdellah, Orem, Elvin, Travel Bee, Adam, Abraham Maslow's, Carl Rogers, Kelly's, Imogene King, etc.

Sources of Knowledge for Theory Development/Research

Ideas are generated in many ways and highly structured and are generally bound by defined rules of process, which includes:

1. **Scientific enquiry:** The scientific method is a body of techniques for investigating phenomena, acquiring new knowledge and integrating previous knowledge is commonly based on empirical or measurable evidence subject to specific principles of reasoning. It involves the inductive and deductive logic.
2. **Critical thinking:** It is a rational unbiased analysis or evaluation of an issue (factual evidence) in order to form a judgment. It is self-directed, self-disciplined, self-monitored, and self-corrective thinking. It entails effective communication and problem solving abilities and will empower one's knowledge and understanding.
3. **Logical reasoning:** In research approach sources of knowledge involves the mental process of logical reasoning using rational, systematic series of steps based on sound ideas with mathematical precision and uses reasoning consistently to come to a conclusion. Problems that involve logical thinking call for structure, for relationships between facts. It involves inductive and deductive reasoning.
4. **Intuition:** It is the ability to acquire knowledge without conscious reasoning and the ability to understand something instinctively. It is frequently used method in problem solving. It can operate one of two ways as a form that closely resembles sensory perceptions, or as an extra sensory experience independent of sensory unit. It includes practical reasoning, all forms of reasoning including scientific reasoning and the production of scientific knowledge.
5. **Trial and error:** Learning by trial and error is another way of gaining knowledge. Making mistakes or repeatedly trying various ways of accomplishing something will result in problem solving. This method of learning is practical but it is unsystematic way of learning. In nursing, student nurses may get exposed to trial and error methods.
6. **Experience:** A person learns through experience without this, a person would have to relearn procedure every time it was performed. Practice leads to the development of routines that help in building skills. Experience makes a person to increase knowledge, work with confidence, and improve the performance of skills.

Theory Development Process

Primarily theory development process involves induction, deduction, and retroduction.

Inductive Approach

This form of reasoning that moves from the specific to the general in inductive logic, a series of particulars is combined into a larger whole or set of things and particular events are observed and analyzed as a basis for formulating general theoretical statements. This is a theory to research approach.

Deductive Approach

It is a form of logical reasoning that moves from general to specific. This process involves a sequence of theoretical statement derived from a few general statements or axioms. It uses two or more relational statements are used to draw conclusions. Abstract theoretical relationships are used to derive specific empirical hypothesis. This is a theory to research approach.

Retroduction

It combines induction and deduction. Theories may be organized according to their form into three categories. These categories include:
a. **Set of laws**: It is an inductive approach that seeks patterns in research findings; these findings are selected and sorted according to degree of empirical support into categories of laws, empirical generalizations, and hypothesis. It may be difficult to organize and interrelate those generalizations. Because the statements are not interrelated, support for one statement does not support another statement. So the research efforts must be extensive.
b. **Axiomatic**: It is an interrelated logical system of concepts, definitions, and relationship statements arranged in hierarchical order. Abstract axioms are at the top and with derived propositions at the bottom. Empirical support for one relational statement also supports the theory.
c. **Causal process**: It increases an understanding through relationship statements that specify cause between independent and dependent. This form also requires concepts, definitions, and relationship statements.

CONCLUSION

There is considerable value in the nursing profession furthering into understanding into models and theories. These are widely applied both in practice and academics.

The use of analogs, constructs, and verbal descriptions of systems, idealization, and graphic representation is wide spread. As nurses become increasingly skillful at developing practice approaches based on sound theoretical information, the usefulness of model will increase.

39 CHAPTER

Nursing Theories

CHAPTER OUTLINE

- Nightingale's Theory
- Henderson's Theory
- Rogers' Theory
- Peplau's Theory
- Abdellah's Theory
- Levine's Conservation Model
- Dorothea E Orem—Self-care Deficit Theory of Nursing
- Dorothy E Johnson—Behavioral System Model
- Imogene King Theory
- Betty Neuman's Systems Theory
- Roy's Adaptation Theory
- Watson's Theory
- Parse's Human Becoming Theory and their Applications.

NIGHTINGALE'S THEORY (FIG. 39.1)

Credentials and Background of the Theorist

- Born on May 12, 1820
- Founder of modern nursing
- The first nursing theorist
- Also known "The Lady with the Lamp"
- She explained her environmental theory in her famous book "Notes on Nursing: What it is, What it is Not"
- She was the first to propose nursing required specific education and training
- Her contribution during Crimean war is well-known
- She was a statistician, using bar and pie charts, highlighting key points
- International Nurses Day, May 12 is observed in respect to her contribution to Nursing
- Died on August 13, 1910.

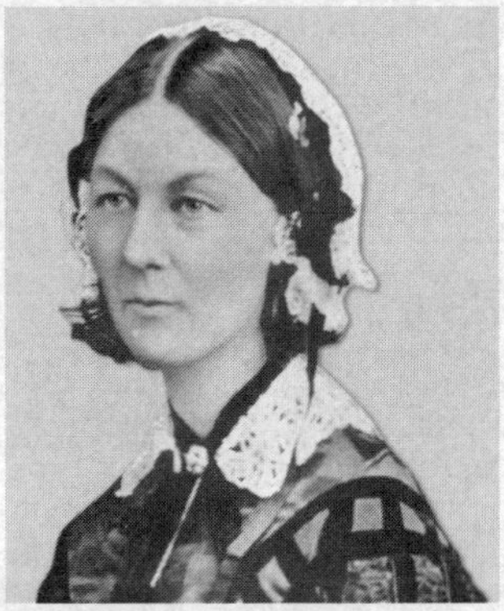

Fig. 39.1: Florence Nightingale.

Definition of Nursing According to Florence Nightingale

"Nature alone cures. And what nursing has to do is to put the patient in the best condition for nature to act upon."

Theoretical Sources

Many factors influenced the development of Nightingale's theory for nursing:

- Individual, society, and professional values where all integral in the development of her work. She combined her individual resources with society and professional resources to produce change.
- The strongest influences on the development of her practice where her education, experience, and observation. This was the logical base for her nursing philosophy.

Use of Empirical Evidence

Nightingale was a devoted statistician she used her careful information to prove the efficacy of her system of hospital nursing and organization during the Crimean war.

Major Concepts of Nightingale's Environmental Theory (Figs. 39.2 and 39.3)

Nightingale's Grand Theory focused on the environment that all the external conditions and influences affecting the life and development of an organism. Her major concepts comprised the components of environment.

- ***Ventilation:*** She believed that healthy surroundings were necessary for proper nursing care. There are five

Chapter 39: Nursing Theories

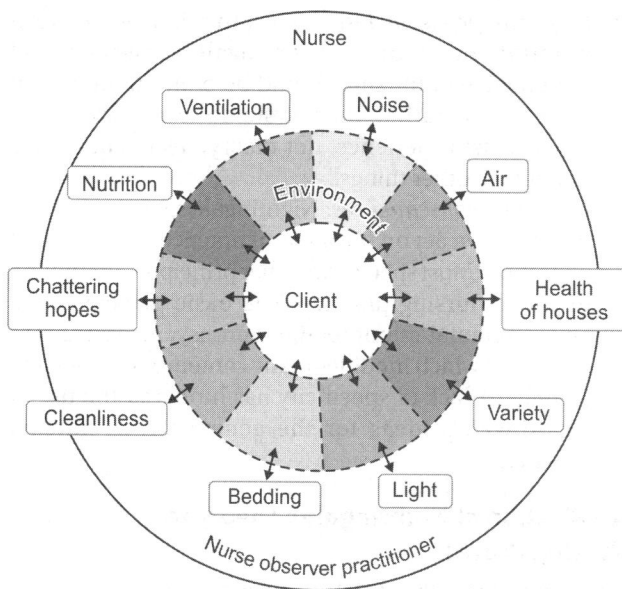

Fig. 39.2: Client and environment in balance.

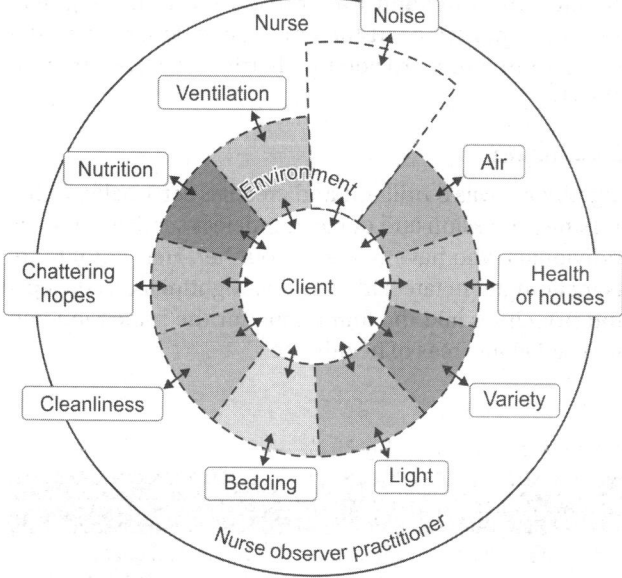

Fig. 39.3: Client expending unnecessary energy by being stressed by environment (noise).

essential points in securing the health of houses—(1) pure air, (2) pure water, (3) efficient drainage, (4) cleanliness, and (5) light. This means the nurse was "to keep the air breathes as pure as the external air, without chilling." She believed pure air was very essential to a patient without which the rest is nothing.

- ❖ **Light:** It is another element of nursing care that Nightingale believed which could not be ignored. She stressed the beneficial aspects of direct sunlight in patient rooms.
- ❖ **Cleanliness:** The need for cleanliness is extended to the nurse and the environment. She stated that, "dirty carpets, walls, dirty sheets, and beds contained large quantities of organic matter and provided a ready source of infection and washed skin interfered with the healing process. Therefore, nurses should wash their hands frequently and keep their patients and surroundings very clean."
- ❖ **Warmth:** Nightingale also believed a nurse should attend to patient's warmth, quiet, and diet. She advised, constantly monitored the patient's body temperature by palpating the extremities to prevent the effects of vital heat loss.
- ❖ **Noise:** It is another environmental element and she believed the nurse should manipulate "unnecessary noise or noise that creates an expectation in mind, is that which hurts a patient."
- ❖ **Diet:** Nightingale was also concerned with the patient's diet. She believed a nurse should not only assess the dietary intake, but also assess the timeline of food intake and its effect on the patient. Observation, ingenuity, and perseverance were the qualities required to distinguish a good nurse.

Nightingale's Theory and Nursing Metaparadigm

Person

The person as the patient is regarded as a human being acted upon by a nurse, or affected by the environment. The person has reparative powers to deal with the disease. Recovery is in the patient's power as long as a safe environment exists.

Environment

The foundational component of this theory is the external conditions and forces that affect one's life and development including everything from a person's food to a nurse's verbal and nonverbal interactions with the patient. She tends to emphasize the physical environment more than the psychological and social environment.

Health

Health is maintained by using a person's healing powers to their fullest extent and by controlling the environmental factors to prevent diseases. It is viewed as a reparative process instituted by nature. Health and disease are the focus of the nurse. Nurses help patients through their healing process.

Nursing

Nursing provides fresh air, light, warmth, cleanliness, silence, diet, and a proper care. The patient's reparative process ensures the best possible environment. Influence of the environment affects health and supports the nursing process.

Theoretical Assertions

- ❖ Nightingale believed disease as a reparative process. She directed that nurse's role was to prevent the reparative

process from being interrupted and to provide optimal conditions for its enhancement.
- Nightingale assumed a person is desirous of health, so that nature and person would cooperate to allow the reparative process to occur.

Logical Form
Nightingale used inductive reasoning to extract loss of health and nursing from her observations and experiences. For example, he/she noticed that diseases fluoresced in confined, dark dam areas and concluded that it was generated from the environment.

Acceptance by Nursing Community
- Practice: Nightingale's nursing principles remain applicable to nursing practice today.
- Education: The Nightingale system was the basis for the origination of many early nurse training schools—St. Thomas Hospital and King's College Hospital in London.
- Research: Nightingale interested was in statistics and her importance in nursing continues to influence nursing research. Gathering information and analyzing the data laid down the introduction of nursing research today. But, her theory lacks complexity and testability. Therefore, it has not generated nursing research.

Critique
- Simplicity: The concepts and their relationships cannot be combined to increase simplicity, but it is simple and logical enough to allow visual representation.
- Generality: Nightingale's attempt was to provide general guidelines to all nurses in all times. So, the generality criterion is met by Nightingale's theory.
- Empirical precision: Little or no provision for empirical examination. Indeed, Nightingale suggested that the practice of nursing should be built on individual observation rather than systematic research. She advised "let experience, not theory, decide upon this as upon all other things."
- Derivable consequences: Nightingale's writings direct the nurses to act on the areas of practice, research and education. Most specific were her principles attempting to shape nursing practice. The basic principles are environmental manipulation and psychological care of patient, which modifies many contemporary nursing settings. A lack of specificity has hindered the use of Nightingale's ideas for the generation of nursing research.

Application of Nightingale's Theory to Nursing Process
Situation (Table 39.1): A 10-year-old girl from rural area was injured in a farm-related machine accident. She had head injury and was conscious. She was not oriented to place and time and was transported to the regional hospital. After triage in the emergency department, she was admitted to a crowded pediatric intensive care unit (PICU).

Conclusion
Nightingale was a brilliant and creative personality in the nursing profession and devoted timeless services to many individuals who have written about her. Her writings are as meaningful in late 20th century. Nightingale's concepts and principles laid the foundation for the profession and are used in all areas of healthcare.

Table 39.1: Application of Nightingale's theory to a client with sleep disturbance (as shown in Fig. 39.3).

Assessment	Nursing diagnosis	Goal	Implementation/nursing intervention	Evaluation
Subjective data: Parents say that primary concern she is unable to sleep and having infected wound. **Objective data:** On observation lights were on 24 h a day, noises from equipment, and visit by her parents were restricted. She looks drowsy, not oriented to place and time and her leg has become infected, requiring IV antibiotics.	Sleep disruption related environmental light/noise and separation from the family.	The female patient will be free from environmental disturbances and sleep well.	Plan for changing the environment to support sleep patterns. Encourage to be awake during day Encourage to listen to her favorite music/watch television and allow her parents to visit more often. Change dressings with aseptic precautions. Reduce volume of alarms, keep dim lights. Keep minimum activities and procedures that would awaken her. Administer antibiotic as prescribed.	After two nights of uninterrupted sleep, normal sounds and parental encouragement demonstrated good sleep, increased orientation to place and identified that she is in hospital.

(IV: intravenous)

HENDERSON'S THEORY (FIG. 39.4)

Credentials and Background of the Theorist

- Born in Kansas City, Missouri, in 1897
- Received a Diploma in Nursing from the Army School of Nursing at Walter Reed Hospital, Washington, District of Columbia in 1921
- In 1929, entered Teachers College at Columbia University for Bachelor's degree
- Master's degree in 1934
- Since 1953, she has been a Research Associate at Yale University School of Nursing
- Died on March 19, 1996.

Theoretical Sources

- First source was she revised the textbook of principles and practice of nursing in 1939.
- A second source was her involvement as a committee member in a regional conference of National Nursing Council in 1946.
- Finally, the American Nurses Association's (ANA) 5 year investigation of function of nurse interested Henderson, who was not fully satisfied with the definition adopted by the ANA in 1995.

Henderson labels her work a definition as a theory and it is not in vogue at that time.

Use of Empirical Evidence

- Henderson incorporated physiological and psychological principles into her personal concept of nursing.
- A correlation with Abraham Maslow's hierarchy of needs is seen in Henderson's 14 components of nursing care, which begin with physical needs and progress to psychosocial components.

Major Concepts and Definitions

Nursing (Fig. 39.5)

Henderson's definition of nursing is in functional terms.

"The unique function of the nurse is to assist the individual, sick or well, in the performance of those activities contributing to health or its recovery (or to a

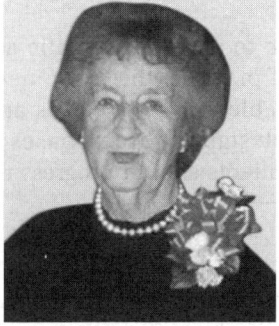

Fig. 39.4: Virginea Henderson.

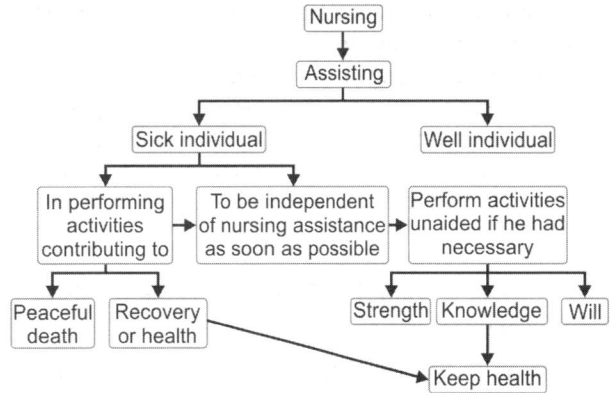

Fig. 39.5: Conceptualization of Henderson's definition.

peaceful death) that he would perform unaided, if he had the necessary strength, will or knowledge and to do this in such a way as to help him gain independence as rapidly as possible."

Health

She views health in terms of patient's ability to perform an unaided the 14 components of the nursing care. It is "the quality of health rather than life itself, than margin of mental physical vigor that allows a person to work most effectively and to reach his/her highest potential level of satisfaction in life."

Environment

Henderson believes that environment as "the aggregate of all the external conditions and influences affecting the life and development of an organism."

Person (patient)

Henderson viewed patient as an individual who requires assistance to achieve health and independence or peaceful death. The mind and body of a person are inseparable. The patient and his/her family are viewed as a unit.

Needs

Henderson identifies 14 basic needs of the patient, which comprise the following components:

1. Breathe normally
2. Eat and drink adequately
3. Eliminate body wastes
4. Move and maintain desirable postures
5. Sleep and rest
6. Select suitable clothes dress and undress
7. Maintain body temperature within normal range by adjusting clothing and modifying environment
8. Keep the body clean and well groomed and protect the integument
9. Avoid dangers in the environment and avoid injuring others

10. Communicate with others in expressing emotions, needs, fears, or opinions
11. Worship according to one's faith
12. Work in such a way that there is a sense of accomplishment
13. Play or participate in various forms of recreation
14. Learn, discover, or satisfy the curiosity that leads to normal development and health and use the available health facilities

Henderson's Theory and Nursing Metaparadigm

Person (patient)

The person must maintain physiological and emotional balance. The mind and body of the person are inseparable. The patient requires help toward independence. The patient and his/her family are a unit. The patient needs are encompassed by the 14 components of nursing.

Health

Henderson viewed health as a quality of life and is very basic for a person to function fully. As a vital need, health requires independence and interdependence. Since health is a multifactor phenomenon, it is influenced by both internal and external factors, which play independent and interdependent roles in achieving health. She also gave emphasis in prioritizing health promotion as more important than care of the sick.

Environment

Environment is important for a healthy individual to control the environment, but as illness occurs, this ability is diminished or affected. In caring for the sick, it is the responsibility of the nurse to help the patient manage the surroundings to protect him/her from harm or any mechanical injury. In assuming this role, the nurse must be educated about safety and must be aware of different social customs and religious practices to assess dangers. Nurses must provide physicians data about the safety needs of the patient, the nurse's observations and judgment regarding these needs as the latter uses this as the basis in prescribing protective devices. It is also the responsibility of the nurse to recommend changes in building construction, purchase of equipment, and maintenance in order for him/her to minimize chances of injury.

Nursing

❖ Henderson asserted that nurses function independently of the physician, but they must promote the treatment plan prescribed by the physician. Although, part of the healthcare team, the nurse must act independently, but in coordination with the therapeutic plan developed by the team.
❖ Another special role of the nurse is to help both the sick and well individual. Care must include people from all walks of life, from the well to the sick, and from the newborn to the dying. The care given by the nurse must empower the patient to gain independence as rapidly as possible.
❖ In the role of the nurse as a health provider, the nurse must be knowledgeable in both biological and social sciences and must have the ability to assess basic human needs of her 14 components of nursing care.

Theoretical Assertions

❖ **The nurse–patient relationship:** The three levels comprising the nurse–patient relationship can be identified, ranging from a very dependent to a quite independent relationship:
  ➢ The nurse as substitute for the patient
  ➢ The nurse as helper to the patient
  ➢ The nurse as partner with the patient
❖ **The nurse–physician relationship:** Henderson insists the nurse has a unique function, distinct from that of physicians such a way as to promote the physicians prescribed therapeutic plan.
❖ The nurse as member of the healthcare team.

Logical Form

Henderson appears to have used the deductive form of logical reasoning to develop her definition of nursing. She deduced her definition of nursing and 14 needs physiological and psychological principles.

Acceptance by the Nursing Community

Practice

Henderson approach to patient care is deliberative and involves decision-making. She believes the nursing process is problem-solving process in the assessment phase nurse would assess the patient in all 14 components of basic nursing care. The planning phase involves making the plan fit individual's needs, updating the plan as necessary, based on the changes, using the plan as a record.

In the implantation phase, the nurse helps the patient to perform activities to maintain health, recovery from illness, and/or to aid in peaceful death. Interventions are individualized, depending on physiological principles and demographic data and evaluation of patient care according to the degree to which he/she performs independently.

Education

Henderson state to use the scientific approach to the improvement of practice, the nurse needs the kind of education available only in colleges and universities. Henderson as designed three phases of curriculum development students should progress through in their learning.

Research

Henderson recommends library reading and surveyed library resources and nursing research at baccalaureate level. The 14 components for basic nursing care of the

Henderson help to pose the question for research. No profession, occupation, or industries in this era evaluate adequately without research. It is the most reliable type of analysis.

Critique

Critique is a grand theory or philosophy in the paradigm stage of theory development in nursing.

Simplicity

Henderson's concept of nursing is complex rather than simple because of the several different descriptions and explanatory relationships. The 14 basic needs are simple as stated, but they become complex when alteration of a need occurs.

Generality

Generality is present in Henderson's definition since it is broad in scope.

Derivable Consequences

She has also influenced curriculum development and made a great contribution in promoting the importance of research in the clinical practice of nursing. She continues to be cited in current nursing literature and publications in all area of nursing practice from holistic to the nursing process.

Conclusion

Henderson was one of the need/problem-oriented theorist. She has placed a philosophical base for nursing profession. The concept of nursing formulated by the Henderson in her definition of nursing and the 14 components of basic nursing care is self-explanatory and simple. Therefore, it guides the present nurses in their nursing practice.

ROGERS' THEORY (FIG. 39.6)

Martha E Rogers—Unitary Being Energy Field Theory

Nursing is both a science and art. The uniqueness of nursing, similar to that of any other science, lies in the phenomenon central to its focus. Nurses long-established concern with people and the world they live in is a natural fore runner of an organized abstract system encompassing people and their environment. The integration of people and environments that coordinate with a multidimensional universe of open systems points to a new paradigm identifies nursing as a science.

Credentials and Background of Theorist

- ❖ Martha E Rogers was born on May 12, 1914, in Dallas, Texas.
- ❖ She began her college education at the University of Tennessee in Knoxville.
- ❖ Where she studied science from 1931 to 1933. She received her "Nursing Diploma" from Knoxville, General Hospital School of Nursing in 1935.
- ❖ In 1937, she received a Bachelor of Science in public nursing from George Peabody, college.
- ❖ Her other degrees include an MA in public Health Nursing Supervision from Teacher's College, Columbia University, New York, in 1945.
- ❖ Master of Public Health (MPH) in 1952. In 1954, she earned her doctorate from John Hopkins University.
- ❖ For 21 years from 1954 to 1975, she was professor and Head of the Division of Nursing at New York University. In 1970, Roger published her book "An Introduction to the Theoretical basis of Nursing."
- ❖ Rogers early nursing practice was in rural public health nursing in Michigan and in Visiting nurse supervision, education, and practice.
- ❖ Her publications include three books and over 200 articles and she lectured in 46 states.
- ❖ She has received citations for "Inspiring Leadership in the Field of Intergroup Relations." "In recognition of your outstanding contribution to nursing" by New York University. "For distinguished service to Nursing" by Teacher's College and many others.
- ❖ She has also been awarded by many awards, funds, and scholarship that have been established in her name.
- ❖ She died on 13 March 1994, at the age of 79.

Theoretical Sources

- ❖ Rogers draws on a knowledge base gained from anthropology, psychology, sociology, astronomy, religion, philosophy, history, biology, physics, mathematics, literature, and sources to create her model of unitary human beings and the environment as energy fields integral to the life process.
- ❖ Several sources influenced Rogers' theorizations during the mid-19th century, Florence Nightingale's proposals and statistical data placed man within the framework of the natural world and the foundation for the scope of modern nursing was laid.
- ❖ In 20th century, Einstein's theory of relativity introduced the four on ordinates of space and time.
- ❖ In 1935, Burr Northrop's "The Electro Dynamic Theory of Life" stated the concepts of the pattern and

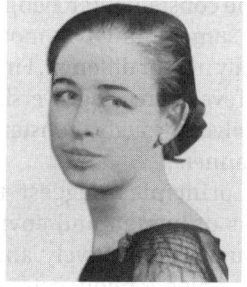

Fig. 39.6: Martha E Rogers.

organization of the electrodynamic field, the outcome of whose activity is wholeness organization and continuity.
- In the 1950s Von Bertalanffy introduced general systems theory, which presented a general science of wholeness and helped her to formulate.

Major Basic Concepts

Roger postulates that human beings are dynamic energy fields integrated with environmental fields. Both human end environmental field are identified by pattern and characterized by a universe of open systems. From these concepts, in her 1983 Paradigm, she populated four building blocks for her model—energy field, a Universe of open systems, pattern and four dimensionality. In 1922, Rogers changed four-dimensionality to pandimensionality. Other concepts that provide clarity to the basic precepts of the Rogerian model include unitary human being, environment, and homeodynamic principles.

Energy Field

An energy field constitutes the fundamental unit of both the living and nonliving. Energy fields are infinite. Two fields are identified—the human field and the environmental field. "Specifically, human beings and environment is energy field." The science of unitary human being (human field) is defined as an irreducible, indivisible, pandimensional energy field identified by pattern and manifesting, characteristics that are specific to the whole and which cannot be predicted from knowledge of the parts. The environment field is defined as an irreducible, pandimensional energy field pattern identified by and integral to the human field. Each environment field is specific to its given human field. Both change continuously and creatively.

An energy field is electrical in nature and consists of waves of electron particles. Every visible object including human is surrounded by a field consisting of waveform. For example, a light bulb is a solid object. When it is lit, it produces both a visible field light and an invisible field heat. Both heat and light are energy forms. The electric flow produced when the lamp is plugged into the electric current, which converts the filament from matter to energy.

Universe of Open Systems

The concept of the universe of open systems holds that energy field is infinite, open, and integral with one another. The human and environment field are in continuous process and are open systems. The human and environmental fields are constantly exchanging energy. There are no boundaries or barriers that inhibit energy flow between fields.

Pattern

Pattern identifies energy fields. It is the distinguishing character of a field and is perceived as a single wave. The nature of the pattern changes continuously and innovatively. Each human field pattern is unique and is integral with its own environment field.

"Manifestations of pattern have been described as unique and refer to behaviors, qualities, and characteristics of the field." The pattern is constantly changing and may manifest disease, illness, or pain.

Pandimensionality

Pandimensionality is defined as "a nonlinear domain without spatial or temporal attributes." The term pandimensional provides for an infinite domain without limit. It best expresses the idea of a unitary whole.

From this conceptual system, Rogers derives the principles of homeodynamics, which postulates a way of perceiving unitary human beings. The principles of homeodynamics are composed of principles of integrity, reasonancy, and helicy.

a. Integrity

In the life process, there will be continuous interactions between human being and environment. Integrity is the "continuous mutual human field and environmental field process." Energy fields pass through one another. The principle of integrity was studied by McDonald (1986), who stated that if there is a continuous mutual human and environmental field process, changes in one field will bring about changes in the other. In the other words, "researchers should be able to demonstrate a relationship between a nurse-initiated modification in a person's environment and an alteration in the person's state of being."

b. Resonancy

The human field and environmental field are identified by wave pattern and organizations manifesting continuous change from lower frequency longer wave patterns to higher frequency shorter wave patterns. The implication of this principle for nursing assessment are that the pattern of the human and environmental field as a whole needs to be assessed from perspective of the rhythmic correlates to human development.

c. Helicy

Helicy is the continuous, innovative, unpredictable, increasing diversity of change in the human environmental field. Because of the constant interchange, an open system never exactly the same at any two moments, rather the system is continually new or different. Finally, the direction of change is toward ever increasing diversity and complexity. The life process evolves through a constant series of change in a rhythmical manner.

Together the principles suggest that the mutual patterning process of human and environmental fields change continuously, innovatively and unpredictably, flowing in lower and higher frequencies.

Conceptual Model (Fig. 39.7)

The Rogerian model provides the abstract philosophical framework from which to view the unitary human being and environmental field. Within the Rogerian framework, nursing is based on theoretical knowledge that guides nursing practice. The Rogerian model, with its implicit assumptions, provides board principles that conceptually direct theory development. Theory can and does emerge from each of the principles, which directs practice. Two theories derived from Rogers' model are mainly used—(1) Bultmeire's theory of Perceived dissonance (1993) and (2) Barrett's theory of Power as knowing Participation in change (1986).

Theory of Perceived Dissonance

The theory of perceived dissonance derived by Bultmeire's from the Rogerian model provides a theoretical perspective for exploring situations of varying resonancy as manifest in healthcare concerns currently labeled as abnormal process. This theory emerges from the principles of resonancy and integrity. The theory provides a mechanism for pattern appraisal of manifestations of the human/environmental field, during times labeled as illness. The theory proposes that resonancy is altered periodically and rhythmically during the evolution of energy fields. The theory of perceived dissonance delineates a human/environmental field process that is perceived as illness in the healthcare system.

People viewed as energy fields embedded in their environmental energy fields. During episodes of varying resonancy, the human and environmental field manifestations may be perceived as nonharmonic and as uncomfortable or unsetting to the person; thus the person views himself or herself as out of harmony or ill.

The theory was of Perceived Dissonance adds clarity to how the nurse can draw on perceptions by the client and have his/her own perceptions to provide nursing care.

The pattern manifestations that emerge during times of variability, labeled as "illness" are crucial in providing a holistic assessment of the unitary human being.

Theory of Power as Knowing Participation in Change

This theory was proposed by Barrett (1986) of Power as knowing participation in change emerges from the Principle of Helicy with in the Rogerian model. This theory provides clear direction for the nurse providing care to the unitary human being. Within this theory, it is proposed that as knowledge increases, so does the capacity to participate knowingly. The theory proposes the capacity of human beings to repattern their human and environmental fields. This capacity can be used by the nurse and by the client during patterning. She specifies that the person must have knowledge in meaningful participation in the repatterning process to occur.

TWO DERIVED THEORIES (FIG. 39.8)

Critical Thinking in Nursing Practice with Roger's Model (Table 39.2)

Within Roger's model, the critical-thinking process can be divided into three components: (1) pattern appraisal, (2) mutual patterning, and (3) evaluation.

Pattern Appraisal

The life process possesses its own unity and it is inseparable from the environment. This holistic appraisal requires the identification of patterns that reflect the whole. The nurse gains a great deal appraisal knowledge during the interview with the client. Pattern appraisal includes multiple lifestyle rhythms such as nutrition, work, exercise, pain, anger, depression, sleep/wake cycles, and safety. During the appraisal, special attention is given to pain and discomfort or areas that the client is uncomfortable or concerned about.

The nurse uses the feeling or sensing level of knowing, often described as intuitive or instinctual. The intuitive knowledge is best realized through reflection, which assists in pattern appraisal.

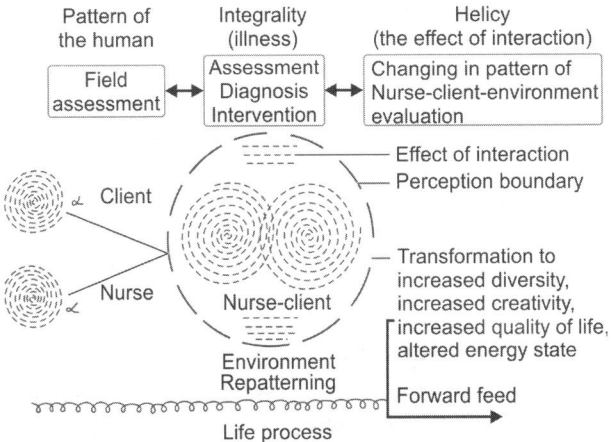

Fig. 39.7: Rogers' conceptual model.

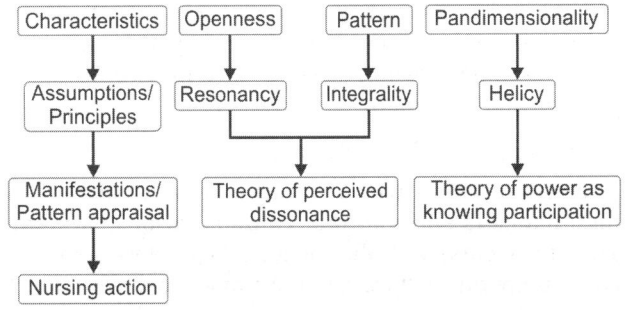

Fig. 39.8: Two derived theories.

Table 39.2: Critical thinking in Roger's model.

Nurse	Client
Pattern appraisal	**Self-reflection**
Comprehensive assessment of: • Human field patterns of communication, exchange, rhythms, dissonance • Environmental field patterns of communication, rhythms, dissonance, harmony intuitive reflection Validate appraisal: • With self • With client	Nutrition Work/Leisure activities, exercise Sleep/wake cycles relationships Discomfort/Pain Fears/hopes
Mutual patterning of human and environmental field	**Patterning activities**
Sharing knowledge offering choices empowering client fostering patterning	Meditation imagery journaling Modifying surroundings
Evaluation	**Personal appraisal**
Repeat pattern appraisal Identify dissonance/harmony Validate appraisal with client	Areas of dissonance Areas of harmony Pattering activities

Mutual Patterning

Once the client/nurse have consensus with respect to the appraisal, then nursing action is centered on mutual pattering of the client human/environmental field. The goal of nursing action is to bring and promote symphonic interaction between human and environment. Barrett defines repatterning as continuous process whereby the nurse, with the client, patterns the environmental field to promote harmony related to the health event. "Change proceeds by the continuous repatterning of both man and environment by resonating waves." Without client participation, patterning is limited and evaluation is difficult.

a. Human field patterning

Patterning activities revolve primarily around noninvasive modalities. Practice modalities concern human life patterning and reflect the wholeness of the unitary human being in "continuous innovative change with the universe." Nurses currently assist clients in the use of meditation, imagery, visualization, and therapeutic touch where there is a primary focus of the patterning of human field. The patterning activities help the client move beyond the physical body to pattern.

b. Environmental field patterning

The environment with its healing quality or lack of dissonance is an important component of treatment. The nurse works with the client in the context of family, community, and cultural group. A supportive environment is needed for harmonious patterning. Color, light, sound, and smell are manifestations of the environmental field. These manifestations can be perceived as dissonant or harmonious.

Evaluation

Evaluation is ongoing and encompasses a repeat of the appraisal process. During the evaluation phase, the nurse repeats the pattern appraisal process to determine the level of dissonance perceived. The perceptions are then shared with the client and family/friends. This process continues as long as the nurse/client relationship continues.

Major Assumptions/Meta Paradigm

The basic concepts common to all nursing models are nursing, man, health, and environment. Rogers used the term "man" refers to person and humankind.

* ❖ *Nursing:* Rogers describes nursing as a learned profession that is both a science dedicated to compassionate concern for maintaining and promoting health, preventing illness and caring for and rehabilitating the sick and disabled. Nursing seeks to promote symphonic interactions between the environment and man, to strengthen the coherence and integrity of the human being and to direct and redirect patterns of interaction between man and his/her environment for the realization of maximum health potential. Nursing is a "science of unitary human being" and is therefore unique because it is the only science that deals with the whole person.
* ❖ *Person:* Rogers defines person as an open system is in continuous process with the open system that is environment. She defines unitary human as an irreducible. Indivisible, pandimensional energy field identified by pattern and manifesting characteristics that are specific to the whole and which cannot be predicated from knowledge of the parts.
* ❖ *Environment:* Rogers defines environment as "an irreducible pandimensional energy field identified by pattern and manifesting characteristics different from those of the parts. Each environment field is specific to its given human field. Both change continuously and creatively."
* ❖ *Health:* It is used by Rogers as a value term defined by the culture or individual. Health and illness are manifestations of pattern and is considered "to denote behavior that are of high value and low value." Events manifested in life process indicate the extent to which man achieves maximum health according to some value systems.

Theoretical Assertions

In 1970, Rogers identified five assumptions that are also theoretical assertions supporting her model derived from literature on man, physics, mathematics, and behavioral science:

- Man is a unified whole possessing his own integrity and manifesting characteristics more than different from; the sum of his parts (energy field).
- Man and environment are continuously exchanging. Matter and energy with one another (openness).
- The life process evolves irreversibly and undirectionally along the space time continuum (helicy).
- Pattern and organization identify a person and reflect their innovative wholeness (pattern and organization).
- Man is characterized by the capacity for abstraction and imagery, language and thought, sensation, and emotion (sentiment and thinking being).

Ten years later Rogers had further developed "Nursing: A science of Unitary Man." The science of nursing seeks to study the nature and direction of unitary human development integral with the environment.

Nursing science seeks to make intelligible knowledge about person and their world that has significance for nursing practice. The phenomenon central to nursing's conceptual systems is man's life process. "The life process in man is a phenomenon of wholeness or continuity, of dynamic and creative change." If the life process in man is to be studied and understood, the normal and the pathological must be treated equally. The life process has its own unity, inseparable from environment, and is characterized as the whole.

Roger's conceptual model of unitary man is a clear, direct statement about the unique focus of nursing, a flexible and creative, individualized and socially oriented compassionate and skillful use of nursing science.

Logical Form

Rogers' model of unitary man is clearly deductive and logical. The theory of relativity, general system theory, electrodynamic theory of life, and many other theories contributed ideas for Rogers' model. The basic building blocks of her models are energy field, openness, pattern, and pandimensionality. These broad generalizations postulate the nature and direction of unitary man's development. The derived theories are intended to explain, predict, and describe phenomena related to the life process on man.

Application to Nursing

Practice

- Based on Rogers' theory, disease conditions must be regarded as manifestations of the total patterns of the individual in interaction with the environment.
- Rogers expects change in nursing practice based on her model, for example, aging process can be perceived not as a decline, but as a growing diversity in field pattern. So, many of the characteristics of the old people, such as sleep disturbances, are not abnormal and do not need interventions. Nursing care should become more individualized to a specific person in their own unique situations, rather than using mass criteria for large "clumps" for individuals.

Education

- Rogers emphasizes structuring the nursing education programs to teach nursing as a science and as a learned profession.
- The education of nurses should be committed to human service. She proposed that the preparation for learned practice in nursing require the baccalaureate degree.

Research

- Rogers model is directly related to research and theory development in nursing science. Rogers expects the theory emerging from her model to ultimately explain, predict, and prescribe about unitary man and life process phenomena. Hence, there is a need for both basic and applied research.
- The theories and hypothesis derived from the model may be subjected to empirical test. Researchers such as Newman (1978), Fawcett (1975), and Fitz Patrick had their research related to Rogers conceptualization.

Critique

Simplicity

Rogers conceptual model is not simple, it is complex. She uses multiple concepts that are not easily understood.

Generality

Rogers model is abstract and is therefore generalizable and powerful. It is usually considered a macro theory. It is broad in scope and attempts to explain everything.

Empirical Precision

Rogers model is deductive in logic and lacks empirical support. The difficulty in understanding the principles, lack of operational definitions and inadequate tools for measurement are the major limitations to effective utilization of this theory. Even though the model lacks empirical support, the theories generated by this model are testable.

Derivable Consequences

Previous studies have implication for guiding nursing practice and education and suggest further research. This differentiates nursing from other profession and basic science. Many ideas for future study have been suggested by Rogers. Based on this, it can be said that Rogers conceptual model is useful.

Conclusion

Rogers abstract conceptual model is broad in scope. It treats the complexity of the single variable the summative unit, "unitary man" the model is not meant to be testable. But theories drawn from it are testable. The abstract conceptual model may not be directly useful to practice. It provides a substantive base for research and theory development, which provides the knowledge base for practice. Rogers model challenges the research, the education and the practitioners to meet their social obligations in creative ways. Her conceptual model of unitary man presents a clear direct statement about the unique phases of nursing and visionary perspective of nursing as science and art.

PEPLAU'S THEORY (FIG. 39.9)

Hildegard E Peplau—Theory of International Relations

Credentials and Background of the Theorist

- Born in Reading, Pennsylvania (1909)
- Graduated from a diploma program in Pottstown, Pennsylvania in 1931
- Done BA in interpersonal psychology from Bennington College in 1943
- MA in psychiatric nursing from Colombia University, New York in 1947
- PhD awarded in curriculum development in 1953
- Published Interpersonal Relations in Nursing in 1952
- 1968—interpersonal techniques: The crux of psychiatric nursing
- Worked as executive director and president of ANA
- Worked with World Health Organization (WHO), National Institute for Mentally Handicapped (NIMH), and nurse corps. Died in 1999.

Theoretical Sources

- Influenced by Harry Stack Sullivan's theory of interpersonal relations (1953).
- Also influenced by Percival Symonds, Abraham Maslow's, and Neal Elgar Miller.

Use of Empirical Evidence

It is empirical evident that Peplau developed her theory describing behavior with in the prospective of psychoanalytic theory, the principles of social learning, the concept of human motivation, and the concept of personality development.

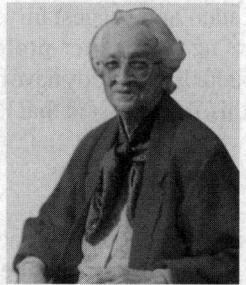

Fig. 39.9: Hildegard E Peplau.

Major Concepts and Definitions

- *Psychodynamic nursing:* Psychodynamic nursing is being able to understand one's own behavior to help others identify. Felt difficulties on to apply principles of human relations to the problems that arise all levels of experience.
- *Nurse–patient relationship:* Peplau describes four phases of the nurse–patient relationship. All though separate they overlap and occur over the time of the relationship (Fig. 39.10).

Orientation Phase (Fig. 39.11)

- Problem defining phase
- Starts when client meets nurse as stranger
- Defining problem and deciding type of service needed
- Client seeks assistance, conveys needs, asks questions, shares preconceptions and expectations of past experiences
- Nurse responds, explains roles to client, helps in identifying problems and uses available resources and services.

Identification Phase

- Selection of appropriate professional assistance.
- Patient begins to have a feeling of belonging and a capability of dealing with the problem, which decreases

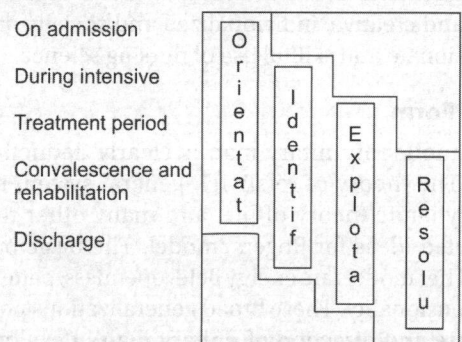

Fig. 39.10: Overlapping phases in nursing.

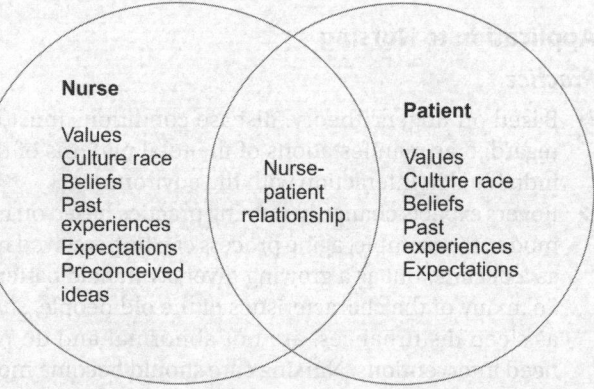

Fig. 39.11: Factors influencing orientation phase.

the feeling of helplessness and hopelessness and provides needed satisfaction.

Exploitation Phase

- Use of professional assistance for problem-solving alternatives.
- New goals to be achieved through personal effort and power shifts from the nurse to the patient delays gratification to achieve newly form goals.
- Individual feels as an integral part of the helping environment.
- They may make minor requests or attention getting techniques.
- The principles of interview techniques must be used in order to explore, understand, and adequately deal with the underlying problem.
- Patient may fluctuate on independence.
- Nurse must be aware about the various phases of communication.
- Nurse aids the patient in exploiting all avenues of help and progress is made toward the final step.

Resolution Phase

- Termination of professional relationship.
- The patients' needs have already been met by the collaborative effect of patient and nurse.
- Now they need to terminate their therapeutic relationship and dissolve the links between them.
- Sometimes may be difficult for both as psychological dependence persists.
- Patient drifts away and breaks bond with nurse and healthier emotional balance is demonstrated and both become mature individuals.

Nursing Roles

Peplau describes six different nursing roles that emerge in the various phases of the nurse-patient relationship (Fig. 39.12):

1. *Stranger:* The nurse and patient are strangers who meet each other in life situations and provide an accepting climate that builds trust.

2. *Teacher:* Who imparts knowledge in reference to a need or interest
3. *Resource person:* One who provides specific health information that aids in the understanding of a problem or new situation.
4. *Counselors:* Helps to understand and integrate the meaning of current life circumstances, provides guidance and encouragement to make changes by integrating other experiences of life.
5. *Surrogate:* Helps to clarify domains both patient and nurse defines areas of dependence, interdependence and independence and acts on client's behalf as an advocate.
6. *Leader:* Helps client assume maximum responsibility for meeting treatment goals in a mutually satisfying way.

Nursing Metaparadigm

- *Nursing:* A significant therapeutic interpersonal process. It functions cooperatively with other human process that makes health possible for individuals in communities. Peplau describes six different nursing roles that will be carried out by the nurse during the phases of developing nurse-patient relationship.
- *Person:* Man is an organism that lives in an unstable equilibrium.
- *Health:* A word symbol that implies forward movement of personality and other ongoing human processes in the direction of creative, constructive, productive, personal, and community living.
- *Environment:* Defines of "existing forces outside the organism and in the context of culture, from which mores, customs, and beliefs are acquired." However, general conditions that are likely to lead to health always include the interpersonal process.

Theoretical Assertions

Peplau makes theoretical relationships that nursing as a maturing educative force uses the experimental learning of both patient and nurse.

Logical Form

Peplau uses an inductive approach to theory building. Empirical generalizations are inductively established. Peplau concepts are organized larger component, forming relationships that are logical and complete.

Interpersonal Theory and Nursing Process

- Both are sequential and focus on therapeutic relationship
- Both use problem-solving techniques for the nurse and patient to collaborate on, with the end purpose of meeting the patient needs
- Both use observation communication and recording as basic tools utilized by nursing (Table 39.3).

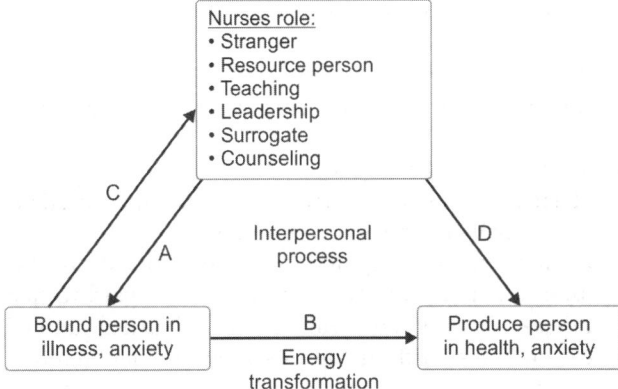

Fig. 39.12: Peplau's model of interpersonal process.

Table 39.3: Application of Peplau's phases and nursing process bring it last after derivable consequences.

Assessment	Orientation
Data collection and analysis (continuous)	Noncontinuous data collection felt need
May not be a felt need	Define needs
Nursing diagnosis planning	Identification
Mutually set goals	Interdependent goal setting
Implementation	Exploitation
Plans initiated toward achievement of mutually set goals May be accomplished by patient, nurse, or family	Patient actively seeking and drawing help Patient initiated
Evaluation	Resolution
Based on mutually expected behaviors May led to termination and initiation of new plans	Occurs after other phases are completed successfully Leads to termination

Application of the Model Nursing Education

❖ Peplau contributed significantly to moving the nursing profession to graduate education. Her model has been used extensively in educating both undergraduates as well as graduate nursing students about a major component of nursing activities the interpersonal relationship.

❖ She has provided theoretically based knowledge for nursing specialization in psychiatric settings where in one-to-one relationship is the primary methodology in nursing.

In Nursing Practice (Fig. 39.13)

A 37-year-old male unmarried was admitted in the psychiatric hospital with a long documented history of schizophrenia. Chief complaints are:

❖ Poor hygiene and grooming
❖ Increased motor activities
❖ Inability to sit in one place
❖ Difficulty in sleeping
❖ Suicidal and homicidal tendency
❖ Auditory and visual hallucinations.

In Nursing Research

❖ Peplau postulated several topics of research today. Her model provides a theoretical framework for research about anxiety and mental health as a whole. The theory can be used for qualitative and quantitative research designs.

❖ Her interpersonal models' operational concepts can be used in explaining the effectiveness of the nursing process in productive patient behavior.

Critique

Simplicity

It is simple because:
❖ Interpersonal relations between patient and nurse are easily understood.
❖ The key concepts are defined.
❖ There is a sequential description of the interpersonal problems.
❖ Roles of the nurse are clearly indicated.
❖ Ideas are taken from specific and applied to general.
❖ Peplau is consistent with established theories and principles.

Generality

❖ Quality of generality is not met for the reason that the theory cannot be applied in all patients.
❖ Peplau has a narrow perception of environment and does not explain the environmental influence on the person but focuses more on the psychological tasks within the person.
❖ In applying theory to clinical practice, there exist limitations in working with unconscious patient as the major concept in the theory is interpersonal relationship, so the theory cannot be applied in senile, unconscious and newborn.

Empirical Precision

Peplau theory can be termed empirically precise because of the following:
❖ Theory is based on reality.
❖ The relationship between the theory and empirical data allows for valuation and verification.
❖ Peplau operationally defines the four phases of the interpersonal process, the nurse with regard to her roles and the patient with regard to his/her state of dependence. With further research, the dependence will increase.

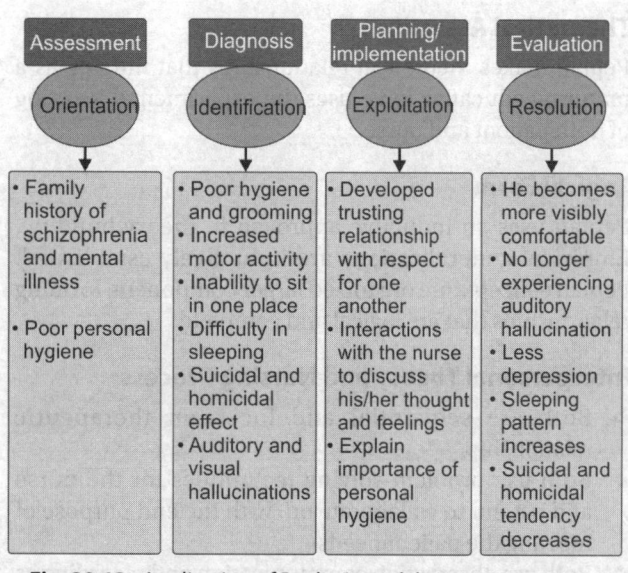

Fig. 39.13: Application of Peplau's model to nursing process.

Derivable Consequences

❖ The evaluative criteria of the derivable consequences have been met.
❖ Peplau's thoughts and ideas have touched many nurses. Peplau's work can be considered pioneering in nursing filed and her work has provided significant contribution to nursing knowledge base. With the help of the theory of interpersonal relations, the client's needs could be assessed.

Conclusion

Peplau's interpersonal concepts in nursing have laid down foundation for theory and practice and these concepts are unique, more applicable in psychiatric clinical settings. Peplau's phases can be compared with the nursing process, it is sequential, and focus on therapeutic interactions. This theory can be applied to a group, family and community.

ABDELLAH'S THEORY (FIG. 39.14)

Faye Glenn Abdellah was one of the most influential nursing theorists and public health scientists in the era. She is the one who has dedicated all her life to the advancement of the nursing profession and accomplished this feat with so much distinction and merit. When she was inducted into the National Women's Hall of Fame in 2000, Abdellah said, "we cannot wait for the world to change". Those of us with intelligence, purpose, and vision must take the lead and change the world. Let us move forward together! I promise never to rest until my work has been completed."

Background of the Theorist

❖ Born on March 13, 1919, New York city
❖ Diploma in nursing in 1942, Fitkin Memorial Hospital, School of Nursing, Neptune, NJ
❖ BS in 1945 and MA in 1947
❖ Doctor of Education in 1955, from Teacher's College, Columbia University, New York City.

Accomplishments

US public health service:
❖ Chief Nurse Officer—1970
❖ Deputy US Surgeon General—1982, Uniformed Services University of Health Sciences

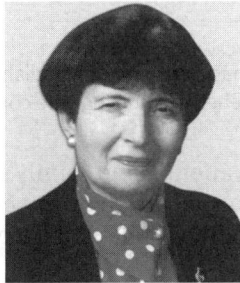

Fig. 39.14: Faye Glenn Abdellah.

❖ Founder and First Dean, Graduate School of Nursing Yale University School of Nursing
❖ Nursing instructor.

Research

❖ Assisted in international nursing research studies during the Korean War (China, Japan, Australia, and Russia).
❖ Abdellah's research findings led to the first federally tested coronary care unit in Connecticut.
❖ Theory and research data led to the establishment of the office of long-term care.

Theoretical Sources

❖ The problem-solving method is the basis for Abdellah's model.
❖ Abdellah states that she was influenced by Virginia Henderson and identifies her as a mentor.
❖ Abdellah as many other theories based Maslow's hierarchy of needs and influenced by Erickson's stages of development.

Empirical Evidence

Empirical evident is the typology that was developed from several studies conducted during 1950s. Nursing also moved toward a philosophy of comprehensive patient catered care. Abdellah and his colleagues conceptualized 21 nursing problems to teach and evaluate students.

Major Concepts and Definitions

Theoretical statement can be derived by using her three major concepts of health, nursing problems, and problem-solving.

Health

Abdellah defined concept of health may be dynamic pattern of functioning whereby there is continued interaction with internal and external forces that results in the optimal use of necessary resources that results in the optimal use of necessary resources that serve to minimize vulnerabilities. By performing nursing services through a holistic approach to the client, the nurse helps the client to achieve a state of health.

Nursing Problem

The client's health needs can be viewed as problems, which may be overt as an apparent condition and covert as a hidden or concealed one. As covert problems can be emotional, sociological, and interpersonal in nature, they are often perceived incorrectly. Such a view of problems implies a client centered orientation.

In her attempt to bring nursing practice into its proper relationship with restorative and preventive measures for meeting total client needs. She seems to saving the pendulum to the opposite pole, from the disease orientation to the nursing orientation, while leaving the client somewhere in the middle.

Problem-solving

Quality professional nursing care requires that nurses be able to identify and solve overt and covert nursing problems. These requirements can be met by the problem-solving approach. The problem-solving process involves:
- Identifying the problem
- Selecting pertinent data
- Formulating hypothesis
- Testing hypothesis through the collection of data
- Revising hypothesis when necessary on the basis of conclusions obtained from the data.

Many of these steps parallel the steps of the nursing process of assessment, diagnosis, planning, implementation, and evaluation. According to Abdellah, the patient will not receive quality nursing care, if the steps of problem-solving are done incorrectly.

Typology of Nursing Problems

- In Abdellah's theory, identification and classification of problems was called typology of 21 nursing problems. Abdellah was motivated to develop her typology by desire to promote comprehensive, client centered nursing care.
- She developed her typology because she realized that nursing needed strong knowledge base to achieve full professional status and autonomy.
- She used the problem-solving approach as base for her typology.
- Typology of nursing problem—first published in 1960.
- In 1973, she refined some of her beliefs about nursing.

The major component of Abdellah's typology is a list of 21 nursing problems, or healthcare needs of the client (Box 39.1).

Abdellah described 21 nursing problems under one of these categories and the three major categories are:
1. Physical, sociological, and emotional needs of clients.
2. Types of interpersonal relationships between the nurse and patient.
3. Common elements of client care.

Ten Steps to Identify the Client's Problems

1. Learn to know the patient.
2. Sort out relevant and significant data.
3. Make generalizations about available data in relation to similar nursing problems presented by other patients.
4. Identify the therapeutic plan.
5. Test generalizations with the patient and make additional generalizations.
6. Validate the patient's conclusions about his/her nursing problems.
7. Continue to observe and evaluate the patient over a period of time to identify any attitudes and clues affecting his/her behavior.

> **Box 39.1:** Abdellah's 21 nursing problems (Fig. 39.15).
>
> **Basic to all patients (four problems)**
> 1. To maintain good hygiene and physical comfort
> 2. To promote optimal activity, i.e. exercise, rest, and sleep
> 3. To promote safety through the prevention of accidents, injury, or other trauma and through the prevention of the spread of infection
> 4. To maintain good body mechanics and prevent and correct deformity.
>
> **Sustenal care needs (seven problems)**
> 5. To facilitate the maintenance of nutrition of all body cells
> 6. To facilitate the maintenance of a supply of oxygen to all body cells
> 7. To facilitate the maintenance of fluid and electrolyte balance
> 8. To facilitate the maintenance of elimination
> 9. To recognize the physiological responses of the body to disease conditions—pathological, physiological, and compensatory
> 10. To facilitate the maintenance of regulatory mechanisms and functions
> 11. To facilitate the maintenance of sensory function.
>
> **Remedial care needs (seven problems)**
> 12. To identify and accept the inter-relatedness of emotions and organic illness
> 13. To identify and accept positive and negative expressions, feelings, and reactions
> 14. To facilitate the maintenance of effective verbal and nonverbal communication
> 15. To promote the development of predictive interpersonal relationships
> 16. To facilitate awareness of self as an individual with varying physical, emotional, and developmental needs
> 17. To create and/or maintain a therapeutic environment
> 18. To facilitate progress toward achievement of personal spiritual goals.
>
> **Restorative care needs (three problems)**
> 19. To accept the optimum possible goals in the light of limitations, physical and emotional
> 20. To use community resources as an aid in resolving problems arising from illness
> 21. To understand the role of social problems as influencing factors in the case of illness.

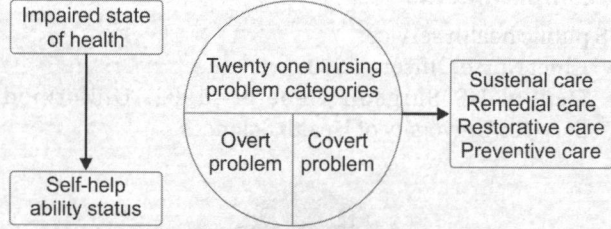

Fig. 39.15: Schematic diagram of Abdellah's problems with comprehensive nursing care concept.

8. Explore the patient's and family's reaction to the therapeutic plan and involve them in the plan.
9. Identify how the nurses feel about the patient's nursing problems.
10. Discuss and develop a comprehensive nursing care plan.

Abdellah's Theory and the Nursing Paradigm

Abdellah does not clearly specify each of the four major concepts:
- Individual or human
- Health
- Environment
- Society
- Nursing

Individual or Human

The recipients of nursing are individuals and families. Her 21 nursing problems deal with biological, psychological, and social areas of individuals and can be considered to represent areas of importance to them.

Health

Abdellah speaks to "total health needs and a healthy state of the mind and body." In her description nursing as a comprehensive service can achieve health.

Environment/Society

Environment/society is least discussed in model, the patient interacts with and responds to the environment and that the nurse is part of that environment. It is also home and community from which client comes (local, state, national, or international).

Nursing

Nursing is broadly grouped into the 21 problem areas to guide care and promote the use of nursing judgement. She considers nursing to be a comprehensive service that is based on an art and science and aims to help people, sick or well, cope with their health needs.
- Making sure the side rails are always up.
- Prevent the spread of infection is through proper disinfection of the equipment.
- **To facilitate the maintenance of elimination:** Providing bedpans or urinals to patients and at times, insertion of Foley catheter when the patient is not able to void.
- **To facilitate the maintenance of a supply of oxygen to all body cells:** When patients manifest breathing problems, oxygen is attached to them, usually via nasal till this.

Application of Abdellah's Theory in Nursing

Nursing Practice (Fig. 39.16)

The most important impact of Abdellah's theory to the nursing practice is that it helped transform the focus of the profession from being "disease-centered" to "patient-centered." It helped bring structure and organization in care.

Nursing Education

To present a comprehensive clinical record for nursing students, thus, provide structure to the nursing curriculum.

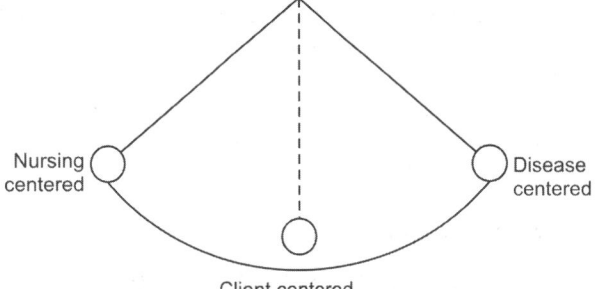

Fig. 39.16: Focus of care pendulum.

Implementation of the model in baccalaureate, associate degree and diploma nursing programs facilitated the move from the medical model to nursing model.

Nursing Research

Her theories continue to guide researchers to focus on the body of nursing knowledge itself, the identification of patient problems, the organization of nursing interventions, the improvement of nursing education, and the structure of the curriculum.

Critique

- **Simplicity:** The concepts of nursing, nursing problem, and the problem-solving process, which is central and described in a simple manner.
- **Generality:** The 21 nursing problems are general and linked to neither time nor environment. The goals of this model vary in generality. The goals are appropriate for nursing.
- **Empirical precision:** The concepts are very specific with empirical referents easily identifiable. Validation of the typology was done by the faculty of 40 collegiate schools of nursing.
- **Derivable consequences:** The emphasis on problem solving is not limited by time or space and therefore provides a means for continued growth and change in the provision of nursing care. The problem-solving process and the typology of 21 nursing problems can be respectively considered precursors of the nursing care process and classification of nursing diagnosis in evidence today.

Application of Typology of 21 Nursing Problems to the Client

To promote safety through prevention of accident, injury, or other trauma and through the prevention of the spread of infection.

Conclusion

Using Abdellah's concepts of health, nursing problems, and problem solving, the theoretical statement of nursing that can be derived is the use of the problem solving approach with key nursing problems related to health needs of people.

From this framework, 21 nursing problems were developed. Abdellah's theory provides a basis or determining and organizing nursing care. The problems also provide a basis for organizing appropriate nursing strategies. It is anticipated that by solving the nursing problems, the client would be moved toward health.

CONSERVATION MODEL

Myra Estrin Levine (1921–1996) (Fig. 39.17)

Credentials and Background of the Theorist

- Born in Chicago Intact, middle-class family, Father influential
- Education and Career—Diploma in 1944
- Private and civilian nurse
- Clinical instructor
- BS 1949
- Surgical supervisor
- Director of Nursing
- Master of Science in Nursing (MSN) 1962
- Chaired Department of Clinical Nursing, Cook County School of Nursing
- Coordinated the graduate nursing program in oncology at Rush University
- Visiting professor at Tel Aviv University, Israel.

Achievements

- Clinical experience in operation theater (OT) technique and oncology nursing
- Civilian nurse at the Gardiner general hospital
- Director of Nursing at Drexel home in Chicago
- Clinical instructor at Bryan memorial hospital in Lincoln, Nebraska
- Administrative supervisor at University of Chicago
- Chairperson of Clinical Nursing at cook country school of nursing
- Visiting professor at Tel Aviv University in Israel.

Theoretical Sources

- Levine learned historical viewpoints of diseases and that the way people think about disease changes overtime from Beland's presentation of the theory of specific causation and multiple factors.

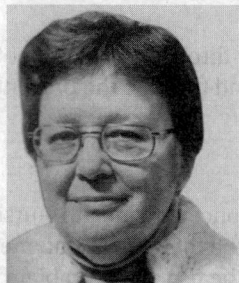

Fig. 39.17: Myra Estrin Levine.

- Levine uses Gibson's definition of perceptual systems, Erik Erikson's differentiation total and whole, Hans Selye's stress theory, and Bates models of external environment.
- Initially, constructed as a teaching framework for medical-surgical nursing based on physical science principles.

Use of Empirical Evidence

Levine believes that specific nursing activities can be deduced from scientific principles. The scientific theoretical sources have been well researched. Much of her work is based on science principles.

Major Concepts of Conservational Principles

- *Holistic:* "Wholeness emphases a sound, organic, progressive, mutuality, between diversified functions and parts within an entirety, the boundaries which are open fluent."
- *Holism:* It means that human beings are more than and different from the some of their parts. Perceiving the wholes depends upon recognizing the organization and interdependence of observable phenomena.
- *Integrity:* It means being in control of one's life.
- *Conservation:* It describes the way complex systems are able to continue to function even when severely challenged. The primary focus of conservation is on the integrity of oneness of the individual. Nursing interventions may deal with one particular aspect and must recognize the influence of the other conservation principle.

Conservation Principles

- *Conservation of energy:* The individual requires a balance of energy to maintain life activities, that energy is challenged by process such as healing and aging.
- *Conservation of structural integrity:* Healing is a process of restoring structural integrity. Nurses should limit the amount of tissue involved in disease by early recognition of functional changes by nursing interventions.
- *Conservation of personal integrity:* Self-worth and a sense of identity are important. Nurses can show patient respect by calling them by name, respecting their wishes, valuing personal professions, providing privacy, and teaching them. The nurse's goal is always to impart knowledge and strength so that the individuals can no longer be a patient or dependent.
- *Conservation of social integrity:* Life gains meaning through social communities and health is socially determined. Nurses fulfill professional roles, provide for family members, assist in religious needs and use interpersonal relationships to conserve social integrity.
- *Adaptation:* It is the process of change by which people maintain their integrity with in the reality of their

Chapter 39: Nursing Theories

environment. Some adaptations are successful and some are not.

- **Environment:** It is where one is constantly and actively involved. The person and is relationship to the environment is what counts. There are three aspects of environment.

  Operational environment consists of those and detected natural forces that impinge on the individual.

  The perceptual environment consists of information that is recorded by sensory organs. The levels of integration that safe guard the end and help the person to maintain his/her integrity or wholeness.

  The conceptual environment is constructed from cultural patterns characterized by spiritual existence, symbols of language, thought, and history.

- **Organismic response:** It is the capacity of individual to adapt to his/her environmental condition. It can be divided into four levels of integration—(1) fight or flight, (2) inflammatory response, (3) response to stress, and (4) perceptual response.

- **Fight or flight:** The most primitive response is the fight or flight syndrome. The individual perceives that he/she is threatened, whether or not a threat does actually exist. The individual response by being on the alert to find the more information and to assure is safety and well-being.

- **Inflammatory response:** This defense mechanism protects the cell from a hostile environment. It is a way of healing. The response uses available energy to remove or keep out unwanted irritants or pathogens.

- **Response to stress:** Selye describes the stress response syndrome to be predictable, non-specifically induced organismic response. The wear and tear of life is recorded on the tissues and reflects long-term hormonal response to life experiences that cause structural changes.

- **Perpetual response:** This response is based on the individual's perpetual awareness.

- **Trophicognosis:** Levin recommended trophicognosis as an alternative to nursing diagnosis. It is a scientific method to reach a nursing care judgment.

Levine's Theory and Nursing Metparadigm

Person

Person is who we know ourself to be or a sense of identity and focus on wholeness of the individual. Human beings are continually adopting in their interactions with their environment. The process adaptation results in conservation. Human beings have need for nursing when they are suffering and accept the services of another.

Health

Health and diseases are patterns of adaptive change. Some adaptations are most successful than others, all adaptations are seeking the best fit with the environment. The most successful adaptations achieve the best fit in the most conserving manner. Health is the goal of conservation.

Nursing

Nursing is a human interaction. The nurse participate actively every patient environment and much of what she does support his/her adjustments as he/she struggles in the predicament of illness. Nursing intervention influences adaptations favorably or toward renewed social well-being. The nurse adds supportive care. The goal of nursing is to promote wholeness.

Theoretical Assertions

Many theoretical assertions can be generated from Levine's work, the important as nursing intervention is based on the conservation of the individual patient's energy, structural, personal, and social integrity.

Logical Form

Levine primarily uses deductive logic. In developing her model, Levine integrates theories and concepts from the humanities and the science of nursing, physiology, psychology and sociology. She uses the information to analyze of nursing practice situations and describe nursing skill and activities.

Acceptance by the Nursing Community

Practice

Levine helps to define what nursing is by giving the scientific principles behind them. Conservation principles have been use frameworks for numerous practice settings in cardiology, obstetrics, gerontology, neonatology, and critical care areas as well as in the homeless community.

Education

- Levine wrote a textbook for beginning students that introduced new material into curricula.
- Introduction to clinical nursing provides an organizational structure for teaching medical surgical nursing, which contains nine models for a teaching beginning students and it serves a background in physical and social science.
- Levin's model is one use as curriculum for several graduate students.

Research

- "All in all Levine's model served as an excellent beginning, a great deal to the overall development of nursing knowledge."
- Many research questions can be generated from the Levine's model. Several graduate students are using the conservation principle as a framework for their research and also use Levine's model for thesis and dissertations.

Critiquing the Theory

- *Clarity:* Levine's model possesses clarity. Her work to be both internally and externally consistent and holistic view of person.
- *Simplicity:* The four conservation principles appear simple, but they contain subconcepts and multiple variables. However, this model is still one of the simple emerging models.
- *Generality:* The four conservation principles can be used in all nursing context, so it meets the criteria of generality.
- *Empirical precision:* Levine used deductive logic to develop her model, which can be used to generate research questions.
- *Derivable consequences:* Various authors disagree to the level of Levine's model. The four conservation principles constituted one of the earliest models and receiving increasing recognition.

Nursing Process According to Levine's Model

Levine's theory initially developed for the organization of content in medical surgical nursing. Her theory inter-relates the concepts of conservation, integrity, and adaptation. This theory has been tested through research and its usefulness demonstrated in clinical practice and education.

Conclusion

Myra Levine's theory has evolved from the medical surgical nursing to facilitate student learning. Her theory interrelates the concepts of conservation, integrity and adaptation. Adaptation is the means of conserving energy by interacting with their environment. This theory has been tested through research and useful in clinical practice and education.

DOROTHEA E OREM (FIG. 39.18)

Self-Care Deficit Theory of Nursing

Credentials and Background of the Theorist

- Born: 1914, Baltimore, Maryland
- Father: Construction, fishing
- Mother: Homemaker, reading
- Youngest of two girls
- Died: June 22, 2007

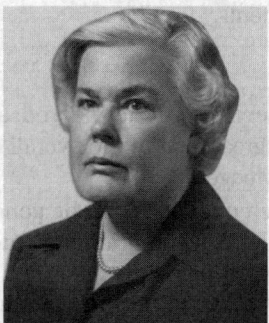

Fig. 39.18: Dorothea E Orem.

Education

- Diploma (1930s), Providence Hospital School of Nursing, Washington DC
- BSN Ed. (1939) and MSN Ed. (1945), Catholic University of America, Washington DC.

Honorary Doctorates

- Doctor of Science (1976) George Town University, (1980) Incarnate Word College in San Antonio, Texas
- Doctor of Humane Letters (1988) Illinois Wesleyan University, Bloomington, Illinois
- Doctor of Nursing Honoris Causae, (1998) University of Missouri, Columbia.

Special Awards

- Catholic University of America Alumni Achievement Award for Nursing Theory (1980)
- Linda Richards Award, National League for Nursing (NLN, 1991)
- Honorary Fellow of the American Academy of Nursing (1992).

Nursing Experiences

- *Directorship (1940–1949):* Both nursing school and department at Providence Hospital, Detroit
- *Indiana (1949–1957):* Division of Hospital and Institutional Services (Indiana State Board of Health)
- *Curriculum consultant (1957):* Office of Education, United States Department of Health, education and Welfare (US DHEW)
- *Project (1958–1960):* Guides for Developing Curricula for the Education of Practical Nurses.

Theoretical Sources

- Orem says her ideas are primarily the result of reflecting upon her experiences and she was not influenced by any one person (Hartweg, 1991)
- Parsons' structure of social action
- Von Bertalnffy's System Theory
- Moderate realism (Kantian Philosophy) and other nursing theories.

Use of Empirical Evidence

In 1958, Orem experienced a spontaneous insight about why individuals required and could be helped through nursing. This knowledge enabled her to formulate and express her concept of nursing.

Major Concepts and Definitions

Orem labels her self-care deficit. Theory of nursing as a general theory composed of three interrelated theories:
1. The theory of self-care—why and how people care for themselves.
2. The theory of self-care deficit—why people can be helped through nursing.

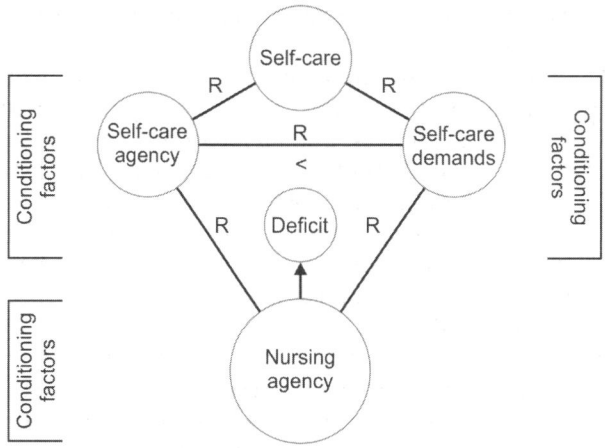

Fig. 39.19: A conceptual framework for nursing. (R: relationship; <: deficit relationship current or projected.
Source: Ann Marriner-Tomey.

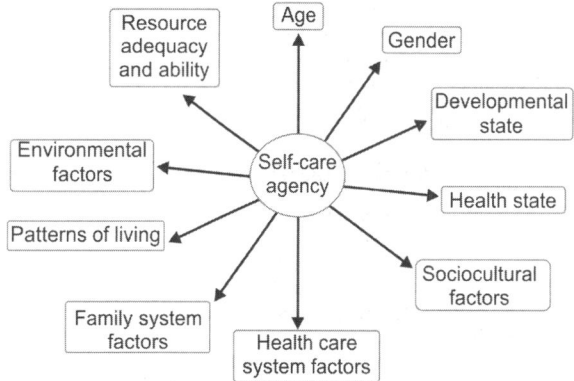

Fig. 39.20: Basic conditioning factors influencing self-care.

3. The theory of nursing systems—describes and explains relationships that must be made and maintained for nursing to be produced (Fig. 39.19).

❖ *Self-care:* The performance of activities that individuals initiate and perform on their behalf to maintain life, health, and well-being.
  ➤ *Self-care requisites:* Self-care requisites means expressions of purposes to be attained, results desired from deliberate engagement in self-care. It consists of three categories.
    i. *Universal self-care requisites:* Requisites/needs that are common to all individuals (e.g. air, water, food, elimination, rest, activity, etc.).
    ii. *Developmental self-care requisites:* Needs resulting from maturation or develop due to a condition or event (e.g. adjustment to new job, puberty).
    iii. *Health deviation self-care requisites:* Needs resulting from illness, injury, and disease or its treatment (e.g. learning to walk with crutches after a leg fracture).

❖ *Therapeutic self-care demand:* The totality of "care measures" necessary at specific times or over a duration of time for meeting an individual's self-care requisites by using appropriate methods and related sets and actions. It is based on the theory that self-care is a human regulatory function.

❖ *Self-care agency:* The individual's ability to perform self-care activities consists of two agents:
  ➤ *Agent:* It is the person taking action
    ♦ *Self-care agent:* The person who provides the self-care
    ♦ *Dependent care agent:* The person other than the individual who provides the care (such as a parent), affected by basic conditioning factors
  ➤ **Basic conditioning factors** influencing self-care are shown in Figure 39.20.

  ♦ *Self-care deficit:* "The condition that validates the existence of a requirement for nursing in an adult is the health associated absence of the ability to maintain continuously the amount and quality of therapeutic self-care in sustaining life and health, in recovering from disease or injury or in coping with their effects." It results when self-care agency is not adequate to meet the known self-care demand.

❖ *The nursing agency:* A complex property of people who are educated and trained as nurses that enables them to act, to know, and to help others meet their therapeutic self-care demands by exercising or developing their own self-care agency.

❖ *Nursing system:* Theory postulates that nursing systems form when nurses prescribe design and nursing that regulates the individual self-care capabilities and meets therapeutic self-care requirements. The five methods of nursing help:
  ➤ Acting or doing for another
  ➤ Guiding and directing
  ➤ Providing physical or psychological support
  ➤ Providing and maintaining an environment that supports personal development.

The three classifications of nursing systems (Fig. 39.21)
1. *Wholly compensatory:* A patient's self-care agency is so limited that she/he depends on others for well-being:
   ➤ Unable to engage in any form of action (e.g. coma).
   ➤ Aware and who may be able to make observations or judgments and decisions about self-care, but cannot/should not perform actions requiring ambulation and manipulative movements (e.g. patients with C3–C4 vertebral fractures).
   ➤ Patients who are unable to take care of themselves and make reasonable judgments about self-care but who can be ambulatory and able to perform some self-care with guidance (e.g. severely mentally retarded).
2. *Partly compensatory:* A patient can meet some self-care requisites but needs a nurse to help meet others;

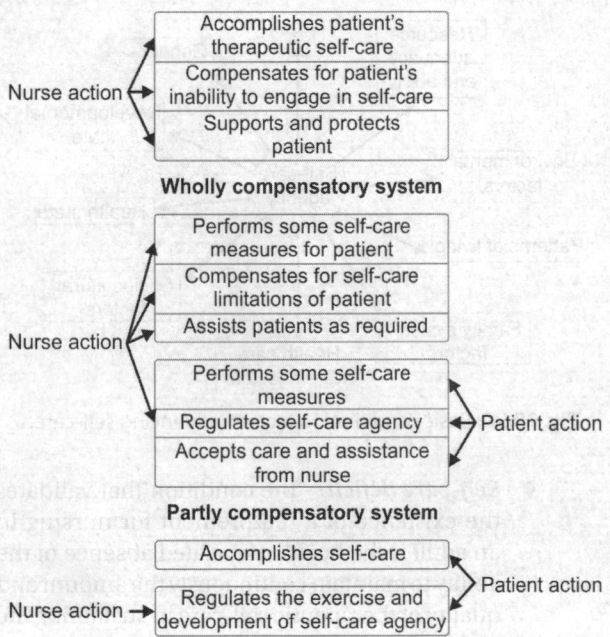

Fig. 39.21: Basic nursing system of Orem's model.

either the nurse or the patient has the major role in the performance of self-care, e.g. a patient with recent abdominal surgery.
3. ***Supportive-educative:*** A patient can meet self-care requisites but needs help in decision-making, behavior control, or knowledge acquisition; the nurse's role is to promote the patient as a self-care agent (teacher/consultant), e.g. a 16-year-old who is requesting birth control information (Fig. 39.21).

Theoretical assertions: The model shows that when an individual self-care capability are less than the therapeutic self-care demand, the nurse compensates for the self-care or dependent care deficits. Self-care, self-care deficits, and nursing systems are related theories/structure.

Logical Form

The generalization of theory is made possible by deductive reasoning. Orem used mathematical logic approach and allowed transformation to computerized nursing information systems.

Acceptance by the Nursing Community

Orem's self-care theory has achieved a greater level of acceptance by the nursing community than the theories of the majority of other theorists.

Practice

❖ Many articles document the use of the self-care theories as a basis for clinical practice. A group of graduate students applied Orem's theory in a nursing home to specific patients and concluded that the employment of the self-care conceptual framework the nurses developed a greater respect for the patient, the patient realized his/her right of choice as a consumer of healthcare.
❖ Orem's self-care concept has been used in work with adolescent alcohol abusers, employees with rheumatoid arthritis, women recovering from radical mastectomies, families and children with cystic fibrosis, patients with congestive heart failure, pre-transfer teaching for cardiac patients, diabetic patients, and patients receiving peritoneal dialysis. It has been related to family centered maternity care, hospitalized children, and hospice care.
❖ Orem's self-care deficit theory has been used in the context of the nursing process to teach patients to increase self-care agency, to evaluate nursing practice and to differentiate nursing from medical practice.
❖ Orem's general theory of nursing has been translated into different languages and been used worldwide. This is applicable to postoperative care was described as wholly compensatory, partly compensatory, and supportive educative. Patient education began immediately after operation, depending on the amount of the assistance required.

Education

❖ Orem's healthcare deficits theory has been the focus of the curriculum in the nursing education at many schools of nursing.
❖ The university is also offering annual self-care deficit theory conferences, nursing research conferences, and annual institutes of self-care theory. Orem's frameworks are used for continuing education courses.

Research

Orem's self-care concept provided the conceptual framework applied for research and Likert scale questionnaire was developed for clinical nursing assessment and studies with adolescents.

Critique

Simplicity

The conceptual framework appears simple. Subconcepts are identified to express the substantive structure of the six broad conceptual elements of the theory.

Generality

The self-care deficit theory of nursing as expressed in universal. It is a theory of nursing as regardless of time or place and at present most commonly applied in the care of adults. It has been applied in the care of both well and sick children.

Empirical Precision

Empirical precision theory identifies concepts, provides definitions, describes relationships, and states assumptions. It can be and has been used for research.

Derivable Consequences

Orem's theory directs nursing practice, the stated goal. Her nursing system provides a framework for nursing practice based on the amount and kind of nursing agency needed. Orem also addresses educational needs for nurses to be able to practice and the use of various levels of nursing practice. Orem's nursing process consists of three steps.

Application of Johnson's Behavioral System and the Nursing Process (Table 39.4)

Step 1: Determine why a patient needs care.
Step 2: Design a nursing system and plan the delivery of care.
Step 3: Management of nursing systems—planning, initiating, and controlling nursing actions.

Application of Orem's Theory to their requirements for universal and health deviation self-care.

Case Study

For Mrs X, she came to the hospital with complaints of pain over all the joints, stiffness, which is more in the morning and reduces by the activities.

She has these complaints since 5 years and has taken treatment from local hospital.

The symptoms were not reducing and came to Hospital for further management.

Patient was able to do the activities of daily living (ADL) by herself, but the way she performed and the posture she used was making her prone to develop the complications of the disease.

She also was malnourished and was not having awareness about the deficiencies and effects.

Nursing Diagnosis

Imbalanced nutritional status less than body requirement related to lack of knowledge regarding nutrition.

Expected Outcome

- Improved nutrition
- Maintenance of a balanced diet with adequate iron supplementation.

Table 39.4: Assessment of a client.

Areas	Patient details
Name	Mrs X
Age	56 years
Sex	Female
Education	No formal education
Occupation	Household
Marital status	Married
Religion	Hindu
Diagnosis	Rheumatoid arthritis
Theory applied	Orem's theory of self-care deficit

Nursing Goals and Objectives

- **Goal:** To achieve optimal levels of nutrition.
- **Objectives:** Mrs. X will:
  - State the importance of maintaining a balanced diet.
  - List the food items rich in iron, which are available in the locality.

Nursing system which she requires

Supportive education.

Method of helping

- Guidance
- Support
- Teaching
- Providing developmental environment.

Implementation

Mutually planned and identified the objectives and the patient were made to understand about the required changes in the behavior to have the requisites met.

Evaluation

- Mrs X understood the importance of maintaining an optimum nutrition.
- She verbalized that she will select the iron rich diet for her food.
- She listed the foods that are rich in iron and that are locally available.
- The self-care deficit in terms of food is decreased with the initiation of the nutritional intake.
- The supportive educative system was useful for Mrs X.

Conclusion

Orem's theory is unique to nursing profession. Self-care deficit theory of nursing continue to evolve, its impact is international and widely used in all fields. Her work contributes significantly to the development of nursing theories.

DOROTHY E JOHNSON (FIG. 39.22)

Behavior System Model

Introduction

- Dorothy E Johnson began her work on the model in the late 1950s.
- The focus of her model is on needs, the human as a behavioral system, and relief of stress as nursing care.

Background of the Theorist

- 1919: August 21st Dorothy was born
- 1942: BSN from Vanderbilt University, Nashville, Tennessee
- 1948: MPH from Harvard University, Boston

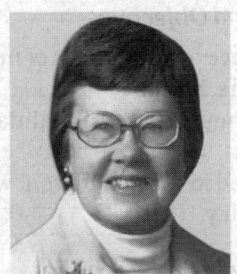

Fig. 39.22: Dorothy E Johnson.

- 1943–1944: She was a staff nurse at the Chatham-Savannah Health Council
- 1949–1978: She was an Assistant Professor in Pediatric Nursing, Associate Professor of Nursing and Professor of Nursing at the University of California in Los Angeles
- 1955–1956: Johnson was pediatric Nursing advisor assigned to the CMC in Vellore
- 1965–1967: She Chaired the committee of the California Nurses' Association
- 1975: Faculty award from graduate students
- 1977: Distinguished Achievement Award from the California Nurses' Association
- 1981: Vanderbilt University School of Nursing Award for Excellence in Nursing
- 1999: She died in February at the age of 80.

Theoretical Sources

Johnson stated that Nightingale's work inspired her model

- She reported that she derived portions of her theory from the works of Selye on stress, Grinker's theory of human behavior, and Buckley and Chin on systems theories.
- Talcott parsons are acknowledged specifically in early developmental writings presenting concepts of the behavioral system model.

Major Concepts and Definitions

Behavior
The output of intraorganism structures and processes as are coordinated and articulated by and responsive to changes in sensory stimulation.

System
A system is a whole that functions as a whole by virtue of organized interdependence of its parts.

Behavioral System
Behavioral system encompasses all patterned, repetitive, and purposeful ways of behaving. These ways of behaving form an organized and integrated functional unit that determines and limits the interaction between the person and environment.

Subsystem
A minisystem with its own particular goal and function that can be maintained in relationship to the other subsystem or the environment is not disturbed.

Johnson Identifies Seven Behavioral Subsystem

Each behavioral subsystem evolves to carry out its own specialized tasks for the system as a whole. A disturbance in one system is likely to have an effect on others. Each subsystem has three functional and structural requirements, which are given below:
- To be protected from noxious influences with which the person cannot cope.
- To be nurtured through the input of supplies from the environment.
- To be stimulated to enhance growth and prevent stagnation.
- ***Attachment or Affiliate Subsystem:*** It is most critical, because it forms the basis for all social organization. It provides survival and security through social inclusion or intimacy and maintenance of strong social bond.
- ***Dependency Subsystem:*** It promotes helping behaviors that calls for a nurturing response designed to get attention, recognition, and physical assistance.
- ***Ingestive/Eliminative Subsystem:*** It fulfills the need to supply the biologic requirements for food and fluids and excrete wastes from the body system.
- ***Sexual Subsystem:*** Serves the biologic requirements of procreation and reproduction.
- ***Aggressive Subsystem:*** Maintains function of self, social protection, and preservation.
- ***Achievement System:*** It attempts to manipulate the environment. Its function is to control or mastery of self or the environment to some standard of excellence.
- ***Equilibrium:*** It is a process of maintaining harmony (stability) with self and environment.
- ***Tension:*** It is a state of being a disturbance in equilibrium. Tension can be constructive in the adaptive change or destructive in the inefficient use of energy.
- ***Stressor:*** Internal or external stimuli that produce tension and result in a degree of instability are called stressor.

Johnson believes that:
- There is organization, interaction, interdependency, and integration of parts and elements of behaviors that to make up the system.
- A system tends to achieve a balance among the various forces operating within and upon it; and that man strive continually to maintain a behavioral system balance and steady state by more or less automatic adjustments adaptations to the natural forces impinging upon him.
- A behavior system, which both requires and results in some degree of regularity and constancy in behavior, is essential to man that is to say, it is

functionally significant in that it serves a useful purpose, both in social life and for the individual.
- System balance reflects adjustments and adaptation that are successful in some way and to some degree.

Johnson's Behavioral Model and Nursing Metaparadigm (Fig. 39.23)

Nursing
Nursing is seen as "an external regulatory force which acts to preserve the organization and integration of the patient's behavior constitutes a threat to physical or social health, or in which illness is found." Primary goal of nursing is to foster equilibrium with in the individual.

Person
Person defined as a behavioral system that strives to make continual adjustments to achieve, maintain, or regain balance through a state of adaptation.

Health
An elusive, dynamic state influenced by biological, psychological, and social factors. It is reflected by the organization, interaction, interdependence, and integration of the subsystems of the behavioral systems. Man attempts to achieve a balance in the system, which will lead to functional behavior. A lack balance in the requirements of subsystems leads to poor health.

Environment
Environment is implied to include all elements of the surroundings of the human system and includes internal stressors. Excessive strong environmental forces disturb the behavioral system's balance and alter the person's stability. The nurse achieves the health goal of the client.

Theoretical Assertion
- This theory addresses to major components the patient and nursing. The patient is a behavioral system with seven interrelated subsystems.
- Each of the subsystem can be described and analyzed in terms of structure and functional requirements. The four structural elements that include:
  - Drive or goal
  - Set, predisposition to act
  - Choice, alternative for actions
  - Behavior
- The nursing is seen as an external regulatory force that acts to restore the balance in the behavioral system.

Acceptance by the Nursing Community
- ***Nursing Practice:*** The goal of the theory is to maintain and restore balance in the patient by helping him achieve a more optimal level of functioning that is valued and acceptable by nursing.
- Used the theory as a model to develop an assessment tool when caring for children.
- This theory is used in the nursing process based on seven subsystems. It is a powerful tool with which used to collect important data. By using these tools, the nurse can discover other choices of behavior will enable the patient to accomplish his goal of health.
- Johnson's suggest that the techniques may include teaching, role modeling, and counseling. The outcome of nursing intervention is behavioral system equilibrium.

Education
Loveland cherry and Wilkerson analyzed Johnson's theory and concluded that it has utility in nursing education applied to the nursing process. In addition to an understanding of systems theory, the student would need knowledge from the social and behavioral disciplines as well as the physical and biological sciences.

Research
- The behavioral system theory leads the researcher in one of two directions. Researcher might investigate the functioning of the system and the subsystems by focusing on the basic sciences, while another researcher might concentrate on investigating, problem-solving activities as they influence the behavioral system.
- Conceptual framework of Johnson's theory used when caring for visually impaired children.

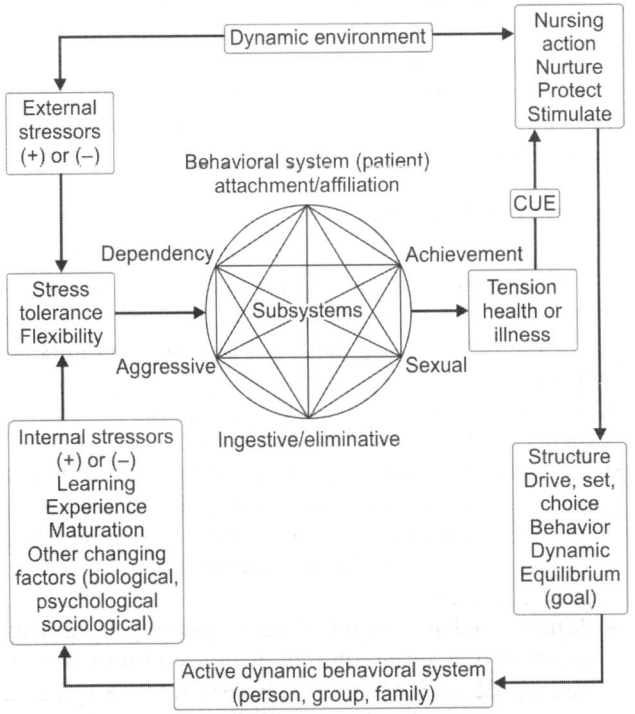

Fig. 39.23: Johnson's behavior model.
(CUE: common usage equipment)

❖ This theory provides researchable questions to conduct research activities on any of the systems.

Critique

Simplicity
Simple in relation based on a number of concepts. However, it is complex due to the possible number of inter-relationships and subsystems.

Generality
Unlimited when applied to sick individuals, but it has not been used with well individuals or groups.

Empirical Precision
Johnson's theory has only a moderate degree of empirical precision because of the highly abstract concepts needs to be better defined.

Derivable Consequences
Johnson's theory could guide and provide conceptual framework for nursing practice, education, and research. The theory has directed questions for nursing research. The theory has potential for continued utility in nursing to achieve valued nursing goals.

Conclusion
Johnson's theory could help and guide the future of nursing theories models, research, and education. By focusing on behavioral rather than biology, the theory clearly differentiates nursing from medicine. But does one need to separate the behavioral from the biological? It can be an asset and it can work, that has been proven by Johnson and some of the followers.

IMOGENE KING THEORY (FIG. 39.24)

Credentials and Background of the Theorist
❖ Born in 1923
❖ Basic Nursing Education from St. John's Hospital School of Nursing in 1945
❖ Bachelor of Science in Nursing and Education with minors in Philosophy and Chemistry from St. Louis University in 1948
❖ Master of Science in Nursing from St. Louis University in 1957
❖ 1961 Doctor of Education from Teacher's College, Columbia University
❖ 1980: Honorary PhD from Southern Illinois University.

Experience of King
❖ As an administrator, an educator and a practitioner
❖ Her area of clinical practice in adult Medical-Surgical Nursing
❖ Director of the School of Nursing at The Ohio State University in Columbus a faculty member at St. John's Hospital School of Nursing.

Basic Function of Nurse
❖ The goal of the nurse is "to help individuals maintain or regain health."
❖ Nursing's domain includes promoting, maintaining, restoring health, and caring for the sick, injured, or dying.
❖ The function of the professional nurse is to interpret information in, what is known as the nursing process, to plan, implement, and evaluate nursing care for individuals, families, groups, and communities.

Theoretical Sources
A book on the theory of nursing to provide a conceptual frame of reference for nursing to be utilized by students, teachers and also by researchers and practitioners to identify and analyze events to specific nursing situations.

A search of the literature in the nursing and the other behavioral science fields, discussions with colleagues, attending in numerous conferences, inductive and deductive reasoning, and some critical thinking about the information gathered, lead to formulate King's own theoretical framework.

Use of Empirical Evidence
❖ King defines theory as a set of concepts, which defined or interrelated and observable in the world of nursing practice. Theory serves to build scientific knowledge for nursing and she has identified two methods for theory.
❖ King's study varies from others, described the nurse patient interaction process that leads to goal attainment.
❖ King also describes her own descriptive, which tested goal attainment and operationally defined a concept of transaction as an integral part of a theory. A system approach is used in the development of the theory of goal attainment.
❖ King's called nursing act as a process stating the nursing process is a series of acts, which connote action, reaction, and interaction. Transaction follows when a reciprocal relationship established by the nurse and patient and both mutually set the goals to be achieved.

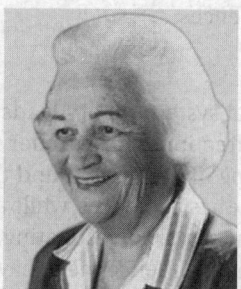

Fig. 39.24: Imogene King.

- A theory of goal attainment was derived from the conceptual framework of interpersonal systems that represents personal, interpersonal, and social systems as the domain of nursing. Each of the three components uses human beings as the basic elements exchange matter/energy/information with other individuals/the environment.

Dynamic Interacting Systems (Fig. 39.25)

Three systems in the conceptual framework are as follows:

Personal System (Individual)

Each individual is a personal system, and the relevant concepts include interaction, perception, communication, transaction, role, stress, growth and development, and time and space (discussed in major concepts).

Interpersonal Systems

Interpersonal systems are formed by human beings interacting with one another:

- Two interacting individuals form a dyad; three form a triad, and four or more form small or large groups.
- The complexity of the interactions increases as the number of people interacting increases. The characteristics of stress are that it is universal dynamic as a result of open systems being in continuous exchange with the environment.
- The nurse's role can be defined as interacting with one or more others in a nursing situation in which the nurse as a professional uses the skills, knowledge, and values identified as belonging to nursing to identify goals with others and help them achieve goals.

Social System

A social system is a group of people in a community/society sharing common goals, interests, and values the roles, behaviors, and practices defined by the system for the purposes of sustaining desirable attributes and for creating methods to maintain the practices and rules of the system. For example, social systems include peers, families, community groups, religious groups, educational organizations, government, and work systems:

- King defines organization as being made up of individuals who have prescribed roles and positions and who make use of resources to meet goals both personal and organizational.
- An organization is characterized by a structure that orders positions and activities and includes formal and informal arrangements of people to gain both personal and organizational goals.
- King defines authority as an active, reciprocal process of transaction in which the actor's experience, understanding, and values influence the meaning, legitimacy and acceptance of those in organizational positions associated with authority.
- King defines status as the relationship of one's place in a group to others in a group or of a group to other groups.
- Decision-making in an organization is defined as a changing and orderly process through which choices related to goals are made among identified possible activities and individual or group actions are taken to move toward the goal; is that nurse and client communicate information, set goals mutually and then act to attain goals.
- King describes the steps of the nursing process as a system of interrelated actions and identifies concepts, provides theoretical basis for the nursing process as a method.

Major Concepts and Definitions

The major concepts in the theory of goal attainment are interaction, perception, communication, transaction, role, stress, growth and development, and time and space (Fig. 39.26):

- ***Interaction:*** King defines interaction as a "process of perception and communication between person

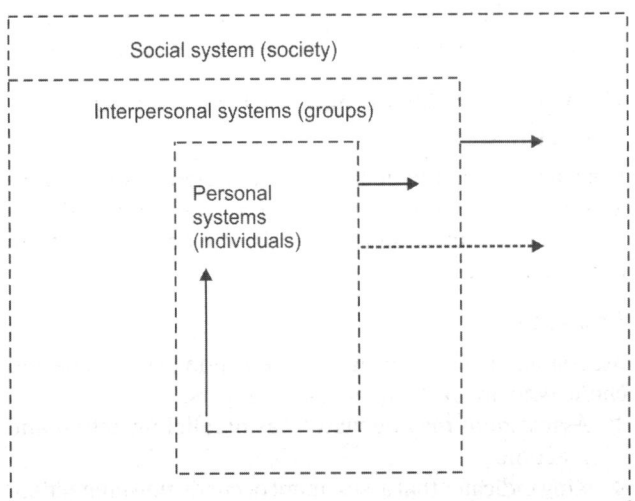

Fig. 39.25: King's open system/conceptual framework.

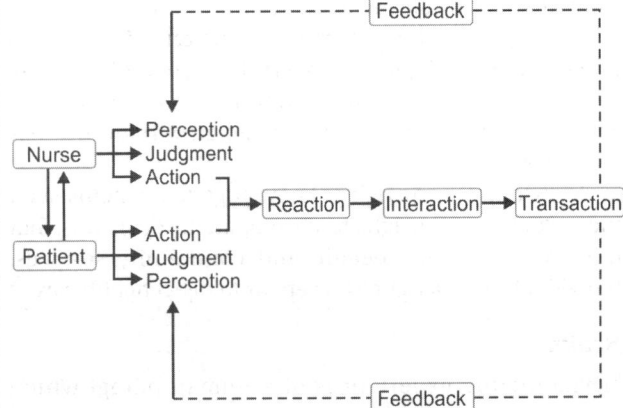

Fig. 39.26: Schematic diagram theory of goal attainment.

and environment and between person and person, represented by verbal and nonverbal behaviors that are goal directed."
- **Perception:** Perception was defined "each person's representation of reality" which includes the import and transformation of energy, and processing, storing, and exporting information. Perception is related to past experiences, concept of self, socioeconomic groups, biological inheritance, and educational background.
- **Communication:** Communication is an information component of the interactions. The exchange of verbal and nonverbal signs and symbols between nurse and client or client and environment is communication.
- **Transaction:** "Transactions are defined as purposeful interactions that lead to goal attainment" which include observable behavior of human beings interacting with their environment.
- **Role:** It is defined as "a set of behaviors expected of persons occupying a position in a social system, rules that define rights and obligations in a position."
- **Stress:** It "is dynamic state whereby a human being interacts with the environment." Stress involves an exchange of energy and information between the person and environment for regulation and control of stressors. An increase in stress may also affect nursing care.
- **Growth and development:** It is defined as "continues changes in individuals at the cellular, molecular, and behavioral levels of activities. Conducive to helping individuals move toward maturity."
- **Time:** "Time is defined as a sequence of events moving onward to the feature. Time is duration between one event and another as uniquely experienced by each human being."
- **Space:** "Space is defined as existing in all directions and is the same everywhere and it is the immediate environment in which nurse and client interact."

King's Theory and Nursing Paradigm

Human Beings

Individuals are "as social, sentient, rational, reacting, perceiving, controlling, purposeful, action-oriented, and time-oriented beings." A concern for nursing is helping people interact with their environment in a manner that will support health maintenance and growth toward self-fulfillment.

Individuals have a right to knowledge about themselves. Individuals have a right to participate in decisions that influence their life, health, and community services. Individuals have a right to accept or to reject health care.

Health

"Dynamic life experiences of a human being, which implies continuous adjustment to stressors in the internal and external environment through optimum use of one's resources to achieve maximum potential for daily living."

Environment

King states that human beings are open systems imply interactions occur between the system and its environment, inferring that the environment is constantly changing. Adjustment to life and health are influenced by an individual's interactions with environment.

Nursing

The goal of nursing is to help individuals maintain their health, so they can function in their roles. Nursing is viewed as an interpersonal process of action, reaction, interaction, and transaction. Perception of nurse and client also influences the interaction process.

Theoretical Assertions

- Perceptual congruence in nurse patient interactions increases mutual goal setting.
- Communication increases mutual goal setting between nurses and patients, and leads to satisfactions.
- Satisfactions in nurses and patients increase goal attainment.
- Goal attainment decreases stress and anxiety in nursing situations.
- Goal attainment increases patient learning and coping ability in nursing situations.
- Role conflict experienced by patients, nurses, or both decreases transactions in nurse–patient interactions.
- Congruence in role expectations and role performance increases transactions in nurse–patient interactions.

Logical Form

There was logical progression of development in the theory. King derived her theory from conceptual framework then organizes elements in the nursing process of nurse client interactions that result in outcomes, i.e., goals attained.

Theory of Goal Attainment and the Nursing Process (Fig. 39.27)

Basic assumption of goal attainment theory is that nurse and client communicate information, set goal mutually and then act to attain those goals, is also the basic assumption of nursing process.

Assessment

Assessment occurs during the interaction of the nurse and client, who are likely to meet as strangers:
- Assessment may be viewed as paralleling action and reaction.
- King indicates that assessment occur during interaction. The nurse brings special knowledge and skills whereas

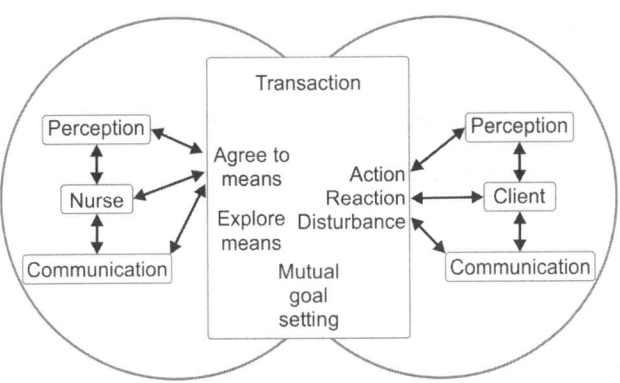

Fig. 39.27: Basic nursing system.

client brings knowledge of self and perception of problems and concern, to this interaction.
- Assessment, interviewing, and communication skills are needed by the nurse as is the ability to integrate knowledge of natural and behavioral sciences for application to a concrete situation.
- During assessment, nurse collects data regarding client (his/her age, sex, education, drug and diet history, growth and development, perception of self and current health status, role and diagnosis of the client, etc.).

Planning

Perception is the basis for gathering and interpreting data thus making it the basis for assessment:
- Communication is necessary to verify the accuracy of perceptions.
- Without communication, interaction, and transaction cannot occur.
- The information shared during assessment is used to derive a nursing diagnosis.
- It is defined by King as a statement that recognizes the distresses, difficulties, or worries identified by the client and for which help is sought.
- After the nursing diagnosis is made, outcomes are identified and planning occurs. King indicates that goal attainment equates to outcomes.
- King says that the concepts involved are decision-making about goals and agreeing to means to attain goals.
- King describes planning as setting goals and making decisions about how to achieve these goals.

Implementation

Implementation occurs in the activities that seek to meet the goals. King stated that implementation is the continuation of the transaction.

Evaluation

- Evaluation involves descriptions of the outcomes identified as goals are attained. According to King's description, evaluation not only speaks to the attainment of the client's goals, but also to the effectiveness of nursing care.
- Although all theory concepts apply throughout the nursing process, communication with perception, interaction, and transaction are vital for goal attainment and need to be apparent in each phase.
- King emphasizes the importance of mutual participation in interaction that focuses on the needs and welfare of the client and of verifying perceptions, while planning and activities to achieve goals are carried out together.

Acceptance by the Nursing Community Practice

- Profession of nursing functions through interactions with individuals groups within the environment.
- Nurses who have knowledge of the concepts of theory of goal attainment are able to accurately perceive and able to suggest approaches for coping with the situations through nursing process.
- The theory and the goal-oriented nursing record useful in practice as nurses to provide individualized plans of care and document effectiveness of nursing care.

Education

- This framework is used by Ohio State University for designing curriculum in the nursing program.
- King's conceptual framework nursing education, practice, and for generating hypothesis for research.
- It provides a systematic means of viewing the nursing profession, organizing a body of knowledge, and clarifying nursing as a discipline.

Research

Research can be designed and conducted to implement this system in a hospital unit in ambulatory care, community nursing, and home care. This information system can be designed for any patient population and for current and future computerization of records in healthcare systems.

King's conceptual framework and her goal oriented nursing record are presently being used in nursing practice and research.

Critique

- *Simplicity:* King's theory presents nine major concepts, thus making the theory complex. The concepts are easily understood because they are defined to show inter-relations in nursing practice.
- *Generality:* King's theory has been criticized for having limited application in areas of nursing where patients are unable to interact competently with the nurse. However, King maintains that she had made transactions with comatose patients, newborns, and applied to psychiatric patients. Its use with groups has not been clarified.

- ❖ ***Empirical precision:*** King has gathered and empirically tested the nurse–patient interaction process that leads to goal attainment by conducting a descriptive study.
- ❖ ***Derivable consequences:*** This theory is useful in nursing practice and focuses on the all aspects of the nursing process.

Application of Theory to Nursing Process

Example: A 50-year-old male client Mr. Y comes to medical outpatient department (OPD) with history of hypertension since 5 years for check. How nurse assists him in controlling blood pressure (BP) through application of King's model concepts.

Assessment

The male patient says he is hypertensive since 5 years; he is feeling giddy and tired on examination his BP is 190/100 mmHg, his weight is 70 kg.

Review oral/written information provides he is on tablet Aten 100 mg od.

Nursing Diagnosis

Knowledge deficit related to disease due to lack of education and ignorance.

Planning

- ❖ Plan for lifestyle modifications
- ❖ Plan for salt free diet
- ❖ Plan for regular exercise
- ❖ Develop good habits

Implementation

Nurse provides health education to the client through interaction to take salt free for diet:
- ❖ Include fiber food
- ❖ Avoid fried food
- ❖ Decrease less fat consumption
- ❖ Exercise 30 min daily
- ❖ Advise brisk walk/jogging/aerobic exercise morning/evening
- ❖ Instruct him to reduce his weight
- ❖ Advise him to take regular medication and check up
- ❖ Advise him to be abstinence from smoking and alcohol and explains the consequences.

Evaluation

Gained in the knowledge and perception related to role of diet and exercise in management of hypertension.

Conclusion

King has presented an open system framework from which she derived a theory of goal attainment, i.e. based on a philosophy of human beings. This theory is applicable widely in nursing practice and applied in the form of a goal-oriented nursing record. The theory is usable, testable, and generalizable as is not situation specific.

BETTY NEUMAN'S SYSTEM THEORY

Credentials and Background of the Theorist

- ❖ Neuman was born in 1924, in Lowel, Ohio.
- ❖ MS in Mental Health Public health Consultation, from UCLA in 1966.
- ❖ PhD in clinical psychology a pioneer in the community mental health movement in the late 1960s.
- ❖ Developed the model, while working as a lecturer in community health nursing at University of California, Los Angeles.
- ❖ The model was published in 1972 as "A Model for Teaching Total Person Approach to Patient Problems" in Nursing Research.
- ❖ It was refined and subsequently published in the first edition of Conceptual Models for Nursing Practice, 1974, and in the second edition in 1980.

Basic Assumptions

- ❖ Each client system is unique, a composite of factors and characteristics within a given range of responses contained within a basic structure.
- ❖ Many known, unknown, and universal stressors exist. Each differs in its potential for disturbing a client's usual stability level or normal line of defense (LOD).
- ❖ The particular inter-relationships of client variables at any point time can affect the degree to which a client is protected by the flexible LOD against possible reaction to stressors.
- ❖ Each client/client system has evolved a normal range of responses to the environment that is referred to as a normal LOD. The normal LOD can be used as a standard from which to measure health deviation.
- ❖ When the flexible LOD is no longer capable of protecting the client/client system against an environmental stressor, the stressor breaks through the normal LOD.
- ❖ The client whether in a state of wellness or illness is a dynamic composite of the inter-relationships of the variables. Wellness is on a continuum of available energy to support the system in an optimal state of system stability.
- ❖ Implicit with in each client system are internal resistance factors known lines of resistance (LOR), which function to stabilize and realign the client to the usual wellness state.
- ❖ Primary prevention relates to general knowledge that is applied in client's assessment and intervention, in identification and reduction of possible or actual risk factors.
- ❖ Secondary prevention relates to symptomatology following a reaction to stressor, appropriate ranking of intervention priorities, and treatment to reduce their noxious effects.

- Tertiary prevention relates to adjustive processes taking place as reconstitution begins and maintenance factors move the back in circular manner toward primary prevention.
- The client as a system is in dynamic, constant energy exchange with the environment.

Major Concepts and Definitions

- *Holistic client approach:* Neuman's systems model is a dynamic, open, systems approach to client care originally developed to provide a unifying focus for nursing problem definition and for best understanding the client interaction with the environment. The client as a system may be defined as a person, family, group, and community.
- *Open system:* A system is open when its elements are exchanging information energy within its complex organization. Stress and reaction are basic components of an open system.
- *Environment:* Internal and external forces affecting and being affected by the client at any time comprise the environment.
- *Created environment:* The created environment is the client's unconscious mobilization of all system variables toward system integration, stability, and integrity.
- *Content:* The five variables (physiological, psychological, sociocultural, developmental, and spiritual of man in interaction with the environment comprise the whole system of the client.
  1. *LOR:* The series of broken rings surrounding the basic core structure are called flexible LOR. These rings represent resource factors that help the client defend against a stressor, e.g. body's immune response system.
  2. *Basic structure:* It consists of all variables as survival factors common to man, as well as unique individual characteristics. The inner circle of the diagram represents the basic survival factors or energy resources of the client.
     - *Process or functions:* The exchange of matter, energy, and information with the environment and the interaction of the parts and subparts of the system of man. A living environment tends to move toward wholeness, stability, wellness, and negentropy.
     - *Input and output:* The matter, energy, and information exchanged between man and environment, which is entering or leaving the system at any point in time.
     - *Feedback:* The process within which matter, energy, and information as output, provides feedback for, corrective action to change, enhance, or stabilize the system.
     - *Negentrophy:* A process of energy utilization that assists system progression toward stability or wellness.
     - *Entropy:* A process of energy depuration that moves the system to illness or death.
     - *Stability:* The client or system successfully hopes with stressors, it is able to maintain an adequate level of health. Functional harmony or balance preserves the integrity of the system.
     - *Stressors:* It is environmental forces that may alter system stability. Neuman's views on stressors are:
       - Intrapersonal forces occurring within the individual, e.g. conditioned responses.
       - Interpersonal forces occurring one or more individual, e.g. role expectations.
       - Extra personal forces occurring outside the individual, e.g. financial circumstances.

     Stressors are stimuli, which might penetrate both the clients flexible and normal lines of defense, the potential outcome of an interaction with a stressor may be beneficial (positive) or noxious (negative).
     - *Wellness:* Exits when the pars of the clients system interact in harmony. System needs are met.
     - *Illness:* Disharmony among the parts of the system is considered illness in varying degrees reflection unmet needs.
  3. **Normal LOD:** It is the models outer solid circle. It represents stability state for the individual, system or the condition following adjustment made to stressors and maintained overtime that is considered uniquely normal.
  4. **Flexible lines of defense:** The models outer broken ring is called the flexible LOD. It is dynamic and can be rapidly altered over a short period of time. It is perceived as a protective buffer for preventing stressors from breaking through the solid LOD. The relationship of the variables physiological, psychological, sociocultural, developmental, and spiritual can affect the degree to which an individual is able to use their flexible LOD against possible reaction to a stressor or stressors, such as loss of sleep. It is important to strengthen this flexible LOD to prevent a possible reaction.
  5. **Prevention as intervention:** Interventions are purposeful action to help the client retain, attain, and/or maintain system stability. They can occur before or after resistance lines are penetrated in both reaction and reconstitution phase. Neuman supports beginning intervention when a stressor is either suspected or identified. Intervention is based on possible or actual degree of reaction, resource, goals, and the anticipated outcome. Neuman identifies three levels of intervention: (1) primary, (2) secondary, and (3) tertiary.
     - Primary prevention is carried out when a stressor is suspected or identified. A reaction has

not yet occurred, but the degree of risk is known. Neuman states the actor or intervener would perhaps attempt to reduce the possibility of the individuals encounter, which the stressor or in some way attempt to strengthen the individuals flexible LOD to decrease the possibility of a reaction.

- Secondary prevention involves interventions of treatment initiated after symptoms from stress have occurred. Both clients' internal and external resources would be used toward system stabilization to strengthen internal LOR, reduce reaction and increase resistance factors.
- Tertiary prevention occurs after the active treatment or secondary prevention stage. It focuses on adjustment toward optimal client system stability. A primary goal is to strengthen resistance to stressors by reduction to help prevention, e.g. avoidance of stressors known to be hazardous to the client.

6. **Reconstitution:** It is the state of adaptation to stressors in the internal and external environment. Reconstitution can begin at any degree or level of reaction and may progress beyond or stabilize somewhat below the clients previous normal LOD. In reconstitution vary with interpersonal, intra- and extra-personal, and environmental factors and inter-related with physiological, psychological, sociocultural, developmental, and spiritual variables.

Neuman's Model and Nursing Paradigm (Fig. 39.28)

Person

Human being is a total person as a client system and the person is a layered multidimensional being. Each layer consists of five personal variable or subsystems:

- ❖ **Physiological:** Refers of the physicochemical structure and function of the body.
- ❖ **Psychological:** Refers to mental processes and emotions.
- ❖ **Sociocultural:** Refers to relationships and social/cultural expectations and activities.
- ❖ **Spiritual:** Refers to the influence of spiritual beliefs.
- ❖ **Developmental:** Refers to those processes related to development over the lifespan.

Environment

- ❖ The environment is seen to be the totality of the internal and external forces, which surround a person and with which they interact at any given time.

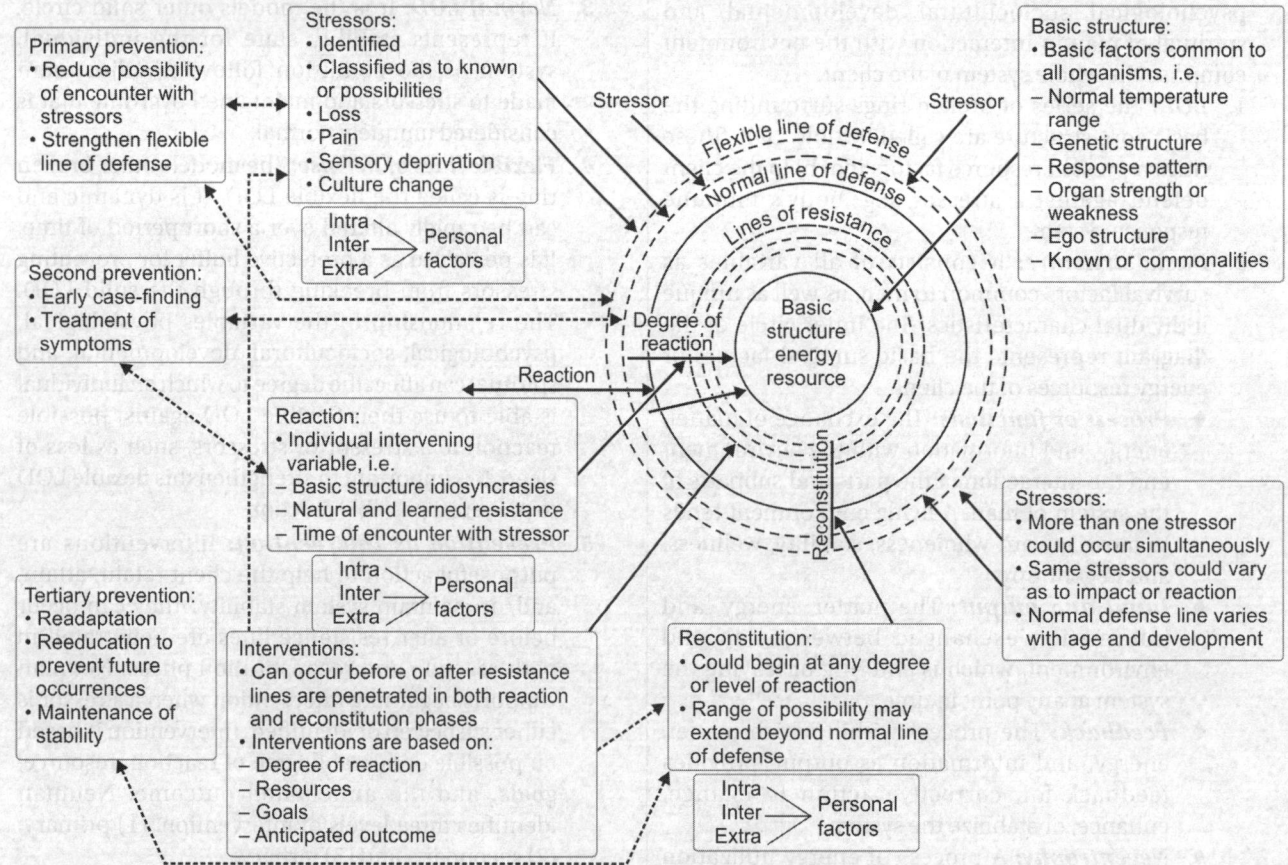

Fig. 39.28: The Neuman's system model.

- ❖ These forces include the intrapersonal, inter-and extra-personal stressors, which can affect the person's normal LOD and so can affect the stability of the system:
  - ➢ The internal environment exists within the client system.
  - ➢ The external environment exists outside the client system.
  - ➢ The created environment is an environment that is created and developed unconsciously by the client and is symbolic of system wholeness.

Health

Health is equated with wellness. Health/wellness is defined as "the condition in which all parts and subparts (variables) are in harmony with the whole of the client (Neuman, 1995)." The client system moves toward illness and death when more energy is needed than is available. The client system moved toward wellness when more energy is available than is needed.

Nursing

Neuman sees nursing as a unique profession that is concerned with all of the variables, which influence the response a person might have to a stressor. The person is seen as a whole and it is the task of nursing to address the whole person:

- ❖ Neuman defines nursing as "action, which assists individuals, families and groups to maintain a maximum level of wellness and the primary aim is stability of the patient/client system, through nursing interventions to reduce stressors."
- ❖ Neuman states that, because the nurse's perception will influence the care given, then not only must the patient/client's perception be assessed, but so must those of the caregiver (nurse). The role of the nurse is seen in terms of degree of reaction to stressors and the use of primary, secondary and tertiary interventions.

Acceptance by the Nursing Community

Nursing Practice

The Neuman's system models have broad relevance for the current and future nursing practice. The model's use in nursing facilities makes it a goal-directed, unified, holistic approach to client care.

Neuman has developed several instruments to facilitate the utilization of the system model:

- ❖ The assessment/intervention helps/assist the nurse in collecting and synthesizing data.
- ❖ Neuman nursing process format to implement the model. It consists of nursing diagnosis, goals, and outcomes.
- ❖ Development of management process too. To implement the model systems approach to the role of nurse administrator.
- ❖ Use of model to organize multidisciplinary assessments and interventions for individuals and families dealing with life-threating and terminal illness.

Nursing Education

The model has been well accepted in academic circles:

- ❖ It is widely utilized as a curriculum guide oriented toward wellness and client care.
- ❖ Development of assessment/intervention tool based on Neuman framework and clinical evaluation tools based on Neuman's model.
- ❖ Selection of the model for baccalaureate programs on the basis of its theoretical and comprehensive perspectives for a holistic curriculum and utilization with the individual, family, small groups, and communities.
- ❖ Use of the model as comprehensive framework for data collection.
- ❖ Use of the model for continuing education in nursing.
- ❖ Use of the model for successful workshop in a clinical setting.

Nursing Research

Neuman's system-based model research is rapidly increasing. Raphealla Sohier, a Neuman trustee, is doing qualitative research in the area of the grieving process of parents of gay men dying of acquired immunodeficiency syndrome (AIDS).

- ❖ Ziegler has derived taxonomy for nursing diagnosis from Neuman's model. He states that nursing diagnosis taxonomy could provide a systematized method for organizing nursing research and for developing nursing theory.
- ❖ Use of the Neuman's model in student nursing research projects, reporting total of 42 studies completed or in process.

Nursing Administration

The utility of the Neuman's system model is nursing service administration is also documented:

- ❖ They presented an innovative Neuman's system management tool that can be used by the administrator to document analysis of management situations, implementation of preventive management, interventions, and evaluation of outcomes.
- ❖ Neuman's system model levels of prevention serve as the framework for nursing intervention.
- ❖ The family system stressor, strength inventory was developed by the use of Neuman's systems model.

Critique of Theory

- ❖ *Clarity:* Neuman presents abstract concepts that are familiar to nursing. Although additional definitions could be helpful, the models concept of client, environment, health, and nursing are all inherent and congruent with traditional values.

- ❖ **Simplicity:** Multiple interactions and inter-relationships comprise this broad systematic model, which are organized in a complex yet logic manner. Neuman states that concepts can be separated for analysis, specific goal settings, and interventions.
- ❖ **Generality:** The Neuman's system model has been used in a wide variety of nursing situations; it is reality adaptable and comprehensive enough to be useful in all healthcare settings, including administration and research. Other related health field can use this framework because of its systematic nature and emphasis on the client system as a whole.
- ❖ **Empirical precision:** Although the model has been completely tested till date, nursing scientists are demonstrating major interest in and use of the model to guide nursing research. Continued testing and refinement will increase the models empirical precision as the research process, analysis, and synthesis of findings from multiple studies are completed.
- ❖ **Derivable Consequences:** Neuman's conceptual model provides the professional nurse with important guidelines for assessment of the whole person, utilization of nursing process, and implementation of preventive interventions. The focus on primary prevention and interdisciplinary care facilities improved quality of care and is futuristic.

Nursing Process by Neuman

Assessment

- ❖ Assess for potential and actual stressors:
  - ➢ Condition and strength of basic structure factors and energy sources
  - ➢ Characteristics of flexible and normal LOD, LOR, degree of reaction, and potential for reconstitution
  - ➢ Interaction between client and environment
  - ➢ Life process and coping factors (past, present, and future) actual and potential stressors (internal and external) for optimal wellness external
  - ➢ Perceptual difference between caregiver and the client.
- ❖ **Nursing Diagnosis:**
  - ➢ Activity intolerance
  - ➢ Ineffective coping
  - ➢ Ineffective thermoregulation
- ❖ **Goal:** In Neuman's systems model, the goal is to keep the client system stable.
- ❖ **Planning:** Planning is focused on strengthening the LOD and resistance.
- ❖ **Implementation:** The goal of stabilizing the client system is achieved through three modes of prevention, which is detailed below.
  - ➢ **Primary prevention:** It is carried out when a stressor is identified or suspected. A reaction has not yet occurred. Actions taken to retain stability.
  - ➢ **Secondary prevention:** It involves interventions or treatment initiated after symptoms from stress have occurred. Actions taken to attain stability.
  - ➢ **Tertiary prevention:** A primary goal is to strengthen resistance to stressors by reduction to help prevent recurrence of reaction or regression. Actions taken to maintain stability.
  - ➢ **Evaluation:** The nursing process is evaluated to determine whether equilibrium is restored and a steady state maintained.

Application of Neuman's Model to Clinical Nursing Practice (Fig. 39.29)

The main use of the Neuman's model in practice and in research is that its concentric layers allow for a simple classification of how severe a problem is for example, since the line of normal defense represents dynamic balance, it represents homeostasis and thus a lack of stress:

- ❖ If a stress response is perceived by the patient or assessed by the nurse, then there has been an invasion of the normal LOD and a major contraction of the flexible LOD.
- ❖ Infection or other invasion of the LOR indicates failure of both LOD.
- ❖ Furthermore each person variable can be operationalized and the relationship to the normal LOD or stress response can be analyzed.

Situation

A female patient aged about 50 years diagnosed as dysfunctional uterine bleeding and admitted to a maternity hospital and undergone abdominal hysterectomy.

Using Neuman's model in the above situation, possible stressors that contributed to that patient is as follows. In this client, the normal LOD has maintained overtime that is considered normal and flexible LOD, i.e. the outer broken ring is rapidly altered over a short period of time it is perceived as protective buffer for preventing stressors from breaking the solid line of defense. The protective line of defense applicable to this patient is the LOR. As she has undergone abdominal hysterectomy, so the flexible LOD and normal life of defense are broken.

Neuman identified three levels of intervention: (1) primary, (2) secondary, and (3) tertiary among this tertiary level of prevention is applicable to that client.

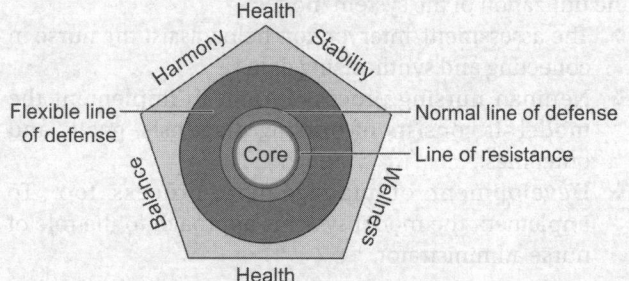

Fig. 39.29: Stressors affecting the system.

Table 39.5: The Neuman's model and the nursing process.

Assessment of stressors	Nursing diagnosis	Nursing intervention	Reconstitution
• **Intropersonal:** A female patient aged 48 years with irregular menstruation since 2 years with weight 48 kg • **Interpersonal:** Marital status G3P3 role expectations altered • **Extrapersonal:** Income 2,500/month coolie • **Social:** No family support • **Developmental:** Irregular bleeding change in regular cycles	• Pain related to soft tissue injury • Imbalanced nutrition related to constipation • Knowledge deficit related to risk for infection	• Primary prevention is carried out when a stressor is suspected or identified • Secondary prevention involves interventions of treatment initiated after symptoms from stress have occurred • Tertiary prevention occurs after the active treatment or secondary prevention stage	• Following strict aspects adaptations • Promote good personal hygiene • Maintain balanced diet • Administer antibiotics • Advice regarding following care

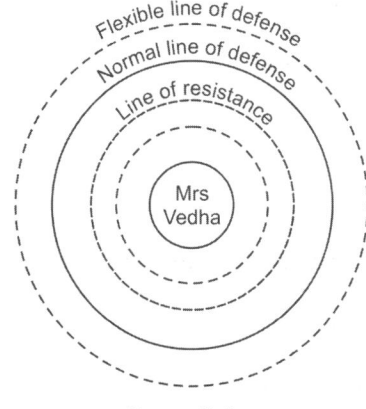

Fig. 39.30: Illustration of interpretation of Neuman's model.

Tertiary prevention is applied to the client by imparting knowledge on various aspects to prevent further complications such as urinary tract, gastrointestinal, and wound infection. Reconstitution is accompanied by maintaining good personal hygiene, taking balanced diet, promoting exercises, maintaining strict aseptic techniques **while performing sterile procedures** and administration of antibiotics (Table 39.5 and Fig. 39.30).

Conclusion

The Neuman's systems model is used equally well with clients as individuals, groups, or communities and it is comprehensive, systemic nature has allowed wide variety of clinical practice, research, and administrative applications worldwide. In her model, Betty Neuman has addressed the effects of stress and reactions to stress on the development and maintenance of health. She states that "person" is a client system, i.e. composed of physiologic, psychological, sociocultural, and environmental variables and "environment" is both internal and external forces surrounding humans at any time. Health or wellness exists if all parts and subparts are in harmony with the whole person. Nursing is seen as unique profession concerned with all the variables affecting an individual's response to stressors.

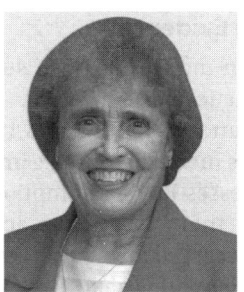

Fig. 39.31: Sister Callista Roy.

ROY'S ADAPTATION THEORY

Adaptation is the process of adjusting to change. The term adaptation implies that a person has effectively coped with accommodation and adjusted to a changed set of date and external conditions.

However, not all adaptations are positive, for example, a young woman diagnosed with diabetes may become suddenly withdrawn and may have permanent response leading to maladaptation.

A fluid appraisal and reappraisal of the causes of stress, the immediate reaction to it and ways of lessening it are hallmarks of natural adaptation. It is portrayed as a balance, an outcome, and the end results of coping efforts.

Credentials and Background of the Theorist

- Sister Callista Roy (Fig. 39.31), a member of the Sister's of Saint Joseph, was born on October 14 1939 in Los Angeles, California
- Bachelor of Arts in Nursing, 1963
- Master of Science in Nursing, 1966
- MA in Sociology, 1973
- PhD in Sociology, 1977

Roy had worked as pediatric staff nurse and began operationalizing her model in 1968. In 1982, she was an Associate Professor and Chair Person of the Department of Nursing. During this time, she conducted research on nursing intervention for cognitive recovery in head injuries.

Roy published many books, chapters, and periodically articles and has presented numerous lectures and workshops focusing on her nursing adaptation theory. She is a member of Sigma Theta Tau, having received the National Founders Award for Excellence in Fostering Professional Nursing Standards in 1981.

Theoretical Sources

- Roy's adaptation model for nursing was derived in 1964 from Harry Helson's work in, psychophysics. In Helson's Adaptation Theory, adaptive responses are a function of the incoming stimulus and the adaptive level.
- According to Roy, more than 1,500 faculties have contributed to the theoretical development of the adaptation model.

Use of Empirical Evidence

- The adaptation model has been supported through research in practice and education.
- Rambo and Randell, Tedrow and Landingham have expanded Roy's model for nursing implementation.
- Tiedeman assesses Roy's assumptions for soundness by classifying them into three according to their foundation—accepted theory (particularly theory with empirical substantiating data).

Major Concepts and Definitions

System

A system is a set of units so related or connected as to function as a whole for some purpose characterized by inputs, outputs, and control and feedback processes.

Adaptation Level

A person's adaptation level is a constantly changing point, made up of focal, contextual, and residual stimuli, which represent the person's own standard of the range of stimuli to which one can respond with ordinary adaptive responses.

Adaptation Problems

Adaptation problems are the occurrences of situations of inadequate response to need deficits or excesses.

A focal stimulus: Focal stimulus is the degree of change or stimulus that may be internal or external stimulus most immediately affecting the system and the one to which the person must make an adaptive response, that is, the factor that precipitates the behavior.

Contextual Stimuli

Contextual stimuli are all other stimuli present that contribute to the behavior caused or precipitated by focal stimuli.

Residual Stimuli

Residual stimuli are factors that may be affecting behavior, but whose effects are not validated.

Regulator subsystem: Automatic response to stimulus (neural, chemical, and endocrine).

Cognator

Cognator is a subsystem coping mechanism, which responds through complex processes of perception and information processing, learning, judgment, and emotion.

Adaptive Modes (Fig. 39.32)

Adaptive or effector modes are a classification of ways of coping that manifest regulator and cognator activity, that is physiological, self-concept, role function, and interdependence.

Adaptive Responses

Adaptive responses are responses that promote integrity of the person in terms of the goals of survival, growth, reproduction, and mastery.

Ineffective Responses

Ineffective responses are responses that do not contribute to adaptive goals that are survival, growth, reproduction, and mastery.

Physiological Mode

Physiological needs involve the body's basic needs and ways of dealing with adaptation in regard to fluid and electrolytes, exercise and rest, elimination, nutrition, circulation, and oxygen regulation, which includes the senses, temperature, and endocrine regulation.

Nurse must be knowledgeable about normal processes five needs (oxygenation, nutrition, elimination, activity, and rest and protection).

Self-concept Mode

Self-concept is the composite belief and feeling that one holds about oneself at a given time. It is formed from perceptions, particularly of others reactions and directs one's behavior. Its components include:

- Physical self, which involves sensation and body image

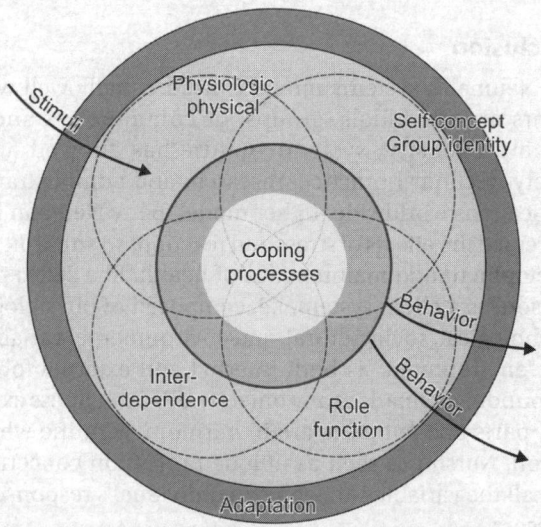

Fig. 39.32: Roy's adaptive modes of intervention.

- Personal self, which is made up of self-consistency, self-ideal or expectancy, and the moral, ethical self.

Role Performance Mode

Role function is the performance of duties based on given positions in society. The way one performs a role is dependent on ones interaction with other in the given situation. The major roles that one plays can be analyzed such as wife, mother, teacher, etc. for a given period of time. Each of these roles is seen as occurring in a dyadic relationship that is with a reciprocal role.

Interdependence Mode

The interdependence mode involves one's relations with significant others and support systems. In this mode, one maintains psychic integrity by meeting needs for nurturance and affection:
- Behavior pertaining to interdependent relationships of individuals and groups
- Focus on the close relationships of people and their purpose
- Each relationship exists for some reason
- Involves the willingness and ability to give to others and accept from others
- Balance results in feelings of being valued and supported by others
- Basic need-feeling of security in relationships.

Model of the Theory (Fig. 39.33)

There are two inter-related subsystems in Roy's model. The primary, functional, or control processes subsystem consists of the regulator and the cognator. The secondary effector subsystem consists of four adaptive modes, i.e. physiological needs, self-concept, role function, and interdependence function.

Roy views the regulator and cognator as methods of coping. Perception of the person links the regulator with the cognator in that input into the regulator is transformed into perceptions. It is the process of the cognator. The responses following perceptions are feedback into both the cognator and regulator.

The four adaptive modes of the second subsystem in the Roy's model provide from manifestations of cognator and regulator activity. Responses to stimuli are carried out. The goal statement should include the behavior to be changed, change expected, and time frame in which the change in behavior should occur.

Intervention

Intervention focuses on the manner in which goals are attained, a nursing intervention is any action taken by a professional nurse that the nurse believes will promote adaptive behavior in a client and they arise from a solid knowledge base and are aimed at the focal stimulus whenever possible.

Evaluation in Roy's Adaptation Model

It is necessary to evaluate whether the person has moved toward the adaptation. It requires analysis, judgment to determine whether the behavioral changes desired in the goal statement have been achieved by the recipient of nursing care.

Roy's Theory and Nursing Metaparadigm

- *Person:* Humans are holistic, adaptive systems. A whole with the parts that function in unity for some purpose. Not limited to just the individual can include:
  - Groups
  - Families
  - Organizations
  - Communities
  - Society as a whole
- *Environment:* Includes all the conditions, circumstances, and influences surrounding and affecting the development and behaviors of the person. Stimuli include can be categorized as focal, contextual and residual. It may be internal and external.
- *Health:* A state and a process of being and becoming integrated as a whole person. Reflection of adaptation that is the interaction of person and environment.
- *Nursing:* Acts to enhance the interaction of the person with the environment to promote adaptation by applying adaptive modes of Roy and practice that expands adaptive abilities and enhances person and environmental transformation.

Application of Roy's Concepts to Nursing Process

Problem-solving approach for gathering data, identifying the capacities and needs of the human adaptive system, selecting, and implementing approaches for nursing care and evaluation the outcome of care provided.
- *Assessment of behavior:* Gathering data about the behavior of the human adaptive system and the current state of adaptation.
- *Assessment of stimuli:* Identification of internal and external stimuli that are influencing the behaviors.
- *Nursing diagnosis:* Formulation of statements that interpret data about the stimuli influencing or not influencing behavior.

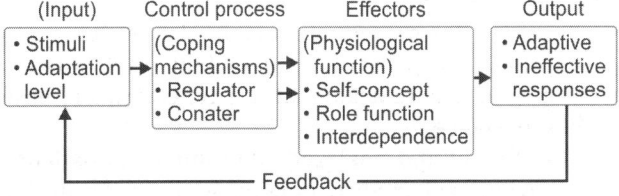

Fig. 39.33: Person as an adaptive system from Sister Calista Roy's Adaptation Model.

- ❖ **Goal setting:** Establishment of clear statements that interpret data about the stimuli influencing or not influencing behavior.
- ❖ **Intervention:** Determination of how best to assist the human system in attaining the previously established goals.
- ❖ **Evaluation:** Judging the effectiveness of the nursing intervention in relation to the behavior of the human system.

Theoretical Assertions

Roy's model focuses on the concept of adaptation of man. Her concepts of nursing, person health, and environment are all inter-related to this central concept. The person continually scans the environment for stimuli so he/she can respond and ultimately adapt. Nursing has a unique goal to assist the person in his/her adaptation effort by managing the environment. The result is attainment of an optimum level of wellness by the person.

Logical Form

- ❖ Roy's adaptation model for nursing is both deductive and inductive. It is deductive in that much or Roy's theory is derived from Helson's psychophysics theory. Roy redefined within nursing to form a typology of factors related to adaptation levels of persons, Roy also uses other concepts and theory outside the discipline of nursing relates these to her adaptation theory.
- ❖ Roy's theory is inductive in that she developed the four adaptive modes from research and the practice experiences of herself, her colleagues, and her students.

Acceptance by the Nursing Community

Practice

Roy's model is useful for practice as it outlines the features of the discipline and provides direction for practice as well as for education and research.

It is valuable theory for nursing practice because it includes a goal that is specified as the aim of activity and prescription for activities to realize the goal. The goal of the model is the person's adaptation in four adaptive modes in situations of health and illness. The prescriptions or interventions are the management of stimuli by removing, increasing, decreasing, or altering them. These prescriptions can be obtained by listing practice related hypotheses generated by the model.

Two-level assessment is unique to this model and leads to the identification of adaptation problems of nursing diagnosis. Intervention is based specifically on the model, but there is a need to develop an organization of categories of nursing interventions.

In 1981, a research study was published that model was applied for problems associated with elderly persons in nursing homes, applicable to treat multiple patient variables and number of healthcare agencies have begun implementing the Roy's model as a basis for nursing practice.

Education

The adaptation model is in use at Mount Saint Mary's College, Department of Nursing in Los Angeles. This program demonstrates the relationship of nursing theory to nursing education. Three vertical strands run through the curriculum. Two theory strands (the adapting person and health-illness) and one practice strand (nursing management). There two horizontal strands in the curriculum-nursing process and student adaptation/leadership. The horizontal strands enhance the theory and practice of the vertical strands. All strands within the curriculum build in complexity from one level to the next. In addition the model allows for increasing the knowledge in both areas of theory and practice.

Research

The Roy's adaptation model is a good conceptual framework applied to many studies in research field. The Roy's model helps to guide to design for research studies, many studies have proved the modes of adaptation were sufficiently comprehensive to permit classification of all data.

Critique

Simplicity

The Roy's model includes the concepts of nursing, person, health-illness, environment, adaptation, and nursing activities. It also includes the sub-concepts of regulator, cognator, and the four effector modes of physiological, self-concept, role function, and interdependence, because this theory has several major concepts and sub-concepts and numerous relational statements, it is complex.

Generality

Roy's model has been classified as a grand theory. The broad scope is an advantage because the model has been used for other theory building and testing in studying smaller ranges of phenomena. Roy's model is generalizable to all settings in nursing practice, but is limited in scope because it primarily addresses the concept of person-environment adaptation and focuses primarily on the client; information on the nurse is implied.

Empirical Precision

- ❖ Because Roy's broad concepts from theory in physiological psychology, sociology, and nursing, empirical data indicate that this general theory base has substance.
- ❖ Roy studied and analyzed 500 samples of patient's behaviors collected by nursing students. From this analysis, she proposed her four adaptive models in man. This is the least supported of Roy's concepts.

Derivable Consequences

The Roy adaptation model has a clearly defined nursing process and can be useful guiding clinical practice. The model is also capable of generating new information through the testing of the hypotheses that have been derived from it.

Application of Theory to Clinical Situation

Debbie is a 29-year-old woman who was recently admitted to the oncology nursing unit for evaluation.

Assessment

- Her complaints of pelvic fullness and noting a watery foul smelling vaginal discharge. A Pap smear revealed a class fifth cervical cancer. She was found to have a stage II squamous cell carcinoma of the cervix and underwent a radical hysterectomy with bilateral salpingo-oophorectomy.
- Her past health history revealed that physical examination had been infrequent. She also reported that she has not performed breast self-examination. She is 164.5 tall and weighs 89 pounds. Her usual weight is about 110 pounds. She has smoked approximately packs of cigarettes a day for the past 10 years. She is gravida 2, para 2. Her first pregnancy was at the age of 16 and her second was the age of 18, since that time she has taken oral contraceptives on a regular basis:
  - Debbie completed the eighth grade.
  - She is married and lives with her husband and two children in her mother's home, which she describes as less than sanitary.
  - Her husband is unemployed; she describes him as emotionally distant and abusive at times.
  - She has done well following surgery, except for being unable to completely empty her urinary bladder. She is having continued postoperative pain and nausea. It will be necessary for her to perform intermittent self-catheterization at home.
  - Her home medications are:
    - Antibiotics
    - Analgesics needed for pain relief
    - Antiemetic as needed for nausea in addition she will receive radiation therapy on an outpatient basis. Debbie is extremely fearful. She expressed great concern over her future and or her two children. She believes that this illness is a punishment for her past life.

Nursing Care with Physiological Adaptive Mode

Assessment of Behavior

Postoperative, Debbie has been unable to completely empty her urinary bladder. She states that she is numb and unable to tell when she needs to void. Catheterization for residual urine revealed that she was retaining 300 mL of urine after voiding. It will be necessary for her to perform intermittent self-catheterization at home. Unsanitary conditions at Debbie's home is a high risk for developing a urinary tract infection. She states that she is scared about performing self-catheterization.

Assessment of Stimuli

It searches for stimuli responsible for the observed behavior. After identified, the stimuli are classified as focal, contextual, or residual. The focal stimuli for the urinary retention are the disease process. Contextual stimuli include tissue trauma resulting from surgery and radiation therapy. Debbie described anxiety as residual stimuli. Infection is a potential problem. The local stimuli are the need for intermittent self-catheterization. Contextual stimuli include altered skin integrity related to surgical incision. A poor understanding of aseptic principles and unsanitary conditions at Debbie's home.

Nursing Diagnosis

From the assessment of behavior and stimuli, the following nursing diagnoses were made:

- Urinary disturbance related to surgical trauma, radiation therapy, and anxiety.
- Potential for infection related to intermittent self-catheterization.
- Impaired skin integrity related to surgical incision, poor understanding of aseptic principles and unsanitary conditions at Debbie's home.

Goal Setting

Goals set mutually were:

- Complete urinary elimination every 4 h as evidenced by correct demonstration of the procedure for intermittent self-catheterization.
- Continued absence of signs of infection of the surgical incision and urinary tract.

Implementation

To attain these goals the following nursing interventions needs implementation:

- ***Altered elimination:*** Urinary related to surgical trauma and radiation therapy. Debbie was taught the importance of performing intermittent self-catheterization every 4 h to prevent damage to the urinary bladder. She was taught relaxation techniques to facilitate voiding solicit it would be necessary for her to catheterize herself as often.
- ***Potential for infection related to self-catheterization:*** Altered skin integrity related to surgical incision, poor understanding of aseptic principles and unsanitary conditions at Debbie's home.

Debbie was taught the importance of washing hands before touching the surgical incision care. The procedure for incision care was demonstrated by the nursing staff and Debbie was asked for a return demonstration after the intermittent self-catheterization procedure was explained and demonstrated.

Evaluation

Evaluation of Debbie's adaptive level was performed each shift significant findings were:

- ❖ It will be necessary for her to perform intermittent self-catheterization at home. Debbie was able to state the importance of performing intermittent self-catheterization on a regular basis. She performed a return demonstration of intermittent self-catheterization before discharge and she was able to adequately adhere to aseptic principles during the procedure. She accurately recorded the time and amount for each voiding and catheterization.
- ❖ Debbie was able to list the signs and symptoms of a wound and urinary infection to state appropriate steps to take, if symptoms occur. She was able to discuss the importance of maintaining adequate oral fluid intake. Debbie was given a thermometer and instructed its use. She correctly demonstrated taking of temperature.

Conclusion

The Roy Adaptation Model makes a significant contribution to nursing knowledge by focusing attention on the nature of the person's adaptation to the changing environment. The Roy Adaptation Nursing Model served a broad conceptual framework.

WATSON'S THEORY

Human Caring Theory

Background of the Theorist

- ❖ Jean Harman Watson was born in Southern West Virginia and grew up during 1940s and 1950s as the youngest 8th children.
- ❖ She earned a MS in Psychiatric Mental Health Nursing in 1966 at the health sciences campus.
- ❖ She earned BS in Nursing in 1964 at the Boulder campus.
- ❖ After moving to Colorado, Watson continued her nursing education and graduation studies at the University of Colorado.
- ❖ In 1978, she initiated Ph.D. program in Colorado.
- ❖ She first published her ideas in nursing—philosophy and science of caring in 1979.
- ❖ She refined her ideas in Nursing science and human care: A theory of nursing in 1985.
- ❖ After her PhD, she became the Dean of the university of Colorado school of Nursing.
- ❖ Watson has also helped to establish the center of human caring at the University of Colorado.
- ❖ Watson is also featured in several national videos on nursing theory, publications, and portraits of excellence—nursing theorists and their work from the ford health trust and theory in practice from the NLN.
- ❖ She redefined her ideas in Nursing science and human care: A theory of nursing in 1985.

Theoretical Sources

- ❖ In addition to traditional knowledge and the works of Nightingale, Henderson, Kreuter, and Hall, Watson acknowledged the work of Leininger and Gadow.
- ❖ Watson attributes her emphasis in the interpersonal and transpersonal qualities of congruence, empathy, and warmth the view of care Rogers. A warm interest from rogus facilitates desire to understand.
- ❖ Seeman's study that describes effectiveness of psychotherapy by mutual affection and respect the therapist and client.
- ❖ Yalom's II curative factors stimulated Watson's thinking about the psychodynamic and human components that could apply to nursing and caring, to her 10 carative factors in nursing.

Use of Empirical Evidence

Empirical evidence incorporates empiricism, but emphasizes methodologies that begin with nursing phenomena rather than the natural sciences.

Major Assumptions

Watson proposes seven assumptions about the science of caring and 10 carative factors of form the framework of her theory:

- ❖ Caring can be effectively demonstrated and practiced only interpersonally.
- ❖ Caring consists of caraitive that result in the satisfaction of certain human needs.
- ❖ Effective caring promotes health and individual or family growth.
- ❖ Caring responses accept a person not only as he/she is now but what he/she may become.
- ❖ Caring is one that offers the development of potential, while allowing the person to choose the best action for himself/herself at a given point in time.
- ❖ Caring is more "healthogenic" than is curing. The practice of caring integrates by a physical knowledge with knowledge of human behavior to generate or promote health.
- ❖ The practice of caring is central to nursing.

Major Concepts and Definitions

Watson bases her theory for nursing practice on the following 10 carative factors. The first three interdependent factors serve as the philosophical foundation for the science of caring:

1. ***Formation of a humanistic—altruistic system of values:*** These values are learned early in life, but can be greatly influenced by nurse educators. This is defined as

Chapter 39: Nursing Theories

satisfaction through giving and extension of the sense of self.

2. ***Instillation faith-hope:*** This factor facilitates the promotion of holistic nursing care and positive health within the client population. It also describes the nurse's role in developing effective nurse client relationships and in promoting wellness by helping the client adopt health seeking behaviors.
3. ***Cultivation of sensitivity to one's self to others:*** The recognition of feelings leads to self-actualization through self-acceptance for both the nurse and client. As nurses acknowledge their sensitivity and feelings, they become more genuine, authentic, and sensitive to others.
4. ***Development of a helping-trust relationship:*** The development of a helping relationship between the nurse and client is crucial for transpersonal caring. It involves:
   - *Congruence:* It involves being real, honest, genuine, and authentic.
   - *Empathy:* It is the ability to experience and thereby understand the other person's perceptions and feelings and to communicate those understandings.
   - *Warmth:* It is demonstrated by a moderate speaking volume, a relaxed, open posture, and facial expressions that are congruent with other.
   - *Communications:* Effective communication as cognitive, effective, and behavior response.
5. ***Promotion and acceptance of the expression of positive and negative feelings:*** Sharing of feelings is a risk taking experience for both nurse and client. The nurse must be prepared either positive or negative feelings. The nurse must recognize that intectual and emotional understanding of a situation differ.
6. ***Systematic use of the scientific problem-solving method for decision making:*** Use of the nursing process brings a scientific problem-solving approach to nursing care, keeping the traditional image of the nurses as "doctor's hand maiden." The nursing process is similar to the research process in that it is systematic and organized.
7. ***Promotion of interpersonal teaching-learning:*** This factor is an important concept for nursing in that it separates caring from curing allows the client to be informed and thus shift the responsibility for one's wellness and health to the client. The nurse facilities the processes by teaching-learning techniques that are designed to enable the client to provide self-care determine personal needs and provide opportunities of their personal growth.
8. ***Provision for supportive, protective, and/or corrective mental, physical, sociocultural, and spiritual environment:*** Nurses must recognize the influence that internal and external environments have on the health and illness of individuals. Concepts relevant to the mental and spiritual well-being and sociocultural beliefs of an individual. In addition to epidemiological variables, other external variables include comfort, privacy, safety, and clean, esthetic surroundings.
9. ***Assistance with gratification of human needs:*** The nurse recognizes the biophysical and intrapersonal needs of self and client. Clients must satisfy lower order needs before attempting to attain higher order ones. Food elimination and ventilation are examples of lower order biophysical needs, whereas activity/inactivity and sexually are considered lower order. Psychophysical needs, achievements, and affiliation are higher order intrapersonal–interpersonal.
10. Allowance for existential phenomenological forces: Phenomenology describes data of the immediate situation that help people understand the phenomenon. Existential psychology is a science of human *existence* uses phenomenological analysis.

Watson believes that nurses have the responsibility to go beyond the 10 carative factors and to facilitate client development in the area of health promotion through preventive health actions (Fig. 39.34).

Watson's Theory and Nursing Metaparadigm

Person or Human being

She adopts a view of the human being as:
- A valued person in and of him or herself to be cared for, respected, nurtured, understood, and assisted in general in general philosophical view of a person as a fully functional integrated self.
- She believes humans are best viewed in a developmental conflicts frame and these conflicts of individuals and their families are necessary for health care. These conflicts based upon Erikson's model and encountered throughout the human life cycle. The nurse must understand human beings when they are sick, under stress.

Health

She acknowledges the WHO definition of health, a state of complete physical, mental, and social well-being not merely the absence of disease or infirmity. She adds the following three elements a high level of overall physical, mental, and social functioning, a general adaptive-maintenance level of daily functioning and the absence of illness. And also health is viewed as subjective state within the persons mind; each person must define a personal state of health.

Environment

One of the variables affects society in today's world. Society provides values. These values are affected by change in the social, cultural, and spiritual arenas. These values affect the perception of the person and can lead to stress.

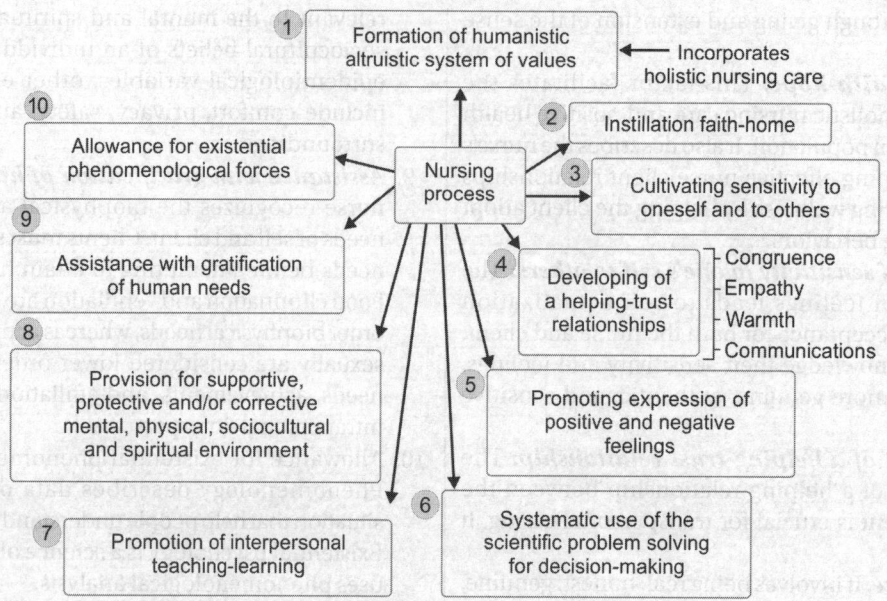

Fig. 39.34: Model of 10 inter-related concepts of Watson's carative factors.

So the practice of caring that nursing can assist in meeting the stress/illness. Such affiliative or affectional needs nursing.

Nursing

Nursing is concerned with promoting and restoring health, preventing illness, and caring for the sick uses the caring process to help a client achieve a high degree of self-harmony to promote self-knowledge, self-healing, or insight into the meaning of life. She sees nurse moving educationally in the two areas of stress and developmental conflicts to provide holistic health care. It combines the research process with the problem-solving approach, enabling a nurse to draw from a database and basic nursing principles to make nursing judgments and decisions.

Logical Form

The framework is presented in a logical form. It contains broad ideas and addresses many situations on the health illness continuum.

Acceptance by the Nursing Community

Practice

- Institutions seeking a holistic approach to nursing care by integrating many aspects of Watson's theory.
- The theory is being clinically validated in a variety of settings and with various populations, for example, nursing journals, articles for reference have incorporated the importance of Watson's theory of caring as an essential domain of nursing.

Education

- Watson has been active in curriculum planning at the University of Colorado. Her framework is being thought in numerous baccalaureates nursing curriculum.

- A study of Watson's framework helped the reader through a thought provoking experience by emphasizing communication skills, use of self-transpersonal growth, attention to both nurse and patient and the human caring process that potentiates and healing.
- Nationally and internationally Watson's work is conducting further testing and implementation of caring into education, research, and clinical practice.

Research

- The abstract framework of Watson is difficult to study concretely. She believes that the essential qualities and subject matter of nursing and the methods used for research.
- Watson hopes that nursing research will incorporate and explore esthetic, metaphysical, empirical, and contextual methodologies.
- Research and practice must focus on both subjective and objective patient outcomes in determining whether caring is the essence of nursing. The development of behaviors and predictors of change is critical for further development of work.

Critique

Clarity

Watson's theory is easily read and uses nontechnical language that provides clarity. The reader's comprehension of her theory is enhanced by an understanding of philosophy.

Simplicity

Watson draws a number of disciplines to formulate her theory. The readers must have an understanding of a variety of subject matters to understand the theory as it is presented.

It is seen as complex when considering the existential-phenomenological nature of her work.

Generality

The theory seeks to provide a moral and philosophical basis for nursing. The scope of the framework encompasses all aspects of the health-illness continuum. In addition the theory addresses aspects of preventing illness and experiencing a peaceful death, thereby increasing generality. The carative factors, described by Watson, have provided important ever, some critics have stated that, the generality is limited due to the emphasis placed on the psychological aspects rather than on physiological aspects of caring.

Empirical Precision

Although the framework is difficult to study empirically, Watson draws heavily on widely accepted work from other disciplines. This solid foundation strengthens her views. Watson describes her theory as descriptive. She acknowledges the newness of the theory. She welcomes input by the others as she continues to develop her theory. The theory does not lend itself to research conducted using traditional scientific methodologies. In her second book, Watson addresses the issue of methodology, nursing as a human science and art can be classified as qualitative, naturalistic, and phenomenological.

Derivable Consequences

Although, further testing is necessary, Watson's theory continues to provide a useful and important metaphysical orientation for the delivery of nursing care. Watson theoretical concepts such as use of self, client identified needs, the caring process and the spiritual sense of human being may help the nurse and their clients find meaning and harmony in a period of increasing complexity.

Application of Watson's Concepts in the Nursing Process

Assessment

Situation: A 14-year-old boy had a slender, almost cachectic appearance. His weight is 38.50 kg and 38.56 inch in height. Both parents were deeply concerned about his weight loss of almost 13.5 kg and were upset by daily battles related to eating. He was equally upset. He was admitted to an adolescent psychiatric unit where the family's problem could be addressed.

On assessment:

- Observed and collected history that he does not have appropriate. Weight to his height, he is not consuming adequate calories in daily menu.
- 24 h diet recall done.
- Physical examination ruled out thin body, skin appeared dry and flank, his bones were clearly visible, no flesh covering his body, and he was restless.
- His food habits were not appropriate.
- Having disinterest in eating.
- His societal and interpersonal relationships are altered that peers are not maintaining good relationship that not accomplishing goals.
- Environmental factors.
- Psychosocial relationships with peers, is starvation retarded to puberty.

Nursing Diagnosis

Disturbance in self-concept related to body image disturbance, powerlessness, impaired social interaction, unresolved independence is dependence.

Planning and implementation by using carative factors of Watson established:

- A caring environment through empathetic understanding.
- Developing a good interpersonal relationship by an encouraging expression—feeling of fear, weight gain, and anger at treatment plan.
- Use warmth, empathy, and congruence to establish open communication.
- Promote interpersonal teaching–learning by involving patient in nutrition plan.
- Teach patient how to deal with conflict, facilitate relationships within the family.
- Encourage identification of stress factors.
- Assist in dealing with sexual identity.
- Encourage patient to assess a social interactions and develop personal stratification.

Evaluation

A patient developing normally in areas of biophysical, psychosocial and interpersonal relationships learned the skills necessary to grow and mature successfully.

Conclusion

Watson provides many useful concepts for the practice of the nursing. She combines many other theories commonly use in the nursing education and this will be helpful to practice nurse or nursing. She is given description of the 10 carative factors can give giddiness to those who wish to employ them in practice or research. Watson's theory can add a dimension to nursing practice that is satisfying and challenging.

PARSE'S HUMAN BECOMING THEORY

Rosemarie Rizzo Parse

Background of Theorist/Introduction

The unfolding of Rosemarie Rizzo Parse's man living health theory is inspectable from the lesser and greater situations that comprise her life. The idea for man living health, Parse recalled began many years ago. When I began to wonder and wander and ask why not? Primarily, through my lived experience in nursing:

- Received her nursing education in Pittsburg.
- Her Master's and Doctorate in Nursing and higher education work earned at the University of Pittsburg.

Major Assumptions

In 1992, using Parse's language revision, the original nine assumptions changed as four assumptions concerning humans and five assumptions concerning are given in Table 39.6.
- She was dean of the school of nursing at Duquesne University in Pittsburg and she developed theory in 1981, a theory for nursing.
- She was motivated to develop her theory from her life experiences and interactions with other.
- Theory defines nursing as a human science rather than one founded in the natural sciences.
- Theory was renamed in 1990 and in 1992, she rephrased her ideas by changing her terminology:
  - The "human" was substituted for "man."
  - "Universe" was substituted for environment.
  - "Becoming" was substituted for "health."

Theoretical Sources

- Major reason of her theory is regarded as unique for nursing by synthesizing the science unitary human beings, as developed by Martha E Rogers, and existential phenomenological thought as articulated by Martin Heidegger, Jean Paul, etc.
- Parse challenges the traditional view of nursing as an emerging natural science.

Use of Empirical Evidence

Nursing does not have practice and research traditions of its own, observed quantitative and qualitative methods of research used to enhance nursing science presently flow from the natural sciences, as a the human science. To enhance her theory using descriptive research methodologies she borrowed human sciences to prove her theory.

Table 39.6: Major assumptions of Parse's theory.

Human	Becoming
The human is coexisting while coconstituting rhythmical patterns with the universe	Becoming is an open process experienced by the human
The human is an open being, freely choosing meaning in situation, bearing responsibilities for decisions	Becoming is a rhythmically coconstituting process of the human universe inter-relationships
The human is a living unity continuously coconstituting patterns of relating	Becoming is the humans pattern of relating value priorities
The human is transcending multidimensionally with the possibles	Becoming is an intersubjective process of transcending with the possibles
	Becoming is human unfolding

Major Concepts and Definitions

From the assumptions of her theory, she drew three thematic elements. She then deduced the three principles of man living health (Fig. 39.35).

Principles of Parse

- **Principle 1:** Structuring meaning multidimensionally cocreating reality through the language of valuing and imaging. The essential concepts of this principle are imaging, valuing, and language.
  - **Meaning:** The thematic element of Parse's first principle "arises from man's inter-relationship with the old. It refers to the both ultimate the meaning moments of everyday life."
  - **Imaging:** The meaning moments of everyday life are those common happenings to which one attaches varying degrees of significance. One does so through the process of imaging. "The cocreating of reality that, by its very nature, structures the meaning of an experience."
  - **Valuing:** "Is man's process of confirming cherished beliefs and is reflective of one's old view. This confirming of beliefs is choosing from imaged options and owing the choices."
  - **Language:** It is expressing valued images of all modes self-presentation including the rhythmical patterns of speech and moment it reflects out the cultural heritage.
- **Principle 2:** Cocreating rhythmical patterns of relating is living the paradoxical unity of revealing-concealing, enabling-limiting, while connecting-separating.
  - **Revealing-concealing:** "It is the simultaneous of disclosing some aspects of self and hiding of others."

Principle 1: Structuring meaning multidimensionally is cocreating reality through the languaging of valuing and imaging

Principle 2: Cocreating rhythmical patterns of relating is living the paradoxical unity of revealing-concealing and enabling-limiting, while connecting-separating

Principle 3: Cotranscending with the possible is powering unique ways of originating in the process of transforming

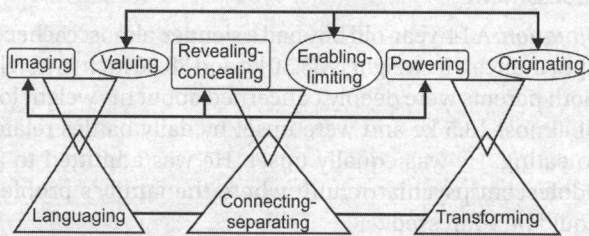

Relationship of the concepts in the squares: Powering is a way of revealing and concealing imaging
Relationship of the concepts in the ovals: Originating is a manifestation of enabling and limiting values
Relationship of the concepts in the triangles: Transforming unfolds in the languaging of connecting and separating

Fig. 39.35: Relationship of principles, concepts, theoretical structures of the theory of human caring.

- > *Enabling-limiting:* "Man cannot be all possibilities of ones and in choosing, one is both enabled and limited."
- > *Connecting-separating:* "It can be recognized as man is connecting with one phenomenon and simultaneously separating from others. In separating from one phenomenon and dwelling with another, a person integrates thought, become more complex and six new unions."
- ❖ **Principle 3:** Cotranscending with the possible is powering unique ways of originating in the process of transforming. The essential concepts of this principle are powering, originating, and transforming.
  - > *Cotranscendance:* The thematic element of third principle "is the process of reaching put beyond self to the not yet."
- ❖ **Powering:** "It is the continuous rhythmical process in carnating one's intentions and actions in moving toward the possibilities." "Powering ways of originating is man distinguishing self from others."
- ❖ **Originating:** Man originates in mutual energy interchange with the environment.
- ❖ **Transforming:** It is man moving toward greater diversity through living new imaged possibilities and transcending present. Transforming as Parse calls transforming "is the changing of change, coconstituting a new in a deliberate way."

Parse's Theory and Nursing Metaparadigm

- ❖ **Person:** It is referred to as "the human" is viewed as an open being who is more than and different from the sum of the parts can choose from option and bears the responsibility for choices. Is in constant, mutual, simultaneous interaction with the environment. Coparticipates with the universe in creating and recognized by these patterns, for example, reaction to the environmental lead to specific values and behaviors.
- ❖ **Environment:** It is referred to as "universe" is inseparable from complementary to and evolving together with the human. Is everything in the person and in the person's experiences constantly interchanges energy with the human as a means of working together toward increasing complexity and diversity.
- ❖ **Health:** It is referred to as "becoming" is an open process of being and becoming experienced by man involves a synthesis of values. Health is rhythmical process resulting from the inter-relationship of the human and universe. It is viewed as a living experience.
- ❖ **Nursing:** It is a human science and art that uses abstract body of knowledge to serve people is responsible for guiding individuals and families in choosing possibilities for changing the health process. Involves innovation and creativity unencumbered by prescriptive rules focuses on the quality of the client's life from the client's perspective; Parse describes the client, not the nurse, as the authority figure and decision maker. Consist of illuminating meaning, synchronizing rhythms, and mobilizing transcendence (dreaming of possibilities and planning to reach them).

Theoretical Assertions

In 1987, the Parse expresses her theoretical structure as practice propositions at the next lower level of abstraction:
- ❖ The first theoretical structure can be stated as struggling to live goals discloses the significance of the situation.
- ❖ The second as creating a new shows ones cherished beliefs and leads in a directional moment.
- ❖ Third as changing views emerging, speaking, and moving with others.
- ❖ She also gives caution that the details of nursing practice is only be specified in the context of particular nurse-person and nurse-group situations.

Logical Form

The inductive-deductive process was central to the creation of man living health. She deductively crafted major components from Roger's science unitary human beings and existential phenomenological thought. Each assumption inter-relates three foundational concepts, each principle as three of Man's livings health's concepts and each theoretical structure a concept from each principle.

Acceptance by the Nursing Community

Practice

- ❖ Parse discussed in detail a family situation and its implications from the perspective of her theory.
- ❖ Mitchell used Parse's theory to guide, care for an elderly woman.
- ❖ Butler used theory to change the health situation of a family facing the loss of it central figure following major neurosurgery.

Education

- ❖ Parse writes for graduate students in nursing, faculty in schools of nursing and nursing administrators in university and major healthcare settings.
- ❖ Parse's theory adopted by masters and doctoral students of nursing to conduct much of the research needed to develop her theory further and will also use her model for curriculum development.
- ❖ She outlines in detail the process base curriculum, including course descriptions and sequencing.

Research

- ❖ Passe's theory and nursing metaparadigm has been validated by six research studies using qualitative methodologies, descriptive, phenomenological, and ethnographic.

- A number of master's theses and doctoral dissertations have been completed and written using Parse's theory.

Further Development
Anticipate the man's living health and continuing evolution. Ongoing research is expected to refine concepts, clarify and lead to higher levels of theory development.

Critique
This theory is an abstract and complex not a model, because its concepts and inter-relationships have received empirical validation.

- *Simplicity:* Parse's use of quotations and references in man living—a theory of nursing rounded out the concepts and rendered them more understandable. An example of Parse's theory was clear and simple. It has the potential to describe, explain, and predict.
- *Generality:* Conceptualization is broad in scope and applicable to individuals, families, communities in change, or crises. It addresses the lived experience of health and at the cutting edge of healthcare.
- *Empirical precision:* Parse's defines man living health's concepts denotatively and at the philosophical level of discourse. Although the concepts are highly abstract and theoretical and they can be observed in situations encountered daily. Linking it and research and practice better understand how man chooses and bears responsibility to the rhythmical patterns of personal health.
- *Derivable consequences:* Parse applied nursing and human sciences and emphasized on human participation. The responsibility of health is timely and this model provides new hope that will be a greater focus in futuristic meaning and quality of life and health that transcends the disease orientation. This theory developed middle range testable theory and most importantly by convincing nurses to replace the scientific method with the humanistic method.

Conclusion
The three elements of Parse's Theory of Human Becoming: (1) meaning, (2) rhythmicity, and (3) co-transcendence. The human (man) and the universe (environment) are viewed as inseparable and in continuous, simultaneous, and mutual interaction with each other. Parse has given great contribution by developing this theory.

CHAPTER 40: A Health Belief Model

CHAPTER OUTLINE
- Health Belief Model [Becker and Maiman's (1975)]
- Advantages

INTRODUCTION

The health belief model was developed to provide a framework for understanding why some people take specific actions to avoid illness, whereas others fail to protect themselves.

The model was designed to predict to use preventive measures and to suggest interventions that might reduce client reluctance to access healthcare. In addition, cues to action such as mass media campaigns, advice from others, reminder postcards from healthcare providers, illnesses of family members or friends, and newspaper or magazine articles may help motivate clients to take action (Salazar, 1991).

Salazar designed three major components and similar to the model presented by Becker.
1. Individual perceptions
2. Modifying factors
3. Variables affecting likelihood of action

Assess the factors which influence the person's behavior. This model provides organized assessment of data about client's abilities and motivation to change their health status. Health education programs can be planned better to meet the needs of the clients.

HEALTH BELIEF MODEL [BECKER AND MAIMAN'S (1975)]

The Health Belief Model by Becker and Maiman's (1975) address the relationship between a person's belief and behaviors. It is a way of understanding and predicting how clients will behave in relation to their health and how they will comply with healthcare therapies (Fig. 40.1). The model is divided into three major components.

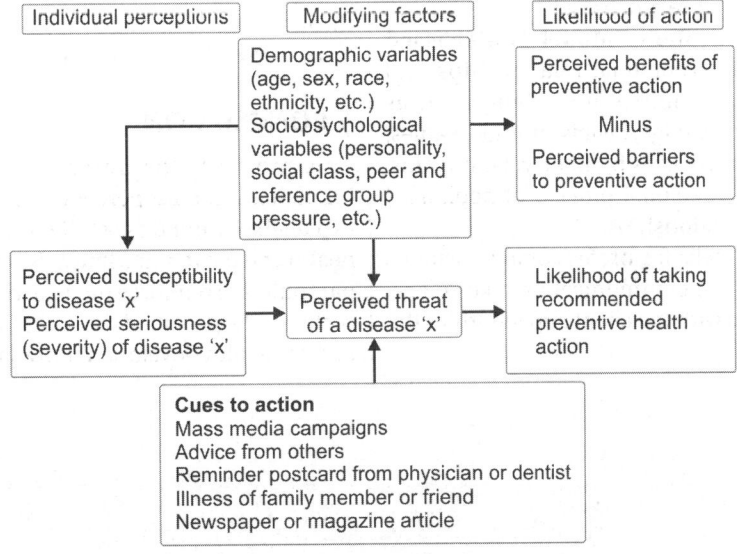

Fig. 40.1: Health belief model.
Source: Modified from Becker MH, Maiman LA. Med Care. 1975;13(1):12.

The first component of this model involves individual perceptions or view susceptibility and seriousness of disease combined to form his or her perceived threat of an illness, e.g. a client needs to recognize the family link for coronary artery disease particularly when one parent and two siblings have died in their fourth decade from myocardial infarction, the client may perceive the personal risk of heart disease.

Second component is the individual's perception of seriousness of illness. This perception is influenced by demographic variables such as age, sex, race and ethnicity as well as personality and pressure from a reference group and cases of action, e.g. mass media campaigned and advice from family friends and medical professionals.

The third component—variables affecting the likelihood of action. The person will take any action influenced by the perceived benefits of action weighed against the barriers of taking action. Preventive actions include, e.g. lifestyle changes, increased adherence to medical therapies, or a search for medical advice or treatment. A client's perception of susceptibility to disease, as well as his/her perception of seriousness (severity) of disease of an illness, helps to determine the likelihood whether the client will or will not take part in healthy behaviors.

ADVANTAGES

- It is useful in health protecting or disease preventing behavior.
- It is useful in organizing information about client's view of their state of health and what factors would influence them to change their behavior.
- Can be used to determine their perceptions, risk of the disease, their knowledge of the disease, and their views of what might benefit or prevent from it.

Application of Health Belief Model is discussed in Peplau's theory of interpersonal relationships and communication process as nurse and client meet as strangers with different knowledge, beliefs, attitude, values, and experience and the nurse tries build up relationships. Through therapeutic interpersonal process of peplau's 4 phases of nurse-patient relationships.

1. **Orientation:** Patient seeks for professional assistance and reciprocal process of communication takes place. Nurse collects the data with the client and identifies the problems/needs.

Table 40.1: The three major components of the Health Belief Model.

Individual perceptions	Modifying factors	Variables affecting the likelihood of initiating actions
Person *beliefs* about his or her own susceptibility to disease **PLUS** The *seriousness* with which he or she views the disease **EQUALS** The perceived of an illness for each person **From Salazar MK:** *AAOHN J*, 39(3):128–35, 1991.	Demographic **Variables** Age Gender Race Ethnicity **Socio-psychological variables** Personality Social class Peer pressure **Structural variables** Knowledge about the disease Prior contact with the disease	Person's *perceived benefits* of action **MINUS** His or her *perceived barriers* to accomplish action **EQUALS** The *likelihood* that person will take action to change his or her behaviors

2. **Identification:** Both must clarify with different needs and perceptions and prepares a plan to meet the needs by mutually set goals.
3. **Exploitation:** New goals to be achieved through personal effort, shifts from nurse-patient delay in gratification. Plans initiated and implementation of care is achieved. Nurse-patient maintains attitude of acceptance, concern and trust. The nurse explore feelings, thought, emotions and behavior. Providing non-judgemental atmosphere and a therapeutic emotional climate.
4. **Resolution:** Collaborative effort between patient and nurse based on mutually established, expected behavior may lead to termination of relationships or initiation of new plans.

Different nursing roles that emerge during the interpersonal process in which problems are solved through role of stranger, resource person, teaching role, leadership role, surrogate and counselor role.

CONCLUSION

This model helps nurses to understand the factors influencing clients' perceptions, beliefs, and behavior and to plan the care and assist clients in maintaining or restoring health and preventing illness. Researchers used educational pamphlets to reinforce preventive health behaviors. Results of the study identified that subjects who perceived a threat to their health developed more preventive behaviors.

CHAPTER 41: Concept of Self-health

CHAPTER OUTLINE

- Self-care in Health
  - Components of Self-care
- Nurses' Role in Self-care Health of People
  - Self-concept
- Components of Self-concept
- Stressors Affecting Self-concept
- Nurses Role

INTRODUCTION

Health is a major public concern. It thus involves the joint efforts of the whole social fabric through the individual, the community, and the state to protect and promote health. Although health is now recognized as a fundamental human right, it is essentially an individual responsibility. It is not a commodity that one individual can bestow on another. No community or state program of health services can give health. In a large measure, it has to be earned and maintained by the individual himself, who must accept a broad spectrum of responsibilities, now known as "self-care."

DEFINITIONS

A recent trend in healthcare is "self-care." It is defined as those health-generating activities that are undertaken by the persons themselves. According to Dorothea E Orem, self-care is "the practice of activities that individuals personally initiate and perform on their own behalf in maintaining life, health, and well-being." It can also be defined as "the process of taking responsibility for developing one's own health potential."

SELF-CARE IN HEALTH

Self-care refers to those activities individuals undertake in promoting their own health, preventing their own disease, limiting their own illness, and restoring their own health. These activities are undertaken without professional assistance, although individuals are informed by technical knowledge and skills. The genetic attribute of self-care is its nonprofessional, non-bureaucratic, non-industrial character, its natural place in social life.

Components of Self-care

- ❖ Comprises observance of simple rules of behavior:
  - ➢ Relating to diet, sleep, exercise, weight, alcohol, smoking, and drugs.
  - ➢ Others include attention to personal hygiene, cultivation of healthful habits and lifestyle.
  - ➢ Submitting themselves to selective medical examinations and screening; accepting immunization and carrying out other specific disease prevention measures.
  - ➢ Reporting early when sick and accepting treatment, undertaking measures for the prevention of relapse or of the spread of the disease to others.
  - ➢ Family planning is added which is essentially an individual's responsibility.
- ❖ Shift in disease patterns from acute to chronic disease makes self-care both a logical necessity and an appropriate strategy. For example, by teaching patients self-care (e.g. recording one's own blood pressure, examination of urine for sugar), the burden on the official health services would be considerably reduced. In other words, health must begin with the individual.
- ❖ Self-care with regard to primary health care: The concept of self-care is proposed as a theory to help healthcare provider how individuals may mobilize their resources for health and well-being.

The goal of primary healthcare to protect, promote, and restore people health requires partnership effort. Just as learning cannot take place in schools without student participation, the goal of primary healthcare cannot be realized without consumer participation. Consumer's involvement in decision-making about healthcare encourages individuals to take responsibility of their own health not just of health professionals.

Some examples of self-care activities at the aggregate levels include community building, safe playgrounds, developing team employment opportunities and providing senior exercise programs.

NURSES' ROLE IN SELF-CARE HEALTH OF PEOPLE

- When people's ability to continue self-care activities drop below their need, they experience a self-care deficit. At this point, nursing may appropriately intervene. However, nursing's goal is to assist clients to return to or reach a level of functioning where they can attain optimal health and assume responsibility for maintaining it.
- Nurses can encourage people to negotiate healthcare goals and practices, develop their own programs; contact their own resources such as support groups or transportation services.
- Identify and implement life-style changes that promote wellness and learn ways to monitor their own health. Client participation is promoted when people serve as partners in the healthcare team.
- The aim of nursing is to collaborate with people rather than to do things for them. As consumers of health services are treated with respect and trust and as a result, gain confidence and skill in self-care, promoting their own health and that of their community.

Self-concept

Self-concept is the aggregate of beliefs and feelings one hold about one self. It is derived from past experiences and interaction with their parents and teachers.

Development of Self-concept

Development and maintenance of self-concept is very important in every individual ace to Erikson's theories of society and environment the influences on the development of self-concept.

Example: During child is illness due to shame she/he may not express the needs.

Components of Self-concept

The self-concept starts developing from birth onwards and continues throughout life. The components are:
1. **Body image or physical self:** It is an individual perception of the shape, size, and mass of her/his body plus psychological experiences of his/her body including feelings and attitudes. Physical and psychological changes occur in adolescence and old age.
2. **Self esteem:** It is closely related to self-concept. Self-esteem is an individual's sense of self-worth, self-acceptances, and one's feeling of personal value. It is developed from others, i.e. in school, working place, and within family.

   Those who are unable to meet self-expectation feel worthless and self-esteem is lowered. Low self-esteem can cause problems like depression.
3. **Role:** Performance is another component of self-esteem. A role is a set of behavior by which a person participates in any social group. Each individual may have many roles.

   For example, a woman may be a mother, wife, and a daughter and she behaves to these roles differently as set of ways and accepted by society.
4. **Identity:** It is also one of the components of self-concept. Identify involves the persistent individuality and sameness of a person overtime and a various circumstances. Ace to Erikson fifth stage of development identity V/s role confusion. A person with a sense of identity will feel integrated rather than diffuse. Self-concept strengthens the sense of identity. If a person behaves in ways that contradict self-concept, she/he experiences anxiety and apprehension.

Stressors Affecting Self-concept

Stressor is a factor; with bring change whether real or perceived response to stressors will depend upon the perception of a stress, which can evoke responses like anxiety, frustration, or mobility to adjust. Hospitalization, illness, and surgery are common stressors. Any of the components of self-concept body image, self-esteem, role and identity may also be affected.

Nurses Role

While planning nursing care, we need to assess the patients altered components of self-concept and its stressors in order to help the patient improve his self-awareness, body image, and self-worth, to formulate realistic goals to adjust new role and to develop coping methods to adapt to changes in body image and role.

CONCLUSION

Development of self-concept has a lot of impact on the development of self-health in later stages of life. We can apply or relate Myra Levine's concepts on conservation of energy, structural integrity, personal integrity, and conservation of social integrity to self-concept, when he maintains above factors body's integrity can be balanced and nurse's role is to promote and help them to maintain positive self-health activities.

CHAPTER 42

Evidence-based Practice Model

CHAPTER OUTLINE

- Features of Evidence-based Practice
- Purposes
- Barriers in Evidence-based Practice
- Types of Evidence and Evidence Hierarchies
- Strategies and Steps for Individual Clinicians

INTRODUCTION

Evidence-based practices (EBPs) have been revolved from the time of Florence Nightingale in nursing. Her concepts of promoting health, prevention of disease, and care of the sick are central components of her system, as well as demonstrated in her theory. EBP is a current trend in all fields and most commonly practiced today. We need to identify, analyze, and select the most appropriate alternative based on evidence and evaluated through EBP and utilize for research.

DEFINITION

- According to Pioneu David Sachett, "EBP is the integration of best research evidence with claimed expertise and patient values."
- According to Sigma Theta Tau International 2008, "it is the process of shared decision-making between practitioner, patient, and others significant to them based on research evidence, the patient's experiences and preferences, clinical expertise or know-how, and other available robust sources of information."

FEATURES OF EVIDENCE-BASED PRACTICE

- As a clinical problem-solving strategy and that it deemphasizes decisions based on custom, authority, or ritual.
- Identifying the best available research evidence and integrating it with other factors.

PURPOSES

- EBP is an approach in which the profession or other decision makers should make decision.
- Its goal is to eliminate unsound or excessively risky practices in favor of these that have better outcomes.
- EBP has contributed a lot toward better patient outcome.

EXAMPLES OF REAL LIFE SITUATION

If a patient is diagnosed with breast cancer today and were faced with the decision about which type of chemotherapy to close, where healthcare provides want to know the evidence regarding the risks and benefits of each therapeutic agent as generated from prior clinical trials with other similar cancer patients. Hopefully answer will be "yes" therefore, essentially it is important clinical decision-making situations.

BARRIERS IN EVIDENCE-BASED PRACTICE

There are many barriers for promoting EBP. Most barriers fall into three categories:
- Quality and nature of the research.
- Resources and evidences influence decision making.
- Organizational factors.
- A lack of professional ability to critically appraise research.
- Lack of time, work load pressures.
- Practice environment may be resistant to changing triad.
- Implementing based practices into practice due to lack of continuing education.
- Introducing newly learned method for improving treatments or patient's health, e.g. new nurses may feel suggest or even feel to superior about newer and more efficient methods/practices available.
- Lack of knowledge of research methods.

TYPES OF EVIDENCE AND EVIDENCE HIERARCHIES (FIG. 42.1)

- What constitutes usable evidence for EBP. There is broad agreement that findings of rigorous research and what qualifies as "best evidence."
- Randomized controlled trials (RCTs) are in fact, very well suited for drawing conclusions about the effects of healthcare practice.

Various Types of Hierarchies

- Strength of the evidence.
- Systematic reviews of RCTs are traditional narrative integration of research findings.
- Integration from multiple RCT using rigorous, methodical procedures.
- Individual RCT studies.
- Merit for ranking of hierarchy evidence depends on some clinical questions, i.e. effects of clinical intervention, e.g. effect of massage therapy for pain in cancer patients.
- For some hierarchy is not the relevant for ranking evidence, e.g. what is the experience of pain in cancer patients?

Narrative reviews of quantitative studies are still common, but a type of systematic review called meta analysis has emerged as an important EBP tool.

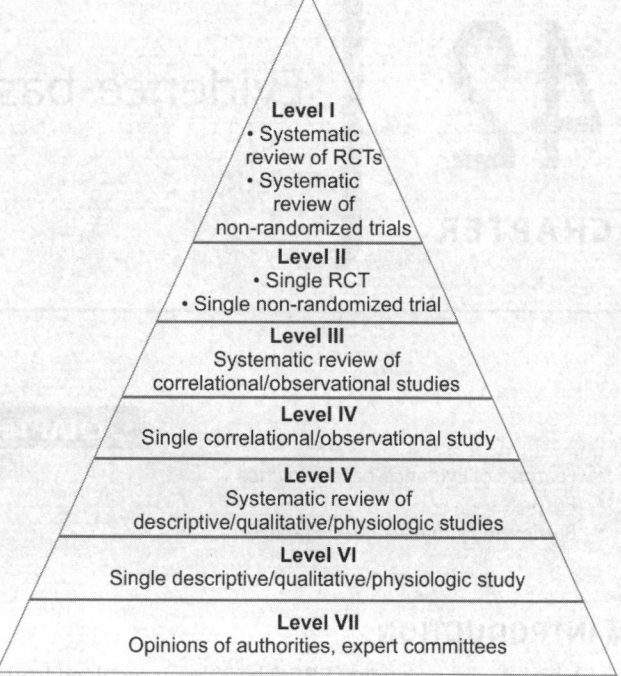

Fig. 42.1: Evidence hierarchy: Levels of evidence regarding the effectiveness of an intervention.

STRATEGIES AND STEPS FOR INDIVIDUAL CLINICIANS

Major steps in EBP include the following (Fig. 42.2):

- ***The first step:*** Formulate a clear question based on clinical problems that can be answered with research evidence. Ideas from different sources but all are categorized in two areas:
  - *Problem-focused triggers:* These are identified by health and staff through quality improvement, risk surveillance, bench marking data, recurrent clinical problems, financial data, and risk management issues.
  - *Knowledge-focused triggers:* This is obtained by reading text materials, listening to scientific papers at research conferences or encounter EBP guidelines published by federal agencies or organizations will guide/phrase clinical questions for quantitative information.

  Acronym used in PICO model is as follows:
  - **P**—the population (characteristics of clients)
  - **I**—the intervention or exposure (what is the potential intervention of interest)
  - **C**—is there a comparison intervention (control group)
  - **O**—the outcome

  For example, pain management, prevention of skin breakdown, brainstorming about ideas, etc.

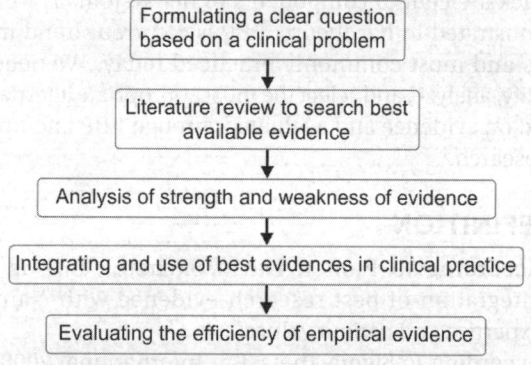

Fig. 42.2: Process of evidenced-based practice.

- ***Searching for and retrieving relevant/best available evidence:*** After selecting a clinical question, the research relevant to the topic must be reviewed of clinical studies, integrative literature reviews, meta analysis, articles, journals, quality of the article theory and clinical. Before reading a critiquing research, it is useful to read about view of nature of the topic and related concepts and then review existing EBP guidelines.

- ***Appraising and synthesizing the evidence:*** Evaluating and analyzing the strengths/weakness of that evidence in terms of validity and generalize ability. Use of rating systems to determine the quality of the research is crucial to the development of EBP. There are several rating systems available in time. The national guideline cleaning course is a database of published EBP guideline abstracts at (http://www.guideline.gov).

Chapter 42: Evidence-based Practice Model

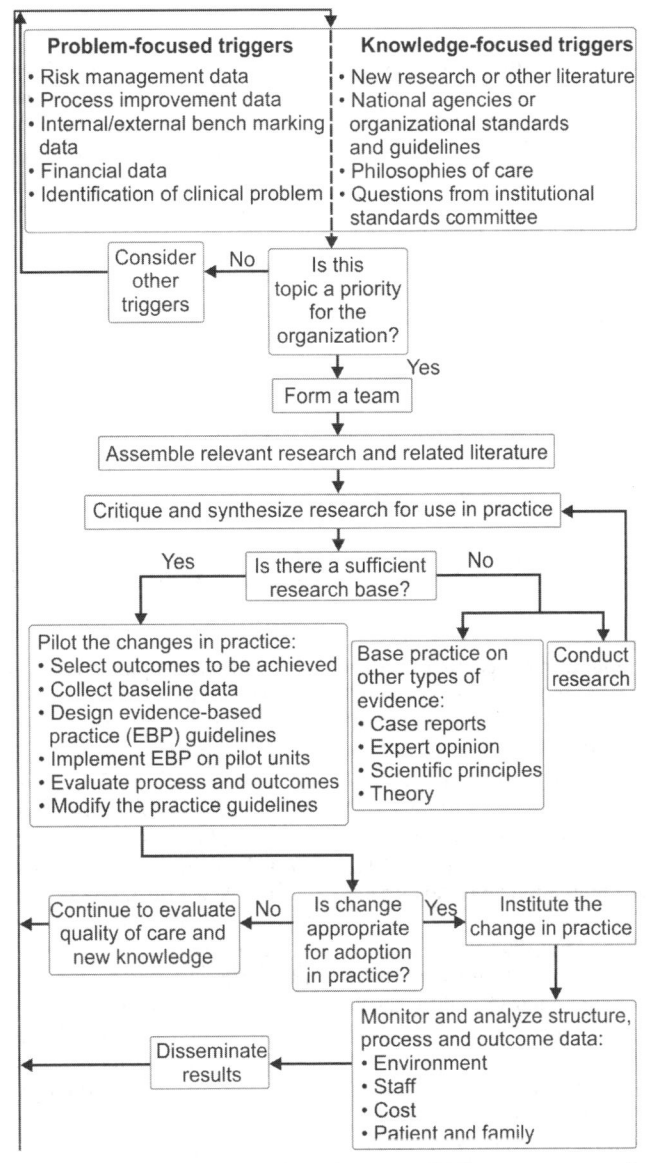

Fig. 42.3: Iowa model of evidence-based practice (EBP) to promote quality care.
Source: Adapted from Titler et al. (2001).

- ❖ ***Implementing useful findings in clinical practice based on valid evidence:*** After determining internal and external validity of the study, a decision is arrived to apply to you research question. It is important to address questions related to diagnosis, therapy, harm, and prognosis. It should be interpreted according to many criteria and should always be shared with other nurses and/or fellow researchers.
- ❖ ***Evaluating efficiency and performance of evidences through a process of self-reflection, audit, and peer assessment:*** After implementation of the useful findings for the clinical practices, efficiency and performance is evaluated through process of self-reflection, internal or external audit, or peer assessment (Fig. 42.3).

CONCLUSION

Evidence-based practice is a newer concept used in claimed research. It is more objective and helps to maintain quality of care in the field of nursing, thousands of EBP projects are undue way in practice settings. Many that have been described in the nursing literatures offer useful information about planning, implementing, and evaluation of the evidences.

SUGGESTED READING

1. Ann Mariner: Tomey. Nursing Theorists and Their Work, 3rd edition. Philadelphia: Mosby Publications.
2. Barbara K, et al. Fundamentals of Nursing Concepts, Process and Practice, 5th edition. Addison, Wesley Publishing Company; 1995.
3. Jacqueline F. Analysis and Evaluation of Conceptual Models of Nursing, 3rd edition. Philadelphia: FA Davis Company; 1995.
4. Joyce PFJ, Ann WL. Conceptual Models of Nursing—Analysis and Applications, Practice. Hall Publishing Co.
5. Julia GB. Nursing Theories, 4th edition. Appleton and Large Publishers, Connect Cut. pp. 229-46.
6. Marilyn PC. Nursing Theories and Nursing Practice. Philadelphia. FA Davis Company.
7. Peggy CL, Maeona KK. Theory and Nursing: A Systematic Approach, 3rd edition. Mosby Year Book; 1991.
8. Perry Potter. Concepts and Practice of Fundamentals of Nursing, 3rd edition. Philadelphia: Mosby Year Book; 1993.
9. Sandra MR, Susan JR, Arlene SM. Nursing Care of Children and Families, 2nd edition, Addison-Wesley Nursing; 1900.
10. Stanhope-Lancaster, Community Public Health Nursing, 5th edition. Mosby Year Book; 2000.

Journal

1. Barret AME. The Theoritical Matrix for Rogerian Nursing Practice 2000, Theoria. Journal of Nursing Theory. Copyright by the Swedish Society of Nursing Theories in Practice, Research and Education.
2. Dhasaradhan Indirani. The Nursing Journal of India, Vol. LXXXXII, Oct 2001.

REVIEW OF SECTION BASED QUESTIONS OF RGUHS

Long Essays

1. Discuss the uses and development of conceptual models in nursing? Explain any one conceptual model in detail? (October 2010)
2. Discuss the humanistic nursing theories and compare the various theories and their relevance to clinical practice? (May 2011)
3. List down the humanistic theories in nursing explain any one in detail. (Nov 2012)
4. Explain the application of Roy's adaptation model to nursing practice with an example? (May 2007, April 2008 and Nov 2012)
5. Discuss the nursing management of a client with myocardial infarction applying Roy's adaptation theory? (May 2010)
6. List five nursing theories? Describe interpersonal theory and its application in adult nursing? (2007)
7. Identify the essential elements of nursing theory? Discuss any one theory and its application in nursing. (2006)
8. Explain the application of Henderson's theory to nursing practice with an example.
9. Explain the application of Roger's theory to nursing practice with an example.
10. Explain the application of Peplau's theory to nursing practice with an example.
11. Explain the application of Abdellah's theory to nursing practice with an example.
12. Explain the application of Orem's theory to nursing practice with an example. (May 2009)
13. Explain the application of Bettyneuman's theory to nursing practice with an example.
14. How to apply evidence based practice model?
15. a. List down the purposes of theories in nursing?
    b. Explain interpersonal theory in detail. (May 2012)
16. a. Explain essential concepts of theory.
    b. Discuss need theory. (May 2012)
17. Identify the criteria necessary for theory? Explain system theory in detail. (May 2011)
18. List five nursing theories? Describe interpersonal theory and its application in adult nursing. (2007)
19. Describe the level of preventive care with reference to Bettyneuman's model. (2000)
20. a. Explain levels of theory?
    b. Write in detail about Abdellah's Typology of nursing problems?
21. Explain the role of adaptation theories in nursing with emphasis on Roy's adaptation model. Give suitable examples. (October 2016)
22. Classify theories? Explain Roy's Adaptation in detail.

Short Essays

1. Health belief model. (May 2010)
2. Health-illness spectrum. (Nov 2012)
3. New trends in theory development in nursing. (Oct 2010)
4. Concepts of self health. (May 2011)
5. Theories of communication.
6. Values and approaches to theories of nursing.
7. Importance of conceptual models in nursing.

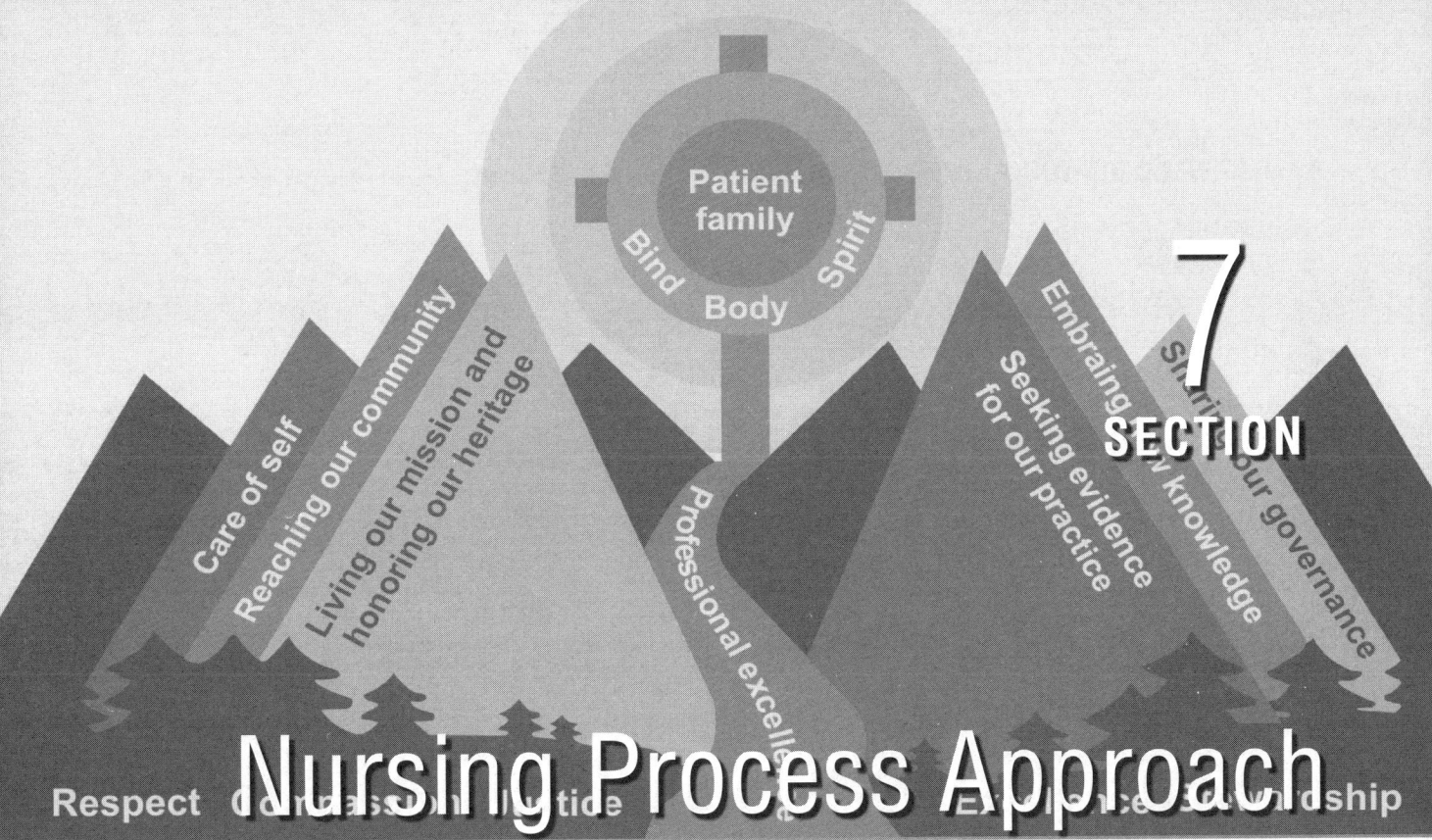

SECTION 7: Nursing Process Approach

Section Outline

43. Health Assessment
44. Methods of Collection, Analysis and Utilization of Data Relevant to Nursing Process
45. Nursing Diagnosis
46. Planning
47. Formulation of Nursing Care Plans, Health Goals, Implementation, Modification, and Evaluation of Care
48. Theory Application in Nursing Process

CHAPTER 43

Health Assessment

CHAPTER OUTLINE

- Equipment Needed
- Techniques
- Psychological Consequences of Illness
  - Illness Behavior

INTRODUCTION

Physical assessment is a component of the first of nursing process. The physical examination is performed in a systematic manner, such as in a head-to-toe manner. Physical assessment is the key means of collecting baseline data and establishing a need for continued focused assessment. The main purpose of physical examination is to identify normal and deviations from normal. Physical assessment offers opportunity for health teaching, for example, breast and testicular self-examination. Accurate assessment requires knowledge of body structure and function (anatomy and physiology) as well as pathologic changes or abnormalities.

DEFINITION

Physical examination is the investigation of the body to determine its state of health using any or all of the techniques for inspection, palpation percussion, auscultation.

EQUIPMENT NEEDED

Instrument needed for the physical examinations are:
- ❖ *Stethoscope:* An instrument with two earpieces connected by flexible tubing to a cone or bell used to listen to and amplify sounds produced by internal organs, e.g. lungs, heart, and intestine.
- ❖ *Otoscope:* It is used to examine the external ear canal and eardrum.
- ❖ *Speculums:* Instruments used to distend or open a body orifice or cavity, permitting visual inspection of the interior, e.g. nasal speculum and vaginal speculum.
- ❖ *Tuning fork:* An instrument to test air and bone conduction, auditory nerve function, and vibration sensation.
- ❖ *Percussion hammer (reflex hammer):* It is an instrument used to test superficial, deep tendon, and pathologic reflexes.
- ❖ *Snellen chart:* It is a chart used to test a person's visual acquity.
- ❖ *Tongue depressor:* A wooden stick used to aid in viewing the pharynx and stimulating the gag reflex.
- ❖ *Safety pins and cotton swabs:* Used to test a person's ability to differentiate dull and sharp pain and sensitivities to touch.
- ❖ *Penlight:* An instrument used to illuminate areas for better viewing and to test pupil constriction.
- ❖ *Sphygmomanometer:* Used to measure blood pressure.
- ❖ *Thermometer:* Used to check the temperature.
- ❖ *Weighing machine:* To check the weight.
- ❖ *Inch tape:* To check the height, head circumference.

TECHNIQUES

Inspection, palpation, percussion, and auscultation are the basic techniques used in physical assessment. The usual sequence of assessment activities is to:
- ❖ Look (inspect)
- ❖ Feel (palpate)
- ❖ Tap or thump (percuss)
- ❖ Listen (auscultate)

This sequence is not used to assess the abdomen. The sequence is inspection, auscultation, percussion, and palpation. Palpation is performed last, because feeling a sensitive abdomen may produce additional symptoms, e.g. suppress early bowel sounds trigger painful spasms.

Inspection

It is an assessment technique in which the examiner observes the body surface. Observe events (e.g. movements), colors, contours, and symmetry or asymmetry.

Good lighting and adequate exposure of the appropriate area facilitate proper inspection.

Palpation

Palpation is an assessment technique in which the examiner feels with his/her fingers and one or both hands. The degree of pressure applied during palpation varies depending on, e.g. the tenderness of the area and the depth of palpation required. Light or deep palpation is used when palpating abdomen. Palpation is difficult to do in people who are anxious or tense, experiencing physical discomfort, obese, or ticklish. During palpation, encourage the person to report feelings of discomfort (e.g. pressure, fullness, tenderness) or pain when you touch.

Purpose of Palpation

- Palpation confirms data gathered by inspection.
- Palpation helps to provide information about structure or function.
- By touching an individual's body with examiners hand can experience various characteristics. For example:
  - Temperature changes.
  - Moisture can feel when stroking the skin.
  - Events (vibrations, such as bruits and voice sounds, crepitus or other movements can be detected by using the fingers and entire palm).
  - Textures can be noted by using fingertips to palpate deep organs such as the kidneys, spleen or liver.
  - Consistencies (hard and soft) are determined with fingertips.
  - Palpation is commonly used to take a pulse and during breast examination.

Percussion

Percussion is an assessment technique in which the examiner taps a body surface with a percussion hammer or the hand or fingers. Percussion assess density (hardness of fullness) can be made from the sound produced by the taping.

Types of Percussion

- ***Direct percussion:*** It is done by the examiner striking the fingers directly against the person's skin.
- ***Indirect percussion:*** The examiner places the terminal phalanx hand of the middle finger of the nondominant firmly against the person's skin and then strikes the phalanx (just behind the finger nailbed) with the end of the middle finger of the dominant hand.

Auscultation

Auscultation is an assessment technique in which the examiner listens to and assess the sound produced by various body organs and tissues such as heart, lung, or bowel.

Sounds of Auscultation

- ***Frequency:*** High pitch, low pitch
- ***Intensity:*** Loud sounds, soft sounds
- ***Quality:*** Difference between two sounds of equal pitch and intensity coming from sources, such as the lungs and bowels
- Duration or length of the sound.

Types of Auscultation

Auscultation can be performed either directly or indirectly.

- ***Direct auscultation:*** It is otherwise known as immediate auscultation. It is less commonly used. The examiner places his/her ear directly against the person's body. This method is limited, because the sounds are too soft, especially with obese people.
- ***Indirect method:*** This is the most common method. It is done with a stethoscope. During auscultation nothing should touch the tubing. Tell the person to remain silent unless following directions from the examiner to speak, cough, or breathe deeply through open mouth.

Promoting Client Comfort during Physical Assessment

- Explain the assessment process to the person.
- Assure the patient that appropriate draping will be provided.
- Before beginning the physical assessment, suggest the person to go to the toilet. This helps the person to relax, facilitates examination of the abdomen, male genitals, vagina, and rectum.
- Keep necessary instruments and equipment assembled, close at hand and ready for use.
- Keep personal exposure to a minimum, expose only the area being exposed.
- Keep the person warm. Elderly, anxious or ill people chill easily. Provide a light weight blanket.
- Examiner's hands should be warm, smooth, and clean.
- Keep fingernails clean, short, and smooth. Wash hands before and after assessment.
- Warm instruments, e.g. warm the bell of a stethoscope by rubbing it between hands before placing it on a person.
- Talk with the person throughout so that activities are not unexpected. I am going to listen to your chest now. Give the person clear instructions. Breathe in and out slowly and deeply through your mouth.
- A relaxed, friendly, yet professional attitude on the examination part help put a person at ease.
- Help the person into required positions.

Conducting the Physical Assessment

When performing the physical assessment, we need to be well organized. Working in head-to-toe manner enables to remember order of the assessment. It is important to compare both sides of the body for symmetry. For example, compare the right upper extremity to the left, the right side of the thorax to the left and the right side of the face to the left side of the face.

Vital Signs

Temperature, pulse, respirations, and blood pressure can be checked at the beginning of the physical assessment or during the examination of specific body systems.

Height and Weight

Height and weight provides data regarding a person's general health and nutritional status. When assessing height, the person should be instructed to remove the shoes. A clean paper towel should be placed on the scale platform. The person is asked to turn and face the direction opposite the balance beam and stand erect on the scale platform. A height measurement rod that is attached to the scale raises up and a level price swings out and over the person's head. Height in inch or centimeter will be displayed at approximately eye level on the measuring rod.

Weight is also assessed, while the person stands on the scale platform. Adjust the weight on the balance beam until the tip of the beam registers in the middle of the mark.

General Appearance and Behavior

Assessment of appearance and behavior begins, while the nurse perhaps the client for the examination. The review of general appearance and behavior includes the following:

- *Gender and race:* Different physical features are related to gender and race. Certains illness are more likely to affect a specific gender or race, e.g. the incidence of skin cancer is 20 times higher in whites than in blacks, and cancer of the bladder is more common in men.
- *Age:* It influences normal physical characteristics. For example, an elderly person may exhibit the normal physiological changes of aging, such as loose, wrinkled skin, kyphosis, and a slowed shift gait.
- *Body type:* Assessment of body type, posture, and gait can provide data related to a person's general level of health. Observe a person's build as thin, average, or obese. Note whether the person assumes an erect or bent posture. Observe the person's style of walking for smoothness and coordination. Posture may reflect mood or presence of pain.
- *Body movements:* Observe whether movements are purposeful and note if there are any tremors involving the extremities. Determine if any body parts are immobile.
- *Hygiene and grooming:* The client's level of cleanliness is noted by observing the appearance of the hair, skin, and fingernails.
- *Dress:* Culture, lifestyle, socioeconomic level, and personal performance affect the type of clothes worn. Depressed or mentally ill persons may be unable to choose proper clothing. An older adult tends to wear extra clothing, because of the sensitivity to cold.
- *Body odor:* An unpleasant body odor may result from physical exercise, poor hygiene, or certain diseases. Poor oral hygiene may cause bad breath.
- *Affect and mood:* Affect is a person's feelings as they appear to others. A person's mood or emotional state is expressed verbally and nonverbally. Note if verbal expressions match nonverbal behavior and observe if the client's mood is appropriate for the situation. For example, the mood is inappropriate if the client seems unusually happy after recently being diagnosed with cancer.
- *Speech:* Normal speech is understandable and moderately paced and shows an association with the person's thoughts. An abnormal pace may be caused by emotions or neurological impairment.

Integumentary System

The integumentary systems serve as a source of protection for the body from the environment, as a body and touch. The layers of the skin tissue are the epidermis, dermis, and subcutaneous tissue. The assessment techniques used with the integumentary system are inspection, palpation, and olfaction. Areas to consider when assessing the skin color, temperature, texture, mobility, lesions, and vascularity.

- *Color:* Inspect the skin for generalized color. Skin color will vary according to body part. A person's race will also affect skin color. Abnormal changes in the skin color include cyanosis, jaundice, and pallor. Cyanosis is a bluish mottled discoloration of the skin, nail beds, and mucous membranes caused by decreased oxygenation of the blood. In persons with darker skin tones, cyanosis may be detected better in palms, soles, palpebral conjunctiva, and nails.
- *Jaundice:* A yellow discoloration of the skin resulting from an increase in bilirubin may be assessed in the bulbar and palpebral conjunctiva, lips, hard palate, and the skin.
- *Pallor:* It is an absence of color in the skin. Pallor is best assessed in the finger nails, lips, mucous membranes, and palpebral conjunctiva.
- *Temperature and moisture:* Skin temperature should remain relatively the same over the entire body. When there is a change in temperature over a body area, it is an indication of a change in blood circulation to that part of the body. Palpation is the technique used in assessing skin temperature. Temperature is assessed using the dorsum or back of the hand. Normally, the skin temperature is warm. Excessive coolness or warmth indicates deviation from normal. Skin moisture is assessed by inspection and palpation. Normally, the skin should be dry to touch with the exception of skin folds and the axilla. Palpate the skin for temperature and moisture.

- **Texture:** The skin's texture should be smooth, soft, and flexible. Some areas such as the palms and the soles possess a thicker texture.

Turgor and Mobility

- **Skin turgor:** It is an indication of hydration status assessed by pinching up the skin and releasing it. It denotes the skin's elasticity. To assess skin turgor, pinch up the skin on the forehead, dorsum of the hand or forearm and release. Note the speed at which the skin returns to its original position quickly. Skin turgor is classified as poor when it takes 3 seconds or longer for the skin to return to its original position. Skin turgor and mobility will be diminished when edema is present.
- **Lesions:** Normally, the skin should be free of lesions. Palpate the lesions to denote mobility (fixed or mobility), contour (flat or raised), and consistency (soft or hard).
- **Vascularity:** Vascularity involves blood circulation of the skin and the appearance of superficial blood vessels. Petechiae minute hemorrhages under the skin and ecchymosis can result from abnormal vascularity. Petechiae are tiny purple or red spots on the skin. Ecchymosis (bruising) is discoloration of an area of the skin. Edema is an accumulation of excessive fluid in the interstitial spaces. As tissue fluid increases, pitting edema will occur.

Head and Neck

- **Head:** When assessing the head, inspect and palpate the hair, scalp, skull, and face.
- **Hair:** Inspect the hair for quality of the hair refers to the texture and color of the hair. Terms used to describe the texture are coarse and fine. A sudden change in dryness, brittleness, or fragility may indicate a bodily dysfunction. An increase in dryness and coarseness of the hair may indicate hypothyroidism. An increase in silkiness and fineness may indicate hyperthyroidism. Observe for nits, which are tiny, white, ovoid eggs of lice. The quantity and distribution of a person's hair will vary with age. Inspect for any area of alopecia (partial or complete loss of hair).
- **Scalp and skull:** Separate the hair and take a thorough look at the skin underlying the hair. Observe for areas of inflammation, cysts, warts, mole, insect bites, flaking, and scaliness. Inspect and palpate the skull for size, shape, symmetry, and tenderness and inspect for dandruff.
- **Face:** Inspect the face for size, shape, symmetry, and any tics or abnormal movements.
- **Eyes:** Areas to be assessed are the position and alignment of the eyes, eyebrows, eyelids, lacrimal apparatus, conjunctiva and sclera and pupils.
  - **Eyebrows:** Inspect the quantity and distribution of the eyebrows. Observe for scarring lesions and hair loss. Hair loss may indicate fungal infection.
  - **Eyelids:** Inspect the eyelids for symmetry, position in relation to the eyeballs, inflammation, lesions (sty), edema, and ptosis (drooping of the eyelid). Inspect the eyelashes, which should be full and extend outward along the entire eyelid. Crusting, scaling, and hair loss are signs of infection.
  - **Lacrimal apparatus:** The puncta are openings located in the inner canthus of the upper and lower eyelid. The major function of this apparatus is to create tears. Tears keep the eyes moist and clean.
  - **Conjunctiva and sclera:** The conjunctiva is a membrane that protects the outer surface of the sclera and the inner surface of the eyelids. Inspect the palpebral conjunctiva and sclera by pulling down the lower lid, while instructing the person to look up. Inspect for lesions, inflammation, and swelling. Palpebral conjunctiva is reddish in color due to tiny blood vessels. Anemia is suspected when the palpebral conjunctiva is pale. When the bulbar conjunctiva is yellow, it is indicative of jaundice.
  - **Pupils:** Inspect the pupils for equality, size, shape, reaction to light and accommodation, normal papillary function is documented as "PERRLA." Pupils equal, round, react to light and accommodation (eyes adaptation for near vision).
    - **Distance visual acuity:** A Snellen's chart is a chart used to test a person's visual acquity.
    - **Near visual acuity:** When testing near visual acuity, a newspaper with various sizes of print may be used.
    - **Color discrimination:** To test color discrimifnation have the person distinguish colors, usually red and green. Observe the lens is free of opacity (cataract) and clouding.

Ears

Inspection and palpation are the techniques used to examine the ear. Areas to be assessed are the external ear (auricle) and ear canal, internal ear canal and tympanic membrane (by performing an otoscopic examination).

- **Auricles:** Inspect the auricle for color, size, location, and angle of attachment to the head. The auricle should be at a level equal to the outer canthus of the eye. Inspect the external ear canal for intactness, general hygiene, a buildup of cerumen (ear wax), discharge, redness, and swelling. The normal ear canal should be clean, dry, free of lesions, and with a minimal amount of cerumen. If discharge is observed, note the color, amount, consistency, and clarity.

Palpate the external ear for nodules and tenderness. The mastoid process is also palpated for tenderness. If the person complains of pain when the auricle is moved up and down, it is an indicative of an external ear infection. If palpation elicits pain in the mastoid process, otitis media is a possibility.

- ❖ **Otoscopic examination:** To inspect the internal ear canal and tympanic membrane, an otoscope must be used. Inspect the internal ear canal for impacted cerumen, foreign bodies, discharge, masses, redness, and swelling. Inspect the tympanic membrane which is usually a shiny pearly gray or light pink. Observe for perforations, abnormal color, bulging or retraction, discharge, fluid or air bubbles behind the tympanic membrane and scars.
- ❖ **Auditory acuity:** Auditory acuity is assessed by the watch and whisper test. The watch test screens high-frequency impairment.
- ❖ **Weber test:** To perform the Weber lateralization test, place the stem of a vibrating tuning fork in the center of the forehead. Ask the person where the sound is heard best. Normally, sound is heard equally well in both ears as it is conducted through the bones. Note any lateralization of sound (sound is heard better in one ear than the other). A person with a unilateral conductive hearing loss will hear the sound best in the impaired ear. This can occur with otitis is heard best in the good ear with a sensorineural hearing loss.
- ❖ **Rinne air and bone conduction test:** The Rinne air and bone conduction test compares bone-conducted sound with air-conducted sound in one ear at a time. Place the stem of the vibrating tuning fork on the mastoid process behind the ear. Quickly move the fork beside the ear canal as soon as the person says the sound is gone from contact with the mastoid bone. Placement beside cars tests air conduction. With a normal (positive) Rinne test sound is heard twice as long by air conduction as by bone conduction.

Nose and Sinuses

The nose is assessed by inspection and palpation. Inspect the external surface of the nose for symmetry in color, shape and size. It is common for one ala nasi to be slightly larger than the other. Inspect the external septum for symmetry and any signs of deviation. Palpate the external nares for tenderness. To assess the potency ask the person to occlude one ala nasi, while breathing through the other.

Nasal cavity: Instruct the person to tilt the head back and then shine the penlight into the nasal cavity. Inspect the mucosa, it should be moist and pink. Note any swelling, lesions, or drainage and also note any pallor, redness, swelling, or polyps. Frontal and maxillary sinuses are palpated for tenderness, swelling, thickening, or secretions. Palpate the frontal sinuses by pressing up on the skull on either side of the nose under the eyebrows. Palpate the maxillary sinuses by pressing up over the lower part of the cheekbones on either side of the nose.

Mouth and Pharynx

The mouth and pharynx are assessed through inspection and palpation. Areas to be assessed include the lips, buccal mucosa, gums and teeth tongue, soft and hard palate, and pharynx.

- ❖ **Lips:** Inspect the lips for symmetry, color, edema, and any surface abnormalities. Palpate the lips for moistness, induration, intactness, and lesions.
- ❖ **Gums and teeth:** Inspect the gums by gently pulling down the lower lip. Repeat the procedure on the upper lips. Normally, the gums are pink in color and free of lesions, inflammation, and bleeding. Palpate the gums for retraction away from the teeth, lesions, and swelling. Inspect teeth for caries, plaque, missing or loose teeth, dentures, and color.
- ❖ **Buccal mucosa:** When inspecting the buccal mucosa, use a tongue blade to displace the cheeks to the side in order to view the mucous membranes with a penlight. Inspect the mucosa for color, pigmentation, ulcers, white patches, and nodules. Normally, the mucosa will be pink, smooth, moist, and free of lesions. In a dark-skinned person, tile mucosa will have patchy brown pigmentation, which is normal.
- ❖ **Tongue:** Note the movement and color of the tongue. Normally, it should be pink, moist, and smooth. Instruct the person to touch the tip of the tongue to the top of the mouth, so that it is easy to examine the floor of the mouth for cyanosis, pallor, and any lesions or nodules. The floor of the mouth is a common site for oral cancer.
- ❖ **Soft and hard palates:** The hard palate is located in the anterior roof of the mouth. It is white or pale pink in color and firm in nature. The hard palate is where jaundice can be readily detected. The soft palate is located posteriorly and is pink in color with a spongy texture. Inspect the hard and soft palate for lesions.

Pharynx

Inspect the posterior wall of the mouth with penlight by asking the person to extend the tongue. A tongue blade is used to press against the person's tongue for better viewing. Normally, it should be pink and free of drainage. The pharynx of a smoker will appear yellowish red with small nodules present. Inspect the tonsils, which are small pink surface growths. Note any enlargement of the tonsils with exudates present. Inspect the uvula, which should be located in the midline. Note any deviation from the midline.

Neck

Inspect the neck for color symmetry, masses, enlargement of the thyroid or lymph nodes, abnormal pulsations, impaired range of motion, lesions, and scars. Instruct the person to move the neck carefully through the entire range of motion, which includes right and left lateral, right and left rotation, flexion, extension, and hyperextension. The neck should move easily without any discomfort. The elderly person may experience some discomfort from neck movement, because of a decrease in range of motion.

Lymph Nodes

Palpate the lymph nodes using the pads of your index and middle fingers. Gently palpate in sequence bilaterally the preauricular, posterior auricular, occipital, tonsillar, submaxillary, submental, anterior cervical, posterior cervical, supraclavicular and infraclavicular lymph nodes. If a node is palpated, note the location, size (in centimeter), shape (usually round), mobility (movable or fixed), consistency (soft, hard, firm), tenderness, and delimitation (discrete or matted together).

Thyroid

Inspect and palpate the thyroid gland for size, symmetry and any masses by instructing the person to swallow water, while extending the neck. Normally, the thyroid gland and the thyroid and cricoid cartilage will rise as the person swallows. An enlarged thyroid gland is called a goiter. Palpate the thyroid gland by standing in front of or behind the person.

Instruct the person to extend the neck, place fingers just below the cricoid cartilage. Ask the person to swallow. Can feel the thyroid isthmus rise beneath your fingers.

Trachea

Inspect and palpate the trachea for any deviation from the midline by placing two fingers over the trachea at the suprasternal notch. Deviation of the trachea from the midline may indicate a mass or respiratory problem such as atelectasis and pneumothorax.

Chest

Examination of the chest involves assessment of the respiratory system (lungs) and the cardiovascular system (heart). A thorough examination of the chest requires you to use the techniques of inspection, palpation, percussion, and auscultation.

Posterior chest

the posterior chest is inspected for any skeletal deformities. Some common abnormalities are kyphosis (an exaggerated curvature of the thoracic vertebrae), scoliosis (a lateral curvature of the spine), and lordosis (an exaggerated curvature of the lumbar vertebrae):

- ❖ Vesicular breath sounds are soft, low pitched, fine resulting sounds located over the periphery of the lung.
- ❖ If the vesicular sounds are decreased over the periphery, this may indicate pneumonia, emphysema, pleural effusion, or atelectasis.
- ❖ Bronchial breath sounds are loud, high-pitched tubular sounds located over the trachea and major bronchi that are heard lower and longer during expiration.
- ❖ Bronchial sounds auscultation over the periphery of the lungs may indicate consolidation or atelectasis.
- ❖ Bronchovesicular breath sounds are moderately pitched sounds located between the scapula posteriorly and on either side of the sternum at the first and second intercostal spaces anteriorly.
- ❖ Bronchovesicular sounds auscultated over the periphery of the lung may indicate consolidation.
- ❖ Adventitious breath sounds and abnormal breath sounds are as follows:
  - ➤ *Crackles:* Are the noises created when air is travelling through vessels containing abnormal moisture.
  - ➤ *Wheeze:* High pitched sounds produced as air passes through a narrowed of defective vessel.
  - ➤ *Rhonchi (gurgles):* Are coarse rattling sounds, louder and lower in pitch than crackers, caused by narrowed airways.
  - ➤ *Friction rubs:* Are crackling, grating sounds produced when two roughened or influenced pleural spaces rub across each other.

Anterior chest

The anterior chest is inspected for any skeletal abnormalities. Some common abnormalities are barrel chest, Pigeon chest.

- ❖ *Barrel chest:* Is a thoracic abnormality characterized by horizontal ribs, slight kyphosis, and a prominent sternal angle.
- ❖ *Pectus carinatum (Pigeon chest):* It is a thoracic abnormality characterized by the forward projection of the sternum.
- ❖ *Pectus excavatum (funnel chest):* It is a thoracic abnormality characterized by the sternum pointing posteriorly, which may cause pressure on the heart.
- ❖ The anterior chest is palpated for areas of tenderness, respiratory excursion, and fremitus.
- ❖ Percuss the anterior and the lateral chest. Normally, resonance is percussed over the entire lung area.
- ❖ Auscultate the anterior chest for vesicular, bronchial, and bronchovesicular breath sounds.

Heart

Inspection, percussion, palpation, and auscultation are techniques used in the examination of the heart.

- ❖ *Inspection:* Position the person in a supine position or lying with the head of the bed at a 35°–45° angle. Inspect the apical impulse or lift heaves. Normally, the only pulsation observable on the chest wall is the apical impulse:
  - ➤ The apical impulse is located over the apex of the heart, at the fifth intercostal space medial to the midclavicular line.
  - ➤ If the heart is displaced or enlarged, the apical impulse may be located lateral to the midclavicular line.
  - ➤ Chest lift: A lift is slight movement, while heave is a vigorous movement. Each one is the result of forceful cardiac action and is considered abnormal.

- ❖ **Palpation:** The precordial points of the chest are palpated for any abnormal pulsations, thrills, lift heaves, apical impulses, and aortic pulsations:
  - ➢ Thrill is a palpable cardiac murmur.
  - ➢ **Apical impulse:** To palpate, place the heel of the hand on the sternum with fingers stretched across the chest, just under the breast area, palpate it with fingertips.
  - ➢ The aortic pulse is palpated in the epigastric area.
- ❖ **Percussion:** Cardiac dullness is located in the third to fifth intercostal spaces. Percussion is no longer used in the assessment of the heart.
- ❖ **Auscultation:** The auscultation techniques assess the normal heart sounds (S_1 and S_2), extra heart sounds (S_3, S_4), and murmurs. Auscultate with diaphragm and bell:
  - ➢ List at each area through several breaths in and out.
  - ➢ Describe the heart sounds according to their pitch, loudness and timing in the cardiac cycle.
  - ➢ Low-pitched sounds are best heard with the stethoscope bell and higher, louder sounds with the diaphragm.
  - ➢ **First heart sounds:** The first heart sound (S_1) is produced by the closure of the mitral and tricuspid heart valves. It is best heard at the apex of the heart.
  - ➢ **Second heart sounds:** The sound heart (S_2) is produced by the closure of the aortic and pulmonic heart valves. It is best heard at the base of the heart (aortic area). S_1 and S_2 are both high-pitched sounds. Note the time between S_1 and S_2 (systole) and between S_1 and S_2 (diastole).
  - ➢ **Third heart sounds:** The third heart sound S_3 (ventricular gallop) is a low-pitched sound heard in the cardiac cycle immediately after S_2 (diastole). It is normal in children and in young adults. It is considered abnormal in adults over 30 years of age. It represents an enlarged ventricle or overly rapid ventricular filling, a sign of left ventricular failure.
  - ➢ **Fourth heart sounds:** The fourth heart sound, S_4 (atrial group) is a low-pitched sound heard in the cardiac cycle just before S_1. S_4 may be normal in children and trained athletes. It is considered abnormal in most adults and is associated with ischemia, coronary artery disease, and aortic stenosis.
- ❖ **Heart murmur:** A heart murmur is a harsh, rumbling, blowing sound caused by blood flow across a defective valve or the shunting of blood through an abnormal passage.

Breast

Inspection and palpations are technique used to do breast examination:
- ❖ The nipple and areola should be inspected and palpated for nodules, swelling, and edema.
- ❖ The males distinguish the breast enlargement from obesity (soft enlargement) and gynecomastia (firm enlargement) through palpation.
- ❖ **Inspection:** Positions assumed when inspecting the breasts are sitting, arms at the sides; sitting, arms raised over the head; leaning forward.
  - ➢ Inspect the breast for size and symmetry, contour, and appearance of the skin.
  - ➢ Inspect the nipples for size, shape, rashes, ulcerations, and discharge.
  - ➢ Observe for any masses, flattening or dimpling of the breasts.
  - ➢ Inspect the skin for color, thickening or edema.
  - ➢ Redness and inflammation indicate infection.
  - ➢ Thickening or edema may be produced by lymphatic blockage.
  - ➢ The skin that resembles an orange peel suggests cancer of the breast.
  - ➢ Nipple inversion is considered a normal variation as it has been long standing. Inversion occurring in a previously erect is suggestive of malignancy.
  - ➢ Nipples should point outward or downward.
  - ➢ If discharge is present, note the odor.
- ❖ **Palpation**
  - ➢ Palpate all four quadrants (right upper, right lower, left upper, and left lower), both areola, tails of breast and axilla for lumps and nodules.
  - ➢ To palpate the breast, gently press the finger pads in rotating movement, progressing slowly across the breast tissue until the total breast is examined.
  - ➢ Maintain continuous finger contact with the tissue rather than lighting the finger up and down to change sites.
  - ➢ If a nodule is detected, note the location, size, shape (round, disk shaped, tubular), consistency (soft, hard, firm), mobility (mobile, fixed).

Axilla

Inspection and palpation are used to assess the axillary area with the person in a sitting position.
- ❖ **Inspection**
  - ➢ Inspect each axilla for rashes, redness, infection, and unusual pigmentation.
  - ➢ Redness and infection originates from the sweat glands.
  - ➢ A change in pigmentation suggests an underlying malignancy.
- ❖ **Palpation**
  - ➢ Palpate the axilla by placing the finger into the apex of the axilla with the person's arm down and the wrist resting in examiner's hand.
  - ➢ Some tenderness occurs high in the axilla during palpation for lymph nodes.

Abdomen

Assessment of the abdomen involves inspection, auscultation, percussion, and palpation. Auscultation is performed after inspection to ensure that the motility of the bowel sounds are not alerted:

- ❖ Ask the person to empty bladder.
- ❖ Assume a supine position with the arms at the side.
- ❖ Instruct the person to flex the knees slightly (this position aids in relaxation of the abdomen).
- ❖ Expose the abdomen from the epigastric area to the symphysis pubis.
- ❖ *Inspection*
  - ➢ Inspect the contour and symmetry of skin, umbilicus and peristalsis.
  - ➢ Inspect the contour of the abdomen (flat, sunken, or protruding).
  - ➢ Are all four quadrants equal in size.
  - ➢ Observe the skin for any scars, striae, or lesions.
  - ➢ Note the contour, location, and any science of inflammation or herniation of the umbilicus.
  - ➢ Peristalsis is usually not visible except in very thin people.
  - ➢ Disease process can cause protrusion of the abdomen and measure the abdominal girth.
  - ➢ Dehydration may cause the abdomen to appear sunken.
  - ➢ Fluid (ascites, masses, or an intestinal obstruction) may cause asymmetry of the abdomen.
- ❖ *Auscultation:* The abdomen is auscultated for bowel sounds, bruits, friction rubs.
  - ➢ Bowels are created by peristalsis and indicate bowel motility.
  - ➢ Bowel sounds within the range of 5–35 per minute are normal:
    - ♦ Hypoactive bowel sounds are fewer than 5 per minute and indicate decreased motility. This may be seen in bowel obstruction, paralytic ileus, and peritonitis.
    - ♦ Hyperactive bowel sounds are greater than 35 per minute and indicate an increase in bowel motility, as seen in gastroenteritis and intestinal obstruction.
    - ♦ Absent bowel sounds may indicate paralytic ileus, peritonitis, or complete obstruction.
    - ♦ A rush of high-pitched tinkling sound may indicate fluid.
  - ➢ Auscultate over the liver and spleen for any possible friction rub. This abnormal rough, grating is present during infection, malignancy or infarction.
  - ➢ A venous hum can be auscultated in the epigastric and umbilical area. It is an abnormal, continuous, medium-pitched sound that suggests hepatic cirrhosis.
- ❖ *Percussion*
  - ➢ The percussion of the abdomen are dullness and tympany.
  - ➢ Dullness is percussed over solid structures (abdominal organs) tympany is percussed over air filled areas.
  - ➢ To percuss upper liver border start at the level of the umbilicus, midclavicular line and percussed upward from tympany to dullness.
  - ➢ The spleen is percussed at the lowest intercostal space in the left anterior axillary line.
  - ➢ When the spleen is of normal size, tympanic sound can be heard. If the spleen is enlarged, tympany will be replaced by dullness.
- ❖ *Palpation:* Light and deep palpation are used to examine the abdomen:
  - ➢ Light palpation is used to assess tenderness, muscle tone, abdominal stiffening, and superficial masses.
  - ➢ Deep palpation is used to distinguish masses, organs, and deep pain.
  - ➢ Begin with light palpation, using the palmar surfaces of the fingertips. Asses all abdominal quadrants. After the competition of light palpation, palpate deeply all the four quadrants. Deep palpation requires more pressure than light palpation. If any masses are palpated, note the size, location, contour, mobility, consistency, and tenderness.
  - ➢ To palpate the liver deeply, place fingertips below the lower border for dullness.
  - ➢ Ask the person to take a deep breath and gently push inward and upward.
  - ➢ Palpate the edge of the liver as the person inhales.
  - ➢ The liver feels smooth, firm, and sharp. If the liver feels hard, this may indicate cirrhosis.
  - ➢ The spleen is not palpable unless it is enlarged.
  - ➢ To palpate, place the right hand below the left coastal margin and palpate it toward the spleen.
  - ➢ The kidneys are usually not palpable, but can feel the lower pole of the right kidney in a thin person.
  - ➢ To palpate the right kidney, place left hand on the person's back of the kidney upward. With the right hand push downward. Ask the person to exhale as slowly release right hand.
  - ➢ Note the size, contour, and any tenderness.

Genitals and Rectum

The genital and rectal areas are examined using inspection and palpation:
- ❖ Keep the person informed of actions.
- ❖ Enhance comfort during the genital examinations by also:
  - ➢ Providing privacy and preventing exposure, e.g. screen, door shut, drapes.
  - ➢ Not prolonging the examination deeply.
  - ➢ Warm the instruments such as vaginal speculum.
  - ➢ Use lubricants when possible to minimize discomfort during insertion, as of gloves.
- ❖ *Male genitalia:* Inspection and palpation of the male genitalia are performed with the person in a supine position and in standing position.

- ❖ *Inspection*
  - ➢ Inspection of the male genitalia includes the penis, scrotum, and inguinal ring and canal.
  - ➢ Observe the penis and testis for size, shape, color, and texture of the scrotal skin and distribution of the pubic hair.
  - ➢ Observe for the presence of lice or nits attached to the pubic hair.
  - ➢ Observe for any lesions, odor, discharge, or inflammation.
  - ➢ The urethra should open in the center of glans tip.
  - ➢ Smegma (cheesy white material) may be observed under the foreskin.
  - ➢ Inspect for any groin masses by asking the person to cough, while observe for any bulging that may indicate inguinal hernia.
- ❖ *Palpation*
  - ➢ Palpate the penis using thumb and the first two fingers. Note any tenderness or induration.
  - ➢ Palpate the testis and epididymis of the scrotum. Note size, shape, consistency, and any tenderness or nodules.
  - ➢ Normally testis feels firm, spongy each testicle is egg [oval] shaped. About 4 cm long and up to 2-2.5 cm wide.
  - ➢ The epididymis is located behind the testicle and is soft spongy.
  - ➢ The spermatic chords are palpated for nodules and swelling.
- ❖ *Female genitalia:* Inspection and palpation are the techniques used to examined the female genitalia:
  - ➢ Instruct the person to empty the bladder.
  - ➢ Female genitalia is examined with the person in a lithotomy position.
- ❖ *Inspection and palpation:* Inspect the external genitalia (mons pubis, labia, and perineum):
  - ➢ Note the character and distribution of the pubic hair.
  - ➢ Separate the labia and inspect the labia minora, clitoris, urethral orifice, and the introitus (vaginal opening).
  - ➢ Observe for inflammation, discharge, ulceration, and nodules.
  - ➢ The pubic hair should be normally distributed. There should be no order and minimal clear discharge.

Rectum

Inspection and digital palpation are performed with the person in a left lateral (Sims) position.

Inspection: The anal area is inspected by gently spreading the buttocks to expose the anus. Observe the anal area for hemorrhoids, rashes, inflammation, and ulcers.

Extremities

The upper and lower extremities are assessed by using inspection, palpation, and auscultation.
- ❖ *Upper extremities:* The upper extremities are inspected beginning at the fingertips and moving toward the shoulder:
  - ➢ Observe size and symmetry, color and texture of the skin and nailbeds, venous pattern, and any edema.
  - ➢ The nail base should be firm with a 160° between the finger nail and nail base.
  - ➢ Observe for any clubbing, an abnormality of the nail in which the nailbed appears spongy (early clubbing) or swollen (late clubbing) and the angle of the nail is 180° or greater. Clubbing may indicate hypoxia or lung cancer.
  - ➢ Blanch the nailbed and note the amount of time required for capillary refill. A capillary refill occurring less than 3-4 seconds is sluggish, and greater than 4 seconds is abnormal.
  - ➢ Observe for spoon nails, beau's line, and paronychia infection.
- ❖ *Lower extremities:* The lower extremities are examined with a person in a supine position:
  - ➢ Inspect for size and symmetry, venous pattern, color and texture of the skin, and nailbeds, hair distribution on lower legs, feet and toes, pigmentation, rashes, scars, ulcers, and edema.
  - ➢ Test the toenails for capillary refill.
  - ➢ Arterial insufficiency will cause pain, decreased peripheral pulses, pale skin color, cool skin temperature, mild edema, thin, shiny skin, loss of hair over the foot and toes, and thickened nails. Ulcers may or may not be present.
  - ➢ Test for Homan's sign, an indicator of deep phlebitis (pain and soreness are present in the calf area when the foot is dorsiflexed).
  - ➢ Assess the patellar, ankle, and plantar reflexes.

Motor System

Assess gait, Romberg's sign, muscle strength, and coordination.
- ❖ *Gait:* It is a person's style of walking. Instruct the person to walk across the room, turn, and walk back. Observe the person's balance and posture. Next instruct the person to walk in a straight line, heel to toe (tandem walking). Inability to do tandem walking reveals ataxia. Ataxia is uncoordinated gait that results from cerebellar disease or intoxication.
- ❖ *Romberg test:* It is a test of sensory equilibrium. Instruct the person to stand with the feet together and eyes open. Note the person's balance. Then tell the person to close the eyes. If the person lose balance, this is considered a "Positive Romberg."

- ➤ **Tests of muscle strength:** Muscles strength is assessed by having the person move against resistance:
  - ♦ Flexion and extension of the elbow are tested by having the person push and pull against your hand.
  - ♦ Extension of the wrist is tested by trying to pull the person's formed fist in a downward motion.
  - ♦ Finger abduction is tested by instructing the person to spread the fingers, while you try to force them back together.
  - ♦ Thumb opposition is tested by instructing the person to touch the thumb to the little finger, while you apply resistance to the thumb.
  - ♦ Hip flexion is tested by applying hand to the person's thigh and instructing the person to raise the leg against resistance.
  - ♦ Abduction of the hip is tested by placing the hands on the outside of the legs of the knee level and instructing the person to spread both the legs against resistance.
  - ♦ Hip adduction is tested by placing the hands on the inside of the person's legs (knee level) and instructing the person to bring legs together.
  - ♦ Knee flexion is tested by placing one hand on the person's slightly flexed knee and the other hand behind the ankle with the person's floor resting on the examination table. Instruct the person to flex the knee against the resistance, without moving the foot.
- ❖ **Tests of coordination:** Coordination is assessed using rapid alternating movements and point-to-point testing:
  - ➤ Instruct the person to touch each finger with the thumb as rapidly as possible. Test each hand separately. Note smooth quick movements.
  - ➤ Movements that are slowed and coordinated may indicate cerebellar dysfunction.
  - ➤ The finger to nose is performed with the person in a setting position and the arms extended forward. Instruct the person to touch the nose with the forefinger, then return the arm to the extended position. Perform this with alternating hands.
  - ➤ Test the person first with the eyes open and then with the eyes closed.
  - ➤ Observe for smooth movements and maintenance of proper body posture. Cerebellar dysfunction is indicated when the person fails to perform this task.

Sensory System

The sensory system is examined through the assessment of pain, temperature, light touch, vibration, and position. In each test, the person's eyes should be closed.

Light touch/superficial pain

- ❖ Using cotton and a safety pin, alternatively touch the distal and proximal portions of the upper and lower extremities.
- ❖ Ask the person to identify the location and the type of sensation (soft or sharp).
- ❖ **Temperature:** The temperature test should be performed only when the person's perception of pain is abnormal:
  - ➤ Fill two tubes with water, on hot and the other cold. Touch all medial and lateral limb surfaces.
  - ➤ Instruct the person to identify whether the sensation is hot or cold.
- ❖ **Vibration:** Vibration is assessed by tapping a tuning fork and placing it firmly on the person's interphalangeal joint of the finger and great toe. Ask the person to describe the sensation (pressure or vibration) and to identify when the sensation ends.
- ❖ **Stereognosis:** Stereognosis is the act of recognizing objects on the basic of touching and manipulating them. Place a familiar object, such as a key, paper clip, or pencil, in the person's hand and ask them to identify the object.
- ❖ **Number identification (graphesthesia):** Trace several numbers on each of the person's palms with the blunt end of a pen or pencil.
- ❖ **Two-point discrimination:** When assessing two-point discrimination, touch the person alternately with one or two safety pins on a particular body part, such as the finger pads.
- ❖ **Point localization:** This is assessed by touching various parts of the person's body with a wisp of cotton. The person is instructed to open the eyes after felt the touch and point to the area.

PSYCHOLOGICAL CONSEQUENCES OF ILLNESS

Introduction

Illness is a state in which a person's physical, emotional, intellectual, social, developmental, or spiritual functioning is diminished or impaired compared to previous experience.

Although nurses must be familiar with different kinds of diseases and their treatments, they are concerned more with illness, which may include disease but also the effects on functioning and well-being in all dimensions.

Illness Behavior

People who are ill generally act in a way that medical sociologists call illness behavior. It involves how people monitor their bodies define and interpret their symptoms, take remedial actions, and use the healthcare system. If people perceive themselves to be ill, illness behavior can be a coping mechanism. For example:

- ❖ Illness behavior can result in clients being released from roles, social expectations, or responsibilities. Parsons (1951) in the new famous theory of sick role behavior suggested that the individual when suffering from an illness may behave in certain ways in order to facilitate recovery.

- They may stay off work or avoid social contacts and normal responsibilities and will normally seek medical alteration. Illness behavior may become abnormal when it is disproportionate to the present problem and that client persists in the sick role (Clark and Smith, 1997).
- A normal sick role during the acute phase following a stroke may be the avoidance of physical activity. This behavior would be inappropriate if it persisted during rehabilitation. Buckingham (1995) believes that or many clients a period of convalescence is necessary after an illness. It is gradual and personal process in which clients recover at their own pace and when healed are able to relinquish the sick role.

Variables Influencing Illness Behavior

Just as health behavior is affected by internal and external variables, so is illness behavior. The influence of these variables, as well as the stage of illness behavior the client may affect the likelihood of seeking healthcare, compliance with therapy, and therefore health outcomes. Based on an understanding of these variables and behaviors, nurses can plan individualized care to assist clients in coping with their illness at various stages of illness. The goal of nursing is to promote optimal functioning in all dimensions through an illness.

Internal Variables

- ***A client's perception of illness:*** If clients believe that the symptoms of their illness disrupt their normal routine, they are more likely to seek healthcare assistance that if they do not perceive the symptoms to be disruptive. If clients believe that the symptoms are serious or perhaps life-threatening, they are also more likely to seek assistance. For example, person awakened by crushing chest pains in the middle of the night generally view this symptom as potentially serious and life-threatening, and they will probably be motivated to seek assistance. However, such a perception can also have the opposite effect. Individuals may fear serious illness, react by denying it, and not seek medical assistance.
- ***Nature of illness:*** Illness either acute or chronic can also affect a client's illness behavior, clients with acute illness are likely to seek healthcare and comply readily with therapy. On the other hand, a client with a chronic illness in which the symptoms may not be cured, but only partially relieved, may not be motivated to comply with the therapy plan. Chronically ill patients/clients may become less actively involved in their care, may experience greater frustration and may comply less readily with care.
- ***A client's coping skills:*** A client's coping skills, as well as his/her or locus of control are other variable that affect the way the client behaves when ill. The ability to cope with illness usually depends on person's experience with similar illness, support systems and overall perception of the illness.

External Variables

External variables influencing a client's behavior include:

- ***Visibility of symptoms:*** It affects the body image and illness behavior. A client with visible symptoms may be more likely to seek assistance than a client without such a visible symptom.
- ***Social group:*** Clients social groups may assist them in recognizing the threat of illness or support the denial of potential illness. Families, friends, and coworkers all may influence client's illness behavior. Client often reacts positively to social support, while practicing positive health behaviors.
- ***Cultural and ethnic backgrounds:*** A person's cultural and ethnic background teaches the person how to be healthy, how to recognize illness, and how to be ill. The effect of disease and its interpretation vary according to cultural circumstances.
- ***Economic variable:*** Economic variables influence the way a client reacts to illness. Because of economic constraints, a client may delay treatment and in many cases may continue to carry out daily activities.
- ***Accessibility of the healthcare system:*** Client's access to the healthcare system is closely related to economic factors. The healthcare system is a socioeconomic system that client's must enter, interact within, and exit. For many clients, entry into the system is complex or confusing and some patients may seek nonemergency medical care in an emergency department, because they do not know how otherwise to obtain health services. The physical proximity of clients to healthcare agency often influences how soon they enter the system after deciding to seek care.
- ***Social support:*** It has been linked to health practices such as seat belt use, exercise, nutrition, smoking cessation, and health screen practices. Research notes that clients react positively to social support during participation in positive health practices. Thus, persons who view themselves as being part of social group and having emotional and personal resources on which they can rely are more likely to practice positive health behaviors.

Impact of Illness on the Client and Family

Illness is never an isolated life event. The client and family must deal with changes resulting from illness and treatment. Each client responds uniquely to illness and therefore nursing interventions must be individualized. The client and family commonly experience behavioral and emotional charges as well as changes in I roles, body image, self-concept, and family dynamics.

Behavioral and Emotional Changes

People react differently to illness or the threat of illness. Individual behavioral and emotional reactions depend on the nature of the illness, the client's attitude toward it, the reaction of others to it, and the variables of illness behavior. Short-term, nonlife-threatening illness evokes few behavioral changes on the functioning of the client or family. For example, A father who has cold may lack the energy to spend time in family activities and may be irritable and prefer not to interact with his family. This is a behavioral change, but the change is subtle and does not last long. Some may even consider such a change as a normal response to illness. Severe illness particularly one that is life-threatening can lead to more extensive emotional and behavioral changes such as anxiety, shock, denial, anger, and withdrawal.

Impact on Body Image

Body image is the subjective concept of physical appearance. Some illness result in changes in physical appearance and clients and families react differently to these changes. These reactions of clients and families to changes in body image depend on the following:

- The type of changes (e.g. loss of a limb or an organ)
- Their adaptive capacity
- The rate at which changes take place
- Support services available.

Then a change in body image occurs such as results from a leg amputation, the client generally adjusts in the following phases:

- ***Shock:*** Initially the client may be shocked by the impending change and may be depersonalize and talk about it as though it were happening to someone else.
- ***Withdrawal:*** Withdrawal is an adaptive coping mechanism that can assist the client on making the adjustment. As the client and family recognize the reality of the change, they become anxious and may withdraw, refusing to discuss it.
- ***Acknowledgment:*** As client and family acknowledge the change, they move through a period of grieving.
- ***Acceptance:*** At the end of acknowledgment phase, they accept the loss.
- ***Rehabilitation:*** During rehabilitation, the client is ready to learn how to adopt to the change in body image through use of a prosthesis or changing lifestyles and goals.

Impact on Self-concept

Self-concept is a mental self-image of strengths and weaknesses in all aspects of personality. Self-concept depends in part on body image and roles, but also includes other aspects of psychology and spirituality.

Self-concept is important in relationships with other family members. A client whose self-concept changes, because of illness may no longer meet family expectations, leading to tension or conflict. As a result, family members may change their interactions with the client.

Nurse's role: In the course of providing care, a nurse is able to observe changes in the client's self-concept (or family members) and develop a care plan to help them adjust to the changes resulting from the illness.

Impact on Family Roles

People have many roles in life, such as wage earner, decision-maker professional child sibling or parent. When an illness occurs, parents and children try to adapt to major changes resulting from a family member's illness. Role reversal is common. If a parent of an adult becomes ill and cannot carry out usual activities, the adult child often assumes many of the parent's responsibilities and in essence becomes a parent to the parent. Such a reversal of the usual situation can lead to stress, confliction, responsibilities for the adult child, or direct conflict over decision-making.

An individual and family generally adjust more easily to subtle, short-term changes. In most cases, they know that the role change is only temporary and will not require prolonged adjustment phases long-term changes however, require an adjustment process similar to the grief process.

The client and family often require specific counseling and guidance to assist them in coping with the role changes.

Impact on Family Dynamics

Family dynamics is the process by which the family functions, makes decisions, gives support to individual members and copes with everyday changes and challenges. Because of the effects of illness, family dynamics changes. For example, if a parent in a family becomes ill, family activities and decision-making often come to a halt as the other family members wait for the illness to pass, or they delay action, because they are reluctant to assume the ill person's roles or responsibilities.

Nurses role: The nurse must view the whole family as a client under stress, planning care to help the family regain the maximal level of functioning and well-being.

Stages of Illness Behavior

Although the behavior of an individual when they become ill are influenced by different factors generally people pass through five stages of illness behavior. Such man in 1965, identify these stages as follows:

- Symptom experience stage
- Assumption of the sick roles
- Medical care contact
- Dependent client role
- Recovery or rehabilitation stage

Stage 1: Symptom Experience

During this initial stage, a person is aware that "something is wrong" he/she usually recognizes a physical sensation or a limitation is functioning, but does not suspect a specific diagnosis. The person's perception of a symptom includes three components.

1. He/she becomes aware of a physical change such as a pain, rash, or a jump.
2. He/she evaluates his/her change and decides that it is a symptom of an illness.
3. The person decides that there may be an illness present. So, he/she shows emotional response.

For example, a woman finds lump in the breast during her self-breast examination. She thinks that it is a symptom of illness, because she knows that lump indicates cancer, she may become anxious or fearful. Once the person acknowledges the presence of a symptom, she may behave in various ways:

❖ If he/she thinks the symptom is mild and not life-threatening (cold), he/she may attempt various self-medication strategies rather than seeking health care. Commonly he/she treats himself/herself with home remedies or over-the-counter drugs.

❖ If he/she regards the symptom a serious or life-threatening one he/she immediately seeks medical care or may deny the symptoms presence or implications. If he/she denies the symptom, he/she delays seeking advice or treatment. Before progressing to the next stage of illness behavior, the person must first acknowledge the presence of symptoms/problems.

Stage 2: Assumption of Sick Role

If the symptom persists and becomes severe, the person assumes the sick role, the second stage. At this stage, the illness becomes a social phenomena and the sick person seeks information from his/her family and social group that he/she is indeed ill and that he/she should be excused from normal duties and role expectations. The social group validates the illness and may support the self-medication. The assumption of the sick role results ill physical and emotional changes. Emotional changes may be simple or complex depending on the severity of illness, degree of disabilities, and the anticipated length of illness.

In case if the illness requires intervention from health professionals that person may deny that such intervention is necessary and delays the contact with healthcare system.

Once the person accepts the sick role he/she seeks contact with the healthcare system and becomes a client, the third stage of illness behavior.

Stage 3: Medical Care Contact

If the symptom persists despite home remedies become severe or require emergency care, the person is motivated to seek professional health services. In stage 3, the client seeks expert validation of his/her illness as well as treatment. In addition, he/she seeks an explanation of the symptoms, the course of illness and the implication of illness for his/her future health.

The client's illness can be validated at any point, on the health illness continuum. A health professional may determine that the client does not have an illness or that illness is in fact present and may be life-threatening. The client then accepts or denies this diagnosis depending on several factors.

First the variable that affects illness behavior in general also influence how the client reacts to his/her illness. If he/she accepts the diagnosis, he/she usually follows through with the treatment plan. If he/she denies the diagnosis, he/she may begin "shopping" within the healthcare system. In such a case, the client consults various healthcare providers until he/she fines one who makes the diagnosis he/she desires or until he/she changes mind and accepts the initial diagnosis. A patient who considers himself/herself ill even if health professionals regard him/her as healthy may explore nontraditional health settings to obtain a desire diagnosis of illness. At the same time, a client who is diagnosed as ill, particularly with a life-threatening illness may seek a different expert to tell him/her that his/her life or health is not threatened.

Stage 4: Dependent Client Role

Once the client accepts the fact of his/her illness and seeks treatment, he/she enters the fourth stage of illness behavior. In this stage, the client depends on health professionals for the relief of his/her symptoms. In the dependent role clients accepts care, sympathy and protection from the demands and stresses of life. A client can adopt dependent role in a healthcare institution, at home or in a community setting.

In the dependent role its socially permissible for the client to be relieved of his/her normal obligations and responsibilities. The more ill the client, the more he/she exempted from his/her responsibilities.

Once the client enters the dependent stage of illness, he/she must also adjust to the disruption of his/her daily schedule. The disruption affects the clients role in his/her occupation, in his/her family and in his/her community and may lead to stress in his/her emotional, intellectual, social, and spiritual dimensions.

Stage 5: Recovery and Rehabilitation

The final stage of illness behaviors, recovery, and rehabilitation can arrive abruptly, such as with the subsiding of fever or long-term care may be required as in the case of fractured leg, before the client is able to resume his/her optimal level of functioning. In case of chronic illness, the final stage may involve adjustment to a prolonged reduction in the level of health and functioning.

Some common effects of illness and hospitalization: Illness brings in its wake, a greater or lesser degree of pain and discomfort, which in turn often prevent rest and sleep and frustrate some of our basic desires. The nurse needs to know this and to realize that the threshold of pain varies from one patient to another. Some patients react to pain with fear, others show resistance, and quite a few give evidence of a sense of desolation and misery. The nurse should assess these emotional reactions and give to each patient the help, which is necessary. The signs, which reveal the presence of pain and be known to him/her, and he/she bout alleviate the pain and discomfort as far as in lies within his/her power or as far as medical and surgical conditions allow.

Illness imposes a certain amount of restriction on the patient regardless of his/her age socioeconomic status of profession. Normal activities have to cease for some time; normal interests and responsibilities have to be given up. All this is enough to produce tensions. In the absence of normal activities and interests, the patient's thoughts may be turned to himself/herself and immediate environment. As such, his/her self-centeredness increases and interferes with quick recovery; hence, the necessity of providing patients with interests and occupations beyond themselves. Restrictions may affect some patients differently. They may begin as they are inadequate, incapable of doing many things. The feelings of inadequacy may prevent them from forming human relationships. They may withdraw from association with other people. They may become apathetic and depressed and try to close themselves off from their surroundings. All this results in increasing their loneliness and feelings of rejection, which arises from the thought that one being ill is different from other people.

Loneliness increases, because the sick are dependent on others to come to them. The feeling of loneliness is accompanied in some patients by a deep sense of guilt. They feel without being consciously aware guilt. They feel, without being consciously aware of it that they are being punished for some failure within themselves.

We have seen that illness produces a feeling of inadequacy and weakens one's self-regard. Some patient's feel the loss of self-regard very acutely and make attempts to restore it. This they do by finding fault with others or they begin to blame other people and their circumstances, which according to them have made them ill. They become critical, complaining, or openly hostile.

Illness may weaken a patient's feelings of security. The factors which cause insecurity are the uncertainty of others, delayed diagnosis and its recovery, the strangeness of the place and of the people surrounding him/her, a complete severance from the human or social environment to which the patient normally belongs to the temporary uprooting from his/her settled social pattern. To some people, the change on daily routine, the unfamiliar bed in a ward full of people whom he/she does not know, the difference in food, meal times, times of waking, and times of setting for sleep-adds to the fear and alarm, which the new and strange situation arouses. It must be noted that much depends on the nature and severity of the illness, as well as on his/her own inner emotional adjustment and basic security. The nurse can lessen these feelings of insecurity by straight forward explanations of hospital conditions and procedures including details of ward routine, by being ward and reassuring in his/her manner and through sincerity of personal interest in the patient.

It has been observed that many patients tend to regress in a prechildish level of behavior, as a reaction to illness. This tendency is shown in the behavior of adult patients, who are highly demanding or fretful or excessively dependent on others. Adult patients who seem to be afraid by taking the treatment and react timidly are also regressing.

The nurse should remember that a certain number of patients use their physical illness as a weapon with which they secure the attention of other nurses, doctors, relatives, or parents. They may complain of many aches and pains and physical discomforts for which no organic cause can be found. Such ailments serve two purposes, first, these reduce the demands made on the patients and recently these coin for them a certain amount of extra sympathy and attention.

For a few patients illness and for that matter, hospitalization may be a boon. Better food, more rest, kind, and sympathetic nurses and doctors make their stay in a hospital very comfortable. The hospital becomes a heaven of refuge from hardships and responsibilities at home. Such patients have to face acute problems during convalescence and at the time of their departure from the hospital. The idea of going back to their work or to their home where they have to fulfill many obligations become disgusting to them in as much as it involves the loss of attention and care they receive from nurses and doctors, and that of freedom from responsibilities, which has characterized the period of sickness in the hospital. These patients become so used to dependence on, and protection from others that they may unconsciously resent being urged to resume responsibility for themselves and being independent.

They may even invent false complaints so that they may continue enjoying attention. The nurse should bear these possibilities in mind and help such patients with proper explanations they should be engaged in some useful activities and occupation during these periods of convalescence as a step toward a normal life of responsibilities and work. The majority of convalescents however are anxious to resume their normal duties and activities as soon as possible and may not realize the necessity of slow process of recovery and longer convalescence. Their patients also need to be helped in a realistic manner.

Child's reaction to illness: Illness or a physical handicap threatens both the physical development of children and the physical of children their sense of trust in other people. Sickness causes pain, restraint of movements, long sleepless periods, and in infants who cannot be fed by mouth, restriction on the fulfillment of their sucking. When they most need their parents, they are without them, unless the hospital has provisions for parents to remain day and night.

Hospitalization is a completely new experience to infants and young children. When they were taken to the private physician's office on the clinic, they made friends with physicians and nurses, but they are too young to understand that personal in the hospitals are also friends. Since parents tend to be anxious they are feeling of far is communicated to their children. It depends in large measures upon how well they were prepared for hospitalization. If they regard the separation from parents as punishment for wrongdoing, they will be able to cope with it they know the real reasons for their hospitalization and something of what to expect after admission.

Infants especially may be emotionally disturbed by hospitalization. Not only are they separated from parents but also they may suffer from sensory and deprivation if the nursing personal do not take time to provide the loving care they need. If infants on the other hand are bright and outgoing, nurses may give them more than the usual amount of cuddling. It is important for nurses to consider each child as an individual, who has basic needs for love and security.

CONCLUSION

There are different methods of health assessment based on the purpose and need we conduct health assessment. The health assessment done on admission of a client is called as comprehensive assessment. Identification of findings, interpretation, and documentation of care accurately are essential aspects.

CHAPTER 44

Methods of Collection, Analysis and Utilization of Data Relevant to Nursing Process

CHAPTER OUTLINE

- Steps of Nursing Process
- Purposes of the Nursing Process
- Characteristics of Nursing Process
- Advantages of Nursing Process
- Nursing Assessment

INTRODUCTION

One of the essentials of any profession is a consensus of what constitutes the core of its practice. The comprehensive analysis of the core of nursing practice is a set of operations called the nursing process. The nursing process is a scientific method used to assist students and practitioners to systematically assess, plan, implement, and evaluate quality individual nursing care.

The nursing process is that which combines the most desirable elements of the art of nursing with the most relevant elements of the systems theory using the scientific method (Shore, 1988). This process incorporates an interactive/interpersonal approach with a problem-solving approach and decision-making process.

DEFINITIONS

- The nursing process is a systematic method of giving humanistic care that focuses on achieving desired outcomes (results) in a cost-effective fashion. Its systematic in that it consists of five steps: (1) assessment, (2) diagnosis, (3) planning, (4) implementation, and (5) evaluation during which deliberate steps are taken to maximum efficiency and attain long-term beneficial results. Its humanism in that it is based on the belief that unique interests ideals and desires of the healthcare consumer (person, family, community) are considered.

  —Alfaro-LeFevre, 1998

- It is a creative systematic logically planned framework if problem-solving approach used its very fine elements of nursing, and systems theory to provide a holistic comprehensive nursing care to the clients family and community to maximize clients capability on the high level of wellness.

STEPS OF NURSING PROCESS (FIG. 44.1)

- **Assessment:** Collect and examine information about health about health status looking for evidence or abnormal function or risk factors that may contribute to health problems (e.g. smoking). Also look for client's strength.
- **Diagnosis (problem identification):** Analyze data (information) and identify actual and potential problems, which are the basis for the plan of care. You also identify strengths, which are essential to developing all efficient plan or care.
- **Planning:** Here you do four key things—determine immediate priorities which problems need immediate attention? Which ones can wait? Which ones will nursing focus on? Which one requires a multidisciplinary approach?
  - *Establish expected outcomes goals:* Exactly what do you expect the patient or client to accomplish and in what time frame?
  - *Determine interventions:* What interventions (nursing actions) will you prescribe to achieve the outcomes?

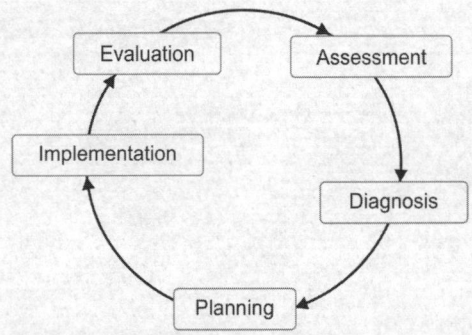

Fig. 44.1: Nursing process of five dynamic interrelated phases.

- ➤ Record or individualize the plan of care: Will you write the own plan or will you adapt a standard plan to meet the patient's specific situation?
- ❖ **Implementation:** Put the plan into action but do not just act. Act thoughtfully:
  - ➤ *Assess the person's current status before acting:* Are there any new problems? Has anything happened that requires an immediate change in the plan?
  - ➤ *Perform the intervention:* Monitoring the person carefully and making changes as needed, without waiting for the formal evaluation period.
  - ➤ *Report and record:* Are there any signs that you must report immediately? What are you going to chart, and where and how are you going to chart it.
  - ➤ *Evaluation:* Determine whether the desired outcomes have been achieved, whether the interventions are effective and whether change need to be made, then change or terminate the plan as needed.

PURPOSES OF THE NURSING PROCESS

- ❖ To provide a systematic methodology for nursing practice.
- ❖ The nurse's roles and functions are defined; communication, collaboration, and synchronization of health team members are enhanced by the nursing process.
- ❖ To identify the healthcare needs, determine priorities, establish goals and expected outcomes of care.
- ❖ Gives direction, guidance, and meaning to nursing care.
- ❖ Provides for continuity of care and reduces omissions.
- ❖ Individualize client participation in care.
- ❖ Promotes creativity and flexibility in nursing practice.
- ❖ Facilitate documentation of data, diagnoses plans.
- ❖ It emphasizes on health promotion, maintenance restoration, or on enhancing a peaceful death depending on client's situation.
- ❖ Evaluate the efficiency and effectiveness of care.

CHARACTERISTICS OF NURSING PROCESS

- ❖ It is goal directed toward client-centered care.
- ❖ It is systematic and provides an organized approach to nursing.
- ❖ It is dynamic by focusing on the changing responses of the client during the ongoing process.
- ❖ It is applicable to individuals, families, and community groups at any level of health.
- ❖ It is adaptable to any practice setting or specialization and the components may be used sequentially.
- ❖ It is interpersonal and based on the nurse–client relationship.

ADVANTAGES OF NURSING PROCESS

- ❖ Provides a theoretical framework to deliver a holistic nursing ease to the client (individual family, community) to solve their problems and to meet their needs.
- ❖ The systems or the nursing process and the well-organized structure helps to focus the nurses attention to identify the problems needs, and the human responses systematically to plan a comprehensive nursing care to meet the needs and to solve the problems.
- ❖ The systems are well organized in such a way to plan and deliver the nursing care so constructively efficiently to avoid errors in delivering nursing care omission of nursing care or repetition of nursing care.
- ❖ It involves the client family and community participation to plan and deliver, which increases the personal responsibilities for the care.
- ❖ It increases the consumer participation in planning nursing care it promotes satisfaction of the client, family, and the community to achieve the expected outcome constructively.
- ❖ It helps to maximize the client capabilities in health promotion maintenance and restoration.
- ❖ It increases the sense of control for a client, family, or community to know what is happening to whole to achieve the expected outcome, and to based the nursing action as for its condition dislikes and likes.
- ❖ It promotes job satisfaction for nurses as the nursing findings and theories concepts.
- ❖ It helps a nurse to use his/her knowledge intuition (creative thinking) and expertize to plan deliver care dynamically as for the conditions of the patient.
- ❖ It helps in nursing research to promote the quality of nursing care.
- ❖ It helps in reimbursement procedures. It serves as a fundamental formula to plan and deliver efficient nursing care in any situation, and in any healthcare settings.
- ❖ It helps in training and supervision of new nursing personnel.
- ❖ It promotes fundamental philosophical values of nursing each individual is unique. Each individual has got right for comparison. Each individual needs should be met based on the hierarchy. Thus, it promotes the high level of being of the patient family and community
- ❖ It is essence of any nursing action, nursing process individually unique in nature. It focuses on human responses to maximize the level of well-being.
- ❖ It serves as a unique communication pattern among health professional such as community of care.
- ❖ It serves as a common language to deliver the care by the health professional.
- ❖ It helps to identify the inadequacies, deficiencies, and malpractice in nursing care.
- ❖ It prevents or legalty of nurses and clients, and serves as a legal implications or legal documents.

NURSING ASSESSMENT

Definition

Nursing assessment is the systematic process of gathering verifying and communicating data about a client. This phase of the nursing process consists of the collection of data and its subsequent analysis as a basic for nursing diagnosis

—Bandman and Bandman, 1995

This is first step in a nursing process systematic organized collection or gathering of data are analyzed verified, organized and validated, and documented or communicated to form a patient diagnosis statement provides information on needs and problems of a client, family, and community to formulate nursing intervention to achieve highest level of well-being.

Collect → Analyze → Organize
Verify → Communicate → Document

Assessment provides consumer participation thereby increases the satisfaction. It provides job satisfaction for the nurses improves standard of nursing care omission and repetition of care is avoided.

Types of Assessment

1. *Initial:* Performed within specified admission to a healthcare agency, e.g. nursing admission assessment. Initial identification of normal functions, functional status, and collection of data concerning actual or potential disfunction. Provides a baseline for reference and future comparison.
2. *Focus or ongoing:* It is integrated with the nursing care, e.g. monitoring hourly intake output in ICU. It determines the status of a specific problem during previous assessment.
3. *Emergency:* During any physiologic or psychological crisis, e.g. rapid assessment of airway breathing and circulation during cardiac arrest. Identification of life-threatening situation.
4. *Time-lapsed assessment:* Several months after initial assessment, e.g. reassessment of clients functional health patterns in home care setting. Comparison of client's current status to baseline obtained previously. Detection of changes in all functional health patterns (after an extended period of time has passed).

Assessment Methods

1. *Observation:* It is a conscious deliberate skill to collect the data systematically g% the senses (auditory hearing, visual, olfactory tactility).
2. *Interview method:* It is a systematic communication established between the interviewer and interviewee (client and a nurse) with certain purpose to evaluate counsel to diagnose or to treat. It is of two types:

   1. *Problem-seeking:* To identify the problem and needs of the patient to solve or to plan intervention effectively.
   2. *Problem-solving:* To solve the problem by nursing intervention with the purpose of solving problem have been identified in problem seeking interview by nursing intervention.

❖ *Focus of interview:*
  ➢ *Directive focus:* Means, it trims to focus on specific problems, e.g. needs straight forward or close questions (questionnaire) (do you have pain? Feeling nausea, yes/no).
  ➢ *Non-directive focus:* It focuses on collecting broad intervention by using open-ended questionnaire successful elements in conducting focus:
    ♦ Have a purpose to conduct an focus
    ♦ Have a preliminary research on interviewer (previous history, medical/surgical and gynecology)
    ♦ Fax an appointment for a interview/request an interview schedule (request the client to give a suitable time to conduct information)
    ♦ Have an interview strategy plan the interview time to go ahead to get a plenty of information
    ♦ Have a rapport with the client to make the client trust to get adequate information
    ♦ *Use in breakers:* It is using certain words or phrases or settling a stage that puts the patient very comfortable relaxed to provide information
    ♦ Come to the business try to get the client to focus on to the problems by avoiding diversion and making him/her concentrate on the interviewer
    ♦ *Be sensitive:* While discussing problems regarding sensitive areas, e.g. taking about HIV, be sensitive (out hurting the client) without hurting the client, but to get maximum information out injuring the feelings
    ♦ *Rebuild the confidence:* Allow the client to recover from the sensitive issues have been talked about
    ♦ *Closure of interview:* Close the interview providing adequate time to conclude or to clarify doubts feeling and ideas.

Phases of Interview

Stages/setups of interview process:
❖ Introduction/orientation
❖ Working on phase
❖ Termination.

Phases establishing a rapport to build a trusting relationship between interviewer and interviewee to the progress to the working phase.

Orientation

Where the actual takes place on the purpose of interview explained. This includes purpose objective for interview, preliminary research interview schedule, and interview strategy.

Working on Phase

The actual data collection regarding the clients present problems (actual problem), and high-risk problems (potential problems/coming problems) and identifying the needs for growth to achieve high level of wellness are all collected g% the interview method to formulate nursing diagnosis to plan interventions to achieve outcome.

Termination

Where the terminator concludes the focus allowing the client to provide about the focus and to clarify his/her doubts ask if and sufficient time is provided for open communication to validate the finding or data collection the closure of focus always helps the validation of data.

In interview there are certain types of questions used:

- **Open-ended questions:** Allows the free common of free exchange of information facilitates collection of wider and broader inform and use non-directive technique.
- **Closed-ended questions:** Provides yes/no information unlimited common straight forward answers and highly structured may not be useful for counseling therapeutic common of free exchange of information, e.g. where do you live? What is your name?
- **Neutral questions:** Neutral does not address any specific problems or needs, but facilitates free flow of inform data, e.g. how do you feel? What is your opinion about this?
- **Leading questions:** Usually problems into the matters and problems where the client feels or hesitates to provide adequate inform for the fear of beings revealed or judged. For example, Do not you think that this injection is painful? Do not you know this STD leads into the infertility?
- **Hypothetical questions:** Frames certain situation and plans the client to decide or to react to that situation, e.g. if you work you feel giddy what will you do? To reveal the knowledge of patient. This question helps for the wellness diagnosis or wellness function.
- **Focus questions:** Points out the options available and does not facilitate free exchange of information, e.g. you are placed in a dark room what will you do?
  - Run away
  - Cry
  - Shout

3. *Physical examination/hands on phase and assessment sequencing*

    Systemic collection of data auditory tactile, olfactory, visual senses by auscultation, percussion, palpation, and inspection

    a. **Inspection:** Direct and indirect observation, verbal and nonverbal common auditory, visual senses, and olfactory.
    b. **Palpation:** Using fingertips to assess the contour shape, size, and movement of the body.
    c. **Percussion:** Probing into the internal structures with knee hammer and by finger tips fluid retention gas, retention solid mass, and reflexes.
    d. **Auscultation:** Hearing noticing and perceiving the stimuli, the auditory sense, and tactile.
    e. **Cephalocaudal approach:** Head-to-toe assessment.
    f. **Body system approach:** Examining all the body systems.
    g. **Review of system approach:** Examine only particular area affected.

Laboratory and Diagnostic Methods

Laboratory and diagnostic methods of data come where the laboratory data or the clinical parameter, invasive and noninvasive diagnostic procedures are collected to validate the findings.

Assessment Process

Data collection, data organization, data validation, and data documentation.

Data Collection

Data collection involves the following:

Nursing health history: Includes biographical information reason for seeking healthcare client's expectation present illness, past health history, family history, psychosocial history, spiritual health, and review of systems.

Types of Data

- **Subjective data:** These are client's perceptions about a health problem. What the patient says expresses perceives verbalizes or feels written as per patient words to prevent error misinterpretation, and to promote accuracy and data is otherwise known as symptoms, e.g. I cannot breath, I cannot walk, I feel pain, I feel like vomiting, patient expresses in his/her own words.
- **Objective data:** These are observations made by the data collector. It is measurable data in quantitative and qualitative terms are all the signs confirms or measures the subjective expression or the symptoms of the clients. For example, patient looks dehydrated skin turns or poor pulses feeble 50 per minute confronting the subjective data objective data.
- **Data organization:** Data collected is organized systematically either by using a nursing models such as Orem's self-care model. Roy's adaptation model, etc., or non-nursing models such as body systems model, Maslow's hierarchy of needs development theories, etc.

- ❖ **Data validation:** It is the act of double checking or verifying data to confirm that they are accurate and factual.
- ❖ **Data documentation:** It is the factual and accurate recording of data, e.g. while recording a patient's food intake it would be appropriate to record as had 100 mL of milk and half slice of bread instead of appetite poor or poor intake, and so on.

CONCLUSION

Nursing assessment is the gathering and verification of data about a client to establish a database. The health history, physical examination, and collection of laboratory data are components of assessment. After collecting data, the nurse validates and sorts out the data and groups the data are preperatory steps to formulation of nursing diagnosis.

45 CHAPTER
Nursing Diagnosis

CHAPTER OUTLINE

- Definition
- Use of Nursing Diagnosis
- Diagnostic Process
  - Components of Nursing Diagnosis
  - Types of Nursing Diagnosis
- Nursing Diagnosis and Medical Diagnosis
  - Advantages of Nursing Diagnosis
  - Limitations of Nursing Diagnosis
  - Definitive Statements of Nursing Diagnosis

INTRODUCTION

The second phase of the nursing process is often referred to analysis as well as problem/identification or nursing diagnosis. Problem identification is a process of data analysis using diagnostic reasoning (a form of clinical judgment) in which judgment decisions and conclusions are made about the meaning of the data collected, in order to determine whether or not nursing intervention is indicated.

DEFINITION

A nursing diagnosis is a clinical judgment about individual family or community responses to actual and potential health problems and life processes. Nursing diagnoses provide the basis for selection of nursing interventions to achieve outcomes for which the nurse is accountable.

—**NANDA (1990), Kim (1997)**

USE OF NURSING DIAGNOSIS

The current North American Nursing Diagnosis Association (NANDA) list of diagnostic labels defines or refines professional nursing activity. There are many benefits, which the use of nursing diagnoses can provide:

- Gives nurses a common language
- Promotes identification of appropriate goals
- Provides acuity information
- Can create a standard for nursing practice
- Provides a quality improvement base.

DIAGNOSTIC PROCESS

The diagnostic process includes decision-making steps the nurse uses to develop a diagnostic statement (Carnevali and Thomas, 1993 Liukkonen, 1992). The diagnosis process uses the critical-thinking skills of analysis and synthesis.

Steps of Diagnostic Process

The diagnostic process has three steps:

Analyzing Data

- Compare data against standards
- Cluster data; generate tentative hypotheses
- Identify gaps and inconsistencies
- Identify health problems, risks and strengths
- Formulating diagnostic statements.

Formulation of the Nursing Diagnostic Statement

- ***Patient diagnostic statement:*** Patient diagnostic statement is a collection of systematically gathered information obtained by observation history taking interview and by physical laboratory diagnostic examination. The basic format for a diagnostic statement is 'problem related to etiology'. However nurses must be able to write one-, two-, three-, and four- part diagnostic statement as well as some variations of each.
- ***One-part statements:*** Some diagnostic statements such as wellness diagnoses and syndrome nursing diagnoses consist of a NANDA label only. As the diagnostic labels are refined, they tend to become specific, so that nursing. Interventions can be derived from the label itself. Therefore, an etiology is not needed. e.g. there are currently one-part NANDA labels reflecting healthy functioning:
  - Rape trauma syndrome, post-trauma response and defensive coping
  - Family coping

- Potential for growth
- Effective breastfeeding
- Anticipatory grieving.

NANDA has specified that any new wellness diagnosis will be developed as a one-part statement beginning with the words potential for enhanced followed by the desired higher level wellness.

❖ **Wellness (one-part statement and positive statements):**
- Improvement in coping
- Improvement in parenting
- Effective breastfeeding
- Positive self-concept
- Positive self-esteem
- Positive coping

Enhance improve positive avoid negative words.

❖ **Basic two-part statement:** The basic two-part statement is used for actual, high-risk and possible nursing diagnosis. It includes the following:
- *Problem (P):* Statement of the client's response.
- *Etiology (E):* Factors contributing to or probable causes of the responses.

The two parts joined by the words related to or associated with rather than due to problem or etiology, for example, noncompliance (diabetic diet) related to denial of having disease, High risk for impaired integrity, High risk for skin impairment related to immobility.

❖ **Basic three-part statement:** The basic three-part statement is called problem, etiology, signs and symptoms (PES) format and include:
- *Problem (P):* Statement of client's response.
- *Etiology (E):* Factors contributing or probable cause of the response.
- *Signs and symptoms (S):* Defining characteristics manifested by the client.

The three-part diagnostic statement includes the problem, the etiology, and the observed signs and symptoms. Actual nursing diagnoses can be documented by using the three-part statement (using related to and as evidence by or as manifested by) because the signs and symptoms have been identified. This format cannot be used for high-risk diagnoses, because the client does not have signs and symptoms of the diagnoses.

For example, self-esteem disturbance related to rejection by husband as manifested by hypersensitivity to criticism; states, I do not know if can manage by myself'. Disadvantage of this method is that it can create very long problem statements.

Four-part statement: Impaired skin integrity, sacral pressure, sore occipital, pressure sore (more than etiology) are the fourth parts very specific to the problem. E.g. impaired skin integrity sacral pressure sore due to immobility secondary to traction accident or cerebrovascular accident (CVA) or cause or labor pain.

Variations of Basic Formats

Variations of the basic one-, two- and three-part statements include the following:

❖ **Writing 'unknown etiology':** When the defining characteristics are present, but the nurse does not know the cause of the contributing factors. e.g. noncompliance (medication regimen) related to unknown etiology.

❖ **Using the phrase 'complex factors':** When there are several etiological factors or when they are too complex to state in a brief phrase. e.g. decisional conflict and chronic low self-esteem related to complex factors.

❖ Using 'possible' to describe either the problem or the etiology. When the nurse believes more data is required about the client's response (problem) or the etiology, the possible is inserted. For example, possible low self-esteem related to loss of job and rejection by family; altered thought processes possibly related to unfamiliar surroundings and possible low self-esteem related to unknown etiology.

❖ Using 'secondary to' divide the etiology into two parts thereby making the statement more descriptive and useful. The part following 'secondary to' is often a path physiologic or disease process as in high risk for impaired skin integrity related to decreased peripheral circulation secondary to diabetes.

❖ Adding a second part to the general response or NANDA label to make it more precise, e.g. the diagnosis impaired physical mobility does not indicate the degree of mobility impairment. To make this label more specific the nurse can add as shown below:

Problem + Descriptor → Related to → Etiology

❖ Impaired physical ability to walk related to knee joint stiffness and pain secondary to muscle atrophy.

❖ Four-part statements are combinations of basic statements and variations four and five are discussed above. For example, the nurse creates a four-part statement by using both variations four and five with a basic two-part statement, as in:
- High-risk for impaired skin integrity
- Pressure sores related
- Immobility
- Secondary to presence of casts and traction.

A four part statement is also created by using the basic three-part statement PES format and adding either variation four or five, for example:
1. Impaired skin integrity.
2. Pressure sore on left heel related.
3. Immobility.
4. A manifested by 2 × 2 cm red excoriated area on the left heel inability to move about in bed.

Collaborative Problems

Some nurse also distinguish between nursing diagnosis, which he/she nurse treats independent and those which the nurse treats collaboratively (jointly shared with the physician). Many nursing diagnoses have both an independent aspect and a collaborative aspect. e.g. there are many measures the nurse may independently use to assist the patient in pain (massage, relaxation techniques) although it is usually a physician prerogative to order a medication. Carpentio (1993) suggested that all collaborative problems begin with the diagnostic label potential complication (PC). For ego potential complication of head injury increased intracranial pressure.

Components of Nursing Diagnosis

A nursing diagnosis has three components:
1. Problem statement.
2. Etiology.
3. Defining characteristics.

Each of these components serves a specific purpose.

Problem Statement (Diagnostic Label)

Describes the client's health problem or response for which nursing therapy is given. It describes the client health status clearly and concisely in a few words. To be clinically useful, diagnostic labels need to be specific; for ego knowledge deficit (medications) or knowledge deficit (dietary adjustment).

Qualifiers are words that have been added to some NANDA labels to give additional meaning to the diagnostic statement:
- Altered (a change from baseline)
- Impaired (made worse, weakened, damaged, reduced, deteriorated)
- Decreased (smaller in size, amount or degree)
- Ineffective (not producing the desired effect)
- Acute (severe or of short duration)
- Chronic (lasting a long time recurring or constant).

Etiology (Related Factors and Risk Factors)

The etiology component of the nursing diagnosis identifies one or more probable causes of the health problem. Etiology may include client's behaviors, environmental factors or interactions of the two.

Defining Characteristics

Defining characteristics are the clusters of signs and symptoms that indicate the presence of a particular diagnostic label.

Major defining characteristics are those that must be present for the diagnosis to be valid.

Minor characteristics may or may not be present. For example, for a nurse to make a diagnosis of activity intolerance, the client would need to exhibit the defining characteristic of 'altered response to activity', which might manifest as dyspnea, shortness of breath, tachypnea or any one of the major symptoms. For most nursing diagnoses, the list of defining characteristics is still being developed and refined.

Types of Nursing Diagnoses

NANDA has identified five types of nursing diagnoses:
1. ***Actual nursing diagnosis:*** An actual nursing diagnosis is a judgment about a client response to a health problem that is present at the time of the nursing assessment. An actual nursing is based on the presence of associate signs and symptoms, e.g. ineffective breathing pattern and anxiety.
2. ***Risk nursing diagnosis:*** A high-risk nursing diagnosis is defined by NANDA is a clinical judgment that a client is more vulnerable to develop the problem than others in the same or similar situation. Identification and analyzing of data in assessment phase indicated the potential or risk problem or needs of an client he/she would be facing in the future or will be subjected in the future and not get manifestated, e.g. high risk for infection to describe the client's health status.
3. ***Possible nursing diagnosis:*** It describes a suspected problem for which current and available data are insufficient to validate the problem. This type of nursing diagnosis such as fluid volume deficit has relevance in that the nurse is directed to gather further data and relevant cue to confirm or eliminate the diagnosis.
4. ***Syndrome nursing diagnosis:*** It is a diagnostic label given to distinct cluster of nursing diagnoses that frequently go together and present a clinical picture (NANDA, 1999). This type of diagnosis a useful and efficient way to describe a complex problem without documenting each component of the problem as a distinct nursing diagnosis, e.g. rape trauma syndrome.
5. ***Wellness nursing diagnosis:*** It is a clinical Judgment about an individual group or community in transition from a specific level of wellness to a higher level of wellness (NANDA, 1999). This type of diagnosis is used when the client wishes to achieve an optimal level of health, e.g. family coping potential for growth related to unexpected birth of twins.

Nursing diagnostic errors can be prevented by:
- ***Using concise wording:***
  - Identify the client's response, not the medical diagnosis.
  - Identify a treatable etiology rather than a clinical sign or chronic problem.
  - Identify the problem caused by the treatment or diagnostic study rather than the treatment or the study itself.
  - Identify the client response to the equipment rather than the equipment itself.
  - Identify the client's problems rather than the nurse's problems.
  - Identify the client problem rather than the nursing intervention.

- Identify the client problem rather than the goal.
- Make professional rather than prejudicial/judgment.
- Avoid legally inadvisable statements.
- Identify the problem and etiology.

In addition, there are three incorrect ways to state the diagnostic label:
1. Statement of nursing diagnoses as medical diagnoses.
2. Use of medical terminology to describe the cause.
3. Statement of the nursing diagnosis as an intervention. These are errors because they shift the focus from the cause to the intervention. As expertise with the diagnostic process is gained, the likelihood of errors is reduced, and the nurse is able to develop nursing diagnoses based on the actual or potential nursing needs of the client. Errors in the diagnostic process result in the development of an incomplete or inappropriate nursing care plan.

NURSING DIAGNOSIS AND MEDICAL DIAGNOSIS

- Nursing diagnosis focuses on and defines the nursing needs of the client (Gordon, 1994).
- The medical focus is on the diagnosis and treatment of the disease.
- Nursing database is global and include in-depth assessment of the physiological, psychological, sociocultural, developmental and spiritual dimensions of the client.
- Medicines database includes the physiological systems and the personal and social system. The personal and social system may be limited to a family medical history and economic, and insurance history of the client (Gordon, 1994).
- The goals and objectives of a nursing diagnosis differ from those of a medical diagnosis.
- The goal of a nursing diagnosis is to direct a plan of care to assist clients and their families to adapt to their illness and to resolve healthcare problems. The goals of a medical diagnosis are to identify and to design a treatment plan for curing the disease or the pathological process.
- The objective of a nursing diagnosis is development of an individualized plan of care so that the client and family are able to cope with changes, and to meet the challenges resulting from health problem. The objective of the medical diagnosis is to prescribe treatment.

Advantages of Nursing Diagnoses
- Nursing diagnose facilitate communication.
- Nursing diagnoses are also used for charting in the progress notes.
- Nursing diagnose can also serve as a focus for quality improvement (Gordon, 1994).
- Nursing diagnosis helps to identify the problems and also helps to identify the high risk or potential (HRP).
- Nursing diagnosis aims for preventive, promotive and rehabilitative aspects by focusing on wellness diagnosis.
- Nursing diagnosis identifies the future problems needs of the client family and community to plan intervention ahead of time.
- It serves as a common language among healthcare professionals.
- It helps to identifies the deficiencies weakness, strength involves to identify the problems promotes clinical research to update the quality of nursing and standard of nursing profession.
- Serves as a continuity of care media.
- Cost effective helps to plan for nursing hours and deligation of responsibility.
- It promotes consumers satisfaction or client satisfaction.

Limitations of Nursing Diagnoses
The continuous evolution of terms and use of nursing diagnoses, the language can occasionally be verbose and contain jargon. This may limit the use of nursing diagnoses to only nursing professionals and result in confusion among other members of the healthcare team. Imprecise language of the diagnosis may incorrectly 'label' a client. The evolving taxonomy can limit nursing practice.

NANDA—Approved Diagnoses New and Revised 2003–2004

New to the 15th Conference
- Communication, readiness for enhanced
- Coping, readiness for enhanced
- Family processes, readiness for enhanced
- Fluid balance, readiness for enhanced
- Knowledge (specify), readiness for enhanced
- Nutrition, readiness for enhanced
- Parenting, readiness for enhanced
- Self-concept, readiness for enhanced
- Sleep readiness, for enhanced
- Sudden infant death syndrome, risk
- Urinary elimination, readiness for enhanced.

Revisions from the 15th conference
- Spiritual distress
- Spiritual well-being readiness for enhanced.

1. ***Communication, readiness for enhanced:*** A pattern of exchanging information and ideas with others that is sufficient for meeting one's needs and life's goals can be strengthened.
2. ***Coping, readiness for enhanced:*** A pattern of cognitive and behavioral efforts to manage demands that is sufficient for well-being and can be strengthened.
3. ***Family processes, readiness for enhanced:*** A pattern of family functioning that is sufficient to support the well-being of family members can be strengthened.

4. ***Fluid balance, readiness for enhanced:*** A pattern of equilibrium between fluid volume and chemical composition of body fluids that is sufficient for meeting physical needs can be strengthened.
5. ***Knowledge of (specify), readiness for enhanced:*** The presence or acquisition of cognitive information related to a specific topic is sufficient for meeting health-related goals and can be strengthened a pattern of nutrient intake that is sufficient for meeting metabolic needs can be strengthened.
6. ***Parenting, readiness for enhanced:*** A pattern of providing an environment for children or other dependent person(s) that is sufficient to nurture growth and development can be strengthened.
7. ***Self-concept, readiness for enhanced:*** A pattern of perceptions or ideas about the self that is sufficient for well-being can be strengthened.
8. ***Sleep, readiness for enhanced:*** A pattern of natural, periodic suspension of consciousness that provides adequate rest, sustains a desired lifestyle can be strengthened.
9. ***Sudden infant death syndrome, risk:*** The presence of risk factors for sudden death of an infant under 1 year of age.
10. ***Therapeutic regimen management, readiness for enhanced:*** A pattern of regulating and integrating into daily living a program(s) for treatment of illness and its sequelae that is sufficient for meeting health-related goals can be strengthened.
11. ***Urinary elimination, readiness for enhanced:*** A pattern of urinary functions that is sufficient for meeting eliminatory needs can be strengthened.

Revisions from the 15th Conference

- ***Spiritual distress:*** Impaired ability to experience and integrate meaning and purpose in life through a person's connectedness with self, others, art, music, literature, nature, or a power greater than oneself.
- ***Spiritual well-being, readiness for enhanced:*** Ability to experience and integrate meaning, and purpose of life through a person's connectedness with self, others art, music literature, nature of a power greater than oneself.

CONCLUSION

Nursing diagnosis is organized based on the priority of the client's needs. There is a standard format for making nursing diagnostic statements laid down by NANDA. Formulation of nursing diagnosis is related to the problem and etiology of the disease and the defining characteristics of the client.

46 CHAPTER

Planning

CHAPTER OUTLINE

- Purpose
- Types of Planning
- Elements of Planning
  - Establishing Client Goals
  - Expected Outcomes

INTRODUCTION

Planning is one of the important step of nursing process. It is very essential component in order to make short term or long term goals and interventions in caring patient needs based on priority.

DEFINITION

Planning is the third step in nursing process in logical systematic organized decision-making process of designing an orderly, detailed program of action to accomplish specific goals and objective.

Marriner has given an equation of planning, that is:

Planning = Setting priorities + Goals + Interventions

PURPOSE

The purpose of planning phase is:
- To determine how to satisfy client needs.
- To prescribe the specific action necessary to meet them.
- Serves to guide the activities of all health workers who are involved in the patients care.

TYPES OF PLANNING

Planning begins with the first client contact and continues until the nurse–client relationship ends, usually when the client is discharged from the healthcare agency.

Initial Planning

The nurse who performs the admission assessment usually develops the initial comprehensive plan of care. Planning should be initiated as soon as possible after the initial assessment especially because of the trend toward hospital stays.

Ongoing Planning

Ongoing planning is done by all nurses who work with the clients more to obtain new information and evaluate the clients' response to care; they can individualize the initial care plan even more.

Discharge Planning

Discharge planning is the process of anticipating and planning for needs after discharge as it has become a crucial part of comprehensive healthcare and should be addressed in each client's care plan.

ELEMENTS OF PLANNING

The elements in planning are as follows:
- Priority setting
- Establishing described patient outcomes
- Selecting nursing interventions
- Writing nursing order
- Communicating the nursing care plan.

Fundamental Principles of Setting Priorities

- Choose a method of assigning priorities and use it consistently, e.g. Maslow's hierarchy of needs.
- Assign a high priority to problems that are contributing factors to other problems.
- The person's perception of priorities.
- The whole picture of problems at hand.
- The person's overall health status and expected discharge outcomes.
- The expected length of stay.
- How standard plans (e.g. critical pathways, guidelines, protocols, procedures, and standards of care) apply to the person's situation.

Applying Nursing Standards

There are guidelines and standards that you must apply to develop the plan. These standards are determined by the following:

- ❖ **The law:** Your state's nurse practice act delineates the scope or nursing practice.
- ❖ The American Nurses Association (ANA).
- ❖ The Canadian Nurses Association (CNA).
- ❖ Specialty professional organizations such as the Emergency Nurses Association and the Critical Care Nurses Association develop standards for specialty practice.
- ❖ The Joint Commission of Accreditation of Healthcare Organizations (JCAHO).
- ❖ The Agency for Healthcare Policy and Research (AHCPR).
- ❖ **The facility where you work:** Each facility usually develops its own unique set of standards (standards of care, guidelines, policies, procedures, critical pathways, standard care plans, and so forth).

Establishing Client Goals/Expected Outcomes

Before delivering any form of nursing care, the nurse must decide what the endpoint of nursing care should be for the client goals, and expected outcomes are specific statements used to indicate anticipated client behavior or response from nursing care.

Definition of Goals

Bulechek and McCloskey define goals has guideposts to the selection of nursing intervention and criteria in the evaluation of nursing intervention are derived from the problem, statement of the nursing diagnosis.

Subject

Who does it

Content Area and Time

The time element answer when, how long, (or) how often the nursing action is to occur, for example, assist client with tub bath at 7 am daily.

Signature

The signature of the nurse prescribing the orders shows the nurse's accountability and has legal significance, for example, (today's date) assist Rao to stand by the side of the bed for 10 minutes twice a day wearing the back brace.

Communicating the Nursing Care Plan

Because the nursing staff is constantly changing, it is important to have written guidelines to promote continuity of patient care.

Steps in Planning

Planning solution to patient problem involves the following steps:
1. Set priorities
2. Research the problem
3. Analyze the patient and the total situation
4. Establish the nursing prognoses
5. Develop goals and expected patient outcome
6. Set deadlines
7. Formulate a plan of action
8. Validating the plan of care
9. Ongoing data collection
10. Documentation.

Format for Care Plans

Although formats differ from agency to agency, the plan is generally organized into five columns or categories:
1. Nursing assessment
2. Nursing diagnosis (or) problem list
3. Planning—goals and expected outcome, nursing interventions
4. Implementation
5. Evaluation.

Advantages

- ❖ Provides a highly client-centered care
- ❖ Follows that all the fundamental philosophical beliefs in nursing are cost oriented
- ❖ Improve standard of nursing care
- ❖ Helps in supervision training accreditation, reimbursement procedures, and the workload of the nurses
- ❖ Helps in patients' classification system
- ❖ Helps to improve nursing practice
- ❖ Provides job satisfaction for nurses
- ❖ Repetition of care is avoided
- ❖ Erosion and malpractice are prevented
- ❖ Helps the nurse to be accountable for the practice
- ❖ Helps in continuity of care.

Selecting Nursing Strategies

Nursing interventions strategies or actions are selected after goals and expected outcomes are established. Nursing strategies or interventions are nursing activities relating to a specific nursing diagnosis that a nurse carries out to achieve client goals.

There are three types of nursing strategies. These are as follows:
1. Independent intervention/nurse-initiated interventions.
2. Dependent intervention/physician-initiated interventions.
3. Collaboration intervention/interdependent interventions.

Guidelines: Determining Nursing Orders

- Determine a baseline of current signs and symptoms of the problem.
- Check the medical orders for nursing interventions related to the problem.
- Use standard plans (e.g. critical path, preprinted plan, and protocol).
- Identify monitoring regimens for potential complications.
- Identify interventions that prevent or minimize the underlying cause(s) of the problem and help achieve the expected outcome.
- If you cannot do anything about the cause, think something to solve the problem.
- Be sure the interventions are congruent with other therapies.
- Consider the person's preferences individualize as much as possible.
- Determine the scientific rationale for planned anions.
- Create opportunities for teaching (e.g. explain rationale for all actions).
- Consult with other professionals when indicated.
- Make your order specific, for example, auscultate lung every 4 hours.

Writing Nursing Orders

Definition

Nursing orders are instructions for the specific activities the nurse performs to help the Diem to meet established healthcare goals. The term order cannot provide a sense of accountability for the nurse who gives the order and for the nurse who carries it out.

Components of a Nursing Order

- **Date:** Nursing orders are dated when they are written and required regularly at intervals that depend on the individual needs.
- **Action verb:** The verbs start the order and needs to be precise.
- **Nonmeasurable verb (do not use)**
  - Know
  - Understand
  - Appreciate
  - Think
  - Accept
  - Feel
  - Learn
  - Observe
- **Conditions/Modifiers:** Conditions/Modifiers may be added to the verb to explain the circumstance under which the behavior is to be performed; they explain what, where, when (how), for example, walks with the help of walker (how).
- **Criteria of desired performance:** The criteria indicates a standard by which a performance is evaluated (or) the level at which the client will perform the specified behavior. These criteria may specify time (or) speed, accuracy, distance, and quality, for example, weighs 15 kg, by April (mine). Lists five out of six signs of diabetes (accuracy).

Target time: When is the person expected to perform the action?

Steps for Deriving Outcomes from Nursing Diagnoses

- Look at the first clause of the nursing diagnosis or problem statement (the word or words before "related"), e.g. risks for impaired skin integrity related to immobility.
- Now restate the first clause in a statement that describes improvement, control, or absence of the problem, e.g. the person will demonstrate no signs of skin irritation or breakdown.

Outcomes are classified into three domains:

1. **Affective domain:** Outcomes associated with change in attitudes, feelings, or values (e.g. deciding old eating habit need to be changed).
2. **Cognitive domain:** Outcomes dealing with acquired knowledge, intellectual skill, e.g. learning the signs and symptoms (if diabetic shock).
3. **Psychomotor domain:** Outcomes dealing with developing motor skills (e.g. mastering how to walk with crutches).

Definition of Outcomes

An expected outcome is the specific step-by-step objective that leads to attainment of the goal and the resolution of the etiology for the nursing diagnosis. An outcome is a measurable change of the client status in response to nursing care and it includes observable client behavior. Several expected outcomes are usually developed for each goal and nursing diagnosis.

Purpose of Goals/Expected Outcomes

- Provide direction for planning nursing interventions that will achieve the desired changes in the client.
- Provide a time span for planned activities.
- To set standards of determining the effectiveness of the intervention.
- Serves as criteria for evaluation of client progress.
- Enable the client and nurse to determine when the problem has been resolved.

- ❖ It helps to motivate the client and nurse by providing a sense of achievement.

Components of Goal/Expected Outcome Statements

To be clear and specific, outcomes must have the following components:
- ❖ **Subject:** The subject, a noun, is the client, any part of the client, (or) some attributes of the client.
- ❖ **Verb:** The verb denotes an action the client is to perform. e.g. measurable verbs (use these to be specific) as shown in Box 46.1.

CONCLUSION

Planning is an important step of nursing process. Planning involves the client's knowledge, abilities of the client, beliefs, and attitude to carry out particular action and prioritizing the needs based on all the plan of action is prepared by the nurse with short-term or long-term goals and expected outcomes.

Box 46.1: Specific measurable verbs used to state goals/expected outcome.

- Apply
- Breathe
- Choose
- Communicate
- Compare
- Construct
- Defend
- Describe
- Design
- Move
- Turn
- List
- Take
- Arrange
- Differentiate
- Discuss
- Drink
- Explain
- Express
- Help
- Identify
- Inject
- Justify
- List
- Name
- Prepare
- Report
- Select
- Share
- Show
- Sit
- Sleep
- State
- Talk
- Transfer
- Verbalize
- Use
- Walk

Chapter 47: Formulation of Nursing Care Plans, Health Goals, Implementation, Modification, and Evaluation of Care

CHAPTER OUTLINE

- Formulation of Nursing Care Plans
- Implementation
- Evaluation
- Documentation

FORMULATION OF NURSING CARE PLANS

Developing Nursing Care Plan

The nursing care plan is a written guide that organizes information about a client's care into a meaningful whole. It includes the actions nurses must take to address the client's diagnosis and meet the standard goals.

Purposes of a Written Care Plan

- To provide directing for individualized care of the client
- To provide for continuity of care
- To provide direction about what needs to be documented on the client's progress notes
- To serve as a guide for assessing staff to care for the client and can make necessary judgments about the client's responses

Writing a Nursing Plan of Care

A nursing plan of care documents the problem-solving process. The ability to create the nursing plan of care has become a standard expected of every nurse. The plan is a critical element in focusing nursing activity. To serve as evaluation criteria and meet the standards of the Joint Commission for Accreditation of Healthcare Organizations (JCAHO), 1996, the plan must be developed by a registered nurse, must be documented in the client's health record, and must reflect the standards of care established by the institution and the profession. Two important concepts that guide a nursing plan of care are as follows:

- The plan of care is nursing centered.
- The plan of care is a step-by-step process.

Keeping the plan of care, nursing centered is essential to identify the scope and depth of nursing practice. By focusing on the treatment of human resources to actual or potential health problems, the nurse remains in the nursing practice domains. A step-by-step process is evidenced by the following. Sufficient data are collected to substantiate nursing diagnoses. At least one goal must be stated for each nursing diagnosis. Outcome criteria must be identified for each goal. Nursing interventions must be specifically designed to meet the identified goal. Each intervention should be supported by a scientific rationale. Evaluation must address whether each goal was completely met, partially met, or completely met.

Guidelines for Writing Nursing Care Plans

- Date and sign of the plan.
- Use the category headings:
  - Nursing diagnosis
  - Goals/outcome criteria
  - Nursing orders
  - Evaluation, and include a date for the evaluation of each goal.
- Use standardized medical or English symbols and keywords rather than complete sentences to communicate your ideas.
- Refer to procedure books or other sources of information rather than including all the steps on a written plan.
- Tailor the plan to the unique characteristics of the client by ensuring that the client's choices, such as preferences about the time of care and the methods used, are included. This reinforces the client's individuality and sense of control.
- Ensure that the nursing plan incorporates preventive and health maintenance aspects as well as restorative.
- Ensure that the plan contains orders for ongoing assessment of the client.
- Include collaborative and coordination activities in the plan.
- Include plans for the client's discharge and home care needs.

Types of Nursing Care Plans

As you care people in various healthcare facilities, you will discover a variety of nursing care plan formats. The documentation of the plan of care is also changing as federal, state, and accrediting agencies examine and modify their standards. It can be written in various ways. The most common formats for care plans include student nursing care plan, individually developed nursing care plan, practice guidelines, critical path or case management plans, and computerized nursing care plans.

Student Nursing Care Plans

Each school of nursing has a care plan format adopted by or developed by the faculty for students use. Because student plans are used as learning tools, they are usually more comprehensive and detailed than the care plans utilized by graduate staff nurses. Student care plans focus heavily on documenting signs and symptoms, and proving the rationale for specific nursing interventions. This information is no less important to the graduate nurse. However, the experienced nurse is capable of high-level assessment and synthesis of data, which are still step-by-step for the student. The components usually include nursing diagnoses, client goals, outcome criteria, nursing interventions, scientific rationale, and evaluation.

Individually Developed Nursing Care Plans

The individually developed nursing care plan is the most traditional and oldest method of documenting the plan of care. It typically consists of three columns, which are labeled according to the setting as nursing diagnoses or problems, outcomes or goals, and nursing interventions or orders. Additional columns may be added to the format to include a spot for the date and initials of the nurse who developed the plan, the date for the outcome achievement and the date of nursing diagnosis was resolved. Individual care plans are intended to focus on the specific needs of the person and are to be updated as the person's condition changes. The individually developed nursing care plan, like the other formats for the plan of care, is usually combined with a Kardex. A Kardex is an abbreviated form that contains the following:

- Basic demographic information about the person, such as name, age, sex, medical diagnoses, surgical procedures, and physician's name.
- Basic care information, such as type of bath, frequency of vital signs, allowable activity, ordered treatments, and so on.
- *Advantages:* The advantages of individually developed nursing care plans include their specificity to a particular person. They contain only the pertinent nursing diagnoses, outcomes, and interventions.
- *Disadvantages:* The primary disadvantage of this is the time-consuming aspect of the development process.

Also, as is true with other formats for care plans, the individually developed nursing care plan may not accurately reflect the person's current problems if it has not been updated.

Standardized Nursing Care Plans

Printed care plans, known as standardized care plans, are developed commercially or by an individual health care facility. They direct nursing care for people with specific medical diagnoses (e.g. myocardial infarction) with certain nursing diagnoses such as pain or anxiety, or who are undergoing special procedures such as cardiac catheterization. These care plans are typed, preprinted, duplicated, and made available to the appropriate units in the healthcare facility. The format is designed to leave space for the nurse to individualize the care plan by filling in specific related factors associated with nursing diagnosis, adding deadlines to the outcomes, and clarifying the interventions with additional details. For example, the interventions could be individualized by adding frequencies, amounts, times, and the client's preferences.

- *Advantages:* Reduced amount of writing needed to record routine nursing interventions and help to the staff by highlighting necessary interventions. These are usually developed by a group of nurses who use their collective expertise and experience to produce a well-researched tool. Particularly helpful to nurses who may be asked to work in an unfamiliar area.
- *Disadvantages:* Nurses may use these care plans without individualizing them for a particular person. Many of the nursing diagnoses, outcomes, and interventions may not be applicable. These may tend to be long. Frustrated by the amount of time it takes simply to read them, some nurses have not found them to be helpful. This problem can be reduced by developing concise standardized care plans that contain only the essential information.

Teaching Plans

Teaching plans are a specialized form of nursing care plans. Individually developed teaching plans may be handwritten or computer generated for individuals with complex teaching needs. An agency may have a variety of standardized teaching plans prepared for people with commonly seen teaching needs. The nurse modifies the standard teaching plan as needed and uses the form to document the outcome of the teaching.

Practice Guidelines

Practice guidelines also called protocols; specify nursing management of broad clinical issues such as maintenance of skin integrity, phases of hospitalization such as postoperative care, or interdependent clinical issues, e.g. management of a person receiving a certain type of potent medication, such as cardiac medication given intravenously in intensive care units (ICUs). Whereas the standardized care plan or individually developed care plan contains information about a variety of nursing diagnoses, the practice guidelines typically addresses one issue, problem, or nursing diagnosis. Practice guidelines are usually developed by experts and reviewed by a group of nurses for validity. When a practice guideline addresses an interdependent clinical issue that includes both medical and nursing management of a particular concern, physician committee review of the medical orders is usually needed. These plans illustrate the manner in which healthcare professionals collaboratively manage treatment. Practice guidelines are used commonly in short stay areas of a hospital, such as emergency departments and postanesthesia care units. Certain commonalities exist among people in these areas, making it possible to manage their care according to practice guidelines.

Advantages

- They clearly specify well-researched and agreed-upon management of certain problems.
- Once the initial work of developing the practice guideline is completed, their use saves much time by quickly transmitting information that does not need to be documented for each person for whom it is applicable.
- Practice guidelines are not considered standards.

Disadvantages

- The temptation to follow uncritically the interventions without individualizing them for a particular person.
- No prepared plan of care, no matter what its format, replaces the judgment and critical thinking of the nurse.

Case Management Care Plans

Case management is a method of delivering care that has evolved from the emphasis on decreasing the length of stay in hospitals and the focus on achieving timely client outcomes. Case management is designed to organize care to achieve certain specific outcomes within a time frame permitted by the reimbursement system.

The case management plan is a standardized care plan that consists of nursing diagnoses, outcomes, deadlines, nursing interventions, and physician interventions. The plan is developed collaboratively by nurses, physicians, and other healthcare professionals, and is reviewed and individualized for a particular person. The comprehensive case management plan is often summarized in the form of a critical path or patient outcome timeline. Critical paths can improve quality of care by:

Allowing healthcare professionals to share knowledge with each other.

- Educating clients by thoroughly explaining the treatment plan.
  Permitting comparison of outcomes or results of various treatment methods.
- Identifying and reinforcing steps critical to the desired outcome.

Advantages

- Easy to identify appropriate steps in achieving the outcomes.
- Resources of the nursing staff and hospital are used more effectively as they become directed at moving the person through the hospitalization.
- The person is actively involved in reviewing the plan of care.
- Nurses are given more authority to make changes in the system to facilitate the achievement of outcomes.

Disadvantages

- A great deal of planning needed to implement this method of delivering care.
- It may be difficult in some instances to gain the cooperation of physicians in defining how to manage certain types of clients and to collaborate with nurses on a professional level.
- Certain people will have preexisting conditions or complications that will prevent the achievement of outcomes at specified time periods.

Computerized Nursing Care Plans

Many software vendors have developed computerized nursing care plans and critical paths. Computerized plans of care are generated from assessment of data entered into a computer about a specific client. The plan is written by experts in the area and the content is similar to that of standardized plan of care. Once the plan is on the computer screen, the nurse has opportunity to customize it for the client. Computers are increasingly being used to create and store nursing care plan. The computer can generate both standardized and individualized care plans. Nurses access the clients stored care plans from a centrally located terminal at the nurses' station.

Advantages

- Legibility
- Reduction in the amount of time needed to develop and update the plan.
- Access to plans developed by expert clinicians.
- Ability to collect information about groups of patients for research.

Disadvantages

- It requires a critical analysis of a preexisting plan to ensure that it is appropriate and current.
- It is critical that all pertinent information be collected and entered into the system.

Nursing Assessment Format

- History taking
- Biographical information (Box 47.1)

Physical Examination

General Appearance

- Body built, nourishment, etc.
- Vital signs—temperature, pulse and respiration (TPR) and blood pressure (BP), pulse pressure
- Height and weight
- Skin and mucous membrane.

Head-to-Foot Examination

- **Head:** Size, shape, hair color and its distribution, symmetry.
- **Eyes:** Conjunctiva, pupils, equal, round and reactive to light, and accommodation (PERRLA) present/absent.
- **Ears:** Appearance, hearing, etc.
- **Nose:** Lesions, patency, sense of smell, and deviated nasal septum (DNS).
- **Mouth:** Teeth intact, gums, oral ulcers, stomatitis, and glossitis.
- **Neck:** General appearance, any lymph node enlargement, thyroid enlargement, and presence of venous arterial pulsation.
- **Breast:** Symmetry, any lumps, lymph node enlargement, areola, etc.
- **Respiratory system:** Respiration, lung size, lung shape, symmetrical movement, abnormal sounds such as wheeze, stridor, rhonchi, etc.
- **Cardiovascular system:** Chest size and shape, jugular vein pulsations, heart sounds, and heart rate.
- **Abdomen:** Shape, bowel sounds, any distention.
- **Back:** Spine and curvature, lordosis, scoliosis, kyphosis, etc.
- **Genitourinary system:** Bladder pattern, any white discharge, any lesions, prolapse of genital organs.
- **Upper extremities:** Range of motion of limbs, edema.
- **Lower extremities:** Any deformities of lower limbs, muscle strength, plantar reflexes, and knee jerk reflexes.
- **Nervous system:** Conscious, looks drowsy, judgmental ability, speech, sensory, and motor function.
- **Reflexes:** Superficial, deep, and visceral reflexes.

Example of Nursing Care Plan (Table 47.1)

Situation: Mrs. Rama 24 years admitted to hospital with history of stress and anxiety for 4 days. On assessment identified nursing diagnosis according to priority.

IMPLEMENTATION

Definition

Implementation: Put the plan into an action/putting the nursing orders into an action.

"Implementation is the initiation and completion of actions to accomplish the defined goals of the optimal wellness for the client." —**Yura and Walsh**

Implementation initiation and completion of nursing actions to meet the nursing goals and expected outcome or carried out in the implementation prove competencies required for implementation individual competence. The nurse should be competent to carry out.

Legal and Ethical: Nursing actions should be based on legal ethical issues.

Implementation Process

The nurse must adequately and thoroughly prepare before implementing the care plan. This preparation ensures efficient, safe, and effective nursing care. The implementing component as the nursing process has five steps:

1. Reassessing the client
2. Reviewing and revising the existing nursing care
3. Organizing resources and care delivery
4. Anticipating and preventing complications
5. Implementing nursing in interventions.

Evidence-based Practice Model for Implementation

Stetler (2001) has defined evidence-based practice as, "an approach to professional nursing practice that basis relevant decisions and practice strategies on best available evidence, including research finding and as appropriate, other credible verifiable facts on information".

Implementation Methods

- Assisting with activities of daily living (ADL)
- Counseling

Box 47.1: Biographical information format.

Name:
Age:
Sex:
IP No.:
Address:
Religion:
Marital status:
Education:
Occupation:
Income:
Date of admission:
Diagnosis:
Chief complaints:
Present history:
Past history:
Family history:
Psychosocial history:
Nutritional history:
Menstrual history:
Elimination pattern: Bladder and bowel movements
Habits:
Environmental history:

Table 47.1: Sample problem of nursing care plan.

Assessment of subjective/ objective data	Nursing diagnosis	Nursing goals	Expected out come	Plan of action	Scientific rational	Implement action	Evaluation
Subjective: I am awakening in the nights. I am unable to sleep during night **Objective:** Looks dull restless, frequent yawning	Sleep pattern disturbance related to hospital environment, pain, newborn care as evidenced by verbal report of sleeplessness and frequent yawning	Induce sleep	• Rama will achieve an improved sense of adequate sleep for 6 hours in night within 2 days. • Client will verbalize adherence to a regular bed time routine within 2 days	• Determine usual sleep habits and changes that are occurring • Provide comfortable bedding and some of own possessions, e.g. pillow • Establish new sleep routine incorporating old pattern and new environment • Promote bedtime comfort regimes, e.g. warm bath and massage, a glass of warm milk • Teach client to use infant nap time as a time for her also to nap • Advise client to limit visitors and activities	• Assesses need for and identifies appropriate interventions • Increases comfort for sleep as well as provides physical and psychological support • When new routine contains as many aspects of old habits as possible stress and related anxiety may be reduced • Promotes a relaxing, soothing effect. Milk has soporific qualities, enhancing synthesis of serotonin a neurotransmitter that helps patient fall asleep faster and sleep longer • This helps to replenish energy and decreases fatigue • Limiting visitors and activities help to avoid fatigue	• Client verbalized interrupted sleep • Provided comfortable bed • Takes one glass of warm milk before going to bed • Advised Rama to use infant nap time as a time for her also to nap • Advised Rama to limit visitors and activities	Rama reported that slept well for 6 hours last night

Chapter 47: Formulation of Nursing Care Plans, Health Goals, Implementation, Modification, and Evaluation of Care

- Teaching
- Providing direct nursing care
- Delegating, supervising, and evaluating the work of other staff members.

Factors that Inhibit the Process of Implementation
- Lack of essential nursing competencies
- Poor levels of nursing staff
- Unclear or ambiguous job description pertaining to a clinical
- Lack of resources
- Unrealistic expectation from colleagues
- Not being graded or financially reward appropriately for the job
- Conflict with nurse manager
- Being used a junior doctor replacement
- Absence or incomplete protocols for some activities
- Opposition to the advanced nurse practice role by medical staff—feeling threatened, resentful, and nonaccepting of the role.

Steps in Implementation
- Assess the patient need and problems.
- The objectives to be stored in terms of behavior and specific skills.
- Consider the situation and the environment.
- Establish common client.
- Globalization/Common other health professional.
- Consider the likes and dislikes of the client.
- Implement the care.

Advantages
- Consumer satisfaction helps to improve professional standards
- Helps in quality of nursing care
- Helps in research
- Reimbursement procedures
- Categorization of patient
- Nursing hours
- Patient classification
- Continuity of care
- Better utilization of care
- Improves common other health professionals
- Cost-effective

EVALUATION

Definition
Evaluation is a planned systematic process of collecting, organizing, analyzing, and comparing the client's health status with the desired expected outcomes and judging the degree of client achievement of the outcome.
—Janer W Kenney

Purpose of Evaluation
- Is to determine the client's progress in the designated expected outcomes.
- Is to judge the effectiveness of the nursing process components in assisting the client to achieve the expected outcomes.
- Used to determine the overall quality of care given to a group of clients through quality improvement and total management programs.

Evaluating the Quality of Nursing Care
Evaluating the quality of nursing care is an essential part of professional accountability; other terms used for this measurement are quality assessment and quality assurance.
- ***Quality assessment:*** It is an examination of services.
- ***Quality assurance:*** It implies that efforts are made to evaluate and ensure quality health care.

Principles of Evaluation
- Evaluation should be a continuous process.
- Should determine to what extent the objectives of care being met.
- Method of evaluation should be selected on the basis of behavior to be measured.
- Adequacy of expertise should be in terms of acquiring skill and quality of life.
- The patient records should reflex with objectives achievement and give evidence to the extent of achievement of those objectives.

Evaluation Criteria and Standards
The five classic elements of evaluation are as follows:
1. Identifying evaluative criteria and standards what we are looking for when we evaluate, for example, expected patient outcomes.
2. Collecting data to determine whether these criteria and standards are met.
3. Interpreting and summarizing the findings.
4. Documenting our judgment.
5. Terminating continuing or modifying the plan.

Approaches of Quality Evaluation/Forms/Type
1. ***Concurrent Outcome Evaluation***
   Judges the client's present health status skills, knowledge, and abilities before services to the client are discontinued, e.g. the client demonstrates crotch walking correctly, are the client's vital signs stable?
2. ***Retrospective Outcome Evaluation***
   Judges the client's health status and behaviors as documented in the chart after services to the client have been discontinued, for example, was the client able to demonstrate activities of daily living?

Tools and Methods for Measuring Quality Care

Measuring the quality of care is a complex talk, and development of tools involves a series of steps:
- Defining and clarifying the nature of nursing.
- Deciding what approach to take (structure, process, and outcome).
- Developing standards and criteria for ego standard IV each client has written nursing care plan.

Process of Evaluation

The evaluation progress has five components:
- Identifying the outcome criteria that will be used to measure achievement of the goals.
- Gathering data related to the identified criteria.
- Comparing the data collected with the identified criteria and judging whether goals have been attained.
- Relating nursing actions to the outcomes.
- Reexamining the clients care plan.
- Modifying the care plan.

DOCUMENTATION

Definition

Documentation is defined as anything written or printed that is relied on as record of proof for authorized persons. Effective documentation reflects the quality of care and provides evidence of each healthcare team member's accountability in giving care.

Purpose of Documentation

Patient records serve many purposes they are as follows:
- **Communication:** The patient record helps healthcare professionals from different disciplines interact with the patient at different times to communicate with one another.
- **Legal protection:** Accurate documentation provides legal protection and is an important defense in a lawsuit.
- **Reimbursement:** Patient records are also used to demonstrate to payers that patient received the care for which reimbursement is being sought.
- **Patient teaching:** Documentation is a source for determining educational needs of the patient and the patient's response to teaching.
- **Education:** Healthcare professionals and students reading a patient's chart can learn a great deal about the clinical manifestations of particular health problems, effective treatment modalities, and factors that affect patient goal achievement.
- **Quality assurance:** Quality of care is formally measured by quality assurance or quality-improvement programs. Licensing or accrediting organizations conduct audits in which nursing document is investigated to determine if care meets minimum standards and the healthcare organization meets standards of accreditation.
- **Statistics/Research:** Statistical information from client records can help an agency anticipate and plan for people's future needs. For example, the number of births and kinds of illnesses can be obtained from records.

Goal of Documentation

The goal of the documentation systems is to:
- Facilitate the delivery of quality patient care.
- Ensure documentation of progress with regard to patient-focused outcome.
- Facilitate interdisciplinary consistency and communicate the progress of treatment goals.

Characteristics of Quality Documentation

Quality documentation and reporting have five important characteristics. They are as follows:
- **Factual:** This record contains descriptive, objective information about what a nurse sees, hears, feels, and smells, for example, the client seems anxious.
1. **Accurate:** The use of exact measurement ensures that a record is accurate, for example, the nurse makes description, such as intake 860 mL of water rather than client drank an adequate amount of fluid.
2. **Complete:** The entry of reports and record should be appropriate and complete to avoid unnecessary words or irrelevant data.
3. **Current:** To increase accuracy and decrease unnecessary duplication, many healthcare agencies bedside records, which helps immediate documentation of information as it is collected from a client. Activities or findings to communicate at the time of occurrence include the following:
   - Vital signs
   - Administration of medications and treatments
   - Preparation for diagnostic tests or surge
   - Change in status
   - Admission, transfer, discharge, or death of a client
   - Treatment for a sudden change in status
- **Organized:** The nurse communicates information in a logical order.
- **Standards:** Current standards require that all clients who are admitted to healthcare instruction have an assessment of physical psychological environmental self-care client education and discharge planning needs, for example, if a nursing department's standards of practice use nursing diagnosis or a framework.

Formats for Nursing Documentation

1. **Nursing Care Plan**
   Nursing care plans are many types of nursing care plans formulated according the need:
   - *Individualized care plan:* Based on client centered the problems of the written form of common all the forms.

Chapter 47: Formulation of Nursing Care Plans, Health Goals, Implementation, Modification, and Evaluation of Care

- *Computerized nursing care plans (Certain nursing diagnosis):* Certain care plans are computerized and use if for the same condition of the other person account to the human responses.
- *Institutionalized care plans:* Certain institutions formulate the care plan as per their philosophic procedure and policies in certain format, for example, Kardex.
- *Traditional care plan:* These forms have three columns: one for nursing diagnosis, second for expected outcomes, and third for nursing interventions.
- *Standardized care plan:* These have traditional care plans, which are written for each client separately. These plans may be based on institution's standards of practice, thereby helping to provide a high quality of nursing care.

Critical Pathways
The critical pathway is a tool that includes intervention for a client with a specific diagnosis.

2. **Kardex**

The Kardex is a form or card that is kept in a portable flipover file or notebook at the nurses' station. Examples are resulted as follows:
- Patient information about the client such as name, room number, age, religion, marital status, admission date, doctor's name, diagnosis, type of surgery, and date of operation.
- List of medications with the date of order and time of administration to each.
- List of intravenous fluids with dates of infusions.
- List of daily treatment and procedures such as irrigations, dressing changes, postural drainage, or measurement of vital signs.
- List of diagnostic procedure ordered such as roentgenography or laboratory tests.
- Allergies.
- Specific data on how the client's physical needs are to be met such as type of diet assistance needed (use of side rails and so on).
- A problem list stated goals and list of nursing approaches to meet the goals and relieve the problems.

3. **Problem-oriented Medical Records**

The problem-oriented medical record (POMR) is a method of documentation that places emphasis on the client problems. Date organized by problem or diagnosis. Ideally, each member of the healthcare team contributes to a single list of identified client problems. This assists in coordinating a common plan of care. The POMR has the following major sections:
- Date base
- Problem list
- Care plan
- **Progress notes:** In this, there are six methods used to write progress notes, they are as follows:
    - Narrative charting
    - Subjective, objective, assessment, and plan (SOAP) format
    - Problem, intervention, and evaluation (PIE) format
    - Flowsheets
    - Focus charting [data, action, and response (DAR)]
    - Charting by exception

Narrative Charting
Narrative charting is a description of information; chronological charting records data in sequence as time moves forward.

Example: Flowsheets, checklist.

Disadvantage: It is difficult for a reader to find all the data about a specific problem without examining all of the recorded information.

SOAP Format
- SOAP format is used for subjective data, objective data, assessment, and planning.
- The acronyms SOAPIE and SOAPIER refer to formats that adds implementation evaluation and revision.
- A more recent format is the assessment, plan, implementation, and evaluation (APIE).

PIE Charting
The PIE charting model is originated from the nursing process and is similar to the SOAP charting. This system consists of client care assessment flowsheet and progress notes.

Focus Charting or DAR
With this method of documentation, the nurse identifies a "focus" based on client concerns or behaviors determined during the assessment. For example, a current client concern or behavior such as decreased urine output.

In flow charting, the assessment of client's status, the intervention carried out, and the impact of interventions on client outcomes are organized under the heading of data, action, and response.
- **D—d**ata both subjective and objective. Subjective or objective information that supports the stated focus or describes the client status at the time of a significant event or intervention.
- **A—a**ction or nursing intervention. Completed or planned nursing interventions based on the nurse's assessment of the client's status.
- **R—r**esponse of the client (i.e. evaluation of effectiveness). Description of the impact of the interventions on client outcomes.

Flowsheets
The flowsheet, a graphic record is used as a quick way to reflex the client's condition. Flowsheets commonly used are as follows:

- Clinical records, for example, body temperature, pulse, and respiration.
- A 24-hour fluid balance record, for example, intake and output chart.
- Medication record, for example, order, expiration date, medication name and doses, etc.
- Daily nursing care record, for example, nursing care plan.

Charting by Exception

Charting by exception is an innovative approach used to streamline documentation. It is a short-hand method for documentation normal findings and routine care based on clearly defined standards of practice and predetermined criteria for nursing of assessment and intervention. For example:
- Admission sheet—specific demographic data.
- Physician order sheet—date, time, and medications.
- Nurses admission assessment—summary of nursing history and physical examination.
- Graphic sheet and flowsheet—record of repeated observation.
- Medical history examinations—results of initial examination.
- Nurses notes—nursing process.
- Medication records administration—accurate documentation all medications to client such as date, time, and dose.
- Physician progress notes—ongoing record of client's progress responses to medical therapy.
- Healthcare discipline's record—summary of client's condition.
- Discharge summary—summary of clients condition, prognosis, rehabilitation, and teaching needs.

Case Management

The case management model of delivering care incorporates a multidisciplinary approach to documenting client care.

CONCLUSION

Although identifying a correct nursing diagnosis requires time to analyze the gathered data and to validate the diagnostic. It is the pivotal part of the nursing process. The time taken to formulate a patient's statement and to plan care results in increased nursing efficiency better use of time for all nursing staff and delivery of appropriate. Documentation of patient care communicates and reflects the individualization of care we provide. Documentation promotes continuity of patient care among the varied healthcare providers and serves as a basis for the evaluation of the care provided. Medical record is a legal document and requires informing describing the care that is delivered to a client.

CHAPTER 48: Theory Application in Nursing Process

CHAPTER OUTLINE

- Application of Nursing Theory into Practice
- Jonson's Behavioral System and Nursing Process
  - Nursing Assessment and Integration of Model Concepts and Nursing Diagnosis
- Application of Theory
  - Planning and Implementation
  - Evaluation

APPLICATION OF NURSING THEORY INTO PRACTICE

"Application of nursing theory into practice" by using Dorothy E Johnson "behavioral system model." Johnson first proposed her model in 1968 to foster the "efficient and effective behavioral functioning in the patient to prevent illness".

In 1980, Johnson published her behavioral system model in "conceptual models for nursing practice".

In Johnson's model, the person is viewed, as a behavioral system comprises of set of organized, interactive, independent, and integrated subsystems. The seven subsystems Johnson identifies as carrying out special functions are the affiliative, dependency, ingestive, eliminative, sexual, aggressive, and achievement subsystem.

According to Johnson, each behavioral subsystem has structural requirements (goal, predisposition to act, scope or action, and behavior) and functional requirements (protection from harmful influences, nurturance, and stimulation to enhance growth and/or event stagnation). The goal of nursing intervention is to restore, maintain, or attain behavioral system balance and stability at the highest possible level of the individual.

JOHNSON'S BEHAVIORAL SYSTEM AND THE NURSING PROCESS

This model easily fits the nursing process model. Grubbs (1980) developed an assessment tool on Johnson seven subsystems, plus a subsystem is labeled as restorative which focus on activities of daily living (ADL). Considering this, Mr. X assessment of subsystems presenting health problems require assistance from the nurse, e.g. a patient who had fractured neck and was admitted for the treatment, applying Dorothy E Johnson's behavioral system model.

ASSESSMENT: Nurse collects the base line data from his family, which includes Mr. X, age: 20 years, education: 10th Std., poor socioeconomic status. Marital status: unmarried.

- ❖ **Stressors:**
  Internal: Fractured neck, situational crisis.
  External: Low income, lack of support from the family members.

The problem of the patient is assessed according to seven subsystems of the theory (Fig. 48.1).

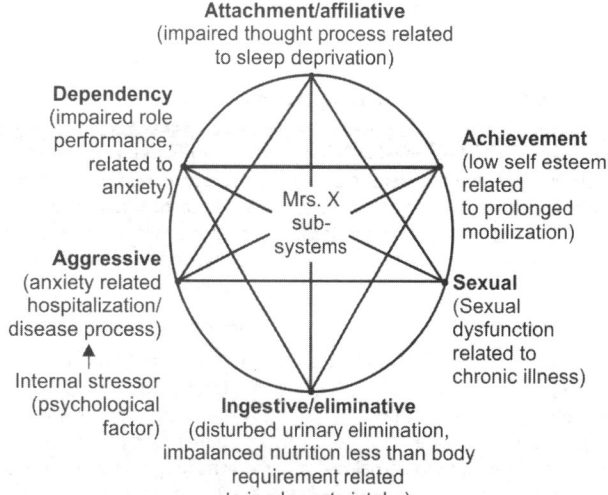

Fig. 48.1: Application of Dorothy E Johnson behavioral model to a client.

Affiliative Subsystems

- *Description:* Promote survival and provide a sense of security.
- *Assessment:* Assessing the stress, illness, lifestyle, sensory impairment, safety, and awareness.
- *Nursing diagnosis:* Altered thought process related to sleep deprivation.
- Impaired home maintenance management related to insufficient finance.
- Risk for injury related to altered mobility.

Dependency Subsystem

- *Description:* Promoting helping or nurturing behavior from others.
- *Assessment:* Assessment of self-identification, self-awareness and body image (is there something about your body you would change? If so what it is?). Self-esteem (what do you feel about yourself?).

Nursing Diagnosis

- Altered role performance related to anxiety
- Body image disturbance related to disease condition
- Ineffective individual coping related to low self-esteem.

Ingestion Subsystem

- *Description:* Involves food intake, results in appetite satisfaction.
- *Assessment:* Body weight, body muscle mass, food intake pattern, gaining of weight, weight loss, fatigue, mouth gum sores, the diet history, habitual intake of food and liquids, etc.

Nursing Diagnosis

- Altered nutrition less than body requirement related to inadequate intake of nutrients in the diet.
- Activity in tolerance related to pre-intake of food.

Elimination Subsystem

- *Description:* Involves behavior surrounding the excretion of waste from the body.
- *Assessment:* Incontinence, pattern of elimination, constipation, and diarrhea.

Nursing Diagnosis

- Altered bowel elimination related to immobility—constipation related to immobility.
- Diarrhea related to stress and anxiety—dietary intake.
- Functional incontinence related to mobility limitation.
- Altered urinary elimination related to sensory motor impairment.

Sexual Subsystem

- *Description:* Involves behavior associated with procreation and sexual gratification.
- *Assessment:* Decreased libido, erectile dysfunction, pain or fatigue, body image change, etc.

Nursing Diagnosis

- Altered sexuality patterns related to depression or separation from spouse.
- Sexual dysfunction related to chronic illness.
- Body image disturbance related to sexual dysfunction.

Aggressive Subsystem

- *Description:* Involves behavior related to self-protection and preservation of the self and society.
- *Assessment:* Appearance, personality traits, problem-solving skills, confidence, competency, independence, etc.

Nursing Diagnosis

- Ineffective individual coping related to chronic illness.

Table 48.1: Sample of a nursing-care plan of Mr X.

Assessment	Nursing diagnosis	Nursing goals	Expected outcome
Sub D: I am feeling tensed, I fear that whether I have to undergo surgery. Obj D: He is anxious, facial tension. A.scale-7	Anxiety related to situational crisis, i.e. hospitalization threat of changes in health status as evidenced by increased tension, fear, worry.	Mr. X relieves anxiety and enhances comfort.	Mr X will identify healthy ways to cope with feelings of anxiety.
Plan of action	**Rationale**	**Implementation**	**Evaluation**
• Assess the level of anxiety, stress and coping situations. • Convey calm, empathetic supportive attitude. • Encourage client to verbalize feeling. • Assist client's family to identify feelings of anxiety. • Explain about labor process.	• Provides a baseline data for further intervention. • Can help client maintain emotional control in response to challenging health status. • Provides opportunity to clarify information and plan for facilitating problem solving. • Reduces the anxiety.	• Assessed the level of anxiety and stress management coping situations. • Provided psychological support. • Encouraged verbalization of feelings. • Explained about labor process and instructed to adopt experience of labor pains.	Mr X verbalizes relief of anxiety by 1 day.

- Fear and anxiety related to hospitalization and disease condition.
- Altered family process related to unexpected illness.

Achievement Subsystem

- *Description:* Involves behavior related to manipulation of the environment to gain mastery. Includes intellectual, physical, creative, mechanical, and social skills.
- *Assessment:* Assesses the feelings and thoughts self-responsibility toward disease condition.

Nursing Diagnosis

- Self-esteem disturbance related to prolonged immobilization.
- Altered role performance related to action toward disease condition.
- Situational low self-esteem related to unresolved grief.

Note: Planning and evaluation for the nursing process can be made according to the nursing diagnosis.

APPLICATION OF THEORY

Planning and Implementation

Nurses' plan is to focus to modify client's behavior and to bring two homeostasis in subsystem based on the assessment of the individual abilities, observable behavior that nurture the subsystem an focus on subsystem's equilibrium. Implementation is based on the nursing diagnosis made during assessment, formulating care plan, and implementing the nursing interventions according to the plan.

Evaluation

It is based on attainment of goal of balance identified in the subsystem, baseline data for the individual, compare with alterations in the behavior that are planned. Mr X was able to cope up with stressors affected on his body system and underwent neck-traction treatment for 3 weeks. Using this model, nurse centered activity with the nurse determining the client's needs and appropriate interventions were carried out. Therefore, he could adapt to the situation, recover, and maintain his subsystems equilibrium.

CONCLUSION

This model covers up many concepts of subsystem in which patient problems are assessed. Each subsystem has observable behaviors, drives and choices need to be included, which nurtures environment and stimulates growth. An imbalance in any of the subsystem results in disequilibrium. Although there is a limitation of this model that nurse is concerned to specific client behaviors.

SUGGESTED READING

1. Bates B, Bickley LS, Hockelmon RA. A Guide to Physical Examination and History Taking, 6th edition. Philadelphia: J.B. Lippincott Company; 1995. pp. 104-8.
2. Bolander VB. Sorensen's and Luckmann's Basic Nursing, A Psychophysiologic Approach, 3rd edition. Philadelphia: WB Saunders Company; 1994. pp. 627-701.
3. Ellis JR, Nowlis EA, Benty PM. Modules for Basic Nursing Skills, 5th edition. Philadelphia: J.B. Lippincott Company; 1992. pp. 62-71.
4. Fuller T, Ayers JS. Health Assessment: A Nursing Approach, 2nd edition. Philadelphia: J.B. Lippincott Company; 1994. pp. 11-62.
5. Gardon M. Nursing Diagnosis Process and Application, 3rd edition. Mosby Publication.
6. Kozier B, et al. Fundamentals of Nursing Concepts, Process and Practice, 5th edition. Addison-Wesley Publishing Company; 1995. pp. 17-21.
7. Lillis T, Lynn L. Fundamentals of Nursing, 7th edition. New Delhi: Wolters Kluwer (India) Pvt. Ltd. pp. 195-319.
8. Perry P. Fundamentals of Nursing, 7th edition. Elsevier. pp. 231-95.
9. Polit DF, Beck CT. Nursing Research Generating and Assessing Evidence for Nursing Practice, 9th edition. New York: Lippincott Williams and Wilkins; Wolters Kluwer; 2012.
10. Stanhope M, Lancaster J. Community Health Nursing. Promoting Health of Regularly Families and Individuals, 4th edition. New York: Mosby Publishing; 1996. pp. 254-5.

REVIEW OF SECTION BASED QUESTIONS OF RGUHS

Long Essays

1. Enlist the components of nursing process of how will you determine the outcome of the nursing care. (Oct 2010)
2. Explain (enumerate) the steps in nursing process and explain any one step in detail. (2006)
3. Evaluate the parts of a nursing diagnosis and how it differs from a medical diagnosis. Identify the errors to be avoided in making a nursing diagnosis. (2000)
4. "Assignment is he first patient care." Discuss applied nursing process approach on a patient with asthma. (April/May 2007)
5. Nursing diagnosis is delivered from nursing assessment. Discuss with examples. (May 2009)
6. Define nursing process. How nursing process is used in providing comprehensive nursing care to patients. (Sep 2007)
7. Nursing process is a "TOOL" for providing quality. Discuss "how." (April 2008)
8. List the steps of nursing process and explain in detail the nursing process of an unconscious patient. (May 2010 and 2011)
9. Discuss nursing assessment in detail and throw light on common errors in formulating nursing diagnosis. (May 2012)
10. Enumerate steps of nursing process and describe nursing diagnosis. (May 2012)
11. Discuss the evaluation phase of nursing process. Discuss its importance in quality patient care. (May 2010)
12. Nursing diagnosis is derived from nursing assessment. Discuss with example. (May 2010)

Short Essays

1. Approaches to health assessment.
2. Approaches to nursing assessment. (2002)
3. Reassessment of client in relation to nursing care plans. (Sep 2007)
4. Nursing assessments. (Oct 2010)
5. Development of protocol for minor illness. (May 2012)
6. Protocol for treatment of diarrhea. (May 2009)
7. Protocol for upper respiratory tract infection. (May 2011)
8. Utility of nursing process. (May 2011).
9. Nursing goals. (Sept 2007)
10. Steps in developing nursing diagnosis.
11. Nursing care standards. (Oct 2016).

SECTION 8
Psychological Aspects and Human Relations

Section Outline

49. Human Behavior, Life Process, Growth and Development, Personality Development, and Defense Mechanisms
50. Communication, Interpersonal Relationships, Individual and Group, Group Dynamics and Organizational Behavior
51. Basic Human Needs, Growth and Development (Conception Through Preschool, School Age Through Adolescence, Young and Middle Adult, and Older Adult)
52. Sexuality and Sexual Health
53. Stress and Adaptation, Crisis and its Intervention
54. Coping with Loss, Death and Grief
55. Principles and Techniques of Counseling

CHAPTER 49

Human Behavior, Life Process, Growth and Development, Personality Development, and Defense Mechanisms

CHAPTER OUTLINE

- Definition of Psychology
- Application of Psychology
- Human Behavior
- Overview of Human Development
- Personality
- Defense Mechanisms

INTRODUCTION

Introduction of psychology will touch on a wide array of factors involved in what we human beings do; it will present major principles underlying human actions. Such principles give us rational basis for understanding human behavior. Psychology is gradually nearing the hoped upon goal of understanding human behavior. It is useless to focus our attention upon one part or one aspect of his/her behavior. We must focus on the individual in his/her situation and see it as whole in detail and without distortion. It is a complicated phenomenon influenced by anatomy, physiology, biochemistry, psychology, and sociology all interacting in such a way that everything is either part of and is some influenced by everything else.

Another necessary environment peculiar to man is the interpersonal social and cultural environment. People cannot live as human beings without maintaining contact with other people and without carrying on an interchange with them. It is helpful to remember that each aspects feeds in to the whole interplay of forces, which influences respect in any situation.

DEFINITION OF PSYCHOLOGY

"Psychology is the science of human and animal behavior. It includes the application of this service to human problems." Another important part of most sciences included is measurement defined as the assignment of numbers to objects or events according to certain rules.

We are all familiar with measurement of physical scales, length, time, temperature, etc. Measurement in psychology directly is more difficult psychologists cannot measure directly on scales, experiments/observations, based number of times a person behaves one way in one situation and another way in another situation.

APPLICATION OF PSYCHOLOGY

The second part of definitions psychology often used to solve real-life problems. Applications of knowledge to practical problems is an art, it is skill or knack for doing things, which is acquired by study, practice and special experience:

- Clinical psychologist
- Psychotherapist
- Educational psychologist.

HUMAN BEHAVIOR

What is Meant by Saying Psychology Studies Behavior?

The word behavior is the definition of psychology. Behavior includes anything a person or animal does that can be observed in some way. Behavior unlike mind or thoughts or feeling can be observed, recorded, and studied.

No one ever heard or saw a mind, but we can see and hear behavior, we can observe and record what a person says (vocal below), mental events are studied.

Definition of Behavior

The term behavior refers to the way in which an organism responds to a stimulus, since we are primarily concerned with human beings. We will be limited to the behavior of people. By stimulus we mean, which brings certain changes within the individual, while response refers to action, covert inferred it is not readily observed, overt readily discern to the outside behavior.

Stimuli may originate in either external or internal environment of the individual. For example, if the room temperature changes from warm to cold and one develops goose flesh.

Varieties of Behavior

For our purpose, three varieties of behavior will be considered:
1. *Reflex action:* It is most simple type of activity that occurs automatically in response to a stimulus, for example, knee jerk for percussion hammer.
2. *Goal-directed activity:* Presupposes existence of two conditions. If there is need present in the individual or change in internal environment, for example, hungry in his/her external environment, which is capable of producing a change in the internal condition and thus satisfying the need such as 8-month-old child hungry given thus satisfying the need.
3. *Response to frustration:* It mainly suggested no specific goal/need.

Brain and Behavior

Man has the capacity for thought. Thought is an interactive activity of the brain. Physiological psychology is the study of relationship between behavior and brain.

Mind is an interactive capacity developed by the brain. Thinking, decision making, memory, intelligence, emotion, control over one's behavior and talk, and awareness. Surroundings are all different functions. Mind is active part of "self" and is sense of our activities. The basic unit of nervous system and the brain is the neuron. The brain is made up of millions of such nerve cells.

1. *The brainstem:* Responsible for the basic or vital functions of the body such as response, heart/pulse/blood pressure (BP), consciousness, etc. damage to brain stem can lead to loss of consciousness and even death.
2. *Limbic system:* Controls emotions and sexual behavior. The limbic system lies beneath the cerebral hemisphere and above the central core. It is highly interrelated structures primarily the hippo campus the amygdala and the septal area ring the tip of the brains central core with it and with cerebral cortex. The limbic system emotional behavior and goal directed behavior feeding, fighting, fleeing, making, etc. pleasure centers have located in limbic system.
3. *Cerebral cortex:* This is responsible for thinking memory social behavior, speech, language, decision making, perception, and other belief. Different parts of the brain cortex are responsible for different functions. Examples are given as follows:
    - *Frontal lobe:* Thinking and social behavior.
    - *Occipital lobe:* Visual perception.
    - *Temporal lobe:* Hearing and smell.
    - *Parietal lobe:* Control movement of the body and sensory perceptions.

The left part of the brain controls thinking, speech, language, ability, and master technologies issues, while right brain is responsible for the ability to the position of articles in space, music, dancing and other artistic abilities, emotions, and spiritual thinking.

Neurotransmitters

The small space or cleft between two neurons is known as synapse; when message reaches the end of nerve cell, it stimulates pockets of a chemical substance and releases it into the synapse. The chemical substance is called neurotransmitter. It acts as a bridge and helps the message to reach the other cell. When an individual thinks, talks, or does anything, many such neurotransmitters are actively involved. When changes in neurotransmitters—changes functioning of mind disturbed. For example:
- Obsessive compulsion disorder (OCD)—decreased serotonin
- Depression—decreased levels of norepinephrine or serotonin
- Anxiety disorder—increased norepinephrine, serotonin and gamma amino butyric acid (GABA)
- Opioid drug addiction—increased endorphins.

Characteristics of Neurotransmitter

- It is manufactured in the presynaptic terminal of a neuron.
- It should be released when a nerve impulse reaches the terminal.
- Its presence in the synaptic gap must generate a biological response in the next neuron.
- If its release is blocked there must no subsequent response.

Following are the neurotransmitters:
- Acetylcholine, serotonin, dopamine, norepinephrine (noradrenalin) epinephrine, (adrenalin), amino acids, and GABA are main inhibitory transmitters in the brain.
- Glutamic acid—the chief excitatory transmitter.
- Neuropeptides—chains of amino acids found in the brain.
- Encephalins—mostly inhibitory as pain relief.
- Beta endorphin—most powerful pain reliever produced in the brain, contained in the stress hormone, and adrenocorticotrophic hormone.

OVERVIEW OF HUMAN DEVELOPMENT

Overview of human development Represents traits from all theorists.

Stages of Growth and Development

There are about nine stages or periods in the total life span. As explained in the previous lesson, those 10 stages are as follows:
1. Prenatal period
2. Neonate
3. Infancy
4. Toddler

5. Preschool age (early childhood)
6. School age (late childhood)
7. Adolescent
8. Adulthood
9. Old age

Prenatal Period—Prenatal Development

Prenatal period ("pre" means before, "natal" means birth; therefore, prenatal is the term used for the period which precedes birth from the time of conception) is from the time of zygote formation or conception to birth. Zygote is a technical term which some of you might have already come across in biology. Zygote is nothing but a fertilized ovum. An ovum comes from the woman and sperms are generated by men. If a sperm fertilizes an ovum, the product is called zygote. New life, therefore, begins with the union of male sex cell (spermatozoa—plural; spermatozoon—singular) and a female sex cell (ovum—singular; ova—plural).

Male and female sex cells have chromosomes. There are genes in each chromosome. Genes are the true carriers of heredity. A gene is a minute particle, which is found in combination with other genes in a string-like formation within the chromosome. There are approximately 3000 genes in each chromosome. These are passed on from parent to offspring.

All sex cells (both male and female) go through preliminary stages of developments. Male sex cells go through two preliminary stages, namely, (1) maturation and (2) fertilization while female sex cells go through three stages, which are (1), maturation, (2) ovulation, and (3) fertilization.

Maturation is the process of chromosome reduction through cell division; one chromosome from each pair goes to a subdivided cell, which in turn splits lengthwise and forms two new cells. The mature cell is called a haploid cell. Maturation of sex cells does not occur until sex maturity has been attained, following the onset of puberty in boys and also in girls.

Ovulation is a preliminary development limited to the female sex cells. The two ovaries alternate in producing a ripe ovum during each menstrual cycle. After being released from one of the follicles of the ovary, the ovum finds its way to the open of the fallopian tube nearest the ovary from which it was released. Once it enters the tube, it is propelled along by a combination of the following factors.
a. Cilia or hair-like cells lining the tube,
b. Fluids composed of estrogen from the ovarian follicles and from the lining of the tube, and
c. Rhythmic progressive contractions of the walls of the tube.

When the length of the menstrual cycle is normal (approximately 28 days), ovulation occurs between the 5th and the 23rd day of the cycle with the average on the 11th day.

Fertilization occurring at the time of conception is the third stage of development, preliminary to the beginning of a new life. It normally occurs while the ovum is in fallopian tube. Fertilization takes place within the first 24 hours after the ovum has entered the tube.

After a spermatozoon has penetrated the ovum, the surface of the ovum changes in such a way that afterward no other spermatozoon can enter. After the sperm cell penetrates the wall of the ovum, the nuclei from the two cells, each containing 23 chromosomes approach, each other. There is a breakdown in the membrane surrounding each nucleus, and this allows the two nuclei to merge. Thus, the species number of chromosomes 46 is restored with one-half coming from the female cell and the other half coming from the male cell.

The normal prenatal period is 10 lunar months or 9 calendar months plus 10 days long. However, this period can vary greatly in length ranging from 180 to 334 days, the legal limit of post maturity. There are approximately three times as many babies born prematurely as post maturely.

Prenatal development is orderly and predictable and so it is possible to give a timetable of the important developments taking place during this period.

The prenatal period is generally divided into three stages as follows:

Fertilization: Period of the ovum (fertilization to end of second week): The size of the zygote (more or less equal to the size of a pinhead) remains unchanged because it has no outside source of nourishment. It is kept alive by yolk in the ovum.

As the zygote passes down the fallopian tube to the uterus, it divides many times and separates into an outer and an inner layer. The outer layer later develops into the **placenta**, the **umbilical cord**, and the **amniotic sac** and the inner layer develops into a new human being. About 10 days after fertilization, the zygote becomes implanted in the uterine wall.

Period of the embryo (end of the second week to and of the second lunar month): The embryo develops into a miniature human being. Major development occurs in the head region first and in the extremities last. All the essential features of the body, both external and internal are established. The embryo begins to turn in the uterus and there is spontaneous movement of the limbs. The placenta, the umbilical cord, and the amniotic sac develop and they protect and nourish the embryo.

Period of the embryo (end of the second week to and of the second lunar month): The embryo develops into a miniature human being. Major development occurs in the head region first and in the extremities last. All the essential features of the body, both external and internal are established. The embryo begins to turn in the uterus and there is spontaneous movement of the limbs. The placenta, the umbilical cord, and the amniotic sac develop and they protect and nourish the embryo.

Period of the embryo (end of the second week to and of the second lunar month): The embryo develops into a miniature human being. Major development occurs in the head region first and in the extremities last. All the essential features of the body, both external and internal are established. The embryo begins to turn in the uterus and there is spontaneous movement of the limbs. The placenta, the umbilical cord, and the amniotic sac develop and they protect and nourish the embryo.

By the end of the fifth lunar month, the different internal organs have assumed positions nearly like the ones they will have in the adult body. Fetal activity increases rapidly up to the end of the ninth lunar month, when it slows down because of crowding in the amniotic sac and pressure on the fetal brain.

By the end of the seventh lunar month, the fetus is well-enough developed to survive, should he be born prematurely. By the end of the eighth lunar month, the fetal body is completely formed, though smaller than that of a normal, full term infant. If anything prevents these developments from taking place at the proper time, the individual will begin his/her postnatal life with a handicap that may cause a lot of hardships for the rest of one's life.

Organogenesis (Figs. 49.1 and 49.2)

❖ 14–15 days: Appearance of primitive streak
❖ 16–18 days: Notochordal process appears; hemopoietic cells in yolk sac
❖ 19–20 days: Intraembryonic mesoderm spread under ectoderm; primitive streak complete, umbilical vessels and cranial folds begin
❖ 20–21: days: Cranial neural folds elevated and deep neural groove established, embryo begins to bend
❖ 22–23 days: Fusion of neural folds in cervical region, cranial and caudal neuropores open widely, heart tube beginning to fold

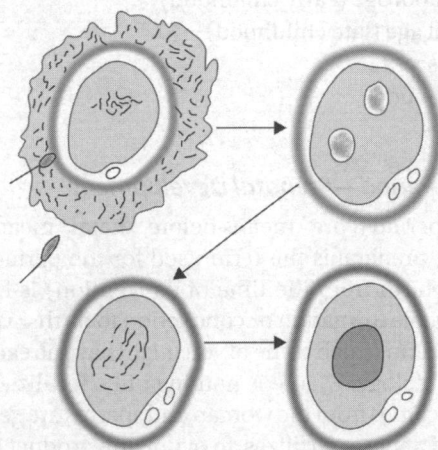

Fig. 49.2: Embryo in 14 days to 8 weeks.

❖ 24–25 days: Cephalocaudal folding under way, optic vessels formed, optic placodes appear
❖ 26–27 days: Caudal neuro pores closing or closed, upper limb buds appear, three pairs of vesicle arch
❖ 28–35 days: Fourth vesicle arch formed, hind limbs buds appear, optic vesicles and lens formed
❖ 36–42 days: Digital rays in hand and feet, external vesicles formed, umbilical herniation initiated
❖ 43–49 days: Pigmentation of retina visible, nipple and eyelids formed, upper lips form
❖ 50–56 days: Limbs long, bent at elbows and knee, tails disappears, umbilical herniation persists.

Birth–3 months (Figs. 49.3 to 49.5)

❖ 4–6 weeks: Limb buds appear, formation of face
❖ 6–8 weeks: All major structures form, complete ventricular septum formed, recognizably human
❖ 8–12 weeks: External genitalia develop
❖ 20 weeks: Skin covered with lanugo, vernix caseosa
❖ 28 weeks: Testes descends to inguinal ring
❖ 36 weeks: One testes descends to scrotum, lanugo disappears
❖ 40 weeks: Both testicle descends to scrotum, nails project beyond finger tips, posterior fontanelle closed.

Neonate: Birth–1 Month

Infancy is the shortest of all the developmental periods. It is also called the period of the newborn. It begins at birth and ends when the infant is approximately 2 weeks old. This is the time when the fetus must adjust to life outside the uterine walls of the mother where he/she has lived for approximately 9 months.

According to medical criterion, the adjustment is completed with the fall of the umbilical cord from the naval; as per the physiological criterion, it is completed when the infant has regained the weight lost after birth; according to psychological criterion, it is completed when he/she begins to show signs of developmental progress in behavior.

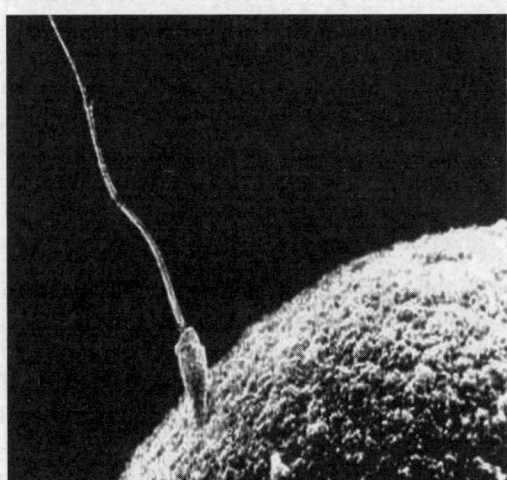

Fig. 49.1: Ovum in 0–14 days.

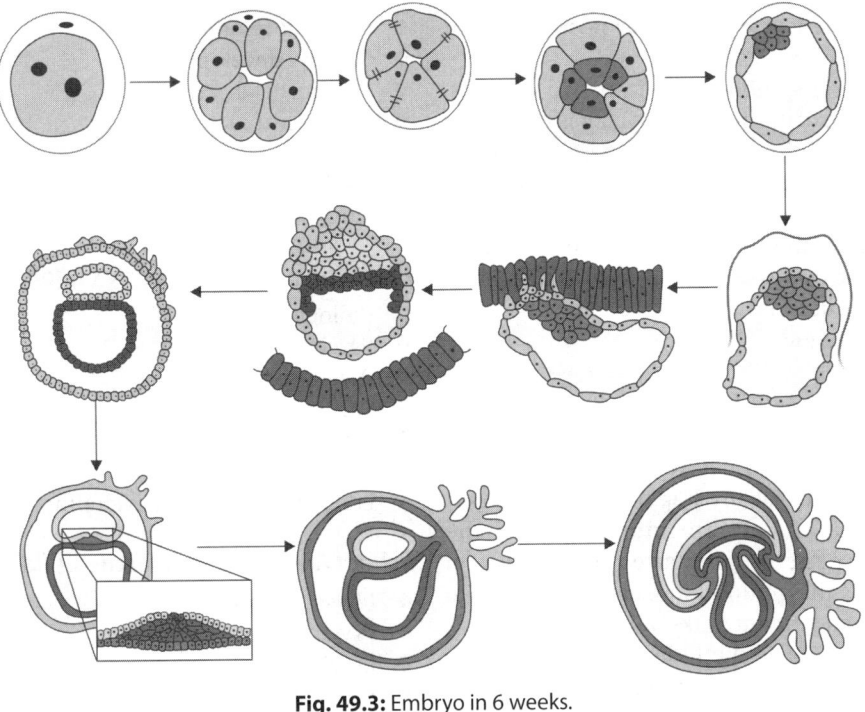

Fig. 49.3: Embryo in 6 weeks.

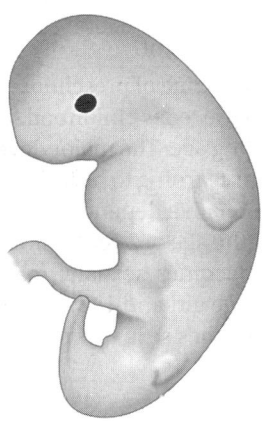

Fig. 49.4: Fetus in 6 weeks.

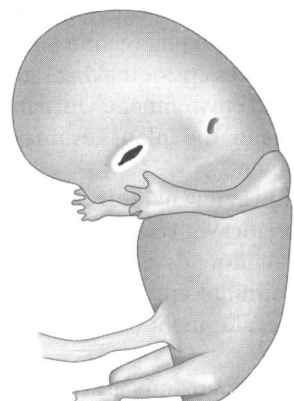

Fig. 49.5: Fetus in 8 weeks.

Unquestionably, one of the most important factors contributing to difficulties in postnatal adjustment is a prenatal environment characterized by prolonged and intense maternal stress. This leads to complications during pregnancy and childbirth.

According to Jeffcoate, birth is the most dangerous journey made by any individual who has to pass through the four inches of the birth canal.

Kinds of birth: There are five kinds of birth, each having certain distinctive characteristics. They are as follows:

1. **Natural or spontaneous birth:** In a natural birth, the position of the fetus and its size in relation to the mother's reproductive organs allow it to emerge in the normal head first position.
2. **Breech birth:** In a breech birth, the buttocks appear first, followed by the legs and finally the head.
3. **Traverse birth:** In a traverse presentation, the fetus is positioned crosswise in the mother's uterus. Instruments must be used for delivery unless the position can be changed before the birth process begins.
4. **Instrument birth:** When the fetus is too large to emerge spontaneously or when its position makes normal birth impossible, instruments must be used to aid in delivery.
5. **Cesarean section:** If X-rays taken during the latter part of pregnancy indicate that complications will result if the infant emerges through the birth canal, he is brought into the world through a slit made surgically in the mother's abdominal wall.

Very few infants are born exactly 280 days after conception. Those who arrive ahead of time, are known as premature—often referred to in hospitals as "premies"—

while those who arrive late are known as postmatures or post-term babies.

Infancy is generally subdivided into two periods, namely, (1) the period of the partunate which is from birth to 15–30 minutes after birth and during this period the infant continues to be a parasite and makes no adjustments to the postnatal environment and (2) the period of the neonate which is from cutting of the umbilical cord to the end of the second week and during this period the infant is a separate independent individual who must make adjustments to his/her new environment.

Infancy: First Year of Life Infancy

Characteristics of infancy:

1. **Infancy is a time of radical adjustments:** Though the human life span legally begins at the moment of birth, birth is merely an interruption of the developmental pattern that started at the time of conception. It is the graduation from an internal to an external environment. Like all graduations, it requires adjustments on the individual part. Infants take approximately two weeks to adjust to their new environments.
1. **Infancy is a plateau in development:** The halt in growth and developmental characteristic of this plateau is due to the necessity for making radical adjustments to the postnatal environment. Once these adjustments have been made, the infant resumes his/her growth and development.
2. **Infancy is a preview of later development:** It is not possible to predict with even reasonable accuracy what the individual future development will be on the basis of the development apparent at birth. However, the newborn's development provides clue as to what to expect later on.
3. **Infancy is a hazardous period:** Physically, it is hazardous because of the difficulties of making the necessary radical adjustments to the totally new and different environment. Psychologically also it is hazardous because it is the time when the attitudes of significant people toward the infant are crystallized. Many of these attitudes are established during the prenatal period and may change radically after the infant is born but some remain relatively unchanged or are strengthened depending on conditions at birth and on the ease or difficulty with which the infant and his parents adjust during the infancy period.
   - Biologic growth, muscular development, sensory development, psychosocial, psychosexual, spiritual, intellectual, moral, language, and play development.

Toddler: 1–3 Years

- Physical growth
- Physiologic development
- Motor development
- Sensory development
- Psychosocial
- Psychosexual
- Spiritual
- Intellectual, moral
- Language, and play development.

Preschool: 3–6 Years (Early Childhood)

- Biologic growth
- Psychosocial
- Psychosexual
- Spiritual
- Intellectual
- Moral
- Language, and play development.

School Age: 6–12 Years (Late Childhood)

- Physical growth
- Psychosocial
- Psychosexual
- Spiritual
- Intellectual
- Moral
- Language development.

Childhood: It is the same of preschool age and school age. Babyhood, which precedes childhood, is a foundation age and a very appealing age. The major developmental task of babyhood involves learning to be independent. Childhood begins when age relative dependency of babyhood is over approximately at the age of 2 years and extends to the time when the child becomes sexually mature at roughly 13 years for the average girl and 14 years for the average boy. After the child becomes sexually mature, he/she is known as an adolescent.

Adolescent: 12–20 Years

- Early adolescent: 12–14 years
- Middle adolescent: 14–16 years
- Late adolescent: 16–20 years.

Adulthood: 30–60 Years

- Early adult: 20–40 years
- Late adult: 40–60 years.

Old Age

60 and Above.

Stages of the Family Life Cycle

- Single young adult
- The newly married couple
- The family young children
- The family adolescents
- The family launching grown children.

PERSONALITY

Nurses should have basic knowledge of human personality development to understand maladaptive behavioral responses commonly seen in psychiatric clients.

Developmental theories identify behavior association with various stages through which individual pass there by specifying what is appropriate or inappropriate at each developmental level.

- ❖ **Specialists in child development:** It is believed that infancy and early childhood are the major life periods for the origination and occurrence of development change. Specialists in life cycle development believe that people continue to develop and change throughout life. Thereby suggesting the possibility for renewal and growth in adults.
- ❖ **History of personality:** In the past, personality was thought to be the personal appearance. About 50 years ago, personality was thought to be God given, and it would remain the same. Hereditary and environment are parts of the personality.

Definition Based on Personality

When psychologists define personality, they tend to refer to qualities in a person or the characteristics of a person's behavior or both.

- ❖ **American Psychiatric Association (APA) 2000:** Personality traits as enduring patterns of perceiving relating to and thinking about the emit and oneself that are exhibited in a wide range of social and personal contexts.
- ❖ **According to Gordon Allport (1937)**
  - ➤ Personality is the dynamic organization in the individual of those psychophysical systems that determine his unique adjustment to his environment.
  - ➤ Personality has been studied in a number of different ways. Some have developed broad theories and makeup of personality, while others have focused only on one or two issues such as the influence of heredity on personality.

The major personality development theories are tabulated as follows:
- ❖ **Theories adopting developmental approach:** Psychosexual theory of Sigmund Freud, psychosocial theory of Erik H Erikson.
- ❖ **Interpersonal theory:** Sullivan's stage.
- ❖ **Cognitive theories:** Intellectual development by Piaget and Bruner.
- ❖ Humanistic theory of personality (personality as the self):
  - ➤ Maslow's self-actualize theory.
  - ➤ Carl Rogers's self-theory.
  - ➤ Kelley's personal construction.
- ❖ **Theories adopting type approach:** Hippocrates, Kretschmer, Sheldon, and Jung.
- ❖ **Theories adopting trait approaches:** Allport, Cattell, and the five-factor model.
- ❖ **Theories adopting type-cum-trait approach:** Eysenck's theory of personality.
- ❖ **Behavior learning theories:** Dollard-Miller early learning theories, B F Skinner, and Bendura's social learning theory.

Psychoanalytic Theory

Sigmund Freud (1856–1939) is a psychoanalyst, is first to identify development by stages. He considered the first 5 years of a child's life to be the most important because he believed that individuals' basic character had been formed by the age of five.

Freud

It is conceptualized according to structure and dynamics of the personality, topography of the mind, and stages of personality development.

Structure of Personality (Fig. 49.6)

Freud organized the structure of the personality into three major components, which are id, ego, and superego.

1. **Id (pleasure principle):** Id is the part of one's nature that reflects basic. It begins between 4 and 6 months of age or innate desires such as pleasure seeking behavior aggression, and sexual impulses.

    It will be present at birth, it endeavors the infant with institutional drives that seek to satisfy needs and achieve immediate gratification. It may be impulsive and may be irrational.

2. **Ego:** These are "rational self" reality, principle, and ego experiences. Reality of the external world adapts to it and responds to it. One of the important is the balancing and mediating force between the id and the superego or mediator, that is, maintain harmony among the external world the id and superego. It may impulsive and may be irrational.

3. **Superego (perfection principle):** This develops between ages 3 and 6 years; internalizes the values and morals set forth by primary caregivers, derived out of a rewards and punishments. Superego two major components self-esteem and conscience behavior becomes ego ideal.

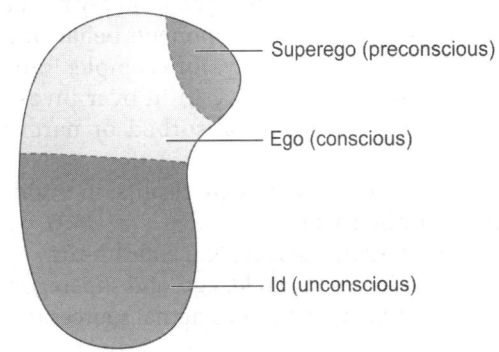

Fig. 49.6: Topography of the mind.

The conscience is formed when the child is punished consistently for bad behavior. The child learns what is considered morally right or wrong from the feedback received from parental figures and from society or culture.

When moral and ethical principles or even internalized ideals and values are disregarded conscience, it generates a feeling of guilt within the individual superego, socialization of the individual because it assists the ego in the control of id impulses. When superego becomes rigid, related to punishment punitive problems with low self-confidence and low self-esteem arise.

Freud classified all mental contents and operations into three categories:
1. **Conscious:** It includes all memories that remain within an individual awareness. It is the smallest of the three categories events and experience that are easily remembered or retrieved within ones conscious awareness, for example, birthdays of self and significant others telephone numbers, some special days.

   The conscious under the control of the ego rational and logical structure of person.
2. **Preconscious:** It includes all memories that may have been forgotten or not in present awareness, but with attention can be readily recalled into consciousness, e.g. telephone numbers and addresses once known, but little used and feedings associate significant life events that may have occurred in past. The preconscious helps to suppress unpleasant or nonessential memories. It is thought to be partially under the control of superego and suppresses unacceptable behavior.
3. **Unconscious:** It is all memories that one is unable to bring to conscious awareness. It is largest of three topographical levels. It consists of unpleasant and nonessential memories that have been repressed and can be retrieved only through therapy hypnosis and certain substances alter the awareness and have the capacity to restructure repressed memories dreams—incomprehensible behavior.

Dynamics of Personality
- If an excessive amount of psychic energy is stored in one of these personality components behavior reflect that part of the personality, for example, impulsive behavior prevails excessive in Id over investment in the ego reflects self- absorbed or narcissistic behavior.
- An excess within superego results in rigid self-deprecating behavior.
- Freud listed terms, cathexis, and anticathexis.

To describe forces within id, ego, and superego that is used to invest psychic energy in external sources to satisfy needs:

- Cathexis is the process by which the id invests energy into an object in an attempt to achieve gratification, for example, individual who instinctively turn to alcohol to relieve stress.
- Anticathexis is the use of psychic energy by the ego and the superego to control id impulses, for example, a person would attempt to drink who is having ulcer, not to drink rational thinking.
- Freud believed that an imbalance between cathexis and anticathexis resulted in internal conflicts producing tension and anxiety.

Freud's Stages of Personality Development (Table 49.1): Freud's described formation of the personality through five stages of psychosexual development. He placed emphasis on first 5 years of life and believed early characteristics developed during these early years have heavily on one's adaptation patterns and personality traits in adulthood.

- ***Oral stage (birth to 18 months):*** The behavior is directed by id and the goal is immediate gratification of needs.

  The focus of energy is the mouth with behavior includes sucking, chewing, and biting. Sense of attachment felt and unable to differentiate self from the person who is mothering.

  Feeling of anxiety mother may be passed on to her infant, leaving the child vulnerable to similar feelings. The infant starts 4–6 months self-development of the ego from the mothering figure. Ability to trust and sense of security derived from the gratification of basic needs during this stage.

- ***Anal stage (18 months to 3 years):*** The major tasks in the anal stage are gaining independence and control with particular focus in excretory function. Freud believed that toilet training may have far facing effects on the child in terms of values and personality characteristics.

  Toilet training is strict and rigid, child may choose to retain feces, constipation retain personality traits

Table 49.1: Freud's stages of personality development.

Age	Stage	Major development tasks
Birth to 18 months	Oral	Relief from anxiety through oral gratification needs
18 months to 3 years	Anal	Learning independence, control, and focus on the excretory function
3–6 years	Phallic	Identification with parent of same sex, development of sexual identity, focus on genital organs
6–12 years	Latency phase	Sexually repressed focus on relationship with same sex peers
13–20 years	Genital	Libido reawakened as genital organs mature focus

influenced by this type of training include stubbornness, stinginess, miserliness, as a result strict child may expel feces is an unacceptable manner inappropriate times. Far reaching of this behavior pattern include malevolence, cruelty to others destructiveness, disorganization, untidiness toilet training is more permissive, and accepting child becomes extroverted productive and altruistic.

- ❖ **Phallic stage (3–6 years):** In this the focus of energy shifts to the genitals area. Discovery of differences as between genders results in a heightened interest sexuality of self and others. This may be manifested in sexual self-exploratory or group exploratory play. Freud proposed development of the Oedipus complex (males) Electra complex (females) occurs during this stage of development.

  He described child's unconscious desire to eliminate the parent of the desire to eliminate the parent of the same sex and to possess the parent of opposite sex for himself/herself. Guilt feelings result with superego during these years. Resolution of this internal conflict occurs when child develops strong identification. With the parent of same sex and that parent is attitudes beliefs and value system are subsumed by the child.

- ❖ **Latency stage (6–12 years):** During elementary school years, the focus changes from egocentrism to more interest in group activities learning and socialization peers. Sexuality is not absent during this period, but remains obscure. The preference is homosexual children of this age show distinct preference for same sex relationships even rejecting members of the opposite sex.

- ❖ **Genital stage (13–20 years):** In this the maturing of the genital organs results in a reawakening of the libidinal drive the focus relationships opposite sex and preparations for selecting mate. The development sexual maternity evolves from self-gratification to belief deemed acceptable by societal norms relationships more genuine pleasure desire rather than more self-serving.

Knowledge of structure of personality can assist nurses who work in the mental health setting. The ability to recognize behaviors associate id, the ego, and superego assist in the assessment of development level understanding use of ego mechanism and determines maladaptive behavior in planning care for clients to assist in creating change or in helping clients accept themselves as unique individuals.

Theory of Psychosocial Development

Erikson (1963) studied the influence of social processes in the development of personality. He described eight stages of the life cycle during individuals struggle with development "crisis" specific tasks associated with each stage must be completed for resolution of the crisis and for emotional growth to occur (Table 49.2).

- ❖ **Infancy (birth to 18 months)—trust and mistrust:**
  - ➢ Achievement task results in self-confidence, optimism, faith in gratification of needs, and desires for future.
  - ➢ Nonachievement results emotional dissatisfaction with self and others suspiciousness and difficulty interpersonal relationship, the task is unresolved when primary care given fails to respond to infants distress signals promptly and consistently.
- ❖ **Early childhood (18 months to 3 years)—autonomy vs shame and doubt:** Achievement results in a sense of self-control and ability to delay gratification and feeling self-confidence to perform.

  This is achieved when parents encourage and provide opportunities for independent activities.
  - ➢ Nonachievement results lack of confidence a lack of pride in the ability to perform sense of being

Table 49.2: Erikson's stages of psychosocial development.

Age	Stage	Major development tasks
Infancy (birth to 1 year)	Trust vs mistrust	To develop a basic trust in the mothering figure and learn to generalize to others
Early childhood (18 months to 3 years)	Autonomy vs shame and doubt	To gain some self-control and independence within the environment
Late childhood (3–6 years)	Initiative vs guilt	To develop a sense of purpose and the ability to initiate and direct own activities
School age (6–12 years)	Industry vs inferiority	To achieve a sense of self-confidence by learning, competing, performing successfully, and receiving recognition from significant others, peers, and acquaintances
Adolescence (12–20 years)	Identity vs role confusion	To integrate the tasks mastered in the previous stages in to a secure sense of self
Young adulthood (20–30 years)	Intimacy vs isolation	To form an intense lasting relationship or a commitment to another person, cause institution, or creative effort
Adulthood (30–65 years)	Generativity vs stagnation	To achieve the life goals established for oneself, while also considering the welfare of future generations
Old age (65 years to death)	Ego integrity vs despair	To review one's life and desire meaning from both positive and negative events, while achieving a positive sense of self-worth

controlled by others and this task remains unsolved care givers restrict independent behaviors both physically and verbally or setup the child for failure with unrealistic expectations.

- ❖ *Late childhood (3-6 years)—initiative vs guilt:*
  - ➢ Achievement of the task results in the ability to exercise restraint and self-control of inappropriate social behaviors. Assertiveness and dependability increase and child enjoys learning and personal achievement.
  - ➢ Nonachievement results in feeling of inadequacy and a sense of defeat not responsible child view himself/herself as evil and deserving of punishment.
- ❖ *School age (6-12 years)—industry vs inferiority:*
  - ➢ Achievement of the sense of satisfaction and pleasure in the interaction and involvement with others. The individual masters reliable works habits and develops attitudes of trust worthiness, feels pride in achievement, and enjoy play but desires a balance between fantasy and real-world activities encouragement is given to activities and responsibilities in the school and community.
  - ➢ Nonachievement results in difficulty interpersonal relationship because of feelings personal inadequacy. Individual neither cooperative and compromise with others in group activities nor problem solve. When discipline harsh and tends to unpair self-esteem and negative feedback.
- ❖ *Adolescence (12-20 years)—identity vs role confusion:*
  - ➢ Achievement results in a sense of confidence emotional stability and new of the self as unique individual commitments are made to a value system to choice of a career and to relationships with members of both genders. Identify experience independence by making decisions that influence their lives.
  - ➢ Nonachievement results in sense of self-consciousness, doubt, and confusion about one's role in life. When independence is discouraged discipline inconsistent harsh or absent. Parental rejection or frequent shifting of parental figures.
- ❖ *Young adulthood (20-30 years)—intimacy vs isolation:* Capacity for mutual love and respect between two people and the ability of one to pledge total commitment to another. Commitment in personal sacrifices are made for another. Intimacy is achieved by oneself to another nonachievement results withdrawal social isolation of aloneness. Unable to form intimacy.
- ❖ *Middle adulthood (30-65 years)—generativity vs stagnation or self-absorption:*
  - ➢ Achievement results in a sense of gratification from personal and professional achievement and from meaningful contribution to others individual are active in service and to society.
  - ➢ Nonachievement results in lack of concern for the welfare of others and total preoccupation the self. He becomes withdrawal isolated and highly self-indulgent with no capacity for giving of the self to others. Not fulfilled and the individual does not.
- ❖ *Late adulthood (65 years to death)—ego integrity vs despair:*
  - ➢ Achievement results in a sense of self-worth and self-acceptance as one reviews life goals accepting that some were achieved and some were not individuals derives sense of dignity from his life experience and does not fear of death. Ego integrity is achieved when individuals successfully completed the departmental tasks.
  - ➢ Nonachievement results in sense of self-contempt and disgust how life has progressed he would like to start over and have a second chance at life. He/She feels worthless/helpless to change, anger depression, and loneliness are evident perceived failures impending death devoid ideas of suicides may prevail.

This theory relevant to nursing practice incorporates sociocultural concepts into the development personality. It provides tasks during each approach and illness. Specific tasks during each stage nurses assist them to achieve these tasks onto a higher depth level.

Interpersonal Theory

Sullivan (1953) believed that individual behavior and personality development are the direct result of interpersonal relationship. He studied and Freud diverted from intrapersonal/interpersonal flavor in which human behavior could be observed in social interactions with others, for example, contentment and pleasure.

Sullivan Major Concepts

- ❖ **Anxiety:** Chief disruptive force in interpersonal relations and manifests development serious difficulties in living.
- ❖ **Satisfaction of needs:** For examples, oxygen, food, warmth, tenderness, rest, activity, and sexual expression.
- ❖ **Interpersonal security:** Relief from anxiety—innate need for interpersonal security.
- ❖ **Self-system:** Collection of experience (good me), positive feedback measuring (bad me) negative feedback adapted by distress, discomfort, and displeasure.

Sullivan's Stages of Personality Development

- ❖ **Infancy (birth to 18 months):** During this stage, major development task for the child is the gratification of needs such as crying, nursing, and thumb sucking.
- ❖ **Childhood (18 months to 6 years):** Child learns interference fulfillment of personal wishes and desires may result in delayed gratification—often last most parental approval reward tools of this stage include the mouth, anus, language, experiment, manipulation, and identification.
- ❖ **Juvenile (6-9 years):** Formation of satisfactory relationships within peer groups. This is accomplished

through use of competition cooperation and compromise learning to form satisfactory relationships.

- **Preadolescence (9-12 years):** Focus on developing relationships with persons of the same sex. One is ability to show love and affection for another person begins at this stage. Learning to form satisfactory relationship with persons of same sex initiating feelings of affection for another person.
- **Early adolescence (12-14 years):** The child is struggling developing sense of identity that is separate and independent from the parents major learning to form satisfactory relationship with members of the opposite sex. Sullivan—biological changes as a major force.
- **Late adolescence (14-21 years):** Tasks association the attempt to achieve interdependence in the society and the formation of a lasting opposite sex genital organs is major development focus of this stage. Establishing self-identity, experiencing satisfying relationships working to develop a lasting, intimate opposite sex relationship.

It has significance to nursing practice. Relationship development major concept of this theory is a major psychiatric intervention.

Knowledge about behaviors association all levels of anxiety and methods for alleviating helps a sense of well-being.

Sullivan—achieves higher degree of independent and interpersonal functioning.

Piaget's Cognitive Development Theory (Table 49.3)

Piaget (1969) has been called the father of child psychology. His work is concerned cognitive development in children is based on the promise that human intelligence is an extension biological adaptation or one's ability to adapt psychologically to the environment. He believed that human intelligence progresses through a series of stages that are related to age, demonstrating at each successive stage a higher-level of logical organization than at the previous stages. From extensive studies in children he discovered four stages of cognitive development.

- **Stage 1: Sensorimotor (birth to 2 years):** From the beginning, the child is concerned only with satisfying basic needs and comforts. The self is not differentiated from the external environment. Sense of differential occurs with nursing mobility and awareness and mental system expanded. The child develops greater understanding regarding objects within external environment and their efforts upon him/her. Knowledge is gained by manipulating objects and experiences with the environment. The sense of object permanence notion that an object will continue to exist when it is no longer present to the senses is initiated.
- **Stage 2: Preoperational (2-6 years):** Piaget believed that preoperative thought is characterized by egocentric. Personal experiences are thought to

Table 49.3: Piaget's stages of cognitive development.

Age	Stage	Major development tasks
Birth to 2 years	Sensorimotor	With increased mobility and awareness, development of a sense of self as separate from the external environment the concept of object permanence emerges as the ability to form mental images evolves
2–6 years	Preoperational	Learning to express self with language development of understanding of symbolic gestures achievement of object permanence
6–12 years	Concrete operations	Learning to apply logic to thinking development of understanding of reversibility and spatiality; learning to differentiate and classify used socialization and application of rules
12–15 years	Formal operations	Learning to think and reason in abstract terms making and testing hypothesis, capability of logical thinking and reasoning expand and are refined cognitive maturity achieved

be universal and the child is unable to accept the differing new points of others. Language development progresses as ability to attribute gestures bringing a story book to mother is a symbolic invitation to have story read. Reality is often given to inanimate objects. Object permanence culminates in the ability to conjure up mental representations of objects or people.

- **Stage 3: Concrete operations (6-12 years):** The ability to apply logic to thinking begins in this stage; an understanding of the concepts of reversibility and spatiality is developed. For example, the child recognizes that changing the shape of objects does not necessarily change amount weight volume or the ability of the object to return to original form. Another achievement classifies objects by any of their several characteristics. For example, he/she can classify all poodles as dogs, but recognizes that all dogs are not poodles.

The concept of a lawful self is developed at this stage as the child becomes more socialized and rule conscious. Egocentrism loses the ability to cooperate in interactions with other children and understanding and acceptance of established rules grow.

- **Stage 4: Formal operations (12-15 years):** At this stage, the individual is able to think and reason in abstract terms. He/She makes and tests hypothesis using logical and orderly problem solving. Current situations and reflections of the future are idealized. Formal operations enable individuals to distinguish between the ideal and the real. He suggests most individuals achieve cognitive maturity. The capability to perform all mental operations needed for adulthood in middle-to-late adolescence. Nurses in psychiatry particularly depressed clients with techniques of cognitive therapy. Individual taught to control thought distortions that are considered to be a factor in the development are considered to be a factor in the development and maintenance of mood disorders.

Humanistic Theories—Personality as the Self

Humanists such as Carl Rogers and Abraham Maslow reject the internal conflicts of Freud's view and the mechanistic nature of behaviorism. They believe that each person is creative and responsible, free to choose, and each strives for fulfillment or self-actualization. Human beings want to grow and develop to their greatest potential. If we stop studying other people behavior for a moment and pause to think about our own we become aware of a set of feelings and attitude and a certain sense of who we are.

A number of theories have focused their work upon this entity known as the self. One set has to do with people's attitudes about themselves and their perceived abilities traits weakness. This collection constitutes what is known as the self-concept or self-image attitudes feelings perceptions and evaluation of self as an object.

Second set of meanings relates the executive functions processes by the individual manage copes thinks remembers perceives and plans. These two meanings self as object and self as process are seen in most theories involving the notion of self.

This theory differs from psychoanalysis and learning theory. It is also called phenomenological theory because once feeling given moment in time. It stresses once individuality ones inherent growth for self-identity and actualization. Problems may cause self-actualizing humanistic stresses, optimism, and creativity. The self is the focus of treatment. Increasing one self-awareness and enhancing one's self-esteem and personal growth is called therapeutic roles.

Abraham Maslow (1954) "Human Needs"

Abraham Maslow emphasized on the development of self. He believed that each person has an essential nature that "presses" to emerge like "press" with in action to become "oak tree" higher-level of needs self-actualize and assume dominant role in our lives after ours.

Maslow broke away from the reward/punishment/observable behavior mentality of behaviorism and developed his humanistic theory. His theory emphasized two things, which are our capacity for growth or self-actualization and our desire to satisfy a variety of needs. Maslow's need hierarchy arranges needs in an ascending order, with biological needs at the bottom and social and personal needs at the top. As needs at one level are met, we advance to the next level.

Maslow believed we should study transcendent people. He worried that exclusive study of emotionally disturbed people as in Freud's theory and others distorted.

Instead, models of self-actualized people who appeared to have fulfilled their basic potentialities Lincoln, Jefferson, and Einstein are optimal people. Priority problems and how clients motivate and balance change during life crisis, for example, a woman having breast cancer 35 years who has to be in the hierarchy of love and belongings frustration.

Level she reduced to safety and security lower order of needs, higher remains unfulfilled.

Carl Rogers Self-theory (1959–1961)

Carl Rogers rejected the psychodynamic approach because it placed too much emphasis on unconscious, irrational forces. Instead, Rogers developed a new humanitarian theory called self-theory. It has two primary assumptions:

1. Personality development is guided by each person's unique self-actualization tendency.
2. Each of us has a personal need for positive regard. Rogers said that the self is made up of many self-perceptions, abilities, personality characteristics, and behaviors that are organized and consistency with one another.

He grew out his client-centered approach to psychotherapy and below change.

Like psychoanalysis, Carl Rogers did not include complex stages of personality development. He emphasized the whole of experiment the phenomenal field. This is individual frame of reference it may or may not correspond to external society.

The self, a self, or self-concept gradually develops central idea in his theory important sense of goal to become his real self or ideal self, for example, perceived self may not match the ideal self. When there are mismatches and this can be disturbing because we need self-esteem/with acceptance:

Personality development as children grow parents other react to their behavior some positive way sometimes with disapproval.

❖ Thoughts and feelings unworthy aspects of self.
❖ Clients are best position to know experiences and make sense of them to regain their self-esteem and to progress toward self-actualization.
❖ Therapist only supportive role rather than directive or expert role because he viewed the client as an expert on his/her life.

Therapist promote self-esteem

❖ Unconditional positive regard nonjudgmental caring
❖ Genuineness or realness
❖ Empathetic understanding
❖ Unconditional positive regard self-esteem and decreases his need for defensive behavior
❖ Self-acceptance grows
❖ Natural self-actualization process continue
❖ Self-improvement and constructive change

If repeated conflicts—loses self-esteem, defensive, and not healthy

Kelley—Personal Construction

Construct is a belief or attitude that remains. He assumed we have various ways in world surrounds us. There always exist an alternative perceptive to choose from to dealing with word. This is called alternative. Man works through transparent and then creates to fit over the realities to which world is composed on Kelley called personal constructs. Therefore, representation of events that is then distinct against reality.

Theories Adopting Type Approach

The theory approached human personality and behavior characteristics using somatic structure, blood type, and secretions.

Types Based on Temperament

Hippocrates (about 400 BC), the father of medicine, classified people into four types as per temperament depending on which one of one's bodily humors or fluids they believe to predominate:
- Sanguine—cheerful, vigorous, confident, optimistic (blood)
- Phlegmatic—calm, slow moving, unexcitable, unemotional (mucus)
- Choleric—irritable, hot tempered (yellow bile)
- Melancholic—depressed, morose (black bile)

Types Based on Body Build
- Kretschmer
- William Sheldon.

  Kretschmer (1925) divided people into three body types:
  1. Asthenic—introvert, tall, thin, sensitive
  2. Athletic—active, aggressive, well-developed muscular body
  3. Pyknic—extrovert, round, fat

  William Sheldon (1954) divided people into three types according to body build:
  1. **Endomorph:** Plumb, soft, fat, round—sociable even tempered and relaxed (such as Santa Claus)
  2. **Mesomorph:** Heavy set and muscular—physically active and noisy
  3. **Ectomorph:** Tall, thin, flat-chested—self-conscious, shy, fond of solitude, and reserved.

  Although a person's physique may have some influence on personality, the relationship is much more subtle. Research has shown little correlation between body build and specific personality characteristics.

  Types A and B based on emotions and stress as classified by health psychologists.

Classification by Psychological Types

On the basis of sociability Dr. Karl G Jung classified people into two main groups namely extroverts and introverts.

Extroverts

Extroverts are people who take more interest in others and like to move with people and are skilled in etiquette. They are friendly and sociable and not easily get upset by difficulties. They are dominated by emotions, whereby they take decisions quickly and act on them without delay. They are realistic and face the problems of life objectively.

Introverts

Introverts are those who are interested in themselves, their own feelings, emotions, and reactions. They are busy in their own thoughts and are self-centered. They are reserved and like to work alone. They are very sensitive and are unable to adjust easily to social situations. They are inclined to worry and easily get embarrassed. Poets, philosophers, scientists, and artists belong to this group.

Ambiverts

Ambiverts are very few people who are pure extroverts or introverts. Majority of the people are ambiverts having the qualities of extroverts and introverts in different proportions.

Trait Theories

In trait approach, the personality is received in terms of traits such as honest, shy, lazy, dull, dependent, etc. Traits are defined as relatively permanent and constant behavior patterns that the individual exhibits in many situations. These behavior patterns are considered as the basic units of personality. If a person behaves honestly on several situations, he/she is called honest. Honesty or laziness becomes a behavior trait of his/her personality.

Gordon Allport (1887–1967)

Gordon Allport was the first personality theorist who adopted trait approach. According to him, an individual develops a unique set of stable tendencies of traits organized around a few primary traits. Personality traits Allport (1961) used different traits to describe the uniqueness of each individual. The most common way to describe people, e.g. a nurse, is to list a number of qualities she should possess, for example, patience, honesty, perseverance, thoroughness, and initiative. These qualities are called personality traits. Groups of personality traits are known as personality factors or dimensions of personality. When traits are analyzed and results are put on a graph, it is called personality profile.

RB Cattell

RB Cattell, the British born American research worker, defined trait as a structure of the personality inferred from behavior in different situations. He described four types of traits:
- Common traits
- Unique traits
- Surface traits
- Source traits.

The theory of Cattell intends to give certain specific dimensions to personality, so that human behavior related to a particular situation can be predicted. Cattell has adopted factor analysis as a technique for his work.

Five-Factor Model or Five Traits Theory

For over 50 years, a major goal of personality researchers was to find a way to define the structure of personality with the fewest possible traits. The search for a list of traits that could describe personality differences among everyone began in 1930s with a list of about 4500 traits and ended in 1990s with a list of only five traits.

The five (traits) factor model traits theory organizes personality traits under five categories (mnemonic "OCEAN"):
- O—**O**penness
- C—**C**onscientiousness
- E—**E**xtraversion
- A—**A**greeableness
- N—**N**euroticism.

These traits that are referred to as the big five traits raise three major issues:
1. First, although traits are stable tendencies to behave in certain ways, this ability does not apply across all different situations.
2. Second, personality traits are both changeable and stable. Most change occurs before age 30 years because adolescents and young adults are more willing to adopt new values and attitudes or revise old ones. Most stability occurs after age 30 years, but adult do continue to grow in their ideas, beliefs, and attitudes.
3. Third, genetic features have a considerable influence on personality traits and behaviors. Genetic factors push and pull the development of certain traits whose development may be helped or hindered by environmental factors.

Traits are useful in that they provide shorthand descriptions of people and predict certain behaviors.

Trait theory says relatively little about the development or growth of personality, but instead emphasizes measuring identifying differences among personalities.

Learning or Behavior Theories

Early learning theory
Early learning theory (Dollard and Miller, 1930) explained individual and social behavior by basic learning principles of approach-avoidance conflict in a variety of human problems. They argued that we may act indecisive and neurotic we are torn between approaching and avoiding a certain course of action. For example, when we want the tooth filled, but we fear pain. In such cases, the tendency to approach (getting filling) is often stronger than the avoidance tendency at first. But as we get closer to the moment of truth, the more likely it is that the approach tendency will miss out and we will retreat from the planned action. We will cancel our dental appointment. Another example is twin analysis of Mrs. A, a woman treated by a physiotherapist in New York for severe depression because of conflict between her sexual (urges), appetite (approach), and her fear of open sex (avoidance).

Social learning theory
Social learning theory developed by BF Skinner (1904-1990), emphasis on learning as a process, whereby individuals, as a result of their experiences, establish an association or linkage between two events, for example, burning stove and a painful burning sensation. This process is called conditioning. Behavior can be divided into units called responses and the environment into units called stimuli. The process by which one strengthens the possibility of another event occurring is called reinforcement. The environment is responsible for development of personality.

The social cognitive theory emphasizes the importance of learning through observation, mutation, and self-reward in development of social skills, interactions, and behaviors. According to this theory, it is not necessary that you perform any observable behaviors or receive any external rewards in order to learn new social skills because many of your behaviors are self-motivated and intrinsic.

When comparing Bendura's, Freud's and Erickson theories, we find that they are complementary because each emphasizes a different process. Social cognitive theory emphasizes learning through modeling and imitating behaviors that you observe in social interactions and situations). Freud's theory focuses on parent–child interactions that can occur in satisfying innate biological needs. Erickson's theory points to the importance of dealing with social needs.

Factors of Personality

- The physical factors include the physique of the individual his size, strength, looks, and constitution.
- The environmental or social factor.
- Mental or psychological factors including motives, interests, attitudes, will and character, intellectual capacities as intelligence, reasoning, attention, perception, and imagination. These traits and factors are assessed by psychological tests. Trait theory is an approach for analyzing the structure of personality by measuring, identifying, and classifying similarities and differences in personality characteristics or traits.

Methods/Techniques of Personality Assessment

Personality testing is done for various reasons. A psychologist may want to identify people for a salesman's job. A clinical psychologist often uses personality tests to evaluate psychological disorders. Personality tests do not have "right" and "wrong" answers. Instead, they seek answers that will reveal people's characteristic tendencies or behavior.

The techniques of personality assessment can be divided into five categories:
1. Where one can see how the individual behaves in actual life situations:
   a. Observation technique.
   b. Situation technique.
2. Where one can find out what an individual says about themselves:
   a. Autobiography.
   b. Questionnaire/Personality inventory.
   c. Interview.
3. Techniques by which one can find out what others say about the individual whose personality is under assessment:
   a. Case history taking, that is, extracting information.
   b. Biography.
   c. Rating scales.
   d. Sociometry.
4. Techniques by which one can find how an individual reacts to an imaginative situation involving fantasy, e.g. projective methods.
5. Techniques by which one can indirectly determine some personality variables in terms of physiological responses by measuring (technical) instruments.

Assessment of Personality

The following are some of the methods used for evaluation and measurement of personality traits:
- Observational methods (the interview).
- Personality inventories (based on trait theories).
- Projective techniques (based on psychoanalytical theory).

Interviews

Interview is the most popular method of observation. Appearance, bearing, and speech can be noticed. Questions can be asked about attitudes and interests. Interviews are used to evaluate a person's personality for the purpose of employment and for education as well as for identifying personality trait. An interview may be informal or unstructured. It can be formal or structured, where specific topics are selected by the interviewer before and the flow of conversation is controlled.

Body language of the client can be observed during an interview. The body language may be posture, movement of the hands, facial expressions, or voice. However, interviews take place under stress and great skill is needed to put the interviewee at ease.

Questionnaires

Questionnaire is the most common written method of measuring personality. A personality interview is a questionnaire in which the person reports his/her feeling in certain situations.

They are very easily checked and scored. More often the answers are scored by machines which eliminate the prejudice of the tester, making the test more objective (Table 49.4).

Table 49.4: Examples of questions used in questionnaires.

Questions	Answers	
Would you rate yourself as a quiet person?	Yes	No
Do you prefer to work alone rather than with others?	Yes	No
Do you frequently feel sad?	Yes	No

Minesota Multiple Personality Inventory

Minesota multiple personality inventory (MMPI) is one of the most commonly used personality test. This test asks for answers of "true," "false," or "cannot say" to 567 statements (one for men and another for women) about different personality traits such as attitudes, emotional reactions, physical and psychological symptoms, and past experiences. The answers are quantitatively measured and personality assessment is done based.

DEFENSE MECHANISMS (TABLE 49.5)

Freud in 1904 used the term defense mechanism to refer to the unconscious process that defends a person against anxiety. When the primitive id drives are in serious conflict with the controls imposed by the ego or the superego, the individual suffers from tension and anxiety. This uncomfortable situation is reflected in the individual behavior some methods of developing a compromise and relieving the tension and anxiety are needed.

Definition

According to Sigmund Freud (1904):
- Defense mechanism is any automatic unconscious response that helps a person reduces painful feelings associated with emotional problems.
- The human being is usually able to relieve the conflict by utilizing certain forms of adaptation, which are called ego defense mechanisms, adjustment mechanisms, or mental dynamism.

Table 49.5: Defense mechanisms can be divided into successful and unsuccessful mechanisms.

Successful	Unsuccessful
• Repression	• Suppression
• Rationalization	• Reaction formation
• Intellectualization	• Displacement
• Compensation	• Denial
• Substitution	• Isolation
• Sublimation	• Projection
	• Regression
	• Conversion
	• Fixation
	• Fantasy

❖ 'The individuals have devices for protecting themselves against psychological dangers and distress. These protective devices are known as ego defenses or defense mechanisms. All of us use defense mechanisms some time or the other in our normal behavior. When used moderately, they are harmless and help us face conflicts and frustrations easily and protect our ego. However, excessive and persistent use of these mechanisms is harmful as they don't solve conflicts and frustrations basically, but only help the individual to make adaptations to distressing experiences.

Groups of Defense Mechanisms

Successful Mechanisms (Table 49.5)

❖ *Repression:* Involuntary and automatic regulation of unbearable ideas and impulses; submersion of these to subconscious real time helps provide a forgetting and protective function for the ego, for example, after recent death of a spouse the surviving spouse can remember the marriage date.

❖ *Rationalization:* In rationalization we "make excuses" giving a reason different from the real one for what we are doing. It is a defense mechanism in which an individual justifies his/her failures and socially unacceptable behavior by giving socially approved reasons.

Purpose is to help raise self-esteem and social approval disguising motivations, for example, students who fail in the examination may complain that the hostel atmosphere is not favorable for study.

A scientist who is unable to carry out research of high order may blame the lack of facilities.

Rationalization is not lying. We believe our explanations it is like a blanket to cover the human weaknesses it operates in two forms:

1. Source grapes
2. Sweet lemon.

Intellectualization: Related to rationalization is intellectualization another defense mechanism, which involves reasoning it is the distancing from an emotional or threatening situation by talking or thinking about it in intellectual terms, for example, a nurse or a doctor worker can't afford to become emotionally attached to each patient. So they use the technique of detaching themselves from emotions through calm abstract statements about the situation. You may speak calmly and intelligently rather than emotionally with patients and their families, for example, if there is a patient who is acutely ill, calmly till the family members rather than saying "I am so sorry," etc.

❖ *Compensation:* An attempt to make up for real or imagined deficiencies. Something given to replace a loss or to make up for a defect). It helps relieve fears of failure in one activity by emphasizing another can result in one sidedness caused by over compensation, for example, a student who fails in his/her studies may compensate by becoming the college champion in athletics.

❖ *Sublimation:* It is the channeling of strong and socially unacceptable drive or urge into a form that is acceptable to society. The most important of these are social desires. It helps channel forbidden instinctual impulses into constructive activities. Sublimation is one of the more positive mechanisms of adjustment and is responsible for much of the artistic and cultural achievements of the civilized, for example, a young man who has lost his lover may turn to write poetry about love.

Unsuccessful Mechanism (Table 49.5)

❖ *Suppression:* Suppression is an intentional pushing away from awareness of certain unwelcome ideas memories or feelings. We merely push them into the basic ground, into our subconscious mind, where they are accessible to us whenever we wish to remember them.

For examples, a student consciously decides not to think about her weekend so that she can study effectively, a patient may refuse to consider.

❖ *Reaction formation:* It is some time possible to conceal a motive from ourselves by giving strong expression to its opposite such a tendency is called reaction formation. For example, the mother of an unwanted child may feel quietly and so become over indulgent and overprotective of the child to assure herself that she is a good mother; an adolescent struggles with hostile feelings, but presents herself in an ingratiating way.

❖ *Displacement:* Redirection of emotional feelings from one idea person or object to another.
  ➢ *Purpose:* Helps the person disguise feelings by using a less threatening object to release feelings. For example, a person who is angry with his boss, but cannot show it for fear of losing the job may fight with his wife and children or on return from the office; a physician berates a nurse and when a visitor enters the client's room. The nurse harshly tells the person to wait for visiting hours.
  ➢ *Denial:* Denial of reality is when refuse to accept or believe the existence of something that is very unpleasant to us. We use denial most often when faced with death serious illness or something painful and threatening. For example, a patient admitted to the psychiatric ward may say that he just needs rest, when some very near and dear one die in the family some people try to keep up the pretence that he is still alive. Denial is quite harmless if practiced in moderation, but can lead to serious difficulties in health and lifestyle if practiced to excess.

- **Projection:** Projection is a frequently used unconscious mechanisms that relieve tension and anxiety by transferring the responsibility or unacceptable ideas, impulsive wishes, or thoughts to another person. For examples, the student who believes that everybody cheats in examinations may also cheat in the same way; an adulterer blames his wife that she is an adulteress. People who are dishonest often attribute dishonesty to others.
- *Regression:* Retreat to an earlier and more comfortable level of adjustment. It helps the person retreat from the present situation and become dependent and less anxious. When faced with the difficulty of life, the individual reverts to a less mature from of behavior where he finds less conflict and hence less anxiety. For example, a 5-year-old child going to school for the first time may have toilet accidents revert to baby talk demand cuddling.
- *Identification:* By this adjustment, the individual feels the personal satisfaction in the success and achievement of other people and groups. A very common age for practicing identification is in the teens. For example, adolescents often will identify with successful people in the movies. Identification with a hero either in fiction or in real life is called hero-worship. Much of the learning process in childhood is through identification. As we grow a little older, we identify with our teachers, legendary fingers, heroes, and idols. Identification is quite normal and healthy. Since it plays a large part in the development of a child's personalities and in the process of acculturation. If the object with which we identify is good, their effect once will be constructive if it is bad, the effects can be destructive.
- *Conversion:* Conversion is exactly what is says strong emotional conflicts are expressed as or converted into physical symptoms. For example, the boy who hates father and is torn between the desire to strike at him and fear of the consequences if the does so develops a paralyzed arm. The conflict is resolved. He cannot strike his father even if he wishes to and the situation carries no threat of relation in addition the boy secures sympathy and attention for his symptoms. The mechanism of conversion also operates wholly on an unconscious level.

Fantasy or Day Dreaming

Fantasy is a kind of withdrawal when faced with real problems of life. The tendency to daydreaming is most pronounced during adolescence. Day dreaming is a pleasant thing. It may help us to escape during times of stress. For example, when one is having financial problem one can escape from them temporarily by planning how to spend an imaginary fortune.

Fantasy may after temporary relief from pressures, but excessive daydreaming may lead to loss of contact with realities and may lead to a psychotic disorder.

Withdrawal

Whenever an individual respects that he is likely to be criticized or disgraced on account of some prior unfortunate experience or failure. Here sorts to withdrawal. Such a person is seen as avoiding all work saying he cannot do this or he cannot do that it is a protective device by which the individual prevents further and damage to his security by withdrawing from people and avoiding all close interpersonal relations it may occur as a temporary pattern. Withdrawal is one of the dominant personality traits in schizophrenics.

CONCLUSION

All of us use defense mechanisms to overcome conflict, anxiety, and stressful situations in our daily life. That is how we are able to adjust in life and maintain the optimum mental health. Thus, it would give an insight to one's own behavior, but when these defense mechanisms are used frequently by the patients and they start interfering with the routine activities of an individual.

CHAPTER 50

Communication, Interpersonal Relationships, Individual and Group, Group Dynamics and Organizational Behavior

CHAPTER OUTLINE

- Definition
- Factors Influencing Communication
- Types of Communication
- Components of Communication
- Barriers of Communication
- Techniques to Improve Therapeutic Communication
- Theories of Communication
- Characteristics of Therapeutic Communication
- Levels of Communication
- Interpersonal (Therapeutic) Relationship
- Development of a Therapeutic Relationship
- Phases of Therapeutic Relationship
- Group Dynamics
- Organizational Behavior

INTRODUCTION

Communication is an essential component of survival for all creatures. Even plants communicate. Research has demonstrated that when a tree is attached by insects, it sends a chemical message to other trees in that area.

Animals communicate in simple and complex ways using both sound and movement, but the master communicator, the user of language, is the human being. The fulfillment of man's basic needs such as food and water requires cooperative effort of the people and cooperation is not possible without communication and understanding. Therefore, communication is very essential to nursing process, because communication is the vehicle for establishing a therapeutic relationship leading to the successful outcome of nursing intervention.

DEFINITION

- Communication refers to the reciprocal exchange of information, ideas, feelings, and attitudes between two persons or among a group of persons.
  —**Taylor (1994)**
- Communication is a two-way process concerned with conveying a message or an idea between two or more individuals.
- Communication is a process by which information is exchanged between individuals through a common system of symbols, signs or behaviors.
  —**Webster's New Collegiate Dictionary**

FACTORS INFLUENCING COMMUNICATION

Situations have several contacted aspects that influence the nature of communication and interpersonal relationships. These include the participants' physical and emotional status, the nature of their relationship, their environment, the situation prompting communication, and sociocultural elements present.

- *Psychophysiological context:* The internal factors influencing communication are as follows:
  - Physiological status (pain, illness)
  - Emotional status (anxiety, anger)
  - Growth and developmental status
  - Unmet needs
  - Attitudes, values, and beliefs
  - Perceptions and personality
  - Self-concept and self-esteem.
- *Relational context:* The nature of the relationship between the participants is as follows:
  - Social, helping or working relationship
  - Level of trust between participants
  - Level of self-disclosure between participants
  - Shared history of participants.
- *Situational context:* Information exchange, goal achievement, problem resolution, and expression of feelings.
- *Environmental context:* Degree of privacy, degree of comfort and safety, noise level, and presence of distraction.

❖ *Cultural context:* Education level of participants, language and self-expression patterns, customs, and expectations.

TYPES OF COMMUNICATION

Communication takes place on several levels. Each person involved in sending and receiving messages is a complete and unique personality who interacts on several levels at one time. These levels can be verbal and non-verbal communications. Communications at each of these levels occur through every person-to-person interaction.

❖ *Verbal communication:* Verbal communication occurs through words, spoken or written. It includes speaking and writing, the use of language and symbols, and the arrangement of words or phrases.
❖ *Non-verbal communication:* Non-verbal communication encompasses everything that does not involve the spoken or written word, including the five senses. It includes one's interpersonal communication—the messages created through body's motions and use of touch, space, and sight. It also refers to the unspoken interpersonal communication and includes behaviors such as eye movements, gestures, body movements, facial expressions, postures, and eye contact.

Meta-communication

Meta-communication refers to role expectation or mode of communication, that is, how the message should be understood by a receiver in the context of verbal and non-verbal communications. For example, the message, "you look fresh and lovely today," is conveyed with wrinkles on the forehead, so the receiver must interpret the sincerity of the sender in giving the compliments.

COMPONENTS OF COMMUNICATION

For a successful communication to occur, five components must be in place—the sender, the message, the receiver, the feedback, and the context (Fig. 50.1), which are explained as follows:
❖ The sender is the one who forms the message and transmits.
❖ The message is the verbal and non-verbal information expressed by the sender to the receiver.
❖ The receiver is the person to whom the message is sent.
❖ The feedback is the responses of each person when messages are being sent and received.

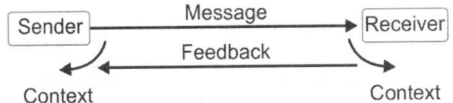

Fig. 50.1: Components of communication.

❖ The context is the setting in which the communication takes place. It includes both physical and psychosocial settings.

BARRIERS OF COMMUNICATION

The barriers of communication are as follows:
❖ Failure to listen
❖ Failure to focus on the ill person's problem
❖ Failure to remain on the topic under discussion
❖ Talking too much
❖ Talking very little
❖ Ineffective reassurance
❖ Probing
❖ Challenging
❖ Advising
❖ Defending.

TECHNIQUES TO IMPROVE THERAPEUTIC COMMUNICATION

The techniques to improve therapeutic communication are as follows:
❖ *Active listening:* An active process of receiving information and examining reaction to the messages received. For example, maintaining eye contact and receptive non-verbal communication.
❖ *Broad openings:* Encouraging the patient to select topics for discussion. For example, "What are you thinking about?"
❖ *Restating:* Repeating the main thought the patient has expressed. For example, "You say that your mother left you when you were 5 years old."
❖ *Clarification:* Attempting to put into words vague ideas or unclear thoughts of a patient to enhance the nurse's understanding or asking the patient to explain what he/she means. For example, "I am not sure what you mean, could you tell me about that again."
❖ *Reflection:* Directing back the patient's ideas, feelings, questions, or content. For example, "You're feeling tense and anxious and it is related to a conversation you had with your husband last night?"
❖ *Focusing:* Questions or statements that help the patient to expand on a topic of importance. For example, "I think that we should talk more about your relationship with your father." Sharing observations, sharing feelings, sharing empathy, using touch, sharing hope, using silence, sharing humor, asking relevant questions, providing information, self-disclosing, clarifying, and confronting.
❖ *Exploring:* Examining certain ideas, experiences, or relationships more freely. For example, "Tell me more about that would you describe it more freely."

- **Informing:** Skill of information giving. For example, "I think you need to know more about how your mediation works."
- **Suggesting:** Presentation of alternative ideas for clients' consideration relative to problem solving. For example, "Have you thought about responding to your boss in a different way when he raised that issue with you? For example, you could ask him if a specific problem has occurred."
- **Silence:** Lack of verbal communication for a therapeutic reason. For example, sitting with a patient and non-verbally communicating interest and involvement. Sharing empathy, sharing hope, sharing feelings, using touch, asking relevant questions, self-disclosing and confronting.

THEORIES OF COMMUNICATION

Transactional Analysis by Eric Berne (1964)

Transactional analysis is the study of communications or transactions that have taken place between people. This approach to personality was developed by Eric Berne (1964), a psychiatrist who made transactional analysis a popular theory through his classic book, "Games People Play: The Psychology of Human Relationships."

The cornerstone of this theory is that each person's personality is made up of three distinct components called ego states. An ego state is a consistent pattern of feeling, experiencing and behaving. The three ego states that make up personality are the parent ego state, adult ego state and child ego state:

The parent ego state: It consists of all the nurturing, critical and prejudicial attitudes, behaviors, and experiences learned from other people, especially parents and teachers.

- **The adult ego state:** It is the reality-oriented part of the personality. It gathers and processes information about the world and is objective, emotionless and intelligent in its approach to problem solving.
- **The child ego state:** It is the feeling part of the personality. In it resides the feelings of happiness, joy, sadness, depression and anxiety. It contains all the feelings the individual had as a child.

Berne's Model of Communication

The Berne's model of communication makes it possible to diagram transactions using these ego states. A transaction/communication (Fig. 50.2) between two people can be complementary, crossed or ulterior.

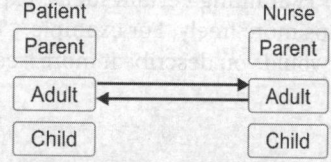

Fig. 50.2: Transaction/communication.

Complementary Transaction

A person responds from the ego state, addressed to the ego state from which message was received (Fig. 50.3). For example:

Patient: I know that when I get mad at my boss, I take it out on my wife and kids, but I don't know what else to do.

Nurse: Do you think you could let your boss know how you're feeling.

Patient: He'll fire me for sure.

Nurse: Perhaps you could talk it with a co-worker.

Patient: I do not have time to chat on the job like that. Besides, no one cares about someone else's life.

Nurse: Sometimes physical exercise helps people get rid of their anger. Have you ever tried it?

Patient: Sure, I work out a lot, but that doesn't help.

Nurse: My wife's tired of "all my talk" as she puts it. She says she wants some action.

The transactional analysis model of communication provides a framework for the nurse to use in exploring the patient's recurrent behaviors, identifying patterns, thinking about causes and planning alternative ways to respond.

Patient: I know that when I get mad at my boss, I take it out on my wife and kids.

Nurse: Are you ready to think about some other ways you can handle your anger?

Crossed Transactions

The person does not respond from the ego state addressed (Fig. 50.4). For example:

Patient: I know that when I get mad at my boss, I take it out on my wife and kids.

Nurse: Man always think that's OK, but the women have to suffer for it.

Ulterior Transactions

Ulterior transactions take place on two levels, the social overt and the psychological/covert level. These transactions

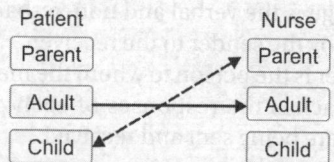

Fig. 50.3: Complementary transaction.

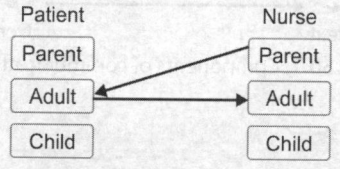

Fig. 50.4: Crossed transactions.

tend to be destructive because the communication conceals their true motivations. Double messages are sent and received.

Ruesch's Theory

A theory of communication that considers communication as the social framework for healthcare was developed by J. Ruesch in the late 1950s. He believed that communication included a broad range of activities that were designed to affect another person.

Communications were viewed as a circular process, whereby messages traveled from within one person to another person and back again. Events within the sender prompt the sending of a message. The message is then transmitted to another who receives it, processes it internally and responds; successful communication occurs when agreement about the meaning of the message has been reached.

Therapeutic communications are distinguished from ordinary communication by the intent of one of the participants to bring about a positive change. According to Ruesch, a therapist seeks to find the nature of clients' distress and develops an understanding of their problems. Then with the use of therapeutic communication techniques, both the client and the therapist agree on the nature of the problem and what should be done about it.

Therapeutic communication is the hallmark of a therapeutic relationship, which is the art and process of reaching the person with messages designed to facilitate health.

Therapeutic relationship refers to interpersonal process between a professional nurse and a client. It fosters and promotes growth of the personality and improves the constructive and protective ways of living.

CHARACTERISTICS OF THERAPEUTIC COMMUNICATION

- ❖ **Acceptance:** Conveying acceptance is an important part of a therapeutic communication. It means you are non-judgmental. Acceptance is a willingness to hear a message or to acknowledge feelings, yet does not mean that you agree or approve. Acceptance includes giving a positive feedback, making sure verbal and non-verbal cues match, using touch, being empathetic, restating and avoiding arguments.
- ❖ **Respect:** It refers to the acceptance of a patient as a person of worth who is valued and accepted without qualification.
- ❖ **Interest:** Nurses' communication interest when they are genuinely curious and express a desire to know another person. Interest is conveyed by asking about these aspects of a person's life that others often reject.
- ❖ **Honesty:** Nurses are honest when they are consistent, open, and frank; nurses do not take refuge behind a professional mask, but instead communicate with the client as an authentic person. Nurses are honest and non-defensive about their thoughts and feelings that they discover through self-assessment.
- ❖ **Concreteness:** Involves using specific terminologies rather than abstractions when discussing the patient feelings, experiences, and behavior. It helps to keep the nurses' responses close to patients' feelings and experiences, to foster accuracy of understanding by the nurse and to encourage the patient attend to specific problem areas.
- ❖ **Assistance:** Nurses assist clients by committing time and energy to the therapeutic relationships.
- ❖ **Permission:** Nurses communicate permission by conveying the message that is acceptable to try new ways of behaving—permission needs to be given to clients to encourage them to see and do things in new ways.
- ❖ **Protection:** Nurses protect clients by ensuring clients' safety and developing effective ways of dealing with problems.

Client: "I am really scared to go home on my pass this weekend? What will people say? How will they expect me to behave?"

Nurse: "I hear that you're scared, and that's very natural for you to feel. Let's work together to try to anticipate what will happen over the weekend and see if, together, you and I can come up with some strategies for dealing with those hot spots."

LEVELS OF COMMUNICATION

Nurses use different levels of communication in their professional role:

- ❖ **Intrapersonal communication:** It is a powerful form of self-talk, self-verbalization, self-instruction, inner thought, inner dialog, and positive self-talk.
- ❖ **Interpersonal communication:** It is a one-to-one interaction between the nurse and another person face-to-face.
- ❖ **Transpersonal:** It is an interaction that occurs in a person's spiritual domain, e.g., prayer, meditation, and religious rituals.
- ❖ **Small-group communication:** It refers to a small number of individuals who meet together—goal directed.
- ❖ **Public communication:** It is an interaction between an audience and a nurse on health-related topics.

INTERPERSONAL (THERAPEUTIC) RELATIONSHIP

The goal of nursing has always been to promote health; mental health is defined as the forward movement of personality and other ongoing human processes in the direction of creative, constructive, productive, personnel, and community living.

The psychiatric nurse needs to recognize that every interaction has the potential to promote the health of the client. Indeed, psychiatric nurses have an obligation to use their skills within a therapeutic relationship to promote and maintain health.

Social versus Therapeutic Relationships

A social relationship is with friends and acquaintances, and it exists for the mutual satisfaction of those involved. Its duration, focus and intensity vary according to the participant's wishes; it is a subjective relationship.

The therapeutic relationship is viewed as a social relationship, where "two people come to know each other well enough to face the problem at hand in a cooperative way." It is unique in the world of interactions with human beings.

Role of a Nurse

Roles are socially expected behavior patterns determined by an individual's position or status in a particular group or relationship. The nurse has been identified to play four roles:

- ❖ *Resource person* is the one who gives specific information to clients, thus allowing them to understand situations or procedures.
- ❖ *Counselor* is the one who listens to the client's experience and assists in clarifying feelings associated with it.
- ❖ *Surrogate* is the one with whom the client casts into roles of past relationships (parents, siblings, spouse and teacher), perhaps needing clarification of feelings.
- ❖ *Technical expert* is the one who can navigate the complexities of the healthcare system.

Aspects of the Therapeutic Relationship

The different aspects of the therapeutic relationship are as follows:

- ❖ *Goal-directed:* The overall goal of any therapeutic relationship is to assist the client to move toward health by becoming more self-responsible. Each individual is unique, however, and specific goals need to be defined for each person.
- ❖ *Client-centered:* It implies that it is focused on the client; it is the goals, reactions, coping strategies and growth that are the center of the relationship.
- ❖ *Objectivity:* It requires nurses to be aware of their feelings and reactions being with clients rather than to just responding to clients on a personal level.
- ❖ *Transference*: It refers to the feelings of the client toward the nurse and the helping relationship. These feelings truly belong to the significant people in the client's life prior to the therapeutic relationship with the nurse and are transferred and played out again in the therapeutic relationship.
- ❖ *Counter transfer:* It is defined as the feelings of the nurse toward the client. These feelings may be positive or negative and are a natural part of therapeutic relationship problem that arises only when the feelings are discounted because they upset, surprise or embrace the nurse in some way.

Preparation for Interactive Therapy

- ❖ Self-awareness
- ❖ Areas for self-assessment
  - ➢ Need to be liked
  - ➢ Being judgmental
- ❖ Responsibility
- ❖ Potential for human growth.

Self-awareness

Self-awareness is clear from the proceeding discussion that the psychiatric nurse needs a strong sense of self or at least the willingness to develop one. The term 'sense of self' refers to self-awareness or self-knowledge. This is necessary because nurses must be able to separate their own subjective belief from the facts. Self-awareness implies recognition of one's thinking, values, conflicts, interactions and attitudes, and an awareness of how these can influence the interaction with the clients.

Areas for Self-assessment

- ❖ *Need to be liked:* It is important to assess the need to be liked. The need to be accepted and valued can be strong that it can paralyze the nurse during interactions. For example, the nurse is at risk for becoming hurt/angry if the client acts in an angry or hostile manner or the nurse may hesitate to comment, for fear that the client would be offended in some way and consequently think less of the nurse. In fact, rapport will develop best when nurses focus on their clients so much that they forget their own need to be liked.
- ❖ *Being judgmental:* Another area to evaluate is being judgmental; judgments are quick stereotyping of people so as to sort them into categories to ease one's own interactive experience. Forming judgments is also a survival skill that allows us to decide issues of emotional safety quickly. Often, these judgments are based on a few life experiences and tend to be generalized in others.

Responsibility

Another critical area is the assumption of responsibility. It is necessary for psychiatric nurses to clarify their own understanding of who is responsible for what in the therapeutic relationship. There are areas of nursing where the outcomes depend solely on nursing performance. For example, the absence of sepsis around a surgical wound, the administration of medication or the proper rate of fluid replacement via an intravenous infusion. All these administrations involve the nurse doing something for the client.

Potential for Human Growth

This also requires the psychiatric nurse to have some confidence in the client's ability to grow, learn, and make changes. Nurses need to assess their own assumptions about the potential for human growth. Nurses can assess these symptoms by evaluating their own personal needs for sympathy and protection. If nurses believe that they need to be protected from life experiences, they may assume that they do not have the capabilities to deal with life and that it is not possible to develop them. Hence, the need for protection exists.

DEVELOPMENT OF A THERAPEUTIC RELATIONSHIP

Establishing a therapeutic relationship is not magic; it requires hard work and the skillful application of knowledge. Beginners in interactive therapy are so often concerned with the content of the session that they overlook the basic concepts at work in every therapeutic relationship. These concepts are boundary development, safety development, and trust development. The concepts apply to the individual therapeutic relationship, as well as the family and group processes, although they are expressed in different ways. These three concepts are tightly interwoven, each affecting the other.

Boundary Development

The term 'boundary' refers to the definition of an entity. The boundaries of a country define its shape, size and location in relationship to other countries. In psychological terms, boundaries refer to the definition and the separation of the self from others. They serve to define the responsibilities and duties of one's self in relationship to others.

Safety Development

Safety is the sense of security within the therapeutic relationship. A clear sense of boundaries is essential in developing a sense of safety in the therapeutic relationship. Safety comes from knowing what the expectations are and what one's responsibilities are in meeting those expectations. Consequently, part of nurses' role in a therapeutic relationship is to enhance safety by acting consistently within the defined boundaries. It is confusing and dangerous for the clients if a nurse should introduce social elements into the therapeutic relationship. In an attempt to be "friendly," nurses should act within the boundaries of their role by assisting the client to focus on the assigned tasks and explore one for growth, healing, and understanding.

Trust Development

As the nurse exercises the concepts of boundary and safety, trust develops within the nurse–client relationship. Trust is the reliance on the truthfulness or accuracy of the relationship. Trust develops when there is congruence between words and actions; for many clients, the relationship with the caregivers may be the most trusting one in their lives. Trust does not develop from doing everything the client asks; trust develops from doing what one said one would do. These three concepts of boundary development and maintenance, safety development and trust development are the foundations of every therapeutic relationship. The nurse constantly works to develop these in each relationship; it is an "invisible work" within the net of three concepts; and the nurse works with the client in a goal-directed and client-centered way, using a variety of skills such as listening and feedback.

PHASES OF THERAPEUTIC RELATIONSHIP

A vital characteristic of the nurse–patient relationship is the sharing of behaviors, thoughts, and feelings. Therapeutic relationship goes through various phases (Fig. 50.5):
- Preorientation phase
- Orientation phase
- Working phase
- Termination phase

Preorientation Phase

The preorientation phase begins before the nurse's first contact with the patient. The initial task of the nurse is self-exploration/self-analysis.

The orientation phase is the first phase of the therapeutic relationship. It occurs when the clients enter the system and are filled with tension and anxiety associated with their own needs, in addition to those generated by exposure to a new and uncertain situation.

The nurse works to assist clients to clarify their impression of the problem, thus defining the scope or boundary of the work. In addition, the nurse assists the client to function within the relationship, to have questions answered, needs expressed and sincerity developed (Peplau, 1952), thus defining the scope or boundaries of the relationship itself.

Tasks of Preorientation Phase
- The nurse reviews available data
- Anticipate health concerns/issues that may arise
- Identify a location and setting that will foster comfortable, private interaction

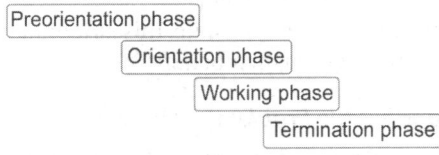

Fig. 50.5: Phases of therapeutic relationship.

Orientation Phase

Goal to Develop Trust

It is during the introductory phase that the nurse and patient first meet. In this phase, the client and the nurse get to know one another, and begin to accept each other as a unique human being. Boundary development is done in specific ways.

Nurses initially approach clients as strangers (Peplau, 1952) and must work to define themselves as allies and helpers. In introducing themselves to clients, nurses must state their purposes clearly. It is important that when speaking with new clients (strangers), nurses say whatever is appropriate for clients to hear, without using slang terms or incomplete remarks (Peplau, 1952). For example, if meeting a depressed client in an inpatient unit, the nurse could say, "Hello, I'm Mary Webster. I'm your nurse. I'll be working with you while you're here to help you get used to the hospital and to look at the areas in your life that are troubling you." This introduction serves to identify the relationship as therapeutic and defines the nurse's role as a helping professional.

There is no clear ending to the orientation phase or beginning of the next phase, the working phase. The phases of the relationship overlap. As the working phase begins, the boundaries of the relationship have been established and the client acts within these boundaries. Safety and trust have also developed to the point that the client is willing to risk further exploration of issues. The nurse and the client have come to know each other well enough to be able to cooperate in dealing with a problem.

Tasks of Orientation Phase

- Establish rapport, trust, and communication
- Gather data
- Formulate a contract
- Set mutual specific goals with the patient.

Working Phase

Most of the therapeutic work is carried out during the working phase. The nurse and the patient explore stressors and promote the development of insight in the patient by linking precipitations, thoughts, feelings, and actions. This insight should be translated into action and change in behavior. The nurse helps the patient to master anxieties, increase independence and self-responsibility and develop constructive coping mechanisms.

There are two parts to the working phase:
1. Understanding the problem
2. Assisting clients to translate this understanding to actions that work to their benefit

Understanding the Problem

Counseling acknowledges that self-renewal, repair and awareness come from within the individual. The function of the nurse counselor is to assist the individual's self-directed learning in ways that promote health and integration of experience (Peplau, 1952).

Necessary skills for this phase of work are careful listening, open-ended and non-judgmental responses. The nursing response to a client's statement must not obstruct the possibility of identifying feelings or thoughts that assist clients in learning about themselves (Peplau, 1952).

To further demonstrate nursing responses that promote the client's understanding of the situation, consider the following example of the suicidal client:

Client: "I just want to die."
Nurse: "You're thinking about death very seriously."
Client: "Yes, It would take care of everything."
Nurse: "You're seeing death as a solution."
Client: "Yes."
Nurse: "I'm not sure I understood. Tell me more."
Client: "About what?"
Nurse: "About death as a solution."
Client: "Well, the insurance money would pay off my debts and my wife would have money to live on."
Nurse: "You're thinking it would be a financial benefit to your wife."
Client: "Yes, She'd probably be happier, too without me. I'm not worth much these days."
Nurse: "You think your wife would be happier if you were to die."
Client: "Yes well, not right away, of course. She'd get over it. Find somebody worthy of her."
Nurse: "It sounds as if you think highly of her."
Client: "Oh, yes, I don't know why she puts up with me, though. I've been terrible to be around."
Nurse: "You sound puzzled that she could love you even during this difficult time."

In this case, the nurse did not argue against the client's solution of suicide, but explored the dynamics behind it. The questions/statements also help to introduce different perspectives to the client (the fact that he is worthy of love even during his depression and the possibility that the depression is time-limited).

Further exploration with both these clients would serve to clarify the patterns of thinking and acting that contribute to their dysphoria. This is crucial information. It is the meaning of the behavior, mood or thoughts perceived by the client that offers the nurse clues to determine which needs must be met (Peplau, 1952). The nurse obtains this information as purely as possible without contaminating it. To do this, the nurse acts as a neutral sounding board so that clients can voice their views in a relationship that is safely defined and non-judgmental (Peplau, 1952).

Translating Understanding into Action

The second part of the working phase is to assist clients to translate their expanded understanding of the situation into behavioral changes or actions that promote health. There are many ways to do this, depending on the client's situation and nurse's theoretical perspective. One aspect common to all client situations is that the behavioral changes are practiced in the "here and now."

The client actually attempts behavioral change in the clinical situation with nursing support. For example, perhaps the suicidal man has learned that his days are much worse when he does not get out of bed in the morning. Together with the nurse, he has identified a behavioral pattern in which he stays in bed isolated from his wife, reflects on his worthlessness and becomes more despondent as the day goes on. This pattern has been repeated in the unit. The client and the nurse have decided to evaluate whether a change in this pattern would effect a change in his self-perception; they decide to test this by having the client get out of bed promptly in the morning and interact with at least one person at breakfast (this would be consistent with a cognitive therapy approach).

Tasks of Working Phase

- Maintain the therapeutic relationship
- Gather further data
- Promote clients' insight and use of constructive coping mechanism
- Encourage the patient to communicate and socialize
- Facilitate behavioral changes
- Evaluate problems.

Termination Phase

Termination is one of the most important phases of the therapeutic nurse–patient relationship. During the termination phase, learning is maximized for both the patient and the nurse. It is a time to exchange feelings and memories, to evaluate mutually the patient's progress, to attain high level of trust and intimacy, and to reflect on the quality of relationship and the sense of loss experienced by both the nurse and patient.

In a more concrete sense, termination is the real loss of the nurse for the client. The relationship ends and the client must face life without the external support of the nurse. But life is nothing if not full of contrasts. At the same time, that ending is being acknowledged, so are accomplishments, growth, and individuality. It is as if the ending of a relationship emphasizes the very being of the individual who created the relationship. The work of the psychiatric nurse during the termination phase is to assist clients to acknowledge both these realities and to integrate them into their personalities. The therapeutic work is the acknowledgement of the formal closure of the boundaries of the relationship and the transfer of safety and trust to the client.

Prior to Termination

As noted earlier, termination work begins during the introductory phase. The nurse defines the time frame for the therapeutic relationship to exist. The inpatient nurse may state, "while you are in the hospital, we will be working together." The outpatient nurse may say, "during the 6 weeks of this program." The nurse defines the time frame of the work during the initial meetings and thus begins to prepare the client for the eventual end of the relationship. In addition, the work of the relationship has been clearly defined during the introductory period, and specific goals have been identified. Thus, the relationship has been defined by time limits and desired outcomes.

As clients begin to do more for themselves, the nurse can transition to the termination phase by spacing contacts incrementally further apart to allow clients more time to "stand on their own" according to their ability to do so. This gives clients the opportunity to support themselves gradually and the nurse acknowledges this.

During the transition to the termination phase (and during termination itself), new or intense topics should not be introduced. This is a time of solidifying gains and acknowledging the work accomplished. If other issues exist, they may be acknowledged as areas for future work. It is unfair to the client to raise issues that cannot be resolved within the time that remains.

Nurse's Role in Termination

As noted earlier, the American culture does not deal with endings well. Consequently, few clients have a frame of reference for handling this crucial aspect of life. The nurse has the unique opportunity to assist the client in a successful separation and ending, allowing the client to transfer this knowledge to the next situation. To do this, the psychiatric nurse must model effective parting for the client. The first step is for the nurse to clearly understand the goal of termination, which is to dissolve the therapeutic relationship, while assuring the client of an improved ability to function independently (Fortinash and Holoday-Worret, 1995).

The second step is for the nurse to have a clear understanding of the dynamics of toss and how these concepts affect the client and the nurse. For instance, it is important that the nurses not respond to the client's anger or regression in a personal manner, but instead continue to work to help clarify the client's feelings and reactions. Nurses, like clients, need to express their own mixed feelings about the separation. For example, "I also feel sad that this relationship is ending, and I am happy about the work we have accomplished," is a statement that helps clients' normalize any reactions they may experience.

Goal: To bring a therapeutic relationship and to nurse–patient relationship.

Tasks of Termination Phase

❖ Establish reality of separation
❖ Review progress of therapy and attainment of goals
❖ Mutually explore feelings of rejection, loss, sadness, and related behaviors.

GROUP DYNAMICS

Introduction

In today's explosion of information technology, communication continues to be a complex process. Group dynamics can be very positive and helpful where team members support each other and do what is best.

Negativity among the members of organization is increasing leading to selfishness. Therefore, the organization/administrator should have a positive attitude and it is important that they counsel individuals exhibiting negative behavior to achieve positive group dynamics.

Definitions

Group:

❖ A group may be defined as a number of individuals who join together to achieve a goal. People join groups to achieve goals that cannot be achieved by them alone.
—**Johnson & Johnson (2006)**
❖ A collection of people who interact with one another, accept rights and obligations as members and who share a common identity.

Group dynamics:

❖ A branch of social psychology which studies problems involving the structure of a group.
❖ The interactions that influence attitude and behavior of people when they are grouped with others through either choice or accidental circumstances.

Type of Groups

❖ **Formal groups:** It refers to those which are established under the legal or formal authority with the view to achieve a particular result.
 Example: Trade unions.
❖ **Informal groups:** Refer to aggregate of personal contact and interaction and network of relationship among individuals.
 Example: Friendship group.
❖ **Primary groups:** They are characterized by small size, face-to-face interaction and network of relationship among members of a group.
 Example: Family and neighborhood group.
❖ **Secondary groups:** Characterized by large size, individual identification with the values and beliefs prevailing in them rather than cultural interaction.
 Example: Occupational association and ethnic group.
❖ **Task groups:** They are composed of people who work together to perform a task but involve cross-command relationship.
 Example: For finding out who was responsible for causing wrong medication order would require liaison among ward in charge, senior sister and head nurse.
❖ **Social groups:** Refers to an integrated system of interrelated psychological group formed to accomplish defined objectives.
 Example: Political party with its many local political clubs and friendship groups.
❖ **Reference group:** One in which they would like to belong or refer by someone from the group.
❖ **Membership groups:** Those where the individual actually belongs.
❖ **Command groups:** Formed by subordinates reporting directly to the particular manager and are determined by formal organizational chart.
❖ **Functional groups:** The individual works together daily on similar tasks.
❖ **Problem-solving groups:** It focuses on specific issues in their areas of responsibility and develops potential solution and often empowered to take action.

Objectives of Group Dynamics

❖ To identify and analyze the social processes that impact on group development and performance.
❖ To acquire the skills necessary to intervene and improve individual and group performance in organizational context.
❖ To build more successful organizations by applying techniques that provide positive impact on goal achievement.

Principles of Group Dynamics

❖ The members of the group must have a strong sense of belonging to the group.
❖ The group arises and functions occurring to common motives.
❖ Groups survive by placing the members into functional hierarchy and facilitating action toward the goal.
❖ The intergroup relations group organization and member participation is emotional for effectiveness of group.
❖ Information relating to needs for change, plans for change and consequences of changes must be shared by members of a group.

Elements of Group Dynamics

Communication

One of the easiest aspects of group process to observe is the pattern of communication. The kinds of observations we make give us clues to other important things which may be going on in the group such as who leads whom or who influences whom.

Content versus Process

When we observe what the group is talking about, we are focusing on the content. When we try to observe how the group is handling its communication, we are talking about group process.

At a simpler level, looking at process really means to focus on what is going on in the group and trying to understand it in terms of other things that have been going on in the group.

Decision

Many kinds of decisions are made in groups without considering the effects these decisions have on other members.

Some try to impose their own decisions on the group, while others want all members to participate or share in the decisions that are made.

Some decisions are made consciously after much debate and voting.

Influence

Some people may speak very little, yet they may capture the attention of the whole group. Others may talk a lot but other members may pay little attention to them.

Task versus Relationship

The group's task is the job to be done. People who are concerned with the task tend to:
- Make suggestions
- Attempt to summarize what has been covered
- Give or ask for facts, ideas, or search for alternative relationship meaning how well people in the group work together.

Roles

Behavior in the group can be of three types:
- **Task roles:** Which help the group accomplish its task.
  - Initiator, information/opinion seeker, information/opinion giver, clarifier and elaborator, summarizer, energizer, coordinator.
- **Relationship roles:** Which help group members get along better.
  - Harmonizer, gatekeeper, encourager, relationship roles, compromiser and follower.
- **Self-oriented roles:** Which contribute to neither group task nor group relationship.
  - Dominator, negativist, aggressor, playboy, story teller and interrupter.

Stages of Group Development

Bruce W. Tuckman is a respected educational psychologist who first described the four stages of group development in 1965. The four-stage model is called Tuckman's stages for a group. Tuckman's model states that the ideal group decision-making process should occur in four stages.

Stage I—forming:

It is the initial stage marked by uncertainty and confusion. The structure of the group is uncertain and unpredictable leadership cannot be implemented effectively.

Stage II—storming:

There is a huge rift created because of various disparities and disagreements between members.

Stage III—norming:

The scopes of the group's tasks or responsibilities are clear and agreed. They now understand each other better and can appreciate each other's skills and experience. Individuals listen to each other, appreciate and support each other, and are prepared to change preconceived views, and they feel they are part of a cohesive and effective group.

Stage IV—performing:

Working in a group to a common goal which is an highly efficient and cooperative basis.

Stage V—adjourning (mourning the adjournment of the group):

This is about completion and disengagement both from the task and the group members. Individuals will be proud of having achieved much and glad to have been part of such an enjoyable group.

Some authors describe stage 5 as "Deforming and mourning" recognizing the sense of boss felt by group members.

M. Scott Peck developed stages for larger-scale groups (i.e., communities) which are similar to Tuchman's stage of group development. Peck describes the stage of a community as:
- Pseudo-community
- Chaos
- Emptiness
- True community.

Group Dynamic Process

Group Formation

The group is able to share experiences to provide feedback to pool ideas to generate insights and provide an arena for analysis of experiences. The group provides a measure of support and assurance.

Participation

Participation is a fundamental process within a group because many of the other processes depend upon participation of the various members. In essence, participation means involvement, concern for the task and direct or indirect contribution to the group goal. If members do not participate, it ceases to exist.

Factors which affect member's participation are:
- The content or task of the group
- The physical atmosphere

- The psychological atmosphere
- Member's personal pre-occupation
- The level of interaction and decisions
- Familiarity between group members

Communication

Communication within a group deals with the spoken and the unspoken, the verbal and non-verbal, the explicit and the implied manages that are conveyed and exchanged relating to information and ideas and feelings.

Two-way communication implies a situation where not only the two parties talk to each other but that they are listening to each other as well. It helps in clarification of doubts, confusions and misconceptions, both parties understanding each other receiving and giving feedback.

Hints for effective communication:
- Circular seating arrangement so that everyone can interact
- Respect individuals
- Encourage and support quiet members to voice their opinions
- Ensure that only one person speaks at time
- Discourage sub-groups from indulging in side-talk

Problem solving

Most groups find themselves unable to solve problems because they address the problem at a superficial level. After that they find themselves blocked because they cannot figure out why the problem occurred and how they can tackle it.

An efficient problem-solving procedure would be to:
- Clearly define the problem
- Try thoroughly to explore and understand the causes behind the problem
- Collect additional information from elsewhere and analyze it to understand the problem further
- The group should suspend criticism and judgement.

Leadership

Leadership involves focusing the effects of the people towards a common goal and to enable them to work together as one. In general, we designate an individual as one. In general, we designate an individual as a leader. Thus, one member may provide leadership with respect to achieving the goal while a different individual may be providing leadership in maintaining the group as a group. The roles can switch and change.

Development of Groups

The development process of small groups can be viewed in several ways. First, it is useful to know the persons who compose a particular small group.
- People bring their past experiences
- People come with their personalities
- People also come with a particular set of experiences.

The priorities and expectations of persons comprising group can influence the manner in which the group develops over a period of time.

Stages

Viewing the group as a whole, we observe definite patterns of behavior occurring within a group. These can be grouped into stages:

First stage: The initial stage in the life of a group is concerned with forming a group. This stage is characterized by members seeking safety and protection, tentativeness of response, seeking superficial contact with others and demonstrating dependency on existing authority figures. Members at this stage either engage in busy type activity or show apathy.

Second stage: The second stage in the group is marked by the formations of dyads and triads. Members seek out familiar or similar individuals and begin a deeper sharing of self. Continued attention to the group and tensions across the dyads/triads may appear. Pairing is a common phenomenon.

Third stage: The third development stage is marked by a more serious concern about task performance. The dyads/triads begin to open up and seek out other members in the group. Efforts are made to establish various norms for task performance. Members begin to take greater responsibilities for their own group and relationship while the authority figure becomes relaxed.

Fourth stage: This is a stage of a fully functional group where members see themselves as a group and get involved in the task. Each person makes a part of the group. Group norms are followed by effectiveness of the group. The group redefines its goals in the light of information from the outside environment and shows an autonomous will to pursue those goals. The long-term viability of the group is established and nurtured.

Facilitating Groups

A group cannot automatically function effectively, it needs to be facilitated. Facilitation can be described as a conscious process of assisting a group to successfully achieve its task while functioning as a group. Facilitation can be performed by members themselves or with the help of an outsider. To facilitate effectively, the facilitator needs to:
- Understand what is happening within the group
- Know how to facilitate and beware of personality.

ORGANIZATIONAL BEHAVIOR

Definition

Organizational behavior is "the study of human behavior in organizational settings, the interface between human behavior and the organization, and the organization itself."

The systematic study and application of knowledge about how individuals and groups act within the organization where they work.

Concepts of organizational behavior:
- The nature of people, i.e., social system and mutual interest
- Individual differences
- A whole person
- Motivated behavior
- Value of the person

Factors Influencing Organizational Behavior
- Individual
- Group
- Organization
- Personality and motivation
- Teams processes relies
- Decision making
- Power and influence on organization
- Stress and its effect on individuals
- Attitude change, group process, and individual culture.

Importance of Organizational Behavior
- Provides road map to our lives in organization
- Uses scientific research to help, understand, and predict organization life
- Organizational behavior helps us influence organizational events
- Helps understand himself and others better
- Helps to understand the basis of motivation
- Useful for maintaining cordial relationship
- Upward trend in economy.

Scope of Organizational Behavior
- *Individual* organizations are the associations of individuals. The study of individuals involves personality, perception, attitudes, values, job satisfaction, learning, and motivation
- *Group of individuals*—Include group dynamics, group conflicts, communication, leadership, power, and politics
- *Organization structure*—Study of organization structure includes structure, culture, change and development.

Flowchart in Elements of Organizational Behavior

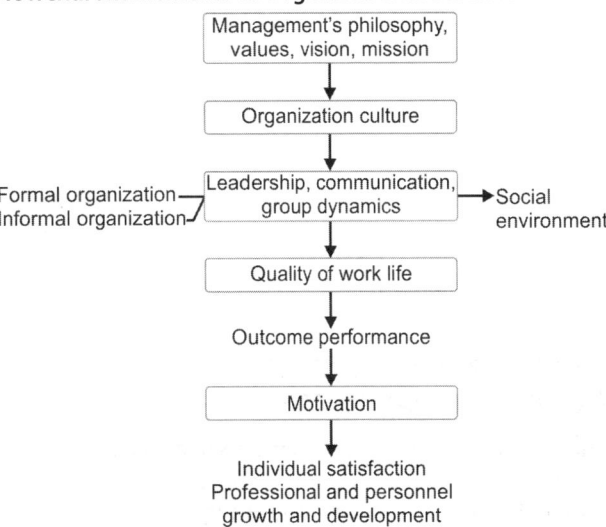

CONCLUSION

Communication is a powerful therapeutic tool and an essential nursing skill used to influence others and to achieve positive health outcomes. Communication is most effective when the receiver and sender accurately perceive the meaning of one another's messages. Effective communication techniques are facilitative and tend to encourage the other person to openly express ideas, feelings, or concerns.

Group dynamics helps to understand the behavior of the people in an organization. To achieve organizational goals, group cooperation, group morale and commitment of the administrator are essential.

51. Basic Human Needs, Growth and Development (Conception Through Preschool, School Age Through Adolescence, Young and Middle Adult, and Older Adult)

CHAPTER OUTLINE

- Abraham Maslow (1954) Basic "Human Needs"
- Growth and Development from Conception to Old Age

ABRAHAM MASLOW (1954) BASIC "HUMAN NEEDS"

The basic human needs are elements necessary for human survival and health (e.g. food, water, safety and love). Although each person has other unique needs, the basic human needs are shared by all people, and the extent to which health needs are met is a major factor in determining a person's level of health and position on the health-illness continuum.

Maslow's hierarchy of human needs is a model (Fig. 51.1) that nurses can use to understand the interrelationships of basic human needs. According to this model, certain human needs are more basic than others; that is, some needs must be met before other needs (e.g. fulfilling the physiological needs before the needs of love and belonging).

The major goal is to restore the client as much as possible to a self-actualized state. This model can provide a basis for nursing clients of all ages in all health settings. However, when the model is applied, the focus of care is on the client's needs rather than strict adherence to the hierarchy.

In all cases, an emergent physiological need takes precedence over a higher-level need. In some situations, it is unrealistic to expect a client's basic needs to occur in the fixed hierarchical order. To provide the most effective care, the nurse needs to understand the relationships of different needs and the factors that determine the priorities for the client.

GROWTH AND DEVELOPMENT FROM CONCEPTION TO OLD AGE

Definitions

Growth: Growth is a process of physical maturation resulting in an increase in size of the body and various organs. It is a quantitative change, which can be measured in inches or kilograms.

Development: Development is the process of functional and physiological maturation of the individual. It is an increase in skill and capacity to function. It includes psychological and social change.

Maturation: Maturation is an increase in competence and change in behavior and ability to function at a higher level depending upon genetic inheritance.

Principles of Growth

- ❖ Cephalocaudal direction
- ❖ Proximodistal direction
- ❖ Normal sequence in development

Principles of Development

- ❖ Development involves change
- ❖ It is the process of maturation and learning
- ❖ Developmental pattern is predictable
- ❖ There are individual differences in development
- ❖ Periods in developmental pattern
- ❖ There are social expectations for every developmental period

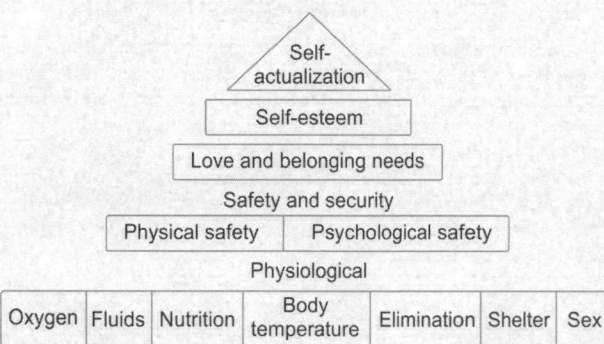

Fig. 51.1: Maslow's hierarchy of "human needs".

- Every area of development has potential hazards
- Happiness varies at different periods of development.

Stages of Growth and Development

Development in Infancy

Neonates are born with abilities to perceive and respond to some parts of their world. In an organized and effective way, for example, reflexes that are in place at birth permit neonates to grope for the breast, to suck when an object is placed in its mouth and to swallow milk and other fluids. Other classes of reflexes, which are obvious adaptive values are breathing, blinking, coughing, sneezing, vomiting and withdrawing from painful stimuli.

Another class of reflexes is attributed to the immaturity of certain parts of the brain, for example, Moro's reflex (when support is withdrawn from the back side of the head, the neonate extends its arms to the sides, extends its fingers and bring its arms inward in a sort of embracing movement); this reflex and other reflexes in this category normally disappear in early infancy as the brain matures if these reflexes persist too long. It may mean that there is a problem with the infants developing central nervous system. Newborn senses are very active that they respond to gustatory, olfactory, auditory, visual and tactile stimuli. Newborn also learn via classical and instrumental conditioning.

Physical growth and development occur at gradually decelerated rates throughout the babyhood while development of psychological functions occurs at a rapid rate. Because muscle control follows the laws of developmental direction, the earliest skills to be learned are the head, arm and hand skills. To be able to communicate, the babies should be able to comprehend what is communicated to them and in turn communicates with others by crying, babbling, gestures and emotional expressions.

Babyhood emotions differ from those of older children, adolescents and adults in that, first, they are accompanied by behavior patterns proportionally too great for the stimuli to give rise to them, and second, they are more easily conditioned in later ages. Early social foundations are important, because the type of behavior babies show in different situations affects the personal and social adjustments and second, once they exist, they persist. Play development follows a pattern that is greatly influenced by the baby's physical, motor and mental development, sensory exploration and motor manipulation.

Development During Early Childhood

Personality development: Early childhood, which extends from 2 to 6 years of age, is labeled by parents as problematic, the troublesome or the toy age; by education as the preschool age and by psychologists as pre-gang age, the exploratory age or the questioning age.

Physical development proceeds at a slow rate in early childhood, but the psychological habits whose foundations were laid in babyhood becomes well established. Early childhood is regarded as the teachable moment for acquiring skills because children enjoy the repetition essential to learning skills; they are adventurous and like to try new things; and they have few already-learned skills to interfere with the acquisition of new ones.

Speech development advances rapidly as seen in improvement in comprehension and in different speech skills. This has a strong impact on the amount of talking young children do and the content of their speech. While emotional development follows a predictable pattern and the variations in this are due to intelligence, sex, family size, child training and other conditions. Early childhood is the pre-gang age; companions play an important role in socialization. Play in this phase is influenced by motor skills, the degree of popularity they enjoy among their age mates, the guidance they receive in learning different patterns of play and socioeconomic status of their families.

Inaccuracies in understanding are common in early childhood because many childish concepts are learned with inadequate guidance and because children are encouraged to view the world in an unrealistic manner to make it more interesting and colorful. Early childhood is characterized by morality by constraint—a time when children learn through punishment and praise to obey rules automatically; it is also the time when discipline differs, with some children subject to authoritarian discipline, while others brought up by permissive and democratic discipline. The common interest in early childhood includes interest in religion and the human body, in self, in sex and in clothes. The important aspects of sex role stereotypes and accepting and playing the sex appropriate games. Different family relationships (parent–child, sibling and relationship with relatives) play roles of different degrees of importance in the socialization of young children and in their development of self-concepts.

Development During Late Childhood

Personality development: Late childhood, which extends from 6 years until children become sexually mature at approximately age 13 for girls and 14 for boys is labeled by parents as sloppy or quarrelsome age and educators call them as elementary school age; psychologists call them as gang age, age of conformity or the age of creativity. Physical growth is slow and relatively at even rate is influenced by health nutrition, immunization, sex and intelligence. The skills of late childhood can be categorized roughly into four major groups—self-help skills, social help skills, school skills and play skills. The help of handedness develops all of these. While the areas of speech pronunciations, vocabulary and sentence structure develop rapidly as does the comprehension, the content of speech starts to deteriorate.

Older children learn to control their overt expressions of their emotions and to use emotional catharsis to clear their systems of the pent-up emotionality caused by social pressure to control their emotions. The gang formation occurs at this age, which confirms to the patterns of behavior and to the values and interests of others. As gang members, children often reject parental standards, develop an antagonistic attitude toward members of the opposite sex, and become prejudiced with non-gang members.

The socioeconomic status of the older children varies from popular to that of social isolate. Once a child's status is established in a group, it is difficult to change whether the status is of a leader, follower or isolate. Play interests of the older children and the amount of time they devote to play depends more on the degree of social acceptance they enjoy than on any other condition. There is a rapid increase in understanding and in accuracy of concepts partly as a result of increased intelligence and partly as a result of increased learning opportunities.

In late childhood, most people develop moral codes influenced by moral standards of the groups in which they are identified and a conscience which guides their behavior in place of external controls needed when they were younger. The interests of older children are broader than those of younger children and include many new subjects like names, clothes, the human body, sex, school, future vocations, status symbols and autonomy.

Sex-role typing is influenced by children's appearance, behavior, aspirations, interests, attitudes towards members of the opposite sex and self-evaluation. The deterioration of family relationships and characteristic of late childhood affect children's personal and social adjustments and have a strong impact on their personalities through its effects on their self-evaluations. This is especially serious when the gap between their ideal and real self-concepts is large because it acts as an obstacle in their search for identity.

There are three stages of puberty—the prepubescent, the pubescent and the postpubescent. The criteria most often used to determine the onset of puberty are the menarche in girls and nocturnal emission in males. Puberty is caused by hormonal changes, which because they are not controllable to date, come at variable times. The average for girls is 13 years and in boys 14–14.5 years.

The time needed to complete the changes during the puberty is 2–4 years. The puberty growth spurt—the time when pubertal changes take place more rapidly—are variable because it is influenced partly by heredity and partly by environmental factors. There are four major changes in puberty, changes in body size, changes in body proportion, development of primary and secondary sex characteristics.

The most rapid growth in body size comes during the year or two before the sex organs begin to function and then tapers off. Changes in body proportion are influenced by the age of sexual maturing. The primary sex characteristics—sex organs grow and develop rapidly during puberty and become functionally mature in approximately in the middle of puberty. The secondary characteristics—the physical features that distinguish from males and females—develop according to predictable patterns, and by the end of puberty, all are at their mature or near-mature levels. Puberty changes the physical well-being of the individuals as well as attitudes and behavior, especially during the early parts of puberty, the two major concerns of puberty are normal and sex appropriateness.

Physical hazards and psychological hazards: Physical hazards of puberty are minor compared with the psychological hazards. The most common is the tendency to develop unfavorable self-concepts; to become underachievers, unwillingness to accept changed bodies or socially approved sex roles and deviant sexual maturing. Because the three A's of happiness, acceptance, affection and achievement, are often violated during the years, puberty tends to be one of the most unhappy periods of the life span, and tends to be habitual.

Adolescence

Adolescence, which is the period extending from sexual maturity to the age of legal maturity (18 years), is divided into early and late adolescence. It is an important period of time. A time of change, a problem age, the time to search identity, a dreaded age, a time of unrealism and the threshold of adulthood—these are the terms used to describe this period of life. Because mastery of the developmental tasks of adolescence requires major changes in children's habitual attitudes and patterns of behavior, many adolescents reach legal maturity before attaining the tasks and hence carry many unfinished tasks to adulthood. Even though physical growth is far from complete, when puberty ends, it slackens during adolescence and much of the changes occur then is internal rather than external.

When physical growth will be complete, it is influenced by sex and age of maturing and thus causing many concerns for the boys and girls. While traditionally adolescence is a period of heightened emotionality, a time of storm and stress, there is a little evidence that this is universal or persistent as popularly believed. The important social changes in adolescence include increased peer group influence, more mature patterns of social behavior, new social groupings and new values in the selection of friends and leaders, and social acceptance.

The most important and universal interests fall into seven major categories: recreational interests, personal and social interests, educational interests, vocational interests, religious and interest in status symbols. The major changes in morality consists of replacing specific moral concepts with generalized moral concepts of right and wrong; the building of moral code based on individual moral principles; and control of behavior through the development of conscience.

Sex interests and behavior, which center around heterosexuality, have two separate distinct elements, the development of pattern of behavior involving the members of the two sexes. The development of attitudes relating to relationship between members of the two sexes. There are a number of effects in the sex-role typing on adolescents, the most important of which are masculine supremacy, sex bias, underachievement in activities regarded as sex inappropriate and fear of success in the part of adolescent girls because of possibility of facing the stigma of sex inappropriateness.

Relationships between adolescents and members of their families tend to deteriorate in the early adolescence though these relationships often improve as adolescence draw to a close especially among adolescent girls and their family members. Most adolescents are anxious to improve their personality with the hope of advancing their status in the social group; many of the conditions influencing their self-concepts are beyond their control.

Physical hazards and psychological hazards: The most common being suicide, there are others as well. Awkwardness, a sex-inappropriate body build and homeliness are too common to be overlooked. The major psychological hazards transcend upon failure to make transition to maturity—which is the most important developmental task of adolescence. It is usually due to obstacles that they have little or no control.

The immaturity in adolescents leads to failure to make the transition to more mature behavior are especially common are social, sexual and moral behavior, and immaturity in family behavior. When immaturity is pronounced, it leads to self-rejection with its damaging effects on personal and social adjustments. Most adults remember adolescence as an unhappy age. Studies of adolescence have revealed that this is truer than of late adolescence.

Adulthood: Development

Adulthood—the largest period of the life span—is usually subdivided into three periods: early adulthood, which extends from 18 to approximately 40 years; middle adulthood or middle age, which extends from approximately 40 to 60 years; late adulthood or old age, which extends till death.

Early adulthood is the settling down or reproductive age, a problem age and one of emotional tension; a time of social isolation; a time of commitments; and often a time of dependency, of value changes, or creativity and of adjustments to new life pattern. There are certain aids to mastering the developmental tasks of early adulthood—physical efficiency, motor and mental abilities, motivation and a good role model. Because many of the interests carried over from the adolescence are no longer appropriate for the adult role, changes in all areas of interests are inevitable.

The greatest change is narrowing down the range of interests. Personal interests in early adulthood include interest in appearance; in clothes and personal adornment; in symbols of maturity and status symbols; in money and in religion. Even though the recreational activities of adults serve much the same purposes as play activities do in childhood, the recreational interests of adults may differ in many respects from the play interests of childhood due to changes in roles and life patterns. The major recreational interests of young adults include talking, entertaining, hobbies and amusements, which most of it is enjoyed at home.

Social activities in early adulthood are often greatly curtailed because of vocational and familial pressures. As a result, many young adults experience, as Erickson says, an isolation crisis, a time of loneliness due to isolation from the social group. During early adulthood, social participation is often limited and changes in friendship, social groupings, and in values placed on popularity and leadership status are inevitable. Social mobility in men comes mainly through their own efforts, while in women it comes mainly through marriage to upper status men, or those who, through their achievements, have been able to climb the social ladder. Most young married women find sex-role adjustment very difficult, especially when they are forced into the traditional roles after playing more egalitarian roles before marriage.

Development in Middle Adulthood

Personality development: Adjustment in the middle adulthood can be difficult due to the foundations laid earlier. There are four important characteristics of middle age:
- It is a dreaded age
- A time of transition and of stress
- A time of achievement and of evaluation
- A time of emptiness and that of boredom

The success of adjusting to physical changes in middle age is aided by camouflaging the signs of aging. Changes in interests are depending upon role changes. Middle-age people as a group have a greater interest in clothing and appearance because of the influence of vocational success. Interest in religion in middle age is usually greater than that in early adulthood and is often based on personal and social needs. Interests in strenuous activity wanes, there is a shift from recreational activities involving large group to those involving only a small number of people.

Recreational activities are adult rather than family oriented as they were in early adulthood; overall, there is a narrowing down of recreational interests. Social interests in the middle age are greatly influenced by social class status, sex and marital status. Vocational adjustments of middle-age men and women are complicated by factors such as social attitudes, increased use of automation, group work, increasing importance of the role of wives, compulsory retirement dominance of big business and necessity for relocation.

Adjustment for single parent is more difficult in women than in men. Adjustment due to the loss of spouse due to death is different from due to other factors such as divorce or extra relationships. Chances of remarriage are slimmer in women as time progresses, while men have no problem with that. However, adjustment approaching retirement and approaching old age should be important developmental tasks.

Physical hazards and psychological hazards: The most important hazards are acceptance of traditional belief about middle age, idealization of youth, unrealistic aspirations and changes in roles, in interests and in value placed on status symbols. An unattractive appearance, lack of social skills, preference for family contacts, financial problem, family pressures and obligation social mobility and a desire for popularity are other hazards. Vocational hazards can be failure to reach earlier goals or decline in creativity, boredom, the growing tendency towards bigness in business and industry. Marital hazards are opposition to child's marriage, sexual adjustments, care of an elderly parent, loss of a spouse and remarriage.

Development in Old Age

Those who do achieve a sense of wholeness and integrity may develop one of the hallmarks of successful aging—wisdom. Many cultures traditionally rely on selected elderly people for advice about complex life problems. One reason may be that older people who have been attentive to their experience often have a perspective on reality that is richer and more informed than the view that most young people take. Some have also suggested that a wise person is one who has a balanced investment in self as well as in others and who combines experience, reflectiveness, and emotional balance.

Retirement: Retirement is a traditional marker of old age. For some people, retirement signifies loss—loss of a familiar day routine, loss of valued social interactions, loss of well-established roles and even loss of income. For many others though, retirement is a welcomed transition, one that offers new opportunities and new freedom. Retirement can alter one's collection of daily acquaintances and it can greatly increase the time husband and wife spends together. Both changes can bring on adjustments and new personal growth.

The individual response to freedom depends on many factors, but two of the most important seem to be job satisfaction and income. People who find their jobs unrewarding often welcomes retirement. So are those people whose postretirement income meets their preretirement living standards. We need to distinguish between scheduled, long anticipated retirement and unscheduled retirement caused by sudden illness or a demand from supervisors that one quit the job. Such unscheduled retirements tend to produce anxiety and depression. Scheduled retirements do not.

Grand parenthood—second round parents: For many, one of the special delights of old age is having grandchildren. The roles played by the grandparent differ from family to family. A typical urban style of grand parenting is the formal style, in which the grandparent takes an ongoing interest in their grandchild and occasionally give the child special treats, but carefully limit their role so as not to interfere with their parents.

The second common role is an informal, playful approach in which grandchildren are seen as a source of leisure activity and mutual fun. The third most common role is the distant figure role, in which grandparents are benevolent, but have only brief, infrequent contact with their grandchildren. Younger grandmothers who have a job and a living spouse emphasize the social orientation and they are not deeply involved in the grandmother's role. Older grandmothers, most of whom are widowed and who do not have jobs, emphasize the personal orientation and are more involved with their grandchildren.

Widows and widowers coping with loss: One of the most painful inevitabilities of intimate relationships in old age is that one partner will lose the other and face the pain of bereavement. As difficult as it is to develop and sustain a warm, intimate relationship with single partner, it can be even more difficult to face life without the partner. Women have a longer life span than men, making them more susceptible to this phenomenon. But women in general cope better than men. Middle-class women with strong investment in their roles as wives report strong disruption after the death of the husband. However, women who, in addition to their marriages, have had active lives in the community or workplace report loneliness, but relatively less disruption in their lifestyles.

CONCLUSION

Abraham Maslow has given great contribution to the human basic needs where the hierarchy of the Maslow's concepts helps nurses to assess the needs of the client and prioritize the problems and provide care. Nurses should have the knowledge about the different stages of growth and development so that the physiological, physical, emotional and social needs can be assessed accordingly and health education and counseling can be planned and referral services are given.

52
CHAPTER

Sexuality and Sexual Health

CHAPTER OUTLINE

- Development of Sexual Identity
- Adolescent Sexuality
- Adult Sexuality

INTRODUCTION

The nurse is expected to provide counseling and guidance to sexually maturing and sexually active individuals as well as to expectant and new parents. New parents often need information about the expected behavior, physical growth and development of the individuals, and their family. This information helps the nurse individualize nursing plans of care. Family members are the first significant others in the child's sexual, cognitive, and personality development. As the child matures and ventures into the wider world, peer, educational and other social groups provide environments that affect development, characterized by a rapid increase in knowledge and technology.

The common myths about reproduction and birth control are:

- ❖ A couple must have simultaneous climaxes (orgasms) if conception is to take place. A woman can become pregnant only through penile penetration or artificial insemination.
- ❖ Urination by the woman after coitus or having sexual intercourse in a standing position will prevent pregnancy.
- ❖ The woman determines the sex of the child.
- ❖ Excessive masturbation is harmful.
- ❖ Sex during menstruation is unclean and harmful.
- ❖ Advancing age means the end of sex.

DEVELOPMENT OF SEXUAL IDENTITY

Sexual identity begins with conception. During conception, through the chance combination of an ovum and a sperm, a person's biologic sex is determined. Thereafter, intrauterine and extrauterine environmental influences both play their part in the realization of each person's sexual potential. Biophysical, psychological, sociocultural and mid-ethical factors all contribute to the molding of an individual's sexuality. Development of a concept of sexual roles and sexual identity begins at an early age, and continues as a series of developmental tasks throughout a person's life span.

Infancy and Childhood

One of the first questions parents ask when their child is born is "is it a boy or a girl?" The answer sets in motion a series of social influences that will be reflected in the child's concept of "who I am" and "what I can do." The developmental tasks relative to forming a sexual identity include developing core gender identity, acquiring prescribed sex role standards, identifying with the parent of the same sex and establishing gender preference.

Core gender identity is the earliest and most stable form of gender identity. From the child's perspective, knowing oneself as either a girl or a boy begins before full realization of the implications of sexual identity. The infant's gender identity is largely accomplished by acceptance of parental labeling, for example, "be a good boy," "that's my girl" and "that is my big boy." By 2 years of age, children can differentiate between girls and boys through awareness of dissimilarities in hair and clothing, and some awareness of anatomic differences. Core gender identity is developed in normal children by the time they have reached 3 or 4 years of age.

The term "sex role standards" refers to the various behaviors, attitudes and attributes that differentiate the roles. Even 2-year-olds are exposed to this conditioning, because parents choose for them the kinds of clothing, toys, and activities that reflect the parents' expectations of sex role standards.

The feelings children develop about themselves as people in general and as sexual people in particular are directly related to their experiences with their bodies, and the attitudes and values they derive from many sources.

One of the most important ways children learn about their bodies is through exploratory sexual behavior (sex play).

Sex play is defined by Kinsey et al. (1948-1953) as "actual genital play." There are four categories of sex play: self-exploration and self-manipulation, same-sex comparison, coital play and exhibitionism.

Self-exploitation and self-manipulation begin by 2-3 months of age. As they grow, infants discover they are able to experience sexual pleasure through self-stimulation. Parents who feel masturbation is harmful will rebuke even young children and forbid them to "play with themselves." Same-sex comparisons provide children with reassurance that their genitals are similar in size and shape to those of other children. Coital play (e.g. when a boy lies on top of a girl) is largely experimental, imitative and exploratory. Children become aware of parental sleeping arrangements, bathing and privacy. They begin differentiating sex role behaviors and will play being "mommy" and "daddy." Exhibitionism consists of showing and handling genitals in public, especially in the presence of companions. Most children engage in sex play activities only sporadically, especially when these activities are ignored by adults. Gender preference implies not only knowledge of one's gender and the appropriate sex role but also a liking for it.

Development of gender preference involves three elements:
- Success in the role
- Liking the same-sex parent
- Reinforcement from family, ethnic group and arid social institutions as to the value of the role:
  - Deep-seated sex preferences on the part of parents can affect initial parent–child relationships if the child is not of the preferred sex. The parenting lag that results can last a day or a lifetime, depending on whether the parent succeeds or fails in resolving conflicting emotions. Certain ethnic groups have welcoming rituals for one sex and not for the other. These seemingly innocuous societal and personal preferences eventually lead a person to make value judgments about the worthiness of her/his sex. As a result, the individual's self-esteem is either increased or diminished.
  - By the time puberty occurs, the person has completed most of the developmental tasks of early childhood. Acceptance of childhood sexual identity will have consequence on self-esteem, peer relations, and selection of skills and interest.

Implications for Nursing

A nurse has many opportunities to help young parents provide a supportive environment for their children's sexual development. Nurses and parents must be careful not to ascribe adult motives to the sexual behaviors of children. To do so would be like calling a child who believes in ghosts and fairies delusional or mentally ill (Katchadourian, Lunde, 1972). Parents may project contradictory messages about the body. For example, parents tell their children to "wash behind the ears" and then remind them to "wash down there." Parents and many health professionals respond to their own insecurities about sex when confronted by the overt, but innocent sexuality of children.

Adolescence

Adolescence, the transitional period between childhood and adulthood, begins with puberty. Biologically, the first visible signs of puberty are the development of the secondary sexual characteristics. Menstruation can be a first indication of puberty. Shortly thereafter, most teenagers experience a rapid increase in linear growth. Concomitantly, emotional changes such as moodiness, tearfulness or withdrawal are suddenly noticeable in a previously serene youngster. It is not until adolescence that the socially and parentally defined sex role is openly questioned. In recent years, changes in the concepts of what constitutes female and male roles have had great impact on teenagers. Conflict can result when the teenager chooses standards consistent with the peer group's attitude rather than with parental expectations.

Developmental Tasks

Erikson (1959) has described the adolescent stage of development as the one in which the major task is achieving identity versus identity confusion. A person's identity has many dimensions, including intellectual, interpersonal and sexual. It is now recognized that the adolescent developmental process proceeds in sequence through three phases. These phases early, middle and late adolescence put a characteristic stamp on the mariner of accomplishing the developmental tasks. The developmental tasks of adolescence may be defined as follows (adapted from Havighurst, 1972):

- ***Achieving awareness and acceptance of body image:*** The body image is well established by about 15 years of age. Adolescents must cope with normal but rapid changes in physical appearance and alterations in functional capacity. They must accept their physique and learn to use their bodies effectively. Deviations from the "norm" are a source of stress, and may or may not be incorporated into the adolescent's body image.
- ***Achieving emotional independence of parents and other adults:*** The movement away from dependence on parents that was begun with the school years is completed in this period of development. A successful accomplishment results in affection and respect for one's parents without a childish dependence on them.
- ***Achieving new and more mature relations with age mates of both sexes:*** Adolescents accomplish a satisfactory social adjustment through social activities and experimentation with the peer group. Here, they learn to behave as adults as they create, on a small

scale, the society of their elders. The influence of the peer group increasingly takes precedence over that of the family.

- *Achieving a feminine or masculine social role:* Although sex is biologically determined, the feminine and masculine roles are culturally established behavior patterns that must be learned.
- *Establishing a lifestyle that is personality and socially satisfying:* This includes the choice of a career as well as contemplation of sexual relationships, marriage, family interdependence, and parenthood.
- *Acquiring a set of values and an ethical system as a guide to socially responsible behavior:* This includes assuming responsibility for her/his own behavior and recognizing the effect that behavior may have on another's welfare.

Early Adolescence

Early adolescence begins approximately between 11 and 13 years and merges with mid-adolescence at 14 or 15 years (Johnson, 1983). It is characterized by an increase in height and the appearance of secondary sexual characteristics. Young adolescents tend to see the world around them only in relation to the effect it has on them. As their capacity for abstract thought increases, they become intensely interested in themselves, their thoughts, ideas, and fantasies, and what effect they have on others.

As a result, they are introspective, self-conscious and easily hurt by real or imagined slights. They feel that everyone is looking at them critically, so they demand privacy. The slamming of the bedroom door, the "no admittance" signs put on retreats and the long periods of self-enforced isolation from the family are typical of this phase.

The major task of early adolescence is acceptance of a new body image. The rapid changes in appearance cause adolescents to spend much time thinking about their bodies and comparing their physiques with those of others. Girls are interested in their developing breasts and often want to wear brassieres before they are needed. They tend to idealize body structure and feel depressed when their skin, hair, and legs do not compare favorably with the "ideal."

Parents are still in control, and the young adolescent is aware of vulnerability and need for dependence. However, parents, brothers, and sisters notice the beginning of the critical appraisal to which they will be increasingly subjected. The adolescent becomes aware of the status of the family in the community and is anxious that his/her family measures up to certain standards. This is the time of intense relationships with members of the same sex and these relationships are used primarily for support and mutual understanding.

Mid-adolescence

Mid-adolescence begins around 14 or 15 years and merges with late adolescence at about age 17. Almost all adolescents have reached their growth peak by mid-adolescence. Many aspects of the body have attained their adult form.

The mid-adolescent phase is characterized by increasing competence in abstract thought (Johnson, 1983). The adolescent is capable of perceiving future implications of current acts and decisions. The ability to think in this manner fluctuates. In time of stress, the adolescent reverts to concrete operations. The major task during this phase is emancipation from the family. Adolescents vacillate between acting as responsible adults and acting as dependent children. Their ability to step into the adult role, even if briefly, increases their resentment of being considered children. Role experimentation becomes a central process in the search for identity.

There is a definite movement away from the family, mid-adolescents are critical of their parents, and the parents' appearance, behavior, dress and social manners are all subjected to intense scrutiny and disparagement. Brothers and sisters are considered as nuisance, and adolescents see themselves as being treated unfairly in terms of other members of the family. An adult outside the family group, for example, a nurse, a physician, a coach, or a school counselor may be taken as a role model. There is increased participation in the adult world. Adolescents become advocates of various ideologies and enjoy debating merits of current ideas.

Many show evidence of leadership potential as they engage in developing their cognitive skills. Rebellion is usually couched in verbal terms rather than physical and is more destructive than constructive. Running away is a common phenomenon for adolescents between ages of 15 and 17 years as an attempt to solve problems, and to prove they are not children. Peer relationships now dominate over family ones.

The adolescent looks to the peer group for definitions of the behavioral code. There is a strong need to affirm the newly developed self-image through the affirmation of peers. Most conflicts with parents reflect this change and communication patterns that were once open may become closed. There is a change in relationship with members of the same sex (homosexual) and with members of the opposite sex (heterosexual relationships or heterosexuality). Adolescents test their ability to attract the opposite sex. They continue to define the parameters of femininity and masculinity.

Late Adolescence

The late adolescent phase extends from age 17 through 21. The upper limit of the phase depends on cultural, economic, and educational factors. The late adolescent is physically mature. Most late adolescents have achieved a stable body image, and the agonizing over this or that real or fancied disability is largely over. They have established abstract thought processes. They are future oriented and capable of perceiving and acting on long-range options.

One of the major tasks confronting the late adolescent is to become a fully independent productive citizen. They become self-supporting or begin their professional education. They have become socially functioning adults. Late adolescents are capable of forming stable relationships. They are ready for mutuality and reciprocity in caring for another, in contrast to the former self-centered orientation. Although young women are now assuming the right to choose careers rather than early marriage, many still suspend the final shaping of a career until after commitments to parenthood are fulfilled.

ADOLESCENT SEXUALITY

The adolescent's heightened sexual awareness brings sexual concerns to the surface. These include myths about masturbation and concerns about possible homosexuality, sexual activity and the presence, frequency and content of sexual fantasies and dreams. Although physically sexually mature, adolescents are trying to cope with emerging sensations and social situations, while they are still psychologically immature.

Masturbation

Young adolescents may fear that any variation from normal, particularly of the genitals, has resulted from masturbation. The adolescent needs to learn that masturbation is a normal, universal behavior that causes neither physical nor mental harm. It is a natural part of learning about human sexuality and can be a useful means of relieving sexual tension (Brookman, 1983).

Masturbation is also a common mode of discharge of tension for adolescents, particularly when alone, unhappy, or frustrated. It serves to fuse psychological and physical sexuality. It is not always associated with sexual fantasies. The value of masturbation may be lessened by the shame and guilt that accompany it. Adolescent boys often fear discovery of evidence of ejaculation and girls often fear changes in their genitals as a result of masturbation. Fears are not limited to discovery by others but also are caused by the expansive experience of orgasm, with the resulting feelings of loss of ego boundaries. If masturbation is used as a continual source of comfort or with inappropriate exposure (exhibitionism), it is indicative of disturbance (Stuart and Sundeen, 1991).

Homosexuality

Homosexual experience to some degree is part of the psychosexual development of many individuals. The adolescent who is over-affectionate with same-sex peers or adults may cause considerable parental concern. This is a result of society's unresolved position on the meaning or acceptance of homosexuality. Fantasies about sexual encounters with members of the same sex can be very disturbing to the adolescent. Memories of early same-sex explorations compound the adolescent's fear of becoming homosexual. The fear is probably a reaction to society's negative valuation of homosexuality.

For many years, the medical profession, including psychiatry, has searched for causes of homosexuality. The message in looking for the cause of a condition is that it is a maladaptive state that can be treated or cured. Today, emphasis is placed on learning more about homosexuality and viewing it as a sexual preference or mode of sexual expression (Kinsey, 1948).

Marmor (1980) defined the homosexual person as one who is motivated in adult life by a definite preferential erotic attraction to members of the same sex and who usually (but not necessarily) engages in overt sexual relations with them. Marmor's definition excludes transitory incidental homosexual activity in adolescence and in primarily heterosexual persons.

The incidence of homosexuality in the United States today has been conservatively estimated at 10%–15% of the population. If these estimates are accurate, nurses come into contact with homosexuals on a daily basis. Despite this incidence of homosexuality, nurses generally know little about homosexuality and almost always assume that all clients are heterosexual (Stuart and Sundeen, 1991).

Sexual Activity

Adolescents are surrounded by mixed messages. Parents, religious groups, teachers, health professionals and others tell them to refrain from sexual contact, to control sexual impulses and to keep away from temptation. Many of these same adults are asking adolescents to refrain from activities they themselves openly practice. At the same time, books, movies, music and advertisements are laden with sexually stimulating messages.

The data were gathered through open-ended interviews that lasted 2–3 hours. The factors that led to the first sexual activity included establishing a trust relationship with their partners, believing they could not get pregnant, relying on their partner for contraception and sacking knowledge about contraception. Family relationship also was a factor and included elements such as much unsupervised time, inconsistency in mother's wishes and daughter's behavior, lack of maternal authority and inability to discuss sex. The critical factors in the decision to maintain the pregnancy included accepting the diagnosis of pregnancy and being aware of available alternatives.

The adolescents denied the pregnancy for several months, which narrowed the choices about maintaining the pregnancy. Although none of the girls married, all received support and involvement from the fathers. All of the girls had friends of their age who were pregnant or were parents. Four of the girls had financial and emotional support from their families.

Approximately, two-thirds of all teenage boys and one-half of all teenage girls have had intercourse at least once; many younger adolescents may use intercourse as a means of conforming to peer group expectations, as a challenge to parents, as experimentation or as a means of relieving loneliness or stress. Some adolescents develop sincere commitments to one another that may persist and lead to marriage. Many have a series of close, committed, single-partner relationships, each lasting weeks, months or longer (Brookman, 1983).

Few adolescents are promiscuous; that is, they do not have multiple partners with little or no commitment, and adolescents are hesitant to talk to adults, especially parents, because the adult often discounts or invalidates their feelings. Some parents are threatened by their adolescent's budding sexuality. They deal with their own uncertainty about sex by ignoring the reality of adolescent sexuality or by becoming hostile and punitive. At times, little attention is given to the teenager who is reluctant to engage in dating at all. The young person who fails to show any interest may need careful evaluation.

Implications for Nursing/Sexual Health

Health professionals need to be knowledgeable and comfortable with their own sexuality to work effectively with adolescents. Glossing over-important issues and making broad generalizations about sexual concerns can be more confusing than helpful. Nurses who counsel young people about specific sexual issues need:

❖ Knowledge of sexual anatomy, physiology and behavior
❖ Recognition of the importance of local peer influences
❖ Understanding of the adolescent's family and ethnocultural background.

The approach to adolescents is based on their intellectual and psychosocial maturation. Provision of privacy and reassurance of confidentiality are essential to building trust and confidence between adolescent and nurse. The adolescent usually is willing to express concerns if the discussions are held in a comfortable and non-judgmental setting. The increased incidence of adolescent pregnancy and the increased number of adolescents with sexually transmitted diseases, including acquired immunodeficiency syndrome (AIDS), make sex education and sex counseling a major task for nurses working with adolescents. Information about their bodies' sexual responses, contraception, pregnancy and sexually transmitted disease can be made available to adolescents to help them become sexually responsible adults.

■ ADULT SEXUALITY

Adulthood encompasses the period from adolescence to a person's death. Three phases are discernible—early, middle and late adulthood.

Early Adulthood

Early adulthood encompasses that portion of the life cycle devoted to parenting, consolidation of relationships whether marital or non-marital and commitment to a life work. The young adult has attained physical and intellectual maturity. Stature and reproductive growth are virtually complete; body image remains a concern for the young adult, particularly in terms of body contour and size (Woods, 1984). Non-acceptance of one's body may inhibit the establishment of sexual relationships. Cognitive powers include the ability to think abstractly, to be future oriented and to act on long-range options (Piaget, 1950). Personality development is related to the task of developing intimacy and solidarity as opposed to existing in isolation (Erikson, 1959). Intimacy involves learning to give and receive love, choosing whether to marry and choosing a sexual partner or partners (Duvail, 1977).

Family ties are important, but the relationship of parent and child takes an adult quality. The young adult is expected to be moving toward financial and social independence from the family. He/she is also expected to choose a vocation and obtain the necessary education for it. Establishing a career and advancing in it are major concerns throughout this part of the life cycle. Social groupings include varying age levels and are often based on similar interests.

The need for strong friendships with peers diminishes as individual friendships assume permanence. Early adulthood has been described as a period of maximum sexual self-consciousness (Offer and Simon, 1976). There is social acceptance and legitimization of sexual experiences. The tasks of sexual development for the young adult include maintaining a commitment to a sexual relationship, reproductive healthcare and making rational decisions about childbearing.

Commitment to a relationship is strengthened by the need to give and receive pleasure. Commitments vary in length and type. For example, some couples remain monogamous throughout their marriage. Others have open marriages, in which the couple agrees that one or both may participate in other sexual encounters. Some couples remain in relationships without formal marriage. Relationships can be terminated by divorce or death.

Finally, serial monogamy is practiced by many people in the United States, and serial monogamy is characterized by repeated marriages and divorces. The person is married to only one person at a time, but is married a number of times throughout his/her life. Responsible reproductive healthcare includes such actions as women have a Papanicolaou smear at prescribed intervals and both women and men avoid sexually transmitted diseases.

Rational decisions about childbearing are important to ensure that every child is a wanted child. The couple is responsible for using reliable contraceptive means when pregnancy is not desired. Unwanted and unplanned children often become targets of abuse and neglect.

Middle and Late Adulthood

These phases of the life cycle represent the greatest maximizing of early potential and then a gradual lessening of biopsychosocial attainment through the normal process of aging. Changes in family structure from events such as children leaving home, death of a spouse or role reversal in dealing with aging parents necessitate major changes in lifestyle.

The critical task for these years is maintaining feelings of self-esteem versus despair. The need to love and be loved, to be successful and to feel meaningful prompts involvement in community service and in leisure pursuits. Cognitive powers continue unabated until physical insults such as Alzheimer's disease or cerebrovascular accident cause a decline. Body image remains an important concern.

Western society's accent on health and youth make grooming, weight, nutrition, and exercise a continuous part of an adult's daily life. Adulthood focusses primarily on adapting to the physical and emotional changes in sexual performance caused by the aging process. The childbearing years are coming to an end. This is a relief for many couples because the possibility of pregnancy can be removed from their lovemaking. Others may mourn the loss of the chance of another child.

The fear of growing older in a youth-dominated society can be a source of depression and anxiety. Bodily changes, lower hormone production and menopause may contribute to anxiety and depression. The research of Johnson (1926) has shown that aging does not decrease libido or the capacity to be orgasmic. Men and women are capable of sexual activity well into their old age. Disinterest and abstinence are probably caused by loss of a partner, boredom, ill health, or cultural attitudes about the appropriateness.

Many older people do not understand the impact of aging on their physical response to sexual stimulation. They see these changes as an indication that they should terminate sexual activity rather than merely as a need to make minor adaptations. For example, vaginal lubrication in women is slower and decreased in amount, and in men erection is slower and erectile firmness is decreased. Love play will probably need to be extended, with more direct genital stimulation to produce lubrication and erection. Women have a shortened orgasmic phase and men's need to ejaculate decreases, resulting in decreased volume of ejaculation. These physiological changes require adaptations in sexual behavior and not cessation of sexual activity.

Mims and Swenson (1980) have stated that sexual fulfillment throughout adulthood and old age is not only possible, but likely. The feeling that older people are not interested in sex (except if they are abnormal the "dirty old man" syndrome) is largely caused by the inability to imagine parents or grandparents as sexually active people. The greatest danger of such attitudes is that they tend to comprise a "self-fulfilling prophecy" (if people believe that sexual interest ceases with advancing age they will find that it does cease). Or if sexual interest persists, people may believe themselves to be abnormal, sinful, or psychologically sick.

Implications for Nursing/Sexual Health

The nurse is in a unique position to help adults with health maintenance and detection of problems concerning sexuality. The role of sex educator is an important one for nurses working with families during the childbearing and child-rearing years. Parents often need help with teaching their children about sex because adults commonly are misinformed about many aspects of reproduction and how their bodies function. Parents therefore need accurate sex information to their children to be healthy, responsible sexual beings.

Besides helping with childhood and adult sexuality, the nurse can help prepare clients for many sexual problems and changes that occur with aging. Many nurses have not been aware of the importance of sex education to older people thinking that the elderly people are no longer interested in sexual dysfunction problems after children are born. The mother, especially nurse, becomes so involved with child-rearing that her relationship with her husband suffers. At the same time, the husband may be actively involved in career development, thereby sparing little time for home life. The nurse needs to be aware of how the demands of parenting can adversely affect the marital relationship. Simple counseling provided during these early years may prevent serious marital problems in later years.

CONCLUSION

The sexuality and sexual health is a concept of recent issues which need discussion so that the appropriate knowledge can be imparted especially to adolescents. Lack of awareness, hesitation, and shyness to discuss problems make it go unreported many times. So nurses can help them in these issues and help identify problems of sex and health and prevent the STDs and HIV/AIDS. There are many helplines available for any sex-related problems.

53 CHAPTER

Stress and Adaptation, Crisis and its Intervention

CHAPTER OUTLINE

- Stressors
- Mediating Processes
- Physiologic Response to Stress
- Stress Theories
- Models of Illness
- Adaptive Coping Strategies (Methods)
- Nursing Management of Stress Assessment

INTRODUCTION

Every person experiences various kinds of stress throughout life; stress can provide the stimulus for change and growth. In this respect, some stress can be positive; however, too much stress can result in poor adjustment, physical or mental illness, and inability to cope with the stressor. Between 1980 and 1990, the number of stress disability claims made by California state workers increased by more than 80%. Job stress, burnout, environmental stress, marital stress, and examination stress are examples that bound in everyday life. Scientists in the field of physiology, psychology, and sociology have developed bodies of knowledge on the subjects of stress, but they have not focused on the possible connections that might exist among these various bodies of knowledge. Recent discoveries and knowledge from studies in the field of psychoneuroimmunology are providing insight into the complex relationship of the domains of psychology (the mind and emotions), neurology (the brain and central nervous system), and immunology (the body's cellular defenses against internal and external invaders). These studies demonstrate ways that the mind and emotions can affect physiological health. The feelings deepen the understanding of the effects of stress on the body.

DEFINITION OF STRESS

- Hans Selye (1956-1976) defined stress as the non-specific response of the body to a demand regardless of its nature. This response included a series of physiologic reactions called the general adaptation syndrome (GAS).
- Lazarus and Folkman (1984) defined stress as an internal state that can be caused by physical demands in the body or by environmental and social situations that are evaluated as potentially harmful, uncontrollable, or exceeding our resources for coping.

DEFINITION OF ADAPTATION

Adaptation is a constant, ongoing process that requires a change in structure, function, or behavior so that the person is better suited to the environment. The process involves an interaction between the person and the environment. The outcome depends upon the degree of fit between the skills and capacities of the person and his/her sources of social support on the one hand and the type of challenges or stressors being confronted on the other.

As such, adaptation is an individual process with each individual having different levels of ability to cope or respond. Adaptation goes on throughout the life span, and during that process, many developmental and situational challenges will be encountered, especially in situations of health and illness. The goal of the encounter is to promote adaptation.

As both stress and adaptation may exist at different levels of a system, it is possible to study these reactions at cell, tissue, and organ levels. Biologists study the subcellular components and the subsystems of the total body. Sociologists study stress and adaptation in individuals, families, groups, and societies, and thus, they speak of the adaptation of the groups, in the sense that a group's organizational features are modified to meet the requirements of the social and physical environment in which they exist. Adaptation is a continuous process of seeking harmony in an environment. The desired end goals of adaptation for many systems are survival, growth, and reproduction.

STRESSORS

A stressor may be defined as an internal or external event, condition, situation, and/or cure that has the potential to bring about or actually activate significant physical or psychosocial reactions.

Types of Stressors

Stressors exist in many forms. They may be classified as follows:
- Physical, physiological, and psychological stressors
- Day-to-day stressors
- Life event stressors
- Time-related stressors

Physical, Physiological, and Psychological Stressors

- Physical stressors include cold, heat, or chemical agents
- Physiological stressors include pain or fatigue
- Psychological stressors include emotional reactions, such as fear of failing exam or not getting a job.

Day-to-day Stressors or Commonly Occurring Frustrations or Hassles

Day-to-day stressors include common occurrences such as getting caught at a traffic jam, experiencing computer downtime, and having argument with a spouse or roommate. These experiences vary in effect; for example, encountering a rainstorm while one is vacationing at the beach will most likely evoke a more negative response than it might at another time. These less dramatic, frustrating, and irritating events called daily hassles have been shown to have a greater health impact than major life events because of the cumulative effect they have overcome. They can lead to high blood pressure (BP), palpitations, or similar physiologic problems. Major complex occurrences involve large groups or even entire nations; for example, events of history such as terrorism and war, which are threatening situations when experienced either directly in the war zone or indirectly through live news coverage. The demographic, economic, and technologic changes occurring in the society also serve as stressors. The stress produced by any stressor is sometimes a result not only of the change itself but also of the speed with which the change occurs.

Life Event Stressors

This group of stressors has been studied most extensively, and it comprises situations that directly affect the individual. This category includes the influence of life events, such as death, birth, marriage, divorce, and retirement. It also includes the psychological crises described by Erickson as occurring in the life cycle stages of the human experience. Some chronic stressors are having permanent functional disability or dealing with the burden associated with providing long-term care to a frail and elderly parent.

Relating life events to illness has been a major focus of psychological studies. Holmes and Rahe (1967) developed life event scales that assign numerical values called life change units to typical life events. By using a life event scale for checking the number of recent events and deriving a total score, one can predict the likelihood of this stressor. The items reflect events and require a change in persons, i.e., patterns of the variable change are important because they require adjustment. The recent life change questionnaire, developed by Tausing (1982), contains 118 items related to events such as death, birth, mania, divorce, promotions, serious arguments, and vacations. The events listed include both desirable and undesirable happenings. Research findings in nursing and other disciplines have demonstrated only weak-to-moderate associations between stressful events and outcomes (Werner, 1993).

Time-related Stressors

Stressors can also be categorized according to their duration. They are as follows:
- ***Acute:*** Time-related stressors, such as awaiting for surgery or a final examination.
- ***Stressor sequences:*** Consist of a series of events over a period of time that results from some initiating events such as job loss or divorce.
- ***Chronic intermittent chronic enduring:*** Sources of stress that persist over time.

Ballard (1981) identified immobilization, isolation, orientation, and sensory deprivation as stressful conditions in a study of patients in a surgical intensive care unit. She observed that nurses could change many of the stressors in the intensive care unit. She also observed that not only illness and major surgery are stressors but also the role changes and financial demands occasioned by the illness are additional stressors. This is an example of the stressor sequence, overtime, when one event lead to others or may have an impact on existing situations.

MEDIATING PROCESSES

Following the recognition of the stressor, the person will consciously or unconsciously react to manage the situation. This is called the mediating process. The theory developed by Lazarus emphasizes cognitive appraisal and coping.

Appraisal and Coping

Cognitive appraisal is a process through which an event is evaluated with respect to what is at stake (primary appraisal) and what might and can be done (secondary appraisal).

Primary Appraisal

Primary appraisal is influenced by the personal goals and commitments or motivation of the individual. For example, how important or how relevant is what is happening? Is it in conflict with what the person wants or desires? Does the situation threaten the person's own sense of strength and ego identity?

As an outcome of the primary appraisal, the situation will be identified as either stressful or non-stressful. If non-stressful, the situation is irrelevant or benign positive. A stressful situation may be one of the three kinds:
- Those in which harm or loss has occurred
- Those that are threatening, in that harm or loss is anticipated
- Those that are challenging, in that some opportunity or gain is anticipated.

Secondary Appraisal

Secondary appraisal is an evaluation of what might and can be done. This includes assigning blame or credit to those responsible for a frustrating event, thinking about whether or not one can do something about the situation (one's coping potential), and determining future expectancy or whether things are likely to change for better or worse (Lazarus). The degree of stress is determined by a comparison of what is at stake and what can be done about it (a sort of risk–benefit analysis).

Reappraisal

Reappraisal occurs and refers to a changed appraisal based on new information.

Emotional Appraisal

Negative emotions such as fear and anger accompany harm or loss appraisals, while positive emotions accompany challenge. To illustrate challenge, unexpected quiz in the classroom might be judged as threatening by the unprepared student; and fear, anger, and resentment might be felt.

Relational Appraisal

Lazarus has expanded his former ideas about stress, appraisal, and coping into a more complex model relating emotions to adaptation. He calls this a negative cognitive–motivational–relational theory with relational standing for a focus or negotiation with a physical and social world.

Coping Appraisal

Coping appraisal consists of the cognitive and behavioral efforts made to manage the specific external demands that tax a person's resources. Coping can be emotion focused or problem focused.

Personal Resources

Appraisal and coping are affected by the internal characteristics of the person—these include health and energy as well as person's belief system including existential beliefs (faith, religious beliefs, commitments or life goals [motivational properties]) and the person's own sense of self including self-esteem control and mastery. They also include knowledge, problem-solving skills, and social skills (ability to communicate and interact with others). Those characteristics that have been studied the most in nursing research include health-promoting lifestyle effect of stressors. From a nursing practice standpoint, this outcome supports nursing's goal of promoting health.

Hardness is the name given to a general quality that comes with rich, varied and rewarding childhood experiences. It is a personality characteristics composed of control, commitment, and challenge. Hardy persons perceive stressors as something they can chance and therefore control. Potential stressful situations are interesting and meaningful (commitment); change and new situations are viewed as an opportunity for growth (challenge).

External Resources

Social Support

Social support is a major external resource. Cobb (1976) defined social support as information belonging to one or more of the following three categories:
- The first category of information adds the individual to believe that he/she is cared for and loved. This appears most often in a relationship between two people in which mutual trust and attachment are expressed by helping one another to meet their needs. Such expressions are sometimes called emotional support.
- The second category of information leads the individual to believe that he/she is esteemed and valued. This is most effective when there is a public announcement that demonstrates the favorable position the individual has in the group. It elevates the person's sense of self-worth. This is called esteem support.
- The third category of information leads the individual to believe that he/she belongs to a network of communication and mutual obligation. Information is shared by the members of the network, they all know what it is, and they are all aware that it is shared.

PHYSIOLOGIC RESPONSE TO STRESS

Interpretation of Stimuli by Brain

The physiologic response to a stressor is a protective and adaptive mechanism to maintain the homeostatic balance of the body. Neural and hormonal actions to maintain homeostatic balance are integrated by the hypothalamus. It integrates autonomic nervous system mechanisms that maintain the chemical constancy of the internal environment of the body.

The hypothalamus and the limbic system regulate emotions and many visceral behaviors necessary for survival (e.g., eating, drinking, temperature control, reproduction, defense, and aggression).

In the stress, afferent impulses are carried from sensory organs (eye, ear, nose and skin) and internal sensors (baroreceptors and chemoreceptors) to nerve centers in the brain. Stress may be perceived by different centers ranging from the cortex down to the brainstem, which in turn relay information to the hypothalamus. The response to the perception of the stress is integrated in the hypothalamus, which coordinates the adjustments necessary to return to homeostatic balance. The degree and duration of response vary—major stress evokes both sympathetic and pituitary adrenal responses.

Neuroendocrine Response

Neural and neuroendocrine pathways under the control of the hypothalamus are activated in the stress response. First, there is a sympathetic nervous system (SNS) discharge followed by a sympathetic–adrenal-medullary discharge, and finally, if the stress persists, the hypothalamic–pituitary system is activated.

Sympathetic Nervous System Response

The SNS is rapid and short lived. Norepinephrine is released at nerve endings in direct contact with their respective end organs to cause an increase in the function of the vital organs and a state of general body arousal. The heart rate is increased. Peripheral vasoconstriction occurs, raising the blood pressure. Blood is also shunted away from abdominal organs. The purpose of these activities is to provide better perfusion of vital organs (brain, heart and skeletal muscles). Blood glucose is increased and supplies more readily available energy. The pupils are dilated, and mental activity is increased. A greater sense of awareness exists.

Constriction of the blood vessels of the skin limits bleeding in the event of trauma. Subjectively, the person is likely to experience cold feet, clammy skin and hands chill, palpitations, and a "knot" in the stomach. Typically, the person appears tense with the muscles of the neck, upper back, and shoulders tightened; respirations may be rapid and shallow, with the diaphragm tense.

Sympathetic–Adrenal-Medullary Response

In addition to its direct effect on major end organs, SNS stimulates the medulla of the adrenal gland to release the hormones epinephrine and norepinephrine into the blood stream. The action of these hormones is similar to that of the SNS and has the effect of sustaining and prolonging its actions. Both epinephrine and norepinephrine also stimulate the nervous system and produce metabolic effects that increase the blood glucose level and the metabolic rate. The effect of the sympathetic and adrenal medullary response is summarized in Table 53.1. This effect is called the "fight or flight" reaction.

Hypothalamic–Pituitary Response

The longest acting phase of the physiologic response, which is more likely to occur in persistent stress, involves the hypothalamic–pituitary pathway. The hypothalamus secretes corticotropin-releasing factor, which stimulates the anterior pituitary to produce adrenocorticotropic hormone (ACTH). ACTH in turn stimulates the adrenal cortex to produce glucocorticoids, primary cortisol. Cortisol stimulates protein metabolism, releasing amino acids; stimulates liver uptake of amino acids and their conversion to glucose (gluconeogenesis); and inhibits the glucose uptake (anti-insulin action) by many body cells, but not those of the brain and heart. These cortisol-induced metabolic effects provide the body with a ready source of energy during a stressful situation. There are some important implications to this effect; a person with diabetes who is under stress, such as that caused by an infection, will need more insulin than usual. Any patient who is under stress (illness, surgery, and prolonged psychological stress) will catabolize body protein and need supplements. Children subjected to stress will have retarded growth.

Table 53.1: The effect of the sympathetic–adrenal-medullary response.

Effect	Purpose	Mechanism
↑ Heart rate	Better perfusion of vital organs	Increased cardiac output due to increased myocardial contractility and heart rate; also increased venous return (peripheral vasoconstriction)
↑ Blood pressure		
↑ Blood glucose	Increased available energy	Increased liver and muscle breakdown; also increased breakdown of adipose tissue triglycerides
↑ Mental activity	Alert state	
Dilated pupils	Increased awareness	
Tension of skeletal muscles	Prepared for activity, decreased fatigue	Excitation of muscles; also increase in the amount of blood shunted to the muscles from the abdominal viscera
Ventilation	Provision of oxygen for energy	
Coagulability of blood	Prevention of hemorrhage in event of trauma	Vasoconstriction of the surface vessels

The actions of catecholamines (epinephrine and norepinephrine) and cortisol are most important in the general response to stress. Other hormones that are released are antidiuretic hormone (ADH) from the posterior pituitary and aldosterone from the adrenal cortex. The ADH and aldosterone promote sodium and water retention, which is an adaptive mechanism in the event of hemorrhage or loss of fluids through excessive perspiration. The ADH has also been shown to influence learning and so may facilitate coping in new and threatening situations.

Growth hormone and glucagons are secreted, and they stimulate the uptake of amino acids by cells, helping to mobilize energy resources. The secretion of other hormones is also affected, but their adaptive function is less clear. The production of endonephrine, an endogenous opiate, is also increased during stress and enhances the threshold for tolerance of painful stimuli. It may also affect mood. It has been implicated in the so-called "high" that long distance runners experience.

Stress and Immune System

Glucocorticoids depress the immune system. When they are present in high concentrations, there is a reduction in the inflammatory response to injury or infection. The steps of the inflammatory process are inhibited, lymphocytes are destroyed in lymphoid tissues, and antibody production is decreased. As a result, the ability of a person to resist infection is reduced. The inhibition of the inflammatory response can be used to advantage pharmacologically in the prescription of cortisol to treat the inflammatory and immune responses in arthritis, asthma, and transplant rejection.

The relationship of stress to the immune response is a subject of new fields of study called behavioral immunology, psychoneuroimmunology, and neuroimmunomodulation. Studies of animals have shown that extreme psychologic stress can have a profound effect on immune competences. Studies in humans have not been conclusive, but investigators believe that the mind influences immune responses with consequences that can be harmful to the host.

STRESS THEORIES

There are three types of theories:
1. Stress is the non-specific response of the body to any demand made upon it.
2. Stress is a stimulus that causes a disrupted response.
3. Stress can be transactional and interactional.

The theory "Stress as the non-specific response of the body to any demand made upon it" is first proposed by Selye. He explains that stress can be physical or emotional, pleasant or unpleasant, as long as they require the individual to adapt; whether the stress was physical in nature, such as a burn, or psychological in nature, such as the death of loved one, it results in a series of physiological responses; Selye called this pattern of response as GAS.

Phases of the General Adaptation Syndrome

Selye described in 1956 the stress of life. He identified three stages or phases of the GAS:
1. Alarm reaction
2. Stage of resistance
3. Stage of exhaustion

Alarm Reaction or Acute Phase

In the alarm reaction of the gas, the individual perceives a stressor physically or mentally and the "fight or flight" mechanism is initiated. When the stressor is of sufficient intensity to threaten the steady state of the individual, it requires a reallocation of energy, so that adaptation can occur. This temporarily decreases the individual's resistance to stress and may even result in death if prolonged and severe.

Physical symptoms of the alarm reaction are generally those of SNS stimulation. These symptoms include an increased rate and force of heartbeat, increased BP and respiratory rate anorexia, nausea, pupil dilatation, and increased perspiration.

Stage of Resistance

Here the individual quickly moves from the alarm reactions to the stage of resistance in which physiological forces are mobilized to increase resistance to stress. It may involve modification of the external and internal environment. There is some resistance to the stressor; the body adapts lower optimal level; this requires a greater than usual expenditure of energy for the individual.

Stage of Exhaustion

The adaptive mechanisms become warm and fail. The negative effect of the stress spreads to the entire organisms. If the stressors removed or counteracted, death will result.

Any experience believed by the individual to be stressful may stimulate a psychological response. The stress does not have to be recognized consciously. If people recognize that they are under stress, they are often unable to connect the cognitive understanding of stress with physical symptoms of the psychophysiological disorder.

Local Adaptation Syndrome

According to Selye's theory, there is also a local adaptation syndrome (LAS). This syndrome includes the inflammatory response and repair processes that occur at the local site of tissue injury. The LAS occurs in small, topical injuries, such as in contact dermatitis. If the local injury were severe enough, the GAS would be activated. Selye emphasized that stress is the non-specific response common to all stressors, regardless of whether they are physiologic, psychologic, or social.

The fact that different demands are interpreted by different people as stressors is explained by the many conditioning factors in each person's environment. Conditioning factors also account for differences in the tolerance of different persons for stress. Some may develop diseases of adaptation, such as hypertension, migraine, and headaches, while others appear to be unaffected.

Indicators of Stress

Indicators of stress and stress response include subjective and objective measures. These signs and symptoms may be observed directly or reported by the person. Some may be psychological, physiological or behavioral:

- ❖ *Physiological indicators of stress*
  - ➢ Elevated BP
  - ➢ Increased muscle tension in neck, shoulders, and back
  - ➢ Elevated pulse and increased respiration
  - ➢ Sweaty palms
  - ➢ Cold hands and feet
  - ➢ Fatigue
  - ➢ Tension headache
  - ➢ Stomach upset
  - ➢ Higher pitched voice
  - ➢ Nausea, vomiting, and diarrhea
  - ➢ Change in appetite
  - ➢ Change in weight
  - ➢ Change in urinary frequency
  - ➢ Abnormal laboratory findings—elevated ACTH, cortisol, and hyperglycemia
  - ➢ Restlessness
  - ➢ Dilated pupils.
- ❖ *Behavioral and emotional indicators of stress*
  - ➢ Anxiety
  - ➢ Depression
  - ➢ Increased use of chemical substances
  - ➢ Change in eating habits, sleep, and activity pattern
  - ➢ Mental exhaustion
  - ➢ Feeling of inadequacy
  - ➢ Loss of self-esteem
  - ➢ Increased irritability
  - ➢ Loss of motivation
  - ➢ Emotional outburst and crying
  - ➢ Decreased productivity and quality of job performance
  - ➢ Tendency to make mistakes
  - ➢ Forgetfulness and blocking
  - ➢ Diminished attention
  - ➢ Day dreaming
  - ➢ Inability to concentrate
  - ➢ Increased absenteeism and illness
  - ➢ Lethargy
  - ➢ Loss of interest
  - ➢ Proneness to accidents and some reflect social behaviors and thought processes.

MODELS OF ILLNESS

There are two types:
- ❖ General model of illness
- ❖ Specificity model of illness

General Model of Illness

General model of illness is based on Selye's theory which basically suggests that any stressor elicits a state of disturbed physiologic equilibrium. If this state is prolonged or the response excessive, it will increase the susceptibility of the person to illness. This susceptibility, coupled with a predisposition in the person (genetic traits, health and age), leads to illness. Selye proposed a list of disorders, which he called diseases of maladaptation. It includes the following:
- ❖ High blood pressure
- ❖ Diseases of the heart and blood vessels
- ❖ Diseases of the kidney
- ❖ Eclampsia
- ❖ Rheumatic and rheumatoid arthritis
- ❖ Inflammatory diseases of the skin and eyes
- ❖ Infections
- ❖ Allergic and hypersensitivity diseases
- ❖ Nervous and mental diseases
- ❖ Digestive diseases
- ❖ Metabolic diseases
- ❖ Cancer
- ❖ Diseases of resistance in general.

Specificity Model of Illness

The specificity model of illness has developed in contrast to the general model. This model flows from the work of Mason and others indicating that there are specific patterns of physiologic response to specific emotions. Specific illness can flow from these patterned disturbances.

Coping with Illness

The five predominant ways of coping with illness identified in a review of 57 nursing research studies were:
- ❖ Trying to be optimistic about the outcome
- ❖ Using social support
- ❖ Using spiritual resources
- ❖ Trying to maintain control either over the situation or over feelings
- ❖ Trying to accept the situation

In all studies, patients and family members both used a combination of emotion-focused and problem-focused coping in dealing.

ADAPTIVE COPING STRATEGIES (METHODS)

General prerequisites for stress management include regular exercise, humor, good nutrition and diet, adequate rest, and relaxation techniques.

Regular Exercise

A regular exercise program improves muscle tone and posture, controls weight, reduces tension, and promotes relaxation. In addition, exercise reduces the risk of cardiovascular diseases and improves cardiopulmonary functioning. In general, for a fitness program to have positive physical effects, a person should exercise at least three times a week for 30–40 minutes.

Everyone should do warm-up exercises before vigorous exercises such as jogging, aerobic dancing, or tennis; warm-up exercises stimulate blood flow to the muscles and increase flexibility; and they reduce the risk of damage to the musculoskeletal system during exercise. Similarly, after vigorous exercises, a person should do cool down exercises rather than stop abruptly. For example, after jogging or aerobic dancing, a person should walk around at moderate pace, gradually slowing down and stopping. Cool down exercise allows the cardiovascular, pulmonary, musculoskeletal, and metabolic systems to gradually return to their resting states.

Exercise programs are effective in decreasing the severity of stress-related conditions such as hypertension, obesity, tension headaches, fatigue, mental exhaustion, irritability, and depression. Exercise promotes the release of endogenous opioids that create a feeling of well-being (Muccubbin, 1993).

Humor

Humor as a therapy has been popularized in the lay literature by Norman Cousins (1979). The ability to perceive fun and laugh alleviates stress. The physiological hypothesis is that laughter releases endorphins into the circulation, and feelings of stress are relieved. Simon (1990) notes that humor can influence an older infant's perception of health and morale; in turn, the ability to observe situational humor is related to successful aging. Through the helping role, nurses can initiate therapeutic activities such as encouraging clients to relate past humorous anecdotes or develop a "humor" scrapbook.

Nutrition and Diet

Nutrition and exercise are closely related. Food provides the fuel for activity and increased exercise, which improves circulation and the delivery of nutrients to body tissues.

Everyone is encouraged to maintain weight according to standard ranges for sex, age, and body built. In addition to avoiding overeating or undereating, a person should be aware of the nutritional quality of the foods. Too much fat, caffeine, salt, or sugar can upset the body's metabolic functioning deficiencies in vitamins, minerals, and nutrients and can also cause metabolic problems. Poor dietary habits can worsen a stress response and make person irritable, hyperactive, and anxious. This impairs the ability to meet personal, family, and role responsibilities.

Rest

An established, habitual pattern of sufficient rest and sleep is also important for managing stress. A person experiencing stress should be encouraged to allow time for rest and sleep. Sleep not only refreshes the body but also helps a person become mentally relaxed.

Relaxation Techniques

Progressive relaxation with or without muscle tension and imaging techniques reduces the physiological and emotional components of stress. Relaxation techniques such as deep abdominal breathing exercises, comfortable relaxed position with legs and feet uncrossed, and arms relaxed and eyes closed are learned behaviors and require training and practice sessions. Changes resulting from the relaxation techniques are:
- Lowered BP
- Lowered heart rate
- Decreased muscle tension
- Lowered metabolic rate
- Improved concentration
- Improved ability to cope with the stressors.

Spirituality

Spiritual activities can also have a positive effect in decreasing stress. Practices such as prayer, meditation, or reading religious material may be meaningful resources for a client.

Music

Music also plays an important role in alleviating stress. Music is provided according to client's taste, considering age and background. The client concentrates on the music and emphasizes rhythm by tapping fingers or patting the thigh.

NURSING MANAGEMENT OF STRESS ASSESSMENT

Many behaviors are associated with psychological disorders; careful assessment is needed so that organic problems are identified and treated. The type of illness should never be dismissed. The primary behaviors observed with psychophysiological responses are the physical symptoms. These symptoms lead the person to seek health care. The most common problems involved; in addition, longer general hospital stays have been reported being associated with greater psychophysiological morbidity, particularly depression and anxiety amongst others. Such research underscores the importance of linking physiological and psychological assessments.

Nursing Diagnosis

Impaired adjustment related to anxiety:
- Internalized feelings of inadequacy, resentment, frustration, anger, and negative self-talk
- Inability to obtain relief from stress and unmet needs

Intervention

Intervention helps to decrease anxiety. It also helps to develop effective steps for decreasing anxiety, given as follows:
- Explore situations that lead to feelings of anger and resentment.
- Discuss possible causes and explore stressors or events that trigger illness.
- Assist client to learn to be in tune with feelings and recognize situations that cause increase in anxiety
- Encourage direct expression of feelings and help client to recognize from when the feelings are internalized
- Examine possible cause–effect relationship between internalizing feelings and somatic symptoms
- Help client recognize the difference between assertive and aggressive behaviors and instruct in assertiveness techniques
- Demonstrate/encourage the use of relaxation techniques, progressive relaxation and meditation
- Use gentle, supportive therapeutic approach to develop a positive rapport
- Explore possible recreational activities to alleviate and rechannel stress productivity, e.g., brisk walk, jogging, volleyball, bowling, and swimming.

Improved Adjustment Related to Ineffective Coping Individuals

- Ineffective individual coping
- Compelling, intense desire to compete and win excessive need to achieve success
- Unrealistic perception.

Develop and Implement Coping Strategies Based on Problem-solving Techniques

- Assist client to identify present coping patterns and consequences, and to evaluate their effectiveness
- Help client identify/understand the unmet needs and understand how the present coping pattern is related to relief of anxiety
- Demonstrate/practice problem-solving techniques to encourage client to think through problems and identify goals for own care
- Ask client to give an example of situations when resentment and anger were felt and were not expressed.
- Discuss/role play alternate ways to handle these situations
- Examine how needs are expressed, passively and aggressively
- Encourage client even though the circumstances cannot always be controlled
- Identify competitive behaviors and explore reasons for feeling a compulsion to achieve/win
- Evaluate the effect that these compulsive feelings have had on physical and emotional health
- Explore how these behaviors have affected interpersonal relationship
- Discuss the importance of leisure time and how to develop and use it.

Feeling of Powerlessness

Feeling of powerlessness is related to:
- Unresolved dependency conflicts, sacrificing own wishes for others
- Feeling of insecurity, resentment, and regression of anger and aggressive feelings.

Provide help to recognize and work through feelings of insecurity resentment:
- Ask client to describe events that lead to feeling inadequate or having no control
- Assess client's attitudes toward making mistakes, for example, able to admit and accept or feel inadequate and worth cost
- Encourage client to do the feared activity and provide support for these efforts
- Ask client to describe significant others' behaviors and how fear of these behaviors can be overcome
- Explain how attack of self-confidence in one's own judgment and abilities can result in feeling powerlessness in stressful situation
- Encourage client to be open and direct in verbal expression
- Discuss causes of difficulty in making own need, known to others, and fears surrounding these issues
- Assist client to think through these concerns and identify ways to deal with them
- Have client identify what will happen and client functions independently.
- Assist client to learn how to use own capabilities.

Self-esteem Disturbance

Self-esteem disturbance is related to:
- Lack of positive feedback and repeated negative feedback, resulting in diminished self-work
- Dysfunctional family system and unmet dependency needs
- Unrealistic expectations of self and others.

Help to demonstrate self-confidence by getting realistic goals activity participating in life situations:
- Assess client's strength and limitations and compare with client's own assessment of self
- Discuss client's goals—are they what the client really wants or are they what the client thinks they should "ought to be?"
- Explore expectations family and significant others hold for client
- Reinforce client's ability to assume responsibility and rely on own ability.

Sleep pattern disturbance related to financial and familial concerns, evidenced by falling asleep and frequent awakening during night.

Planning

Treatment plans for these patients may be lengthy. The nurse must offend to all the patient's biopsychological needs. Most patients, while having need in all areas, have their most urgent needs in a limited area of functioning. Physical disorders are usually disabling and may be life-threatening. Psychological problems will hinder recovery from physical illness and onset also be given immediate attention.

Help the client to interact appropriately with each other, providing support assistance as indicated:

- Explore fast relationship and feelings about successes and failures
- Discuss precipitating stresses regularly, real and feared threats to significant personal relationships
- Determine the extent of enabling behaviors evidenced by family members, explore with family/client
- Assist to develop communication skills that enable needs to be met by using assertive expressions
- Explore possible negative feelings or fears caused by feeling compelled to meet demands of others
- Discuss handling troublesome situations by using newly learned coping skills
- Give positive feedback for efforts toward using newly learned coping skills
- Refer to support groups, family therapy, if indicated.

Evaluation

- Verbalize understanding of relationship between feelings of anxiety and physical symptoms:
  - Develop effective methods for decreasing anxiety
  - Experience marked decrease in somatic complaints
- Develop and implement coping strategies based on all problem-solving techniques:
  - Use assertive techniques in place of passive, aggressive, and maladaptive behaviors
  - Verbalize understanding of health tasks.

CONCLUSION

Stress is the most common problem to every individual, family, and community. Adaptation to stress is one of the coping strategies through which man responds to the stimuli. Adaptation differs from individual to individual; number of stressors affecting the system and the time of encounter all these trigger a person to cope with the situation. Therefore, nurse should have an understanding of the concepts of the above and help to identify the problems and treat accordingly.

54 CHAPTER

Coping with Loss, Death and Grief

CHAPTER OUTLINE

- Loss
  - Problems of Loss
  - Meaning and Definitions
  - Categories of Loss
  - Types of Loss
- Grief and Bereavement
  - Definition
  - Stages of Grief
- Types of Grief
- Theories of Grief
- Symptoms of Grief (The State of Grieving—Bereavement)
- Spirituality and Grief
- Stages of Grief (Kubler-Ross)
- Stages of Grief (Bowlby)
- Stages of Grief (Engel)
- Nanda Diagnoses for Acute Grief

LOSS

Introduction

Birth, loss and death are universal and individually unique events of the human experience. Life is a series of losses and gains, a child beginning to walk, gains independence with mobility. An older person with visual and hearing changes may lose self-reliance. Illness and hospitalization frequently causes loss. A nurse works with many clients who experience different types of loss. Coping mechanisms determine people's ability to face and accept loss. Grief is a natural response to loss. The nurse assists clients in understanding and accepting loss so that life can continue. When clients do not grieve after a profound loss, serious emotional, mental, and social problems can occur.

Humans can anticipate death. This causes anxiety, planning, denial, love, loneliness, achievement, and lack of achievement. Death can be an overwhelming experience that affects dying persons and their families, friends, and caregivers. When a person becomes terminally ill, others can be reminded of their mortality. The style of dying reflects a person's style of living and attitudes about death depend on a person's beliefs and emotional strengths.

Problems of Loss

Depression, manifestation, recognition, and intervention.

Meaning and Definitions

Loss is an integral part of human experience. It may be defined as a state of being without something that has or could have had meaning for an individual or family. Loss has many meanings because each individual has a distinct life history of contact, with loss and beliefs about loss that reflect life experience.

Loss is one of the most important issues any person has to adjust during his/her lifetime. The emotional energy invested in an object originates with the pleasure-seeking and aggressive drives. For the young child, his/her original objects are his/her parents or other important caregivers. He/she forms affectionate bonds and attachments with them. As he/she matures, he/she is able to form relationships with others, the strength of which is based on the ability he/she demonstrated to form attachments with his/her parents. The strength of a person's attachment to an object will determine his/her reaction to the loss of that object. The human beings' normal goal is to establish bonds and relationships.

Accordingly, human behavior, from infancy through adulthood, is directed toward the goal of forming, maintaining and defending against the loss of relationships.

Psychoanalytic theorists believe that only human beings can be classified as "objects." The energy invested in another person, the ability to relate to the other person and the quality of that relationship is considered object relations. Other theorists consider any entity in which emotional energy is invested, not only other people to be objects. For example, a person can invest emotional energy in a job, a body that responds normally, a well-functioning heart, hair, a perfect baby, unmarked skin, working kidneys, or the ability to talk. In any case, whether the emotional investment is in another person, an aspect of one's self that is concrete or abstract, a job or any other important entity actual or threatened loss through the impact of illness can cause a maladaptive reaction.

Loss is a change in status of a significant object. The loss can be actual or threatened; either way, the personality will organize itself to defend against its effects. A loss can be any change in the person's situation that reduces probability of achieving implicit or explicit goals. These can be abstract, such as being able to marry, to obtain a promotion, or to have a well-functioning attractive body.

Categories of Loss

Five categories of loss are—(1) loss of external objects, (2) loss of a known environment, (3) loss of a significant other, (4) loss of an aspect of self and (5) loss of life. Nurses may encounter a client who has experienced more than one type of loss. For the hospitalized chronically ill adult, Lewis (1983) describes many potential permanent losses. Loss threatens self-concept, self-esteem, security, and sense of worth. The nurse must recognize the meaning or each loss to the client and its impact on physical and psychological functioning.

Loss of External Objects

Loss of an external object involves any possession that is worn out, misplaced, stolen, or ruined by disaster. For an adult, it may be jewelry or an article of clothing. The extent of grieving a person feels for a lost object depends on its value, the sentiment the person attaches to it and the object's usefulness.

Loss of a Known Environment

The loss associated with separation from a known environment includes leaving a familiar setting for a period or relocating permanently. Examples include moving to a new neighborhood or city, taking a new job, or hospitalization. Loss through separation from a known environment may occur through maturational or situational circumstances and through injury or illness.

Loss of Significant Other

Significant others include parents, spouses, children, siblings, teachers, clergy, friends, neighbors, and work associates. Entertainment figures and well-known athletes may be significant others for young people. Research shows that many people regard pets as significant others. Loss occurs as a result of separation, moving, running away, promotion at work, and death.

Loss of an Aspect of Self

The loss of an aspect of self may include a body part, physiological function, or psychological function. Loss of a body part may include a limb, eye, hair, teeth, or breast. Loss of physiological function includes loss of urinary or bowel control, mobility, strength, or sensory function. Loss of psychological function includes loss of memory, humor, self-esteem, self-confidence, power, respect, or love. The loss of these aspects of self may result from illness, injury, or developmental and situational changes. Such a loss lessens the individual's well-being. A person not only experiences grief over the loss, but may also experience permanent changes in body image and self-concept.

Loss of Life

Persons who face death—live, feel, think, and respond to events and to people around them until the moment of death. Concern is often not about death itself, but about pain and loss of control—although most people are afraid of and anxious about death, the same issues will not be equally important to each person. Each person responds differently to death. For people who have lived alone and suffered long terminal illnesses, death may be a relief. Some perceive death as an entry into an after-life to be reunited with loved ones in paradise. Others fear separation, abandonment, loneliness, or mutilation. The threat of death often causes individuals to become dependent. The helplessness and shame of dependence experienced by some clients create a challenge for the nurse.

Types of Loss (Fig. 54.1)

Personal Loss

Personal loss is significant loss of someone or something that can no longer be seen, felt, heard, known or experienced through the grieving process. Personal losses can include tangible and intangible components, such as perceived beauty, roles, pleasure, and satisfaction with life in general. It is an individual interpretation of the value of the person or object that makes it personal or unique.

Actual Loss

Actual loss is any loss of a person or object that can no longer be felt, heard, known, or experienced by the individual. The tangible loss is usually understood by all who are aware of its value to the grieving client. Examples could include the loss of an arm, hair, youth, child, spouse, relationship, object, known environment, body functions, and role changes. Lost objects that have been valued by a client include any possession that is worn out, misplaced, stolen, or ruined by disaster. A child may grieve over a familiar toy or blanket. A widow may grieve over the loss of the smell of her deceased husband's pipe on his clothing.

Valuing is unique to each person, but the concept of loss is common or understood by others. The moving of an individual into an assisted living facility represents the loss of familiarity and independence.

Perceived Loss

Perceived loss is any that is less tangible and uniquely defined by the grieving client such as the loss of confidence or prestige. By individual interpretation, no actual loss may need to take place. Examples could be the parents'

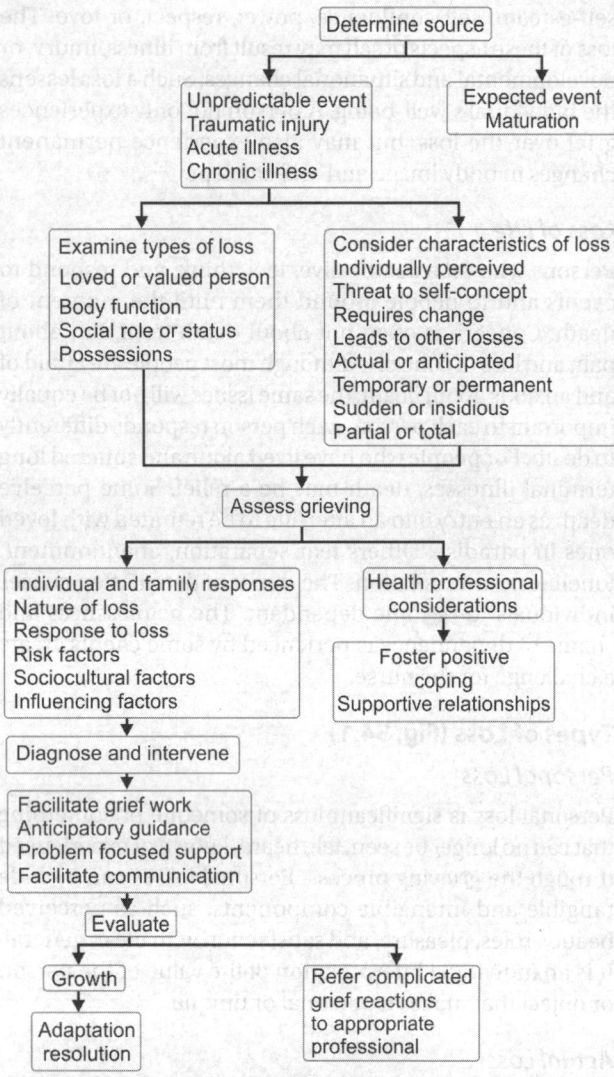

Fig. 54.1: Assessment of loss.

expectation of a tall blonde girl and the actual situation when a fat-faced red-headed boy is born.

Despite the fact that the red hair is not a death sentence and the child is healthy, it is the expectation of the blonde-haired child, idealized during the pregnancy that is the perceived loss. Therefore, the loss is in the eye of the beholder; other examples of perceived loss can include a minor scar or gaining two pounds, which may be major disasters to someone, who values personal good looks. Individual interpretation makes a difference in how the loss is really uniquely valued and the response that one will have during the grieving process.

Maturational Loss

Maturational loss includes any change in the developmental process that is normally expected during a lifetime. One example would be the feeling of loss as the child goes to school for the first time. Another would be the loss of dependence felt when the child stops breastfeeding or the empty nest syndrome felt by the parents whose last child has finally left home. These events are expected, but the feelings of loss persist, as grieving occurs to adapt to the change.

Situational Loss

Situational loss includes any sudden, unexpected, and definable event that is not predictable. Often this type of loss includes multiple situational losses rather than a single loss. A hurricane or massive flooding that has removed houses, possessions, livelihood, the things of the past and the hopes for tomorrow is one type of situational loss. An automobile accident may leave the driver paralyzed, but the grief of causing the death of another person may be a greater loss than the driver's own injury.

Conclusion

Loss is experienced throughout the life cycle. Each person responds to loss in a different way by asking, "What is happening to me? How can I live through this? How can I get over my loss?" While death is viewed as the ultimate loss other losses produce grief reactions as intense and painful as those of the death experience. Theories of loss and grief developed by practitioners in a variety of disciplines provide a basis for understanding the process an individual goes through in the work of grieving and mourning a loss. Working with clients responding to loss can be both difficult and rewarding for the nurse. Loss is painful and can be viewed as a crisis in people's lives. Changes required in adjusting to the loss can influence the successful resolution of the loss. Knowledge and understanding of the grieving process offer the nurse the potential for self-growth as well as the opportunity to provide effective nursing care for clients responding to loss.

GRIEF AND BEREAVEMENT

Introduction

Various emotional and psychological responses occur when one experiences a loss. These emotional experiences are termed as grief. Mourning occurs when an individual expresses sorrow with outward signs of grief as a result of a perceived or threatened loss.

Definition

Grief is defined as the emotional response that occurs as a response to loss.

Stages of Grief

West Berg (1979) described 10 stages of grief.

Stage 1: State of Shock

During the first stage, the grieving person experiences a state of temporary anesthesia that may last anywhere from a few minutes to a few days. If the stage of shock lasts over a week or two, it is a sign of unhealthy grief and professional help should be obtained before maladaptive behavior occurs. Caregivers should be near and available during this stage of grief, but are advised not to take tasks that the person can perform. Self-care is therapeutic and enables the person to proceed to the next stage.

Stage 2: Expressing Emotion

In this stage, people are encouraged to express pent-up emotions after a significant loss occurs. Members of the healthcare team should encourage the expression of emotions and should not be ashamed to cry with the patients.

Stage 3: Depression and Loneliness

During this stage, the person experiences feelings of utter depression and isolation. The caregiver is advised to "stand by" in quiet confidence and reassure the grieving person.

Stage 4: Physical Symptoms of Distress

Physical symptoms such as insomnia, chest pain, abdominal pain, shortness of breath may occur when someone stops at one of the stages of grief process. If no one helps the person to explore the reason for emotional and physical complaints associated with unresolved grief, an illness can develop. The physical consequences of distress resulted in death.

Stage 5: Panic (a Period of Anxiety/Fear)

During the fifth stage, the person is unable to think of anything except the loss. Concentration and productivity are impaired because of obsessive thought, causing the person to think he is "losing his mind." The helping person should encourage the grieving person in this stage to develop new and different interest and interpersonal relationships rather than to stay at home and prolong grief work.

Stage 6: Guilt Feelings

The person who says that he/she will never forgive himself/herself and continually berates his/her actions out of proportion to the real situation is exhibiting symptoms of guilt. Such people should be encouraged to talk about guilt feelings so that they begin to handle them effectively and resume living.

Stage 7: Anger and Resentment

Once the grieving person overcomes guilt feelings and is unable to express emotions, stronger feelings such as anger and resentment may emerge. During this stage, the person may blame anyone or everyone for the loss. Such feelings are a normal part of grief and can be overcome in time.

Stage 8: Resistance

During this stage, grieving persons resist returning to normal daily living. They are intent on keeping the memory of a loved one or thing alive. Returning to normal activities may be too painful for some people because they experience emptiness in the world around them. Friends and relatives are encouraged to help keep the memory of the loss alive because this facilitates progress toward the stage of hope.

Stage 9: Hope

After a few weeks or many months of grief, hope generally emerges. Life does go on; opportunities do exist for change or improvement in one's life in spite of the recently experienced loss. Friends can gradually help one find meaning again in life.

Stage 10: Affirming Reality

Grieving persons generally realize that life will never be the same again, but they begin to sense that there is much in life that can be appreciated and enjoyed. People who have a mature faith or belief in God often demonstrate an inner strength that helps them to face a serious loss without feeling that they have lost everything.

Types of Grief

Types of grief include anticipatory grief, acute grief and dysfunctional grief.

Anticipatory Grief

Anticipatory grief or pre-mourning is defined as grief associated with anticipation of a predicted death or loss. This is generally viewed as an adaptive process that can help to resolve relationships and prepare survivors to some extent for the loss.

Acute Grief

Acute grief is usually simply referred to as a grief, be the prototypical painful experience after a loss. There is agreement that acute grief is time limited, but many factors other than culture and religion affect the length and intensity of grief such as the nature of the relationship, manner of death survivor involvement in the care, length of illness and the presence or absence of hope.

Dysfunctional Grief

Dysfunctional grief has been described in multiple ways. They are absent or inhibited grief, characterized by no expression of grief following significant loss. Suppressed or repressed grief may manifest as chronic physical illness such as ulcerative colitis or psychological disability such as depression.

- ❖ **Distorted grief:** Characterized by distortion, usually exaggeration, of one or more components of grief especially guilt or anger. This grief may result in psychosocial disability.
- ❖ **Converted grief:** Similar in nature of a conversion disorder, which preoccupation with the deceased may be exaggerated to the extent at the survivors' exhibits symptoms or characteristics of the deceased.

- *Chronic grief:* Unending grief, the symptoms of which may intensify over time. Chronic grief occurs in response to a loss while chronic sorrow occurs in response to an ongoing loss.

Chronic Sorrow

Chronic sorrow is a form of grief that may include characteristics of other forms of grief, but differs in several other aspects. First, chronic sorrow is a response to ongoing loss. Second, persons experiencing chronic sorrow seldom experience physical or mental disability. A person at risk of chronic sorrow includes parents with children who have mental retardation, schizophrenia or other chronic illness.

Theories of Grief

- *Lindemann:* Grief is manifested by predictable psychological and somatic symptomatology. Acute mourning is characterized by somatic distress, preoccupation with the deceased person's image, guilt, hostile reactions and loss of patterns of conduct. The duration of grief and the development of dysfunctional grief largely depend on the success with which the mourner works through grief.
- *Elizabeth Kubler-Ross:* Kubler Ross's stages of dying are often applied to grief. The initial response to loss may include denial, anger and bargaining. Denial is characterized by refusal to accept the loss. Anger may initially be directed at the healthcare staff and later in the process, at the person who died. Depression tends to be the lengthiest phases and in dysfunctional grief may become chronic. Acceptance of the grief is a gradual process, and as the grief work progresses, acceptance increases.
- *Bowlby:* Grief and loss are characterized first by numbness in which the loss is recognized, but not necessarily felt as real. Yearning and searching in which the loss is not fully realized follow numbness. In the third phase, disorganization and despair, the loss is real and intense emotional pain and cognitive disorganization occurs; reorganization is the final phase and is characterized by a gradual adjustment to life without the deceased.
- *Engel:* The initial response to loss is shock and disbelief. Awareness of the loss and the meaning of loss develop during the first year of mourning.
- *Shneidman:* Conceptualizing less structure or stages than other theorists in regard to grief, he views the expression of grief as dependent primarily on an individual personality or style of living. An individual who goes through life feeling depressed and guilty is likely to grieve similarly. One who avoids emotional investments with others will also tend to avoid grief.

Symptoms of Grief (the State of Grieving—Bereavement)

- *Physical manifestations* of grief include weakness, anorexia, feelings of choking, shortness of breath, tightness in the chest, dry mouth, and gastrointestinal disturbances. Fatigue, exhaustion and insomnia are common. Additionally, grief is seldom a direct cause of illness or death; there is a direct link between grief and depression and heart disease.
- *Cognitive symptoms:* Cognitive manifestation centers on preoccupation with the image and thoughts of the deceased. Overtime, preoccupation usually diminishes, although link with the deceased may be maintained for years in the form of remembrances such as treasured things or negotiated relationships with the deceased. Other common symptoms are difficulty concentrating, such as complete lapses of focus or even orientation to time and place. Seeking and longing for the lost person is universally experienced. Some grieving people experience hallucinations that are most often described as momentary glimpses of the person who died, or brief auditory messages perceived to be spoken by the deceased.
- *Behavioral and relating symptoms:* This includes disruptions in patterns of conduct, ranging from an inability to perform even basic activities of daily living, to draining through daily activities, to a restless, disorganized behavior that includes searching for that which is lost the survivor can no longer perform well. Many people who are bereaved cry with little apparent provocation, which often results in discomfort for the mourner and others.
- *Affective symptoms:* Affective manifestations of grief are often overwhelming with sadness, guilt and anger among the most common. Sadness, loneliness and hopelessness tend to predominate along with other symptoms. Grief accompanied by sustained loss of self-esteem and ambivalence about living is an indication that suicide risk is increased and help is needed. Anger is common and may be directed toward the person who died, family members, healthcare staff, God or turned inward to self. People who are bereaved soon learn that nobody wants to hear your sad story.

Bereavement Care (Prevention)

- *Prevention prior to loss:* Grief is a universal experience that may come with or without warning and occurs, many times and with varying intensity throughout the life. The factors that significantly influence grief are a psychiatric history prior to the loss, inadequate social support, multiple losses and lengthy terminal illness; supportive and healthy families are less likely to experience dysfunctional grief's primary promotion of mental health and preventive mental programs to families are likely to promote healthier grief experience among members.

- ❖ **Prevention when loss is expected:** Second point at which health promotion or disability prevention should be elation to grief work in the case of terminal illness or other anticipated losses. Interventions in these situations include assisting individuals and families in working toward personal interpersonal and spiritual reconciliation. The means for intervention at this point includes individual informal or formal counseling in acute care settings, family support groups, hospice care and support from religious institutions.
- ❖ **Prevention after the loss:** This is known as post-prevention, often simply called grief therapy. Intervention at this point may be preventive, directed towards addressing existing problems that are interpersonal in nature or related to normative or dysfunctional grief. Preventive grief therapy includes hospice programs, grief workshops, etc.

Spirituality and Grief

All basic spiritual needs or issues may be threatened by the grief experience; meaning hope, relatedness, forgiveness, and transcendence may fall away and leave the mourner in a spiritual vacuum. The nature of God and previously held beliefs, including any easy answers to life's problems are called into question and may not support the reality of the current feelings.

Stages of Grief (Kubler-Ross)

Denial

A person's reaction may be shock and disbelief after receiving word of an actual or potential loss. Typically, after receiving a terminal diagnosis, notification of a death or other serious loss statements such as "this cannot be happening to me" or 'this cannot be true" are common. This initial stage of denial serves as a buffer in helping the individual or family mobilize alternative defenses.

Anger

The loss is resisted and the anger, behaviorally described as acting out, is often directed toward family and healthcare providers.

Bargaining

This stage is an attempt to formulate an agreement to postpone the reality of the loss. A secret bargaining is made with God in which the individual is willing to do anything to postpone the loss or change the prognosis. Model behavior or being a good patient is the individual's plea for an extension of life or the chance to make everything right with family and friends.

Depression

This stage occurs when the full impact of the actual or perceived loss is realized. The depression stage allows the individual to prepare for the impending loss by working through the struggle of separation. Grieving over what cannot be is manifested behaviorally either as taking freely about the loss or withdrawal.

Acceptance

This stage is reached by some individuals who are dying. When the dying person has reached peaceful acceptance, the stage is almost void of emotion. The struggle is past and the emotional pain is gone. If the loss is of a loved one or other valued object, the bereaved individual begins to come to terms with the loss and resumes activity with an air of hopefulness for the future.

Stages of Grief (Bowlby)

Bowlby divided the grief process into three phases:

Protest

- ❖ Lack of acceptance of loss
- ❖ All energy is directed toward protesting the loss
- ❖ Feelings of anger toward self and others
- ❖ Feelings of ambivalence toward lost object
- ❖ Crying and angry behaviors characterize this phase.

Despair

- ❖ Behavior becomes disorganized
- ❖ Despair mounts as efforts to deny the loss compete with acceptance of permanent loss
- ❖ Crying and sadness, coupled with a desire of the lost object to return
- ❖ Result is disorganized thoughts as the reality of the loss is recognized.

Detachment

- ❖ As the permanency of the loss is realized and attachment to the lost object is gradually relinquished
- ❖ A reinvestment or energy occurs
- ❖ Both the positive and negative aspects of the relationship are remembered
- ❖ Expressions of hopefulness and readiness to move forward are characteristic of this phase.

Stages of Grief (Engel)

Acute Stage

Lasts for 4–6 weeks

- ❖ **Shock and disbelief (1–2 days):** The first phase of acute stage beginning immediately after receiving the news of loss. The initial response is that of denial, which may occur in order to cope with the overwhelming pain.

- **Developing awareness:** This second stage develops as the denial fades. As the finality of the loss becomes a reality, pain and anguish begins to surface. Crying is the most frequently observed behavior. Anger, guilt and blame surface.
- **Restitution:** In this stage, the institutionalization of mourning occurs. Friends and family gather to support the bereaved through participation in the rituals dictated by the culture.
- **Long-term phase:** After a period of restitution, the mourner begins to come to terms with the loss of interest in people and activities are renewed in this phase. The lost relationship is put in perspective as the bereaved person begins to form new relationships. This phase may last up to 1–2 years (Table 54.1).

Bereavement and Mourning

Grieving mourning and bereavement are the processes one uses to work through the response to loss and are healthy responses to loss.
- **Bereavement:** The state of grieving due to loss
- **Mourning:** Process (grief work) by which grief is resolved. The process of mourning is a distinct psychological process and is a normal reaction to a real perceived loss (Table 54.2).

NANDA Diagnoses for Acute Grief

Assessment

Nursing assessment of a bereaved person is based on knowledge of:
- Normal and pathologic aspects of the grief process
- Influences on the grief process
- Persons resources.

Table 54.1: Differences between grief and depression.

Grief	Depression
Grief is a disturbance in mood; it is normal	Depression is a disturbance in mood; it is the pathological elaboration of grief
Universal and necessary in individual's life experience	Depression is the reaction to the actual threatened or imagined loss of a valued object tangible or intangible
Grief is a reaction to the real loss of highly valued object that may be tangible or intangible	Depression is not self-limiting and goes beyond grief in duration and intensity
Grief is self-limiting and gradually diminishes over a period of about a year	Depression is prolonged, severe and increasingly incapacitating in all areas of individuals life
Phases of normal grief includes shock and disbelief; developing awareness and restitution	Depression does not enter the phase of restitution; professional help is needed

Assessment includes the following:
- The grief experience of the mourner
- Factors that inhibit or promote working through the grief process
- The mourner's ability to mobilize cognitive, behavioral and emotional coping strategies and supports.

Nursing Diagnosis
- Personal identity disturbance
- Situational low self-esteem
- Impaired social interaction
- Dysfunctional grief
- Risk for violence self-directed
- Grieving, dysfunctional: Unexpressed
- Caregiver role strain.

Outcome Criteria

It focuses on:
- Enhancement of emotional coping skills or methods
- Cognitive and behavioral coping skills.

Outcome identification of grief includes:
- Verbalize absence of suicidal ideations
- Express any guilty or angry feelings related to the death
- Express both positive and negative feelings about the deceased versus idealizing the qualities of the deceased
- Explore the relationship with the deceased in a multifaceted way that includes both positive and negative aspects
- Formulate and implement reasonable plans for adapting life
- Participate in at least one social or community activity each week.

Planning

The plan of care for a person with acute grief consists primarily of:
- Supporting mobilization of the providing normative data about the grief process
- Supporting the person in her/his grief process.

Implementation

Nursing interventions
- Assess any intent to harm self or others. To ensure safety and prevent violence.
- Promote a therapeutic alliance with the client to encourage healthy expression of grief.
- Follow through on all obligations and care with consistency to promote an orderly predictable environment for the client who is experiencing grief.
- Facilitate the expression of feelings related to the loss to help the client understand and accept his/her grief responses.

Table 54.2: Phenomena experienced during mourning.

Symptoms	Examples
Sensation of somatic distress	
Tightness in the throat, shortness of breath, sighing, "mental pain," exhaustion. Food tastes like sand, things feel unreal. Pain or discomfort may be identical to the symptoms experienced by the dead person. Normally symptoms are brief.	A woman whose husband died of a stroke complains of weakness and numbness on her left side.
Preoccupation with the image of the deceased	
The bereaved brings up and thinks and talks about numerous positive memories of the deceased. The bereaved may also take on many of the mannerisms of the deceased through identification.	A man whose wife just died states, "I just can't thinking about my wife. Everything I see reminds me of her. We picked this sea shell on our honeymoon." His friends noticed that when he talks, his hand gestures and expressions are very like those of his recently deceased wife.
Guilt	
The bereaved reproaches himself/herself for real or fancied acts of negligence or omissions in the relationship with the deceased	Should have made him go to the doctor sooner. Should have paid more attention to her, and been more thoughtful.
Anger	
The anger the bereaved experiences may not be toward the object that gives rise to it, but the anger is displaced on to the medical or nursing staff. The anger at its highest during the first month, but is often intermittent throughout the first year	The doctor did not operate in time, if he had, many would be alive today. How could he leave me like this?
Change in behavior (depression, disorganization and restlessness)	
The person may exhibit marked restlessness and an inability to organize his/her behavior. Routine activities a long time to do, depressive mood is common. Loneliness and aimlessness are most pronounced 6–9 months after the death	Six months after her husband died, Mrs. Rama stated, "I just can't seem to function. I have a hard time doing the simplest task. I can't be bothered with socializing. I feel so down …. so … so empty."
Reorganization of behavior directed toward a new object or activity	
Gradually, the person renews his/her interest in people and activities. The grieving thus releases the bereaved from one interpersonal relationship, and new ones are free to take its place	Twenty months after her husband's death, Mrs. Rama tells a friend, "I'll be away this weekend I'm going for a holiday trip with my brother and his friend."

- Introduce the possibility of other feelings related to the loss such as anger, frustration, and despair. To help the client acknowledge feelings that may be part of the grief process in order to deal with them.
- Help the client understand the relationship between self and the lost object/person. To assist the client in moving beyond grief responses.
- Discuss meanings within the relationship. To view the content of the relationship in a realistic manner.
- Promote interactions with others. To avoid spending prolonged periods of time alone.

Evaluation

The nurse evaluates the client's increasing ability to express feelings and to develop effective coping strategies. It is important that the client should express the full spectrum of feelings that:

- Associated with the loss
- Related to the relationship with the deceased may be reluctance by the grieving individual to discuss these experience and feelings with family, friends or clergy.

NANDA Diagnoses for Acute Grief

- Personal identity disturbance
- Situational low self-esteem
- Impaired social interaction
- Dysfunctional grief
- Risk for violence; self-directed
- Grieving, dysfunctional: unexpressed
- Caregiver role strain.

CONCLUSION

Grief is a normal human reaction to loss, and the feelings associated with grief are normally painful. The key to successful grief work depends on the individual's understanding of the relationship with the deceased persons in the family.

Principles and Techniques of Counseling

CHAPTER 55

CHAPTER OUTLINE

- Guidance and Counseling
- Guidance
- Counseling

GUIDANCE AND COUNSELING

Introduction

The pattern of movement in counseling since the end of World War II has been toward expansion of the counseling and guidance concepts into education industry, the armed services, religious settings, and vocational rehabilitation work as well as other areas.

Professional organizations have expanded after getting changed titles in order to accommodate a broader scope of interest in counseling and guidance. The professional counselor has strongly supported the use of the term "counseling" as referring to a distinctively professional activity. In this context, guidance seems to be considered a mere inclusive activity one which is contributed by a number of practitioners with varied status (e.g. teacher, administrator and nurses).

While counseling has more professional distinctiveness even in the schools, which is believed that all guidance workers are not counselors, but all counselors are guidance workers as they support a broader program of education through guidance without precipitation personnel meeting.

GUIDANCE

Definition

Guidance assists the individual in the process of self-understanding, acceptance, appraisal of his/her present and possible future socioeconomic environment and integration of these two variables by choices and adjustments that further both personal satisfaction and socioeconomic effectiveness (Failor, 1957). The help given by one person to another in making choices and adjustments, and in solving problems and it aims at aiding the recipient to growing its independence and ability to be responsible for himself/herself (Jones, 1971).

To guide means (synonyms):
- To indicate
- To point out
- To show the way
- To lead
- To direct
- To seek

Characteristics

- It is a process as it helps every individual to help himself/herself to recognize and use his/her inner resources:
  - To set goals
  - To make plans
  - To work out his/her own problems of development.
- It is a continuous process: Guidance has to be provided throughout the life cycle of the individuals. For example, early childhood, adolescence, adulthood, and old age.
- Choice and problem points are the distinctive concerns of guidance. The individual's unique world of perceptions interacts with the external order of events in his/her life context.
- It is assistance to the individual in the process of development rather than a direction of that development.

Aim: To develop the capacity for:
- Self-direction
- Self-guidance
- Self-improvement.

Guidance is a service meant for students not only for awkward situations and abnormal students but also to meet the needs of all students.

- It is both generated and a specialized service:
  - Generalized service: Every one, for example, teachers, advisers, deans, and parents play a part in the program.

> Specialized service: Specialized qualified personnel such as counselors, psychiatrists and psychologists join hands to help the individual to get out of the problem.

COUNSELING

Counseling is a specialized service of guidance and basically an enabling process, designed to help an individual come to terms with his/her life and grow to greater maturity through learning to take responsibility and to make decisions for himself/herself.

Basically, counseling involves understanding and working with the individual to discover his/her unique needs, motivations and potentialities and help him/her appreciate them (Bernard and Fuller, 1972).

Counseling is an accepting, trusting and safe relationship in which clients learn to discuss freely what upsets them, to define their goals, to acquire the essential social skill and to develop the courage and self-confidence to implement desired new behavior. Cormier and Hackney (1987) defined it as the helping relationship that includes:
- Someone seeking help
- Someone who is willing to give help
- Capable/trained to help

The process of counseling can be defined on the means by which one person helps another to clarify his/her life situation and to decide further lines of action.

Concept

An accepted, trusting and safe relationship will be formulated in which clients will learn to discuss openly their problems, to acquire the social skills, courage, self-confidence and to implement denied new behaviors.

Characteristics

- It is a purposeful learning experience for the counselor
- It is a purposeful oriented and private interview between the counselor and counselee
- Based on mutual confidence, satisfactory relationship will be established
- Counseling process is structured around the felt needs of the counselor
- Main emphasis in the counseling process is on the counseling self-direction and self-acceptance.

Characteristics or the Qualities of a Counselor

- Inter-personal relationship
- Personal adjustment
- Scholastic potentialities and education, and background
- Health and personal appearance
- Leadership
- Philosophy of life
- Professional dedication
- Faith in the spiritual quality of the world respects universal principles of religion
- Had a high sense of morality.

Process

- Giving guidance or assisting the client in problem-solving. The family members and significant or influencing personalities will be included in the counseling session
- Counseling varies with situation to situation
- Everyone participating in the counseling situation must feel comfortable
- It is a process initiated by diseased client or student who is having a problem. It is a two-way interaction between provider and the client
- Situations support will be provided for the client
- Correct information will be given, encourages the client, the freedom of choice and changes available as it facilitates client to make proper decision
- Helps the counselor to focus and identify themselves for their immediate and long-term needs, and propose realistic actions suitable for meeting their needs.
- Assist the clients to accept reality
- Helps the client to accept the problem and provide information on all the aspects of problem (e.g. technical, social and legal) and its correction.

Steps

- **G:** **G**reet the clients
- **A:** **A**sk clients about themselves
- **T:** **T**ell clients or give information of strategies of coping mechanisms
- **H:** **H**elp the client to use a method
- **E:** **E**xplain how to use a retired
- **R:** **R**eturn for follow-up.

Supportive Behavior of Counselor

- Verbal behavior
- Uses language which is understood by the client
- Clarifies client's statements
- Explains clearly and adequately
- Advising, preaching and moralizing
- Reassuring
- Summarizing
- Respond to the client to speak
- Gives needed information.

Non-judgmental; does not criticize or censure the clients or thoughts:
- **C:** **C**larity
- **L:** **L**isten
- **E:** **E**ncourage
- **A:** **A**cknowledge
- **R:** **R**eflect and repeat

Does not speak too quickly or too slowly.

Non-verbal Behaviors

- **R:** **R**elax
- **O:** **O**pen and approachable
- **L:** **L**ean towards client
- **E:** **E**ye contact
- **S:** **S**mile and sit comfortably.

Uses tone of voice similar to that of client. Maintains eye contact; occasionally nods the head—maintains suitable distance.

RELATIONSHIP BETWEEN GUIDANCE AND COUNSELING

- Guidance is an organized service to identify and develop the potentialities of pupils. Comprehensive information about every (all the) pupil is collected with the help of different tests/tolls, resources, recorded and interpreted.
- This then is communicated to the individual to help them understand themselves. Pupils are also given information about educational and vocational opportunities available to them, and are helped in their career planning and development.
- Guidance thus comprises information given to the pupils for their all-round development, in counseling, and in guidance more often than not, information is given to solve their problem. While informer is also given in counseling, all information given is not counseling.
- Guidance is preventive, whereas counseling is therapeutic.
- Guidance information makes the basis for counseling sessions. Any guidance worker may do guidance. Whereas counseling requires high level of skill as well as special professional training.
- Guidance may be given in any normal setup whereas counseling requires a special setup (room to conduct interviews).
- Guidance is an integral part of education and assists it in fulfilling its aims, whereas counseling is needed in all the fields.
- In guidance, decision-making operates at intellectual level, whereas in counseling it operates at emotional level.

PRINCIPLES OF GUIDANCE AND COUNSELING

- It is concerned with the whole individual and not just with his/her intellectual life alone.
- It is not only concerned with special or problem students therefore have adequate evidence before designating a person as abnormal.
- It is more than just the activity of a specialist, and hence involves the whole school staff (faculty).
- It is concerned with developing students' self-understanding and self-determination.
- It accepts that problems have causes and are inter-related, so a deep knowledge of causes is essential.
- It is a continuous and a slow process.

Types of Counseling

Supportive Counseling

Supportive counseling is when we are asked to support people. This may take the form of action as a sounding board for their ideas, plans and suggestions. The primary skill in action in this way is the skill of listening. It also calls for the capacity to imagine how the world seems to the other person. It is the empathetic understanding (Rogers 1983).

Social exchange theory offers the cynical view that there is always a payoff, in human relationships; states that secret of human exchange is to give to the other man behavior that is more valuable to him than it is costly to us and to gel from him behavior that is more valuable to us than it is costly to us and get from him behavior that is more valuable to us than it is costly to him. For example, doctor, nurses and various healthcare professionals use this counseling in a variety of healthcare settings.

Informative Counseling (Fig. 55.1)

Professionals develop considerable amount of knowledge about the domain in which they work. Some of this form the knowledge (learnt from book, lectures, etc.) and lot of it from experiential or personal knowledge that is gained through the process of living and working with people. For example, informative counseling in the field of HIV and AIDS a student/teacher gives in a community/hospital. This type is best-restricted situations when expert information makes a direct contribution to the person's well-being and enhance comfort.

Educational Counseling (Fig. 55.2)

- Many of the caring professions operate an apprenticeship type of training in which work in the field is combined with blocks of study, e.g. nursing profession. People who work in education capacity frequently find themselves in the role of personal tutor to one/more students. Such tutoring combines both the educational aspects of students' life and the personal. The use of contract is helpful here where the tutor negotiates the

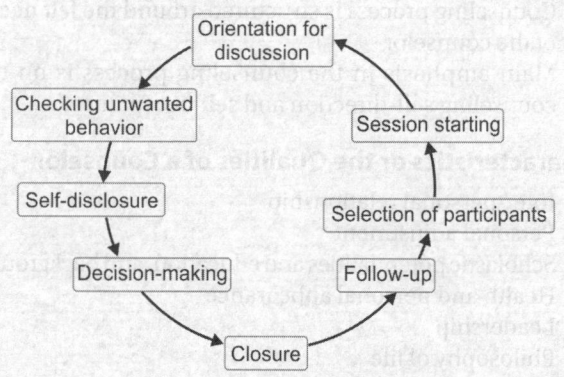

Fig. 55.1: Group counseling.

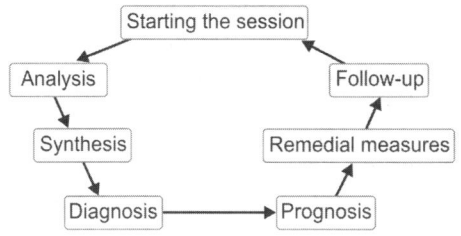

Fig. 55.2: Individual counseling.

following with the student: The amount of time that they will spend together (e.g. 1 hour/week)
- The type of counseling relationship that is required (e.g. academic/personal)
- Whether some academic counseling will take place in small groups to include other personal tutors (to economics time)
- Both tutor's and student's expectation of the outcome of the process.

Who can move freely between academic work and persons issues, while retaining certain objectivity about course work.

Other Types of Counseling

- Management counseling, e.g. at administration level
- Counseling in crisis, e.g. panic attacks sudden death, etc.
- Post-trauma counseling, e.g. disasters and personal tragedies
- Counseling in spiritual distress in situations of total inability to invest life with meaning
- Counseling in emotional distress (brings to the surface a great deal of bottled-up feelings).

Individual Counseling

- Directive counseling
- Non-directive counseling (Fig. 55.3).

Phases of Counseling (Fig. 55.4)

The phase may overlap each another, e.g. the assessment may begin even while the phase of establishing the relationship is still going on. Goal setting may start, while

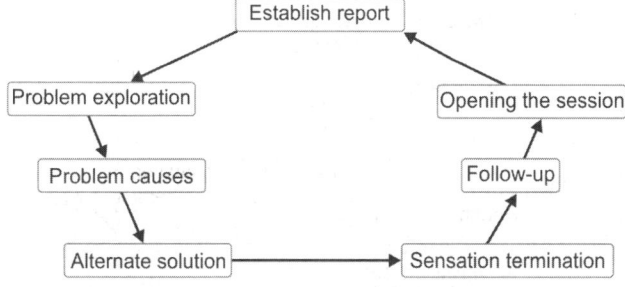

Fig. 55.3: Non-directive counseling process.

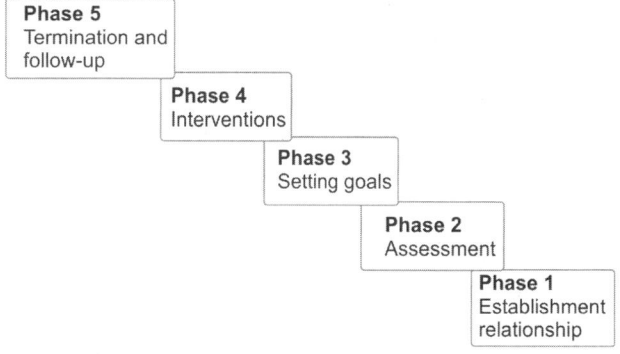

Fig. 55.4: Phases of counseling.

assessment is still going on. These phases are in progressive movement and collectively describe the counseling process.

Techniques of Counseling

- Interview
- Testing
- Observation
- Cumulative record
- Rating scales.

Knowing various problems of students, teachers may use appropriate counseling approaches in educational settings (Table 55.1).

Areas of Counseling in Nursing Education

- *Educational:* This function of counseling helps the pupils to get maximum benefit out of education and solve their problems related to education, classroom or clinical; specifically, the following functions are performed:
  - To help pupils to orient themselves to the new purposes and philosophy of nursing education
  - To help pupils identify the need of education planning

Table 55.1: Application of counseling in nursing and education.

Clinical with the client	Academic with curriculum
Helping to plan nursing care	Talking through course work and academic problems
Identifying the patients' needs and wants	Helping students to write essays and dissertations
Coping with dying and bereaved people	Vocational guidance
Reassuring relatives and colleagues	Pastoral work (spiritual/identity of one's own life)
Handling other people's anger and fear	
Helping student to work through projects	
Managing health service trusts	

- To help pupils make an appraisal of their own abilities and interest
- To help pupils develop study habits most appropriate for the study of nursing
- To orient pupil with clinical field and methods of clinical learning
- To orient pupil with library and other facilities which are available to them in a school of nursing and outside
- To help pupils choose specialization according to the needs and interest
- To give information about higher education and stimulate them to consider them carefully.

❖ *Vocational:* To help the students to understand their abilities, interest, values and goals:
- To provide information of occupations—rewards, conditions of employment, opportunities for advancement and equipment for success in it
- To help them know about the various programs of financial assistance scholarships, fellowships for improving their prospects.

❖ *Health and living conditions:* The purposes of counseling in this area are:
- To develop referral services for health guidance, society, mental and physical
- To provide sex education
- To help the authorities in the supervision and maintenance of proper sanitation in and around the hostel, and/or to help authorities in providing satisfactory living conditions along with food to the students
- To help students develop interest in games and other activities, which will promote health.

❖ *Personal:* Provides advice on personal problems:
- Provides at the right time, hints or suggestions to improve personal appearance
- Helps pupils develop inter-personal skills
- Helps pupils to accept themselves and others.

❖ *Moral, religious and social:* Providing and developing learning experiences to inculcate right ideals and conduct of living:
- Providing training in correct social convictions
- Enabling the pupils to inculcate and prorate their values that would be beneficial to them and the society.

❖ *Leisure:* Counseling function in the area helps the pupil to and opportunities for creative use of their leisure time. Counseling function in this area provides opportunities—curricular, cocurricular, and extracurricular—to develop their interest, which provide avenues for recreation, organization of guidance and counseling in schools/college of nursing. For organizing guidance and counseling program in schools of nursing, the following steps are to be taken:
- Formulate philosophy
- Outline your objective
- Formulate institutional policy
- Formulate committee, which is headed by the principal of the school/college
- Decide the type of services that are going to be provided, e.g. orientation program career, counseling, group counseling, etc.
- Identify the referral systems
- Chalk out the facilities, e.g. separate room provision of letter box.

Prepare the records that will be maintained like:
❖ Cumulative record
❖ Critical incidence record
❖ Anecdotal records
❖ Case history.

The coordination and organization of faculty advising may proceed out of the office, of dean, of students or of the academic dean.

Organization and coordination of the work faculty counselors may be assigned to:
❖ A single individual in either the student personnel or an academic area
❖ Several individuals within an area or from different areas working in conjunction
❖ A board committee or council
❖ A counseling center
❖ An individual aided by a committee.

Identify resources for short courses in counseling and guidance teachers.

Following is a conceptual model for organization, guidance and counseling program in schools of nursing (adapted from the National Workshop on Organizing Guidance and Counseling for Nurses Educators at RAK, CON) (Figs. 55.5 and 55.6).

Responsibilities of the Nurse Administration in Student Guidance and Counseling Services

While student personnel services are mainly serviced and coordinated by individuals other than nursing personnel, the nurse administration has a wide variety of responsibility in promoting student welfare. Selection of student's cooperation with other administrative personnel in promoting student welfare keeping a student records selecting and guiding nursing faculty who will participate

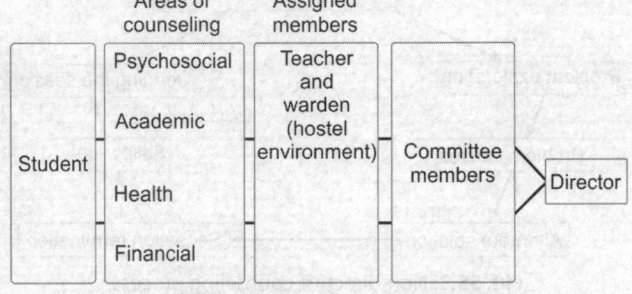

Fig. 55.5: Faculty counselors.

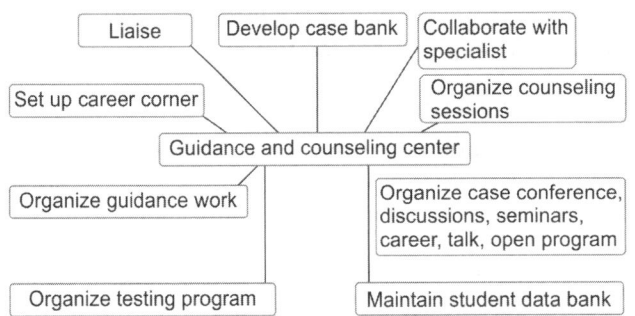

Fig. 55.6: Activity spectrum of the guidance and counseling center.
Source: Barki BG, Mukhopadhyay B. Guidance and Counseling: A Manual. Sterling Publications; 1989.

in the counseling process, and counseling nursing students so that they can make more effective use of student personnel services are among the responsibilities of the administrator.

Recruitment of Students

❖ The administrator participates in the overall college recruitment program. The administrator is responsible for the recruitment, selection and preparation of competent professional nurses.
❖ The administrator participates in campus career day functions as part of the overall college recruitment program. On these occasions, the administrator has an opportunity to disseminate information about the nursing program; faculty members have an opportunity to contact future nurses.
❖ The administrator disseminates information about the collegiate nursing program or her educational institution the administrator nor studies the geographical areas from which students in the nursing program have been drawn. The information should deal with admission requirements, such as recommended high school subjects, desired rank in high school, the range of extracurricular activities, which may be of students, fees and other costs, educational and vocational opportunities in nursing, how students may make application availability or scholarships and loans, extracurricular activities, campus facilities and other pertinent information about the nursing program.

The administrator counsels the faculty on methods working with future nurse club members and other individuals in the presence of recruitment of students, he/she expects his/her faculty in establishing and maintaining good public relations and to assist in the dissemination of information.

Selection of Students

The administrator is responsible for selecting capable students who will, with all probabilities, complete the program, successfully write tile licensing examination and have a successful career in nursing. Selection of high- quality candidates tends to strengthen the collegiate nursing program.

At the time of the interview, the administrator can determine the student's emotional stability, social maturity, speech, physical potential and motivation, as well as the more tangible qualification from records.

The college admissions committee uses these records in selecting students for admission to the college. Students who have the potential may then be presented for further consideration to an admissions committee or the nursing unit. This committee, appointed by the administrator, functions in selecting the best qualified students for admission.

Retention Selection

Selection continues throughout the period in which the student is enrolled in planning. During this period, nursing faculty and other faculty members are testing and guiding the student. Academic progress, personality and health development are evaluated.

Orientation

The administrator cooperates with student service personnel in planning an orientation program. In addition to orientation to the college residence and activities, the nursing student needs to be oriented to nursing facilities, activities of the student nurse association, the laboratory and clinical facilities utilized by the nursing unit and any other specific requirements. The administrator plans with the personnel service office in coordination with the activities of the nursing with the orientation activation of the college.

Improving Students' Welfare

❖ The administrator works in harmony with the chairman of other administrative units in matters that support the concept that student welfare current philosophy supports the concept that student personnel services and instrumental program completion and supplement each other. Thus, any change in policy, either in student personnel service or in the academic area, may affect the student's welfare. The nurse administrator should be informed of any anticipated policy changes, and be given an opportunity to study, discuss and evaluate the proposition.
❖ The administrator seeks support from other administrators for peer recommendations and for changes in policies, which may affect welfare of students. He/she supports the colleagues and inmates, which is intended to improve the effectiveness of student personnel or instrumental services. When policies have been adopted, he/she accepts and supports them. He/she interprets and gains the support of nursing facility members for the college policies and practices.
❖ The administrator promotes the development of good student health services, which emphasize preventive,

curative and rehabilitative aspects of physical, mental and social health.

- ❖ The administrator works with testing and guidance with central administration, nursing faculty and the business office in establishing policy for the use and administration of achievement tests.
- ❖ Like all other functions, tests must be scheduled. The administrator plans schedules for achievement tests.
- ❖ The administrator participates in committees and conferences with other administrators to consider policy issues, which affect student welfare. To discuss with individual students, to discuss till progress of a group of students in a particular project or to plan a new course the college may offer.
- ❖ The administrator participates in committees and conferences to review case studies in an attempt to learn about students, their problems and how to best utilize the student personnel services for the students' benefit.
- ❖ The administrator solicits funds and establishes criteria for nursing scholarships and grants-in-aid for his/her contacts with people in the community, gives him/her an opportunity to inform civic groups of the need for nurses and the need for scholarship to attract old, more capable students in nursing. Certain groups in a community prefer helping those who are in financial need. The administrator appeals to these groups for funds to establish grants-in-aid.

The administrator works with groups that plan to contribute to the scholarship or grants-in-aid fund.

- ❖ The administrator is a good informer; he/she is familiar with the various sources of scholarships and loans—college, community, state and national.

Educational, Vocational and Personal Counseling

The administrator works closely with students, personnel, service workers, with other administrators and with academic advisers to assist students in selecting the curriculum best suited to their abilities, in making a vocational choice and in personal counseling. Some students need help in selecting a major. The administrator assists students in selecting the nursing program best suited to their abilities. Vocational counseling takes place prior to admission during the students' enrolment in the program and upon graduation.

The administrator counsels and encourages students to develop their potentials through the effective utilization of student guidance and counseling services. The administrator encourages student to participate in college activities.

Academic Counseling

Academic counseling is the responsibility of faculty members. The administrator selects nurse faculty members who are competent and who have ability, interest and personality suitable for counseling students.

Students Record System

Personnel records service may have purposes. Perhaps one of the most important purpose of records is that of aiding faculty and counselors in understanding student as he/she has contact with different phases of college life.

Records serve as a basis for counting in the registers and the accounting offices they are used in selection of students, for counseling of student and as a guide in coordinating the effort of faculty advisors, counselors and others who are concerned with student welfare. Records are useful in evaluating the present programs and for future planning of student personnel or instructional services. Records may be deposited in a central office or in several offices according to the policies of the institution.

Administrator Maintains a System of Records for the Nursing Unit

In order to counsel students, the administrator and faculty must keep records. A file should be kept for each student enrolled in the nursing program. This file should contain:

- ❖ ***Admission records:*** A copy of the student's high school transcript, preadmission test results, and preadmission interview report.
- ❖ ***Records of the student, while enrolled in the program:*** Progress reports, scholastic achievement records, plan of studies, copies of examinations, academic standing, anecdotal record, records of behavior, records of academic achievement, financial status, honors, and offices held.
- ❖ Final counseling record including future occupational plans and the student's achievement on the licensure examination. The administrator keeps a record of each student enrolled in the nursing program.

CONCLUSION

The need for guidance and counseling is linked with the need of an individual to know themselves, their environment and fit them into this environment. A counselor helps three types of student problems, namely educational, vocational and personal or emotional.

Testing makes an important technique in the process of counseling besides interviews, observation rating scales and the creative work of the counselor. Guidance involves certain basic principles and the matching qualities required for an individual to make a good counselor. Organization of guidance services requires integration within the college system and the cooperation between different departments.

SUGGESTED READING

1. Fortnish, Holoday–Worret. Psychiatric Mental Health Nursing. Philadelphia: Mosby; 1999. pp. 503-514.
2. Gail W Stuart, Michele T Lanaia. "Principles and Practice of Psychiatric Nursing," 7th edition. Published by Mobby Inc. Missouri; 2001. pp. 15-47.
3. Louise RS. Basic Concepts of Psychiatric-Mental Health Nursing, 2nd edition. Philadelphia: JB Lippincott Co.; 1990. pp. 229-243.
4. Michelle Morrison. "Foundations of Mental Health Nursing" Mosby-Inc, Missouri; 1997. pp. 128-159.
5. MS Bhatia. "Textbook of Psychiatry". Published by CBS, New Delhi.
6. O Briew, Kenntlly, et al. Psychiatric Nursing. McGraw Hill, New York; pp. 16-19.
7. Patricia A Potter, Anne Griffin Perry. "Basic Nursing Essentials for Practice", 5th edition. Published by Mobby. St Louis; 2003. pp. 114-131.
8. Rawlins PR, Williams RS, Beck K. Mental Health – Psychiatric Nursing, A Holistic Life Cycle Approach, 3rd edition.
9. Wesley Nursing, California, 1996.

REVIEW OF SECTION BASED QUESTIONS OF RGUHS

Long Essays

1. What are needs of preschool children? Explain the growth and developmental changes taking place in them.
2. What are the theories of stress an adaptation. Explain in detail the management of stress.
3. Principles and techniques of counseling.
4. Explain about the crisis intervention. (May 2012)
5. Differentiate between stress and stressor, and discuss the impact of stress on health and illness. (November 2012)
6. a. Explain the essentials of communication.
   b. Discuss the importance of communication in nursing. (October 2016)
7. Discuss the principles and techniques of counselling you will follow while counselling a HIV Positive client.

Short Essays

1. Sexuality and sexual health.
2. Group dynamics.
3. Organizational behaviours.
4. Defense mechanism.
5. Communication in inter-personal relationships.
6. Care of death and grieving process.
7. Role of a Nurse in grieving process. (October 2016)
8. Therapeutic communication. (May 2013)

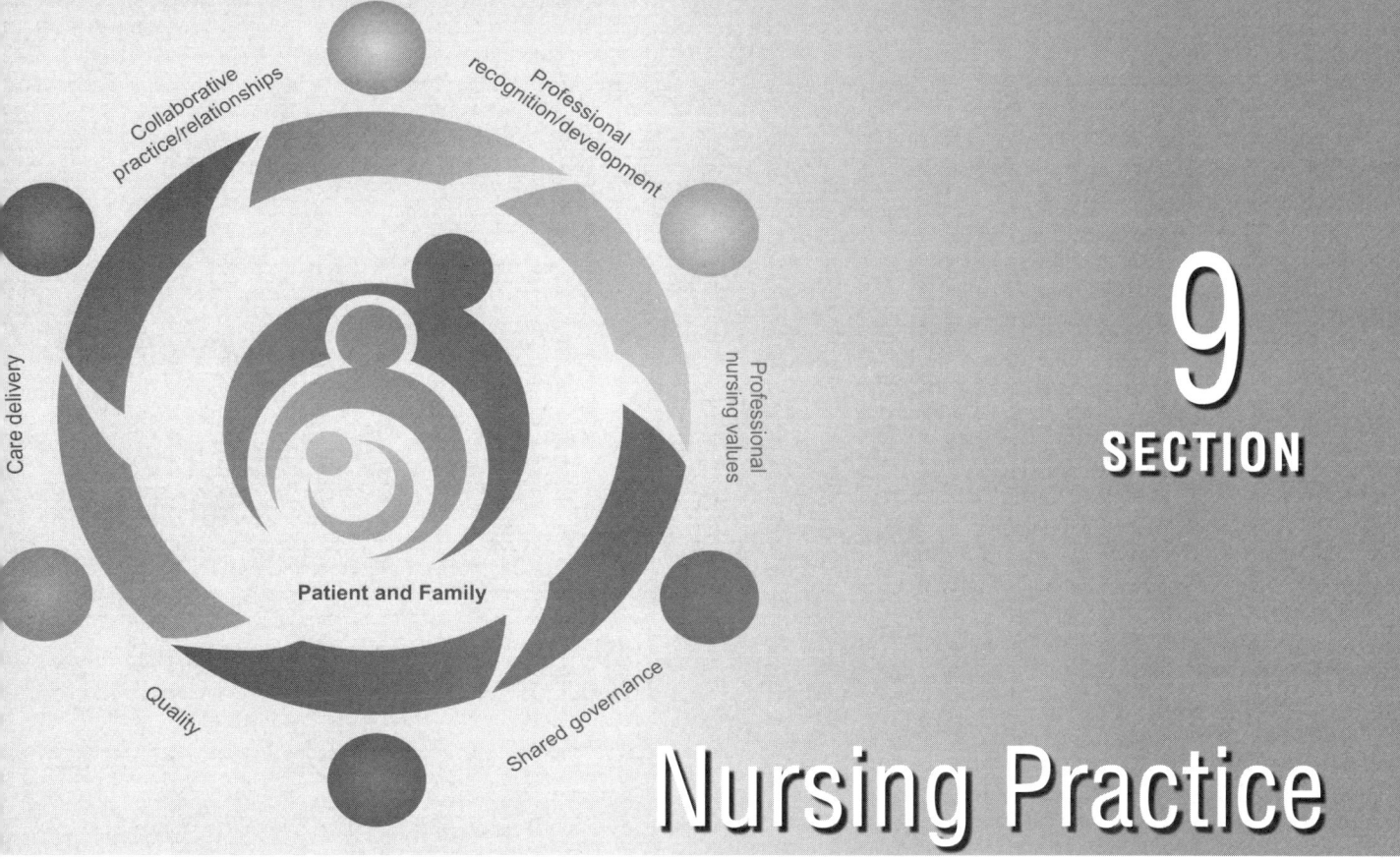

SECTION 9

Nursing Practice

Section Outline

56. Framework, Scope and Trends
57. Alternative Modalities of Care, Alternative Systems of Health and Complimentary Therapies
58. Extended and Expanded Role of the Nurse in Promotive, Preventive, Curative and Restorative Healthcare Delivery System in Community and Institutions
59. Health Promotion and Primary Healthcare
60. Independent Practice Issues—Independent Nurse Midwifery Practitioner
61. Collaboration Issues and Models Within and Outside Nursing Models of Prevention
62. Family Nursing, Home Nursing
63. Gender Sensitive Issues and Women Empowerment
64. Disaster Nursing
65. Geriatric Considerations in Nursing
66. Evidence-based Nursing Practice: Best Practice
67. Transcultural Nursing
68. Innovations in Nursing

56 CHAPTER
Framework, Scope and Trends

CHAPTER OUTLINE
- Definition
- Framework
- Trends/Scope in Nursing Practice
- Trends in Nursing Practice
- Models of Quality Management

INTRODUCTION

When we think about the profession of nursing, a set of words and images come to mind—tender, loving, care, compassion and an expectation of clinical competence. To understand the source of female nurse represented by qualities, we can understand the guided development of today's practice of nursing. In 1859, Florence Nightingale published notes on nursing, this small, but incredibly important volume to establish nursing as a profession.

Society and its healthcare needs are always evolving. As a result, healthcare today faces many challenges, including rising costs, shortages of professionals, an aging population, the introduction of new technology and difficulties with access to care. The demand for collaborative, innovative clinical practitioners to act as leaders in healthcare has never been stronger. Nurses in advanced nursing practice are well positioned to respond to the evolution of healthcare. In particular, advanced nursing practice plays a key role in meeting the health needs by building nursing knowledge, advancing the nursing profession and contributing to a sustainable and effective healthcare system.

DEFINITION

A loosely organized set of complex ideas which provides the overall structure of a curriculum—Peterson (in context to curriculum).

FRAMEWORK

- ❖ A conceptual framework is a means of looking at or describing reality.
- ❖ A nursing conceptual framework is a means of seeing nursing in its relationship with the broader reality of giving a meaning to nursing in the context in which it operates.
- ❖ Once individuals have studied and accepted a conceptual framework as their "way of thinking" about nursing, they should achieve a more efficient acquisition and application of knowledge.

TRENDS/SCOPE IN NURSING PRACTICE

- ❖ The scope of practice is not limited to specific tasks, functions or responsibilities but includes direct caregiving and evaluation of its impact, advocating for patients and for health, supervising and delegating to others, leading, managing, teaching, undertaking research and developing health policy for healthcare systems.
- ❖ Furthermore, as the scope of practice is dynamic and responsive to health needs, development of knowledge, and technological advances, periodic review is required to ensure that it continues to be consistent with current health needs and supports improved health outcomes.

Background

- ❖ The scope of practice is defined within a legislative regulatory framework, and communicates to others the roles, competencies (knowledge, skills and attitudes) and the professional accountability of the nurse.
- ❖ The practice and competence of an individual nurse within the legal scope of practice is influenced by a variety of factors including education, experience, expertise, and interests as well as the context of practice.
- ❖ **Nursing practice in different settings:** Individual registered nurse's responsibility:
  ➢ The registered nurse is responsible and accountable, professionally and legally, for determining his/her professional scope of nursing practice.

- Since the role and responsibilities of nurses, and consequently, the scope of nursing practice, is ever changing and increasing in complexity, it is important that the nurse makes decisions regarding his/her own scope of practice.

❖ **Mobile nursing practice:**
- In 1984, a need was seen to offer more extensive home healthcare for local residents who preferred to receive needed care in their own homes.
- This enabled many to reduce costs and remain in their homes, at least for a longer period of time.
- Each registered nurse is responsible and accountable for making decisions and practicing in accordance with his/her educational background and experience in nursing within the statutory parameters of the Nurse Practice Act.

❖ **Nurse manager and nurse:**
Executive's responsibility:
- The nurse manager makes decisions regarding the roles and responsibilities of nurses within the institution or agency in order to provide quality care.
- The nurse executive, in a changing and complex health delivery system, is knowledgeable regarding changes in rules and regulations, accreditation standards and standards of care and practice, in addition to evaluation of the boundaries specified in the Nurse Practice Act.
- It is the largest and oldest home healthcare system in the area, except for public organizations, and it has had a favorable competitive effect on those resulting in overall improved care for the area residents from a variety of public and private sources.

❖ **Military nursing services:**
First World War:
- The Military Nursing Service (MNS) has its origin from the Army Nursing Service formed in 1881 as a part of the Royal Army.
- After the war on 1 October 1926, the nursing services were granted permanent status in the Indian Army.

Rank structure:
- Commissioned Officers
- Major General
- Brigadier
- Colonel
- Lieutenant Colonel
- Major
- Captain
- Lieutenant

❖ **Nursing robot:**
- "Development of a Nursing Robot System" included the development of a mobile robot system (the nursing robot) to help physically handicapped people.
- The nursing robot system comprises three major components, i.e. a self-propelled vehicle, a robotic arm mounted on it and a communications post (workstation) next to the disabled person's bed.

Second World War:
- With the outbreak of Second World War, nurses once again found themselves serving all over the world.
- During the middle of the war in 1943, the Indian Army of the nursing services was separated through Indian Military Nursing Service Ordinance, 1943, and redesignated it, thereby constituting the MNS in its present form.

❖ **Telenursing:**
- Refers to the use of telecommunications and information technology for providing nursing services in healthcare, whenever a large physical distance exists between patient and nurse, or between any numbers of nurses.
- As a field, it is part of telehealth and has many points of contacts with other medical and non-medical applications, such as telediagnosis, teleconsultation, telemonitoring, etc.

❖ **Nursing in occupational health:**
Occupational health nurses:
- Are registered nurses who independently observe and assess the worker's health status with respect to job, tasks, and hazards. Using their specialized experience and education, these registered nurses recognize and prevent health effects from hazardous exposures and treat workers' injuries/illnesses.
- Have special knowledge of workplace hazards and the relationship to the employee health status.
- Understand industrial hygiene principles of engineering controls, administrative controls and personal protective equipment.
- Have knowledge of toxicology and epidemiology as related to the employee and the work site.

School health nurses' responsibility:
- Promoting healthy lifestyles and schools
- Child and adolescent mental health
- Chronic and complex healthcare needs in children and young people
- Vulnerable children and young people.

❖ **Legal regulation:**
The professional nurse is responsible and accountable for making decisions that are based upon the individual's educational preparation and experience in nursing. Behaviors and activities of the nurse relating to the scope of practice could lead to disciplinary action.

❖ **School health nurses:**
School nurses are primary care nurses for school children. They work with individual children, young people and families, schools and communities to improve health and tackle inequality. In addition, they

are recognized as contributing to raising education standards.

- *Space nursing society*
  - Space nursing society (SNS) is an international space advocacy organization devoted to space nursing and the contribution to space exploration by registered nurses. SNS is an affiliated, non-profit special interest group associated with the National Space Society.
  - The SNS provides a forum for the discussion and exploration of issues related to nursing in space and its impact upon the understanding of earthbound nursing through conference participation and its newsletter expanding horizons.

TRENDS IN NURSING PRACTICE

Trends in nursing are closely tied to what is happening to healthcare in general. Trends are fascinating phenomena, but they do not exist in vacuums. Most are interrelated; one trend often spawns another.

Broadening focus:
- The focus of nursing has broadened from the care of the ill person to the care of the people in illness and from care of only the patient to care of the client, the family, and in some instance, the community.
- In the past nursing like medicine was oriented towards disease and illness.
- Today, there is increasing recognition of people's need for healthcare as distinct from illness care and of the nurses' independent functions in this area.

Scientific basis:
In the past, nursing largely was either intuitive or relied on experience or observation rather than on research. Through trail and error, the individual nurses discovered with measures would assist the client and many nurses became highly skilled in providing care through experience.

Renewed focusing caring:
The increasing use of technology in hospitals and homes has created an increasing need to humanize. Nursing has traditionally been a caring and humanizing profession.

Indicators of this trend:
- The increasing number of professionals, articles and books about balancing of caring and technical skills
- Many studies regarding caring as an aspect of nursing
- Increasing recognition in nursing of needs of clients in technology and environment
- Another aspect of the broader nursing focuses on the movement of nursing practice into the community. In a sense, there is a return to the beginning of nursing, that is, before it became a recognized occupation
- The nursing activity not only assists those who are ill but also helps those who are healthy to maintain or continue their health.

Technology:
Technology or mechanization is being applied in the health field extensively. Certain areas of a hospital are more technologic than others. Nurses find themselves in the midst of this rapidly changing, increasingly technologic environment in hospital and in client's homes.

Expansion of employment opportunities:
Nursing practice trends include a growing variety of employment setting in which nurses have greater independence, autonomy and respect as member of the healthcare team. Nursing roles continue to expand and develop, broadening the focus of nursing care and providing a more holistic, and all-encompassing domain.

Nursing's public perception:
- Any member of society who has been ill, hospitalized or visited an emergency department has experienced nursing campaign. Note everybody needs a nurse.
- Nursing is a pivotal healthcare profession; as frontline healthcare providers, nurses' practice in all healthcare settings constitutes the largest number of professionals.

Changing trends in nursing:
The present-day nurse provides care for the people in health and illness. Nursing is one of the health services which contributes to the well-being of an individual, family, and community. Therefore, nursing is defined as a humanistic science dedicated to maintain and promote health, preventing illness, care for and rehabilitation of the sick and disabled persons.

Role of professional nurse care provider:
- The goal of nurse in this role is to convey understanding about what is important and to provide care.
- The nurse supports the client by attitude and actions that shows concern for the client's welfare and acceptance of the client as a person, not merely a mechanical being.
- Caring is central to most nursing interventions and an essential attribute of the expert nurse.

Nursing's impact on politics and health policy:
- Nurse's involvement in politics is receiving greater emphasis in nursing curricula, professional organizations and healthcare settings.
- Professional nursing organizations have employed lobbyists to urge state legislatures to improve the quality of healthcare.
- Nursing process includes doing, thinking, and interacting component. It is mainly and basically a problem-solving approach of nursing cares. The nursing process consists of four steps, i.e. assessment, planning, implementation and evaluation. Each step of a nursing process leads to the next one, which makes it a continuing cyclic process.

Communicator:
- Communications shape the relationships between nurses and clients, nurses and support persons, and nurses and colleagues.

- ❖ Communications facilitate all nursing actions.
- ❖ Nurses communicate pertinent information verbally—at change of shift reports, when clients' are shifted to another unit, at clients rounds and when clients are discharged to another healthcare agency.

Teacher:
It is an interactive process between a teacher and one or more learners in which specific learning objectives or desired behavior changes are achieved. The focus of the behavior change is acquiring a new knowledge or technical skills.

Client advocate:
- ❖ Advocacy involves concern for and defined actions on behalf of another person or organizing to bring about a change.
- ❖ It involves promoting what is best for the client, ensuring that the clients' needs are met and protecting the clients' right.

Manager:
- ❖ Management is planning, giving direction, developing staff, monitoring operations, giving rewards fairly and representing both staff members and administrations as needed.
- ❖ The nurse manages the nursing care of individuals, groups, families, and communities.
- ❖ The manager delegates nursing activities to ancillary workers and other nurses and supervises and evaluates their performance.

Counselor:
- ❖ It is the process of helping the client to recognize and cope with stressful psychological or social problems, to develop improved interpersonal relationships and to promote personal growth.
- ❖ It involves providing emotional, intellectual, and psychological support.
- ❖ The nurse encourages the client to look at alternative behaviors, recognize the choices and develop a sense of control.

Leader:
- ❖ Nursing leadership is defined as a mutual process of interpersonal influence, although a nurse helps client to make decision in establishing and achieving goals to improve the client's well-being.
- ❖ To improve the health status and potential of individuals or families.
- ❖ Increasing the effectiveness and level of satisfaction among the professional colleagues providing care.

Researcher:
Nurse who will engage in research; there is a growing expectation that all nurses will be able to critically appraise research reports and will utilize scientific studies as a basis for making decisions in their work.

Expanded nursing roles:
An expanded role is one that a nurse assumes by virtue of education and experience. The nurse who assumes an expanded role has increased responsibility and usually greater autonomy. Nurses are assuming expanded roles in both hospitals and community settings.

Nurse clinician:
The clinicians provide bed side or direct care in a specialty area. They may or may not have advanced educational preparation.

Nurse specialist:
- ❖ The nurse specialist has advanced knowledge and skill in a particular area of nursing.
- ❖ This nurses practice in hospitals or communities. In hospitals, such nurses give direct client care, advice other nurses, and coordinate nursing given by others.
- ❖ The clinical nurse specialists are a role model and are expected to keep abreast of new developments in the field.

Nurse generalist:
The American Nurses Association (ANA) conducts nurse generalists' certification programs that issue certificates in 11 areas, i.e. general nursing practice, medical-surgical nursing, gerontologic nursing, pediatric nursing, perinatal nursing, college health nursing, school nursing, community health nursing, psychiatric and mental health nursing, continuing nursing education and staff development, and home health nursing.

Nurse practitioner:
- ❖ The role of nurse practitioner is an extension of the nurses' basic caregiving role. It prepares nurses for an expanded role in the provision of primary care.
- ❖ The nurse practitioner may be generalists, e.g. family nurse practitioners or specialists or geriatric nurse practitioners.
- ❖ Nurse practitioner in a community employed in health maintenance organizations, health centers, schools, and physician's office.

Each nurse must determine his/her own individual scope of practice. To determine one's scope of practice, the nurse must understand his/her own evolving set of competencies. A nurse's scope of practice will change over time, with additional experience and education. Determining scope of practice is an obligation and responsibility jointly shared by individual nurses, nurse managers, nurse executives and educators, as well as the regulatory agencies and professional organizations.

■ MODELS OF QUALITY MANAGEMENT

Upwardly Spiraling Feedback Loop Model

This model takes the ANA model one step further. It adds a feedback loop that makes the process dynamic and subject

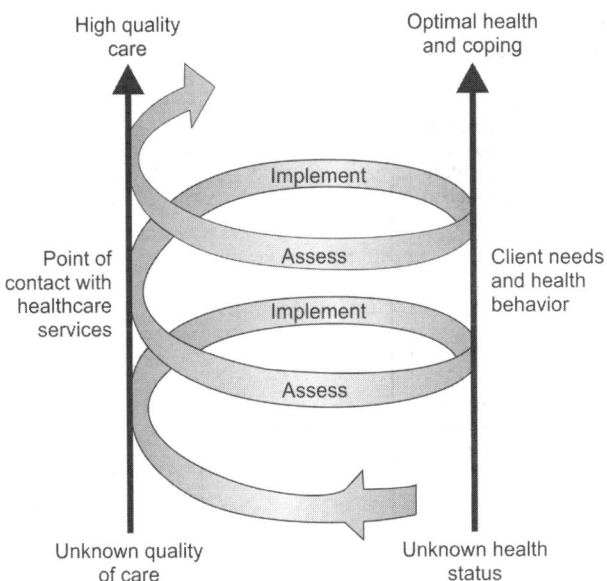

Fig. 56.1: Upwardly spiraling quality assurance feedback loop.

to change in response to ongoing feedback, which is used to assess and then implement revisions in care or plans. The model in Figure 56.1 illustrates this idea graphically. The right pole of the model represents the continuum of a client's health needs and personal health behaviors from a client's current status to optimal health and coping.

The left pole depicts the contact between clients and the healthcare system. The spirals movement from pole to pole demonstrates the quality assessment activities that nurses use to assess their clients, revise nursing care or plans and implement changes. Any changes are assessed again at a future date as part of the ongoing review process.

This ongoing and repetitive process should result in improvements in the quality of care and the client's health. The model makes two basic assumptions; first, that specific nursing activities are known to maintain and promote health, and second, that positive results are brought about by positive interventions.

This model shows the distance between the two poles of client needs and behaviors, and contacts with the healthcare delivery system. It demonstrates that nurses should step back from the everyday demands of direct client care, and assess that care and the desired outcomes. More specifically, stepping back from the process prompts nurses to do the following:

- ❖ Identify and prioritize the health problems and needs of the population served.
- ❖ Determine the systems, nursing actions or outcomes in terms of client behaviors that are facilitated by the nurse.
- ❖ Examine the success or failure of nursing efforts with a specific group.
- ❖ Adjust nursing care, systems or client goals as needed.
- ❖ Plan for future quality assessments.

Hoesing and Kirk Quality Management Model (Fig. 56.2)

A final model focuses on the "big picture" and provides the clarity needed to manage quality, and to monitor and evaluate the results (Hoesing and Kirk, 1990). The model is designed for supervisory and administrative personnel as well as for the individual professional nurse. The model begins with defining the major nursing responsibilities within the agency. If nurses know what is desired and expected of them, they will also have direction and knowledge of what it is they are working toward in achieving goals, as well as objective measures to monitor and evaluate results (Hoesing and Kirk, 1990).

The key to this quality management model is identifying measurable and verifiable indicators and being able to easily access timely and accurate information about them. Hoesing and Kirk use concepts of standards of care, practice and finance (Kirk and Hoesing, 1991).

Information gathered from monitoring the major responsibility areas is collected, organized and analyzed. From that data, it can be determined whether the indicator is being met or exceeded and the appropriate action to take. The next step in the process is to communicate feedback, information, then praise, and then to go on to develop even higher targets to promote a higher level of improved quality. For example, within a community health agency, a practitioner performance indicator might be that nurses complete client assessments during the first home visit 95% of the time. If that 95% goal or indicator is met, feedback in the form of praise is shared with the staff and a higher target can then be implemented (97.5%). Agencies might use that model to determine whether it would ever be practical to expect 100% compliance with an indicator. For instance, would it ever be possible to expect 100% of the assessments completed on the first home visit. There may be the circumstances beyond the nurse's control, and such a crisis may occur in the home at the time of visit or the client may be aphasic and the caretaker may be unavailable at the time.

An example of a client results indicator might be that on a scale of 1–10, client satisfaction should be at least 8. If that is not met because the results are 7.2, then these data are shared, some praise may be in order, especially if previous surveys indicated that client satisfaction had been 6. However, discussion may lead to changes in any or all parts of the program to achieve a higher level of client satisfaction. The more that successes, problems and information are shared with agency staff, the greater the potential for quality improvement.

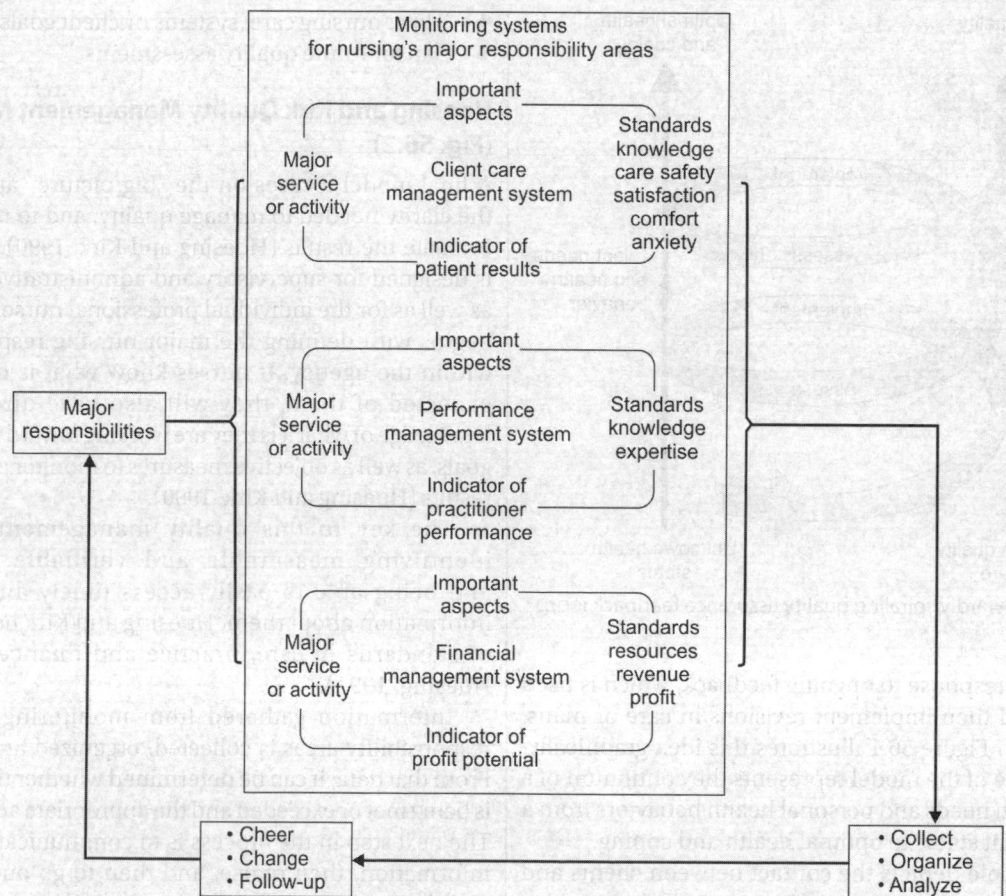

Fig. 56.2: Quality management model.
Source: Adapted from Hoesing H, Kirk R. Common sense quality management. Journal of Nursing Administration. 2010;11.

CONCLUSION

The scope of practice refers to the change of roles, functions, responsibilities and activities, which registered nurse/midwife is educated and competent to practice. Each nurse determines his/her own individual scope of practice. A nurse's scope of practice will change over time, with experience, competence and education. Determining scope of practice is an obligation and responsibility jointly shared by individual nurses, nurse managers, nurse executives and nurse managers.

57 CHAPTER
Alternative Modalities of Care, Alternative Systems of Health and Complimentary Therapies

CHAPTER OUTLINE

- Alternative Medicine
- Alternative Modalities of Care
- Alternative Systems of Health

ALTERNATIVE MEDICINE

Alternative medicine does not fall in the realm of conventional medicine. It is based on historical or cultural traditions rather than on scientific evidence.

In the 1998 systematic review of studies—13 countries concluded that 31% of cancer patients use complementary and alternative medicine (CAM).

❖ Austria and Germany—CAM is mainly in the hands of physicians

Definition

Complementary medicine or integrative medicine in general refers to the same interventions when used in conjunction with mainstream techniques, under the umbrella term CAM.

Alternative medicine methods base themselves as traditional, folk language, spiritual beliefs or newly conceived approaches of healing.

Characteristics of CAM

❖ Focus on individualizing treatments
❖ Treating the whole person
❖ Promotes self-care and self-healing
❖ Recognizing the spiritual nature of each individual
❖ Good nutrition and preventive practices.

Limited Experimental and Clinical Study

❖ Claims about efficacy of alternative medicine tend to lack evidence, repeatedly fail while testing, evidence base—problematic.
❖ The National Center for Complementary and Alternative Method (NCCAM) terms all medicines generally used to describe independent practices or in place of conventional medicine.
❖ CAM is primarily used to describe practices employed in conjunction with or to complement conventional medical treatments.
❖ Integrative medicine is not synonymous with CAM. It has meaning and mission in that it calls for restoration of the focus of medicine on health and healing, and emphasize centrally of patient–physician relationship.

Classifications

The NCCAM has developed one of the most widely used classification systems for the branches of CAM. It classifies complementary and alternative therapies into five major groups, which have some overlaps:

Whole medical systems: Cut across more than one of other groups; examples include traditional Chinese medicine (TCM), naturopathy, homeopathy, and Ayurveda.

Mind–body medicine: Takes a holistic approach toward health that explores the interconnection between the mind, body, and spirit. It works under the premise that the mind can affect bodily functions and symptoms.

Biology-based practices: Use of substances found in nature include herbs, foods, vitamins, and other natural substances.

❖ ***Manipulative and body-based practices:*** Features manipulation or movement of body parts, such as done in chiropractic and osteopathic manipulation.
❖ ***Energy medicine:*** It is a domain that deals with putative and verifiable energy fields. Biofield therapies are intended to influence energy fields that it is purported, and that surround and penetrate the body. No empirical evidence has been found to support the existence of the putative energy fields on which these therapies are predicated. Bioelectromagnetic-based therapies

use verifiable electromagnetic fields, such as pulsed fields, alternating-current or direct-current fields in an unconventional manner.
- Acupuncture is the practice of inserting very thin needles in specific acupuncture points or combinations of points on the body.
- **Alternative medical system is the name of a NCCAM[I]** classification for those forms of alternative medicine that are built upon a complete system of ideas and practice. It can include:
  - Ayurveda
  - Chiropractic
  - Homeopathy
  - Naturopathic medicine
  - Osteopathy
  - TCM
- Anthroposophical medicine is a holistic and salutogenic approach to healing developed in the early 20th century by Rudolf Steiner and Ita Wegman. Practitioners supplement the uniquely anthroposophical approach with conventional, and homeopathic therapies, and remedies. Anthroposophical doctors must have a recognized medical degree (MD or equivalent).
- Anthroposophic pharmacy is the discipline related to conceiving, developing, and producing medicinal products according to the anthroposophic understanding of man, nature, substance and pharmaceutical processing. Anthroposophic medicinal products are used within anthroposophic medicine.
- **Aromatherapy** is the use of essential oils and other aromatic compounds from plants to affect someone's mood or health.

ALTERNATIVE MODALITIES OF CARE

Aromatherapy uses plant materials and aromatic plant oils, including essential oils, managed into the skin, inhaled or used in the bath and other aromatic compounds for improving psychological or physical well-being.

Aromatherapy massage relieves tension and improves circulation and can reduce anxiety in short-term settings such as intensive care. A trial of "melissa" (lemon balm) aromatherapy shows highly significant effects in reducing agitation and increasing social interaction in dementia patients (Fig. 57.1).

Aromatherapists, who specialize in the practice of aromatherapy, utilize blends of therapeutic essential oils that can be issued through topical application, massage, inhalation or water immersion to stimulate a desired response.
- **Attachment therapy** is a form of therapy aimed at children with alleged "attachment disorders," usually fostered or adopted children. It is substantially based on outdated notions of suppressed rage due to early adverse experiences. Traditionally, it uses a variety of confrontational and physically coercive techniques

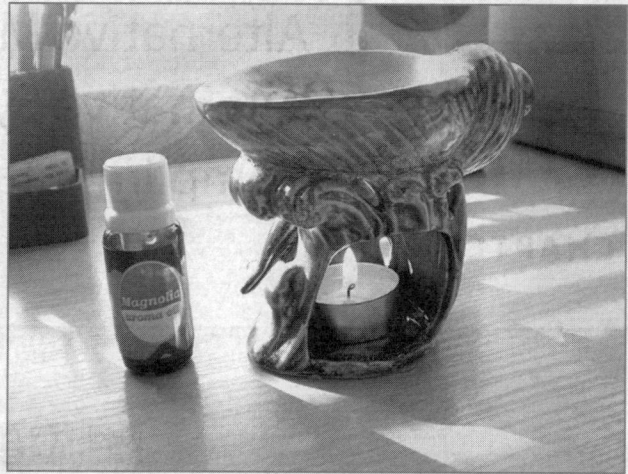

Fig. 57.1: Aromatherapy.

of which the most common form is holding therapy, accompanied by parenting methods, which emphasize obedience. Following implication in a number of child death and maltreatment cases in the United States of America, there has been a recent move away from coercion by some leading theorists and practitioners. It is largely unvalidated.

Bates method is an alternative approach to eyesight improvement and maintenance. It is based on the belief that errors in visual accommodation are due to mental strain and that vision may be improved by appropriate relaxation techniques.

"Biologically based therapies" is the precise name of a NCCAM classification, for alternative treatments that use substances found in nature and/or some other natural therapy. It can include:
- Chinese food therapy
- Fasting
- Herbal therapy
- Macrobiotic lifestyle
- Natural health.

Natural therapy:
- Diet and food
- Dietary supplements
- Exercise
- Naturopathy
- Orthomolecular medicine
- Urine therapy.

CAM is an acronym for complementary and alternative medicine, an umbrella term for a large range of treatments and of theories on the nature of health and illness, many of them unrelated, and is not commonly employed by the conventional medical establishment.

List of branches, famous people in alternative medicine and history of alternative medicine.

Chelation therapy is the use of chelating agents such as ethylenediaminetetraacetic acid to remove heavy metals from the body. While in conventional medicine, chelation therapy is used only to treat heavy metal poisoning, and some alternative practitioners advocate the use of chelation therapy to treat coronary artery disease.

Chinese medicine: The group of philosophies embodied by Chinese medicine are, more accurately, referred to as oriental medicine with roots in many different Asian countries. This millennia-old Asian medical tradition works to bring balance to the body through acupuncture, massage, eastern herbalism, diet and lifestyle changes such as martial arts and meditation.

The practice of chiropractic is a manual therapy involving the manipulation of the vertebra subluxation to restore proper motion biomechanics and nerve flow from the brain to the body (Fig. 57.2).

Chiropractic is a form of alternative medicine mostly concerned with the diagnosis and treatment of mechanical disorders of the musculoskeletal system, especially the spine.

Christian Science is a small denomination which teaches that Christian healing as practiced by Jesus of Nazareth and his followers for several centuries after him was in fact not a short-term dispensation to induce faith, but had an underlying principle (specifically God) and method. While its practice is regarded within the denomination as incompatible with medical care, it also respects the philanthropy of the medical faculty and is uncondemningly noncompulsory. Resort to Christian Science may be private or involve the care of a Christian Science practitioner.

Color puncture is an alternative medicine practice asserting that light can be used to stimulate acupuncture points for the purpose of balancing energy in the body and promoting healing and better health. It is also called color light acupuncture in North America. It is a form of color therapy.

Complementary medicine refers to treatments that are used alongside ("complementary to") conventional medicine.

Diet-based therapy uses a variety of diets in order to improve health and longevity, to control weight, as well as to treat specific health conditions like high cholesterol:
- Breatharian
- Fruitarianism
- List of diets
- Living foods diet
- Macrobiotic lifestyle
- Okinawa diet
- Ovo-lacto vegetarian
- Raw foodist
- Vegan
- Vegetarianism
- Low-fat diet
- Low-carbohydrates diet (zone diet, Atkins diet)

Eclectic medicine was a 19th-century system of medicine used in North America that treated diseases by the application of single herbal remedies to effect specific cures of certain signs and symptoms.

Energy medicine is the name of an NCCAM classification for alternative treatments that involve the use of veritable (i.e., which can be measured) and putative (i.e., which have yet to be measured) energy fields. It can include:
- Jin Shin Jyutsu
- Magnet therapy
- Medical qigong
- Reiki
- Shiatsu
- Therapeutic touch
- The WISE method (holistic integrated spiritual energy)
- Eden energy medicine approach developed by Donna Eden
- Exercise-based therapy uses a variety of traditional forms of physical movement, in order to improve health and longevity, to increase, lengthen and tone muscle mass, gain flexibility, as well as to treat specific health conditions and to relieve stress. It can include:
- Active isolated stretching
- Aerobic exercise
- Aerobics
- Bodybuilding
- Feldenkrais method
- Martial arts
- Physical culture
- Pilates
- Proprioceptive neuromuscular facilitation
- Stretching
- Some forms of qigong
- Walking
- Weight training
- Yoga
- Feldenkrais method is an educational system centered on movement, aiming to expand and refine the use of the self through awareness

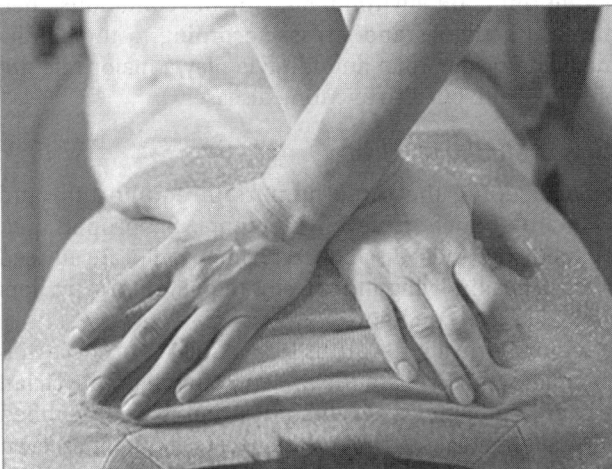

Fig. 57.2: Chiropractice.

- ❖ Flower essence therapy is regarded by some as a subcategory of homeopathy, which uses homeopathic dilutions of flowers. This practice was begun by Edward Bach with the Bach flower remedies, but is now practiced much more widely
- ❖ **Folk medicine** is the collection of procedures traditionally used for the treatment of illness and injury, aiding in childbirth and maintenance of wellness.

Herbalism is the practice of making or prescribing herbal remedies for medical conditions.

Heroic medicine is any medicine or method of treatment that is aggressive or daring in a dangerously ill patient. It is generally used to refer to the prescientific treatments of 18th-century doctors, such as bloodletting.

Holism is the study and advocacy of wholeness in health, science, politics or any other area of life.

Hydrotherapy is the external use of water in the medical treatment of disease, such as through the use of baths, the application of hot and cold compresses or sheet packs and shower sprays. These applications typically use water as a medium for delivery of heat and cold to the body, capitalizing on the thermoregulatory properties of the body for therapeutic effect.

ALTERNATIVE SYSTEMS OF HEALTH

Ayurveda

Definition

Ayurveda is a system of healing based on homeopathy and naturopathy, with an extensive use of herbs.

Ayurveda (Devanagari, the "science of life") is a system of traditional medicine native to the Indian Subcontinent originated >5000 years ago and practiced in other parts of the world as a form of alternate medicine. In Sanskrit, the word Ayurveda consists of the words ayus, meaning "life," and veda, meaning "related knowledge" or "science." Evolving throughout its history, Ayurveda appeared during the Vedic period in India. The Sushruta Samhita and the Charaka Samitha were influential works on traditional medicine during this era, which detail the prevention and treatment or disease has a prominent place in treatment, including restructuring a patient's lifestyle to align with the course of nature and four seasons to guarantee complete wellness Ayurvedic practitioners also identified a number of medicinal preparations and surgical procedures for curing various ailments and diseases.

Aims of Ayurveda

- ❖ To remove the cause of disorders, prevent illness and harmonize body, mind and consciousness
- ❖ Ayurveda aids in maintaining good health, increasing longevity and overall quality of life

Alternate Ayurvedic treatments and self-help regimes include—nutrition, herbal remedies, aromatherapy, lifestyle recommendations, massage treatments, color/sound therapy, meditation, Panchakarma (detoxification), Yoga, meditation and rejuvenation. Ayurveda empowers the individual to take control of their own health and well-being.

For Example

Terminalia arjuna is useful in alleviating the pain of angina pectoris and in treating heart failure and coronary artery disease. *Terminalia* may also be useful in treating hypercholesterolemia.

Siddha

The Siddha medicine is a form of South Indian Tamil traditional medicine and part of the trio Indian medicines—Ayurveda, Siddha, and Unani. However, Lord Sri Akshunna, a master of northern siddha tradition, says there is use of siddha medicine in the North Indian part or rather in Himalayan region as jhur phuk and siddha buti (medicine) tantra. This system of medicine was popular in ancient India; due to antiquity of this medical system, the siddha system of medicine is believed to be the oldest medical system in the known universe.

The system is believed to be developed by the 9 nath and 84 siddhas in the north and 18 siddhas in the south called siddhar. They are the ancient supernatural spiritual saints of India and the Siddha system is believed to be handed over to the Siddhar by the siddhars, the followers of Lord Shiva (saivam). Siddhar's total numbers are 18 in which themagathiyar is the first siddhar. Siddhars believed in the concept that a healthy soul can only be developed through a healthy body. So, they developed methods and medication that are believed to strengthen their physical body and thereby their souls. Men and women who dedicated their lives into developing the system were called Siddhars. They practiced intense yoga, including years of fasting and meditation and are believed to have achieved supernatural powers and gained the supreme wisdom and overall immortality.

It is assumed that when the normal equilibrium of three humors (vatha, pitha and kapha) is disturbed, disease is caused. The factors, which are assumed to affect this equilibrium, are environment, climatic conditions, diet, physical activities and stress. According to the siddha medicine system, diet and lifestyle play a major role not only in health but also in curing diseases.

Aims of Siddha Medicine

- ❖ At keeping the three humors in equilibrium and maintenance of seven elements. So proper diet, medicine and a disciplined regimen of life are advised for a healthy living and to restore equilibrium of humors in diseased condition.
- ❖ Saint Thiruvallur explains four requisites of successful treatment. They are the patient, attendant, physician and medicine. When the physician is well qualified and other agents possess the necessary qualities, even severe diseases can be cured easily. The treatment should be commenced as early as possible after assessing the course and cause of the disease.

Treatment is classified into three categories

- ❖ Devamaruthuvum (divine method); manuda marthuvum (rational method); asura maruthuvum (surgical method). In divine method, medicines like parpam, chendooram, gur, kuligai made of mercury, sulfur and pashanams are used. In the rational method, medicines made of herbs like churanam, kudineer and vadagam are used. In surgical method, incision, excision, heat application, bloodletting, and leech application are used.
- ❖ According to therapies, the treatments of siddha medicines could be further categorized into categories, such as purgative therapy, emetic therapy, fasting therapy, steam therapy, oleation therapy, physical therapy, solar therapy, bloodletting therapy, yoga therapy, etc.

Unani and Tibbi

This is one of the alternative forms of medicine. Unani has found favor in Asia, especially in India. In India, these Unani practitioners can practice as qualified doctors, as the Indian government approves their practice. Unani medicine is very close to Ayurveda. Both are based on the presence of the elements (in Unani, they are considered to be fire, water, earth and air) in the human body. (The elements, attributed to the philosopher Empedocles, determined the way of thinking in Medical Europe.) According to followers of Unani medicine, these elements are present in different fluids and their balance leads to health and their imbalance leads to illness.

All these elaborations were built on the basic Hippocratic theory of the Four Humors. The theory postulates the presence in the human body of blood, phlegm, yellow bile and black bile. Each person's unique mixture of these substances determines his temperament—a predominance of blood gives a sanguine temperament; yellow bile, bilious (or choleric); and black bile, melancholic. As long as these humors are in balance, the human system is healthy, and its imbalance can result in disease.

Homeopathy (Fig. 57.3)

Integrative medicine as defined by NCCAM combines conventional medical treatments and CAM treatments for which there is some claimed scientific evidence of their safety and effectiveness. Integrative medicine also adopts the term "integrative health," which incorporates mental, spiritual and community wellness with personal health.

Iridology (also known as iridodiagnosis) is an alternative medicine technique whose proponents believe that patterns, colors and other characteristics of the iris can be examined to determine information about a patient's systemic health. Practitioners match their observations to iris charts, which divide the iris into zones corresponding to specific parts of the human body.

Life extension is a movement, the goal of which is to live longer through intervention, and to increase maximum lifespan or average lifespan, especially in mammals. Researchers of life extension are a subclass of biogerontologists known as "biomedical gerontologists." See also the list of life extension-related topics.

- ❖ Lifestyle describes the particular attitudes, habits or behaviors associated with an individual.
- ❖ Lifestyle diseases are diseases that appear to increase in frequency as countries become more industrialized and people live longer.
- ❖ Manipulative and body-based methods is the precise name of an NCCAM classification, for alternative treatments that are based on manipulation and/or movement of one or more parts of the body. It can include:

Manual lymphatic drainage is a type of gentle massage, which is believed by proponents to encourage the natural circulation of the lymph through the body.

The mind-body connection idea says that the causes, development and outcomes of an illness are determined as much from the interaction of psychological and social factors as they are due to the biological factors of health. Many mind-body therapists take the definition of mind-

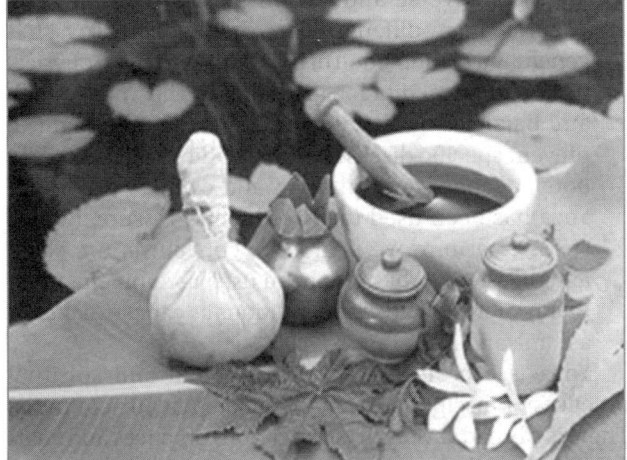
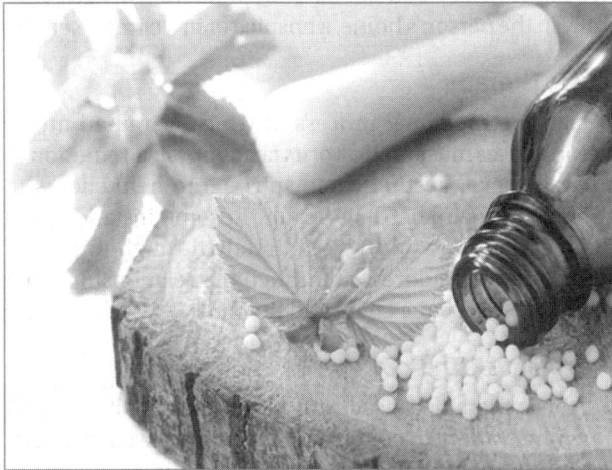

Fig. 57.3: Homeopathy.

body connection further and state that the root cause of illness is actually in the mind and spirit, and that for complete and permanent eradication of an illness, the cause must be addressed and cure focused there.

NCCAM has classified complementary and alternative therapies into five different categories or domains:
1. Whole medical systems
2. Mind–body intervention
3. Biologically based therapy
4. Manipulative and body-based methods
5. Energy therapy.

Qigong is an exercise aspect of Chinese medicine. Qigong is mostly taught for health maintenance purposes, but there are also some who teach it, especially in China, for therapeutic interventions. There are hundreds of different schools, and it is also an adjunct training of many East Asian martial arts.

Reiki is a form of treatment developed by Mikao Usui in Japan around 1922. Practitioners use their hands on or above the patient in order to control, increase or open up a postulated energy, "ki," in the body. Training is usually through short courses after which one can become certified as a "Reiki master."

Reflexology

Massage therapy along with manual pressure applied to specific areas of the foot. These areas are believed to correspond to different organs or body systems via miridians. Stimulation of these areas eliminates the blockage of energy responsible for pain or disease.

Thalassotherapy

Is the use of seawater as a form of therapy. Thalassotherapy was popular in England during the second half of the 18th century, with Doctor Richard Russell credited as playing a significant role in its popularity.

Therapeutic Music

The music played live at the bedside of persons who are faced with physical, emotional and spiritual challenges, generally in the person's home, a hospice or in a clinical setting.

Music Therapy

It is an interpersonal process in which a trained music therapist uses music and all of its facets physical, emotional, mental, social, aesthetic and spiritual to help clients to improve or maintain their health. In some instances, the client's needs are addressed directly through music; in others, they are addressed through the relationships that develop between the client and therapist.

Uses of Music Therapy

❖ Music therapy is used with individuals of all ages and with a variety of conditions, including psychiatric disorders, medical problems, physical handicaps sensory impairments, developmental disabilities, substance abuse, communication disorders, interpersonal problems and aging.
❖ To improve learning, build self-esteem, reduce stress, support physical exercise and facilitate a host of other health-related activities.

Music therapists are found in nearly every area of the helping professions. Some commonly found practices include developmental work (communication, motor skills, etc.) with individuals with special needs, song-writing and listening in reminiscence/orientation work with the elderly, processing and relaxation work and rhythmic entertainment for physical rehabilitation in stroke victims. It is considered as one of the expensive therapies.

Traditional Chinese Medicine (TCM)

TCM is a system of health care, which is based on the Chinese notion of harmony and balance inside the human body as well as harmony between the body, and its outside environment. TCM can include or address the following components:

❖ Uropathy is a specialized branch of alternative medicine, including any sort of oral or external application of urine for medicinal or cosmetic purposes (refer urine therapy).
❖ **Water cure (therapy)** in the therapeutic sense is a course of medical treatment by hydrotherapy. In the 19th century, the term "water cure" was used synonymously with "hydropathy," which itself is the 19th-century term for hydrotherapy. Conceptually, water cures include a broad range of practices essentially any therapeutic uses of water.
❖ Wellness has been used in CAM contexts since Halbert L. Dunn began using the phrase "high level wellness" in the 1950s, based on a series of lectures at a Unitarian Universalist Church in Arlington, Virginia. Wellness is generally used to mean a healthy balance of the mind–body and spirit that results in an overall feeling of well-being.
❖ **Yoga** is a diverse and ancient East Indian practice. There are many different styles and schools of yoga. It is generally a combination of breathing exercises, physical postures and meditation that calms the nervous system, and balances body, mind and spirit. It is thought to prevent specific diseases and maladies by relaxing the body, deepening respiration and calming the mind. Yoga has been used to lower blood pressure, reduce stress and improve flexibility, concentration, sleep and digestion. It has also been used as supplementary therapy for such diverse conditions as cancer, diabetes, asthma and AIDS (Fig. 57.4).

Yoga is a group of physical, mental and spiritual practices or disciplines which originated in ancient India. There is a broad variety of yoga schools, practices and goals in Hinduism, Buddhism and Jainism.

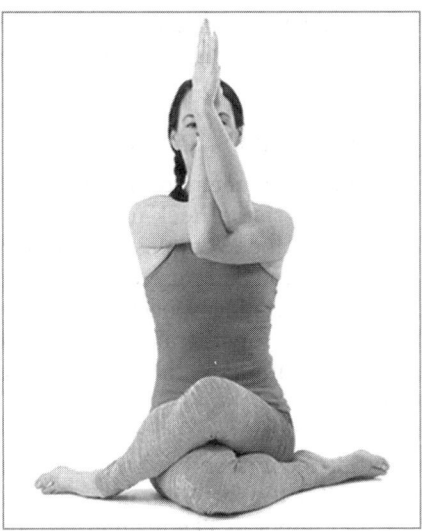

Fig. 57.4: Yoga.

Other Therapies

Curanderismo

It is a cultural healing tradition found in Latin America and among many nations in the United States. Although it is traditional healing system, it utilizes western biomedical belief, treatment and practices. Three levels of care are practiced among curanderos (man) and curanderas (women)—the material level, the spiritual level and mental level. Healers have the gift for working at only one of these levels. The majority of healers work at the material level and most combine spiritual healing, herbal medicine and first aid techniques.

Spiritual Therapy

Spiritual therapy is a regimen designed to heal one's spirit and psyche as well as the body. In many traditions, it is believed if one's spirit is ailing, one's whole being suffers. This is where spiritual therapy comes in. It treats the whole being, especially the spirit to promote a healthy whole person.

Faith and Prayer

Faith is the confident belief or trust in the truth or trustworthiness of a person, idea or thing. The word "faith" can refer to a religion itself or to religion in general. As with "truth," faith involves a concept of future events or outcomes and is used conversely for a belief "not resting on logical proof or material evidence." Informal usage of the word "faith" can be quite broad and may be used in place of "trust" or "belief."

- Faith is often used in a religious context, as in theology, where it almost universally refers to a trusting belief in transcendent reality or else in a Supreme Being and/or this believes in the role in the order of transcendent, spiritual things.
- Prayer is the act of addressing a God or Spirit for the purpose of worship or petition. Specific forms of this may include praise, requesting guidance or assistance, confessing sins, as an act of reparation or an expression of one's thoughts and emotions. The words used in prayer may take the form of intercession, a hymn, incantation, words of gratitude or a spontaneous utterance in the person's praying words. Praying can be done in public, as a group or in private.

Baha'i Faith

In the Baha'i, faith is ultimately the acceptance of the divine authority of the manifestations of God. In the religion's view, faith and knowledge are both required for spiritual growth. Faith involves more than outward obedience to this authority, but also must be based on a deep personal understanding of religious teachings.

By faith is meant, first, conscious knowledge, and second, the practice of good deeds.

Humor and Laughter

Laughing is found to lower blood pressure, reduce stress hormones, increase muscle flexion and boost immune function by raising levels of infection-fighting T-cells, disease-fighting proteins called gamma-interferon and B-cells, which produce disease-destroying antibodies. Laughter also triggers the release of endorphins, the body's natural painkillers and produces a general sense of well-being.

Laughter is infectious. Hospitals around the country are incorporating formal and informal laughter therapy program into their therapeutic regimens. In countries such as India, laughing clubs in which participants gather in the early morning for the sole purpose of laughing are becoming as popular as Rotary Clubs in the United States.

Benefits of Laughter

- Laughter activates the immune system
- Laughter decreases "stress" hormones

Laughter brings in positive emotions that can enhance well-being but cannot replace conventional treatments. Hence, it is another tool available to help fight the disease.

Humor

Humor is the tendency of particular cognitive experiences to provoke laughter and provide amusement. Many theories exist about what humor is and what social function it serves. People of all ages and cultures respond to humor. The majority of people are able to be amused, to laugh or smile at something funny and thus they are considered to have a "sense of humor."

The sense of humor is the ability to experience humor; although the extent to which an individual will find something humorous depends on a host of variables, including geographical location, culture, maturity, level of education, intelligence, and context. For example, young children may favor slapstick, such as Punch and Judy puppet shows or cartoons such as Tom and Jerry. Satire may rely more on understanding the target of the humor and thus tends to appeal to more mature audiences. Non-satirical humor can be specifically termed "recreational drollery."

Bioelectromagnetic Therapy

Bioelectromagnetic therapy (BT) is the application of electromagnetic fields to treat and prevent disease and promote health and longevity. Electromagnetism is a powerful clinical tool, simple to apply yet complex in its biological effects.

Whenever current (I) passes through a wire, it includes a magnetic field. Although the electricity itself remains confined within the wire, the magnetic field induced moves outside.

What makes this treatment so remarkable is that living tissue is especially transparent to magnetic fields. When a varying electromagnetic field is placed close to a conductive medium such as the human body, it will induce electrical currents. BT may be new to the reader, but it has been applied clinically almost from the moment we learned to send electricity over wire. It is the standard practice in Eastern Europe and it has been studied systematically for many years. Positive results are documented in a lengthy list of conditions and thousands of studies have been performed.

Some of the documented effects of electromagnetic fields include:
- Accelerated healing, greater cellular energy (increased ATP), vasodilatation/increased blood flow
- Reduced inflammation and edema, muscle relaxation, cell membrane changes, enhanced movement of calcium, sodium and other ions, bone formation, improved oxygenation, better sleep, lysis of clots
- Reduction in platelet adhesion, increased fertility, enhanced cognitive ability
- Improved central and peripheral nerve function, reduced stress and better mood.

Photo Energy Therapy

Photo energy therapy devices emit near infrared light (NIR Therapy) typically at a wavelength of 800 nm. This wavelength is believed to stimulate the release of nitric oxide, an endothelium-derived relaxing factor into the bloodstream, thus vasodilating the capillaries and venules in the microcirculatory system. This increases circulation and is effective in various clinical studies.

Detoxification Therapy

Detoxification therapy involves the removal of toxic substances. Our body naturally eliminates or neutralizes toxins. But due to industrial revolution, the accumulation of toxins (food additives, chemicals, anesthetics and residue of pharma drugs, pesticides and heavy metal) surpasses its elimination.

Methods of Detoxification Therapy

- There are a number of methods of detoxification
- First, a brief physical check-up is made, X-ray is taken, urine and blood samples are sent for analysis, sometimes sweat and hair may be analyzed.
- Colonic irrigation, fasting, special diets, hyperthermia, other hydrotherapy treatments, lymphatic stimulation and nutritional supplements are some methods of detoxification.
- Nutritional supplements–intake of massive quantities of vitamin C is recommended for people undergoing detoxification treatment. Vitamin A, vitamin B and vitamin E and minerals like magnesium, potassium, selenium and zinc are also suggested. Herbs such as cayenne, echinacea and garlic are also included.

Benefits of Detoxification Therapy

- Food additives, preservatives, environmental pollutants and many synthetic chemicals have bad effects and interfere with normal functioning of our bodies and cause serious damage to adrenal glands, liver, kidney and thyroid.
- A chemical free home and workplace and healthy diet is insufficient to fully undo the damage caused by years of toxic build-up.
- And only detoxification programs are found beneficial in these cases. But some experts argue that many of the recommended treatments are ineffective and dangerous as well.

Contraindications for Detoxification Therapy

- Weak or underweight, elderly, pregnant and nursing mothers; people suffering from ulcers and diabetes should avoid all forms of detoxification
- Ulcerative colitis, Crohn's disease, any other type of bowel inflammation or hemorrhoids, diverticulitis, tumor of large intestine or rectum
- Liver or kidney problems
- High or low BP, heart disease, epilepsy, multiple sclerosis or asthma
- Lung problems or TB, heart problems, advanced cancer or diabetes
- People with a history of blood clots

CONCLUSION

The trend is that people are rushing to alternative systems of care. Because of limited side effects, people are more oriented towards preventive knowledge and seek advance care. There is much research being undertaken to prove that alternative system of modalities is beneficial.

58. Extended and Expanded Role of the Nurse in Promotive, Preventive, Curative and Restorative Healthcare Delivery System in Community and Institutions

CHAPTER OUTLINE

- Extended Roles of the Nurse
- Extended Care Facilities
- Common Expanded Roles of Nursing
- The Roles of Nurse related to Medical Surgical Nursing Area
- Expanded Roles of Nurse in Child Health Nursing Area
- Expanded Roles in Community Health Nursing
- Expanded Roles in Psychiatric Nursing

INTRODUCTION

Nursing today is a fast-changing profession that is influenced by increasing knowledge about causes of diseases, rapid advances in science and technology, and lengthening of life expectancy. As changes occur constantly in the healthcare field, nursing is continuing the process of defining and describing its role. Nursing personnel are the most widely distributed group and they have the most diverse roles, functions, and responsibilities. Nurses provide healthcare to individuals, families, groups, and communities. Their care includes health promotion, disease prevention as well as treatment of common diseases, acute care, and rehabilitation. In hospitals, they could take more leadership roles in assessing patients during planning, implementing, and evaluating care, organizing, and leading the work of others.

Meaning of Role

Role is a set of expected behaviors associated with a person's status or position and includes behavior, rights, and responsibilities. Nurses perform a variety of roles every day. Often, roles overlap which may lead to a conflict in expectations or responsibilities.

Importance of Roles of Nursing in Healthcare Delivery System

- During the last five decades, nursing profession made significant progress toward developing a body of scientific knowledge and establishing the credibility of nursing science.
- Nursing practice changes in response to consumer demands for accessibility and evolvement in decision-making, new technology, changes in healthcare delivery systems, and public policy.

Some Predominant Nursing Roles

Nurses assume a number of roles when they provide care to clients. Contemporary nursing requires that the nurse possess knowledge and skills in a variety of areas. In the past, the principal role of nurse was to provide care and comfort. But changes in nursing have expanded the role to include increased emphasis on health promotion and illness prevention as well as concern for the client as whole.

EXTENDED ROLES OF THE NURSE

A nurse practitioner integrates health maintenance, disease diagnosis, treatment of common episode and chronic problems in primary healthcare with equal emphasis on health, teaching, and disease management.

EXTENDED CARE FACILITIES

- Extended care facilities, formerly called nursing homes, are now often multilevel campuses that include independent living quarters and assisted living facilities for seniors, skilled nursing facilities and extended care facilities that provide all levels of personal care for those who are chronically ill or are unable to take care of themselves without assistance.
- Traditionally, extended care facility provided care for elderly clients of all ages who require rehabilitation or custodial care.
- An extended care facility is an institution providing intermediate and long-term medical, nursing, or custodial care for clients recovering from acute illness or clients with chronic illness or disabilities.
- Nurses in extended care facilities assist clients with their daily activities; provide care when necessary and coordinate rehabilitation activities.

❖ These nurses have increased responsibilities and autonomy, and they are supposed to provide care in a variety of settings such as hospital, community, etc.

Health Promoter

Health promotion is an important aspect of nursing practice. It is a way of thinking that revolves around philosophy of wholeness, wellness, and well-being. Many people are aware of the relationship between lifestyle and illness and are developing health promoting habits. The role of the nurse in health promotion is to work with the people to act as a facilitator for the process of assessing, evaluating, and understanding health.

Caregiver role includes those activities that assist the client physically and psychologically while preserving the client's dignity. Nursing actions may involve full or partial care for the client and supportive educative care to assist client in attaining their highest possible levels of health and wellness. Specific activities of the caregiver include feeding, bathing, and administering medical treatment.

Protector and Client Advocate

As protector, the nurse helps to maintain a safe environment for the client and takes steps to prevent injury and protect the client from possible adverse effects of diagnostic or treatment procedures and takes informed consent.

A client advocate is a person who speaks or acts on behalf of the client. In the role of client advocate, the nurse protects the client's human and legal rights and provide assistance in assessing those rights if need arises. The nurse may also defend client's rights in a general way by speaking out against policies or actions that endanger client's well-being or conflict with their rights.

Counselor

When acting as a counselor, the nurse assists the clients with problem identification and resolution. Counseling is done to help clients increase their coping skills. Effective counseling is holistic in that it addresses individual's emotional, psychological, spiritual, and cognitive dimensions.

Learner and Teacher

Nurses have both learning and teaching responsibilities. They must continue to learn so that they can maintain their knowledge and skills amid the many changes in the healthcare. Teaching is an intrinsic part of nursing. The nurse views each interaction as an opportunity for education. As a teacher, the nurse helps clients learn about their health and the healthcare procedures they need to perform to restore or maintain their health. Nurses also share their expertise with other nurses and health professionals.

Leader and Manager

Today's professional nurses assume leadership and management responsibilities regardless of the activity in which they are involved. A leader influences others to work together to accomplish specific goal. The leader role can be involved in different levels—individual, client, family, groups of clients, colleagues, or the community.

As a manager, the nurse manages the nursing care of individuals, families and communities. The nurse manager also delegates nursing activities to ancillary workers and other nurses, supervises and evaluates their performance.

Research Consumer

Nurses often use research to improve client care in nursing. According to the American Nurses Association, all nurses share commitment to the advancement of nursing science. Nurses in clinical practice identify the problem in need of investigation and collaborate with nurse researcher who designs studies to address the problem and analyze data, and clinician will determine appropriate application of those finding to practice.

Clinical Decision-Maker

To provide effective care, a nurse uses critical thinking skills throughout the nursing process. Before understanding any nursing action, the nurse plans the action by deciding the best approach for the client. The nurse makes these decisions alone or in collaboration with the family and in consultation with other healthcare professionals.

Political Advocate

Nurses are actively participating in political processes to promote change within the profession and to influence the policy-making regarding nursing and healthcare policy issues.

Colleague and Collaborator

Changing models of healthcare have created a need for modification of traditional roles. Collaboration among healthcare professional involves recognition of the expertise of the others within and outside one's profession and referral to those providers when appropriate. Collaboration also involves some shared functions and common focus on the same overall mission.

Telehealth/Telenurse

Nurses engaged in telenursing practice used technologies such as Internet, computers, telephones, digital assessment tools and telemonitoring equipment to deliver nursing care. In India, 10 hospitals are having telemedicine departments.
Example: Narayana Hrudayalaya, Chaitanya Medical Foundation, etc.

Prison Nurse

A nurse who is recruited by the government, semi-government, or private agencies, self-help groups and social service agencies, to serve for prisoners. She is responsible for the health of prisoners and also responsible to give counseling services to prisoners.

Qualification: Basic or Master's in Nursing and trained to carry out the counseling or diploma in social service.

Extended Role and Functions of the Nurse

Caregiver

In this role, nurses assess the clients and analyze collected information to determine clients' needs, develop nursing diagnosis, plan nursing care and carries out the plan, and evaluates the care given. As a caregiver, the nurse provides physical care through skills such as taking vital signs, changing dressings, or administrating medications. The nurse also implements psychological intervention such as encouraging the client to discuss concerns or offering measures to reduce the client's anxiety. Nurses assist each person to achieve the maximum level of wellness possible.

Educator

Client education is a large part of nursing care. The nurse tries to improve health by providing information on health promotion, disease, illness, and specific treatment. As educators, nurses work with individual's clients as well as with family members or other caregivers.

Care Coordinator or Manager

A variety of healthcare team members provide client care. Although the physician is usually considered the head of the healthcare team, the nurse serves an important role in coordinating the efforts of all team members (i.e. nutritionists, physical therapists, etc.) in meeting the client's goals.

Discharge Planner

Discharge planning involves an assessment of the client's health needs before his/her discharge. A large part of this process is assessment of the home or other setting to which the client is discharged for available resource, support systems and equipment, if needed. The nurse then teaches the client how to continue one's self-care after discharge.

Change Agent

The professional nurse serves as a change agent within the work setting and with the profession. The role of change agent involves planning and implementation of a system to change the client's health-related behaviors. In the work, setting the nurse assess health behaviors of the client and family to identify those who need altering. The most important factor in this process is to assess the client's readiness to change. Within the community, nurses serve as role models and assist consumers in bringing out changes to improve the environment and affect health.

Communicator

A nurse documents client care and the client's response. Nurses record information in daily flow sheets or nursing notes. They record medications and treatment. They communicate with other healthcare team members in daily reports and team meetings to maintain continuity of care.

COMMON EXPANDED ROLES OF NURSING

- It prepares graduates for expanded role in provision of primary care to children and adolescents.
- It focuses on clinical and theory application related to promotion of health, growth and development assessment, pathophysiology, pharmacology, and management of chronic and acute conditions.
- It has a family-centered approach.

Expanded Role

Expanded role implies any enlargement of the nurse's role within the boundaries of nurse education, theory and practice, thereby expanding their role around the needs of the patient rather than simply taking on delegated medical tasks.

The nurse who assumes an expanded role has increased responsibilities, and usually greater autonomy nurses are assuming expanded roles in both hospital and community settings. Expanded roles include:

- Nurse specialist
- Nurse practitioner
- Nurse clinician
- Nurse generalist
- Primary nurse.

Nurse Specialist

The nurse specialist has advanced knowledge and skills in a particular area of nursing. An educational prerequisite is Master's degree in nursing. Nurses practice in hospitals or communities. In the hospital, such nurses give direct client care, advise other nurses and coordinate nursing given by others.

The clinical nurse specialist functions as a client care provider, educator, consultant and researcher, manager to plan and improve quality care provider to client and family.

Nurse Practitioner

The role of the nurse practitioner is an extension of the nurse's basic caregiving role; it prepares nurses for an expanded role in the provision of primary care. A pediatric nurse practitioner provides healthcare to infants and children. The nurse practitioner who is also a certified nurse midwife may independently deliver infants. Nurse practitioners in a community may be employed in health centers, schools, and physician's offices. They are usually skilled at making nursing assessments, performing physical assessments counseling, teaching, and treating minor illness. Nurse practitioners in hospitals are often employed in specialty areas.

Qualification

A nurse who has an advanced education is a graduate of nurse practitioner program. The nurse practitioners are employed in healthcare agencies or in community settings and deals with non-emergency acute or chronic illness and provide primary ambulatory care. Nurse practitioners are currently recognized as critical component of healthcare reform.

Job responsibilities include:
- Taking client history
- Conducting physical examination
- Ordering, performing and interpreting diagnostic tests
- Prescribing pharmacologic agents
- Treatment and therapies for management of client's conditions
- Providing primary care
- Consultant for individuals, families and communities

The major nurse practitioner categories are:
- **Adult nurse practitioner**—who provides primary ambulatory care to adults with non-emergency, acute, or chronic illness and some settings in tertiary care.
- **Family nurse practitioner**—who provides primary ambulatory care for families in collaboration with family care physician.
- **Pediatric nurse practitioner**—Qualification: Basic B.Sc (N) and M.Sc (N) and passed in NCLEX—RN.
 This program prepares nurses to assume an expanded role in providing total healthcare to children in offices of private pediatricians and in areas with inadequate health services. Nurses provide care to healthy children, and identify, appraise and manage, acute, and chronic conditions of a sick child. This program has resulted in realignment of function performed by physician and nurses, so that each of them can assume responsibility of patients' needs.
- **Geriatric nurse practitioner**—who provides ambulatory or inpatient care to older adults. Their activities include interventions for health maintenance, illness prevention or health restoration.
- **Acute care nurse practitioner**—An acute care nurse practitioner functions in settings where critically ill patients reside. This type of nurse provides special expertise. The certification includes physiology, advanced assessment, pathophysiology, pharmacology, and advanced therapeutics.
- **Cardiac nurse practitioner:**
  - *Nurse clinician:* The term nurse clinician was first used by Frances Reiter in 1966. The nurse clinician role was an attempt to increase involvement of senior nurses in patient care responsibilities and to create opportunities for advancement in the clinical nursing area.
  - *Nurse generalist:* Nurse generalist is a certification program that issues certificates in 11 areas—general nursing practice, medical surgical nursing gerontology nursing, pediatric nursing, perinatal nursing, college health nursing, school nursing, community health nursing, nursing continuing education and staff development, and home health nursing. The certification designation is registered nurse (RN) certified.
  - *Primary nurse:* Primary nurse is the nurse who plans, implements and evaluates the total care of an individual from admission to discharge.
  - *Critical care nurse: Qualification* of critical care nurses are basic B.Sc degree or diploma in nursing and advanced preparation in critical care nursing. Critical care is progressed from a "do the best you can" approach into a specialty based on a solid body of scientific knowledge and intricate skills. The critical care nurse uses the primary nursing delivery system which allows a certain degree of independence and also serves as a full pledged team member in patient management.
    - These nurses provide care to patient with life-threatening problems, by performing high-intensity therapies and interventions. Critical care nurses monitor patients closely and are skilled in neonatal, adult, pediatric and nursing practice.
    - They are responsible for assuring that acutely ill patients and their families receive optimal care and support.

Functions include:
- Monitoring balloon angioplasty, pacemaker, hemodynamics, intra-aortic balloon pumping, bedside hemodialysis, advance neurological and surgical procedures.
- Teaching physicians primarily interns and residents in teaching hospitals about caring for critically ill patients.
- Help design products and techniques for practice.
- Manages patient total care.
- Performs defibrillation.
- Interprets diagnostic tests.

- *Nursing educator:*
  - Nurse educators are employed in nursing programs at educational institutions and in hospital staff development department of healthcare agencies and client education departments. Nurse educators usually have a baccalaureate degree or more advanced preparation. A faculty member in a school of nursing prepares students function as a nurse and are responsible for teaching current nursing practice theory and necessary skills in laboratories and clinical settings.

Chapter 58: Extended and Expanded Role of the Nurse in Promotive, Preventive, Curative and Restorative...

- Nurse educators in staff development department provide educational programs for nurses within their institution. As nurse educator in client educator department, she/he teaches ill or disabled client and families to provide care in home.
- *Nursing administrator:* The nurse administrator manages client care, including the delivery of nursing service. The functions of nurse administrators include budgeting, staffing and planning programs. The *educational preparation* for nurse administrator is at last a baccalaureate degree in nursing and frequently a Master's or doctoral degree.
- *Nurse researcher:*
  - A nurse tries to solve any public problem in a very scientific and methodological way.
  - Minimum educational qualification is doctorate with at least a Master's degree in nursing. The nurse researcher investigates problems to improve nursing care and to further define and expand the scope of nursing. They may be employed in an academic setting, hospital or independent professional or community service agency.
- *Nurse anesthetist:* A nurse anesthetist is an RN who received advanced training in an accredited program in anesthesiology.

  Functions:
  - Carries out postoperative visit and assessments.
  - Administration of general anesthetic agent for surgery under the supervision of anesthetist.
  - Assessment of postoperative status of the client.
- *Nurse dietician:* Community health nurses not only participate in MCH clinics or family planning services but also give vitality to nutrition and especially of special groups like under five children or a pregnant woman; therefore, she calculates required amounts of calories per day and plans diet for each age group. Health education regarding exclusive breast feeding (EBF), weaning, and supplementary nutrition.

  She should be certified with dietician courses along with the basic or Master's degree in nursing.
- *Nurse entrepreneur:* An entrepreneur is an individual who organizes, operates and assumes the risk of business ventures. Such businesses include independent nursing practice consultant services. The nurse may be involved in education, consultation, research, etc.
- *Nurse author:* Nursing knowledge must be disseminated as widely as possible to nursing practice to keep pace with the health needs of the community. The quality of journals which publish materials concerning nursing issues depends on quality of material submitted. It is a responsibility of nurses to attempt to publish any new knowledge they gain.
- *Nurse informaticist:*
  - Nurse informaticist is defined as a combination of computer science, information science for the management and processing of nursing data, information and knowledge to support the practice of nursing and delivery of nursing care.
  - They are involved in the design, development, implementation, education and evaluation of clinical information system in various healthcare settings. These systems are then used to provide information to nurses and other healthcare professionals to assist in their decision-making capabilities. Because of their nursing knowledge, informatics nurses are essential to the successful design and implementation of healthcare system.
- *Nurse premier answerer:* A nurse who is a dedicated contributor and who spends a bulk of her time in researching and answering questions. Here, the nurse should have Master's degree and she should be an experienced worker in community setting.
- *Nurse statistician:* As a part of expanded role, public health nurse involves herself in collecting data, compile them and submits their nursing statistics to the concerned authorities.

  Nurse statistician should have Master's degree in nursing and she should be capable and experienced to carry out the statistical issues.
- *Nurse philosopher:* Community health nurse formulates the preventive, promotive or curative and also associates with higher authorities to determine the philosophy and objectives of community health program.

  Nurse should be qualified with MSc (N) associated with university. She takes training for framing curriculum.
- *Budget nurse:* The nurse connects between the higher and lower health authoritative members that think logically about the resources and very specifically about finances on whole. He/she prepares budget for the nursing services to be effective.

  Qualification includes basic or Master's degree in nursing with certified course in health economics.

THE ROLES OF NURSE RELATED TO MEDICAL SURGICAL NURSING AREA

Ambulatory Care Nurse

These nurses are RNs who provide preventive care and treat patients with a wide variety of illness and injuries. The day of an ambulatory care nurse is diverse and unpredictable as the work depends on what illness patients present with.

The main duties include:
- Providing healthcare to patients with varying illness or injuries
- Promoting healthcare and health maintenance to patients
- Educating patients on how to manage their injury or illness at home
- Providing healthcare either face-to-face or over the phone or Internet
- Assisting patients preventing and managing illness.

Catheterization Laboratory Nurse

Cardiac catheterization laboratory nurses are RNs working in the field of diagnosis of heart diseases. They administer interventional procedures to patients including cardiac catheterization, angioplasties, and valvuloplasties. They assist doctors in the implantation of pacemakers and implantable cardioverter defibrillator.

Main duties include:
- Providing care to patients in ICU, cardiac care units and Cath lab until they are discharged
- Acquiring and maintaining patient record and updating patient charts
- Organizing patient for medical procedure
- Operatory treatment equipment, administering IV therapy
- Medicating patients according to physician's instructions
- Conducting and participating in cardiac specific research projects
- Educating other healthcare professionals about cardiac catheterization.

Addictions Nursing

Provides care for the patients seeking help with addictions such as alcohol, drugs, tobacco, etc.

Main duties include:
- Promoting recovery
- Providing therapy and counseling to patients
- Educating patients and their families
- Facilitating group therapy session
- Working closely with social workers, doctors, community groups, etc.
- Spending long period of time with individual patients.

Diabetes Management Nurse

These nurses are RNs who assist patient to manage diabetes. These nurses often work in outpatient clinics and often travel to hold clinics in regional areas.

The main duties include:
- Dealing with complications of patient diagnosed with diabetes mellitus
- Working closely with physicians, pharmacists, and other healthcare professionals
- Educating patient of the best practices in improving their health
- Providing advice on diet and exercise
- Advising on injecting medications
- Administering tablets/insulin if the patient is unable
- Monitoring blood glucose level.

These nurses can work at hospitals and outpatient clinics in regional areas.

Emergency Trauma Nurse

These nurses are RNs who work in hospitals or stand-alone emergency department. They provide care to the patients who have suffered serious and sometimes life-threatening physical injuries.

For example, car accidents, work-related injuries, suicidal attempts, etc.

These injuries can potentially result in secondary complications such as respiratory failure, shock and death.

The main duties include:
- Providing care to patients in an emergency situation
- Administering emergency procedures, e.g. cardio-pulmonary resuscitation (CPR)
- Acting fast and decision making abilities
- Handling complex and difficult situation
- Operating healthcare machines.

Emergency trauma nurses provide an initial assessment of patients with potentially life-threatening conditions. They can become transport nurses. They can work at casuality department and emergency rooms of public and private hospitals.

Certified Registered Nurse Anesthetist

It is one of the advance practice nursing specialties. Certified registered nurse anesthetists are highly skilled and educated registered nurses who have qualified to carry out the same anesthesia services as an anesthetist.

The main duties include:
- Working with other healthcare professionals, i.e. anesthetists, dentists, and surgeon
- Providing preoperative, intraoperative, and postoperative care to patients
- Administering anesthesia to patient
- Assisting with pain relief in the delivery of baby
- Monitoring patients postoperatively to ensure recovery from anesthesia.

Geriatric Nurse

Geriatric nurse is a RN who specializes in gerontology. They provide healthcare to geriatric population.

Main duties include:
- Providing healthcare to the residents of long-term care units and nursing homes
- Education and supporting the families of elderly patients

- ❖ Assess the clients' ability to perform assisted daily living
- ❖ Working with patients with dementia and other illness affecting the elderly
- ❖ Diagnosing and managing diseases
- ❖ Promoting good health
- ❖ Operating healthcare machines
- ❖ Administration of first aid services.

Forensic Nurse

Forensic nurses are the RNs who provide care to the victims of violence. They also assist police investigations by collecting evidences and giving consultation services to other medical personnel, law agencies and the courts.

There are many career paths within the forensic nursing. They are:
- ❖ Forensic Clinical Nurse Specialist
- ❖ Forensic Nurse Investigator
- ❖ Forensic Psychiatric Nurse
- ❖ Nurse Coroner
- ❖ Sexual Assault Nurse
- ❖ Legal Nurse Consultant
- ❖ Forensic Gerontology Specialist
- ❖ Correctional Nursing Specialist.

A forensic nurse can work at laboratories, police departments, etc.

Hospice and Palliative Care Nurse

Qualification: Basic or diploma in nursing with certified course on hospice and palliative care. These nurses are RNs and they work in collaboration with other community and healthcare providers.

Example: Social workers, physicians, etc.

Together they work to meet the needs of the patient and family facing terminal illness bereavement and trained to give care to critical and terminal ill patients in homely environment.

The main difference between this and other specialization is that the medications that hospice nurses administer and the symptoms they record are not intended to aid a patient's recovery but to make the remaining days of the patient as comfortable as possible.

Duties include:
- ❖ Observing patients and recording their symptoms
- ❖ Liaison with physicians and social workers
- ❖ Supporting patient/family emotionally
- ❖ Ensuring that the final days of the patient are as comfortable as possible.

Legal Nurse Consultant

These nurses are highly experienced RNs who offer a consulting service to attorneys, insurance companies and other healthcare professionals on medical-related legal cases. This specialization is ideal for a very experienced nurse who is looking for new challenges while using their nursing qualification.

The legal nurse consultant will have expertise in ready medical records and understanding medical terminology.

The main duties include:
- ❖ Working alongside of attorneys and insurance companies to assist with complex medico legal cases
- ❖ Research
- ❖ Examining medical records
- ❖ Reporting on injuries or illness
- ❖ Communicating with expert witness
- ❖ Testifying in court case as medical experts
- ❖ Identifying codes of practice
- ❖ Organizing medical records
- ❖ Educating attorneys/lawyers and other non-medical professionals on medical issues.

Rehabilitation Nurse

They are RNs who work in long-term patient care facilities and hospitals. They care for individuals of all ages who have permanent or temporary disability.
- ❖ Rehabilitation is the process by which individuals return to maximum level of functioning after illness, accidents or other disabling events. Rehabilitative and restorative activities range from teaching client with crutches to helping client cope with lifestyle changes after associated with chronic illness.
- ❖ They can work in inpatient and outpatient settings and also help a patient's family adjust to changes brought about by disability.
- ❖ The most important role of rehabilitation nurse is education. She teaches the client to perform self-assessment, and makes decision about beginning/continuing self-care measures. She performs everyday activities and evaluates his/her progress and recovery.

Occupational Health Nurse

Occupation health nurses are fully qualified RNs who observe working conditions and hazards in a workplace. They work in many industries including manufacturing, mining, construction, and office work.

The main duties include:
- ❖ Recognizing and preventing hazards in the workplace
- ❖ Treating injuries encountered by workers
- ❖ Educating employer and employees on personal protective equipment
- ❖ Documenting illness and injuries
- ❖ Educating employers on the law in relation to occupational health.

Nurse Oncologist

Advance oncology nursing practice is defined as expert competency and leadership in the provisional care to

individuals with an actual or potential diagnosis of cancer.
* These are qualified RNs who provide healthcare for patients with cancer
* They assist the oncologist/radiologist with administration of radiation and chemotherapy
* They will also provide follow-up monitoring and support for patient after treatment
* Educate public on the risks of developing cancer
* Provide assistance to those surviving cancer.

Medical Surgical Nurse

Qualification needed is B.B.Sc (N) and certification in specialization of care of patients admitted with non-surgical and surgical condition.

Role: Care of patient with non-surgical cases such as stroke and surgical cases such as appendectomy.

Dialysis Nurse

Degree in nursing and dialysis nurse training from a recognized institution and she needs to pass licensure exam (NCLEX-RN).

Roles: Provides care for patients with acute or chronic illness related to kidney failure.

This includes:
* Blood product transfusion
* Monitoring vitals
* Monitoring lab values
* Removal of excess fluid
* Effort to normalize or reduce elevated electrolyte levels.

Tuberculosis Nursing

Tuberculosis (TB) nurse was originated in the United States in 1903 to provide home care and instruction to TB patients. By the 1930s, TB nursing has become a part of generalized practice of nurses employed in the health department.

Functions
* Care of patients with advanced disease
* Conducting tuberculin skin testing
* Health education about preventive action.

HIV/AIDS Nurse

HIV/AIDS nurses are registered nurses with specialist education in HIV/AIDS. They educate individuals on preventing the spread of HIV, and also help those who are infected cope with the physical, social, and psychological aspects of their diseases.

They also provide education and support to the families and friends of individuals infected with the disease. HIV/AIDS nurses need to have strong interpersonal skills and an ability to cope with death.

Intellectual and Developmental Disability Nurses

Intellectual and developmental disability nurses, also known as special needs nurses, are registered nurses who provide care for the patients suffering from a number of intellectual and developmental disabilities, that is, mental retardation, pervasive mental disorders, autism spectrum disorder, Rett's syndrome, etc. These nurses work in many settings from hospitals to home help providing unique healthcare and social need assistance to their patients.

Operating Room Nurse/Circulating Room Nurse

Qualification: The nurse should have a B.Sc (N) + CPR certificate + course in operating room nursing care.

Role: These nurses provide care for the patient immediately before and during a surgical procedure.

She monitors patients' vital signs, warmth and safe positioning, prepares operating room with supplies, equipment and instrument, and answers as the communication liaison to family, other departments and members of the operating team.

When patients are admitted before or after surgery, the operating room nurse monitors patients' progress from the time he/she enters the operating room until he/she is dismissed to the attending staff nurse. She also performs preoperative assessment, prepares the patient for surgery, setup for surgery, assists the surgeon during the surgery and manages patient recovery.

Orthopedic Nurse

Qualification: The nurse should have basic B.Sc (N) and an additional orthopedic nurse certification.

Role: Manages the care of patients before and after surgery involving musculoskeletal system.

Monitors, fraction, splint, or cast care and other orthopedic equipment.

Cardiac Care Nurse

These nurses choose a variety of specializations including:
* Cardiac Catheterization Nurse
* Cardiac Rehab Nurse
* Vascular Nurse
* Telemetry Nurse
* Cardiac Nurse Practitioner
* Cardiac Clinical Nurse Specialist.

Role: These nurses work in taking care of patients and handle instruments in their specialized area.

Recovery Room Nurse/PACU (Post-Anesthesia Care Unit Nurse)

A recovery room nurse must have an RN license with at least two or more years of nursing experience with an associate degree (AD)/associate degree registered nurse (ADRN).

Role: She provides care for the patient immediately following an anesthesia-induced surgical procedure. This stage is a critical stage and needs quick response.

Transplant Nurse

They are RNs who provide preoperative, intraoperative and postoperative care to patients receiving organs by means of transplant surgery.

They are also responsible for providing healthcare to living donors.

Wound, Ostomy, Continence Nurse

They treat patients with wounds caused by injuries, ulcers, diseases, etc. They provide support and postoperative care for the patients who need alternative methods of bodily waste elimination. They are also responsible for treating patients with urinary and fecal incontinence.

Perioperative Nurse

These nurses are RNs who assist surgeons during surgery. They can work as a scrub nurse who passes instruments to the surgeon or as circulating nurse who take care of overall nursing care during surgery. Perioperative nurses can choose to specialize in certain fields of medicine such as cardiac care or plastic and reconstructive surgery.

They work closely with surgical team consisting of circulating/scrub nurse, anesthetists, surgical assistant and other assistive personnel.

Perioperative nurses are also responsible for providing preoperative and postoperative care to the patient.

EXPANDED ROLES OF NURSE IN CHILD HEALTH NURSING AREA

Advanced Neonatal Nurse Practitioner

This program was introduced in the United Kingdom in 1992 in the context of extending roles in a range of specialties. She should be skilled in interpersonal communication and technical expertise.

Qualification: Basic B.Sc (N)/M.Sc (N)/certificate in neonatal nursing/four years' experience.

Pediatric Oncology Care

The evolution of pediatric nurse practitioner in oncology specialization in care of cancer survivors is described in certain aspects of role solidified. The early concept of role includes three interdependent functions:
- Clinician/care given
- Education
- Research.

Pediatric Critical Care Nurse

She should be an expert in caring critically ill patients, emergency care, expert in CPR, assisting in emergency procedures.

Qualification: B.Sc (N)/Diploma (N)/associate diploma nurse should have a license of NCLEX and RN certification in certified critical care registered nurse.
- **Clinical nurse leader:** Policy development of children
- **Nurse advocate:** Preservation of universal right of children, child laws, including the child in planning care

  Qualification: B.Sc (N)/M.Sc (N).

Clinical Nurse Leader

Role: Participates in policy development for children.

Recovery Room Nurse/PACU Nursing

Provides care for patients following surgery or anesthesia.

Qualification: B.Sc (N)/M.Sc (N) + License for ADRN.

Child Psychiatric Nurse

Role: Care of child with mental retardation, behavioral and learning disorders.

Rehabilitation Nurse

Role: Care of child with mental disorders and permanent disabilities.

Neonatal Nurse Clinician

Acts as a consultant for care of neonatal-related disease conditions.

Clinical Nurse Specialist Hemophilia

Care of child with hematological disorder and hemophilia.

EXPANDED ROLES IN COMMUNITY HEALTH NURSING

Community Health Nurse

Community health nurse functions within the communal framework. She serves the health needs of the portion of public assigned to her and delivers care to the community as a whole. The goal of the community health nurse is to improve community health by identifying people who are at risk for illness, disability or death. The community health nurse maintains records of patient's progress and healthcare needs and makes assessments, provide health education and provide referral if necessary.

Home Healthcare Nurse

It describes a system in which healthcare and social services are provided to disabled people in their homes rather than medical facilities. Home health is the largest employer of nurses within community-based nursing roles.

Occupational Health Nurse

It is a branch of public health nursing. Occupational health nurses work in traditional manufacturing, industry service, construction sites and government settings. In this space, the nurse provides for and delivers health and safety programs and service to workers, worker dependents and community group.

The nurse should have industrial nursing training certificate along with the Basic or Master's degree in Nursing.

Functions:
- Worker/workplace assessment and surveillance
- Primary care
- Case management
- Counseling
- Health promotion and protection
- Research
- Administration and management
- Community orientation
- Legal and ethical monitoring.

School Health Nurse

Here, nurse specializes the well-being of student to achieve academic success. The nurse accesses a consultant, direct care given in a school. The goal is to support the educational process by helping students keep healthy and by teaching students and teacher's preventive practices.

Regular monitoring of height and weight growth and developmental delays, care of child with accidents, immunization, conducting school health program, care of under-fives.

A school nurse is responsible for providing healthcare to a child or young person attending a school/college.

Some large schools will have school nurse working full time.

Main duties include:
- Develop healthcare plan for the school
- Training school-based staff in first aid, dealing with epilepsy and asthma
- Educating teachers and students on different health issues
- Educating parents on the importance of nutrition and exercise
- Testing hearing, eyesight and monitoring the height and weight of the child
- **Disaster nurse:** Nurse whose service is based on disaster management which extends from emergency management till rehabilitation of affected people. She takes part completely in all aspects of disaster management.
- **Qualification:** Basic or diploma in nursing with certified course on disaster management.
- **Flight nurse:** Nurse with experience and degree qualification and license to practice care in the flight during emergency and as a routine.

EXPANDED ROLES IN PSYCHIATRIC NURSING

Registered Psychiatric Nurse

She provides psychiatric mental health nursing care to individual, families and groups to enable them to function at an optimal level of psychological wellness through more effective, adoptive behaviors and increased reliance to stress. She must be able to provide safe, basic care, have a wide understanding of psychological and developmental problem and their treatment, and have a highly developed level of communication skills.

She works with children, adolescents, adults and elderly with dysfunctional behavior patterns and developmental handicaps.

A register psychiatric nurse works in an independent entity. She works in various kinds of inpatients facilities and community settings.

Nurse Psychotherapist

She can take up psychotherapy role as an individual therapy, group therapy and counseling. She should have a certificate course in therapies in addition to Basic or MSc in psychiatric nursing training.

Psychiatric Nurse Educator

The main function is planning and changing curriculum according to the needs of the society and learner. The Indian Nursing Council include psychiatric nursing as compulsory for qualifying BSc from 1965 and even in Diploma Nursing from 1986.

Psychosocial Rehabilitation Nurse

It is concerned with helping the people with chronic mental illness to lead independent and satisfactory lives in the community.

Child Psychiatric Nurse

She identifies emotional and behavioral problem in the children and provides comprehensive care.

Deaddiction Nurse

These units identify psycho social problems and maintain the factors in addicts. She also provides the various therapies to the addicts and their family members.

Neuro Psychiatric Nursing

Psychiatric nursing is extended to patients who are suffering from neuropsychiatric disorders such has dementia, epilepsy, brain tumor, head injury with behavioral problems, HIV infection with behavioral problems, etc.

Gerontological and Geriatric Nursing

Gerontological nursing provides emotional support to those people who have retired from services, who have no financial sources and helps them in understanding these situations and in developing new coping mechanism.

Geriatric nursing is expanding these psychiatric nursing practices to aged people who have been affected by emotional and behavioral disorders such as dementia, chronic schizophrenia, delirium, etc.

Community Psychiatric Health Nurse

It is the application of nursing in preventing mental illness, promoting and maintaining mental health of the people. It includes early diagnosis appropriate therapy referrals, care and rehabilitation of mentally ill people.

Forensic Psychiatric Nurse (Legal)

Qualification: Diploma in forensic psychiatric nursing.

Responsibilities

- First aid
- Screening
- Follow-up
- Control of communicable diseases
- Immunization
- Teaching health classes
- Transmitting knowledge that supports healthful behaviors
- Conducting health-related studies
- Responding to calls from other schools
- Referral

Psychiatric Consultation Liaison Nurse

Psychiatric consultation liaison nurse has arisen in response to the increased recognition of the importance of psycho-physiological interpersonal relationships and their impact on physical illness, recovery, and wellness.

Nurse Psycho-pharmacologist

One of the latest roles is that of the nurse psycho-pharmacologist, the psychiatric clinical nurse specialist with prescriptive authority.

CONCLUSION

Hence, to conclude, nurses' roles are not limited to the hospital alone but they have both extended and expanded roles in practice. These roles are independently practiced in the United States of America and some of the other developed countries. However, in India, due to lack of autonomy, some roles have not come into practice, but in future, there is hope for the existence of roles due to development in nursing education and practice.

59 CHAPTER
Health Promotion and Primary Healthcare

CHAPTER OUTLINE

- Health Promotion Model
- Promotion of Health through Pender Model in Nursing Practice
- Nurses' Role in Health Promotion
- Primary Healthcare
- Concept of Health for All
- Indian Health System Infrastructure for Primary Healthcare Institutions and Tiers of Delivery

INTRODUCTION

The concepts of health promotion, wellness, and illness in practice overlap to some extent. Health promotion is an emerging field with proactive attempts to prevent illness or disease. Nola J. Pender has introduced a model for health promotion in 1982. Nurses in all areas of practice often have an opportunity to assist clients. Primary prevention may be accomplished by measures designed to promote general health and well-being, and quality of life of people or by specific protective measures. Pender has also highlighted that nurses need to understand the variables influencing clients' health beliefs and practices. Internal and external variables can influence thoughts and actions. Understanding the effects of these variables allows the nurse to plan and deliver individualized care (Pender, 1990; Palank, 1991).

HEALTH PROMOTION MODEL

Pender's (1982, 1984) health promotion model (HPM) was introduced as a complementary counterpart to models of health protection. Health promotion seeks to increase a client's level of well-being (Pender, 1987). The model focuses on the client's cognitive-perceptual factors, modifying factors and participating in health promoting behaviors. It identifies factors that enhance or decrease health promotion activities. It also organizes cues into a pattern to explain the likelihood of a client's development of health promotion behaviors (Pender, 1990). The model has been tested with many populations and is a reliable indicator of health promotion (Fig. 59.1).

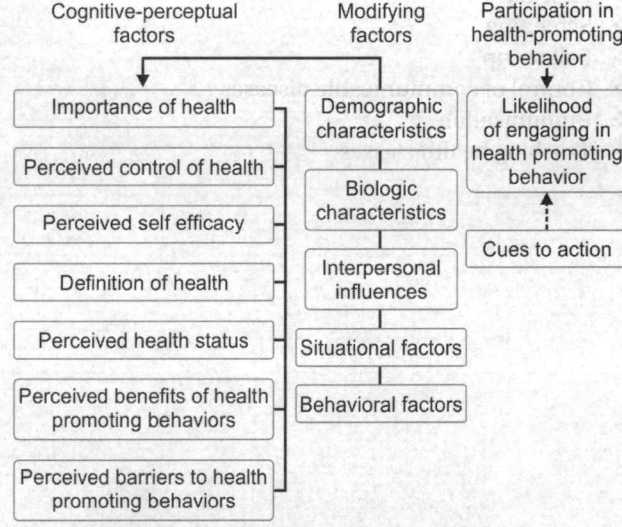

Fig. 59.1: Health promotion model (Pender NJ).

Source: Used with Permission from Pender NJ, khojier text book and stanhope text also. Health Promotion in Nursing Practice. New York: Appleton-Lange. 1987. p. 58.

Credentials and Background of the Theorist (Fig. 59.2)

- Noja J Pender was born in Lansing Michigan in 1941.
- She received her Diploma in Nursing in 1962 from Michigan Hospital.
- In 1964, Pender completed her BSN at Michigan State University in East Lasting.
- In 1965, she earned her MA in human growth and development from Michigan State University.

Chapter 59: Health Promotion and Primary Healthcare

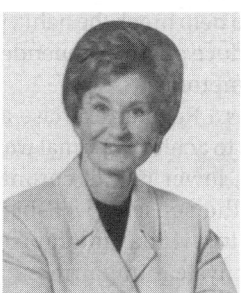

Fig. 59.2: Noja J Pender.

- In 1969, she completed her PhD in Psychology.
- In 1975, Dr Pender published a conceptual model to preventive behavior.
- In 1982, she published a text health promotion in nursing practice.

Nola Pender has provided important leadership in development of nursing research in the United States.

- She promoted scholarly activity in nursing through her involvement with sigma theta tau.
- In 1990, she became the Director for the Center for Nursing Research at the University of Michigan School of Nursing and published numerous articles; she is an expert speaker and consultant on some topics.

The model focuses on the following three areas:
- Cognitive perceptual factors (individual perceptions)
- Modifying factors (demographic and social)
- Participation in health promoting behavior (likelihood of action).

Major Concepts and Definitions

- ***Cognitive perceptual factors (individual perceptions):*** This includes the activities related to health promotion:
  - *Importance of health:* Individuals who value health highly are more likely to seek it.
  - *Perceived control of health:* The individual's perceptions of his/her own ability to change his/her health can motivate his/her desire for health.
  - *Perceived self-efficacy:* The individual's strong belief that a behavior is possible can influence the occurrence of that behavior.
  - *Definition of health:* The individual's definition of health means ranging from absence of disease to high level well-being can influence behavior changes.
  - *Perceived health status:* The current state of feeling well or ill can determine the likelihood of health promoting behavior will be initiated.
  - *Perceived benefits of behaviors:* The individuals may be more interested to begin or continue health promoting behaviors considered high positive outcomes that will occur from health behavior.
  - *Perceived barriers:* The individual's belief that an activity or behavior is difficult or unavailable may influence his/her intention to engage in it.
- ***Modifying factors (demographic and social):*** Modifying factors such as age, gender, education, income, family patterns of healthcare behaviors and the expectations of significant others, family patterns of healthcare and interactions with health professionals. These modifying factors are seen having indirect influence on behavior, with the cognitive perceptual factors bearing directly on behaviors.
- ***Participation in health promoting behavior (likelihood of action):*** Participation in health promoting behavior in the HPM signifies variables affecting the likelihood of action depending on internal and external cues such as whatever to feel good, mass media, health messages, e.g. that regular exercise helps to prevent heart disease or conversation with others.

Assumptions of the HPM

- Individuals seek to actively regulate their own behavior.
- Individuals in all their biopsychosocial complexity interact with the environment, progressively transforming the environment and being transformed overtime.
- Health professionals constitute a part of the interpersonal environment, which exerts influence on persons throughout their lifespan.
- Self-initiated reconfiguration of person–environment interactive patterns is essential to behavior change.

Acceptance by the Nursing Community

- The concept of health promotion is a popular one in practice.
- This model has been tested with a variety of population, because it is a reliable indicator of health promotion.
- The use of the HPM has not been established in nursing education.
- The HPM is primarily a tool for research.

PROMOTION OF HEALTH THROUGH PENDER MODEL IN NURSING PRACTICE

Definition of Health Promotion

Health promotion is defined as an action taken to develop a high level of wellness and is accomplished by influencing individual behavior and the environment in which people live. Health promotion is the process of enabling people to increase control over and to improve health.

Selected Areas of Health Promotion/Interventions

Counsel patients on the topics of proper nutrition, smoking cessation, exercise, relaxation and sexual health to promote health:
- Health education
- Environmental modifications
- Nutritional interventions
- Lifestyle and behavioral changes

Health Education

Health education is one of the most cost-effective interventions. A large number of diseases could be prevented with little or no medical intervention if people were adequately informed about them and if they were encouraged to take necessary precautions in time. The WHO's constitution states that "the extension to all people of the benefits of medical, psychological and related knowledge is essential to the fullest attainment of health."

Environmental Modification

A comprehensive approach to health promotion requires environmental modifications such as provision of safe water, installation of sanitary latrines, control of insects and rodents, improvement of housing, etc.

Nutritional Interventions

Nutritional interventions comprise food distribution and nutrition improvement of vulnerable groups, child feeding programs, food fortification, nutrition, education, etc.

It is projected that 35% of all cancer could be prevented with an improved diet recommended by National Cancer Institute. A low-fat, high-fiber diet is recommended. Fat should not account for more than 30% of calories. More servings of fruits and vegetables should be included daily. If weight loss is desired, have the patient weigh in monthly and review the diet, weight reduction program in obesity, etc.

Lifestyle and Behavioral Changes

The action of prevention is one of the individual and community responsibilities for health, the physician and each health worker acting as an educator than a therapist. Health education is a basic element of all health activities. It is important in understanding risk factors, behavior, risk factor modification and behavior modification changing the views, behavior and habits of people.

- ❖ *Smoking prevention/cessation:* Smoking is a risk factor for hypertension, heart disease, peripheral vascular disease and cancer of lungs, colon, larynx, oral cavity, etc. Not smoking promotes health by increasing exercise tolerance, enhancing taste bud function and bad breath. Smoking cessation can be accomplished through an individualized multidimensional program including information on the short- and long-term health effects of smoking, practical behavior modification to help break the habit, use of medications designed to reduce physical dependence and minimize withdrawal symptoms.
- ❖ *Exercise/fitness:* Regular exercise as part of a fitness program helps to achieve optimal weight, control blood pressure (BP), lower risk of coronary artery disease and improve the sense of well-being. Plan exercise according to individual tolerance, time allotment, interest and physical impairment. Suggest walking, jogging, bicycling, swimming, water aerobics, etc. Exercise program should include 5–10 minutes warm-up and cool down periods with stretching activity to prevent injuries. Advice patient to stop if pain or shortness of breath, dizziness, palpitation or exercise sweating is experienced.
- ❖ *Relaxation/stress management:* Stress is a change of environment that is perceived as a threat, challenge, or harm to the person's dynamic equilibrium. A limited amount of stress can be a time motivator to take action. Excessive or prolonged stress can cause emotional discomfort, anxiety and illness. In times of stress, sympathetic nervous system is activated and leads to high BP, arteriole sclerosis, cardiovascular disease, acute asthma attack, peptic ulcer, migraine headache and other illness. Identify patients' physiological and psychological stress.

Relaxation therapy is advised:
- ❖ *Relaxation breathing:* Breath slowly and deeply until relaxation therapy is achieved.
- ❖ Progressive muscle relaxation.
- ❖ *Autogenic training:* It can help relieve pain and induce sleep.
- ❖ *Imagery:* Uses imagination and concentration to take a mental vacation.
- ❖ *Distraction:* Uses the patient's own interest and activities to divert attention from pain or anxiety and include listening to music, watching TV.
- ❖ *Assist the patient with relaxation therapy:* Encourage the patient to combine techniques such as relaxation, breathing before and after imaginary or progressive muscle relaxation along with autogenic training to achieve better results.

Sexual health:
- ❖ Education about sexual activity should begin during school age, heighten during adolescence and continue through adulthood.
- ❖ Teach about normal reproduction, unwanted pregnancy, contraception, sexually transmitted diseases, mode of transmission, prevalence, signs and symptoms, and method of prevention.

Specific Protection

Health protection is defined as the provision of conditions for normal mental and physical functioning of human being individually and in group. It includes promotion of health, prevention of sickness and curative and restorative medicine in all its aspects.

Primary prevention is a holistic approach. It relies on measures designed to promote health or to protect against specific disease agents and hazards in the environment. Primary prevention has become increasingly identified with "health education" and the concept of individual and community responsibility for health. The following are some of the currently available interventions aimed at specific protection:
- Immunization
- Use of specific nutrients
- Chemoprophylaxis
- Protection against occupational hazards
- Protection against accidents
- Protection carcinogens
- Avoidance of allergens
- The control of specific hazards in the general environment, e.g. air pollution and noise control
- Control of consumer product quality and safety of foods, drugs, cosmetics, etc.

Information, education and communication activity: Provide educational programs, literature and posters of the food pyramid in schools, work sites, food stores and other public places to promote awareness. Encourage restaurants to offer healthy menu items.

NURSES' ROLE IN HEALTH PROMOTION

Nurses have played key roles in prevention in areas such as prenatal care, immunization, occupational health and safety, cardiac rehabilitation and education and public healthcare finding and early intervention:
- Meet health promotion needs of the patient whether practice is in the hospital, clinic, patient home's health maintenance organization, etc.
- Health promotion is primarily accomplished through patient education.
- Health promotion should occur through the life cycle with topics focused for infancy, childhood, adolescence, adulthood and old age.
- *For infancy:* Teach parents about the importance of prenatal care, basic care of infant's breastfeeding, nutrition, and infant safety.
- *For childhood:* Teach about immunization, proper nutrition, and safety practices.
- *For adolescence:* Motor vehicle safety, avoidance of drugs, alcohol and tobacco use, sexual decision-making, contraception and prevention of suicide.
- *For adulthood:* Teach about nutrition, exercise, and stress management to help them feel better. Also teach cancer-screening techniques such as breast and testicular self-examination and risk factor reduction for leading causes of death, heart disease, stroke and cancer.
- *For older age:* Stress on nutrition and exercise to help them live longer and stay fit.

PRIMARY HEALTHCARE

Introduction

Health has been declared as a fundamental human right. Millions of people in the world today, particularly in the developing countries, have a poor state of health. More than half of the population in the world does not have the benefit of proper healthcare. National governments all over the world are striving to expand and improve their healthcare services. The present criticism against healthcare services is that they are predominantly urban oriented, mostly curative in nature and accessible mainly to a small proportion of the population. Tile present concern is not only to reach the whole population with adequate healthcare services but also to secure an acceptable level of health for all through the application of primary healthcare programs.

CONCEPT OF HEALTH FOR ALL

The disparities in health and socioeconomic conditions between rich and poor within countries and between countries and the concern of members of WHO regarding the health and deterioration of existing health services lead to new thinking in provision of healthcare in order to narrow this gap and finally eliminate it.

So, there was felt a need among health planners administrators for evolving in healthcare approach that would answer the problems and needs of underprivileged. Thus, the 30th World Assembly resolved in May 1977 that the main social target of governments and WHO in the coming decades should be the attainment of Health For All (HFA) in the year 2000 AD. The fundamental principle of HFA strategy is equity, i.e., an equal health status for people and countries ensured by an equitable distribution of health resources. Further, there are several other experiences and developments, which led to the evolution of goal of HFA by the year 2000.

Meaning of Health for All

Health for all means that health is brought within reach of everyone in a given country. It does not mean that in the year 2000, doctors and nurses will provide medical cure for everybody in the world for all their existing ailments, nor does it mean that in the year 2000 AD, nobody will be sick or disabled. It does mean that:
- Health begins at home, in school and in factories.
- People will use better approaches for preventing diseases and alleviating unavoidable illness and disability.
- There will be an even distribution among the population of whatever health resources are available.

- Essential healthcare will be accessible to all individuals and families in an acceptable and affordable way and with their full involvement.
- The international goal of "Health For All" by the year 2000 was mooted in the World Health Assembly in 1977, and was later adopted by WHO in 1981.

Definition of Health for All

Health for all has been defined as the attainment of a level of health that will enable every individual to lead a socially and economically productive life.

National Strategy for Health for All 2000

As a signatory to the Alma Ata Declaration in 1978, the Government of India is committed to taking steps to provide health for all to its citizens. In 1983, the Government of India evolved a national health policy, which has laid down the goals mentioned in Table 59.1.

The 21st Century

Health for all in the 21st century is a continuation of the HFA process. It aims to realize the vision of health for all launched at Alma Ata conference in 1978. It sets out goals to achieve for the first two decades of the 21st century.

Goals of HFA in the 21st Century

- An increase in life expectancy and quality of life
- Improved quality in health between and within countries
- Access for all to sustained health systems and services.

Targets

Ten global targets are identified to guide the implementation of HFA policy in the 21st century. These can be broadly classified into three groups:
- **Health outcomes:**
  - Percentage of children under five years, who are stunted, should be less than 20% in all countries and in specific subgroups within countries by the year 2020 AD
  - Maternal mortality ratio less than 100/1 lakh births by the year 2020
  - Infant mortality ratio less than 45 per 1,000 live births by the year 2020
  - Life expectancy at birth over 70 years by the year 2020
  - Eradication of measles by 2020
  - Elimination of leprosy, neonatal tetanus by 2010 and trachoma by 2020
  - Elimination of vitamin A and iodine deficiency before 2020.
- ***Intersectoral action for the determinants of health:***
The provision of safe drinking water, adequate sanitation, food, and shelter in sufficient quantity and quality by 2020.
- **Health policies and systems:**
  - Promoting health enhancing lifestyles
  - Develop implement and monitor HFA policies
  - All people will have access throughout their lives to high quality, comprehensive, essential healthcare by 2010
  - Enhance health information and surveillance system
  - Support research for health by 2010.

All policy lays stress on the preventive, promotive, community health and rehabilitation aspects of healthcare and points to the need or establishing comprehensive primary healthcare services to reach the population in the remotest areas of the country. The health strategies include restructuring the health infrastructure, developing manpower and research development. With increasing recognition of failure of existing health services to provide healthcare, alternative ideas and methods to provide healthcare have been considered and tried. Discussing these issues at the joint WHO–UNICEF International Conference in 1975 in Alma Ata, the governments of 134 countries and many voluntary agencies called for a revolutionary approach to healthcare. Declaring that the existing groups inequality in the health status of people particularly between developed and developing countries as well as within countries is politically, socially, and economically unacceptable. This conference called for acceptance of the WHO goal of health for all by 2000 AD and proclaimed primary healthcare as the key approach for achieving "Health For All."

Development of Primary Healthcare Concept

The concept of primary healthcare was born in India as it may be recalled during the post-independent era when:
- In 1946, the Bhore Committee brought its recommendations of integrating preventive health activities along with curative services in offering healthcare to people in rural areas through the network of primary health centers (PHCs) and creation of public health nurses.

Table 59.1: Indicators for health for all (HFA) and achievement.

Parameter	Target for 2000	Existing level
Infant mortality rate	Below 60	64
Life expectancy at birth		
Male	64 years	64.8
Female	64 years	63
Crude birth rate	21	25
Crude death rate	9	8.9
Net reproduction rate	1.00	1.4
Potable water supply	100.1	76.6%

Chapter 59: Health Promotion and Primary Healthcare

- In 1962, Mudaliar Committee recommended greater use of anxiety personnel for carrying out routine duties rather than by highly trained doctors. Manpower development by training of professional and auxiliary nurses at different levels of service.
- In 1973, Kartar Singh Committee recommended multipurpose health workers scheme integrated approach towards delivery of health services by introducing health worker scheme and utilization of services of supervision and increase in the auxiliary nursing personnel.
- In 1974, Shrivastav Committee recommended creation of bands of paraprofessional and semiprofessional health workers from within community itself, e.g., school teachers, postmasters and gram sevaks to provide simple promotive, preventive, and curative health services needed by the community.
- *Fifth Five Year Plan (1977):* Establishment of one PHC for each community development block and one subcenter for 10,000 population, provision of drugs upgradation of one PHC in every four PHCs to 30-bedded hospital known as community health center. In modern period, the primary healthcare movement started officially in 1977. The concept of primary healthcare was adopted by the member countries of WHO as the key for achieving the goal to health for all by 2000 AD. Primary healthcare is a new approach to healthcare, which integrates at the community level all the factors required for improving the health status of the population (Fig. 59.3):
  - Conceptualization of basic health services accessibility and availability of health services in rural population
  - International conference on primary healthcare Alma Ata declaration
  - Concept of primary healthcare
  - Re-examination and evaluation of health services correlating health with economic development
  - Shift of emphasis on preventive approach from curative approach. Urban to rural privileged to underprivileged and unipurpose to multipurpose workers.

Alma Ata Conference (1978) defined primary healthcare as follows:

Essential healthcare based on practical, scientifically sound and socially acceptable methods and technology made universally accessible to individuals and families in the community through their full participation and at a cost that the community and country can afford to maintain at every stage of their development in the spirit of self-reliance and self-determination.

Characteristics of Primary Healthcare

- It is an essential healthcare, which is based on practical, scientifically sound and socially acceptable methods and technology.
- It should be rendered universally, acceptable to individuals, and the families in the community through their full participation.
- Its availability should be at a cost, which the community and country can afford to maintain at every stage of their development in a spirit of self-reliance and self-determination.
- It requires joint efforts of the health sector and other health-related factors, namely education, food and agriculture, social welfare, animal husbandry, housing, rural reconstruction, etc.

Elements of Primary Healthcare

According to Alma Ata Declaration, primary healthcare includes at least eight elements which are to be implemented in an integrated manner. They are:
- Education about prevailing health problems and methods of preventing and controlling them
- Promotion of food supply and proper nutrition
- An adequate supply of safe water and basic sanitation
- Maternal and child health (MCH) care including family planning
- Immunization against major infectious diseases
- Prevention and control of locally endemic diseases
- Appropriate treatment of common diseases and injuries
- Provision of essential drugs.

Principles of Primary Healthcare

The primary healthcare approach is based on principles of social equity, nationwide coverage, and self-reliance; intersectoral coordination and people's involvement in planning and implementation of health programs in pursuit of common health goals. This approach has been described as "Health by the People" and "Placing people's health in People's hands."

The main principles of primary healthcare are:
- Equitable distribution
- Community participation
- Intersectoral coordination

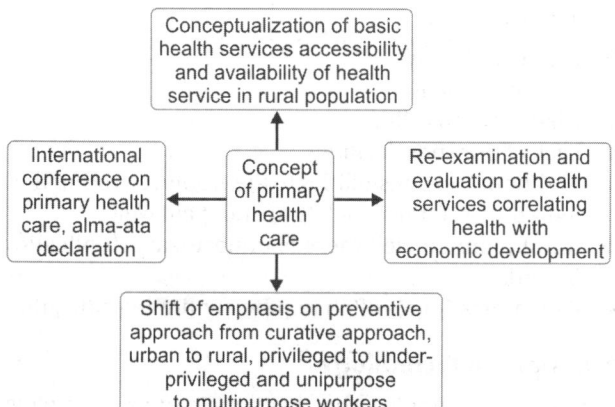

Fig. 59.3: Concept of primary healthcare.

- Appropriate technology
- Focus on prevention.

Equitable Distribution

The first key principle in primary healthcare strategy is equity or equitable distribution of health services, i.e., health services must be shared equally by all people irrespective of their ability to pay and all (rich or poor, urban or rural) must have access to health services. At present, health services are mainly concentrated in the major towns and cities resulting in inequality of care to the people in rural areas. The worst hit is the needy and vulnerable groups of the population in rural areas and urban slums. This has been termed as social injustice. The failure to reach the majority of the people is usually due to inaccessibility. Primary healthcare aims to redress this imbalance by shifting the center of gravity of the healthcare system from cities (where three-quarters of the health budget is spent) to the rural areas (where three-quarters of the people live) and bring these services as near people's homes as possible.

Community Participation

Community participation is the process by which individuals, families and communities assume responsibility in promoting their own health and welfare. There must be a continuing effort to secure meaningful involvement of the community in the planning, implementation and maintenance of health services, besides maximum reliance on local resources such as manpower, money and materials. One approach that has been successfully tried in India is the use of village health guides (VHGs) and trained dais. They are selected by the local community and trained locally in the delivery of primary healthcare to the community they belong, free of charge.

Advantages

- Community participation is a cost-effective method.
- People begin to view health more objectively. Then they are more likely to accept preventive approaches in healthcare.
- Health awareness becomes an integral part of the village life and activities.
- Health worker gets greater support of people.
- People become more self-reliant in their ability to prevent diseases, promote positive health.
- Health services become more relevant to the health needs of the community.
- Health planning is done at the most peripheral and gross root level. WHO sponsored meeting on community participation in health held at Brioni (Yugoslavia) in 1985, discussed about two broad approaches of community involvement:
  - Ensuring easy access to information and knowledge about health service programs and projects
  - Creating awareness and understanding regarding the causes of poor health.

This approach helps involvement of community in:
- Solving their health needs
- Assessing their health needs
- Taking responsibility for mobilizing local resources
- Suggesting new approaches and solutions to their problems.

Drawbacks

- Lack of political commitment
- Lack of support to the community in managing health projects
- **Inadequate inputs:** People are not satisfied with improper allocation of resources
- Health is neither a commodity nor a service, but a process of living, participating and being
- Attitude of community is apathy
- People who are involved are politically and socially weak and continued to be neglected
- Community is not one entity. It is difficult to organize it
- **Rigid professional:** Behavior of healthcare providers
- Wrong assumption by health staff that community does not know what is good for them
- Decision in health services is generally taken by the professional staff and not by the community.

Intersectoral Coordination

There is an increasing realization of the fact that the components of primary healthcare cannot be provided by the health sector alone. The declaration of Alma Ata states that primary healthcare involves in addition to the health sector, all related sectors and aspects of national and community development in particular agriculture, animal husbandry, food industry, education, housing, public works, communication and other sectors. To achieve such cooperation, countries may have to review their administrative system, reallocate their resources and introduce suitable legislation to ensure that coordination can take place.

Drawbacks

- Lack of publicity
- Unemployment
- Hike in commodities
- Lack of transport facilities
- Additional responsibilities to the employees other than their duties, for which they are not paid well
- If not planned well there is unnecessary duplication of work
- Para professionals often require continuing education.

Appropriate Technology

Appropriate technology has been defined as technology that is scientifically sound, adaptable to local needs and acceptable to those who apply it and those for whom it is used, and that can be maintained by the people themselves in keeping with the principle of self-reliance with the resources the community and country can afford.

The term appropriate is emphasized because in some countries large, luxurious hospitals that are totally inappropriate to the local needs are built, which absorb a major part of the national health budget, effectively blocking any improvement in general health services. This also applies for using costly equipment, procedures and techniques when cheaper, scientifically valid, and acceptable ones are available, namely oral rehydration fluid.

Drawbacks

- There is a wide gap between what we are saying and what we are doing
- Expensive hospitals, which are inappropriate to local needs are being built.

Focus on Prevention

The emphasis is on prevention. It runs through all the elements of primary healthcare.

Role of Nurses in Primary Healthcare

In 1981, an informal meeting was convened by WHO to consider the role of nursing in contributing to the achievement of the goal of HFA/2000 through primary healthcare. The following five basic strategies have been proposed by the WHO–ICN meeting by nurses (Table 59.2 and Fig. 59.4).

WHO Expert Committee in 1984 defined the role of nurses in primary healthcare as follows:

- Assessing the health status of individuals and communities
- Mobilizing community involvement
- Providing integrated healthcare including the treatment of emergencies and making referrals
- Maintaining epidemiological surveillance
- Training and supervising health workers
- Collaborating with other development sectors
- Monitoring progress in primary healthcare.

With regard to the role of nurses and primary healthcare, WHO study group (1985) identified four main self-explanatory roles of the nurses as given below:

- ***Nurse as a direct care provider:*** Since a nurse has been trained in such a way to provide care to all individuals, he/she can provide direct care to individual, who seeks medical help. For example, control communicable disease, MCH care, family planning activities, etc.
- ***Nurse as a teacher and educator:*** Community health nurse can play an important role in educating the people on prevailing health problems. She will play

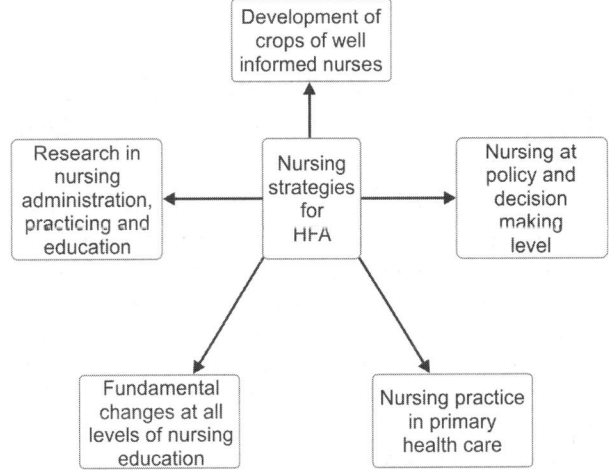

Fig. 59.4: Nursing strategies for health for all (HFA).

Table 59.2: Conceptual model of nursing for attainment of health for all through primary healthcare.

Strategies	Action proposed
• Develop a corps of nurses that is well informed about PHC and ready to bring necessary changes in nursing system • Inclusion of nursing personnel at all levels of policy-making and administration so that the profession can contribute to determine the action to be taken • Involvement of nurses and use of their skills in initiating and extending primary healthcare • Fundamental changes at all levels of nursing education to ensure that the priority needs are functionally integrated into education and into nursing practice • Research into nursing administration, practice, and education that will demonstrate the need for nursing contribution primary healthcare, clarify the implications, evaluate the services	• Arrange series of workshops • Develop texts, guides and communication slides • Planning training program • Orient nurses in legislative and political processes • Creation of administrative positions in nursing at all levels of government • Establishing systems for information on the supply and training of nurses as per community need • Preparation of nurses to assume responsibility for the provision of first level care in community • Encourage nurses for the practice of primary healthcare • Provide facilities for nurses working at periphery • Utilize approaches to close the gap between nursing, education and services • Obtain administrative support • Re-orientation in nursing education • Re-orientation in post-basic nursing education • Organizing continuing education • Include research in postgraduate program • Find government to the intersectoral support • Develop projects to demonstrate usefulness of research in nursing practice

her role as a teacher and an educator in relation to individual and family about a healthy lifestyle and the community on the primary prevention of ill-health as well as preventive and suggestive health measures.

❖ **Nurse as a supervisor and manager:** Since, the nurse is an active member of the health team, she can possess and exercise some kind of leadership, while supervising other personnel in providing care, planning health service in conjunction with other members of the health team and organizing and administering health services.

Nurse as a researcher and evaluator: At present, we are living in the dynamic world, which demands healthcare system to be dynamic as it deals with human being's well-being. So, nurses are also needed to be dynamic in their services to being about changes and innovations in the healthcare provided. These can be achieved based on a role of a researcher and evaluator, and nurses have to play for providing better services to the community.

INDIAN HEALTH SYSTEM INFRASTRUCTURE FOR PRIMARY HEALTHCARE INSTITUTIONS AND TIERS OF DELIVERY

Keeping in view Government of India's commitment to achieve the goal of HFA through primary healthcare approach, the National Health Policy has laid down a plan of action for reorienting and shaping the existing rural health infrastructure within the framework of five-year plans. At present, in India, the health infrastructure is based on a three-tier system of services provided at three levels as given below (Fig. 59.5):

❖ Primary healthcare
❖ Secondary healthcare
❖ Tertiary healthcare.

Primary Healthcare

Services are being rendered through the PHC, subcenters and village health centers as follows:

Facilities at village level: In a village, with a population of about 1,000, there will be one VHG and one trained "dai" or traditional birth attendant, both will be selected from the community. VHG Scheme was introduced in 1977, with the idea of securing people's participation in their own healthcare.

Local dais introduced under the rural health scheme (1975) based on the principles of placing health in people's hand is an extensive program to train all trained birth attendants in the country to improve their knowledge in the simple concepts of MCH services.

And also, these is one more functionary, i.e., Anganwadi worker introduced under the integrated child development scheme for 1,000 population. She is also selected from the community, and has to undergo training in various

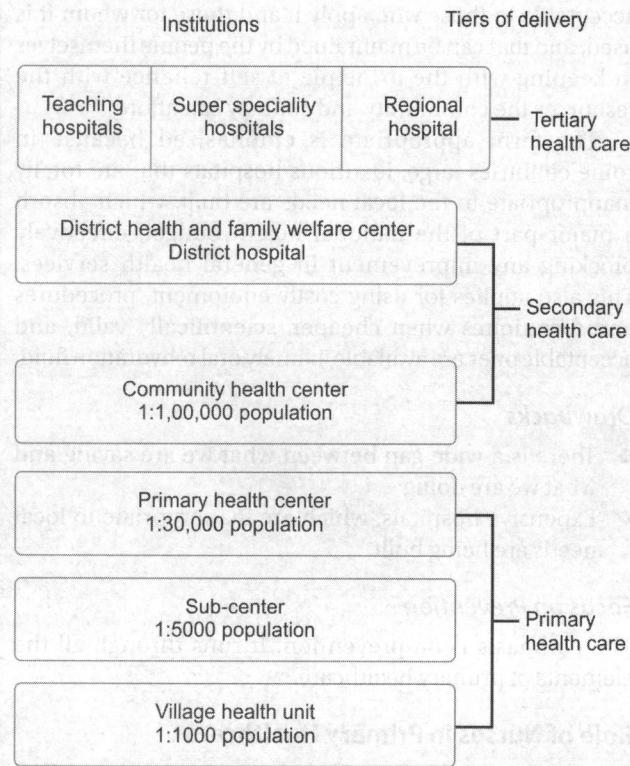

Fig. 59.5: Diagrammatical representation of 3 tier of healthcare delivery system.

aspects of health, nutrition, and child development for 4 months. After that, she has to provide service to the people of the village, which includes taking part in health check-up, immunization, supplementary nutrition, and health education in matters related to mothers and children of 6 years age.

Facilities at subcenter level: Subcenter is one of the important peripheral health units manned by one male and one female health worker. They are being established on the basis of one subcenter for every 5000 population in general and every 2500–3000 population in hilly, tribal, backward areas. The functions of subcenter are limited to MCH, family planning, immunizations and other relevant simple and referred services.

Facilities at primary health center level: The concepts of PHC was emphasized by the Health and Survey and Development Committee (1946) to provide integrated health services in the rural population, which includes preventive, promotive and curative aspects of health. PHCs were started in 1952 as part of community development program. Now, we are expected to have one PHC for 30,000 population.

The functions of PHCs in India cover all the essential elements included in the primary healthcare as follows:
❖ Medical care
❖ MCH and family planning
❖ Safe water supply and basic sanitation

- Prevention and control of locally endemic diseases
- Collection and reporting of vital statistics
- Education about health and nutrition
- National health programs—as relevant
- Referral services
- Training of health guides, health workers, local dais and health assistants
- Basic laboratory services.

CONCLUSION

The challenge that exists today in many countries is to reach the whole population with adequate healthcare services and to ensure their utilization. The large hospital, which was chosen either for the delivery of health services, has failed in the sense that it serves only a small part of the population, that too, living within a small radius of the building and the services rendered are mostly curative in nature. Therefore, it has been aptly said that these large hospitals are more ivory towers of diseases than centers for the delivery of comprehensive health services. Rising costs in the maintenance of these large hospitals and their failure to meet the total health needs of the community have led many countries to seek alternative models of healthcare delivery with a view to provide healing care services that are reasonably inexpensive and have the basic essentials required by rural population, which can be accomplished successfully through primary healthcare approach.

CHAPTER 60

Independent Practice Issues—Independent Nurse Midwifery Practitioner

CHAPTER OUTLINE

- Independent nursing practice
  - The concept of autonomy and independent practitioner roles in India
  - Certified nurse midwife
  - Women health nurse practitioner
  - Neonatal nurse practitioner
  - Genetics nurse
- Maternity nurse practitioner
- Family nurse practitioner
- Maternity clinical specialist
- Critical care obstetrician
- Obstetric and gynecologic nurse practitioner

INDEPENDENT NURSING PRACTICE

Historically, the concept of independent nursing practice has evolved from the nurse practitioner (NP) movement. The role of NP was developed in response to the rapidly growing need for primary health care. The focus of the role was not only congruent with the medical model but also consistent with nursing concepts. Initially, in the early 1970s, the NP was tied to the physician or an agency, the nurses realized that while they function interdependently with physicians, the mechanism for providing services could be in a setting not reliant on an agency or medical practice. In the early 1970s, NPs were the first nurses known to hangout their struggles and open private nursing practices.

Independent nurse practice refers to nurses who are self-employed and although they are still bound by all nursing legislation and standards, they face some unique challenges in their practice. Independent nurses must maintain high standards of nursing care and uphold the public trust that has been bestowed upon the nursing profession. There are many advanced practice roles, which supports autonomy for nurses as case manager, clinical educator, clinical researcher, clinical consultant, corporate practitioner, nurse generalist, nurse clinician, NP, nurse specialist, etc.

Autonomy and Independent Practice Roles in India

In India, nursing professionals are the most widely distributed group and they have the most diverse roles, functions, and responsibilities. Nurses provide health promotion and disease prevention as well as treatment of common diseases and rehabilitation to individuals, families, and groups. There are many advanced practice roles, which supports autonomy for nurses such as case manager, clinical educator, clinical researcher, clinical consultant, corporate practitioner, nurse generalist, nurse clinician, NP, nurse specialist, etc.

In India, private NP is quite unheard to general public. There can be "a practicing medical man," but a practicing nurse is a highly controversial issue to the health community; and also the nursing community has curious and doubtful views about the scope and prospects of independent nursing practices. However, in India, given the limited authority and autonomy, the ability to be independent, adept and expand nursing practice remains unlimited.

In 1977, in India, the Ministry of Health and Family Welfare in consultation with the Indian Nursing Council (INC) has developed a project for specialist midwifery NP under the Indo-Australia Training Program. This program has been taken up on a pilot basis in the states of Himachal Pradesh, Madhya Pradesh, and West Bengal, the duration of the course is 18 months which includes 6 months internship for graduate nurses with 2 years clinical experience within community health center where no gynecologist is available. Practice settings nurses are increasingly taking an independent role in nurse run clinic, collaborative practice and advance practice settings.

Independent Nurse Midwifery Practitioner

The expanded roles of the obstetric nurse are as follows:
- ❖ Certified nurse midwife (CNM)
- ❖ Women's health nurse practitioner (WHNP)
- ❖ Neonatal NP.

Certified Nurse Midwife

Certified nurse midwife is an advanced practices nurse who has specialized education and training in both nursing and midwifery. These professionals serve childbearing women in homes, hospitals, birthing centers, and ambulatory care arenas. CNMs teach their clients well-women health care, the management of pregnancy, health promotion, and antepartum and postpartum care.

- ❖ *Education:* They are required to possess a minimum degree of Master of Science in Obstetrics and Gynecology Nursing or postmaster's certificate midwives should also possess an active registered nurse (RN) license in the state, which they practice.
- ❖ *Practice setting:* CNM practice in hospitals and medical clinics and also may conduct delivery in birthing centers and attend at home births.
- ❖ *Functions*
  ➢ They are able to prescribe some medication.
  ➢ They provide medical care to women from puberty through menopause including care for their new born.
  ➢ For women, they provide antepartum intrapartum postpartum and nonsurgical gynecological care.
  ➢ They also provide care to the male partner in areas sexually transmitted diseases and reproductive health of their female patients.
  ➢ They also work in collaboration with an obstetrician and gynecologist who provides consultation to patients who develop complications.

Women Health Nurse Practitioner

A women health NP is an RN who has advanced education and clinical experience in women's healthcare. She is considered as a specialist who delivers comprehensive healthcare to women throughout their life span.

- ❖ *Qualification:* A women health NP requires a minimum degree of Master of Science in nursing. They are also qualified to practice in a variety of subspecialty areas such as infertility, urogynecology, high-risk pregnancy and to perform advanced technical procedures such as limited ultrasounds.
- ❖ *Practice settings:* Women health NP works in a variety of outpatient care long-term care and community-based settings as well as in hospitals. Settings include primary care clinics, community health centers, hospital antepartum triage units, school and college health clinics, employee health settings, and nursing homes.
- ❖ *Functions*
  ➢ The women health NP is well qualified to provide well-woman care prenatal and postnatal care.
  ➢ Care for women experiencing episodic acute or chronic illness.
  ➢ Care of men who have selected reproduction health needs or problems.

Neonatal Nurse Practitioner

Neonatal NP is the provision of nursing care for newborn, infant up to 28 days after birth.

- ❖ *Qualifications:* Neonatal nurses are RNs with Bachelor of Science (BSc) in nursing degree. Some countries or institutions may also require a midwifery qualification. A neonatal NP is required to hold a postgraduate degree in neonatal nursing.
- ❖ *Functions*
  ➢ Their competency includes management of high-acuity patients requiring ventilator support surgical care resuscitation.
  ➢ Low-acuity care associated with premature infants such as their nutritional needs, phototherapy, or administering antibodies.

Genetics Nurse

- ❖ *Qualification:* BSc(N)/MSc (N) + certification course in genetics. Genetics clinical nurses are RNs with special education and training in genetics. They provide care and treatment to patients who have genetic disorders such as Alzheimer's disease, cancer, diabetes, cystic fibrosis, Down syndrome, hemophilia, Huntington's disease, etc. The main duties of the genetics nurse include:
  ➢ Screening patients for genetic disorders
  ➢ Identifying potential risks
  ➢ Working with patients and treatment of diseases
  ➢ Genetic counseling family-centered care of child with genetic disorders.

Maternity Nurse Practitioner

She provides prenatal care for uncomplicated pregnancies in conjunction with a physician consultant. She takes a health and pregnancy history performs the physical and obstetric examinations, interprets laboratory and other diagnostic in conjunction with the physician, and assesses family relationships and psychological needs. Throughout the pregnancy, the maternity NP sees the women an antepartum visits, sometimes alternate with the physicians, evaluates the progress of the pregnancy, and manages minor physical problems.

- ❖ She provides information and counseling related to pregnancy and childbirth and assessment of the couples adjustments and family problems.
- ❖ She is skilled in provision of contraception and can select appropriate methods for the client including oral contraceptives, intrauterine devices, etc.

Family Nurse Practitioner

Who provides primary ambulatory care for families in collaboration with family care physician. Family NP apart from the responsibilities if maternity NP provides postdelivery care for baby as it grows thus providing continuity through the reproductive process during the intrapartum phase.

Maternity Clinical Specialist

Advanced study of maternal nursing after graduate and master degree. Care of high risk pregnancy and breast-feeding mothers. She undergoes advanced study of maternity nursing at the graduate level and is able to provide in-depth intervention for adaptation and psychological problems encountered in maternity care.

❖ She will have an area of expertise within the specialty field as maternity clinical specialist with special expertise in the care of pregnant diabetics, breast-feeding mothers, parents experiencing neonatal death, and so on.
❖ These nurses with Master's degree will act as consultants to other maternity nursing staff assisting them in planning care for difficult problems or special situations observed.
❖ They may be involved in staff education direct client services using a high degree of knowledge, skills, and competence in their area of specialty.

Critical Care Obstetrician

They deal with especially high risk cases and critical can postpartum. Now they are not much in number of high risk clients and the high tech equipment it is expected that this specialized people will increase in number.

Obstetrics and Gynecological Nurse Practitioner

Provides ambulatory care for women seeking obstetrical or gynecological health care and conducts delivery independently.

Responsibilities include:
❖ Providing independent care for women during normal pregnancy, labor, and delivery caring for newborn
❖ Family planning
❖ Routine Papanicolaou smears
❖ Treatment for minor vaginal infections
❖ Routine breast examinations.

CONCLUSION

In the present era, the nurse cannot limit her role in patient care by totally depending on the physician's order. Today, the education and knowledge acquired through various certificate courses and degree courses, masters and postgraduate, in nursing help nurses gain confidence to work independently. In India, there are nurses with these qualifications and with sufficient experience, but for a nurse to practice independently the law of the country should permit it, for which amendments have to be made, a bill has to be passed and an Act has to be made. Lack of sufficient nurse leaders, lack of motivation, and insufficient efforts from the existing nurse leaders can also be considered reasons for the delay. Therefore, in my view, nursing today requires many better nurse leaders who can take initiative and fight for our rights in governmental forums and join hands with the law makers in order to get the bill passed. Once the bill is passed, the nurse will attain and gain greater freedom to practice independently.

CHAPTER 61

Collaboration Issues and Models Within and Outside Nursing Models of Prevention

CHAPTER OUTLINE

- Health
  - Collaboration Issues
  - New Philosophy of Health
  - Concept of Prevention
  - Health Belief Model
  - Health Promotion Model
  - Travi's Wellness Model
  - Maslow's Hierarchy of Human Needs
  - Health-Illness Continuum Model
- Hall's Core Care and Cure Model
- Roy's Adaptation Model
- Agent, Host, and Environment Model
- Holistic Health Model
- Dunn's High-level Wellness Grid
- Wellness–illness Model
- Precede-proceed Model
- Clinical Model
- Role Performance Model

INTRODUCTION

A model is a theoretical way of understanding a concept or idea. Models represent different ways of approaching complex issues. Health beliefs are a person's ideas, convictions, and attitudes about health and illness because health beliefs usually influence health behavior which can positively or negatively affect a person's health. Prevention of illness is a positive health behavior; common positive health behaviors include immunizations, proper sleep patterns, adequate exercise and nutrition; there are different health models.

Preventing tensions is one aspect of wellness care that focuses on detection or prevention of disease. Primary prevention focuses on the health of a person or population; secondary prevention includes screening for those diagnosed early in the process for prompt treatment; tertiary prevention occurs when diagnostic of a long-term disease desperately has already been made the goal is to minimize complication and maximize function many ways possible for these clients.

HEALTH

- According to Traditional medicine health is thought to be absence of disease.
- Health is a state of complete physical, social, and mental well-being and not merely the absence of disease or infirmity to make secondary and economically productive.
  —**WHO, 1948–2011**

- State of well-being where person uses purposeful adaptive response to maintain relative statutory and comfort strive for personal objectives cultural goals.
  —**Marry and Zentuer**

Collaboration Issues

Models of Collaboration Between Nursing Education and Service

Introduction

The nursing profession is faced with increasingly complex healthcare issues driven by technological and medical advancements, an aging population, increased numbers of people living with chronic disease, and spiraling costs.

Meaning

The collaboration/collaborate is to "work jointly with others or together." Collaboration is an intricate concept with multiple attributes. Attributes identified by several nurse authors include sharing of planning, making decisions, solving problems, setting goals, assuming responsibility working together cooperatively, communicating, coordinating openly.

Definition

It is a process in which members of various disciplines or agencies share their expertise. Accomplishing this requires these individuals to understand and appreciate what it is that they contribute to the whole.

Collaboration/collaborative care as a partnership relationship between doctors, nurses, and other healthcare providers with patients and their families.

—**Virginia Henderson**

Collaboration is nurses and physicians co-operatively working together, sharing responsibility for solving problems, and making decision to formulate nursing care plan.

—**Baggs and Schmitt, 1988**

Objectives

1. Provide client directed and client centered care using a multidisciplinary, integrated, participative framework.
2. Enhance continuity across continuum of care.
3. Improve client and family satisfaction of care.
4. Provide quality, cost-effective, and research-based care.
5. Develop interdependent relationships.

Principles of collaboration

1. Assertive and positive attitude
2. Accountability
3. Agreement
4. Acknowledgment
5. Achievement
6. Reciprocal benefits
7. Respects
8. Responsibilities
9. Time and timings
10. Tact and talent
11. Trust

Types of collaboration

1. Interdisciplinary
2. Multidisciplinary
3. Transdisciplinary
4. Interprofessional collaboration

Common barriers in collaboration

- Lack of communication
- Lack of understanding and appreciation for what the others contribute to the team
- Inability to work together
- Lack of mutual trust
- Lack of respect
- Misconceptions
- Overlap of responsibilities and expertise
- Unresolved conflicts
- Unwillingness to share autonomy and responsibility.

Types of collaborative partnerships

1. Networking partnership—informal partnering, e.g. professional conference meetings with new or established partners.
2. Coordinated partnership—partnering to achieve common purpose. e.g. clinical rotations are altered to meet service demands, while achieving student educational level.
3. Cooperative partnership—partnering to share resources and information and alter activities for mutual benefits, e.g. use of joint appointments from service in academic classes.

Continuum of collaboration

Highest level
→ Referral
→ Co-management
→ Consultant
→ Co-ordination
→ Information exchange
→ Parallel functioning
→ Parallel communication

Lowest level

Types of relationship among health professionals

1. **Complementary relationship**
   - One person is dominant and the other is submissive.
   - Control is not divided equally between two participants

   Physician (dominant)
   ↑↓
   Nurses (submissive)

2. **Symmetrical relationship**
   - Control is more evenly distributed between the two participants.
   - Free to express their opinions.

   ↓↓   ↑↑
   (Both submissive)   (Both dominant)

3. **Parallel relationship**
   - Control moves back and forth between the participants.
   - Participants take turns by holding and giving control, depending on the circumstances.
   - Effective and flexible communication.

   Nurse/physician
   ↑↓
   ⇄
   Nurse   Physician
   Physician/nurse

Collaborative models within nursing

1. **Nursing institutional collaboration model (Fig. 61.1)**
   a. *Collaboration at clinical practice level:* At the clinical practice level, the staff nurse may collaborate with clinical instructor to develop the plan of care, provide care in an integrated and comprehensive manner, and evaluate the outcome of the care.
   b. *Collaboration with a nursing educator/nurse specialist:* The nurse educators work with clinical nurse specialist to develop a curriculum that is more appropriate to healthcare needs and day-to-day clinical practice situations.

Chapter 61: Collaboration Issues and Models Within and Outside Nursing Models of Prevention

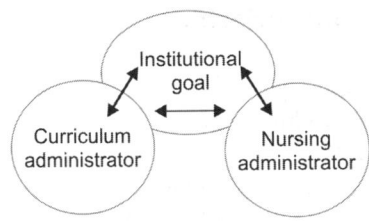

Fig. 61.1: Nursing institution collaborative relationship.

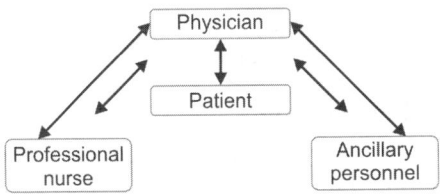

Fig. 61.2: A collaborative practice model.

c. *Collaboration with nurse researcher:* Collaboration between nurse researcher and nurse educator/nurses in clinical practice helps to approach and solve problems and issues systematically.

2. **Nurse physician collaborative practice model**
 And nurse also collaborates with hospital staffs and other health personnel of the profession and with patients and community.

3. **Collaboration with multidisciplinary health care team (Fig. 61.2)**
 Nurse
 - Patient
 - Registered nurse
 - Advance practice nurse
 - Licensed vocational nurses
 - Nurse extenders } Multidisciplinary team
 - Physicians
 - Occupational therapist
 - Social workers
 - Pharmacist

4. **Collaboration in a community-based nursing (Fig. 61.3)**
 In a community, health nurse has to carry out variety of extended roles with skills and comprehensive quality care to be provided by assisting with clients and families.

5. **Public health nurse model (Fig. 61.4)**
 In public health nurse model, there is communication among all members.

6. **Traditional practice model (Fig. 61.5)**
 - Minimal communication between team members and the patient.
 - Minimal evaluation of the care.
 - Comprehensive and quality of care is questionable

7. **Collaborative learning unit model (British Columbia, 2005)**
 In this model, the staff, student, and faculty work to create a positive learning environment and provide

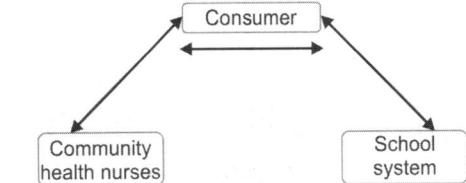

Fig. 61.3: Collaboration in a community-based nursing.

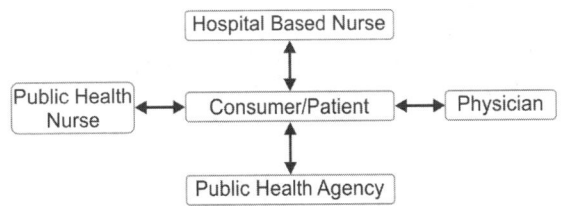

Fig. 61.4: The public health nurse model.

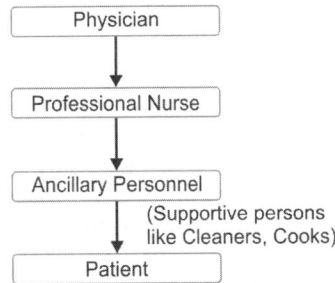

Fig. 61.5: The traditional practice model.

high-quality patient care. Increase the nursing students' opportunities and exposure to clinical situations.

Bridge the gap between academic and clinical expectations.

Provide increased professional development and socialization.

Increase instructor availability and staff on the clinical unit.

Collaboration outside the nursing

i. **Practice research model:** It is an innovative collaborative partnership agreement between Fremantle Hospital and Health Service and Curtin University of Technology in Perth, Western Australia. The partnership engages academics in the clinical setting in two formalized collaborative appointments.

It is an innovative collaborative partnership agreement between Hospital and Health Services and the University. The partnership engages academics in the clinical setting in two collaborative appointments. This partnership not only enhances communication between education and health services, but also fosters the development of nursing research and knowledge. This type of partnership is practiced in Western Australia.

ii. **The collaborative approach to nursing care (CAN care) model 2006 (Fig. 61.6):** The essence of CAN care model is the relationship between nurse learner

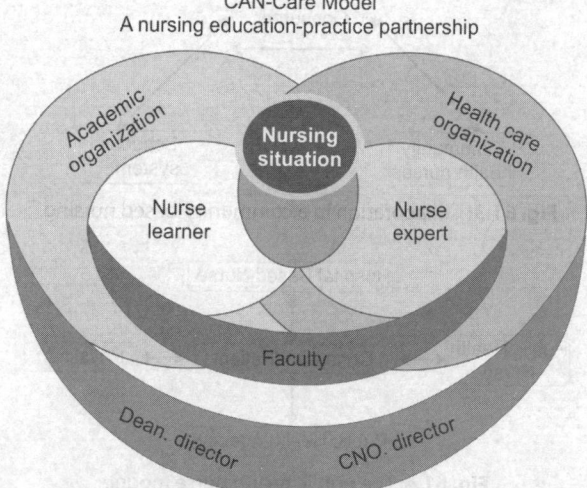

Fig. 61.6: A collaborative approach to nursing care.

(student) and nurse expert (unit based nurse) within the context of each nursing situation. Through this model, the student comes to know the organization context of nursing practice the multifaceted role of professional nurses and assumes responsibility for coming to know the meaning of nursing in each unique situation.

This model emerged as academic and practice leaders acknowledge the need to work together to promote the education, recruitment, and retention of nurses at all stages of their career. The idea partnership model emerged when the Christine E Lynn College of Nursing, Florida Atlantic University was established.

Nurse learner plus nurse expert: Learner role is to engage in learning process and play an active role in establishing a dyadic learning partnership with nurse expert. In this model, the healthcare organization becomes an active participant in creating environment contributing learning activity.

Prof. Dr K Reddamma, Ex Dean Behavioral Sciences, NIMHANS, Bangalore viewed and stated regarding collaboration issues in web source that there is a bridge between the theory and practice, due to lack of collaboration between education and services in India. To improve the quality care, collaboration model of services should be adopted by the organizations.

NIMHANS, Bangalore, and CMC, Vellore, are institutions adopted/practicing dual role of education and practice model. This improves the quality of nursing education and nursing care to patient and community at large.

The Government of India conducted a pilot study on collaborative partnerships, bridging the gap between education and service in selected institutions like one ward of AIIMS. This project was successful, patients and medical personnel appreciate the move but it required financial resources to replicate this process.

New Philosophy of Health

Health is:
- ❖ Fundamental right
- ❖ Essence of productive life
- ❖ Intersectoral
- ❖ Integral part of development
- ❖ Central to the concept of quality of life
- ❖ Involves individual state and international responsibilities
- ❖ Word code social goal
- ❖ Major social investment.

Concept of Prevention

- ❖ Prevention is any activity, which reduces the burden of mortality or morbidity from disease
- ❖ The act of preventing or impeding
- ❖ A hindrance an obstacle.

Health Belief Model (Fig. 61.7)

The health belief model was developed to provide a framework to explain why some people take specific actions to avoid illness whole other fail to protect them:

- ❖ This model was designed by Hochbaum (1958) modified and used by Kegeles (1965), Rosenstock (1974), Becker (1974).
- ❖ The model addresses the relationship between a person's belief and behavior. It provides a way of understanding and predicting how clients will behave in relation to their health how they are company to healthcare therapy.

The model is divided into three major components:
1. Individual perception
2. Modifying factors
3. Variables affecting the likelihood of imitating actions.

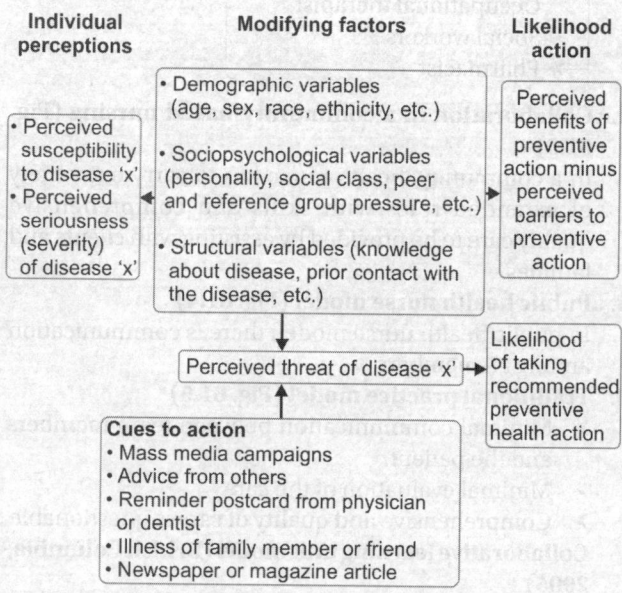

Fig. 61.7: The Health Belief Model (from Becker M, 1974).

Individual Perceptions

Individual perceptions or view of susceptible to disease and seriousness of the disease combine to form his or her perceived threat of an illness, e.g. a client needs to recognize the family link for coronary artery disease particularly when one parent and two siblings have died in their forth decade from myocardial infraction the client may perceive the personal risk of heart disease.

Contributory Factors

Contributory factors include such demographic variables as age, sex, race, and ethnicity as well as personality second class and pressure from a reference group and cases of action, e.g. mass media campaigned and advice from family friends and medical professionals.

Variables Affecting the Likelihood

Third component is variables affecting the likelihood that the person will take any action influenced by the perceived benefits of action weighed against the barriers to acting, e.g. barriers are inconvenience costs, unpleasantness or how much change it requires, e.g. lifestyle changes increased adherence to medical therapies or a search for medical advice or treatment.

Advantages

- It is useful in health protecting or disease preventing behavior.
- It is useful in organizing information about clients view of their state of health and what factors would influence them to change their behavior.
- Can be used to determine their perceptions risk of the disease their knowledge of the disease and their views of what might be the advantage and disadvantages of being immunized.

Travi's Wellness Model (Fig. 61.8)

Travi is a pioneer in the field of wellness who popularized the theoretical concept of wellness through development and teaching of the model. The impact of the model resulted in the recognition that wellness requires attention and it does not happen automatically.

The medical model represented on the left side of Figure 61.8 brings the client back from illness or disease to neutral point. The right side represents the potential for high-level health and wellness.

The objective of the model is to determine and demonstrate how people can move from the point of illness or neutrality into the realm of high-level wellness and to reduce the occurrence or recurrence of illness and disease (Fig. 61.8).

Maslow's Hierarchy of Human Needs (Fig. 61.9)

Abraham Maslow (1968-1984) developed a hierarchy of human needs. In this theory, he assigned priorities to basic needs this hierarchy of human needs arranged the basic human needs in five level of priority as follows—self-actualization, self-esteem (recognition), social affecting (love and belonging) safety, and security physiology needs.

Physiological Needs

According to this model, human needs are localized at the base of the hierarchy of needs that are very essential to life and therefore they are placed in the top priority when unsatisfied and remain as having higher probity centers satisfied they are:

- **Basic needs:** Air, water, food, clothing, shelter, elimination, sexuality, physical activity, and rest.
- **Physiological needs:** Oxygen, fluid, shelter, rest, elimination they are actually physical needs, which involve physiological and homeostatic process in the body.

Safety and Security Needs

Safety and security needs are involved with self-preservation physical safety and psychological safety and security.

- **Physical safety:** It means protecting a person from potential or actual harm.
- **Emotional safety:** It involves trusting others and being free from fear anxiety and apprehension.

Love and Belongings

Love and belongings are the needs or social affiliation in which person expects meaning from interpersonal relationship group acceptance and love belonging.

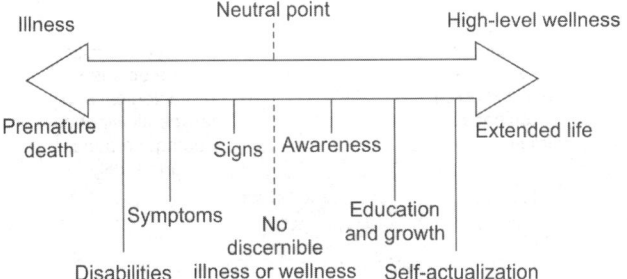

Fig. 61.8: Travi's wellness model.

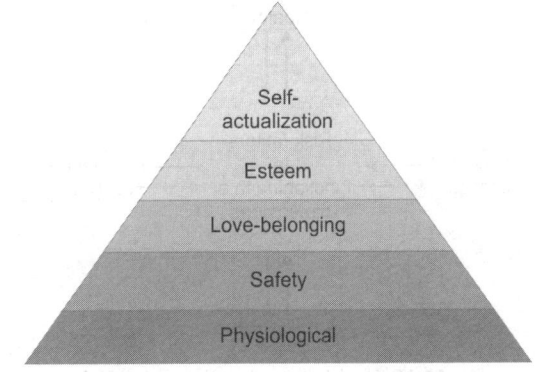

Fig. 61.9: Maslow's hierarchy model.

Self-esteem Needs

Self-esteem need is the need for a person to feel good about himself/herself to feel pride and a sense of an accomplishment and to believe that others also hold one is high regard. If gives the individual confidence and independence.

Self-actualization Needs

Self-actualization is the need for an individual to reach his/her potential through full development individual unique capabilities. Self-actualization is a state of having reached ones fullest potential and being able to cope with problems in others words it is a state fully achieving potential, and having ability to solve problems, and cope realistically with life situation.

Characteristics of Self-actualization

- Solves his own problem
- Assists others in problem solving
- Accepts suggestion from others
- Has a broad interest work and social topic
- Possess good communication skills as listeners communication
- Manages stress and assets others
- Enjoys privacy
- Seeks new experience and knowledge
- Shows confidence in abilities and decision
- Anticipates problems and success
- Works self.

Health Illness Continuum Model (Fig. 61.10)

According to health illness continuum model, health is a dynamic state that influence fluctuates as a person adapts to changes in the internal and external environments to master a state of physical emotional intellectual social development and spiritual well-being. Illness is a process in which the functioning of a person is diminished or improved in one or more dimensions when compared whether persons previous condition.

High-level wellness and severe illness are at opposite of the continuum according to Neumann (1990) health is a continuum is the degree of client wellness that at any point in time ranging from an optimal wellness condition with available energy at one maximum to death, which represents total energy depletion central at the model are risk factors, which are important in identifying the level of health, which include genetic and physiological variables each as age lifestyle environment.

The way clients view their levels of health depends their attitudes toward health values beliefs and perceptions their physical emotional intellectual social development and spiritual well-beings.

Advantages

- The health illness continuum as most effective when used to compare a client's present level of health with the clients own previous level of health.
- It is useful as the nurse helps the client set goals to attain a future level of health.

Drawback

It is not always easy to describe a client's level of health to terms of point between two extremes.

Hall's Core Care and Cure Model (Fig. 61.11)

Hall's nursing model practices provide a basis for nursing care. She formulated her model at a time when health care has dominated by the practice of medicine her ideas of nurses controlling nursing care her model consisted of three interlocking circles—(1) the core circle, (2) care circle, and (3) cure circle.

Core Circle

It refers to patient and involves developing in interpersonal relationship with a patient, which allows the patient to

Person, environment and health are not specifically

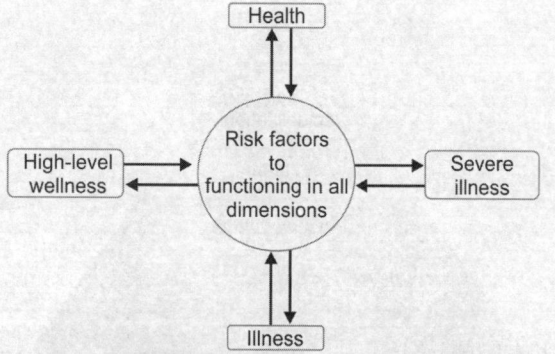

Fig. 61.10: Health-illness continuum model.

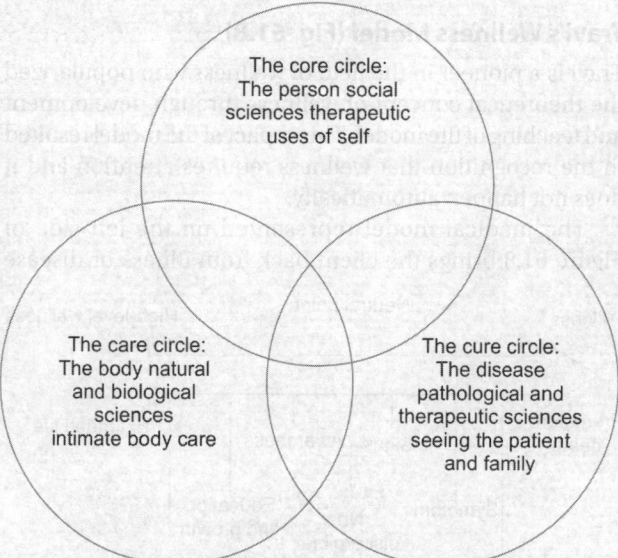

Fig. 61.11: Hall's core, care, and cure model.

express feeling about disease and further patient maturity and self-identity.

Care Circle

It refers to the patient's body and presents the nurturing aspects of nursing care. It also involves intimate body care such as bathing and feeding a nurse uses knowledge of natural and biological sciences as a basis for this care.

Cure Circle

It refers to pathological processes or the disease. It involves helping a patient and family members through the medical surgical and rehabilitative measures instituted by the physician it includes an active role as patient advocate from the patient's view point. The nurse role in the cure circle may take on the negative qualifying of avoiding pain rather than the positive quality of providing comfort.

Advantages

- It involves interacting with a patient in a complex process of teaching and learning.
- It strives to form a relationship that helps the patient Develop self-idea.
- It combines knowledge of medical procedures and diseases with teaching and learning skills to provide the patient with individual care.

Drawbacks

- Person environment and health are not specifically defined by hall.
- The core circle the person social sciences therapeutic uses of self.
- The care circle the body natural and biological sciences intimate body care.
- The cure circle the disease pathological and therapeutic sciences seeing the patient and family.
- Hall's core, care, and cure model.

Agent, Host, and Environment Model (Fig. 61.12)

The agent, host, and environment model of health, and illness also called the ecological model originated as the community health work of Leavens and Clark (1965) and has been expanded into a general theory of multiple causes of disease. The model is used primarily in predicting illness rather than in promoting wellness although identification of ask factors that result from the interactions of agent, host and environment, and helpful in promoting, and maintaining health.

Agent

Any environment factor or stress (biological, chemical, mechanical, physical, or psychosocial) which by its presence or absence (e.g. lack of essential nutrients) can lead to illness or disease.

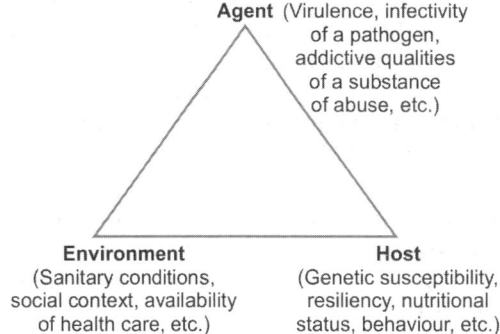

Fig. 61.12: Agent host-environment model.

Host

Persons who may or may not be at risk of acquiring a disease family history age and lifestyle labels influence the host's reaction.

Environment

All factors external to the host that may or may not predispose the person to the development of disease; physical environment includes climate living conditions sound levels, economic level; social environment includes interactions and other life events such as death of a spouse.

Holistic Health Model

Edelman and Mandle 2002: Holeson acknowledges and respects the interaction of a person's mind body and spirit within the environment. Smuts saw holism as an antidote to the atomistic approach of contemporary science. An atomistic approach takes thing apart examining the person place by place in an attempt to understand the larger picture. Holem is based on the belief that people (or their parts) cannot be fully understood if examined solely in pieces apart from their environment. Holism sees people as ever-changing systems of energy.

In this model, nurses using the nursing process consider clients the ultimate experts regarding their own health and respect clients' subjective experience as relevant in maintaining health or assessing in healing. In holistic model of health, clients are involved in their healthy process there by assuming some responsible for health maintenance. Nurses using the holistic nursing model recognize the natural healing abnormal of the body and incorporate complementary and alternative interventions such as music therapy, reminiscence relaxation therapy, therapeutic touch, and guided imagery because they are effective economical noninvasive, nonpharmacological complements to traditional medical care.

Dunn's High-level Wellness Grid

Dunn (1959) described a health good in which a health axis and an environment axis interest. The good demonstrates the interaction of the environment with the illness-wellness continuum. The health axis extends from peak wellness to death and the environmental axis extends from very favorable to very unfavorable.

- **High-level wellness in a favorable environment:** *An example is a person who implements healthy lifestyle behaviors and has the biopsychosocial spiritual, and economic resources to support this lifestyle.*
- Emergent high-level wellness in an unfavorable *environment:* An example is a woman who has the knowledge to implement healthy lifestyle practices, but does not implement adequate self-care practices because of family responsibilities, job demands or other factors.
- *Protected poor health in a favorable environment:* An example is an ill person whose needs are met by the healthcare system and who has access to appropriate medications diet and healthcare instruction.
- *Poor health in an unfavorable environment*: An example is a young child who is starving in a drought stricken country.

Wellness–Illness Model

Jenson and Allen (1993) propose a wellness–illness model that describes the relationship between health disease wellness and illness as distinct parts of a process involving the changing person in the changing world. In this model, wellness–illness is affected by interpersonal, intrapersonal health disease related, and extrapersonal factors.

- *Intrapersonal factors:* Include personality past experience emotional state.
- *Interpersonal factors:* Include social support and relationship.
- *Health and disease-related factors:* Include health promotion orientation functional status visibility of disease health and severity and prognosis of disease.
- *Extrapersonal factors:* These are social, cultural, and economic wellness–illness is viewed as the human experience of actual or perceived function dysfunction states that are influenced by the way, the individual perceives or views the experience of health disease.

Precede-Proceed Model

Precede-proceed model focuses primarily on planning and evaluating community health education programmed. It involves the client in a problem-solving approach to provide health education for an identified area of need the precede-proceed model focuses on helping communities to change their behavior. It begins by assessing the environment in which the group lives and considering the social factors that influence health behavior. Net the model examines both the internal and environment factors of the group that predispose at (precede) to certain behaviors or health problems the model than asks for the identification of factors that were here the groups in adopting health actions priorities are set the program developed implemented and finally evaluated (proceed).

Table 61.1: Precede-proceed model.

Phase	Title	Description
I	Social diagnosis	The social concerns of community are identified
II	Epidemiological diagnosis	Epidemiological date care used to suggest health problems
III	Behavioral and environment diagnosis	Behavioral and environmental risk factors that seem to affect health care are identified
IV	Educational	Predisposing reinforcing and enabling factors are identified organization diagnosis
V	Administrative	Planning related to health education and policy regulation occurs policy diagnosis
VI	Implementation	The health education program is implemented
VII	Process evaluation	The education process is evaluated in an ongoing fashion
VIII	Impact evaluation	The immediate effect of objectives of the educational program is evaluated
IX	Outcome evaluation	The short-term and long-term effects of the educational program are evaluated

The precede-proceed model is easy to use its steps area checklist for ensuring that all stages of the problem-solving process are followed (Table 61.1).

Clinical Model

In this model, the absence of signs and symptoms of disease indicates health. Illness would be the presence of signs and symptoms of disease. People who use this model of health to guide their use of healthcare services may not seek preventive health services or they may work until they are very well to seek care clinical model is the conventional model of discipline of medicine.

Role Performance Model

Here, health is indicated by the ability to perform social roles. Role performance includes work family and social roles performance based on societal expectations illness would be the failure to perform a person's roles at the level of others in society. This models is bases for work and school physical examination, and physician excused absences the seek roles in which people can be excused from performing their social roles, while they are used as a vital component of the role performance model, e.g. maternal role attainment model.

CONCLUSION

Nurses have developed this health models to understand the client's attitudes and values about health, and illness so that effective health care can be provided; these nursing models allow nurses to understand and product client's health behavior including how they use health services and adhere to recommended therapy.

62 CHAPTER

Family Nursing, Home Nursing

CHAPTER OUTLINE

- Use of Coping Index and Family Process
- Family Nursing Process
- Home Nursing

USE OF COPING INDEX AND FAMILY PROCESS

Assessment of the Family Coping Ability

The family healthcare depends not just on the identified needs and problems of the family, but is based on the assessment of the coping ability of the family and their utilization of available material, e.g. manpower resources within the family and outside the family circle. One of the tools used to assess this family coping ability is the coping index.

Family Coping Index

The purpose of the family coping index is to provide a basis for estimating the nursing needs of a particular family.

Nursing Need

A family nursing need is present when the family has a health problem they are unable to cope, e.g. disease or disability there is reasonable likelihood that nursing will make a difference in the family ability to cope.

Nature of Nursing Needs

- Concept of nursing needs can be defined from nursing terms, i.e. in relation to nursing interventions. Medical and social conditions make demands on the family may or may not give rise to nursing needs.
- The health problem, attitudes and knowledge of the family, and the availability of medical and hospital resources will determine in some measure the amount of nursing skills required by a particular family at a particular time.
- Different problems, e.g. diabetics, school and unmarried problems may require quite different patterns of nursing care although all patterns will be made up of same elements of nursing practice, physical care, therapeutics measures, education, family counseling, etc.
- One family in which diabetes is a problem will need extended direct service and education, modification of the family attitudes sand behavior and referral services.

Relation of Coping to Nursing Need

Coping may be defined as dealing with problems associated with healthcare with reasonable success. To maintain health, the individual or family must be able to:

- Deal with problems by participating in preventive, curative, or rehabilitative measure.
- To make social adjustments those are required by the health situation.
- To make wise decisions in relation to seeking and using health services.
- To contribute in whatever ways they can toward maintaining the health of others.

This capacity to deal with the situation or cope is central to health competence of the family. Coping has been selected as an index of nursing need because the particular contribution of nursing to healthcare is to strengthen or supplement the capacity of the individual or family, or family in its encounters with the stress of illness or the opportunity to prevent disease or promote health. When the family is unable to cope with one or another aspect of healthcare, they may be said to have a coping deficit.

A coping deficit in a family cannot be equated as nursing need according to the definition. The likelihood that nursing will make a difference in coping must also enter into the equation:

If a family is coping poorly, family health maintenance and diet is poor and use of preventive measure is resisted, one must think the use of educational and supportive efforts of nursing care likely to result in changes.

The form is designed to record family rather than individual capacity in community health nursing (CHN), the family cannot be seen as individual patient. In patient's family, the health of some helper is influenced by another.

Guidelines for Using Scale

Coping index consists of two parts a point on the scale a justification statement:
- ❖ The scale enables one to place the family in relation to their ability to cope with nine areas of family nursing at the time observed.
- ❖ A point scale is rated in 3 months or at the time of discharge when each nine categories has been rated, the result will be a profile of family coping capacity in relation to the family nursing required and changes occur in the course of nursing service. The index should be completed for each new family admitted for more than incidental services, i.e. one family makes more than three visits.

The evaluation should be repeated in:
- ❖ At 3 months intervals if family needs help for a longer period of time.
- ❖ Whenever drastic change, in short. For example, sick member goes to hospital—chronically ill patient develops acute episodes at discharge.

General Considerations

- ❖ It is coping capacity and not the underlying problems, i.e. being rated.
- ❖ It is the family, i.e. rated if a man fails to realize importance of nature, i.e. being rated if man is unable to care for himself/herself due to severe disability, but the necessary care is being provided by members of the family coping is adequate even though the individual himself/herself not able to manage severe stress other members feel deprived of the needed case the family is not coping even though the individual patient conditions is good.

Scaling Cues

The following description statements are cues to help one as he/she rates family coping. They are limited to three points no competence, moderate competence, and complete competence:
- ❖ *Physical independence:* Ability to move out from bed, grooming, walking even individual is dependent, family is able to compensate this to provide personal care to its family members.
- ❖ *Therapeutic competence:* It includes all of the procedures or treatments prescribed during care of illness such as giving medications, using appliances (crutches), dressings, exercises and relaxation, special diets, etc. Family either not carrying out or do it unsafely.
- ❖ *Knowledge of health conditions:* The particular health condition, for example, knowledge of the disease or disability, communicability of family uninformed conditions, has some knowledge of diseases.
- ❖ *Application of principles of hygiene:* Maintaining family nutrition securing adequate rest and relaxation for family members carrying out accepted prevention measures such as immunization, medical appraisal, safe home making foods, family diet, grossly inadequate unbalanced necessary immunization not secured for children keeping dirty. Failing to apply some general principles of hygiene and household runs smoothly.
- ❖ *Health attitudes:* This category is concerned when family feels healthcare is general includes preventive measures and services, care of illness, and entry health measures:
  - ➢ Family resists, resents healthcare
  - ➢ Accepts healthcare to some degree
  - ➢ Understands and recognizes need for health case in illness.
- ❖ *Emotional competence:* Maturity and integrity, which the members of the family are able to meet the usual stress, and problems of life:
  - ➢ Family does not face relatives
  - ➢ Unwanted pregnancy lack in emotional control
  - ➢ Family members usually do fairly well
  - ➢ All members of the family able to maintain reasonable degree of emotional calm face.
- ❖ *Family living:* Is largely concerned with interpersonal or group aspects of family life and how they get along with the one another:
  - ➢ Family consists of group of individual indifferent or hostile to one another.
  - ➢ Family gets along, but has habits or customs that interfere with effectiveness as a family.
  - ➢ Family cohesiveness means doing things together and each member acts as good member of the family.
- ❖ *Physical environment:* With home and community, and work environment as it affects family health:
  - ➢ House in poor condition unsafe unscreened poorly ventilated
  - ➢ House needs some sound repair and painting
  - ➢ House in good repair provides
- ❖ *Use of community facilities:* This has degree to which the family knows about the available use of only resources for health education and welfare:
  - ➢ Family using the following they need appropriately and promptly.

FAMILY NURSING PROCESS

Definition

- ❖ Family health nursing process is a systematic approach to help family develop and strengthen its capabilities to meet its health, and solve health process facilities standardized nursing actions to achieve family health nursing goals and objectives.

Chapter 62: Family Nursing, Home Nursing

- Family health nursing process is a problem-solving process and follows systematic steps to analyze health problems, and find their solutions whether the problem is simple or complex, e.g. poor health status, poor environment, ignorance.
- The process helps in providing systematic need-based comprehensive healthcare services to the entire family within the resources available their active involvement. It helps in achieving desired goals of health promotion prevention and control of health problems.

There are four distinct phases of patient nursing process, which are sequential:
1. Assessment phase
2. Planning
3. Implementation
4. Evaluation.

Planning for Data Collection

- Health assessment—health deficits
- Family structure, characteristics, lifestyle, culture, social economic factors, health and medical history and health behavior, and environmental factor
- Primary sources—family members
- Secondary from extended for friends, neighbors, and the colleagues.

Data Collection Methods and Techniques

Requires professional skills:
- Observation
- Questioning
- Discussion
- Listening
- Review of family health record
- Examination
- Making judgment
- Effective common investing and measurement.

Investigation

- Data should be systematic
- Do not force to get information
- Explain reasons for seeking information
- Ensure confidentiality
- Be polite and tactful
- Make them comfortable
- Sympathize and listen attentively
- Record the data as planned on interview schedule.

Analysis of Data

Organized into revised categories for coping the norms and standards of fly health Ruth freeman explained.

Health Deficits/Health Threats

Foreseeable crisis situation or stress points: These are interdependent and overlap when the process is in action. The arrows in a diagram show ongoing orderly and cyclic pattern of the phase.

Family Nursing Diagnosis

Once the data is processed and analyzed to describe the fly profile, make family diagnosis to communicate these findings to family and concerned health personnel to take further action.

Planning Phase

- Analysis of health problems and assess of family's abilities:
  - Ability to recognize the presence of health problem and make decisions for appropriate health action
  - Ability to provide desired care to the sick
- Community health nurse plays very important role to resolve health problems:
  - Development of nursing intervention—education, guidance, and counseling
  - Facilitate nursing intervention—improve family physical facilities and psychosocial environment and mobility
  - Supplemental nursing interventions—give direct nursing care service, which the family is not able to give.
- Establishing priorities:
  - Type of health problem—health deficit/health threat and forcible crisis
  - Severity of the consequences of problems—nature and magnitude
  - Modifiability of the problem, nursing intervention
  - Family perception evaluation of preventive potential prevalence eradicating
- Setting goals and objectives provide need-based care:
  - Client focused goal—malnutrition
  - Nurse focused goal—to educate malnutrition:
    - To asses nutrition status
    - To arrange for medical the help family to carry out treatment

After the nursing intervention, the mother will be able to provide need-based care to malnourished children. After nursing intervention, the family will plan and prepare balanced meals for children within available resources, feed children according to agreed upon balanced list.

Factors Influencing Goals and Objectives

- Intellectual property right (IPR)
- Family perception of its problem
- Family felt need
- Family percepts and seriousness of existing problem
- Family ability to face the reality

Selecting Appropriate Interventions

Resources such as family, community, and health facility resources will compile and prepare schematic format.

- ❖ ***Implementation (action) phase:*** Implementation phase is concerned the interaction of community health nurse with the family to put plan into action to achieve family health goals and objectives:
  - ➢ Review of plan and mobilization of resources—regular and periodical contacts should be arranged review of plan.
  - ➢ Implement and documentation.

  Plan as it is or modified. It depends upon the resources available and family readiness to participate family conditions.
- ❖ ***Evaluation phase:*** Evaluation is the last step of nursing process. Community health nurse compasses actual outcomes, expected goals and objectives.

  These goals and objectives serve as the evaluation standards and criteria against family's progress:
  - ➢ Structure evaluation
  - ➢ Process evaluation
  - ➢ Outcome evaluation

Examples of Family Problems

- ❖ Suspected case of pulmonary tuberculosis (TB) and spread of TB in infection to family members
- ❖ Two children 5 and 3 years with:
  - ➢ Malnutrition
  - ➢ Underweight
  - ➢ Look pale
  - ➢ Lethargy and weak
- ❖ Newborn baby (anticipated period of unusual demands)
- ❖ Large family size husband with four children and mother

Format of Family Nursing Care Plan

- ❖ Health problem/family nursing problem/goals and objectives
- ❖ Nursing intervention/evaluation/feedback

HOME NURSING

Introduction

Visiting the sick people at their home and giving them nursing care has been a tradition since early times. At present, in the field of CHN, the importance of home nursing is increasing day by day, especially due to nonavailability of health services, their uneven distribution, and the lack of resources. These has made home nursing an essential feature for achieving the objectives of home nursing practice.

Home healthcare nursing is defined as "the delivery of specialized nursing care services in the home healthcare setting."

Objectives

- ❖ Protection against diseases
- ❖ Providing essential treatment
- ❖ Providing comfort and relief from pain to the patient
- ❖ Giving a support and empathy to the patient and his family
- ❖ Using domestic equipment for the nursing
- ❖ Identification of communicable and noncommunicable diseases and making referral to the hospitals
- ❖ Providing health education
- ❖ Giving as much respect as possible to the faiths and beliefs of the family during the procedure.

Role of Community Health Nurse in Home Nursing

- ❖ Participating and coordinating with all the health programs operated by health and family welfare department of concerned states
- ❖ Providing maternal and child healthcare (MCH) services and prompt referral
- ❖ Recording the history of family to ascertain the cause and duration of illness
- ❖ Providing treatment and related care
- ❖ Demonstrating the nursing procedure to educate the family members
- ❖ Giving medicines as per the standing orders and providing essential nursing care in emergency situations
- ❖ Supervising the nursing procedures provided by family members
- ❖ Including the patient in taking care of himself/herself in chronic illness (heart, arthritis, cancer, diabetic patients, etc.) and giving them mental support
- ❖ Preparing plans to carry the patient to the hospital or clinic and then bringing him back to his/her home.

General Instructions for Home Nursing

- ❖ While nursing the patient at home, one should remember what Florence nightingale said; first objective of home nursing is to provide nursing, second is to keep the patient and his room in the nursing order, and the third is to remove all those shortcoming of cleanliness, which can cause the illness or death.
- ❖ Try to include the aspects of general nursing in the home nursing.
- ❖ It is essential to make family independent in taking care of their health, so their activities should be carefully monitored.
- ❖ As far as possible, home nursing should not affect the daily life and normal activities of the family and their mental strength should be enhanced.
- ❖ In home nursing, it is necessary to take care of the patient's age, his hierarchy to the family, financial condition, educational background, etc.
- ❖ In case of chronic and fatal diseases, diversional or recreational and occupational therapy should be used.
- ❖ In home nursing, there should be maximum utilization of family resources and items available in home.
- ❖ To increase the participation of family in home nursing, the class sessions should be preplanned. These sessions

should be separately organized for women, men, and children.
- For home nursing, the nurse should have a thorough knowledge of the diagnosis, etiology, sources of infection, course of disease, treatment, complications arising from the disease, surgery, and aseptic techniques.
- In the home nursing, it is necessary to pay attention to social, psychological, and emotional aspects, because they influence the isolation treatment and the process of nursing.
- In home nursing, the nurse should follow her professional standard and code of conduct (ethics).
- All principles of home visit should be followed in home nursing.

Principles of Home Visit

Home visit is the process of providing nursing care to patients at their doorsteps. The goal of home visit is to provide appropriate nursing care leading to wellness of the patients. When carrying out home visits, the community health nurse should follow certain basic principles given below.
- Home visits should be planned with purpose and should be beneficial to patients.
- The purpose of home visits should be clear and must meet the needs of the patients. It should include surveys and statistics, MCH services, home nursing in cases of illness, including health teaching.
- Home visits should be regular and flexible according to the needs of the patients.
- Home visits should be educative, i.e. it gives excellent opportunities for health and education.
- Home visits should give excellent opportunities for nurses to demonstrate hygienic principles.
- Home visit should be convenient, acceptable and educative to the patients.
- The nurse should make an attempt to include each family member while using nursing process.
- The nurse and the family must develop positive interpersonal relationship in their work to achieve the goal.
- The nurse must be flexible and must respect the patient's rights to accept or reject care and to participate in goal-setting and goal-achievement.
- Home visits should be recorded in the diary and family folder.

Advantages of the Home Visits

- Home visit provides an excellent opportunity to implement the nursing process.
- Home visits provide an opportunity to study the home and family situation.
- Home visits provide an opportunity to render services to the family members at their own surroundings.
- Prompt and proper home visits create a good understanding between nurse and family and builds good image of nurse.
- Home visits clarify the doubts raised by the family members.
- Home visits help to observe family practices and progress of care given by nurse and others.
- Home visits help to prevent and handling the problems.
- Home visits help the nurse and family members to modify the ways of their care.
- Home visits are convenient for the patients.
- Home visits facilitate patient control of the setting.
- Home visits are the best option for patients unwilling or unable to travel.
- Home visits provide natural environment for the discussion of concerns and needs.

Components of Home Visit

As it has already been stated that home visit provides an opportunity to implement nursing process in the community. The home visit itself can be viewed in a process in which the nursing activity may be initiation phase, pre-visit phase, activities during home visit phase, post-visit phase of visit, or transfer phase of visit.

The activities of a nurse in each phase are discussed here briefly.

Initiation phase

In this phase, the community health nurse clarifies the source of referral for visit and purpose of visit and also share information on reason and purposes for home visits with family.

Pre-visit activities

When the nurses are assigned to home visit, they must know certain prior information regarding the home and the family which includes location of the house and its distance, and address and some information on need for visit. Pre-visit is the part of assessment phase in which the nurses gather information about the patient, investigates community resources assembles supplies, and plans for the first patient contact. The information may be obtained from family-folders care agencies regarding age, sex, family culture and values, problems, care given, and appropriate steps during the visit to meet the needs of the patient and also help to make initial planning. In brief, in this phase, the CHN initiates contact-with the family, establishes shared perceptions of purpose with family, determines family willingness for home visit, and reviews referred and/or/family record.

Activities during home visit

The community health nurse have to use their talents, to make family to be receptive to their visit, for which they have to begin to develop trust and rapport, which are the basis for positive inter-personal relationship. The nurse–patient relation is the basis for providing possible health services to the community. Here, the nurse introduces herself to family, shows professional identity, and establishes nurse–patient relationship.

Nurse–patient relationship is defined as "a professional relationship that occurs when the nurse and another person have entered into an agreement to interact to achieve some mutually determined health-oriented goals that are consistent with nursing professional obligation."

The society has assigned the nurse the responsibility for assisting the patient as unified whole, to adjust his activities of daily living so that his steady state is maintained or regained while he is moving to higher level of wellness. The health-oriented goals are delineated by the nurses professional obligations that are determined by the society. In order to fulfil this assignment, the nurse–patient relationship should have the following characteristics:

* One person must have knowledge and skills from which another can benefit.
* The needs or requirements of the person to be assisted must take priority over those of helping person.
* The relationship is self-limiting by virtue of the goals to be achieved.
* The person to be helped must need and utilizes the assistance.
* The assistance must be given competently.

The conditions imposed on the nurse-patient relationship evolve from the rights and obligations attached to each of the complementary counter positions of nurse and of patient, the behaviors of the nurse which helps to establish positive interpersonal relationship including creativity, flexibility, follow-through, respect, and good communication.

The nurse should explain the purpose of visit and acknowledge each family member and seek cooperation from them for their care. Then the nurse should use their effective communication skills to implement the nursing process. During visit, nurse assesses the family's needs and plans the nursing care. During home visits, nurse practices a variety of roles when intervening in patient care. The community health nurse has to take a role of collaborator, consultant, co-coordinator, preventer of disease, promoter of health, health educator, and an epidemiologist and takes steps to implement nursing process.

Termination phase of visit

Termination of visits occurs when:

* Nurse–patient goals are reached, health is restored, and the patient can function without nursing actions.
* A patient changes his residence or leaves the home to go to another home.
* The nurse transfers the patients care to another nurse or other members to provide healthcare.

In addition, the nurse has to review visit with family and plan for future visits.

Post-visit activities

Post-visit activities include recording and reporting. The nurse records the important events in the family and reports the necessary materials to the higher authorities and discusses the problems of the family with the colleagues and other members of health teams and make plans accurately to meet the needs of the family. The records are kept with them. The nurse conducts the activities such as analyzing community resources and preparing for the next visit. In brief, at this stage, nurse records the visit and plans for the next.

Nursing procedures/care to be carried out by the community health nurse are:

* Identification of noncommunicable diseases or conditions such as fever, nutritional disorders, diabetes, hypertension, deficiency disorder due to lack of vitamins, iron, and iodine, protein energy malnutrition, cancer patients, simple trauma and skin diseases, and follow-up of family planning services.
* Prevention of communicable diseases such as TB, dengue syndrome, chickungunya, malaria, filarial, etc., identification of these conditions and making referral treatment and care at home.
* Simple home nursing procedures such as hand washing, thermometer disinfection, dressing, disposal of sputum and feces.
* Screening of antenatal mothers and early registration, antenatal care, immunization activities at the center and community, postnatal care, conducting deliveries and making referral, participating in national programs, implementation of all national programs, attending to monthly meetings at urban district, reporting of MCTS and immunizations and human management services of the center and community, participating in school health program and anganwadi, immunization of school children, conducting health education programs at school and anganwadi, implementing the Indra dhanush immunization program at high risk areas and coordinating to activities of the center, documentation, and reporting.

Home Healthcare Nurse

It describes a system in which healthcare and social services are provided to disabled people in their homes rather than medical facilities. Home health the largest employer of nurses within community based nursing roles.

CONCLUSION

Family and home nursing is a growing emphasis on providing nursing and care of chronically ill peoples in their homes to enable them to live as long as possible in their own homes. Implementing sound, rational infection control practices in home care has been challenging since guidelines, standards, and most references have been developed for the acute care setting. Such practices include handwashing, home infusion therapy, respiratory care, wound care, urinary tract care, and isolation precautions. Assessment of the home care environment, cleaning and reprocessing of equipment, surveillance, implications for occupational health

63 CHAPTER
Gender Sensitive Issues and Women Empowerment

CHAPTER OUTLINE

- Gender
  - Men in Nursing—Advantages
  - Problems and Facts
  - Misconceptions
- Women Empowerment
  - A Reality or Myth
  - Definitions
- Reason for Women Empowerment
- Status of Women in Current Reality
- Indicators Reflecting the Status of Indian Women
- Women and Political Participation
- Women Empowerment Strategies.
- Men in Nursing

GENDER

Introduction

Gender consciousness is everywhere; we enforce gender specific roles consciously or unconsciously. For example, when we console a crying boy by saying "don't cry like a girl," we are doing gender. That is we are expecting and at the same time imposing different set of values on the basis of sex. Gender influences on how we think, act, feel, and communicate.

Definition

Gender refers to the difference between women and men within the same household, and within and between cultures that are socially and culturally constructed, and change overtime. These differences are reflected in roles responsibilities. Access to resources, constraints, opportunities needs perception views, etc., here by both women and men. The gender is not a synonym for women, but considers both women and men, and their interdependent relationship.

—Moser C, 1993

Gender Awareness

The recognition that life experience, expectations, and needs of women and men are different that many times they involve in equity and that they are subject to change. In development and relief work, gender awareness refers to the perception, and realization of the ways in which women and men participate in the development process. How they are affected by it and how they benefit from it.

Gender Bias

Gender bias refers to the actions against women (or men) based on the perception that the other sex is not equal and does not have the same rights.

Gender Equality

A term, which reflects an equal sharing of power between women and men is their equal opportunity for education, health, administrative, and managerial positions; equal pay for work and equal value, and equal seats in parliament among others.

Gender Equity

Gender equity refers to the distribution of resources and benefits between women and men according to cultural norms, and values. This concept has different implications in different countries because it is based on different cultural standards. It is usually based on the traditions, perceptions that women and men do not necessarily have the same needs, and rights.

Gender Role

Socially determined behavior takes responsibilities for women and men based on socially perceived difference that define how women and men should act. Gender roles change over time through individual choice or with social or political change such as economic crisis, natural disasters, and the resulting emergencies, and postwar situation in which the decision-making power and responsibilities of women and men may vary.

Example: During post-war situation, women often become the sole providers of food for children, the sick, and the elderly as men are absent. At the same time, they often lack the necessary resources and sometimes the experience to make decisions for the entire house hold. They may also be expected to revert to their former traditional roles despite their new skills. Consequently, the physical and psychological stress on the women is enormous.

Gender Sensitivity

Gender sensitivity means recognizing the difference in male and female communication pattern.

Male

- Males grow up using communication to achieve goals establish individual status and authority and compete for attention and power.
- Men typically prefer to talk about topics that do not expose personal feelings.
- Men find closeness in doing things.
- Men tend to speak directly, while giving criticism or orders. A male nurse may say to his colleagues "Help me turn Jeremy."
- Men are more banter teaching and playful put down. They sometime hesitate to ask overaction for fear of appearing unknowledgeable.
- Men usually want others to know of their accomplishment.

Female

- Females grow up using communication to build connections with others and cooperate, respond to show interest in, and support others.
- Women enjoy discussing feelings and personal issues.
- Women find closeness in dialog (Wood, 1996).
- Women speak indirectly concealing criticism and commands in praise or vagueness to avoid causing offence or hurt feelings. A female nurse might say "Jeemy needs to be turned" expecting her colleague to understand the implied reaction for help.
- Women are questions to elicit information.
- Women may tend to down play their achievements; research has shown that gender difference also influences the way male and female nurse use the silence touch and humor their practice (Perry, 1996).

Gender Insensitive Communication

Gender insensitive communication means a nurse of one gender interprets or reacts to message differently than they were intended by the other gender and includes conversation with sexual innuendoes gender denigrating jokes and male–female stereotyping.

Anger and Gender

According to Thomas, the sometimes oppreceive underfunded healthcare work place can create justifiable anger among nurses. Taking frustrations and anger out on the other nurses is often seen as safer than hostility toward employees or management females were seen as "anger suppressors," while males were seen and "anger venters" Thomas suggested that women need to learn that relationship does not end when anger is honestly described and men need to consider the consequences of too regular hostile aggressive behavior.

Mentor and Women

Literature suggests that historically there have not been enough mentors for women who want one Bolton (1980) described four reasons why women do not have enough mentors:

1. Lack of emphasis on team sports for a girl during childhood could reduce her effectiveness later in life on a business or professional team.
2. Solidarity activities such as cooling and piano lessons are more common to young girls.
3. Boys are still traditionally encouraged to participation in football, bare ball, and basket ball developing expertise to use in a team effort.
4. It may be as a result of low number of women in top-level management who are both willing and available to be mentors to other women besides "belonging" is still associated with feminine socialization "achieving" is often the focus of socialization for men fortunately mentoring opportunities for women are increasing.

Gender Diversity in Nursing

Diversity goal in nursing are not just directed at ethnicity they also frequently include increasing the number of men in nursing. Despite the increase in number of men in nursing progress in this regard has been slow. Stereotypes of male nurse are being different or gay due to their working relationship with women play a role and there are few male faculty role models in nursing many nursing text books refer to the comforting caregiver nurse as she and make no mention of the male gender except as sickly demanding patients. There stereotypes suggest that male nurses are incapable of or less capable of caring compassion and nurturing than female nurses.

Nursing Gender Specific

Many think that nursing is only a profession for female and male sometimes join the course due to family pressure. People feel that traditionally, males are doctors and female are nurses. Everywhere, in every profession, females are dominated by males. The only profession where females take the upper hand is missing.

Why Nursing is Considered as Female Profession

Medical doctors are often the leaders of a team providing services. Often, carry patriarchal values that influence their professional actions and thereby gender in equity for many years nurses were considered the hand maids of the physicians.

Religious explanations: They declare women's bodies to be inherently inferior and sinful, and fit to be controlled by men. A woman is a derivation and as much is included in man. All religious groups worship mother are a model woman who is self-sacrificing and essentially noble, while they support the concept of men as superior to women. The role of a doctor is predominantly a male role; the female role is subsidiary as nurse and helper.

Why Men do not Choose Nursing Profession?

Nursing is about nurturing and caring—essential qualities of a female. From birth, boys are brought up by enforcing gender specific values and roles. As they grow up, boys find out that everything around them communicates and expect sex roles. Even if they take some of the female roles, they are scolded teared or punished. The public and even the nurses would hesitate admitting their sons in nursing courses.

Male Advantage in Nursing

In contract the three arguments Kleinman suggest that the minority status of men in nursing often insult in advantages including hiring and promotion that help rather than hinder their careers. Unlike women in male dominated professions. In addition, managers tend to select men over women for advancement role in the hospital settings. Although sex role stereotyping may limit the recruitment of male into nursing men have been socialized if issues orders assign task and provide a sense of direction whereas women suggest support, and carry out orders. Similarly although male and female nursing students seek empowerment female students want to empower other whereas male students want to empower themselves.

Men in Nursing—the Problems and Facts

Classroom Prejudice

In classroom setting, male nursing students have encountered gender discrimination in the every textbook, some textbooks will make no mention of male gender other than as a patient every picture seemed to identify the nurse as a caring female individual. While the patient was always a male in need of care. Instructors sometimes refer to nurses as if they are all women, which lead to unconscious expectation that men are not supposed to be nurses.

Work Place Prejudices

In the work place, male nurses are being stereotyped as the typical male who may be viewed as insensitive and sloppy. Some male nurses feel that they are held to a higher standard than their female colleagues and that peers may resent them because they are men in a traditionally female role. When male nurse makes in to the supervisory rank gender discrimination become more apparent against as some female nurses resent taking orders from males. Gender discrimination is also apparent with the male nursing teachers in hospital as they are not allowed in certain areas of hospital such as labor room and postpartum area.

Misconception of Men in Nursing

Most people consider nursing to be women's work. Male nurses have been stereotypes as feminine like and nonachievers. They are considered so as they have chosen as a profession so profoundly dominated by female and because they have not conformed to a traditional male occupation. They are labeled lazy nonachievers for going into nursing rather than becoming doctors, engineers, or other masculine profession.

One of the biggest misconceptions is that men are not capable and should not be nurses. Society tends to view nursing as a profession for women. However, their misconceptions are not true and unfair as men belong in the profession as much as women do.

Do Men Really Make a Difference in Nursing?

- "What a nurse brings to the table is not because of hormones or genes."
- Pamela Kidd, Associate Dean for Graduate Programs and Research, Arizona.

If a nurse has mastered the art and science of nursing, people do not care if a nurse is a man or a woman. While female nurses say they do not see any difference male nurses say they have helped, changed nursing relationship with physicians and patients "male nurses have been less tolerant of verbal abuse than women have been in the past." This attitude might have opened the eyes of the doctors that it is not ok to treat any nurse with disrespect.

Traditionally, men tend to choose aggressive areas such as intensive care unit (ICU), cardiac care units, emergency trauma units, etc. Men are usually drawn to the technological aspects of acute care specialties and are challenged by the machinery in those units. Men also have not experienced much gender discrimination

Men in nursing also have an economic advantage national sample survey of registered nurses reported that male nurses averaged approximately 12% more of earnings than female.

Hidden Advantages for Men in Nursing

- They will be viewed as traditionally breadwinner of the families and are considered more permanent reliable employee.
- Better opportunities to employ leadership process and develop leadership skills.
- Better opportunities for personal and professional growth in a profession with few competitive from own sex.
- Better opportunities to choose aggressive areas nursing is not gender it is a profession today there is no domain of work which men or women can claim to be their and

their only society is slowly becoming more comfortable with men as nurses.

Although people may feel a little uncomfortable at first sight, they will quickly come to trust and respect him for his professionalism. When more men join nursing, the relationship with other profession will improve including the public image. The days soon will come when the concept of nurses as helper and only females join in nursing will completely vanish.

WOMEN EMPOWERMENT

Introduction

Women's empowerment is a process in which women gain greater share of control over resources material human and intellectual such as knowledge information ideas, and financial resources such as money and access to money, and control over decision-making in the home community society and nation, and to grow power.

According to the country report of Government of India "empowerment means moving from a position of enforced powerlessness to one of the power."

The Government of India has made empowerment of women as one of the principal objectives of the Ninth Five-year Plan (1997–2002) and also declared 2001 are the year of "women empowerment" to focus on a vision where women are equal partners like men. These issues of gender equality are dismissed in world conference, national and international conferences, etc. Our constitution has conferred and guaranteed equality before law universal adult franchise and equal opportunities for men, and women as fundamental rights. The imperative of gender partnership institutional mechanisms and interventions have been consciously built into the development design.

Separate institutions for women and child development departments at the central, and state level creation of the national commission for women and also state commission for women in several states are some of the important developments for the betterment, and prosperity of women. The launching of Rashtriya Mahila Kosh, Indira Mahila Yojana, Mahila Samridhi Yojana serving of one-third of the number of seats in panchayats and the local bodies are programs launched with a view of improve, and empower women socially, economically, and in political frontiers.

In ancient India, women enjoyed a very high position, but gradually their position degenerated into merely objects of pleasure meant to serve certain purpose. They lost their individual identity and even their basic human rights.

Women Empowerment—A Reality or Myth

The most common explanation of women's empowerment is the ability to exercise full control over one's actions. The last decades have witnessed some basic changes in the status and role of women in our society. There has been shift in policy approaches from the concept of "welfare in the 70s to the 'development' in the 80s and now to empowerment in the 90s." This process has been further associated with some sections of women becoming increasingly self-conscious of their discrimination in several areas of family and public life. They are also in a position to mobilize themselves on issues that can affect their overall position. The latest news items regarding violence committed against women reveal that women's position has worsened.

The discrimination and deep-rooted gender bias still exists in all sectors on the basis of act. Based on community, religious affiliation and class, the Constitution of India grants equality to women in various fields of life, yet a large number of women are either ill equipped or not in a position to propel themselves if they are traditional, unsatisfactory socioeconomic conditions. They are poor, uneducated, and insufficiently trained. They are often absorbed in the struggle to sustain the family physically and emotionally, and rules are discouraged from taking interest in affairs outside home. Oppression and atrocities on women are still rampant. Patriarchy continues to be embedded in the social system in many parts of India denying a majority of women to decide on how they live.

Definitions

Empowerment

* A process though which women and men in disadvantage position increase their access the knowledge resources decision-making power, and raise their awareness of participation their communities in order to reach a level of control their own environment.
* The expansion in people's ability to make strategic life choices in a context where the ability was previously denied to them.
* It is the process of challenging existing power relations and of gaining greater control over the sources of power.

Women Empowerment

* The manifestation of redistribution of power that challenges patriarchal ideology and male dominance.
* It is a social process that neutralizes women's oppression women's decision to empowered.
* Altering relations of power, which constrain women options and autonomy and adversely affect health and well-being.
* A process where by women become able to organize themselves to increase their own self-reliance to assert their independent night to make choices and to control resources, which will assist in challenging, and eliminating their own subordination.

Reason for Women Empowerment

* Willingness to be empowered by women
* Intention to develop one's potential
* Interest to lead meaningful life productivity

- Need of stronger positions to support other and to make substantial contributions to society
- To face the facts of their at all levels of social organization.

Qualitative Indicators

- Increase in self-esteem knowledge on women health nutrition, reproductive rights, legal rights literacy, etc.
- Change in role of responsibilities in the family and in the community
- Changes in social customs, e.g. child marriage, dowry discrimination
- Visible increase or decrease in levels of domestic and other forms of violence
- Increase participation in public meetings and training programs
- Formation of women groups, self-help groups, etc.
- Positive changes in social attitude among the community members
- Women's economic contributions in sharing family responsibilities
- Increased decision-making process related to work, income, and expenditure in her control.

Quantitative Indicators

- Demographic trends
- Number of women participating in different development programs political processes at local level
- Assess and control over community resources, and government scheme
- Visible changes in health with nutritional status changes in literacy.

Status of Women of Current Reality

There is growing importance of establishing gender equality around the world. The United Nations Development Fund for Women (UNIFEM) was established and a separate fund within the United Nations Development Program (UNDP) in 1984. At that time, the general assembly instructed it to ensure women's involvement with mainstream activities.

The platform of action resulting from the 1995 Beijing world conference on women expanded this concept calling, i.e. "gender main streaming." The application of gender perspectives to all legal and social norms, and standards to all policy development, research planning, advocacy development, implementation and monitoring as mandatory for all member states.

Achieving gender equality, however, is a grindingly slow process since it challenges one of the most deeply established of all human attitudes. Despite the intense efforts of many agencies and organizations, and numerous inspiring success, the picture is still disheartening as it takes the more than changes in law or stated policy to change practice in home, in community, and in the decision-making environment:

- In many parts of the world, rape is not considered a crime goes unpunished and continues to be used as a tool of war. Even in highly developed countries, violence against women of all kinds is routine and often condoned.
- Female sexual slavery and forced prostitution are still terrible "facts of life" of poor women.
- Genetic testing for defects of the unborn is used in some parts of the world to determine the sex of the fetus so that females can be aborted.
- While in some countries female infants are buried alive. Forced marriage and bride burning are still prevalent in the Asian subcontinent.
- A pregnant woman in Africa is 180 times more likely to die of pregnancy complications than in western Europe.
- Women mostly in rural areas represent more than two-third of the world's illiterate adults.
- In United States, 90% of Acquired Immunodeficiency Syndrome (AIDS) cases under 20 years of age are girls.
- In many developed countries where basic gender equality appears to have been achieved, the battle front has shifted to removing the more intangible discrimination against working women.
- Women still hold only 15.6% of elected parliamentary seats globally.

Indicators Reflecting the Status of the Indian Women

Sex ratio: The number of females per 1000 males is a significant indicator of the status of women. The ratio is as shown in Table 63.1 reflects a continuous decline except in 2001.

Life Expectancy at Births

Life expectancy at birth tends to be a good summary measure of women's health status. Normally women outlive men. Countries with high outcome women on an average live longer by 6 years than men. Countries with lower income they live only 2 years longer. The life expectancy birth for women has shown a steady rise in the country from 39 to 74 years in 1961 to 66.9 years in 2001–2006 reflecting the achievements made in the health sector.

Table 63.1: Sex ratio in all over India.

Year	No. of women/1,000 men
1951	946
1961	941
1971	930
1981	924
1991	927
2001	933
2011	943
2014	939

Literacy Rate

Education is a potent remedy for most of the ills of the society. Education is the main instrument for transformation in any society. By educating women, a country can reduce poverty, improve productivity ease population pressure, and offer its children a better future. A package approach is required for developing female education. There is a wide disparity between male and female literacy rates. As per 2001 census, the literacy rate was 55% and 75% for female and male respectively in the country. There also exists a rural urban gender divide in literacy rate across the country. This indicates that specific intervention may be required for developing the literacy rates of the female population especially, the privileged clause, in rural areas.

Employment and Work Participation Rate

The work participation rate indicates to a great extent the economic empowerment of women in the society. The status of women is intimately connected with their economic position, which in turn depends on the opportunities for participation in economic activities. Education along with participation of women in work force has been universally recognized as an important element in the adoption of small family norms, which is essential for family planning.

Women and Political Participation

Political equality to all children regardless of birth sex color is one of the basic premises of democracy political equality includes not only equal right to franchise but also more importantly the right to access to the institutionalized centers of power. Women's political empowerment is premised on three fundamental and non-negotiable principles:

- The equality between women and men
- Women's right to the full development of this potentials
- Women's right to self-representation and self-determination.

In Panchayati Raj Institution (PRI), women are increasingly coming to the force and are providing leadership at the grass root level. This has profound social implication, which gives paves way in addressing gender-related discrimination in development:

- Sex ratio: 1000:940
- Mortality rate: 48/1000 lives
- Birth rates: 20.97/1000 lives birth

The male domination of society and government are often seen for the purpose of serving male interests, and in the continued subordination of women.

Levels of Women Empowerment Framework

- **Welfare:** An improvement in socioeconomic status such as improved nutritional status shelter or income, which is the zero level of empowerment where women are the passive recipients of benefits that are given from on high.
- **Access:** To resources and services stands for the first level of empowerment since women improve their own status relative to men by their own work, and organization arising from increased access to resources and services.
- **Conscientization:** As the process by which women collectively urge to act to remove one or more of the discriminatory practice that impede their access to resources. Here, women form groups to understand the underlying causes of their problems and to identity strategies for action for gender equality.
- **Mobilization:** This is the action level of empowerment by forging links with the larger women's movement to learn from the success of women similar strategic action elsewhere and to connect with the wider struggle. The experts on gender issues hold that women's advancement involves the process of empowerment and define it as a process by which women achieve increased control over public decision-making.
- **Control:** It is the level of empowerment when women have taken action so that there is gender equality in decision-making over access to resources so that women achieve direct control over their access to resources.

Women Empowerment Strategies

The United Nations Development Program, Millenium development goals.

Goals 1 and 2

- Eradicate extreme poverty and hunger.
- Achieve universal education.
- Promote gender equality and promote women equality.
- Reduce child mortality.
- Improve maternal health.
- Combat AIDS, malaria, and other diseases.
- Ensure environmental sustainability.
- Global partnership for development.

Promote Gender Equality and Empowers Women

Indicators

- To eliminate gender disparity in primary and secondary education preferably by 2005 and at all levels by 2015:
  - 3:1 ratios of girls to boys in primary, secondary, and tertiary education
  - 3:2 ratios of girls to boys in primary employment in the nonagricultural sector
  - 3:3 proportion of seats held by women in National Parliament
- The Ninth Five-Year Plan commits to empower women through creating an enabling environment where common women can freely exercise their rights both within and outside their homes as equal portions along with men. This is planned to be realized through the national policy for empowerment of women with definite goals targets. Policy prescriptions along

with a well-designed gender development index to monitor.
- United Nations 1995 fourth world conference on women held in Beijing with 20,000 participants. It focused on rights of women to acquire:
  - Education
  - Economic power
  - Inclusion in leadership
  - Involvement in decision-making
  - The nodal department of women and child development for empowering women formulate policies and programs to amend legislation concerning women and reviews guides, and coordinates effort of governmental and nongovernmental organizations.
  - The department implements a few innovative programs, which include:
    - Empowering strategies
    - Employment and income generation
    - Welfare and support services
    - Awareness generation and gender sensitization
    - Other enabling measures.

MEN IN NURSING

The proposition of men in nursing is now showing gain.

Historical Perspectives of Men in Nursing

Historical perspectives of men in nursing relationship to the current nursing shortage and nursing education:
- During the time of Aristocrat and Socrates about 2500 BC, men and women had separate healthcare facilities. Men were cared for by male nurses and women were cared for by female nurses.
- Around 250 BC, the first nursing school was started in India where only men were considered pure enough to become nurses.
- Characteristics include "good behavior" distinguished for purity, possess cleverness and skill imbued with kindness.
- The Order of Santo Spirit (Holy Ghost)—1070 AD
- The Hospital Brothers of St. Anthony—1090 AD
- Knights Hospital—1206 AD
- St. Francis of Assisi founded three orders—1211 AD
- The Teutonic Knights
- The Tertiaries
- The Knights of Lazarus
- In 1859, Florence Nightingale wrote in her notes that every woman is a nurse.

That is reflected in most nursing histories, which state that women are the primary care providers:
- During the civil war from 1861 to 1865, both sides had military men, who served and was paid as nurses.
- Women usually served in general hospital in the major cities.
- In 1888, the Mills School of Nursing and the St. Vincent Hospital School for Men were started.
- In 1914, the Pennsylvania Hospital opened a school for men to study nursing.
- In 1898, during the Spanish-American war, more female nurses were recruited to aid the male nurses.
- In 1901, the army nurse coop was formed and only women could serve as nurse.
- The American Nurses Association was formed in 1919 and only white female could belong.
- During World War I and II, there was a nursing shortage women.
- It was not until after the Korean War (1966) that men were permitted to serve as nurses in the military.
- In 1980, the Supreme Court ruled against Mississippi University for Women which had refused to admit a male student.
- In US until 1982, men were forbidden to attend some government-sponsored nursing school, the Supreme Court ruled against that it was illegal to discriminate against men who wanted to become nurses.
- In 1974, the Michigan Male Nurse Organization was formed
- In 1976, it became the American assembly for men in nursing.
- Mission: To provide a forum for men in nursing in which supporters come together to discuss issues and research related to men in nursing, and men's health in general. To encourage men and boys to become nurses.
- Number of men in nursing in 1960: 5%
- Number of men in nursing in 1996: 5%
- Number of men in nursing in 2000: 5.4%
- Job satisfaction for men who are new to nursing: 67%
- Job satisfaction for women who are new to nursing: 75%
- Established nurses report even less job satisfaction: 69% women and 60% men
- Opportunities in nursing for men to consider nurse anesthesia, psychiatric/mental health, public health, home care, school nursing, rural health, geriatric, genetics, acute care, women health nurse, midwifery, cardiovascular nursing care, management educator nurse, lawyer nurse, entrepreneur consultant, researcher, wellness health promotion.
- One key concept is to let boys know, as early as possible, that nursing is a challenging profession.
- Let boys and men know that nursing has a strong scientific background, and a concern to help people.
- Change curriculum and teaching styles.
- Appoint a male faculty to serve as a role model and mentor
- Advertise in gender neutral sections of newspaper for nursing students
- Today's nursing cannot ignore 50% of the population

❖ Encourage people who have the ability and qualification to become good nurses regardless of gender, sexual orientation, race or religion.

Develop forums at nursing schools for males to attract more male candidates.

CONCLUSION

In earlier generation, women were not given a chance to study, work, or take/hold any post, but now the trend has changed completely where women are treated equal to men in all aspects such as in work areas to a seat in the parliament.

In today's generation, there is a lot of difference in the gender male and female, and there is a lot of changes that are occurring in today's generation. In every profession like males and females are also equally involved, and competent males. So there is a gender bias both male and female. They try to suppress the female by over dominating them.

Even in nursing there is a competition where even it is a job that is usually opted by females even in this profession the males are entering and dominate them there causing interrelationship within the profession.

64 Disaster Nursing

CHAPTER OUTLINE

- Definition
- Phases of Disaster Management
- Disaster Syndrome
- Rehabilitation

INTRODUCTION

Disaster may be natural or man-made; disaster can happen at any time anywhere in the world. A common denominator in the disaster and emergency situation in nursing immediate response; legislation has been enacted to provide federal assistance to individuals and communities to aid recovery from devastation caused by disaster to human life and property.

DEFINITION

A disaster is any man-made or natural event that causes destruction and devastation that cannot be alleviated without assistance. Disasters are sudden catastrophic events that disrupt a pattern of life and in which there is possible loss of life and property in addition to multiple injuries. Disaster can be either natural phenomena or caused by people.

PHASES OF DISASTER MANAGEMENT

The phases of disaster management are as follows (Fig. 64.1):
- Mitigation
- Preparedness
- Response
- Recovery

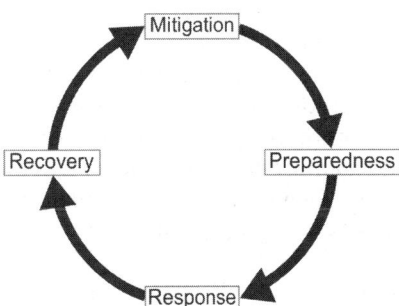

Fig. 64.1: Phases of disaster management.

Mitigation

Disaster mitigation includes any activity that prevents a disaster, reduces the chance of disaster happening, or reduces the damaging effects of unavoidable disaster.

Nurses have a key role in disaster mitigation by working with local, state, and federal agencies in identifying disaster risk and developing disaster prevention strategies through extensive public education in disaster prevention and readiness. Effective mitigation includes recognizing and preventing potential technological disasters and being adequately prepared should such events occur.

Preparedness

Personal Preparedness

Great stress is placed on the nurse with client responsibilities who also become victim. The community health nurse, who will be assisting in disaster relief efforts, must be as healthy as possible both physically and mentally. Personal preparedness can help ease some of the conflicts that will arise and allows nurse to attend to client needs sooner than one may anticipate. The American Red Cross and the Federal Emergency Management Agency (FEMA), the two well-known authorities on disaster preparedness and recovery, have devised a personal checklist to help individuals and families organize for disaster before they strike.

Professional Preparedness

Professional preparedness requires that nurses become aware of and understand the disaster plans at their workplace and community. The more adequately prepared nurses are, the more they will be able to function in a

leadership capacity and assist others toward a smoother recovery phase. Personal items that are recommended for any nurse preparing to help in disaster include:
- A copy of their professional license
- Personal equipment, such as stethoscope
- A flash light and extra batteries
- Cash
- Weather appropriate clothing
- Record-keeping materials
- Pocket-sized reference book

All workers are certified in first aid and cardiopulmonary resuscitation.

Community Preparedness

The level of community preparedness for a disaster is only as good as the people, and organizations in the community make it. If possible, it is also important to review the disaster history of the community, including how past disasters have had an impact on the community health care system and how their particular organization fits into the plan. Understanding these aspects of past disasters has planning implication for further disasters. A solid disaster plan requires multidisciplinary talents and coordination and cooperation of many different organizations. Many community, organizations, and professionals are involved in disaster work including the clergy, morticians, police, fire and rescue, the mayor, and other city officials and the media.

Some people mistakenly believe that past experience with a particular type of disaster is enough to prepare for the next one. In this situation, face-to-face encounter with law enforcement personnel or authority is often necessary to convince individuals to leave their homes and retreat to safer quarters.

Role of the Community Health Nurse in Disaster Preparedness

The role of community health nurse in disaster preparedness is to facilitate preparation within the community and place of employment within the employing organization. The nurse can initiate or update disaster plan, provide educational program and material regarding disaster specific to the area, and organize disaster drills. The community health nurse is also a unique position to provide an updated record of vulnerable people. The community health nurse should also have an understanding of what community resources will be available after a disaster strikes and most importantly how the community will work together. A community wide disaster plan will guide the nurse in understanding what should occur before, during, and after response and his/her role within the plan.

Response

The response is determined by the level of disaster. Levels are not determined by the number of casualties per se, but by the amount of resources needed:

- ***Level 3 disaster:*** This level requires activation by the local emergency medical system in cooperation with local community organizations, for example, one family fire.
- ***Level 2 disaster:*** It requires more of a regional response necessitating several casualty protocol, for example, one building collapse.
- ***Level 1 disaster:*** In this level, a federal emergency has been declared, because of widespread destruction, for example, hurricane.

Federal Response Plan

Once a federal emergency has been declared, the federal response plan (FRP), also known as public law, may take effect depending on the specific need of the disaster. Within the FRP, there are 12 emergency support functions (ESFs), and each is headed by a primary agency. Each primary agency is responsible for coordinating efforts in a particular area with all its designated support agencies. Sheltering, feeding, giving emergency first aid, providing disaster welfare information system, and coordinating bulk distribution of emergency relief supplies constitute mass care of ESFs of which the American Red Cross is the primary.

The National Disaster Medical (NDMS) is part of the ESFs of health and medical services. In a presidentially declared disaster, including overseas war, public health service (PHS) can activate disaster medical assistance teams (DMATs) to an area to supplement local and state medical care needs. Teams of specially trained civilian, physician, nurses, and other healthcare personnel can be sent to a disaster site within hours of activation. DMATs can provide triage and continuing medical care to victims, until they can be evacuated to a national network of hospitals.

Role of the Community Health Nurse in Disaster Response

The role of community health nurse during disaster depends greatly on the nurse post experience, role in the community and institution preparedness, specialized training, and interest.

Triage is the process of separating casualties and allocating treatment based on the potential for survival. Highest priority is always given to victims, who have life-threatening injuries, but who have a high probability of survival once stabilized. Second priority is given to victims, who have injuries with systemic complications that are not yet life-threatening, but who can wait up to 45–60 min for treatment. Last priority is given to those victims, who have local injuries without immediate complications and who can wait several hours for medical attention. Community health nurses working as members of an assessment team have the responsibility of feeding back accurate information to relief managers to facilitate rapid rescue and recovery. Many times nurses are required to make home visit to gather needed information.

Types of information included in initial assessment include:
- Geographical extent of disasters impact
- Population at risk or affected
- Injuries and death
- Availability of shelter
- Current level of sanitation
- Presence of continuing hazard
- Status of healthcare infrastructure.

Recovery

The stage disaster known as recovery occurs as all involved agencies pull together to restore the economic and civic life of the community.

Role of the Community Health Nurse in Disaster Recovery

The role of the community health nurse in the recovery phase is as varied as in the preparedness and response phase of disaster. The community health nurse must be alert for environmental health hazards during the recovery phase of a disaster. Home visit may lead the nurse to uncover situations such as faulty housing structure, lack of water supply, or lack of electricity. Nurse must be attentive to the dangers of live or dead animals and rodents that might be considered harmful to a person's health. An example of this would be finding snakes in and around homes once the water from a flood start to recede (Table 64.1).

DISASTER SYNDROME

The behavior of victims after the impact of disaster can be characterized by progressing through phase of shock, awareness, euphoria, and anger.
- ***Shock phase:*** It may last only a few minutes or for several hours after impact. The victim is dazed and unable to comprehend what is occurring and cannot follow simple direction.

Table 64.1: Types/causes of disaster.

Natural	Man-made
Air • Hurricanes • Tornados • Hailstorms • Cyclones • Blizzards • Hurricane Water • Floods • Mud slides • Tidal wave • Avalanches • Drought Earth • Earthquakes • Volcanic eruptions • Lightening includes forest fires	• Conventional warfare • Nonconventional warfare (nuclear attack, chemical) • Transportation—air, water, land • Structured collapse • Explosions/bombing • Fire-housing, forest • Toxic materials • Pollutions • Civil unrest (riots) • Communicable disease epidemics

- ***Awareness phase:*** It may last up to several days, victim becomes aware of survival and tries to help others. During this stage, guilt feeling may arise because others died and they survived. The victim can follow simple direction, but cannot carryout problem-solving effectively.
- ***Euphoria phase:*** It may last for several weeks. The victim feels a sense of brotherhood with the community and participates willingly in helping others with plans for recovery.
- ***Anger phase:*** This occurs because of the experienced loss. The anger often projected against helping persons, who are not personally affected by the disaster. The nurse who may be assisting victims during the recovery phase to understand that anger is part of the loss experience. As the victim copes with the situation, then the anger will disappear.

Role of Nurses in Disaster Preparedness

Nurses in disaster preparedness facilitate preparation within the community and place of employment. She can:
- Help initiate and update the disaster plan
- Provide educational programs and material regarding disaster specific to the area.

Organize Disaster Drills

- She could recruit people who have demonstrated flexibility, decisiveness, stamina, endurance, and emotional stability (O Nerman, 1990) for the help required during disaster.
- She can help keep a safe environment. Recalling that disaster is not only natural but also man-made.
- She needs to assess and report environmental health hazards of the community.
- She can choose to work with agencies such as the Red Cross.

The following steps are required to get activity involved after disaster training:
- Join a local disaster action team (DAT)
- Act as a liaison with local hospitals
- Determine health related for shelter sites.
- Plan with pharmacies, opticians, morticians, and other health personnel to facilitate service for disaster victims
- Plan for and retain needed supplies
- Teach disaster nursing in the community.

Mass casualty drills and mock disaster are valuable components of any preparedness plan. The objectives are:
- Promote confidence
- Develop skills
- Coordinate activities
- Coordinate participants.

It is especially important that the drill leader have special skills in disaster management and the ability to coordinate many organizations at one time.

Agencies Involved in Disaster Preparedness
- American Red Cross
- Other voluntary organizations
- Labor business organization
- Local government.

Common Reactions to Disaster by Adults
- Extreme sense of urgency
- Pain and fears
- Disbelief
- Discrimination and numbing
- Reluctance to abandon property
- Difficulty in making decision
- Need to help others
- Angered blaming
- Blaming and scapegoating.

Delayed Reactions
- Insomnia
- Headaches
- Apathy and depression
- Sense of powerlessness
- Guilt
- Moody and irritable
- Jealousy and resentment
- Domestic violence.

Children
- Regressive behaviors (bed bathing, thumb sucking, crying, clinging to patients)
- Fantasies that disaster never occurred
- Nightmares
- School-related problems, including an inability to concentrate and refusal to go back to school.

REHABILITATION

Introduction
Rehabilitation means retraining or restoring. Rehabilitation care helps the disabled patient to return to their normal life. Rehabilitation also helps in building confidence in the disabled people. Rehabilitation process starts at the onset of illness and includes not only the curing of illness but also the method of preventing further disability.

Definition
Rehabilitation is a dynamic process of maximizing an impaired person's potential by utilizing competencies and altering deficit to achieve the best quality of life possible. It involves prevention of further injury, stabilization and restoration of function, compensation, and adaptation to disability. Rehabilitation means retraining or restoring in contrast to the word habilitation, which refers to the initial capacity for learning. For example, when the baby first learns to walk, the process is habilitation, but when an individual learns to walk again, it is rehabilitation.

Rehabilitation Process
During the acute phase of illness, therapy and nursing care are directed toward assisting the patient to recover from disabling disease or injury with a minimum impairment, social, psychological, and physical. The prevention of secondary disabilities and provision of emotional security are equally important.

The restorative and retraining phase of rehabilitation follows when the patient's immediate life-saving needs have been met. The rehabilitation program requires measure to improve general physical condition, correction of deformities when indicated, passive and active exercise, and teaching the patient how to resume self-care. Therapy for specific disability includes speech therapy; training in the use of mechanical devices such as braces, crutches, and prostheses; and also teaching the family members how they may accept and help the patient.

Aims
The basic aims of rehabilitation are:
- Prevention of further limitation of body function
- Maintenance of existing abilities
- Restoration of as much function as possible

Components
Components of rehabilitation:
- Rehabilitation team
- Rehabilitation plan
- Rehabilitation outcome.

Rehabilitation Team
The team consists of a group of people working toward a common goal. Early rehabilitation teams were called multidisciplinary with each specialty having separate goals and approaches. This method offered the benefit or input from many specialties to the patient plan of care, but each discipline has individual goals.

The latest evolution in team dynamics is the transdisciplinary team in which mutual goals are formed. The distinguishing character in this model is that each member is responsible for sharing observation about all aspects of patient rehabilitation. Discipline may approach therapeutic treatment together rather than individually, as in the past. Physical and occupational therapies have joint therapy sessions with the patient to establish the most appropriate custom wheelchair for proper positioning. A speech pathologist, occupational therapist, and rehabilitation nurse may schedule a mealtime session with the dysphagic patient for assessment and establishment of approaches to feeding.

Composition of the Team

The team is composed of everyone, who has input to the rehabilitation plan. The number can range from 3 to 25 persons. The essential member of the rehabilitation team is the patient. It is the responsibility of the professionals on the team to help the patient to understand his/her active role on the team. In many rehabilitative settings, patients are called client to indicate the cooperative investment in recovery between the injured person and the rehabilitation professionals. The rehabilitation team evaluates the patient's need for rehabilitation and develops a plan to give maximum assistance in achieving rehabilitation goals. The success of the plan partially depends on the patient's attitude; therefore, the nurse should be guided by considering that the patient is a member of the team.

Rehabilitation Plan

Thorough assessment and evaluation of rehabilitation potential are the initial steps toward rehabilitation. Although it is difficult to predict a final outcome after trauma, there are parameters that help to determine the amount and rate of a patient's potential progress. Factors that influence rehabilitation potential are patient's age, length of time since injury, and availability of resources.

Factors That Represent Patient's Strength and Weakness

- **Physical factors:** For some injuries, there are well-established physical limits owing to normal anatomy and physiology. The limits change as technology and expertise increase. About 20 years ago, a C6 quadriplegic patient would not have been able to become functionally independent. Today, this is possible; perhaps in the future, there will be no physical limits because medical technology will be able to replace, rebuild, or stimulate the growth of a new spinal cord. It is important that rehabilitation professionals maintain their awareness of current research so that their patient can achieve maximum physical outcomes.
- **Cognitive psychosocial factors:** Cognitive factors include the patient's affinity for learning, ability to process and understand information, ability to make appropriate judgment and decisions, educational level, readiness to learn, and prior experience.
- **Psychosocial factors:** These include income, family system, outside stressors, roles, relationship, personal identity, and coping ability.

Evaluating Rehabilitation Potential

The evaluator first defines the rehabilitation outcome that would be typical for patient injury. Then, the potential was further defined by assigning a portability factor or percentage of predicted success to the estimated outcome. A candidate who has had a typical below knee amputation may have excellent potential for return to work and former lifestyle with prosthesis. However, if the evaluator factors include that the candidate is 53 years old and mildly mentally retarded, lives alone and has sustained multiple infections, then the candidate potential for success may drop to 70% of typical outcome.

Rehabilitation Outcome

An example of good outcome measurement includes measurement of function done during rehabilitation, admission, and discharge, followed by measurements done at 6 months and 1 year after discharge.

Nurse's Role as a Member of the Rehabilitation Team

The nurse may stimulate motivation through an attitude of respect for the patient and confidence in his/her ability to return to the highest level of independence possible. The longer contact the nurse has with the patient often provides the opportunity to act as a coordinator in planning the patient's day, thus enabling other team members to schedule their special rehabilitation services more effectively for the welfare of the patient.

CONCLUSION

Rehabilitation is a process that can be accomplished only through the coordinated efforts of all aspects of health and welfare disciplines. The meaning of rehabilitation is to restore capacity and ability, and to make satisfactory social adjustments. However, rehabilitation is a skilled job requiring patience, understanding, and genuine interest in people.

CHAPTER 65
Geriatric Considerations in Nursing

CHAPTER OUTLINE

- Concepts of Aging
- Demography: Myths and Realities
- Theories of Aging
- Age-related Body System Changes
- Pharamacokinetics
- Common Health Problems and Nursing Management; Concept of Old Age
- Disorders More Common in Older People
- Geriatric People Problems
- Psychosocial and Sexual Changes
- Abuse
- Role of Nurse for Caregivers of Elderly
- Use of Aids and Prosthesis (Hearing Aids Dentures)
- Provisions and Programs for Elderly: Privileges, Community Programs, and Health Services
- Home and Institutional Care

CONCEPTS OF AGING

Meaning of Geriatric, Gerontology, Gerontic

- "Geriatric" comes from the Greek words geras (old age) and iatro (relating to medical treatment)
- "Gerontology" comes from Greek, gero (old age) and ology (study)
- "Gerontological Nursing" coined by Gunter and Estes in 1979 define nursing care the service provider to older adults

1. **Geriatrics:** Geriatrics is the study of old age that includes the physiology, pathology, diagnosis, and management of the disorder and disease of older adults.
2. **Gerontology:** Gerontology is the combined biological, psychological, and sociologic study of older adults within their environment.
3. **Geriatric nursing:** It is the field of nursing that related to the assessment, nursing, diagnosis, planning, implementation, and evaluation of older adults in all environment, including acute intermediate and skilled care as well as within the community.
4. **Preventive geriatric:** It is the art and science of preventing disease in the geriatric population and promoting their health and efficiency.

Definition of Aging

Aging is defined as a genetic physiological process associated with morphological and functional changes in cellular and extracellular components aggravated by injury throughout life and resulting in a progressive imbalance of the control regulatory systems of the organism, including hormonal, neuroendocrine, and immune homeostatic mechanisms.
—King 1988

Normal Aging Process

Aging is a multidimensional process and refers to the process of "..accruing maturity with the passage of time." It begins with conception and continues throughout life until death occurs. Aging is progressive, ubiquitous, and inevitable to all living things.

Normal aging and diseases associated with aging are two separate entities. Normal aging refers to those normal deteriorative process that all human beings will experience if they live long enough, such as decreased bone mass, osteoarthritis, and lens cataracts. Diseases that are associated with aging, but not caused by aging and do not occur in all persons (i.e. probabilistic aging) include dementia, hypothyroidism, stroke, and congestive heart failure (CHF); while they are common they are not inevitable to all persons, and not all seniors will have them.

Landmarks of Geriatric Nursing

- 1950—First geriatric textbook published
- 1952—First geriatric nursing study published
- 1961—American Nurses Association (ANA) recommends specialty group for geriatric nurses
- 1966—Duke opens first Master's Clinical Nurse Specialist (CNS) program
- 1970—ANA Stands or Practice
- 1973—First Certification exam

Chapter 65: Geriatric Considerations in Nursing

- 1975—Journal of Gero Nursing by Slack, Inc.
- 1979—First national gero nursing conference
- 1981—ANA scope of practice
- 1984—National gerontological nursing association established
- 1988—First PhD program
- 1992—Nurses Improving Care for Healthsystem Elders (NICHE) established at New York University (NYU)
- 1996—John A Harford Foundation Institute of Geriatric Nursing established at NYU
- 1998—ANA certification available for advanced practice nurses (APNs).

DEMOGRAPHY: MYTHS AND REALITIES

Demographic of Aging in India

The elderly population (aged 60 years or above) account for 7.4% of total population in 2001. For males, it was marginally lower at 7.1%, while for females, it was 7.8%. Among states, the proportion varies from around 4% in small states like Dadra and Nagar Haveli, Nagaland Arunachal Pradesh, Meghalaya to more than 10.5% in Kerala.

- Both the share and size of elderly population is increasing over time. From 5.6% in 1961, it is projected to rise to 12.4% of population by the year 2026.
- The sex ratio among elderly people was as high as 1028 in 1951 but subsequently dropped to about 938 in 1971 and finally reached 972 in 2001 and 939 in 2014.
- The life expectancy at birth during 2002-06 was 64.2 for females as against 62.6 years for males. At age 60, average remaining length of life was found to be about 18 years (16.7 for males and 18.9 for females) and that at age 70 was less than 12 years (10.9 for males and 12.4 for females).
- There is sharp rise in age-specific death rate with age from 20 (per thousand) for persons in age group 60-64 years to 80 among those aged 75-79 years and 200 for persons aged more than 85 years.
- The old-age dependency ratio climbed from 10.9% in 1961 to 13.1% in 2001 for India as a whole. For females and males, the value of the ratio was 13.8% and 12.5% in 2001.
- About 65% of the aged had to depend on other for their day-to-day maintenance. Less than 20% of elderly women but a majority of elderly men were economically independent.
- Among economically dependent elderly men 6-7% were financially supported by their spouses, almost 85% by their own children, 2% by grandchildren, and 6% by others. Of elderly women, less than 20% depended on their spouses, more than 70% on their children, 3% on grandchildren, and 6% or more on others including the nonrelations. Of the economically independent men, more than 90% as against 65% of women were reported to have one or more dependents.
- Among the rural elderly persons, almost 50% had a monthly per capita expenditure level between ₹ 420 and ₹ 775 and among the urban elderly persons, almost half of aged had monthly per capita expenditure between ₹ 665 and 1500 in 2002.
- Nearly 40% of persons aged 60 years and above (60% of men and 19% of women)
- Were working in rural areas 66% of elderly men and above 23% of aged women were still participating in economic activity, while in urban areas, only 39% of elderly men and about 7% of elderly women were economically active.
- Even in 2007-08, only 50% men and 20% of women aged 60 years or more were literate through formal schooling.
- In rural areas, 55% of the aged with sickness and 77% of those without sickness felt that they were in a good or fair condition of health. In urban areas, the respective proportions were 63% and 78%.
- The proportion of elderly men and women physically mobile decline from about 94% in the age group 60-64 years to about 72% for men and 63-65% for women of age 80 or more.
- Prevalence of heart diseases among elderly population was much higher in urban areas than in rural parts.
- About 64 per thousand elderly persons in rural areas and 55 per thousand in urban areas suffer from one or more disabilities. Most common disability among the aged persons was loco motor disability as 3% of them suffer from it.
- In age groups beyond 60 years, the percentage of elderly women married was markedly lower than the percentage of men married.
- More than 75% of elderly males and less than 40% of elderly females live with their spouse. Less than 20% of aged men and about half of the women live with their children (Tables 65.1 and 65.2).

Incidence of Geriatric Population

- 1980—5.3%
- 2000—7.7%
- 2025—13.3% (1.2 billion)
- 71%—Developing World
- 70 million population in India—2001
- 177 million population—2025
- 40% below poverty line
- 73% illiterate.

Categorizing the Aging Population

55–64	Older
65–74	Elderly
75–84	Aged
>85	Extremely aged

Or

60–74	Young old
75–84	Middle old
>85	Old old

Present Geriatric Problems (Current Scenario) in India

- Cataract and visual impairment—88%
- Arthritis and locomotion disorder—40%
- Cardiovascular disease (CVD) and hypertension (HT)—18%
- Neurological problems—18%
- Respiratory problems including chronic bronchitis—16%
- GI tract (GIT) problems—9%
- Psychiatric problems—9%
- Loss of hearing—8%.

Aim of Geriatric Nursing

- Maintenance of health in old age by high levels of engagement and avoidance of disease
- Early detection and appropriate treatment of disease
- Maintenance of maximum independence consistent with irreversible disease and disability
- Sympathetic care and support during terminal illness (Flowchart 65.1).

THEORIES OF AGING (FIG. 65.1 AND TABLE 65.1)

Biological Theories

Biologic views, aging is defined as the progressive loss of function. This age-related decreased occurs along with decreasing fertility and increasing mortality.

No one knows why we age, and the upper limits of the human life span, about 120 years, have not altered over the interval of recorded history despite advances in preventative health care and medicine that have occurred over the last few centuries. While many more persons can live longer today because of these advances (the so-called "rectangularization" of the survival curve. Due to increased survival and concentration of deaths around the mean age at death to older ages.

Using the tools of molecular and cellular biology along with modern genetics, various investigators have proposed a variety of hypotheses for why we age. Below you can find some of these current theories of aging, and none of them are mutually exclusive (Fig. 65.2).

Table 65.1: Theories of aging.

Theory	Concept
DNA damage theories	Various cellular mechanisms constantly repair ongoing occurring DNA damage (i.e. caused by radiation, mutation). The repair efficiency is positively correlated with life span and decreases with age
Oxidative damage/free radicals	Life span is inversely proportional to the extent of oxidative damage caused by unstable and reactive chemical compounds and directly proportional to antioxidant activity
Error catastrophe	Faulty DNA/RNA transcriptional and/or RNA translational processes produce ineffective or toxic proteins
Programmed aging	Cells are programmed with a specific, finite number of divisions and cell death occurs when this number is achieved (i.e. the "Hayflick limit" of 50 doubling of cells seen in tissue culture for fibroblasts). Telomeres (proteins that act like plastic ends of shoelaces to seal the ends of chromosomes, shorten with each division; once the telomere is gone, the end begins to "fray"). This has been suggested as the biological "clock" for aging
Apoptosis	Programmed cell death induced by extracellular signals or "gerontogenes" that tag a cell for removal by phagocytosis
Cross link theory	Chemical bonds form between and within molecules and effect function (e.g. cross-linking in collagen causes loss of elasticity in blood vessels)
"Wear-and-tear"	Ordinary insults and injuries of daily living accommodate and decrease the organism's efficiency to subvital levels.
Immunological theories	Damage to the immune-system makes the body vulnerable to disease. B and T cells are less effective and less numerous as we age
Neuro-endocrine theories	Failure of cells with specific integrative functions (in the pituitary, thyroid, adrenal, pancreas, and gonadal glands) bring about gradual homeostatic failure
Age versus cancer theory (Jan 2002)	Aging may be a side effect of the natural safeguards that protect us from cancer. Over expression of tumor suppressor genes in transgenic mice causes premature aging

Stochastic theory: According to this theory, aging is due to chance.

Nonstochastic theory: According to this theory, aging is not chance.

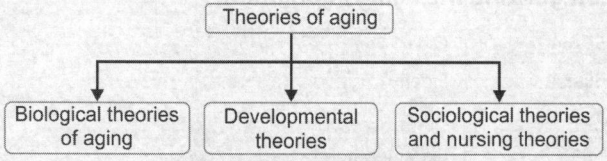

Fig. 65.1: Theories of aging.

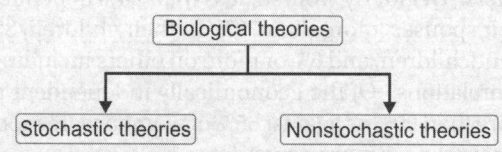

Fig. 65.2: Biological theory.

Stochastic Theories

1. **Error theory:** Aging is due to accumulation of metabolic product in cells.
2. **Somatic theory:** According to this theory, body cells spontaneously develop mutations in the same way germ cells do subsequent cell division perpetuate the mutations until organs become inefficient and ultimately fail.
3. **Intrinsic mutagenesis:** Based on this theory, increased in mutational cells occurs because of a breakdown of the genetic regulatory mechanism.
4. **Free radicals theory:** According to Harman 1956, a free radical is highly reactive atom or molecule that carries an unpaired electron and thus seeks to combine with another molecule causing oxidative process.
5. **Cross link theory:** This theory postulates that over time results of exposure to chemicals and radiation in the environment cross link lipids, proteins, and carbohydrates, as well as nucleic acids. These cross links result in decreased flexibility and elasticity and decreased rigidity in tissues.

Nonstochastic Theories

1. **Programmed theory of cell death:** It is proposed that there is an impairment in the ability of cell to continue dividing, a more recent theory of aging is the telomere-telomerase hypothesis.
2. **Neuroendocrine theory:** It proposed that aging occurs because of functional decrements in neurons associated hormones.
3. **Immunologic theory:** It proposes declining functional capacity of the immune system as the basis for aging as given in Table 65.1.
4. **Developmental theory:** It is proposed by Erikson in the year of 1963.
   According to this theory, the person life consists of eight stages, each representing a crucial turning point in life stretching from birth to death.
5. **Sociological theories:** According to this theory, aging attempts to predict and explain the social interaction and roles that contribute to successful adjustment to old age in old adults.
6. **Nursing theory:** It is proposed by Miller in the year 2004. Miller suggests that nurse can alter that outcome for patients through nursing intervention that address the consequences of these changes.

AGE-RELATED BODY SYSTEM CHANGES

Many normal changes can lead to clear clinical consequences. Not all these changes with aging are necessarily bad; for example, autoimmune disease may "burn out" in later life. However, you should be aware of some general themes, which may explain why disease presentation in the elderly can be a typical (i.e. diminished perception of acute pain may alter the presentation of pancreatitis, or myocardial infarction, etc.), and older adults are more likely to die because of a pneumonia (decreased immune system, decreased respiratory function and reserve) (Table 65.2).

Table 65.2: Age related body system changes.

System	Problems	Needs
Cardiovascular	• Decreased cardiac output • Diminished ability to response to stress • Heart rate and stroke volume do not increase with maximum demand • Increase blood pressure	• Exercise regularly: Pace activities; avoid smoking, low salt diet participation in stress reduction activities • Checked blood pressure regularly • Medication compliance • Weight control
Respiratory	• Increased in residual volume • Decreased in vital capacity • Decreased gas exchange and diffusing capacity • Decreased cough efficiency	• Exercise regularly • Avoid smoking; take adequate fluids to liquefy secretion • Receive yearly influenza immunization • Avoid expose to upper respiratory tract infection
Integumentary system	• Decreased protection against trauma and sun exposure • Decreased protection against temperature extremes • Diminished secretion of natural oils and perspiration	• Avoid solar exposure • Dress appropriately for temperature; maintain a safe indoor temperature • Shower preferable to tub • Lubricate skin
Reproductive	Female: • Vaginal narrowing and decreased elasticity • Decreased vaginal secretion • Decreased size of penis and testes male and female—slower sexual response	• May require vaginal estrogen replacement • Gynecology/urology follow-up • Use lubricate with intercourse
Muscular skeletal	• Loss of bone density • Loss of strength and size • Degenerated joint cartilage	• Exercise regularly • Eat high calcium diet • Limit phosphorus intake • Take calcium and vitamin D supplementation

Contd...

Contd...

System	Problems	Needs
Genitourinary	• Male: Benign prostate hyperplasia • Female: Relaxed perinea muscles, detrusor instability, urethral dysfunction	• Seek referral to urology specialist • Ready access to toilet • Wear easily manipulated clothing • Drink adequate fluids • Avoid bladder irritants • Pelvic floor exercise
Gastrointestinal	• Decreased salivation • Difficulty in swallowing food • Delayed esophageal and gastric emptying • Reduced gastrointestinal motility	• Use ice chips • Mouth wash • Brush, floss, and massage gum daily • Receive regular dental care • Eat small and frequent meal • Sit up and avoid heavy activates after eating • Limit antacids • Eat high fiber • Low fat diet limit laxatives • Toilet regularly • Drink adequate fluids
Nervous system	• Reduced speed in nerve conduction • Increase confusion with physically illness and loss of environmental cues • Reduced cerebral circulation	• Pace teaching; with hospitalization • Encourage visitors • Enhance sensory stimulation • With sudden confusion look for cause • Encourage slow rising from a resting position
Special senses	Vision: • Diminished ability to focus on close objects • Inability to tolerate glare • Difficulty adjusting to changes of light intensity • Decreased ability to distinguish colors	Vision • Wear eyeglasses • Use sunglasses outdoors • Avoid abrupt change from dark to light • Use adequate indoor lighting with area lights and highlights • Use large print books • Use magnifiers for reading • Avoid night driving • Use contrasting color for color coding • Avoid glare of shiny surface and direct sunlight
	Hearing • Decreased ability to hear high frequency sounds	• Recommend a hearing examination • Reduced background noise • Face person enunciate clearly • Speak with low pitched voice • Use nonverbal cues
	Taste and smell • Decreased ability to taste and smell	• Encourage use of lemon, spices, herbs

Oral Cavity

❖ 40% of those >65 are edentulous, mostly because of neglect rather than any natural age-related process.
❖ Risk of caries increases with age as a result of gingival recession and loss of jaw bone density.

Voice

❖ Ossification of the laryngeal cartilages causes stiffness; prevents vocal cords coming together while speaking, resulting in a weaker, breathy voice.
❖ In males, the vocal cords become thin and atrophied with age, resulting in a higher pitched conversational voice.
❖ In females, loss of hormonal influence leads to vocal cords becoming more edematous after menopause, resulting in a lower pitched voice.

Eyes

❖ Presbyopia (loss of lens accommodation) due to hardening and thickening of the lens (making it opaque) and decrease in muscle tone
❖ Decreased visual acuity (VA) because of narrowed pupil, fewer rods (cones spared) so poorer night vision; there is also the need for more light to reach the retina (on average, an older person needs 4× more light than a younger person); additional problems with depth and color perception
❖ Flattening of the corneal surface (with diminished refraction) and clouding of lens.

Ears

❖ Presbycusis; high sound frequencies lost and impaired speech discrimination

Chapter 65: Geriatric Considerations in Nursing

- More prone to excess cerumen (ear wax) occlusion of ear canal, which becomes narrower and more tortuous.

Respiratory System
- Age-related changes resemble emphysema
- Loss of elastic recoil
- Early airway closure (and more dead space where you are ventilating nonperfused lung)
- Decreased arterial PO2 (-4 mm/decade)
- Decreased flow rates, FEV 1, and vital capacity
- Stiffer chest wall and weak muscles
- Increased dead space.

Endocrine System
- Progressive decline in carbohydrate tolerance and increasing insulin resistance
- Decreased aldosterone, renin, calcitonin, and growth hormone
- Slightly decreased (or no change) in thyroid hormones T3 and T4, cortisol, insulin, epinephrine, parathyroid hormone (PTH), and 25-hydroxy vitamin D
- Increase in follicle-stimulating hormone (FSH), luteinizing hormone (LH), and norepinephrine
- In women, decreased estrogen (postmenopause) and prolactin
- In men, decreased testosterone in some (so-called andropause).

Cardiovascular System
- Arterial wall stiffening (true and "pseudohypertension")
- Increased L atrial size and prevalence of S4 heart sound
- Reduced left ventricular (LV) compliance caused by increased myocyte size, increased LV mass, and increased posterior wall thickness (infiltration with lipids, collagen, fat, amyloid)
- Cardiac output decreases at rest/exertion; maximal HR decreases (predicted max is 220—age in years), much less in physically active elders with disease.

Gastrointestinal System
- Reduced lower esophageal sphincter (LES) tone
- Decreased acid production (leading to decreased emptying, less calcium absorption, and differential medication absorption)
- Reduced intrinsic factor
- Decreased liver mass and blood flow leading to reduced oxidative metabolism of some drugs (but not acetylation) and protein synthesis
- Increased transit time
- Increased rectal resting tone and decreased contracting pressure.

Genital/Sexual System
As a rule of thumb, "Everything slows down!".

Male
- More intense stimulation needed for erection
- Erections less firm
- Ejaculation takes longer, less volume and intensity
- Longer refractory period.

Female
- Estrogen-dependent changes [vaginal lubrication slower atrophy (thin epithelium, honeymoon cystitis)]
- Slower reaction of clitoris
- Prolonged refractory period.

Hematologic and Immune Systems
- T-cell: Numbers decrease, delayed hypersensitivity reaction m decreased, fewer natural killer and suppressor cells
- B-cell: Numbers stable, but make fewer antibodies.

Renal System
- Smaller kidneys (cortical renal mass decreases—20%)
- Renal blood flow (RBF) decreases
- Glomerular filtration rate (GFR) progressively decreases; average decline is 50% from age 20–80, but those 80+ show little decline
- More prone to develop syndrome of inappropriate antidiuretic hormone secretion (SIADH).

Musculoskeletal System
- Weight decreases, body fat increases, height decreases (in women especially)
- Sarcopenia (up to 80% decrease in skeletal muscle mass and quality in non-active seniors)
- Osteopenia (decrease in bone mass)
- Total body calcium and potassium stores decreases.

Dermatological System
- Flattening of the dermal–epidermal junction, leading to more thin and fragile skin susceptible to tearing and sheer forces
- Dermal atrophy, and progressive loss of elastic tissue subcutaneous fat leading to lines and wrinkling and problems with thermal regulation
- Loss of melanocytes, and retreat of the dermal plexus leading to pallor and increased vulnerability to sum damage and skin cancer
- Hair graying and hair loss.

Neurological System
- Decrease in brain mass and selected loss of cortical neurons (1% per year loss after age 60)
- 20% decrease in cerebral blood flow from age 30 to 70
- Decreased smell and taste perception
- Reduced perception of acute pain
- Impaired postural reflexes

- Increased reaction time (up to 30% longer)
- Alterations of neurotransmitter levels
- Increased monoamine oxidase (MAO) levels
- Decreased dopamine (and binding sites), norepinephrine, and a slight decline in gamma-aminobutyric acid (GABA) levels.

Sleep
- Less sleep required, but sleep latency increased.
- Reduced slow-wave sleep (sleep stages 3 and 4)
- Increased rapid eye movement (REM) but shorter; decreased REM latency (may compensate)
- Increased night awakenings and sleep fragmentation.

PHARAMACOKINETICS

Medication of Elderly Patient
Older people use more medication than any other age group.

Goal of Drugs in Elderly
- Improve the health and well-being of older people by relieving pain and discomfort
- Treating chronic illness
- Curing infectious.

Polypharmacy—Multidrug and Intervention
Altered pharmacokinetics: Alteration in absorption, metabolism distribution, and exacerbation occur on result of normal aging may also result from drugs and food intervention.
- Due to decreased gastric pH
- Due to decreased body water
- Decreased blood flow of liver and renal and cardiac output.

Steps for Improving Medication Compliance
- Explain the purpose adverse effects.
- Provide medication schedule.
- Encourage the use of standard contains without safety side.
- Remove old, unused medication.
- Encourage the patient to keep a list all medication.
- Review medication schedule periodically.
- Suggest use of multiple day multi dose medication.

Absorption
Unaltered in patients with an intact gastric mucosa.

Distribution
- Decreased body water content: Increased serum concentration + longer activity of water soluble drugs.
- Increased body fat: Longer pharmacological activity of highly lipid soluble drugs.
- Decreased scrum albumin: More free drug available with high protein bounds drugs.
- Increased alpha glycoprotein (an acute phase reactant); enhanced binding of basic drugs (lidocaine).

Metabolism
- Function of the microsomal mixed-function oxidative system declines with age, resulting in decreasing metabolism of drugs.
- Conjugative process does not appear to be altered.
- Decreased hepatic size and blood flow may reduce drug metabolism even if liver function tests (LFTs) are normal.

Elimination
- Beginning in the fourth decade of life, there is a 6–10 reduction in GFR and in RBF every 10 years.
- A decline in muscle may mask the reduction in GFR.
- Reduced tubular excretion.
- HT is common and can reduce real function.
- Drugs eliminated primarily by renal excretion should be dosed differently; for every X% clearance reduction, dose often decreased by X% and interval increased by X%.
- Common drugs eliminated primarily by the kidneys such as Digoxin beta-blockers, angiotensin-converting-enzyme (ACE) inhibitors, aminoglycoside antibiotics, lithium, nonsteroidal anti-inflammatory drugs (NSAIDs).

Pharmacodynamics
- Increased tissue sensitivity to drugs acting on the central nervous system (CNS)
- Decreased beta-receptors sensitivity to agonists and antagonists.

Optimal Pharmacotherapy
To be informed of
- Presenting symptoms
- Detailed medication history and allergies
- Patients finical situation drug benefit coverage
- Patient views on taking medication
- History of dysphagia.

Medication Information Needed
Clinical pharmacology and side effects of the drug.

Other Principles
- Educate the patients and the caregiver about the medication
- Have a simple treatment regimen
- Prescribe liquid formulations when necessary
- Review medication regularly (discontinue if unnecessary)
- New symptoms and illness may be caused by a drug.

Drugs to Avoid in the Elderly

Amitriptyline (Elavil)
Use less anticholinergic agent; change to nortriptyline (same dose), or use a selective serotonin reuptake inhibitor (SSRI) antidepressant instead.

Benztropine (Cogentin)
Used to treat EPS side effects of older neuroleptics, as well as in Parkinson's, but itself can cause confusion and delirium itself, taper gradually and observe.

Cimetidine
Use a less anticholinergic H2 blocker (i.e. Ranitidine). Ask, do they need it, and if the need is established, consider an alternative.

Dimenhydrinate (Gravol)
Too anticholinergic (and a major cause of delirium in older adults); try using Domperidone instead for nausea.

Fluoxetine (Prozac)
Very long half-life; try newer SSRI antidepressants.

Indomethacin (Indocid)
Safer agents less likely to cause NSAID gastropathy are readily available, such as COX-2 inhibitors (or Acetominophen if noninflammatory pain).

Long-acting Benzodiazepines (Valium, Dalmane, Librium)
Use short-acting agents (i.e. Lorazapam, Oxazepam) as they can cause excess sedation and cognitive impairments. Avoid entirely, if possible.

Methyldopa
Safer agents available for controlling blood pressure.

Pentazocine (Talwin)
Safer, more effective agents available.

Propranolol
Other beta-blockers cause fewer central CNS effects (i.e. atenolol).

Theophylline
Can cause nausea, vomiting, and seizures in seniors, especially if liver impairment. Other safer asthma medications are available.

The term elderly mistreatment (EM) is used to describe acts of commission (elderly abuse) or (omission or elder neglect). The harm or threaten to harm an older adults welfare or health.

COMMON HEALTH PROBLEMS AND NURSING MANAGEMENT; CONCEPT OF OLD AGE

Old age consists of ages nearing or surpassing the average life span of human beings, and thus the end of the human life cycle. Euphemisms and terms for old people include seniors (American usage), senior citizens (British and American usage), and the elderly. As occurs with almost any definable group of humanity, some people will hold a prejudice against others in this case, against old people. This is one form of ageism.

Old people have limited regenerative abilities and are more prone to disease, syndromes, and sickness than other adults. For the biology of aging, see senescence. The medical study of the aging process is gerontology and the study of diseases that afflict the elderly is geriatrics.

Health Problems in Old Age Patients

- ❖ Heart disease like coronary artery disease, myocardial infraction, HT
- ❖ Cancer
- ❖ Stroke
- ❖ Alcohol abuse
- ❖ Smoking
- ❖ Nutritional problems
- ❖ Sensory impairment
- ❖ Pain
- ❖ Dementia
- ❖ Urinary incontinence.

Role of Nurse and Nursing Process Application

List of Nursing Diagnoses

Risk for dehydration
Older patients are at greater risk for dehydration and malnutrition during hospitalization

Intervention
- ❖ Getting the patient out of the bed
- ❖ Encouraging patient to take more fluids
- ❖ Monitoring level of hydration
- ❖ Administering small and frequent diet
- ❖ If severe dehydration administering intravenous (IV) fluids.

Risk for urinary incontinence
Due sphincter muscle dysfunction patient cannot able to control urination.

Intervention
- ❖ Monitoring patient's intake and output chart
- ❖ Catheterization of patient
- ❖ Catheter care given daily to prevent urinary tract infection (UTI)
- ❖ Apply any pads if patients cant cooperate
- ❖ Restricted mobility
- ❖ Avoiding diuretics medication.

Risk for skin breakdown
The increased risks of skin breakdown changes in aging skin and to situation that arise in the acute care setting.

Intervention
- ❖ Applying water gloves in pressure points

- ❖ Applying Vaseline gel to prevent skin breakdown
- ❖ Giving bed bath and back care to reduce pressure sore
- ❖ Provided air or water bed
- ❖ Bed making without wrinkles.

Risk for falling

Due to memory impairment and improper coordination, the patients are high risk for falling.

Intervention
- ❖ Putting side
- ❖ Assisting the patient to getting out of bed or doing other activities
- ❖ Monitoring patients
- ❖ Allowing the visitors to staying with patients
- ❖ Putting fall leaf in patient bed.

Common Nursing Diagnosis

Impaired Physical Mobility
- ❖ Increase participation in physical mobility
- ❖ Maintain normal physical and anatomic function and structure
- ❖ Remain free from joint contractures and foot drops
- ❖ Maintain or increase strength and mobility using assistive devices.

Activity Intolerance

Nursing interventions

1. Identify the prescribed activity level
2. Continue to assess strength and joint mobility
3. Perform physical mobility activities in conjunction with daily care
4. Provide good body alignment and frequent position changes
5. Avoid unnecessary restraints that limits physical mobility
6. Consult with the physical therapist to determine a suitable activity/exercise plan to maintain muscle strength and joint mobility
7. Verify that the individual is suitably dressed for activity and that he or she has the proper footwear
8. Provide pain medication in a timely manner so that maximal benefits from the medication occur when greatest physical effort is expected
9. Verify that individual knows the correct method for using assistive devices and that he or she does in fact use them for activity
10. Encourage wheelchair bound patients to move by using their arms or feet whenever possible
11. Provide adequate assistance during ambulation.

Nutritional Imbalanced Nutrition: Less than Body Requirement

- ❖ Imbalanced nutrition—more than body requirements
- ❖ Risk for imbalanced nutrition
- ❖ Readiness for enhanced nutrition
- ❖ Assessment
  - ➤ Appetite
  - ➤ Nutritional intake
  - ➤ Social and cultural factor
  - ➤ Laboratory values: Hb, hematocrit, blood urea nitrogen (BUN), electrolytes
- ❖ Nursing goal/outcome management
  - ➤ Maintain body weight within normal limit
  - ➤ Obtain adequate nutrients to maintain healthy tissue
  - ➤ Identify internal and external cues that influence eating patterns
  - ➤ Adhere to a prescribed therapeutic diet.

Interventions

1. Assess the individual carefully to determine the causes of a problem
2. Schedule weekly weight checks
3. Keep a dietary record of the amount, type, and frequency of food intake
4. Explain the importance of nutrition to overall health or disease control
5. Determine food like and dislikes
6. Monitor laboratory values
7. Assess the condition of the skin, hair, nails, and mucus membrane
8. Consult dietician
9. Institute measures to increase or decrease nutritional intake
10. Complete a thorough documentation of nutritional status, including assessment, interventions, referrals, and patient response.

Communication
- ❖ The most effective way to bridge the gap between the generations is good communication
- ❖ Provide a conducive environment to establish good rapport with elderly
- ❖ Be an empathetic listener
- ❖ Give importance to nonverbal communication.

Nonverbal communication
- ❖ Major communication comes from nonverbal forms:
  - ➤ Verbal: 7%
  - ➤ Nonverbal: 93% (paralinguistic cues – 38%; tone, pitch, volume of voice + 55% from body cues)
- ❖ Consider cultural background of patient.

Symbols:

For example, in health care settings, uniform styles and colors help patients distinguish the various caregivers.

Tone of voice:

For example, whisper, shout, whine.

Chapter 65: Geriatric Considerations in Nursing

Body language:
Different body positions.

Space, distance, and position:

- Space: The use of personal space in communication is called as proxemics
- Distance:
  - Public space: 12 feet
  - Social space: 4–12 feet
  - Personal space: 18 inch to 4 feet
  - Intimate space: <18 inch
- Position: Gestures
  - Facial expressions
  - Eye contact
  - Pace or speed of communication
  - Time and timing
  - Touch
  - Silence
  - Informing
  - Direct questioning
  - Open-ended questioning
  - Confronting
  - Social communication.

Selfcare Deficit

- Bathing/hygiene
- Dressing/grooming
- Toileting.

DISORDERS MORE COMMON IN OLDER PEOPLE

A number of disorders are more common in older adults than in younger persons. They are not caused by aging itself, and do not occur in all older adults.

There is insufficient space to list a few of the more common disorders here (more trans-system problems can be found in the section of Geriatric Giants), and readers are advised to consult their favorite and trusted.

Anemia

- Using World Health Organization (WHO) criteria (Hb < 120 g/L in women and <130 g/L in men), the prevalence of anemia in the elderly ranges from 8% to 44%, with the highest prevalence in men 85 years and older
- A cause can be found in 80 percent of elderly patients
- The most common causes of anemia are anemia of chronic disease and iron deficiency, but Vitamin B12 deficiency, folate deficiency
- GI bleeding and myelodysplastic syndrome are also common causes.

Atrial Fibrillation

- The prevalence of atrial fibrillation increases with age, about 3% in those in their early 60s, and is up to 10% in those older than 80.
- Atrial fibrillation is associated with a higher risk of cardiovascular death, CHF and peripheral embolic stroke in older patients.

Cardiovascular Disease

- CVD is the leading cause of death in older
- HT, the best predictor of coronary artery disease, increases dramatically in prevalence with aging; isolated systolic HT occurs in 34% of men and 38% of women aged 65–74
- 50% of Canadian seniors are on no treatment at all for HT
- CHF is the most common cause of hospitalization among those aged 65+ in the US.

Management

The current standard of therapy for HF includes diuretics, angiotensin converting enzyme inhibitors, and digoxin.

- Several large studies have also indicated that carefully monitored, low-dose beta blocker and spironolactone can decrease mortality
- Cardiovascular health can be promoted by regular exercise
- Proper diet
- Weight control
- Regular blood pressure measurements
- Stress management
- Smoking cessation to avoid lightheadedness, fainting, and possible falls caused by orthostatic hypotension
- The older person should be counseled to rise slowly to avoid straining when having a bowel movement
- To consider having five or six small meals each day
- Hard work should be limited to not more than 20 min on hot summer days
- Exposure to wind to cold weather should also be avoided because of the risk of dizziness of falling.

Cancer

- Lung cancer is the most common cause of cancer-related deaths in both men and women; 68% of cases occur in people over 65
- >50% of breast cancer patients are older than 65 at diagnosis
- Prostate cancer is the most commonly diagnosed cancer among elderly.

Cerebrovascular Disease (Stroke)

- One Canadian study estimated 4.1% of people aged 65+ in the community are living with the effects of stroke
- Seniors who experienced stroke more often reported their health to be "poor" or "fair" than seniors who had not (69% versus 25%).

Respiratory System

- Osteoporotic collapse of vertebrae resulting in kyphosis

- Calcification of the costal cartilages and reduced mobility of the ribs
- Diminished efficiency of the respiratory muscles
- Increased rigidity or loss of elastic recoil in the lung results in increased residual lung volume and decreased vital capacity.

Health Promotion Activities Include
- Regular exercise
- Appropriate fluid intake
- Pneumococcal vaccination
- Yearly influenza immunizations
- Smoking cessation and frequent hand hygiene are prudent health practices
- Hospitalized older adults should be frequently reminded to cough and take deep breaths.

Chronic Obstructive Pulmonary Disease (COPD)
- COPD is the fourth-leading killer diseases of the elderly in Canada.
- Cigarette smoke is the underlying cause in 80-90% of cases.
- Prevalence of COPD for those aged 65-74 years is 5.0%; and for those over 75 years is 6.8%.

Pneumonia
Influenza/pneumonia is a major contributor to deaths and hospitalization in the elderly and is the leading cause of death from infectious disease.

Gastrointestinal System
- Periodical decrease leading to tooth decay and loss of teeth is common
- The older person may experience a dry mouth
- Major complaints often center on fallings mobility may decrease, resulting in delayed emptying of stomach contents
- Diminished secretion of acid and pepsin reduced the absorption of iron calcium, and vitamin B12
- Absorption of nutrients in the small intestine also appears to diminish with age
- The incidence of gallstones and common bile duct stones increases progressively with advancing years
- It may also develop from dysfunction of the striated and smooth muscles of the GIT
- Aspiration of food or fluid is the most serious complication.

Dementia
Alzheimer's disease (AD) is the leading cause of dementia.

Diabetes Mellitus (DM)
- Diabetes has a prevalence of 13% in persons over 65
- Type II DM is the most common form of diabetes in the elderly, accounting for about 92% of cases, and is the sixth leading cause of death in men over 65
- The consent of Type II DM occurs 40% of the time after the age of 60, and there is often a long delay before diagnosis
- Long-term studies have shown that 35% of seniors with diabetes suffer from retinopathy 18% from CVD, 30% from peripheral vascular disease, and 12% from nephropathy.

Hypothyroidism
- One US survey of community dwelling elders found 7% of women and 3% men between 60 and 89 years of age with this hormone deficiency
- The Canadian Study on Health and Aging (CSHA) found 9% of their study population had subclinical hypothyroidism.

Osteoarthritis
Estimates from the Osteoporosis Society of Canada suggest that 1.4 million Canadians have osteoporosis, a leading risk factor for bone fractures and death or morbidity after a fall.

Parkinson's Disease (PD)
- Roughly 1/100 persons in North America are affected
- Average age of diagnosis is 60; the rates rise in persons >70
- Dementia, a feared complication, increases in prevalence with age; it occurs in approximately 30% of patients with advanced PD.

Prostate Disease
Symptomatic benign prostatic hypertrophy (BPH) is very common, affecting 40-50% of men aged 51-60 years, and 80% of men by age 80.

Skin Disease
- US datum show that 20% of all GP visits for those 65+ are motivated by a skin problem (i.e. rash, pruritus, photo aging, cancer)
- Surveys show that two-thirds of those 65+ have at least one dermatological disorder. Physiological changes in aging skin when combined with immobility and incontinence predispose elderly persons to have pressure ulcers; prevalence rate in acute care range from 3.5% to 30% and in long term care facilities from 2.4% to 23%.

Integumentary System
- Changes occur that affect the function and appearance of the skin.
- The epidermis and dermis become thinner.
- Elastic fibers are reduced in number and collagen becomes stiffer.
- Subcutaneous fat diminishes, particularly in the extremities.
- Decreased numbers of capillaries in the skin result in diminished blood supply.

- Hair pigmentation decreases resulting in gradual graying.
- The skin becomes drier and susceptible to irritations because of decreased activity of the sebaceous and sweat glands.

Strategies to Promote Healthy Skin Function Include

- Avoiding exposure to the sun
- Using a lubricating skin cream
- Avoiding long soaks in the tub
- Maintaining adequate intake of water.

Sexual Dysfunction

- Erectile dysfunction (ED) is the most common form of sexual dysfunction in elderly men, affecting nearly 70% of men age 70.
- The prevalence of sexual dysfunction in elderly women is largely unknown, but reduced libido, inhibited orgasm, and dyspareunia are the most common disorders, and are largely due to the decline of estrogen production.

Reproductive System

Changes Occurring in the Female Reproductive System Include

- Thinning of the vaginal wall, along with narrowing in size and loss of elasticity
- Resulting in vaginal dryness, itching, and decreased acidity
- Involution of the uterus and ovaries
- Decreased pubococcygeal muscle tone, resulting in a relaxed vaginal bleeding and painful intercourse.

In Older Men

- The penis and testes decrease in size, and levels of androgens diminish.
- ED may develop with concomitant CVD, neurologic disorders, diabetes, or even respiratory disease.
- Sexual desire and activity decline but do not disappear.
- The use of vacuum penile pumps, local injection or placement of medication into the urethral opening has proved effective for some patients.

UTIs

- Prevalence of asymptomatic bacteriuria in the elderly range from 15% to 60% depending on the study, with twice as many females as men affected.
- The annual incidence of symptomatic bacterial UTIs is estimated to be as high as 10% in those over 65.

Genitourinary System

Changes in Kidney Function Include

- Decreased filtration rate
- Diminished tubular function with a less efficiency in reabsorbing

- Concentrating the urine older women often suffer from stress or urge incontinence or both
- Benign prostatic hyperplasia which is a common finding in older men causes a gradual increase in urine
- Older women often suffer from stress or urgent incontinence or both
- Prostate cancer, a slow-growing cancer, is most often seen in men older than 70 years of age
- Kidney and bladder cancers are most frequently seen after the age of 50 years.

Musculoskeletal System

- A gradual, progressive decrease in bone mass begins before the age of 40 years
- Excessive loss of bone density results in osteoporosis, which affects both older men and women
- Its typical form is associated with inactivity, inadequate calcium intake, and a history after cigarette smoking
- Osteoporotic changes of the spine, kyphosis, and flexion of the hips and knees
- The muscles diminish in size and lose strength flexibility and endurance with decreased activity and advanced age
- Beginning in middle age, the cartilage of joints progressively deteriorates
- Calcium supplements, vitamin fluoride, estrogens, and weight-bearing exercises are often prescribed for the person who is at high risk.

Nervous System

- The loss of nerve cells contributes to a progressive loss of brain mass
- The synthesis and metabolism of the major neurotransmitters are also reduced
- The autonomic nervous system performs less efficiently and postural hypotension, which causes the person to lose consciousness
- Homeostasis is more difficult to maintain
- Mental function is threatened by physical or emotional stressors
- Slowed reaction time places the older person at risk for falls and injuries, including driving errors.

Vision Loss

- Thirteen percent of Canadians over age 65 have some form of visual impairment
- Almost 8% of seniors over 65 (and 11% if over 80) have impairment (blindness in both eyes) sufficient to meet the legal definition of blindness (VA less than 20/200)
- 11% of Canadians between 65 and 74 years of age and 30% of persons over the age of 75 have age-related macular degeneration (ARMD), the most common cause of irreversible vision loss in seniors
- Diabetic retinopathy accounts for 35% of all cases of blindness; prevalence increases with age and the duration of the disease

- The prevalence of lens cataracts sufficient to impair vision (VA less than 20/30) rises from 1% by age 50 to 100% by age 90
- Glaucoma is present in less than 1.5% of those under 65, 2–3% in those aged 65–74 and between 2.5% and 7% for those over 75.

GERIATRIC PEOPLE PROBLEMS

Health Problems

1. Joint problems
2. Impairment of special senses
3. Cardiovascular disease
4. Hypothermia
5. Cancer, prostate enlargement, diabetes, and accidental falls.

Psychological Problems

1. Suicidal tendency
2. The predominant causes of intellectual impairment in older patients are delirium, dementia, and depression.
3. Evidence of dangerous behavior should also be sought (e.g. leaving the stove on wandering, getting lost), usually in elderly with Alzheimer's.

Social Problems

Poverty, loneliness, dependency, isolation, elder abuse, generation gap.

PSYCHOSOCIAL AND SEXUAL CHANGES

Psychosocial Changes in Elderly

The multitude of physical changes that occur with aging are accompanied by numerous psychosocial changes. As adults age, the nature of their daily lives change along with their bodies. Major life events such as retirement, changes in social relationships and roles, changes in living arrangements, and dealing with loss are usually experienced during the later years of life and can affect an individual's health status and outlook on life.

Retirement

An individual's view of retirement is a product of many factors, including overall life attitude, support of significant others, and personal expectations. For individuals who, during their adult years, defined themselves and their success according to their work contributions, retirement is likely to produce feelings of uneasiness and anxiety. An individual who views retirement as the end of the productive years will dread the change in life pattern and social status and may fear being a burden to others, both socially and financially.

Many adults, though, look forward to retirement as their reward for years of hard work and contributions and fill their newly freed days with activities, travel, new skills or hobbies, and interests that time constraints had prohibited them from pursuing during their earlier years. These individuals typically led more balanced lives during their working years, viewing their value as a combination of many factors including work, family, and community involvement; they adjust more easily to the loss of employment status by balancing this change with other positive aspects of their lives. Also, individuals who have planned for retirement and made arrangements (financial, housing, social) ahead of time tend to adjust more readily to this change in work status.

Social Relationships and Roles

Relationships and roles change over time as an individual grows and develops. For the older adult, these changes may take on even more meaning because activities and involvement in other areas of life may change or diminish. Changes in relationships and roles typically occur in conjunction with major life events, such as marriage, divorce, birth, death, relocation, and change in employment status. For instance, the older adult who has been a husband for 40 years will find his life and his roles greatly changed when he becomes a widower. The birth of his children's children will bring him new status as a grandparent, and his retirement will remove him from the full-time work force and present opportunities for the development of relationships with new friends.

A key to successful aging is staying connected to others. Volz (2000) cites a definite link between social support and health: older people "do better if they continue to engage with life and maintain close relationships." One type of relationship that many older adults experience is grandparenthood. This relationship may be the source of pride and happiness, or it can become a negative stressor. For many older Americans, grand parenting has become a full-time responsibility, as they are the sole caretakers of grandchildren. Over 2.4 million families in the United States were maintained by grandparents in 1998. This is a 19% increase since 1990 (Davidhizar, Bechtel, and Woodring, 2000). The changing role of grand-parenthood "causes caregiver stress, adversely affecting child health, and ultimately diminished family functioning" (Davidihizar, Bechtel, and Woodring, 2000, p.24).

However, not all grandparents are overwhelmed by the role of childrearing for the second generation; many find it rewarding (Davidhizer, Bechtel, and Woodring, 2000).

Listed below are some of the factors that have contributed to the increasing numbers of grandparents who are raising their grandchildren on a full time basis:
- Divorce
- Unemployment
- Teen pregnancy
- Death of a grandchild's parent

- ❖ Abuse and/or neglect of the child
- ❖ Substance abuse.

Nurses should be knowledgeable about potential areas of stress imposed by the additional responsibilities of the new grandparenthood role. Also, knowledge of community resources is essential for appropriate referral. Some grandparents may also need information about current childhood problems that were not as prevalent during their years of parenting their own offspring (e.g. cyber-porn, school violence).

Living Arrangements

Advancing age often brings with it changes in living arrangements. The older client has many living options depending on income, health status, activity level, level of independence, and family or other support systems.

A change in living arrangements is a significant event for any individual, but for older adults, this change may mean leaving family, friends, neighbors, and routines that have been a part of life for decades. Most older adults prefer to remain in their homes or dwellings, in a familiar environment and with familiar routines. In some cases, older adults may move in with their grown children and their families or have the grown children and their families or have the grown children move in with them. The degree of physical, psychological, and financial independence of the older adult, and the status of the relationship with the children, will likely determine the success of this arrangement. Larsen (1998) reports.

Coping with Loss

Loss is an inevitable part of live, and the longer a client lives, the more losses will be experienced. Losing a lifetime partner is one of the most stressful loss experiences an individual can face, and many older clients will face.

Loss through death of a spouse at some point in their lives. As the years pass, deaths of children and friends may leave older adults grieving and feeling as if everyone they have known and loved has died before them.

Feelings of isolation and hopelessness may arise; these can be compounded if the individual suffers multiple losses at once or within a short period of time. Losses are magnified in older adults who are socially isolated.

Fleming (2000) states: Sexual Changes

Changes in Men

As men age, the testes become softer and smaller as a result of decreased concentration of testosterone in the bloodstream. The production of sperm is inhibited or decreased and ejaculations are less forceful. Sexual dysfunction increases in prevalence with aging; however, it is not an inevitable result of the aging process.

According to Sheehy (1999), "40% of normal healthy males remain completely potent at age 70." Several factors contribute to the possible development impotence.

Changes in Women

The older woman experiences a decline in the serum levels of estrogen. As a result, the vaginal walls thin and vaginal secretions decrease. The vulva and external genitalia shrink because of loss of subcutaneous body fat.

Postmenopausal changes, such as vaginal dryness, may cause the woman to experience pain during intercourse. The nurse needs to inform the older woman about using water-soluble lubricants to relieve the pain and discomfort that may occur during intercourse. Elders need companionship.

- ❖ Maintain and improve function and independence for the elderly.
- ❖ Multidisciplinary team see patients either at home or on site.

Acute in patient services

- ❖ Short team diagnostic investigation and treatment
- ❖ Multidisciplinary team addresses medical and social issue
- ❖ Core team meets regularly to discuss clinical cases and program development.

Outreach program

- ❖ Assessment of home or long care facility
- ❖ Suitability and safety
- ❖ Attitudes of other people in home or long term care facility
- ❖ Emergency assistance arrangements
- ❖ Nutritional; alcohol, hygiene habits
- ❖ Ability to perform activities of daily living (ADLs) and instrumental ADLs (IADLs)
- ❖ Effective use of outreach program avoids unnecessary hospital admission.

Day hospitals

- ❖ Multidisciplinary team and patient can undertake investigation rehabilitation, medical treatment and maintenance care
- ❖ Aid in transition to full home discharge of patients
- ❖ Prevent early readmission.

Outpatient clinics

Clinics that specialize in specific disorder associated with aging, e.g. memory clinics, continence clinics, osteoporosis clinics.

ABUSE

Physical and Sexual Abuse

Any act of violence or rough treatment, whether or not actual physical injury results, i.e. slapping, punching, kicking, pinching, burning, restraints.

Emotional and Psychological Abuse

Any act that diminishes dignity and self-worth, i.e. confinement, isolation, verbal assault, humiliation, and infantilization.

Financial Abuse and Material Exploitation

Any improper conduct that results in monetary or personal loss for the older adult.

Abandonment and Neglect

- Active neglect—intentional (deliberate) withholding of basic necessities and/or care for physical or mental health.
- Passive neglect—not providing basic necessities and care. There is no conscious attempt to inflict distress.

Medical Abuse

Any medical procedure or treatment done without the permission of the older person or their power of Attorney or substitute decision maker.

Who are the Abusers? Three Categories:

1. Domestic elder abuse (maltreatment by a caregiver in two-thirds of all cases, financial abuse by a distant relative in 90% of cases)
2. Institutional elder abuse (abuse in a residential facility)
3. Self-neglect or self-abuse.

Reasons for Abuse

- Caregiver stress/burnout and social isolation
- Impairment of dependent elder (i.e. dementia)
- Transgenerational "Cycle of Violence"
- Material or other gain.

Abuse Indicators

- Unexplained physical injuries—burns, cuts, bruises, grip marks, rope marks, burns, cuts, head injuries pain, bruising, or bleeding in the genital area
- Unexplained malnourishment or decubitus ulcers
- Unkempt appearance (inappropriate clothing, signs of infrequent bathing or incontinence, a lack of glasses, hearing aids, or dentures when they are needed)
- Failure of a medical condition to improve or the continued presence of pain that might indicate under medication
- Fear of certain family members, friends, or caregivers
- The older person is largely ignored or treated passively by caregivers or others
- Caregivers who are entirely ignorant of the medical problems or treatments for the older person they are directly caring for (Table 65.3).

Geriatric Team consists of

- Geriatricians
- Nurses
- Physiotherapist
- Social worker
- And Health worker.

Table 65.3: Types of elderly abuse.

Types	Characteristics
Physical abuse	Slapping, striking incorrect positioning, over sedition
Physical neglect	Withholding food, water medications, clothing, hygiene, and physical aids
Psychological abuse	Berating verbally, harassment, threaten
Psychological neglect	Failing to provide social stimulation, leaving alone for long period of time
Sexual abuse	Touching inappropriately, sexual contact
Financial abuse	Denying access to personal abuse, stealing money
Violation of personal rights	Denying right to privacy

ROLE OF NURSE FOR CAREGIVERS OF ELDERLY

Caregiver

Caregiver is someone who provides supervision and direct care and coordinates services.

Prevalence of Caregiver

Six to seven million people US provide care to a family members or friends above age 65.

Task of Caregiver

- Assisting with ADLs and IADLs
- Providing emotional and social support
- Managing health care.

Challenges Faced by Caregivers

- Lack of respite or relief from care giving
- Conflict in the family unit related to decisions about care giving
- Lack of understanding of the time and energy needed for giving
- Inability to meet self-care needs such as socialization
- Inadequate information of specific task of care giving
- Financial depletion.

Role of Nurse for Caregivers

- Nurse should consider the caregiver as a patient and plan behaviors to reduce caregiver's role strain.
- Nurse should communicate a sense of empathy to the caregiver while allowing discussion about burden and joys of caregiving.
- The caregiver can be taught about age-related changes techniques.
- The nurse should encourage attendance at a support group.
- Nurse should monitor the caregivers for indications of declines health, emotional distress and role strain.

Chapter 65: Geriatric Considerations in Nursing

Roles of Geriatric Nurse

- Provider of care
- Teacher
- Manager
- Advocate
- Research consumer.

USE OF AIDS AND PROSTHESIS (HEARING AIDS DENTURES)

Hearing Aids in Elderly People

Definition

A hearing aid is a small electronic device that you wear in or behind your ear. It makes some sounds louder so that a person with hearing loss can listen, communicate, and participate more fully in daily activities. A hearing aid can help people hear more in both quiet and noisy situations. However, only about one out of five people who would benefit from a hearing aid actually uses one.

A hearing aid has three basic parts—a microphone, an amplifier, and a speaker. The hearing aid receives sound through a microphone, which converts the sound waves to electrical signals and sends them to an amplifier. The amplifier increases the power of the signals and then sends them to the ear through a speaker.

Uses of hearing aids

Hearing aids are primarily useful in improving the hearing and speech comprehension of people who have hearing loss that results from damage to the small sensory cells in the inner ear, called hair cells. This type of hearing loss is called sensorineural hearing loss. The damage can occur as a result of disease, aging, or injury from noise or certain medicines.

A hearing aid magnifies sound vibrations entering the ear. Surviving hair cells detect the larger vibrations and convert them into neural signals that are passed along to the brain. The greater the damage to a person's hair cells, the more severe the hearing loss, and the greater the hearing aid amplification needed to make up the difference. However, there are practical limits to the amount of amplification a hearing aid can provide. In addition, if the inner ear is too damaged, even large vibrations will not be converted into neural signals. In this situation, a hearing aid would be ineffective.

Indication of hearing aids

- Hearing loss
- Old age with diminished or loss of hearing ability.

Types of hearing aids

- **Behind-the-ear** (BTE) hearing aids consist of a hard plastic case worn BTE and connected to a plastic earmold that fits inside the outer ear. The electronic parts are held in the case BTE. Sound travels from the hearing aid through the earmold and into the ear. BTE aids are used by people of all ages for mild to profound hearing loss.

    A new kind of BTE aid is an open-fit hearing aid. Small, open-fit aids fit BTE completely, with only a narrow tube inserted into the ear canal, enabling the canal to remain open. For this reason, open-fit hearing aids may be a good choice for people who experience a buildup of earwax, since this type of aid is less likely to be damaged by such substances. In addition, some people may prefer the open-fit hearing aid because their perception of their voice does not sound "plugged up."

- **In-the-ear (ITE)** hearing aids fit completely inside the outer ear and are used for mild to severe hearing loss. The case holding the electronic components is made of hard plastic. Some ITE aids may have certain added features installed, such as a telecoil. A telecoil is a small magnetic coil that allows users to receive sound through the circuitry of the hearing aid, rather than through its microphone. This makes it easier to hear conversations over the telephone. A telecoil also helps people hear in public facilities that have installed special sound systems, called induction loop systems. Induction loop systems can be found in many churches, schools airports, and auditoriums. ITE aids usually are not worn by young children because the casings need to be replaced often as the ear grows.

- **Canal** aids fit into the ear canal and are available in two styles. The in-the-canal (ITC) hearing aid is made to fit the size and shape of a person's ear canal. A completely-in-canal (CIC) hearing aid is nearly hidden ITE canal. Both types are used for mild to moderately severe hearing loss.

    Because they are small, canal aids may be difficult for a person to adjust and remove. In addition, canal aids have less space available for batteries and additional devices, such as a telecoil. They usually are not recommended for young children or for people with severe to profound hearing loss because their reduced size limits their power and volume.

Dentures

Introduction

Dentures, also known as **false teeth,** are prosthetic devices constructed to replace missing teeth; they are supported by the surrounding soft and hard tissues of the oral cavity. Conventional dentures are removable (removable partial denture or complete denture). However, there are many different denture designs, some which rely on bonding or clasping onto teeth or dental implants (fixed prosthodontics). There are two main categories of dentures, the distinction being whether they are used to replace missing teeth on the mandibular arch or on the maxillary arch.

Uses of Dentures in Old Age

Dentures can help patients though:
- Mastication, as chewing ability is improved by replacing edentulous areas with denture teeth.
- Esthetics, because the presence of teeth gives a natural appearance to the face, and wearing a denture to replace missing teeth provides support for the lips and cheeks and corrects the collapsed appearance that results from the loss of teeth.
- Pronunciation, because replacing missing teeth, especially the anteriors, enables patients to speak better. There is especially improvement in pronouncing words containing sibilants or fricatives.
- Self-esteem, because improved looks and speech boost confidence in the ability to interact socially.

Types

Removable partial dentures

Removable partial dentures are for patients who are missing some of their teeth on a particular arch. Fixed partial dentures, also known as "crown and bridge" dentures, are made from crowns that are fitted on the remaining teeth. They act as abutments and pontics and are made from materials resembling the missing teeth. Fixed bridges are more expensive than removable appliances but are more stable.

Another option in this category is the flexible partial, which is widely considered to be the most comfortable. The final restoration can now be made very quickly with innovations in digital technology. Flexible partials are becoming much more popular due to their aesthetic qualities. While the cost may be higher than a partial made with visible metal clasps, the results of the flexible partial are beautiful, with high levels of satisfaction. Flexible partial fabrication involves only noninvasive procedures, and serves as a virtually invisible tooth replacement option.

Complete dentures

Complete dentures are worn by patients who are missing all of the teeth in a single arch [i.e. the maxillary (upper) or mandibular (lower) arch]

Prosthodontic principles

Support

Support is the principle that describes how well the underlying mucosa (oral tissues, including gums) keeps the denture from moving vertically toward the arch in question during chewing, and thus being excessively depressed and moving deeper into the arch. For the mandibular arch, this function is provided primarily by the buccal shelf, a region extending laterally from the back or posterior ridges, and by the pear-shaped pad (the most posterior area of keratinized gingival formed by the scaling down of the retro-molar papilla after the extraction of the last molar tooth). Secondary support for the complete mandibular denture is provided by the alveolar ridge crest. The maxillary arch receives primary support from the horizontal hard palate and the posterior alveolar ridge crest. The larger the denture flanges (that part of the denture that extends into the vestibule), the better the stability (another parameter to assess fit of a complete denture). Long flanges beyond the functional depth of the sulcus are a common error in denture construction, often (but not always) leading to movement in function, and ulcerations (denture sore spots).

Stability

Stability is the principle that describes how well the denture base is prevented from moving in a horizontal plane, and thus sliding from side to side or front to back. The more the denture base (pink material) is in smooth and continuous contact with the edentulous ridge (the hill upon which the teeth used to reside, but now only residual alveolar bone with overlying mucosa), the better the stability. Of course, the higher and broader the ridge, the better the stability will be, but this is usually a result of patient anatomy, barring surgical intervention (bone grafts, etc.).

Retention

Retention is the principle that describes how well the denture is prevented from moving vertically in the opposite direction of insertion. The better the topographical mimicry of the intaglio (interior) surface of the denture base to the surface of the underlying mucosa, the better the retention will be (non-removable partial dentures, the clasps are a major provider of retention), as surface tension, suction, and friction will aid in keeping the denture base from breaking intimate contact with the mucosal surface. It is important to note that the most critical element in the retentive design of a maxillary complete denture is a complete and total border seal (complete peripheral seal) in order to achieve "suction." The border seal is composed of the edges of the anterior and lateral aspects and the posterior palatal seal. The posterior palatal seal design is accomplished by covering the entire hard palatal seal design is accomplished by covering the entire hard palate and extending not beyond the soft palate and ending 1–2 mm from the vibrating line.

Prosthodontists use a scale called the Kapur index to quantify denture stability and retention.

Implant technology can vastly improve the patient's denture wearing experience by increasing stability and preventing bone from wearing away. Implants can also aid retention. Instead of merely placing the implants to serve as blocking mechanism against the denture's pushing on the alveolar bone, small retentive appliances can be attached to the implants that can then snap into a modified denture base to allow for tremendously increased retention. Available options include a mental "Hader bar" or precision balls attachments.

Fit, maintenance, and relining

Generally speaking partial dentures tend to be held in place by the presence of the remaining natural teeth and complete dentures tend to rely on muscular coordination and suction to stay in place. The maxilla very commonly has more favorable denture bearing anatomy as the ridge tends to be well formed and there is a larger area on the palate for suction to retain the denture. Conversely, the mandible tends to make lower dentures less retentive due to the displacing presence of the tongue and the higher rate of resorption, frequently leading to significantly resorbed lower ridges. Disto-lingual regions tend to offer retention even in highly resorbed mandibles, and extension of the flange into these regions tends to produce a more retentive lower denture. An implant supported lower denture is another option.

Dentures that fit well during the first few years after creation will not necessarily fit well for the rest of the wearer's lifetime. This is because the bone and mucosa of the mouth are living tissues, which are dynamic over decades. Bone remodeling never stops in living bone. Edentulous jaw ridges tend to resorb progressively over the years, especially the alveolar ridge of the lower jaw. Mucosa reacts to being chronically rubbed by the dentures. Poorly fitting dentures hasten both of those processes compared to the rates with will-fitting dentures. Poor fitting dentures may also lead to the development of conditions such as epulis fissuratum.

When dentures no longer fit well, the correct action is to seek follow-up care. Using denture adhesive may improve the fit, but it tends to work better when only a small amount is used as covering the denture fitting surface in adhesive makes it stay in less well. Adhesives may compensate for gradual loosening of a denture, but it is only a temporary solution; it does not solve the problem. Fortunately, dentures can often be relined with relining materials to restore the proper fit, and this process costs less than creation of new dentures. Overall, a well made denture should last about 5 years or more.

Nursing management

- Educating the patient to daily cleaning of dentures is recommended.
- Instruct the patient Plaque and tartar can build up on false teeth, just as they do on natural teeth.
- Demonstrating the patient how cleaning can be done using chemical or mechanical denture cleaners.
- Dentures should not be worn continuously, but rather left out of the mouth during sleep. This is to give the tissue a chance to recover, and wearing dentures at night is likened to sleeping in your shoes. The main risk is development of fungal infection, especially denture-related stomatitis.

Ethical Issues in Elderly

Ethical Principles

Clinical ethics is the identification, analysis, and resolution of moral problems that arise in the care of patients, four widely accepted prima facie principles that characterized the ethical concerns of clinical practice are autonomy, beneficence, nonmaleficence, and justice. Autonomy refers to the duty to respect person and their rights of self-determination. Beneficence refers to the duty to do good, whereas nonmaleficence refers to duty prevent or do no harm—justice refers to the duty to treat individuals fairly (free of bias and based on medical need). When caring for elderly individuals, clinicians may find these ethical principles at odds with each other.

Common ethical dilemmas in elderly patients

Respect for patient autonomy is the ethical principle that underlies informed consent for patient to be autonomous when making health care decisions, clinicians must adequately inform them about their illness and treatment options.

Legal dust to obtain consent for medical interventions was established in American law during the early 20th century.

However, the term informed consent was:

a. **Informed consent:** Informed consent is that the physician conveys the necessary information to the patient (e.g. the nature of the illness, the proposed intervention, and the risk and benefits of and alternatives to the proposed intervention) and has confirmation of the patient's decision making capacity, understanding of the information, and voluntary agreement to the intervention.

b. **Decision making capacity:** Clinicians commonly care for elderly persons who have conditions (e.g. dementia) that impair decision making capacity, however patients must have decision making capacity to be autonomous and participants in informed consent. Decision making capacity includes the ability to communication a choice, understand the nature and consequences of the choice, manipulate rationally the information necessary to make the choice and reason consistently with previously expressed values and goals.

c. **Promoting advanced care planning and use of advanced directives (ADs):** The AD promotes autonomy of patients who lack, but once possessed, decision making capacity. Clinicians should regard the AD as an extension of the fully autonomous patient; in general, there are two forms of AD—(1) the living will and (2) the durable power of attorney for health care, the living will lists intervention and other actions that should or should not be taken in specific circumstance (usually when the patient is terminally ill). Living wills can be highly detailed or give vague instructions that make their interpretation difficult. The durable of attorney for health care identifies the surrogate decision making in the event the patient lacks decision making capacity, in the case example, the clinician should obtain informed consent for intervention from the child is identified in the AD as the surrogate decision maker.

d. **When withdrawing and withholding life sustaining intervention is appropriate:** Both patients and clinicians see room for improving end of life care should adequately managing pain and symptoms avoiding a prolonged process of dying, achieving a sense of control, relieving burden, and strengthening relationship with loved ones. Dying patients may refuse or request the withdrawal of any or all intervention. However, clinicians may be reluctant to grant such request for fear of litigation or prosecution for unlawful death; nevertheless, the right to refuse, or request the withdrawal of medical intervention is ethical legal. Withdrawal of life sustaining intervention (e.g. mechanical ventilation, hemodialysis, and artificial nutrition) from patients with advanced medical conditions is practiced widely.

   The ethical principles of autonomy underlie the right to refuse, or request the withdrawal of unwanted medical intervention. Patients also have the right to decline previously consented to intervention if their health care values and goals have changed. If a clinician begins or continues as intervention that a patient has refused legally the clinician is committing battery.

e. **Use of cardiopulmonary resuscitation (CPR) and do-not resuscitate orders:** In practice to CPR is presumed and clinicians must perform CPR unless a do-not resuscitate order (to which the patient or surrogate has consented) exists slow codes, nevertheless, CPR is a low yield procedure.

f. **Responding to request for intervention:** Patients frequently make request for medical interventions. Many requests are reasonable, and clinicians should honor request if they are within the standard of care. However, clinicians are not obligated to grant request for intervention that are clearly ineffective or request that violate their conscience.

   Controversies related tom patients request for intervention frequently are due requests of questionable efficiency [e.g. prostate-specific antigen (PSA) screening in elderly men] that support an uncontroversial end (e.g. patient health). These requests often reflect the gap between clinical evidence and clinical practice also patients values goals and experiences of ten prompt these request.

g. **Allocating health care resources:** The elderly population accounts for a disproportionately high percentage of health care spending. Thus, it is not surprising that some have called spending. Thus, it is not surprising that some have called for health care rationing based on age. Clinicians are under increasing pressure from third parties (e.g. health maintenance organizations) to control health care spending.

   Avoiding ethical dilemmas through effective patient clinician communication.

➢ Effective patient–clinician communication maximizes patient autonomy.
➢ However, effective communication goes beyond informed consent and maintaining confidentiality.
➢ Clinicians have an ethical duty to treat patients in a dignified, courteous and respectful manner.

PROVISIONS AND PROGRAMS FOR ELDERLY: PRIVILEGES, COMMUNITY PROGRAMS, AND HEALTH SERVICES

Community Care in Elderly

Care in the community may be provided "informally" through kinship networks, by friends, neighbors, and volunteers or "formally" by statutory social services. Thus, it is possible to distinguish between:

a. Informal care provided by neighbors, friends, and more particularly by families and relatives
b. Formal and quasi-normal care provided by voluntary organizations
c. Formally organized care provided by health boards and local authorities

The notion of "community care" in the Irish context usually embodies a combination of all three. Informal care is not necessarily more desirable than formal care. Both may be narrowly or expansively conceived and operated, they may enhance or reduce dependency, deny or facilitate rights, and restrict or enhance freedom. In each instance, however, the aim is to maintain the elderly person living in the community and in so doing to lessen the need for institutional care.

It is likely that a substantial minority of elderly persons currently in institutions would be able to care for themselves in the community with adequate support.

In this context, it should be noted that 28% of all persons in long-stay geriatric units in this country are there for "social" reasons.

In addressing this issue, it should be recognized that care in the community, while ideologically desirable, is only better for a particular elderly person if it is in fact better care. In many instances when elderly people become ill and dependent, their needs can only be adequately met through some form of institutional care.

Community Care in Practice

In practice, community care can be said to be about very practical and personal matters. It is about loneliness and isolation, illness, and incontinence; help with climbing stairs and distress; aid with preparing meals and housework. It is also about the provision of appropriately designed houses with suitable aids and adaptations and all of this in the context of maintaining and ensuring the elderly person's independence and enhancing their potential for self-care.

Elderly people living at home and particularly if living alone may need special support to enable them to cope with their infirmities and to prevent their isolation from society. As their capabilities diminish, they will more often need home help laundry services, meals-on-wheels, and chiropody. Loss of mobility brings the need for social visits, transport to social clubs, day centers, day hospitals, and arrangements for holidays if social isolation is to be avoided. When illness is added to other infirmities, they may need more nursing, night care and help generally in the home.

In terminal illness, an elderly person may for a limited period need considerable help from many of the community care services.

HOME AND INSTITUTIONAL CARE

Institutional Care Elderly

Introduction

By other hospital and institutional care for the elderly, which is the subject of this section, is meant care at present provided in various settings:

- Geriatric long-term care units associated with specific general hospital departments
- Geriatric hospitals, which were often former old country homes
- Long-stay district hospitals
- Welfare homes (an increasing number of welfare home residents are in need of nursing care)
- Voluntary and private institutions and nursing homes
- Psychiatric hospitals.

The Council believes that:

i. In the past, too often decisions have been taken to place elderly people and particularly the very old, in institutions on a long-term basis without assessment, without their consent, and without consideration of the various alternatives to support them in continuing to live outside institutions, at least on a part time basis.
ii. The general perception regarding many of these institutions is that they are places to commit old people who have, for one reason or another, become a care problem in the family or wider community, places where, once admitted, they remain permanently until the end of their days.
iii. It is necessary to re-structure institutional care for the elderly as we know it. This requires that existing institutions and services for elderly people be adapted and developed in a manner which offers flexible systems of care and a real choice to elderly people and to those caring for them.

Research studies have demonstrated that residential institutions for the elderly very often involve a loss of independence and liberty and do not adequately meet the physical, psychological, and social needs of the elderly living in them.

In the Council's view, there is an urgent need to develop a more adequate and flexible philosophy of care for elderly persons than exists at present. This requires us to address a number of fundamental questions as follows:

a. Do all elderly persons at present admitted to long-stay hospital or institutional care actually need this form of care?
b. Is such care required on a permanent basis?
c. What are the processes and pathways by which elderly persons are admitted to long-term institutional care?
d. What alternative forms of care should be provided?
e. What are the preferences of elderly people themselves in relation to long-term care?

In posing these questions, the Council recognizes that, despite a very good rehabilitation program, some elderly persons will fail to make a full functional recovery after illness and will require continuing nursing care, some on a 24-h basis. For some elderly persons, this may be for a protracted period of time; for others, it will be terminal care and may be for a shorted period.

Management

Health Promoting Activities

- Adequate consumption of fluids is important to reduce the risk of bladder infections and urinary incontinence.
- Avoidance of bladder irritating substances such as caffeinated carbonated and acidic beverages.
- Nutria sweet and alcohol will greatly reduce urinary urgency and frequency.
- Pelvic floor exercises, first described by legal (1948), can also be extremely useful in reducing the symptoms of stress and urge incontinence.
- Teaching the patient how to do the exercises to stop voluntarily the follow of urine without contracting the abdomen, buttocks, or inner thigh muscles.
- As menopause approaches, a woman's circulating estrogen decreases.
- The pelvic floor is deprived of its needed blood supply and nutrients.
- The use of biofeedback assisted pelvic muscle expensing an individual can successfully regain bladder function.
- Constipation can be major factor contributing to urinary incontinence.
- The patient is encouraged to eat a high-fiber diet and drink added fluids.
- Increase mobility to promote regular bowel function.
- Eat small, frequent meals.
- Avoid heavy activity after eating.
- Eat a high-fiber, low-fiber diet.
- Ingest an adequate amount of fluids establishing regular bowel habits.
- Avoid the use of laxatives and antacids.

Nutritional Health

- Decreased physical activity and a slower metabolic rate reduce the number of calories needed by the older adult to maintain an ideal weight.

- Lack of taste discrimination also contributes to suboptimal nutrient intake.
- Health promotion teaching includes fats and high in vegetables, fruits, and fish.
- Reducing salt intake is also advocated.
- Sodium reduction has been shown to correct HT in some people.
- Simple sugars should be avoided and complex carbohydrates encouraged.
- Potatoes, whole grains, brown rice, and fruit provide the person with minerals, vitamins, and fiber and should be encouraged.

Sleep

- The elderly often experience variations in their in normal sleep–wake cycles.
- The lack of napping during the day.
- The nurse can recommend prudent sleep hygiene behaviors such as avoiding daytime napping.
- Eating a light snack before bedtime.

For Skeletal Health, the Nurse can recommend the Following

- A high calcium intake, 1500 mg/day
- A low-phosphorus diet
- Weight bearing exercise
- Reduction of caffeine and alcohol
- Selective estrogen receptor modulators, such as Raloxifene to preserve bone mineral density
- The bisphosphate drugs
- These drugs bind to mineralized bon surfaces to inhibit orthocastic activity and promote bone formation.

Medications and Elderly

- Older patients are two or three times more likely to have adverse drug reactions.
- Drug clearance is often markedly reduced due to
  - A decrease in renal plasma flow
  - Decreased GFR
  - Reduced hepatic clearance
- Reduced hepatic clearance in elderly is due to
  - A decrease in activity of the drug metabolizing microsomal enzymes
  - And an overall decline in blood flow to the liver with aging
- The volume of distribution of drugs is also affected
  - Since the elderly have a decrease in total body water
  - And a relative increase in body fat
- Water-soluble drugs become more concentrated.
- Fat-soluble drugs have longer half-lives.
- Serum albumin levels decline, particularly in sick patients, so that there is a decrease in protein binding of some drugs (e.g. warfarin, phenytoin), leaving more free (active) drug available.
- Older patients have altered responses to similar serum drug levels, a phenomenon known as altered pharmacodynamics.
- They are more sensitive to some drugs (e.g. opiates, anticoagulants) and less sensitive to others (e.g. β-adrenergic agents).
- The older patient with multiple chronic conditions is likely to be taking several drugs, including non-prescribed agents.
- Thus, adverse drug reactions and dosage errors are more likely to occur, especially if the patient has visual, hearing, or memory deficits.

CONCLUSION

Old age is a one of the important stage of life in which all the changes takes place structurally and physiologically and potential for health complications. So nurse should be knowledgeable regarding the concepts of care and problems in order to provide comprehensive care to the clients in her care settings.

CHAPTER 66

Evidence-based Nursing Practice: Best Practice

CHAPTER OUTLINE

- Definitions
- What is Evidence?
  - Purposes
- Resources to Facilitate Evidence-based Nursing
- Steps for Process of Evidence-based Practices
- Barriers or Challenges in Evidence-based Practices

INTRODUCTION

Evidence-based nursing (EBN) is a systematic process that uses current evidence in making decisions about patient care, including evaluation of quality and applicability of existing research, patient performance, costs, clinical expertise, and clinical settings. Everyone uses evidence from a variety of sources both in their daily personal lives and in professional practice. However, the term evidence-based practice (EBP) has been used synonymously with "evidence-based practice" or "evidence-based care" in the National Health Services (NHS) since the early 1990s.

Evidence-based clinical practice is an approach to health in which the clinician uses current research to help guide client care decisions the practice of evidence-based care means integrating individual clinical expertise with the best available external evidence from systematic research in simple words we apply this evidence-based research to our clinical practice.

DEFINITIONS

It is the conscientious, explicit, and judicious use of current best evidence in making decisions about the care of individual patients.

The practice of evidence-based nursing means integrating individual clinical expertise with the best available external evidence from systematic research.

—**Dr David Sackett**

The evidence-based practice is about making decisions about a group of patients, or populations and basing such decisions on careful appraisal of the best evidence available on a more practical level.

—**Muir Gray (1997)**

WHAT IS EVIDENCE?

It is a fact available as a proof. Everyone uses evidence from a variety of sources both in their daily personal lives and in professional practice. Different types of evidence include the information gained from tradition, rituals, experiences, institution, authorities and experts, patients and families, research, audit, and guidelines.

Sources of the Problem Areas

Tradition and Ritual

Learning traditions and rituals is important for transmitting knowledge to students or practitioners from effective colleagues who practice safely and on the basis of best evidence this can be a very useful for sharing knowledge and good practice. However, relying on traditional knowledge may also lead to the transmission of outdated information and practice, putting both nurses and clients at risk.

Experience

Practitioners have their own or experience of others to inform decisions they make about nursing practice. However, whole experience brings confidence and ability to make professional judgment. There is also a risk that experimental knowledge is based on a limited range of events or practice situations to which practitioners have been exposed.

Intuition

It is defined as a way of knowing and behaving that is not based on rational or conscious reasoning.

Authorities and Experts

Often practices in healthcare and nursing care determined by the knowledge and opinions of those members of the healthcare team in positions of authority. Knowledge is considered true because the person who states it has authority or is considered an expert. Whole experts may possess high levels of knowledge in relation to best practice, at times conflicts may arise when one expert or person in authority holds differing views or opinions from one another.

Service Users and Their Families
Patients often feel that they are not involved enough in their own care and are not asked about what services they think should be offered by NHS. As such, they should be able to make decisions and choices about what happens to them. It is important to ascertain the views of people and their families.

Research Studies
Knowledge derived from research is crucial to evidence-based practice.

Audit
Clinical audit can provide knowledge about nursing care and highlight where improvements are needed. Audit is an important link within the evidence-based practice cycle.

Guidelines
Practitioners may also use guidelines as a source of knowledge from which to base case that they provide guidelines are written after the best available evidence. Thus, knowledge is derived from many different sources and used in combination, can ensure that the care and treatment is an effective as possible.

Purposes
1. To provide the highest quality and most cost efficient nursing care as much as possible.
2. To provide advanced quality of nursing care from the professional nurses.
3. To increase satisfaction of patient.
4. To focus on nursing practice away from habits and tradition through evidence and research.

Resources to Facilitate Evidence-based Nursing

Evidence-based Journals
Rather than publishing original research, the objective of these journals is to summarize those studies that are valid and clinically useful. Currently, these journals consist of ACP journal club, evidence-based medicine, evidence-based cardiovascular medicine, evidence-based health policy and management, evidence-based mental health, and evidence-based nursing.
- EBP websites
- Clinical practice
- Guidance, etc

Who Are the Users of Evidence-based Practice?
- Nurses (RN, NP)
- Nursing assistant
- Physicians
- Respiratory therapists
- Physical therapies
- Pharmacists
- Others

Steps for Process of Evidence-based Practices
All of the definitions advocate the use of evidence to support decision making, there is an assumption that evidence is easily used in every day practice. The process of EBP always starts with a question about practices the answer to which will guide the practitioner and reveal whether their current practice is evidence based.

To help practitioners underpin their practice with evidence, assess of steps have been developed this process of events ensures that up-to-data practices are carried out and good standards of clinical practice are maintained. These steps reflect models of evidence-based practice to help practitioners ensure that their practice is evidence based and include the following:
- Questioning practice
- Refining the question into a workable search question
- Finding the evidence
- Appraising the evidence
- Implementing the evidence
- Evaluating or auditing practice.

1. Questioning Practice
The first step toward EBP is the ability of practitioners to question their own practice to do this practitioners will need to identify why they make decisions in a particular way and acknowledge what or who has informed the decision. Too often decisions are based on ritual and custom rather than a reliable evidence base. In order to make effective clinical decisions in practice practitioners need to be able to ask questions about the care or treatment they are providing.

Questioning practice involves thinking about the appropriateness of the care being provides. For example, is it the right treatment? How do practitioners know that treatment works? How do different treatments compare? Is the treatment cost effective?

2. Refining the Question into a Workable Search Question
If decisions are based on tradition or ritual then there is a need to think about finding out of there is more reliable evidence to support decisions about practice to accomplish this, it is useful to formulate a structured question to guide the search for evidence.

Menlyk and Fine Overholt recommended putting the clinical question into PICO format.
P: Patient/population
I: Intervention
C: Comparison
O: Outcome

"P" represents patient or population under consideration

"I" represents intervention or treatment under consideration

"C" represents comparison intervention

"O" represents clinical outcome

3. Finding the Evidence

Once the question has been formulated, the next steps to find the evidence. In today's electronic environment, computer skills and resources are essential tool for nurses. At a minimum, the nurse must possess the skill to search relevant and credible websites as well as access electronic libraries and databases. Librarians (esp. medical) information technology (IT) support, online and telephone helpdesk services, and faculty in computer education are some of the experts who can aid in developing the skills needed for locating the evidence.

Librarian resources

These is perhaps no more valuable asset in the search for evidence than a medical reference librarian; these librarians complete specialized education in healthcare information, they are knowledgeable about each of the many healthcare databases and can provide valuable insight in search strategies.

Electronic databases

These are web-based tools that allow one to search, navigated and personalize searches for thousands of text books, journals, and articles.

Examples include the following:
- Medicine: Literature in the fields of medicine, nursing, dentistry, veterinary, and preclinical sciences.
- Cochrane database of systematic reviews.

Internet resources

Internet recourses provide the most efficient and effective way to find research evidence internet resources not only include websites about EBP and specific problems or practices but also databases such as PubMed and Ovid. These websites serve four purposes:
- To learn about EBP in general
- To identify the processes and tools for EBP
- To provide links to evidence in the form of clinical guidelines
- To provide links to databases in which the nurse can search for evidence on a specific topic.

4. Appraising/Analyzing the Evidence

When the research evidence has been located, it must be critically appraised to make sense of the evidence and decide whether it is believable and robust. We can appraise the evidence by using the following guidelines such as:
- EBP guidelines
- Systematic reviews
- Meta-analysis
- Randomized clinical trial (RCTs)

EBP guidelines

They provide the strongest level of support to guide practice, as they are based on rigorous reviews of the best research on specific topic areas.

Systematic reviews

It is a summary of evidence on a particular topic that uses a various process for retrieving, critically appraising, and synthesizing studies in order to answer a question about burning clinical issues. The COCHRANE database is perhaps the most outstanding resource to identify and retrieve systematic reviews.

Meta-analysis

It is a type of data analysis where the results of several studies are combined.

Randomized controlled trials (RCTs)

The RCTs is considered the "gold standard" of research methods when evaluating the strength of study findings RCTs are an important quantitative method and considered to be very valuable. It is a type of study that establishes cause and effect of treatments and tries to manipulate variable within control. As a result they reduce researcher be as introduce control and limit the confounding variables. It is believed that RCTs are a good type of evidence based because they are reliable.

5. Implementing the Evidence

Following the appraisal of evidence and once the practitioner is satisfied that the evidence is reliable and trust worthy and then they need to think about how to use this evidence in practice implementing evidence-based findings is no easy task but with support from qualified staff and students should be able to make comprehensive plans to help them include the evidence in practice.

The final step in the process of evidence-based nursing is to consider the research evidence in light of clinical experience and patient-related factors and preferences. A decision then can be made about whether to reject, implement, or adapt the intervention for the population of patients and the setting.

Clinical experience: There are numerous nursing interventions that are standard nursing practices but are based in tradition rather than on research evidence. Nurses are thus challenged to ask questions about their practices and search for existing evidence to support the best nursing care and promote optimal outcomes for patients. When no research evidence exists, nurses must evaluate a practice in light of what is believed to be the current standard of practice and also what benefits are believed to exist for patients with the current standards and what consequences (risk) are likely if the practice is not implemented. Even then, a nurse's decision to implement an intervention can be overruled by a patient and his or her performances or wishes.

Patient preferences: Patients often have preferences that influences the types of nursing activities implemented. For example, a patient who has been managing a colostomy stoma for many years in a certain fashion may struggle to change to a new care system despite evidence that the new system is more effective or easier to use thus nurses have to work realistically with patients to select the interventions and activities that are most likely to work for the patients and promote positive or the best outcomes.

Making a decision: Integrating the research evidence, clinical experience, and patient's preferences to make a decision about a practice change can be an enormous undertaking. But by considering all the aforementioned, a decision should be made or a change in practice should be implemented by following all the necessary steps which are supposed to be taken or when a decision has been made regarding a recommendation for practice, the next step is to identify a strategy for presenting the recommendation and implementing the intervention or practice change.

6. Evaluating the Practice is Outcome

Finally, once practitioners have introduced the evidence into practice, there is a need to reflect on and evaluate their work and whether it is safe and effective for the patient or client under their care. Practitioners may find that they need to continuously audit their practice to ensure that it is based on "best evidence." Whatever the situation, the important message is to be able to continuously improve practice by questioning the decisions that practitioners make about patients or client care needs.

Barriers or Challenges in Evidence-based Practices

There are many barriers to promoting evidence-based practices; some of the significant ones are discussed as follows:
- Lack of professional ability to initially appraise research
- Lack of time, workload pressures, and competing priorities of patient care can impede use of evidence-based practices
- Lack of knowledge of research methods
- Lack of support from professional colleagues and organizations and lack of confidence and authority in the research arena
- Practice environment can be resistant to changing tried and true conventional methods of practice
- Lack of continuing education programs
- Another barrier to introducing newly learned methods for improving treatments or patient's health is the fear of stepping on one's toes
- Organizational pressures
- Lack of high-quality research to guide practice
- Inadequate literature searching critical appraisal skills.

Role of a Nurse

To implement the evidence into practice nurse alone does not a play a crucial role but there are many people involved to bring the evidence into practice, that is, it requires the involvement of the individual practitioner, nursing team and the organization. To bring about the EBN into practice, there is a need to create on organizational culture that supports EBP.
- Nurse executives and nurses in leadership positions are responsible for creating this culture
- Need to incorporate EBN expectations into performance expectations
- Recognize the successful effort of nurses who choose to implement evidence in their practice
- Nurses should be taught and supported to practice EBN
- Nurses need to be empowered to evaluate the evidence and make practice changes.

CONCLUSION

EBP acts as a bridge between evidence and nursing practice. EBP is viewed as a means to challenge ritualistic practices by encouraging practitioners to be more questioning of their works and care deliverymen is an existing new concept that will lead to improved quality of patients care. It is based on research, but is more EBN is a logical blending of quality research, nursing expertise, client's preference, and the healthcare reality. Everyone benefits from the practice of EBP the patient, the nurse, other healthcare providers, and the healthcare environment. EBP with all healthcare professionals working in concept will advance nursing into a new era of quality healthcare.

CHAPTER 67: Transcultural Nursing

CHAPTER OUTLINE

- Terminologies Used
- Concept of Culture
- Definitions
- Historical Perspectives
- Goals of Transcultural Nursing
- Transcultural Nursing Model or Sunrise Model
- Role of Nurse in Transculture Nursing
- Research Abstract

INTRODUCTION

The English word "culture" has been used in various concepts in common literature. Culture means social charm and intellectual excellence. Some sociologists have also accepted cultured people as leaders of society. According to Sorokin and McIver, culture stands for the moral, spiritual, and intellectual attainments of man. In the words of Bogardus, "culture is composed of integrated customs, behavior patterns of human groups."

The word culture has had a number of meanings. Originally it referenced to the art and humanities. The cultured man was one who was well-versed in drama, philosophy, and the arts. Nurses have always been contender with the whole person including the physical, emotional, psychological, spiritual, and developmental dimensions. The culture incorporates not only customs, but beliefs, values, and attitudes shared by a group of people and passed down through generations.

TERMINOLOGIES USED

- **Culture**—broadly defines set of values, beliefs, and traditions that are held by a specific group of people and handed down from generation to generation. Culture is also beliefs, habits, likes, dislikes, customs, and rituals learn from one's family (Specter, 1991).
- **Religion**—is a set of beliefs in a divine or super human power (or powers) to be obeyed and worshipped as the creator and ruler of the universe. Ethical values and religion system of beliefs and practices, difference within the culture and across culture are found.
- **Cultural identity**—the sense of being part of an ethnic group or culture.
- **Material culture**—refers to objects (dress, art).
- **Nonmaterial culture**—refers to beliefs, customs, languages, social institutions.
- **Subculture**—composed of people who have a distinct identity but are related to a larger cultural group.
- **Bicultural**—a person who crosses two cultures lifestyles, and sets of values.
- **Diversity**—refers to the fact or state of being different. Diversity can occur between culture and within a cultural group.
- **Ethnic group**—shares a common social and cultural heritage that is passed on to successive generation. Example: Indian culture, American culture (Christians will go to Church on Sunday).
- **Race**—the classification of people according to shared biologic characteristics, genetic markers, or features. Not all people of the same race have the same culture. For example: Indian race, African race, etc.

CONCEPT OF CULTURE

- Culture is learned by each generation through both formal and informal life experiences. Language is primary through means of transmitting culture.
- The practices of particular culture often arise because of the group's social and physical environment.
- Culture practice and beliefs are adapted over time but they mainly remain constant as long as they satisfy needs.

DEFINITIONS

According to the American Nurses Association (1976), "Consideration of individual value systems and lifestyles should be included in the planning and health care for each client. Nursing curriculum recognizes the contribution nursing to the health care needs of a diverse and multicultural society lifestyle may reflect cultural heritage."

According to Leininger, the transcultural nursing is described as that which incorporates all aspects of a person's culture in planning and providing care.

According to Madeleine Leininger (2002), comparative study of cultures to understand similarities (culture universal) and differences (culture specific) across human groups.

HISTORICAL PERSPECTIVES

- ❖ The transcultural nursing has its roots in the early 1900s when public health nurse cares for immigrants from Europe who came from a wide range of cultural background and had diverse health care practices.
- ❖ During the 19th century, the words come to be used almost interchangeably with civilization. This civilization or culture was something achieved as society is evolved people who were cultured or primitive peoples of the world.
- ❖ In the late 1940s, Dr. Madeleine Leininger held the belief that "care is essence of nursing and the central dominate and unifying focus of nursing." She then began to see the importance of nursing care that was beginning to understand the importance of nursing care that was based on the client's cultures that has unique values.
- ❖ Beliefs, practices and life ways passed down from one generation to next. The idea that culture and care are inextricably linked, led her to study other cultures and she becomes the first nurse to obtain a doctorate in anthropology.
- ❖ Transcultural nursing is a body of knowledge and practice for caring the people from other cultures. Many nurse leaders and educators have embraced the need for culture specific care, and various approaches to gaining this knowledge have been developed.

GOALS OF TRANSCULTURAL NURSING

- ❖ According to Leininger, the goal of transcultural nursing care is to preserve, accommodate or repattern the cultures of the patient.
- ❖ When cultural beliefs and values do not have negative effect on care, nursing must make every effort to help the patient preserve his or her culture.
- ❖ In some situations, it may be necessary to make accommodations to preserve the culture of the patient and the family.
- ❖ Repeating the culture of the patient requires the patient to essentially change his or her life.

TRANSCULTURAL NURSING MODEL OR SUNRISE MODEL (FIG. 67.1)

Purpose and Goal of the Theory

The purpose and goal of the theory is to use research findings to provide culturally congruent, safe, and meaningful care to clients of diverse or similar cultures.

Sunrise Model: A Conceptual Guide to Knowledge Discovery

A sunrise model was developed to give a holistic and comprehensive conceptual picture of the major factors held as important to the theory of culture care diversity and university. The model is a conceptual visual guide depicting multiple factors predicted to influence culturally congruent care with people of different culture. The model essentially serves as a cognitive guide for the researcher to visualize and reflect on different factors predicted to influence culturally based care in the discovery process. The sunrise model has also been used as a valuable guide for doing culturological health care assessment of client's health needs.

As the researcher used the model, the different factors depicted in the model are kept in mind in relation to discovering culture care phenomena. Gender and sexual orientation, race, class factors, biomedical condition, and the extent of acculturation are all an integral part of the model and theory. The factors tend to be embedded in social structure; worldview and other dimensions identified in the sunrise model and are usually not quickly identifiable. Hence, they are not isolated variables but are lodged in their nature and meaningful culture context, yet are important discovery areas within the theory.

According to the researcher's interests and skills, one can being the discovery at any place in the model except with the three modes of action and decisions, which are studied last or after drawing upon collected in the upper part of the model. All factors in the model need to be studied to obtain comprehensive or holistic data in order to arrive at an accurate picture of culturally based care. Some researchers may want to start with generic and professional care, whereas others may being with the worldview and social structure dimensions. There is flexibility in the discovery process to fit the information's interested and level of comfort as well as the researcher's goals, domains of inquiry, and research skills.

Because three modes of action and decision (in the lower part of the model) are studied and formulated with informants after the researcher has obtained data in the upper part of the model, the nursing actions or decision become evident. The researcher involves informants in the discussion to arrive at appropriate actions, decisions, or plans. Throughout this discovery process, the researcher holds his or her own etic views, presuppositions, and

Chapter 67: Transcultural Nursing

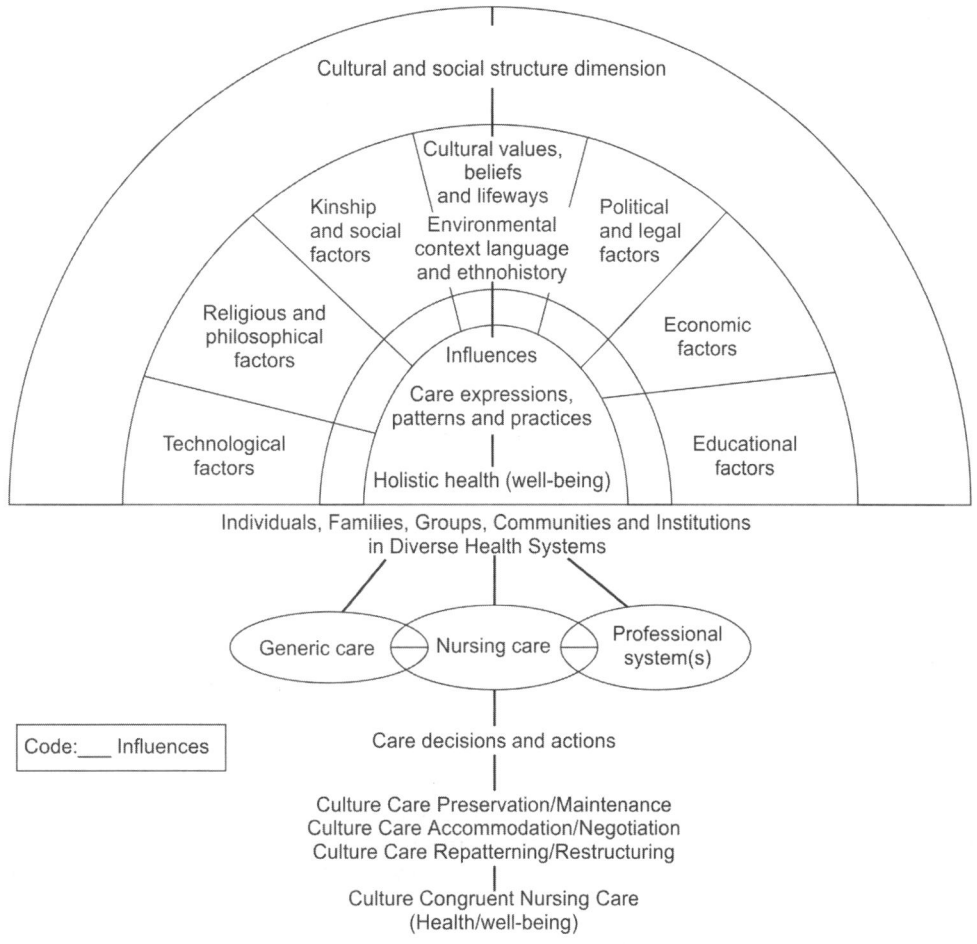

Fig. 67.1: Leininger's sunrise model to depict theory of cultural care diversity and universality.

biases in abeyance, so that the informants cultural ideas will come forth, because they rather than the researcher's view are important and are the reason for the study. Transcultural nurses are taught, guided, and mentored in ways to withhold and deal with their biases and prejudices through formal courses and clinical experience in transcultural nursing.

As the researcher carefully documents the different factors influencing care, he or she focuses on a specific and explicit domain of inquiry (DOI). For example, the researcher may focus on a DOI such as "culture care of Mexican-American mothers caring for their children in their home." Every word in the domain statement is important to study, using the sunrise model and theory tenets. The researcher may have hunches about the domain, but holds them back until all data have been studied with the theory tents. Full documentation of the informant's viewpoints, experiences, and actions is pursued. Generally, informants select what they first want to talk about with the researcher and then the researcher move with informants to cover all aspects of the model and theory tenets. During the in-depth study of the DOI, all areas of the model are covered and discussed and confirmed with the informants. The informants remain active participants throughout the discovery process and in a manner that they feel is their unique and rich contribution.

The sunrise model was developed with the idea of "letting the sun enter the researcher's mind and discovering generally unknown care factors in nurses related to the cultural values and care needs cultures. The model depicts letting the sun "rise and shine" to get fresh and new insights. A wealth of new and unexpected nursing knowledge can be the covered with the model that has never been known and used in traditional nursing for present-day nursing and medical services.

Cultural competent care is the ability of the practitioner to bridge cultural gaps in caring, work without cultural differences, and enable clients and families to achieve meaningful and supportive care. Culturally competent care requires specific knowledge, skills, and attitude in the delivery of culturally congruent care and awareness.

Nursing Decisions

Leininger (1991) identified three nursing decision and action modes to achieve culturally congruent care. All three modes of professional decisions and actions are aimed to assist, support, facilitate, or enable people of particular cultures.

The three modes for congruent care, decisions, and actions proposed in the theory are predicted to lead to health and well-being, or to illness and death.

1. **Cultural preservation or maintenance:** Retain and or preserve relevant care values so that clients can maintain their well-being, recover from illness, or face handicaps and/or death.
   Example: Nutritional practice like malt to protect from protein-energy malnutrition (PEM), etc.
2. **Cultural care accommodation or negotiation:** Adapt or negotiate with the others for a beneficial or satisfying health outcome.
   Example: Kasaya.
3. **Cultural care repatterning or restructuring:** Records, change or greatly modify client's life ways for a new, different and beneficial health care pattern.
   Example: While sleeping head should not be put in north side.

Purposes of Knowing the Patient's Culture and Religion for Health Care Personnel

Cultural background affects a person's health in all dimensions, so the nurse should consider the client's cultural background when planning care. Although basic human needs are the same for all people, the way a person seeks to meet those needs is influenced by culture.

- To heighten awareness of ways in which their own faith system. Provides resources for encounters with illness, suffering, and death.
- To foster understanding, respect, and appreciation for the individuality and diversity of patients beliefs, values, spirituality, and culture regarding illness, its meaning, cause, treatment, and outcome
- To strengthen in their commitment to relationship-centered medicine that emphasizes care of the suffering person rather than attention simply more to the pathophysiology of diseases, and recognizes the physician as a dynamic component of the relationship
- To facilitate in recognizing the role of the hospital chaplain and the patient's clergy as partners in the health care team in providing care for the patient
- To encourage in developing and maintaining a program of physical, emotional, and spiritual self-care introduce therapies from the East, such as Ayurveda and pancha karma.

Status of Traditional Practices

Many traditional practices are used to prevent and a redemptive practice used to prevent illness and harm treat, illness, including objects and substances and religious practices (Morgenstern, 1966).
Example: Circumcision helps to protect men from acquired immunodeficiency syndrome (AIDS).

Use of Protective Objects

Protective objectives can be worm or carried or hung in the home. Amulets are objective with magical powers, for all walks of life and cultural and ethnic backgrounds is example, charms worn on a string or chain around the neck, wrist, or waist to protect the wearer from the evil eye or evil spirits. Amulets exist in societies all over the world and are associated with protection from trouble (Budge, 1978).
Example: Thayatha.

Use of Substances

Substances are ingested in certain ways or amounts regimen, an effort must be made to determine if they are worn or hung in the home. This practice uses diet and consists of many different observances. It is believed that the body is kept in balance or harmony by the type of food eaten, so many food taboos and combinations exist in traditional belief systems. For example, it is believed that some food substances can be ingested to prevent illness. People from many ethnic backgrounds eat raw garlic or onion in an effort to prevent illness or wear them on the body or hang them in the home.

Jews also believe that milk and meat must never be mixed or eaten at the same meal.

Religious Practice

Sanother traditional approach to illness prevention female centers around religion and includes practices such as from a divine source the burning of candles, offering gold and silver to God, rituals of redemption, and in many instances, orthodox religious persons would always prefer to pray. Religion strongly affects the way people attempt to prevent illness, and it plays a strong role in rituals associated with health protection. Religion dictates social, moral, and dietary practices designed to keep a traditional healer (Kaptchuk and Croucher, 1987).

Traditional Remedies

The admitted use of folk or traditional medicine increasing and the practice is seen among people from all walks of life and cultural ethic back ground. Use of folk medicine is not a new practice among heritage consistent people, so many of the remedies have been used and passed on for generations. The pharmaceutical must be made to determine properties of vegetation plants, roots, tested stems, flowers, seeds, and herbs have been studied, tested, cataloged, and used for countless centuries. Many of these plants are used by specific communities. Others cross ethnic and community lines and are used in certain geographic areas in the person's country of origin.

When patients do not adhere to a pharmacological regimen, an effort must be made to determine the remedy if they are taking traditional remedies. Frequently, the active ingredients of traditional remedies are unknown. If a client is believed to be, taking them an effort must be made to determine the remedy as well as its active ingredients often, these ingredients can be antagonistic or synergistic to prescribed medications. Over dose may occur.

Healer

In the traditional context, healing is the restoration of the person to a state of harmony between the body, within a given community; specific people are known to have the power to heal. The healer may be male or and is thought to have received the gift of healing. In many instances, a heritage consistent person may consult a traditional healer before, instead of, or in conjunction with a modern health care provider. Many differences exist between the Western physician and the Eastern. A broad range of health and illness beliefs exist many of these beliefs have roots in the culture, ethnic, religious, or social back ground of a person family, or community. "When people anticipate fear or experience an illness or crisis, they may use a modern or traditional approach toward prevention and healing."

Immigration

Every immigrant group has its own cultural attitudes ranging beliefs and practices regarding these areas. Health and illness can be interpreted in terms of personal experience and expectations. There are countless ways to explain health and illness, and people base their responses on cultural, religious, and ethnic background. The responses are culture specific, based on a client's experience and perception.
Example: The people who came from the Pakistan follow the same cultural beliefs, and tradition as in India; the distance is thousands of kilometers, then they also follow the same things.

Traditional Beliefs about Mental Health

In the traditional belief system, mental illness is caused by a lack of harmony of emotions or sometimes, by evil spirits. Mental wellness occurs when psychological and physiologic functions are integrated. Some elderly Asian Americans share the Buddhist belief that problems in this life are most likely related to transgressions committed in a part life. In addition, our previous life and our future life are as much a part of the life cycle.

Economic Barriers

Several economic barriers, such as unemployment, underemployment, homelessness, lack of health insurance and poverty prevent people from entering the health care system. Poverty is by far the most critical factor. Poverty is a relative term and changes from time and place. In the United States, poverty is pervasive and found extensively among people in certain norms geographical areas, such as rural populations, the elderly migrant workers, and illegal aliens. Poor health, crippling diseases, drug and alcohol abuse, poor education are contributing social causes of poverty.

Several programs, both governmental and private, aid people with short and long term problems. It is important for the nurse to be aware client's needs and financial resources available in the local community.

ROLE OF NURSE IN TRANSCULTURE NURSING

- ❖ The nurse should begin the assessment by attempting to determine the client's cultural heritage and language skills. The client should be asked if any of his health beliefs relate to the cause of the illness or to the problem. The nurse should then determine what, if any, home remedies the person is taking to treat the symptoms.
- ❖ Nurses should evaluate their attitudes toward ethnic nursing care. Some nurses may believe they should treat all clients the same and simply act naturally, but this attitude fails to acknowledge that cultural differences do exist and that there is no one "natural" human behavior. The nurse cannot act the same with all clients and still hope to deliver effective, individualized, holistic care.
- ❖ Sometimes, inexperienced nurses are so self-conscious about cultural differences and so afraid of making a mistake that they impede the nursing process by not asking questions about areas of difference or by asking so many questions that they seem to try into the client's personal life.
- ❖ The process of self-evaluation can help the nurse become more comfortable when providing care to clients from diverse backgrounds.
- ❖ Culture is the sum total of mores traditions and beliefs about how people function encompasses others products of human works and thoughts. Specific to member of an intergenerational group, community, or population.
- ❖ Nurses have a responsibility to understand the influence of culture, race, and ethnicity on the development of social emotional relationship child rearing practices and attitude toward health.
- ❖ Socioeconomic influences play major role in ability to seek opportunity for health promotion for wellness.
- ❖ Religious practices greatly influence health promotion belief in families.
- ❖ Many ethnic and cultural groups in country retain the cultural heritage of their original culture.
- ❖ How culture influences behaviors, attitudes, and values depends on many factors and thus is not the same for different members of a cultural group.

- The nurse should have an understanding of the general characteristics of the major ethnic groups, but should always individualize care rather than generalize about all clients in these groups.
- Before assessing the cultural background of a client, nurses should assess how they are influenced by their own culture
- The nursing diagnosis for clients should include potential problems in their interaction with the health care system and problems involving the effects of culture.
- The planning and implementation of nursing interventions should be adapted as much as possible to the client's cultural background.
- Evaluation should include the nurse's self-evaluation of attitudes and emotions toward providing nursing care to clients from diverse sociocultural backgrounds.
- When nurses provide care to clients from a background other than their own, they must be aware of and sensitive to the client's sociocultural background, assess and listen carefully to health and illness beliefs and practices, and respect and not challenge cultural, ethnic, or religious values and health care beliefs. The nursing process enables the nurse to provide individualized care.
- The client's the nursing process; educational level and language skills should be considered when planning teaching activities.
- Explanations of and practices into nursing therapies; aspects of care usually not questioned by acculturated clients may be required for non-English speaking or nonacculturated clients to avoid confusion, misunderstanding, or cultural conflict.
- The nurse may have to alter her usual ways of interacting with clients to avoid offend ignore alienating a client with different attitudes toward social interaction and etiquette. A client who is modest and self-conscious about the body may need psychological preparation before some procedures and tests.
- The nurse can find out what care the client considers appropriate by involving him and his family in planning care and asking about their expectations. This should be done in every case, even if the nursing care cannot be modified. Because both the nurse and the client are likely to take many aspects of their cultures for granted, questions should be clear and explanations should be explicit.
- Discussing cultural questions related to care with the client and family during the planning stage helps the nurse understand how cultural variables are related to the client's health beliefs and practices, so that interventions can be individualized for the client.
- The nurse evaluates the results of nursing care for ethnic clients as for all clients, determining the extent to which the goals of care have been met.

RESEARCH ABSTRACT

A study was conducted to explore how nurses responded to the cultural needs of their clients among registered nurses ($n = 126$) who were invited to complete questionnaires pertaining to cultural care at University of Nottingham, Faculty of Medicine and Health Sciences, School of Nursing, Queen's Medical Centre. From the transcultural point of view, health care providers must deliver a service that is culturally sensitive and appropriate. However, for a variety of reasons, there is growing concern that the cultural health care needs of minority ethnic groups are not met adequately. This study was done to outline nurses' activity in transcultural care. The findings suggest that most respondents felt that patient's cultural needs should be given consideration. Cultural aspects of care seem to be a feature of the overall nursing picture within a multicultural context of health care. Some felt that patient's cultural needs are adequately met; such needs are perceived as religious practices, diets, communication, dying, prayer, and culture. This study offers some insights into transcultural health care practice, and in accordance with the findings, identifies strategies for improving these practices for nursing and nurse education.

CONCLUSION

Nurses need to be aware of and sensitive to the cultural needs of clients. The body of knowledge relevant to this sensitive area is growing, and it is imperative that nurses from all cultural backgrounds be aware of nursing implications in this area. The practice of nursing today demands that the nurse identify and meet the cultural needs of diverse groups, understand the social and cultural reality of the client, family, and community, develop expertise to implement culturally acceptable strategies to provide nursing care, and identify and use resources acceptable to the client (Boyle, 1987).

CHAPTER 68: Innovations in Nursing

CHAPTER OUTLINE

- Steps in Innovation
- Factors Preventing to Attempt Innovation
- Factors Needed for Innovation
- Factors Leading to Change
- Factors in Organizational Change

INTRODUCTION

The only constant feature in this world is "change." All change may not lead to progress; there can be no progress without change.

To innovate means to introduce something new; to be creative. Changes are imperative in swiftly moving economy, political scene, science, and technology including the expectations of the people. Innovation is a social value of immense proportions.

STEPS IN INNOVATION

Innovation is brought about by a series of processes. It starts with thought. Imagination is the workshop of our mind. It is the act of constructive thinking, grouping knowledge, skills, and attitude into new original and rational ideas. Old ideas and established facts are reassembled into new combinations and put to new uses. Imagination is both interpretive and creative. It can receive impressions and form new combinations and build them into ideas. These ideas are then translated into plans and then into activities. Creative thinking requires keeping our minds open and in a state of expectancy to achieve our objectives. Our minds are compared to parachutes; they function only when they are open.

FACTORS PREVENTING TO ATTEMPT INNOVATION

- Afraid of failures, of opposition, of the unknown, lacking adequate and correct information; reluctant to experiment bound by custom and tradition, and unaware of our strengths for achievement.
- To be innovative, one has to be something of a dreamer and a doer. Even if one does not possess these qualities, one can introduce innovations.

A successful innovator or change agent:
- Identifies opportunities for improvement or overcoming major problems.
- Has readiness to accept change.
- Creates a climate for innovation.
- Supports and sustains the change effort.
- Evaluates, reviews, and modifies activities appropriate for effective change.
- Continues the effort till the desired goal is achieved.

FACTORS NEEDED FOR INNOVATION

- ***A definite purpose:*** To be success, there should be definite aim and purpose. Work out objectives and it should be clear.
- ***Initiative:*** Opens door to opportunity.
- ***Knowledge of facts:*** Get as much information as possible to produce the desired change.
- ***Self-confidence:*** If one thinks one can, one will succeed most of the time.
- ***Persistent efforts:*** One does not succeed, because one gives up at the least difficulty or resistance. One has to be persistent and put up even greater efforts when faced with resistance.

FACTORS LEADING TO CHANGE

- ***Dissatisfaction with status quo:*** Dissatisfaction arises from our desire to do better, to bring improvement over the existing situation. The external and internal environment of organization changes. It may be in:
  - Client needs
  - Technology
  - Competition
- ***Opportunities:*** Newer developments in science, technology, financing, management, etc., may provide opportunities for improvement.

- *A shared vision:* Critical mass of persons within organization for change gives drive and encouragement.
- *Knowledge of first steps:* The first steps are important to get acceptance of the idea by others in organization. It requires knowledge, skills, and attitude to take acceptable first steps.
- *Change has high costs:* The change process the old systems have to continue along with new ones. It produces a dilemma in organization. While introducing innovation there is need to guarantee efficiency, a proper balance has to be maintained.

FACTORS IN ORGANIZATIONAL CHANGE

- A common shared sense of purpose
- Improved quality and reliability of information
- Commitment and sense of responsibility
- Flexible and informal systems, procedures, and practices
- Encouragement and support to initiatives and experimentation
- Teamwork, coordination, and good communication
- Delegation of authority and responsibility
- Open style of managing differences and conflicts
- Willingness to tackle problems and persistence
- Active learning environment
- Valuing individuals and individuality.

An important requirement for innovation is learning from experience. The administrator encounters a situation where something is happening, which was not expected to happen or was not wanted.

The administrator thinks about the problem, and then starts to analyze the problem, its cause, and result. After analysis, objectives are set looking into means and ends, again involving all the persons and winning their consent. The administrator directs, instructs, persuades, negotiates, monitors, and evaluates. The entire organization learns from experience—success or failure.

When introducing a innovation:
- Define the goals and time frame
- Link the activities to goals
- Be specific and integrated; think of the effect on the entire organization
- Sequence the plan
- Be adaptable and acceptable to the people.

Management on change:
- *Technology:* It is changing fast all the time. It is necessary to choose appropriate technology. Improved, suitable technology must be adopted, considering efficiency and benefit ratio. The cost includes not only the cost of machinery and know how but also of retraining personnel and gaining acceptance of the change.
- *Political:* There are problems of allocation of resources. Changes in legislation can affect the function of organization. The management must do these changes adequately and in time.
- *Cultural:* People hold beliefs. It is difficult to change custom and tradition.

The values held by various groups of people in the organization affect acceptance of change.

An innovative organization:
- Accepts uncertainties and risks
- Is willing to face temporary instability
- Allocates sufficient resources for research and development
- Delegates responsibility and authority
- Has dynamic structure to be able to adopt to the changes in future and is flexible
- Uses scientific and technological advances optimally
- Encourages creative thinking.

Readiness to change:
Some individuals and organizations are more ready to effect changes than others. This depends often on degree of felt security. It depends on the culture and climate for innovation, tolerance to ambiguity, possibility of success or failure, and the desire to learn. If there is optimal feeling of security, the individuals and the organization respond to changes if the feeling of security is too high or too low the response to change will not be present.

The scope of health or change in the health has been enormous and the role at which changes occur continues to accelerate. Today's technology and therapeutics were in conceivable even a few decades ago. Over the time, the growth of the health profession has been influenced by those new technologies and therapeutics and there were many other factors and forces like appearance of the new diseases was and consequences of sociocultural issues, religious changes, changing economic, political and legal issue, and changes in the education in nursing.

Definition:
According to Advanced Learner's Dictionary, innovation is defined as the "Introduction of something new."

Development of Innovative Strategies in Nursing Education

Innovations can occur at all levels of an educational organization. Support for innovation in education may begin at the top of the organization or be developed and implemented at a program or individual class levels. Success is enhanced when administrators and the faculty member work side by side to plan strategically and implement changes to improve the educational milieu (Woods, 1998).

Nursing education has gone through innovation. Nildred Montags introduction of associate degree program in nursing developed through the research to meet the assured needs changed the landscape of nursing education. The introduction of the nursing practitioners program also created a revolution in nursing profession.

The introduction of the distance learning in all health professions is the latest revolution and is growing rapidly offering students different choices that is unfettered by the barrier of geography. A successful innovation does not come simply and require creativity, planning, and evaluation.

Process of Innovation

The process of innovation may include several steps. They are as follows:

1. Assessment

It is the first step of the process and it requires a look at both the strength and the problems. Educator must focus on what the expected learning outcome should be with the awareness of learning theory and must student learning styles and need. Specific content requires changes often in health care as new technologies and research bring new knowledge needs with the overwhelming amount of information available in today's healthcare world. It is not possible to include everything the students need. They will need to have appropriate resources to supplement class room/clinical teaching. The instructor must decide what and how much the content to be learned it is so important to consider the students learning needs an understanding and diversity in learning needs to provide a foundation for the development of the effective strategy.

2. Defining Objectives

It is the second step. The literature should be searched for technique that could address the identified needs. Asking students or other faculty members for the suggestion is also helpful. This is the place where the creativity reigns. It is important to look at many different ways to address the learning objectives before selecting one.

3. Planning

Once a strategy has been selected, the third step planning is all important. Understand who the stakeholders are and what their investment is in the present situation or any changes can be helpful in planning the strategies to bring them on the board. May stakeholders including the students do not like the changes and will resist the new approaches. The responsible person can demonstrate the needs and provide information that can make resisters more amenable to changes. Some strategies will require curriculum changes, which is a complex process and one that needs to be started early to avoid immediate delays. It is important to take time to develop a support for the strategy. In more complex strategies, it may be important to bring other faculty members or administrators.

Some strategies may require help from the technical specialist, who may be able to offer support or may give instructions for using and required equipment. Time must be allotted for adequate instructions to enable faculty members and students to reach level, technical staffs may be available to solve the problems, which are bound to occur as a part of planning for evaluation strategy. This is the time to decide what need to be evaluated and how it should be done. This can range from how the strategy will be used in grading to evaluate the learning outcomes for the class as a whole and needs to be developed to allow students and faculty input for the future development. This can also be the time to develop an educational research project if appropriate.

4. Gaining Support for the Innovations

Some strategies require little or no resources to implement whereas others require significant physical and/or financial resources. If resources are needed, then gaining support for the acquisition of those resources is essential grant can provide good funding sources, but require time and effort to secure and may be for a limited time. Administrators may also be excellent resources to tap the discussion for potential funding or acquisition of the physical resources.

Preparing students for innovations
Student instruction needs to be clear and specific. It is the time for motivating the students to want to try this process and for gaining their support. Students need to know how to address the problems especially when technology is involved will not be punished for there mistakes as part of learning process. Evaluation methods or grading must be made clues.

Preparing of faculty members for innovations
Faculty members also need preparation for the innovations for some strategies, rehearsal time may be required or additional education may be required. Planning sufficient for those activities will increase every ones comfort level with this process. This is the time when everyone agrees how the strategy will be run use of perception, validation and clarification can be a valuable tool, e.g., continuing nursing education (CNE) program.

5. Implementation

In this step, it is hoped that the things will be going well, but flexibility may be required if problem arises. Sometimes unintended consequences such as surfacing of emotional issues can occur. Instructors should be alert to need for the follow-up or referral if problem arises.

6. Evaluating the Outcomes

It is the final step of the process learning may continue to occur as the implementation of the strategy. It may be possible to measure short-term attainment of learning outcomes, but it may not be possible to explore the long-term goal. A strong evaluation process provides an opportunity to participate in the educational research. It is important to have evidence-based practice (EBP) in nursing education.

Innovation and Creativity

Innovation and creativity is defined as the introduction of something new by a person, who displays the originality. There are the concepts basic to leadership and any change process. Change innovations and creativity are companion teams but also differentiated changes occur when the system is disrupted. Innovations use changes to create different approaches to solve an issue and develop new products or procedures (Hubber, 1996).

Systemic innovations require willingness to look on changes as an opportunity. Innovations do not create change. Successful innovations are accomplished by exploiting the change not forcing it. The innovative person will look for occasions to be creative and bring new solutions to old problems seven sources for innovative ideas have been identified (Drucker, 1992).

The four sources, which are found internally within the institutions, are:
1. *Unexpected outcomes:* Situations present themselves that require different methods to be adopted knowing what is happening in an institution allows an individual to prepare for the impending changes.
2. *In congruous circumstances:* Disruptions occur that require changes to be made and to eliminate the difference exist between the reality as it is and the reality as it is assumed to be.
3. *Innovations made on the process needs:* Procedures and policies need to be altered to respond to the new regulations, policies, or law.
4. *Changes in structure:* Organizational changes require change in the method of operation.

Three sources are outside the institution:
1. *Changes in the demographics:* Alteration in the community statistics such as age and income levels affects the organizational operations.
2. *New information or knowledge:* New technologies or knowledge requires change in practice.
3. *Changes in perception taste and meaning:* Shifts in demographics, technologies, and social needs create different ways of looking at the situations.

Skills needed for a leader to be an effective innovator
- Looks beyond the immediate situation into the broad world for data on what is happening in other similar areas.
- Finds out the information that is needed to be an effective leader in a specific work situation assumes responsibility for finding information of own needs, uses a variety of different data sources.
- Maintain learning as a lifelong process, incorporate ways to maintain current and up-to-date knowledge.

There are many opportunities for innovations. It is important to be aware of what is going on and recognize the opportunity to be innovative.

Nurses who provide care in a creative and innovative are highly valued by patients. Nurses who are creative give nursing care in a way that is individualized unique and in tune with the circumstances surrounding the patient problems.

Creativity and Innovations in Nursing Practice

Change is inevitable. The individual who looks upon changes as an opportunity to be creative and innovative is to be envied. Having the ability to look beyond the immediate situation and envision the future is the basis for the new and innovative approaches to give the nursing care. Nursing are in all profession is in need of individuals, who have the ability to develop new ways and methods of the care of the problems creative nurse seize the opportunities when presented to try different approaches to solve all the problems.

Flexibility, curiosity, and commitment are needed to try new ways of practicing nursing care, but the students will also need to develop a few characteristics to foster creativity and innovations. Practicing in situations where transits are valued allow the talents to be fostered and nourished. The nursing profession should emphasize the importance of recognizing and rewarding the creative individual.

Having the information about leadership change and innovations allow the nurse to understand the happenings in the clinical area. The knowledgeable nurse will be able to participate and contribute at higher level of performance.

CONCLUSION

World is changing day-by-day with more advancements. All fields are coming up with new innovations. Even nursing has come across many innovative ways in the clinical field and also in the education field. It is the responsibility of every individual to make these contributions, which improves the standard of the profession. Individual as well as the patient will be benefitted out of this.

SUGGESTED READING

1. George Julia B. Nursing Theories: The Base of Professional Nursing Practice, 3rd edition. Norwalk, CN: Appleton and Lange; 1990.
2. Kozier B, Erb G, Barman A, Synder AJ. Fundamentals of Nursing: Concepts, Process and Practice, 7th edition; 2001.
3. Leninger M, McFarland M. Transcultural Nursing: Concepts, Theory, Research and Practice, 3rd edition. New York: McGraw-Hill Professional; 2002.
4. Potter A, Perry G. Basic Nursing :Theory and Practice, 3rd edition. Mosby Company.
5. Kathleen Koerning Blais, et al. Professional Nursing Practice: Concept and Perspectives, Low Price edition, 5th edition; 2007. pp. 373-96.
6. Parker M. Nursing Theories and Nursing Practice. Philadelphia: FA Davis Company; 2001. pp. 365-72.
7. Ackley B, Ladwig G, Swan BA, Tucker S. Evidence-Based Nursing Care Guidelines, 1st edition, Chapter 3: Implementing evidence-based nursing in health care; pp. 3-26.
8. Booker C, Waugh W. Foundations of Nursing Practice, Chapter 5: Evidence-based practice and research; pp. 123-45.
9. Pilot DF, Tatanobeck C. Nursing Research Principles, 7th edition, Chapter 27: Utilizing research; pp. 671-81.
10. Misiaszek BC. Geriatric Medicine Survival Handbook, revised edition, 2008. Michael G. DeGroote School of Medicine at McMaster University.
11. Goldlist B. Geriatric Medicine, 12th edition. MCCQE 2000 Review notes and lecture series.
12. Burke M, Sherman S. Geronotological Nursing, 1st edition. New York: National League for Nursing Press.
13. Bhattacharjee T. Geriatric Nursing, 1st edition. CBS Publishers and Distributors Pvt Ltd.
14. Gomez LM. Geriatric Nursing, 1st edition. Jaypee Publication; 2009.
15. Harrison's Principles of Internal Medicine, 16th edition. New York: McGraw-Hill Medical Publishing Division; 2005.
16. Lewis SM. Medical Surgical Nursing, 7th edition. New Delhi, Mosby Publication; 2002.
17. Block JM. Medical Surgical Nursing, 6th edition. New York: WB Saundars Publication; 2002.
18. Brunner and Suddarth's Textbook of Medical Surgical Nursing, 11th edition. New Delhi: Lippincott and Williams and Wilkins; 2008.
19. Cherry B, Susan RJ. Contemporary Nursing: Issues, Trends and Management, 2nd edition 2 USA: Mosby Publications; 2002. pp. 551-8, 543-4.
20. Potter PA, Perry AG. Fundamentals of Nursing, 6th edition. Toronto: Mosby Company; 2007. pp. 223-5.
21. Stanhope M, Lancaster J. Community and Public Health Nursing, 5th edition. Mosby. Toronto; 2000. pp. 932-42.
22. Jarvis P. The practitioner-researcher in nursing. Nurse Education Today. 2000; 20(1):30-34.
23. www.telenursing.com
24. www.RNcasemanager.com
25. Stanhope M, Lancaster J. Community Health Nursing, 4th edition. New York, Missouri: Mosby; 1996. pp. 230-50.
26. Park K. Preventure and Social Medicine, 21st edition. Jabalpur: Bhanot Publishers.
27. Basavantappa BT. Nursing Research. New Delhi: Jaypee Publishers.
28. Polit DF, Beck CT. Nursing Research Generating and Assessing Evidence for Nursing Practice, 9th edition. New York: Lippincott Williams and Wilkins; Wolters Kluwer; 2012.
29. Basavanthappa BT. Community Health Nursing, 1st edition. Jaypee Publications; pp. 66-96.
30. Grumbach K, Miller J, et al. How much public health in public health nursing practice? Public Health Nursing. 2004; 21(3):266-76.

Journal

1. Malik A. Associate Professor, Qualitative research in Work Practice, volume 21, No.1.
- Narayanasamy A. Transcultural nursing: how do nurses respond to cultural needs? Br J Nurs. 2003 ;12(3):185-94.
- www.nursingcareers>eduction.com
- www.uptodate.com
- www.medscape.com/drupinfo
- www.scribd.com
- www.nursescribe.com
- www.nursing.journals.com
- http:www.uptodate.com
- cochranelibrary.com
- onlinelibrary.wiley.com

REVIEW OF SECTION BASED QUESTIONS OF RGUHS

Long Essays

1. What is the extended and expanded role of nurse? How can it be applied to health care delivery system? Explain in detail about the extended and expanded role of nurse in health care delivery system. (May 2010)
2. Explain in detail about primary health care.
3. What is the role o nurse in disaster management?
4. How innovations in nursing g can be applied to practise?
5. Collaboration issues and models – within and outside nursing.
6. Discuss the issues on independent practise in nursing. (May 2012)
7. Explain the approach o clinical nursing practise through nurse clinician and nurse practitioners. (November 2012)
8. Apply the ethical decision process to specific ethical issues, encountered in nursing practice. (May 2011)
9. Analyze the current concepts of nursing care. Articulate a new vision of nursing practice based on changing technology. (May 2011)

10. Explain the concepts of primary health care and role of nurses in providing primary health care. (October 2010)
11. List three concepts of nursing practise. Explain the advantages and limitation of any one concept. (September 2007)
12. Enumarate the extended and expanded role of the nurse while caring for the patient with CVA. (October 2010)
13. Discuss on the extended and expanded role of the nursing. (May 2010)
14. Explain the concept of primary health care and discuss the problems related to resources in present system of healthcare in India. (May 2009)
15. Research is the key for the future of nursing - Explain.
16. Discuss the importance of research in nursing. Explain two ethical issues of nursing profession. (September 2007)
17. Define, disaster management and discuss the role of nursing during disaster. (April/May 2007)
18. Discuss in detail, the level of prevention healthcare. (2006)
19. Explain, what is primary healthcare and role of nurses in providing, primary healthcare. (2006)
20. Discuss the role of nurse as a nurse clinician in healthcare delivery system. (September 2005)
21. List the extended and expanded role of nurses in our country. Describe the extended nurse's role in basic physical and psychosocial assessment. (September 2005)
22. What is evidence based nursing? Discuss the present status of evidence based nursing in India. (May 2013)

Short Essays

1. Transcultural nursing.
2. Philosophy of nursing practice. (2005)
3. Primary nursing. (September 2005)
4. Nurse clinician. (September 2007)
5. Clinical nurse specialist. (April 2008)
6. Ethical issues in nursing. (May 2010)
7. Women empowerment. (November 2012)
8. Nurse in extended care facilities. (October 2010 and May 2012)
9. Ethical issues in nursing. (2006 and May 2012)
10. Alternative modalities of care.
11. Concept of primary health care and self care. (May 2011)
12. Independent practice issues.
13. Geriatric considerations in nursing. (November 2012)
14. Team Nursing. (May/October 2010)
15. Dimensions of Nursing care. (April 2008, October 2010 and November 2012)
16. Innovations in nursing.
17. Disaster nursing. (May/October 2010)
18. Politics in Nursing. (May 2010)
19. Advanced Nurse practitioner. (May 2009)
20. Primary Nursing. (April/May 2007)
21. Common ethical dilemmas in nursing. (April/May 2007)
22. Expanded and role of nurse. (2006)
23. Independent nurse practitioner. (May 2013)
24. Extended and expanded role of a nurse. (May 2013)

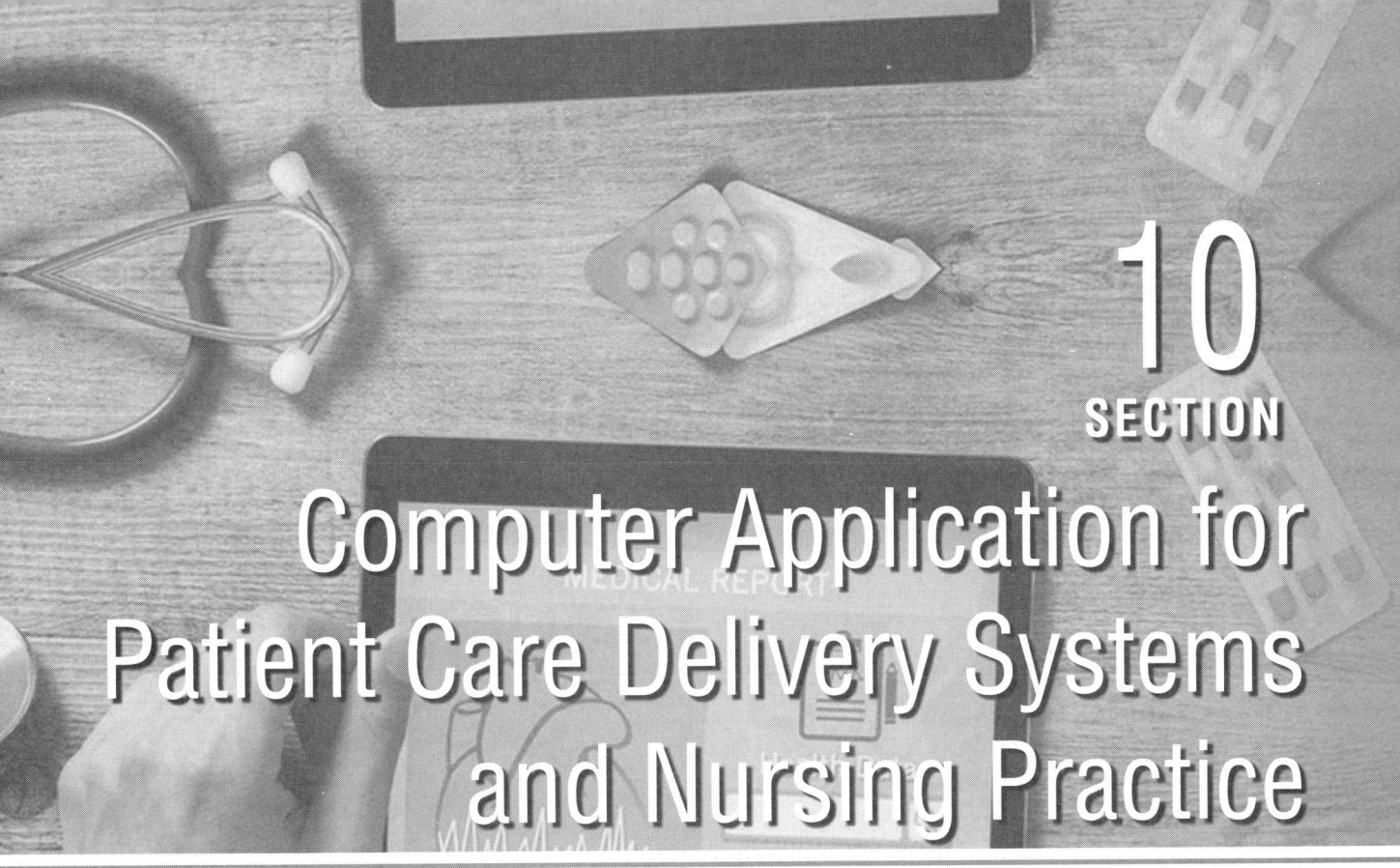

SECTION 10
Computer Application for Patient Care Delivery Systems and Nursing Practice

Section Outline

69. Use of Computers in Teaching, Learning, Research, and Nursing Practice
70. Windows, MS Office, Word, Excel, PowerPoint/Operating Systems of a Computer
71. Internet Literatures Search
72. Statistical Packages
73. Hospital Management Information System Software

69 CHAPTER
Use of Computers in Teaching, Learning, Research, and Nursing Practice

CHAPTER OUTLINE

- Uses of Computers
  - In Clinical Practice
  - In Teaching and Learning
  - In Nursing Research
  - In Nursing Administration

INTRODUCTION

Computers influence every sphere of human activity and bring many changes in education, health care, scientific research, medical transcription, and in social sciences. In developed countries, computers have become part of every man's life, whereas in India, it is limited to certain fields. Use of computers in healthcare system will economize energy, and help the nurses to provide quality nursing care and save time. "Microcomputers in the classroom" is a hands-on course for educators wishing an overall orientation, their operation software and rudimentary concepts of programming. This course is offered three to four times per year; students from all disciplines are eligible.

USES OF COMPUTERS

In Clinical Practice

- Admission and transfer system allows nurses to obtain basic biographical information about the clients before they arrive to the ward/unit.
- When a discharge or transfer is entered in the computer, all the appropriate departments will be notified, e.g. Pharmacy, Dietary, Housekeeping, Census and Client's location in the unit, etc., everything will be readily available, thus it saves the time of the nurses.

Nursing Documentation

Computer typing is very legible. Nursing process, care plan, implementation of activities, nursing notes, and discharge plans can be computerized. It can be stored in a format determined by the institution. Through computers drug calculations, flow rates can be done more accurately and easily. Multiple program choices can be chosen for application of nursing theories in implementation of nursing care activities. Communicate Physician's order, monitor clients' values, and also receive laboratory test results and patient's information to the respective wards, but maintain invasion of privacy.

In Teaching and Learning

Computer-assisted instruction programs are very useful in self-paced learners who will interact with computer (as it takes the role of a teacher).

Drill and Practice

- Most common and least complex method.
- A learner is presented with a series of questions or problems about materials, e.g. drug dosage calculations, drip rate calculations, and terminology.
- Writing of textbooks; collection of education materials.

Library Maintenance

- Tutorial programs
- Display new material
- Tutorial information.

Feedback

- Simulations, the real life situations will be presented to assist learners in problem-solving and decision-making skills in a safe environment.
- Interactive video instruction (IAV) can provide learners with true-to-life simulation.
- Video pictures, graphics can be incorporated in the design of software.

In Nursing Research

- Review literature or search for related articles, e.g. Internet, Med line, pubmed search, etc.

- Tool for data collection.
- Dissemination of findings and results.
- Tabulations or statistical analysis and description of tables.
- Preparation of research reports, project report.

In Nursing Administration

Computerized patients classification system can be used to assign nursing staff based on how severely ill the clients are:
- Clients are classified on the basis of their abilities or need for nursing care.
- Computerized inventory system keeps track of supplies received and disbursed.
- Client billing system.

Diagnosis or Reports

General computer application software, e.g. word processing, electronic spread sheets, database management sheets.

Budget Planning

- Maintenance of individual records.
- Calculation of number of nurses required on each unit (nurses with clients ratio).
- Computers are one of the leading innovations in the present world and are most useful in the field of medicine and nursing.

Computers for Teacher's Activities at the University Level

- Availability of technical support.
- To meet the needs of students, teachers and administrators.
- To assist with operational programs.
- To maintain high standards for professional development and practice.
- To nurture appropriate interest in research.
- To increase knowledge about teaching and learning process.
- Action-oriented research.
- Training and support activities.
- Professionals should get involved in planning for collecting and interpreting data to aid in decisions in their schools.
- Resources of colleges and universities, training and support offered to teachers through colleges should take the advantage of the special resources available there.

Microcomputers are used throughout the university in many different ways:
- Information systems
- Process control
- Laboratory equipment
- Specialized graphics, etc.:
  - Students should have the opportunity to learn about current and future uses of microcomputers
  - Exploration of microcomputers applications open doorways onto the entire world of computing
  - To give appropriate attention to matters of learning and teaching

CONCLUSION

Computers are one of the leading innovations in the present world and are most useful in the field of medicine and nursing.

CHAPTER 70

Windows, MS Office, Word, Excel, PowerPoint/Operating Systems of a Computer

CHAPTER OUTLINE

- Microsoft Windows
- History of Microsoft Windows
- Future of Windows
- Microsoft Office (MS office)
- Microsoft Office Excel
- Microsoft PowerPoint

MICROSOFT WINDOWS

Introduction

Microsoft is a series of operating systems produced by Microsoft.

Microsoft first introduced an operating environment named Windows on November 20, 1985 as an add-on to MS-DOS is response to the growing interest in graphical user interfaces (GUIs). Microsoft Windows came to dominate the world's personal computer market, overtaking Mac OS, which had been introduced in 1984. As of October 2009, Windows had approximately 90% of the market share of the client operating systems for usage on the internet. The most recent client version of Windows is Windows 7; the most recent server version is Windows Server 2008 (Fig. 70.1).

HISTORY OF MICROSOFT WINDOWS

Microsoft has taken two parallel routes in its operating systems. One route has been for the home user and the other has been for the professional IT user. The dual routes have generally led to home versions having greater multimedia support and less functionality in networking and security, and professional versions having inferior multimedia support and better networking and security. The first version of Microsoft Windows, version 1.0, released in November 1985, lacked a degree of functionality and achieved little popularity, and was to compete with Apple's own operating system. Windows 1.0 is not a complete operating system; rather, it extends MS-DOS. Microsoft Windows version 2.0 was released in November 1987 and was slightly more popular than its predecessor. Windows 2.03 (release date January 1988) had changed the OS from tiled windows to overlapping windows.

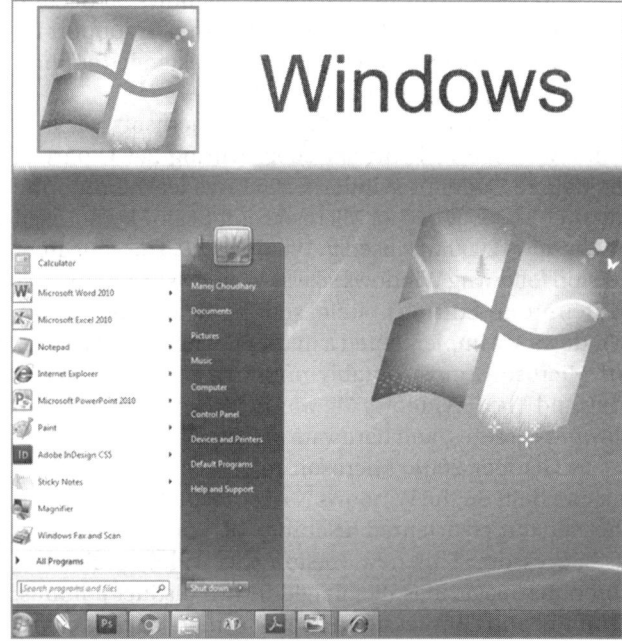

Fig. 70.1: Microsoft windows.

The result of this change led to Apple Computer filing a suit against Microsoft alleging infringement on Apple's copyrights.

Microsoft Windows version 3.0 released in 1990 was the first Microsoft Windows version to achieve broad commercial success, selling 2 million copies in the first 6 months. It featured improvements to the user interface and to multitasking capabilities. It received a facelift in Windows 3.1, made generally available on March 1, 1992. Windows 3.1 support ended on December 31, 2001.

In July 1993, Microsoft released Windows NT based on a new kernel. Windows NT 3.1 was the first release of Windows NT. NT was considered to be the professional OS and was the first Windows version to utilize preemptive multitasking. Windows NT would later be retooled also to function as a home operating system with Windows XP.

On August 24, 1995, Microsoft released Windows 95, a new and major consumer version that made further changes to the user interface, and also used preemptive multitasking. Windows 95 was designed to replace not only Windows 3.1 but also Windows for Workgroups and MS-DOS. It was also the first Windows operating system to use plug-and-play capabilities. The changes Windows 95 brought to the desktop were revolutionary as opposed to evolutionary, such as those in Windows 98 and Windows Me. Mainstream support for Windows 95 ended on December 31, 2000, and extended support for Windows 95 ended on December 31, 2001. The next in the consumer line was Microsoft Windows 98 released on June 25, 1998. It was followed with the release of Windows 98 Second Edition (Windows 98 SE) in 1999. Mainstream support for Windows 98 ended on June 30, 2002, and extended support for Windows 98 ended on July 11, 2006.

As part of its "professional" line, Microsoft released Windows 2000 in February 2000. During 2004, part of the Source Code for Windows 2000 was leaked onto the Internet. This was bad for Microsoft as the same kernel used in Windows 2000 was used in Windows XP. The consumer version following Windows 98 was Windows Me (Windows Millennium Edition). Released in September 2000, Windows Me implemented a number of new technologies for Microsoft; most notably publicized was "Universal Plug and Play." Windows Me was heavily criticized due to slowness, freezes, and hardware problems.

In October 2001, Microsoft released Windows XP, a version built on the Windows NT kernel that also retained the consumer-oriented usability of Windows 95 and its successors. This new version was widely praised in computer magazines. It shipped in two distinct editions, "Home" and "Professional," the former lacking many of the superior security and networking features of the Professional edition. Additionally, the first "Media Center" edition was released in 2002, with an emphasis on support for DVD and TV functionality including program recording and a remote control. Mainstream support for Windows XP ended on April 14, 2009. Extended support will continue until April 8, 2014.

In April 2003, Windows Server 2003 was introduced, replacing the Windows 2000 line of server products with a number of new features and a strong focus on security; this was followed in December 2005 by Windows Server 2003 R2. On January 30, 2007, Microsoft released Windows Vista. It contains a number of new features from a redesigned shell and user interface to significant technical changes, with a particular focus on security features. It is available in a number of different editions and has been subject to some criticism.

On October 22, 2009, Microsoft released Windows 7. Unlike its predecessor, Windows Vista, which introduced a large number of new features, Windows 7 was intended to be a more focused, incremental upgrade to the Windows line with the goal of being compatible with applications and hardware which Windows Vista was not at the time. Windows 7 has multitouch support, a redesigned Windows shell with a new taskbar, referred to as the Super bar, a home networking system called home group and performance improvements.

FUTURE OF WINDOWS

Windows 8, the successor to Windows 7 is currently in development. Microsoft has posted a blog entry in Dutch on October 22, 2010, hinting that Windows 8 will be released in 2 years. Also, during the pre-Consumer Electronics Show keynote, Microsoft's Chief Executive Officer (CEO) announced that Windows 8 will also run on architecture reference manual (ARM) central processing units (CPUs). Since ARM CPUs are usually in the form of systems on chip (SOCs) found in mobile devices. This new announcement implies that Windows 8 will be more compatible with mobile devices such as netbooks, tablet personal computers, and smartphones.

MICROSOFT OFFICE (MS OFFICE)

Microsoft office is a group of software programs designed to help you to create documents, collaborate with co-workers and track and analyze information. Each program is designed so that you can work quickly and efficiently to create professional-looking results. You use different office programs to accomplish specific tasks, such as writing a letter or producing sales presentation, yet all the programs have a similar look and feel. Once you became familiar with one program, you will find it easy to transfer your knowledge to the others. This unit introduces you to the most frequently used programs in office, as well as common features they all share.

Microsoft Office Word

When you need to create any kind of text-based documents, such as memos, newsletters, or multipage report, word is the program to use. You can easily make your documents look great by inserting eye-catching graphics and using formatting tools such as themes. Themes are predesigned combinations of color and formatting attributes one can apply and are available in most office programs (Fig. 70.2).

Parts of a Word Window

Title bar: This lesson will familiarize you with the Microsoft Word screen. We will start with the Title bar, which is located at the very top of the screen (Fig. 70.3). On the Title bar, Microsoft Word displays the name of the document on

Chapter 70: Windows, MS Office, Word, Excel, PowerPoint/Operating Systems of a Computer

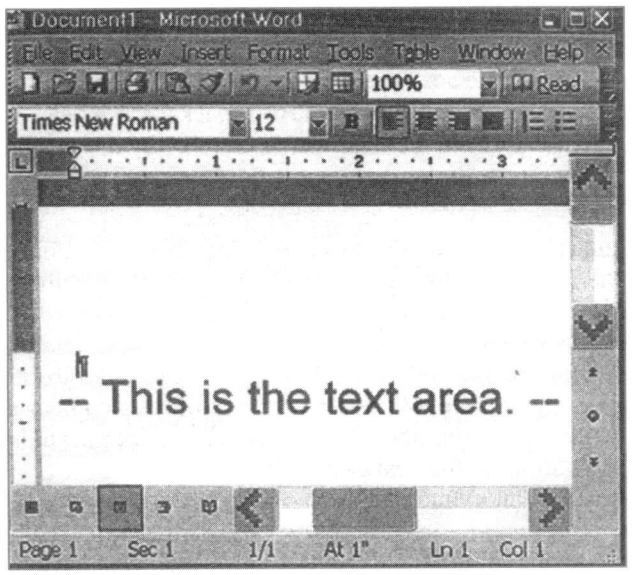

Fig. 70.2: Microsoft word.

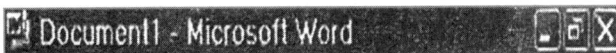

Fig. 70.3: Title bar.

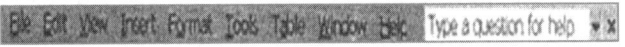

Fig. 70.4: Menu bar.

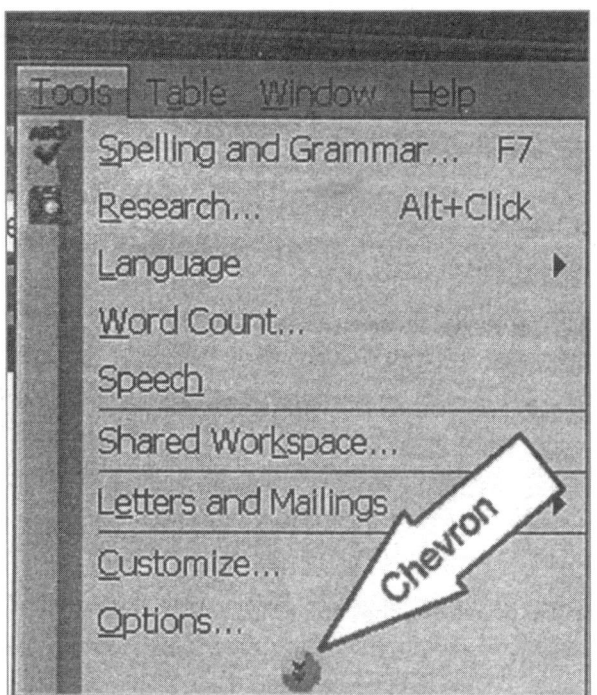

Fig. 70.5: Spelling and grammar.

which you are currently working. At the top of your screen, you should see "Microsoft Word- Document1" or a similar name.

Menu bar: The Menu bar is generally found directly below the Title bar. The Menu bar displays the menu. The Menu bar begins with the word File and continues with Edit, View, Insert, Format, Tools, Table, Window, and Help. You use the menus to give instructions to the software. Point with your mouse to a menu option and click the left mouse button to open a drop-down menu. You can now use the left and right arrow keys on your keyboard to move left and right across the Menu bar options. You can use the up and down arrow keys to move up and down the drop-down menu (Fig. 70.4).

The most frequently used menu options appear on the menu list. A chevron appears at the bottom of the list. Click the chevron to display additional menu options (Fig. 70.5).

To select an option, click the option or use the arrow keys to move to the option on the drop-down menu and press Enter. An ellipse or a right arrow after a menu item signifies additional options; if you select that menu item, a dialog box appears. Items in gray are not available. You can customize your screen so that all of the menu options display when you click a menu item. This tutorial assumes that your menu is set to display all menu options (Figs. 70.6 and 70.7). To customize your menu to display all of the menu options:

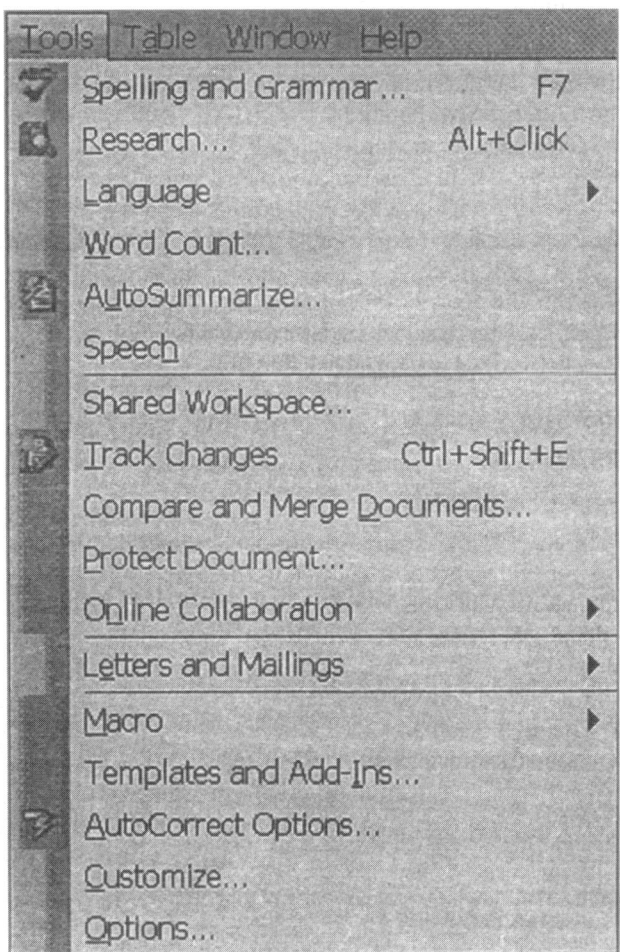

Fig. 70.6: Tools.

Section 10: Computer Application for Patient Care Delivery Systems and Nursing Practice

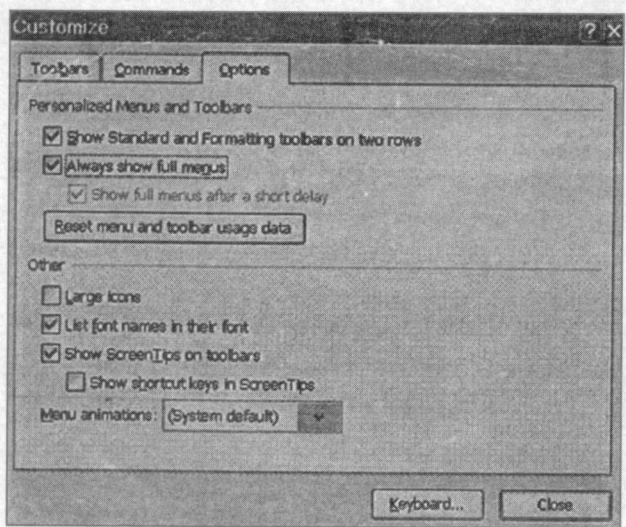

Fig. 70.7: Customize.

- Click "Tools" on the "Menu" bar.
- Click "Customize" on the drop-down menu. The "Customize" dialog box opens.
- Click the "Options" tab.
- Click in the check box to select "Always Show Full Menus."
- Click Close.

Exercise 1: Do the following exercise. It demonstrates using the Microsoft Word menu:
- Click File on the Menu bar.
- Press the right arrow key until Help is highlighted.
- Press the left arrow key until Format is highlighted.
- Press the down arrow key until Styles and Formatting are highlighted.
- Press the up arrow key until Paragraph is highlighted.
- Press Enter to select the Paragraph menu option.
- Click Cancel to close the dialog box.

Toolbars

Standard Toolbar (Fig. 70.8)

Formatting toolbar

Toolbars provide shortcuts to menu commands. Toolbars are generally located just below the Menu bar. Before proceeding with this lesson, make sure the toolbars you will use—Standard and Formatting—are available. Follow these steps:
- Click View on the Menu bar.
- Highlight Toolbars.
- Standard and Formatting should have check marks next to them. If both standard and Formatting have check marks next to them, press Esc three times to close the menu.
- If they do not both have check marks, click Customize.
- Click the Toolbars tab.
- Point to the box next to the unchecked option and click the left mouse button to make a check mark appear. *Note:* You turn the check mark on and off by clicking the left mouse button.
- Click Close to close the dialog box.

Ruler: The ruler is generally found below the main toolbars. The ruler is used to change the format of your document quickly. To display the ruler (Fig. 70.9):
- Click View on the Menu bar.
- The option Ruler should have a check mark next to it. If it has a check mark next to it, press Esc to close the menu. If it does not have a check mark next to it, continue to the next step.
- Click Ruler. The ruler now appears below the toolbars.
- *Document view:* In Word, you can display your document in one of five views: Normal, Web Layout, Print Layout, Reading Layout, or Online Layout.
- *Normal view:* Normal view is the most often used and shows formatting such as line spacing, font, point size, and italics. Word displays multiple-column text in one continuous column.
- *Web layout:* Web layout view enables you to view your document as it would appear in a browser such as Internet Explorer.
- *Print layout:* The Print Layout view shows the document as it will look when it is printed.
- *Reading layout:* Reading Layout view formats your screen to make reading your document more comfortable.
- *Outline view:* Outline view displays the document in outline form. Headings can be displayed without the text. If you move a heading, the accompanying text moves with it.

Before moving ahead, check to make sure you are in normal view.
- Click View on the Menu bar.
- The icon next to Normal should have a box around it. If the icon next to normal has a box around it, press Esc to close the menu. If the icon next to Normal does not have a box around it, continue on to the next step.
- Click Normal. You are now in Normal view.

Text area: Just below the ruler is a large area called the "Text Area." You type your document in "text area." The blinking vertical line in the upper left corner of the text area is the cursor. It marks the insertion point. As you type, your work shows at the cursor location. The horizontal line next to the cursor marks the end of the document (Fig. 70.10).

Exiting word: You have completed Lesson 1. Typically, you would save your work before exiting. This lesson does not

Fig. 70.8: Toolbar.

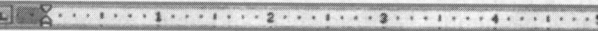

Fig. 70.9: Ruler.

Chapter 70: Windows, MS Office, Word, Excel, PowerPoint/Operating Systems of a Computer

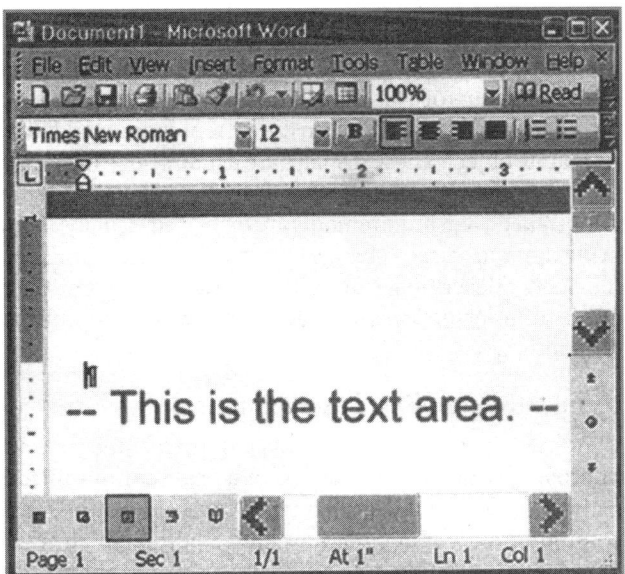

Fig. 70.10: Text area.

require you to enter any text, so you might have nothing to save. To exit word:
- Click File.
- Click Exit, which can be found at the bottom of the drop-down menu.
- If you have entered text, you will be prompted: "Do you want to save changes to Document 1 ?" To save your changes, click Yes. Otherwise, click No.
- Specify the correct folder in the Save In box.
- Name your file by typing lesson1.doc in the File Name field.
- Click Save.

MICROSOFT OFFICE EXCEL

Introduction

Excel is the perfect solution when you need to work with numeric values and make calculations. It puts the power of formulas, functions, charts, and other analytical tools into the hands of every user, so you can analyze sales projections, figure out loan payments, and present your findings in style. The Excel automatically recalculates results whenever a value changes, the information is always up to date. A chart illustrates how the monthly expenses are broken down.

Microsoft Excel is a commercial spreadsheet application written and distributed by Microsoft for Microsoft Windows and Mac OS X. It features calculation, graphing tools, pivot tables, and a macroprogramming language called Visual Basic for Applications (VBA). It has been a very widely applied spreadsheet for these platforms, especially since version 5 in 1993 and it has almost completely replaced Lotus 1-2-3 as the industry standard for spreadsheets. Excel forms part of Microsoft Office. The current versions are 2010 for Microsoft Windows and 2011 for Mac OS X (Fig. 70.11).

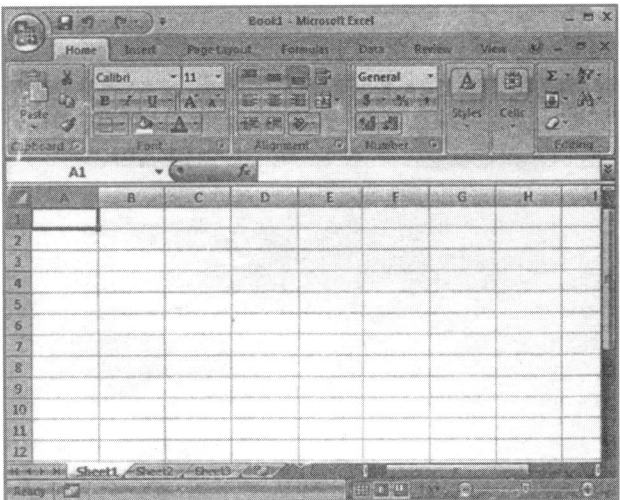

Fig. 70.11: Microsoft excel.

Features of Microsoft Excel: Microsoft Excel has the basic features of all spreadsheets, using a grid of cells arranged in numbered rows and letter named columns to organize data manipulations similar to arithmetic operations:
- It has a battery of supplied functions to answer statistical, engineering, and financial needs.
- It can display data as line graphs, histograms, and charts, and with a very limited three-dimensional graphical display.
- It allows sectioning of data to view its dependencies on various factors from different perspectives (using pivot tables and the scenario manager).
- It has a programming aspect, VBA, allowing the user to employ a wide variety of numerical methods, e.g. for solving differential equations of mathematical physics and then reporting the results back to the spreadsheet.
- Finally, it has a variety of interactive features allowing user interfaces that can completely hide the spreadsheet from the user, so the spreadsheet presents itself as a so-called application or decision support system (DSS), via a custom-designed user interface, e.g. a stock analyzer or in general, as a design tool that asks the user questions and provides answers and reports. In a more elaborate realization, an Excel application can automatically poll external databases and measuring instruments using an update schedule, analyze the results.
- Make a Word report or PowerPoint slide show, and e-mail these presentations on a regular basis to a list of participants.
- Microsoft allows for a number of optional command-line switches to control the manner in which Excel starts (Fig. 70.12).
- The Windows version of Excel supports programming through Microsoft's VBA, which is a dialect of Visual Basic. Programming with VBA allows spreadsheet manipulation that is awkward or impossible with standard spreadsheet techniques. Programmers may

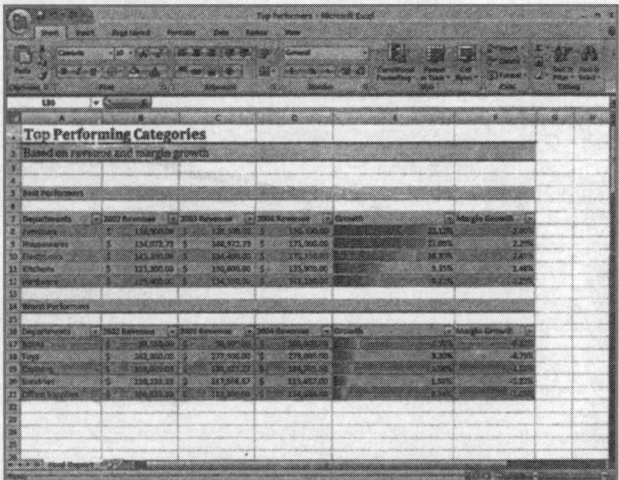

Fig. 70.12: Features of Microsoft Excel.

write code directly using the Visual Basic Editor (VBE), which includes a window for writing code, debugging, and code module organization environment.
❖ The user can implement numerical methods as well as automating tasks such a formatting or data organization in VBA and guide the calculation using any desired intermediate results reported back to the spreadsheet.

VBA Programming

VBA was removed from Mac Excel 2008 as the developers did not believe that a timely release would allow porting the VBA engine natively to Mac as X. VBA was restored in the next version, Mac Excel 2011. A common and easy way to generate VBA code is by using the macro recorder. The macro recorder records actions of the user and generates VBA code in the form of a macro. These actions can then be repeated automatically by running the macro. The macros can also be linked to different trigger types such as keyboard shortcuts, a command button, or a graphic. The actions in the macro can be executed from these trigger types or from the generic toolbar options. The VBA code of the macro can also be edited in the VBE. Certain features such as loop functions and screen prompts by their own properties, and some graphical display items, cannot be recorded, but must be entered into the VBA module directly by the programmer. Advanced users can employ user prompts to create an interactive program, or react to events such as sheets being loaded or changed.

VBA code interacts with the spreadsheet through the Excel Object Model, a vocabulary identifying spreadsheet Objects, and a set of supplied functions or methods that enable reading and writing to the spreadsheet and interaction with its users (for example, through custom toolbars or command bars and message boxes). User-created VBA subroutines execute these actions and operate like macros generated using the macro recorder, but are more flexible and efficient.

Charts

Excel supports charts, graphs, or histograms generated from specified groups of cells. The generated graphic component can either be embedded within the current sheet or added as a separate object. These displays are dynamically updated if the content of cells changes. For example, suppose that the important design requirements are displayed visually; then, in response to a user's change in trial values for parameters, the curves describing the design change shape and their points of intersection shift, assisting the selection of the best design.

Using Other Windows Applications

Windows applications such as Microsoft access and Microsoft Word, as well as Excel as can communicate with each other and use each other capabilities. The most common are dynamic data exchange: although strongly deprecated by Microsoft, this is a common method to send data between applications running on Windows, with official MS publications referring to it as "the protocol from hell." As the name suggests, it allows applications to supply data to others for calculation and display. It is very common in financial markets, being used to connect to important financial data services such as Bloomberg and Reuters. Object Linking and Embedding (OLE): Allows a Windows application to control another to enable it to format or calculate data. This may take on the form of "embedding" where an application uses another to handle as task that it is more suited to, for example, a PowerPoint presentation may be embedded in an Excel spreadsheet or vice versa.

Quirks

A major complaint is finding relevant assistance from the associated help system. Contributing to this issue is the Excel 2007 menu system, which adapts to the users history of use. That adaptivity means that there may be no unique or perhaps even straightforward, way to explain how to do a particular task.

Other errors specific to Excel include misleading statistics functions, mod function errors, date limitations, and the Excel 2007 display error.

Statistical Functions

The accuracy and convenience of statistical tools in Excel has been criticized, as mishandling missing data, as returning incorrect values due to inept handling of round-off and large numbers, as only selectively updating calculations on a spreadsheet when some cell values are changed, and as having a limited set of statistical tools. Microsoft has announced some of these issues are addressed in Excel 2010.

Graphing

The menus related to graphs and graph formatting have been changed completely in Excel 2007. Some common activities in using graphs are less transparent than previously. For example, to add a curve to a graph, one can right click on the graph and choose "select data" from the drop-down menu or use the "chart tools/design" tab. However, when there are other drop-down menus open, this menu does not appear and the "select data" option is grayed out (unavailable) from the tool bar. That facet of the menu system must be "discovered" by the user. These quirks and other nontransparent features contribute to a long learning curve, and to annoyance if one returns to Excel after an absence long enough to forget these little "tricks" of the menu system.

Excel MOD Function Error

Excel has issues with modulo operations. In the case of excessively large results, Excel will return the error warning NUM instead of an answer.

Date Problems

Excel includes January 0, 1900, and February 29, 1900, incorrectly treating 1900 as a leap year. The bug originated from Lotus 1-2-3, and was purposely implemented in Excel for the purpose of backward compatibility. This legacy has later been carried over into Office Open XML file format.

Filenames

Microsoft Excel will not open two documents with the same name and instead will display the following error:
- A document with the name "%s" is already open. You cannot open two documents with the same name, even if the documents are in different folders. To open the second document, either close the document that is currently open or rename one of the documents.
- The reason is for calculation ambiguity with linked cells. If there is a cell =[Book1.xlsx] Sheet1 !G33, and there are two books named "Book1" open, there is no way to tell which one the user means.

Numeric Precision

Despite the use of 15-figure precision, Excel can display many more figures (up to 30) upon user request. But the displayed figures are not those actually used in its computations, and so, for example, the difference of two numbers may differ from the difference of their displayed values. Although such departures are usually beyond the 15th decimal, exceptions do occur, especially for very large or very small numbers. Serious errors can occur if decisions are made based upon automated comparisons of numbers (for example, using the Excel if function), as equality of two numbers can be unpredictable.

In the figure, the fraction 1/9000 is displayed in Excel. Although this number has a decimal representation that is an infinite string of ones, Excel displays only the leading 15 figures. In the second line, the number one is added to the fraction and again Excel displays only 15 figures. In the third line, one is subtracted from the sum using Excel. Because the sum in the second line has only 11 1's after the decimal, the difference when "1" is subtracted from this displayed value is three 0's followed by a string of 11 1's. However, the difference reported by Excel in the third line is three 0's followed by a string of thirteen 1's and two extra erroneous digits. Thus, the numbers Excel calculates with to obtain the third line are not the numbers that it displays in the first two lines. Moreover, the error in Excel's answer is not just round-off error.

Excel works with a modified 1985 version of the IEEE 754 specification. Excel's implementation involves an amalgam of truncations and conversions between binary and decimal representations, leading to accuracy that sometimes is better than one would expect from simple fifteen digit precision and sometimes much worse. See the main article for details. Besides accuracy in user computations, the question of accuracy in Excel-provided functions may be raised. Particularly in the arena of statistical functions, Excel has been criticized for sacrificing accuracy for speed of calculation.

As many calculations in Excel are executed using VBA, an additional issue is the accuracy of VBA, which varies with variable type and user-requested precision.

Versions

Microsoft Windows

- 1987 Excel 2.0 for Windows
- 1990 Excel 3.0
- 1992 Excel 4.0
- 1993 Excel 5.0 (Office 4.2 and 4.3, also a 32-bit version for Windows NT only on the x86, PowerPC, Alpha, and MIPS architectures)
- 1995 Excel for Windows 95 (version 7.0) included in Office 95
- 1997 Excel 97 (version 8.0) included in Office 97 (for x86 and Alpha). This version of Excel includes a flight simulator as an Easter Egg
- 1999 Excel 2000 (version 9.0) included in Office 2000
- 2001 Excel 2002 (version 10) included in Office XP
- 2003 Office Excel 2003 (version 11) included in Office 2003
- 2007 Office Excel 2007 (version 12) included in Office 2007
- 2010 Excel 2010 (version 14) included in Office 2010.

MICROSOFT POWERPOINT

Microsoft PowerPoint is a full-featured desktop presentation program. It is part of the Office suite and can be purchased separately. A presentation can be a collection of slides relating to a specific topic, which may be shown while the topic is discussed or may be shown as a continuous show. From the presentation slides, handouts, speaker notes, or outlines can also be prepared. PowerPoint contains graphic tools and many kinds of pictures and graphs to be imported. A Macintosh version is available which functions almost identically to the Windows version. Presentations created in either platform can be run from the other without any conversion needed. Using the PowerPoint, it is easy to create powerful presentations complete with graphics, transitions and even a sound track. Using professionally designed themes and clip art, you can quickly and easily create dynamic slide shows such as the one shown in the figure.

Hints for Good Presentations

The following are some general tips and suggestions for preparing presentations, creating materials, and giving presentations.

Microsoft PowerPoint Presentation-I (Fig. 70.13)

Preparing for the Presentation

- ❖ **Consider the theme:** What is the purpose of the presentation?
- ❖ **Know the audience:**
  - ➢ Gear the information to what is known about the audience.
  - ➢ Try to take the audience's perspective.
- ❖ **Select materials:**
  - ➢ What is the best way to present the theme?
  - ➢ What is the time frame?
  - ➢ How much time to prepare?
  - ➢ How much time for the presentation?
  - ➢ What materials are needed?
  - ➢ What will the materials cost? Is it cost-effective?
  - ➢ Will there be visual elements such as photos, logos, etc.?
  - ➢ Will they need to be scanned?
- ❖ Always be yourself.

Preparing the Materials

Many desktop publishing tips hold true when creating materials for presentations. The following are some of the things to be considered:

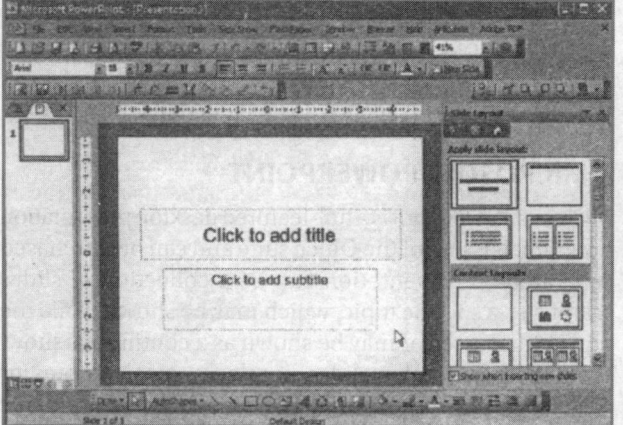

Fig. 70.13: Microsoft PowerPoint presentation-I.

- ❖ **Contrast:**
  - ➢ Use dark text on a light background when producing overhead transparencies.
  - ➢ Use light text on a dark background when producing slides for a computer slide show (yellow text on dark blue background works well).
- ❖ **Balance (proportion):**
  - ➢ Each slide should be balanced within the slide, just like a written document should be balanced, to make it easier to read.
  - ➢ Text with bullets should be left-justified.
  - ➢ Graphics should be off-center to leave room for text. This helps to lead the eye to the text.
  - ➢ Center titles only and an occasional quote.
- ❖ **Capitalization:**
  - ➢ Use in moderation.
  - ➢ Seldom use all caps, except in short titles.
  - ➢ Capitalize the first letter of important words for a more formal look.
  - ➢ Capitalize the first letter of each line for a less formal, more open look.
- ❖ **Simplicity:**
  - ➢ Six to eight words to a line
  - ➢ Six to eight lines per slide
  - ➢ No more than two fonts per page (avoid the "Ransom Note" affect)
  - ➢ Use Sans serif fonts when using projection
  - ➢ Use large font sizes (32, 24 points).

Fontnotes

There are two types of fonts: Serif and Sans Serif. Serif fonts have little "wings" on the characters (such as the font this document is written in). Sans serif fonts do not have "wings" (this is a Sans Serif font called Arial). Serif fonts are easier to read, because the wings allow the eye to follow the flow of characters and should be used when there is a lot of text (the best serif font to use is Times New Roman when dealing with a lot of text. This is a font used by most newspapers for the main body of text). Serif fonts are good headlines, effects and for projection. When choosing a font, think about the following: esthetics (how it looks); who the audience is; what kind of impression or idea is to be achieved; and, how much text is involved.

- ❖ **Emphasis:**
  - ➢ Never underline, unless necessary.
  - ➢ Use italics to emphasize a single word or passage of text or for showing humor or irony.
  - ➢ Use bold for headings, to add emphasis and authority to a word or phrase, or to add contrast of light and dark.
  - ➢ Use color, if possible.

Colornotes

- ❖ Color draws attention to and increases a willingness to read the information. It also helps to increase motivation and participation. When using color,

stick to a common set of colors throughout the entire presentation and limit the number of colors used. Lighter colors on a dark background work well when using projection facilities.
- ❖ Dark blue conveys a conservative, but credible feeling. Blue is a soothing color and can reduce the viewer's blood pressure and heart rate. The combination of a blue background with yellow or white foreground text and graphics is the easiest to read.
- ❖ Red or orange backgrounds heighten emotions. These colors can signal excitement or alarm and increase blood pressure and heart rate. However, reds and oranges do not translate well to the TV screen. Use them with caution. They cause images to "bleed" on the screen. Maroon or burgundy might be a better choice.
- ❖ Green stimulates interaction. Deep forest green, olive green, or teal green will illicit opinions and is useful in education and training oriented presentations.
- ❖ Gray is neutral. Neutrality may be advantageous or not depending on the content and context of the visual.
- ❖ *Graphics:*
  - ➤ Graphics should be off-center to leave room for text. This helps lead the eye to the text.
  - ➤ Charts and graphs should be large enough to read from anywhere in the room.
  - ➤ To show trends, use a line graph.
  - ➤ To compare information, use a bar graph.
  - ➤ To compare parts of a whole, use a pie chart.
  - ➤ When using charts and graphs, use six or fewer items to be compared per chart.
- ❖ *Authoring:* There are many software applications called "authoring" or presentation packages that can be used to create presentations. Many of the packages come complete with graphing and charting capabilities; a built-in outliner; and, print capabilities for the screens to be used by the author or the audience. With a computer and a projection device, transparencies are not necessary. The presentation can be driven by a keyboard, mouse, or set to run automatically at specific timed intervals. Some of the more widely used applications are Microsoft PowerPoint, Harvard Graphics, Asymetrix Tool book, and Gold Disk Astound. Netscape and word processors, such as Microsoft Word and Word perfect, can also be used.
- ❖ *Notes:*
  - ➤ Notes to assist in a presentation can be written on the paper parts of the transparencies or on printouts of the software application presentation screens.
  - ➤ Always print out copies of each "slide" on paper to test the view.
  - ➤ When using transparencies, number them in order of their use.
- ❖ *To create "slides/transparencies":* Slides may be defined as overhead transparencies, computer screen pages, or actual camera slides. Transparencies may be created by printing directly to a transparency created for use with a laser or inkjet printer; by printing the information onto a piece of paper and using a transparency maker or by obtaining transparencies created for a copy machine and using a copier.
- ❖ *Be consistent:* From slide to slide and in everything throughout the presentation, be consistent.

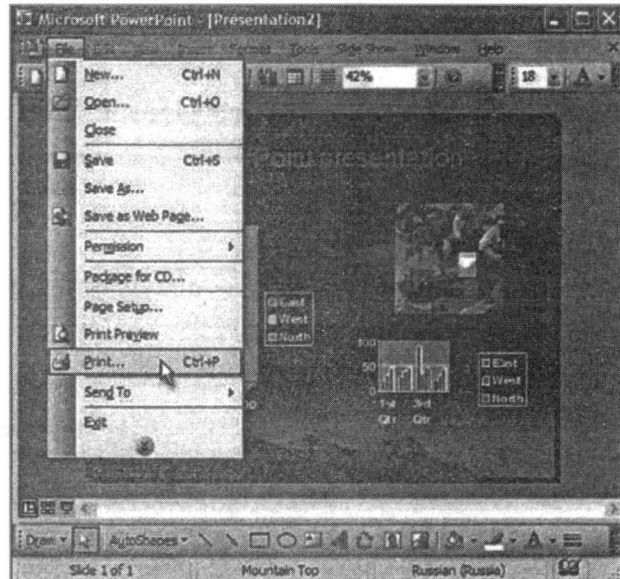

Fig. 70.14: Microsoft PowerPoint presentation-II.

Presentation of the PowerPoint (Fig. 70.14)

- ❖ If possible, test run the presentation in the room it is to be given with all of equipment necessary.
- ❖ Review the topic before beginning the presentation.
- ❖ Maintain eye contact with the audience.
- ❖ Keep the lights on as much as possible.
- ❖ Keep the presentation as interactive as possible.
- ❖ Do not read the visual to the audience—the audience should be able to read.
- ❖ Control with the visual:
  - ➤ Use color.
  - ➤ Reveal one point at a time, if possible.
  - ➤ When using an overhead, turn off the projector to get attention.
- ❖ Review what has been covered to end the presentation.

CONCLUSION

Windows, MS office, Word, Excel, and PowerPoint are the computer operating systems widely used in all fields of nursing. The nurse and nurse educators should have knowledge about these operating systems and undergo basic training on computers. So, that it will help in effective implementation of database in the hospital as well as in the teaching institutions.

CHAPTER 71: Internet Literatures Search

CHAPTER OUTLINE
- Types of Computer Networks
- Sources of Internet Medical Literature
- World Wide Web

INTRODUCTION
The internet is the electronic highway that interconnects tens of thousands of networks around the world over telephone lines. By connecting to the internet through a local service provider or university or through one of the online information services, a user can send email messages, chat online, search database, receive or send files, and share information with others throughout the world.

DEFINITION
The internet is the largest computer network in the world connecting millions of computers. A network is a group of two or more computer systems linked together.

TYPES OF COMPUTER NETWORKS
Series of high-speed communication links are the backbone of the internet such as the one maintained by the US National Science Foundation, unlike every network no person or organization is responsible for the internet.

There are two types of computer networks:
- Local area network (LAN)
- Wide area network (WAN).

Local Area Network
A LAN is two or more connected computer sharing certain resources in a relatively small geographic location, e.g. within/single building.

Wide Area Network
A WAN typically consists of two or more LANs. The computers are further apart and are linked by telephone lines or radio waves. The internet is the largest WAN in existence.

All computers on the internet can be lumped into two groups, which are servers and clients. In a network, clients and servers communicate with one another.

A web server has software running on it that allows it to serve web-related services. WANs are used to tap online information services such as America online, CompuServe, Prodigy, and GEnie.

SOURCES OF INTERNET MEDICAL LITERATURE
First, we should identify the web sources. Some of the medical literature popularity available sources in certain journals documents can be browsed directly and downloaded.
1. The Medline Database. This developed by the US National Library of Medicine (NCM) and is widely recognized as the premier some for bibliographical coverage of the biomedical literature. MEDLINE incorporates information from Index medicines, International Nursing and other sources. It covers more than 3600 journals and contains more than 8.5 million records.
   Under this provides free access include:
   - *PubMed (http://www.ncbi.nlm.nih.gov/pubmed)
   - *Health gate http://www.healthgate.com
2. CINAHL and MEDLINE

WORLD WIDE WEB
World Wide Web (www) is the hottest part of the internet and has become the centerpiece of internet activity. The www facility on the internet links resources, e.g. documents, graphic images, and video clips around the world providing an information exchange of unfathomable proportions. The

internet uses an addressing scheme called uniform resource locator (URL). Basic URLs are used as an initial address to access the homepage of a www, which is a server on the internet that contains documents. The first part (prefix) of any URL is a keyword that indicates the internet protocol that must be used.

For examples, the full URL for the American Nurses Associations "Nursing World" page is: http//www.nursingworld.org, although the internet is currently being used by researchers primarily supportive of the research process the internet also have potential as a resource for data collection.

CONCLUSION

Internet is the fastest means of advanced communication with wide variety of modes through which anyone can access the information which has made wonders in day today world. Internet search is used all over the world in all fields which connects people and organization.

CHAPTER 72

Statistical Packages

CHAPTER OUTLINE

- Major Statistical Software Packages
- Using a Packaged Program

INTRODUCTION

Computers have clearly created numerous opportunities for researchers and nowhere is this apparent than in relation to data analysis. Many statistical procedures are now routinely performed. Some of the calculations are done using manual computations. Readymade programs for the statistical analysis of research data are widely available.

Computer centers at universities are particularly likely to have a variety of software packages available to their users. Most computer centers have a professional staff that is accessible for consultation concerning the computer library of programs sophisticated programs for performing statistical analysis available for both mainframes and personal computers (PCs).

MAJOR STATISTICAL SOFTWARE PACKAGES

Most widely used statistical software packages on mainframe and PCs include the statistical package for the social sciences (SPSS) and statistical analysis system (SAS). Both of these packages contain programs that handle a broad variety of statistical analysis and these packages are updated, refined, and expanded frequently.

Readers are advised to check with personnel at their computer facility for any modifications to the description and listings provided.

Statistical Package for the Social Sciences

The SPSS was developed by researchers at the University of Chicago and National Opinion Research Center to assist researchers in the analysis of social science data. The SPSS represents a highly flexible program with a syntax that is not technically oriented. For people with limited statistical and computer backgrounds, SPSS is relatively easy to learn.

The SPSS has a mainframe version, but the desktop version is adequate for performing analysis of all, but largest data sets. The current version of SPSS for PCs is SPSS 8.0 for Windows, which offers such features as pop-up definition of statistical terms:

- ❖ The SPSS also has a data entry program that can be used to create data files for subsequent analysis.
- ❖ The SPSS can perform all of the basic descriptive and inferential statistical analysis such as t-test, analysis of variance (ANOVA), correlation analysis, and a wide range of nonparametric procedures. The SPSS can also perform most widely used multivariate analysis including multiple regression analysis of covariance (ANCOVA), discriminant function analysis factor analysis multivariate analysis of variance (MANOVA), canonical correlation, logistic regression life-table analysis, proportional hazards modeling, and structural equation modeling.

Statistical Analysis System

The SAS is a computer package that was developed at the North Carolina State University. The SAS is an integrated set of data management tools that includes a complete programming language as well as modules for multiple functions including spreadsheets, project management, scheduling, and mathematic engineering and statistical applications. The SAS's analytic programs are generally considered to be somewhat more sophisticated from a statistical point of view than those of SPSS.

Like SPSS the base SAS system is fairly easy to learn even for those without a strong statistical or computer background. The SAS is also available in both a mainframe and a PC version. The SAS statistical package includes all basic descriptive and inferential, statistical plus additional programs for cluster analysis, Guttman scalogram analysis, multiple regression factor analysis, discriminant function analysis, canonical correlation logit/probit analysis, and psychometric analysis.

Further information about the SAS system is available through the SAS institute in Cary, North Carolina, or through the internet. The URL for SAS is **www.sas.com**.

USING A PACKAGED PROGRAM

Researchers using packaged programs do not need to know a programming language, but they still must be able to communicate to the computer such as some basic information about what their variables are and how the data are to be analyzed. This is accomplished by means of certain commands that are unique to each software package. We can illustrate some aspects of the process using concepts from the menu-driven windows version of SPSS.

The first step is to get your data file into SPSS through the open command on the file menu. The SPSS can read most spreadsheet files, dBASE files, and ASCII text files (ASCII files are created through database and word processing programs, but are stripped of any proprietary codes leaving only 'plain vanilla' ASCII numbers and text). Alternatively the data into SPSS, you will in most cases need to define variable names and data formats.

For example, if your data were in a text file in fixed format, once all the data have been defined, any needed data transformations can be performed through various data transformation dialog boxes accessed through the transform menu. Then through the statistics menu, a statistical procedure can be specified. For any specified statistical procedure, the variables in the data file would be displayed and the relevant variables can be selected through standard mouse-clicking procedures. Finally, the procedure would be run and the results would be displayed in SPSS's output navigator. In the output navigator window, you could browse the output results and could readily access whichever part of the output you wanted to see. Output files can be edited saved transferred to another application and printed.

We hope that this brief discussion has made it clear that a researcher need not be a statistical expert or computer whiz to make use of computer for quantitative analysis (Fig. 72.1). The new graphical and menu driven environments of SPSS and SAS are designed to be easy to learn by people with limited computer skills.

CONCLUSION

Statistical packages are widely used in research to organize, analyze, and compare the collected data. As a nurse with advanced education and practice, they should be familiar with the some of the statistical packages. It helps them to apply in the field of research and in effective utilization and dissemination of the research findings.

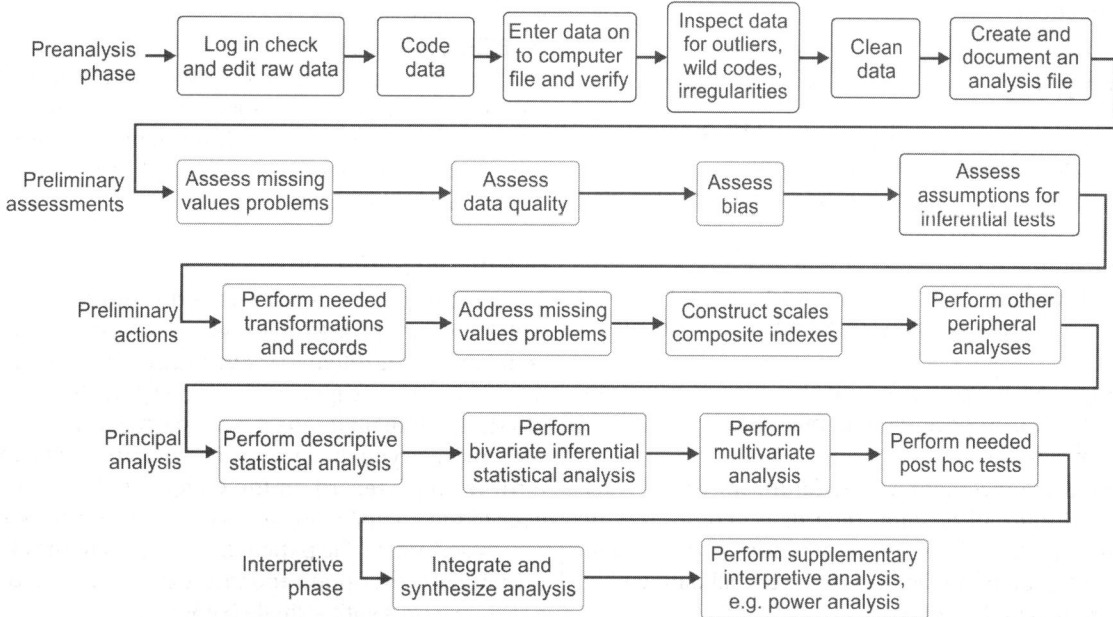

Fig. 72.1: Flow of tasks in analyzing quantitative data.

CHAPTER 73

Hospital Management Information System Software

CHAPTER OUTLINE

- Computerization of Hospital and Nursing Homes
- Electronic Hospital Management Software
- Computers in Medicine and Health Care
- Hospital Information System

INTRODUCTION

The present manual hospital management system requires daily updating of a number of registers. Different registers have to be maintained for recording different patients, visiting doctors, types of diseases, types of treatments, and time it will take for recording bill payment, and payment due. There is an increased risk of error in the manual system. In view of the above, a proposed computerized hospital maintenance application for the hospital management is strongly needed.

OBJECTIVES

The objective of the proposed system would be to overcome the problems faced in the manual system:

- Updating records would not be a problem and also crosschecking of records in the proposed system would not be required.
- Mathematical, accounting, and logical errors would get automatically rectified in the proposed system.
- Reports can be generated on the click of a button. Design of the proposed system must take the following into consideration.
- Hospital management will be future software, which will maintain all hospital records on computers no matter whether it is prescription of doctor or treatment sheet of patient, medicine, employees all data will be maintained in this software.
- Fully networked based and will be managed by the latest technology tools. Software will be easy to use and fully graphical interface will be provided to the end user. This software will make your hospital "WPP" that means without paper and pen.

COMPUTERIZATION OF HOSPITAL AND NURSING HOMES

Nursing homes and small as well as medium-sized hospitals can computerize various areas of their working depending on the size, number of patients, etc. In addition to the clinical applications, the following administrative tasks should be computerized:

- Patient records
- Reports of investigations
- Inventory
- Billing and accounts.

Computerized medical records are much more efficient and as compared to manual records. It is far easier to retrieve any record and the information is presented in a systematic and pattern. The record can be available at various points in a where it is needed.

Additional Computers

Today's computers are very powerful and single machine, which can perform all the tasks for any small hospital. If your job is in the different room and the computer is in front office, computer capacity and time spare, but it becomes physically difficult for the lab people to use computer.

Suppose you have a clerk who first registers and retrieves their record on the computer. The patient then goes to the doctor, who enters the clinical details and also the prescription. The patient then returns to the clerk for a printout of prescription and to pay the fees. Obviously such a system works with a single computer.

Network

Larger hospitals can have a networked hospital management software, which is available throughout the hospital and specialized clinical software separately for each department. If you want to share resources, such as printer and importantly if you want to share information, then you should use local area network (LAN) to link up the computer.

Software

Most software developers are not familiar with medical terminology and speak a totally different language from doctor. So why buy software from a company, which makes stock exchange software. A good program should first be intended to help to understand requirements of most people. Second, it should be flexible enough to be modified to individual requirements, by the user themself.

Operator

Doctors and existing staff are usually the best people to operate the computer. Moreover, the people who are already working in your institution are familiar with procedures, staff, and your way of working.

Electronic Medical Record Software

For most doctors, one of the most time-consuming functions is to go through a patient's medical history. This could include the patient's previsits, family, and social history and recommended medication. After this, the doctor proposes a treatment plan and records the entire process for transcription. What if all these functions could be taken care of with an electronic medical record system that would not only speed up the doctor's interaction with the patient chart but also ensures better care for patients?

Electronic medical record software does exactly this. More than just a medical practice management software, it is a hospital information system (HIS) that simplifies the way patient charts are managed in the doctor's office.

Benefits of Electronic Medical Records Software

This software application facilitates input, storage, transfer, and retrieval of medical information within a practice and enables interfacing with other data.

The significant financial benefits include savings on transcription and recording.

This allows doctors to spend their valuable time with new patients without paying for transcription.

This provides the doctor to capture super bill details for hospital visits, ensuring that no billing information of a patient is lost.

This also allows the doctor to track appointments, while on the move.

The electronic medical record solution also uses the charts database to optimize claim documentations, thus ensuring higher returns for each claim.

Features of Electronic Medical Record Software

- Electronic medical records or electronic health record software provides an application service provider (ASP) solution for managing a practice and maintaining health records.
- The electronic health record system facilitates input, storage, transfer, and retrieval of medical information within a practice.
- It also acts as healthcare logistics software by enabling interfacing with other data providers outside the practice.

Elements of Electronic Medical Record Software

The contents of the electronic healthcare software system are briefly explained below.

- *Appointment scheduling—daily scheduler*
  - Appointment scheduling for physicians, physician assistants, nurse practitioners, equipment, and rooms.
  - Simplifying the process of organizing care by integrating workflows customizable to each of the practice needs.
  - Simplifies the process of scheduling by pre-configuring physician's preference of availability and unavailability through user-friendly wizards.
- *Authorization manager:* Verifies the status of authorization and requests the same, if it has expired. Once the authorization is received, the patient shall be notified and books an appointment for consulting.
- *Medical billing:* The acts as a medical billing software and performs billing operations. With this, users can capture the charges and prepare claims. The software personalizes the electronic claim keeping in tune with different regulations and practices of the insurance providers from state to state. Electronic superbill where in the data captured in superbill is translated into charge entry supports batch claims. The system preprocess all prepared claims to rectify erroneous data has supporting comprehensive reporting capability.
- *Reports:* System reports shall display set of default reports. Reports can be configured and customized depending on the access levels of the user. This shall display any data as per the selection and access levels of the user.
- *Administration/security:* The administration section will have the following functionalities:
  - Create and delete users
  - Create and delete groups
  - Create rank list, where the users can be arranged in different levels. This is required when routing an order/task from one user to another.
- *Starting hospital management software:* To start electronic healthcare or hospital management software from the desktop screen of windows just double click the icon, you will see the main screen given in Figure 73.1.
- *Password protection (Fig. 73.2):* Password protection is the screen that is used for the security purpose. Any

Section 10: Computer Application for Patient Care Delivery Systems and Nursing Practice

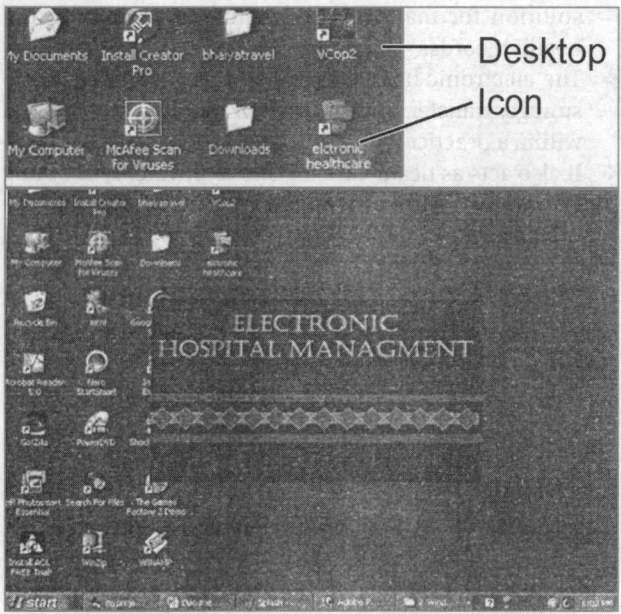

Fig. 73.1: Beginning of hospital management.

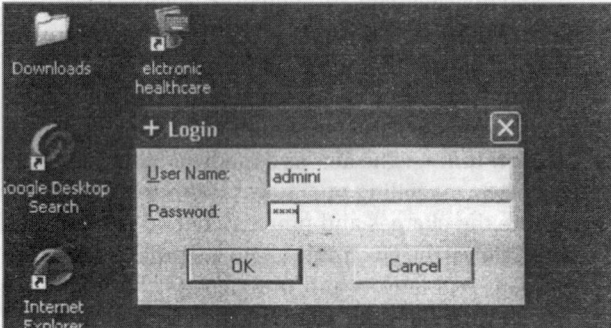

Fig. 73.2: Password protection.

user wishing to use the application has to pass through the login form. The login form is a common gateway for the normal users and administrator. The administrator and the user have their own different password and user name. This can be used during the process of login. The users enter their User ID in the user name box and password in the password box. If the user ID is valid and the password entered is correct, then the user is logged in.

- ❖ **Validity checks**
  - ➢ Empty spaces in a text box are not allowed.
  - ➢ It is checked whether a normal user or the administrator has logged on.
  - ➢ It is validated whether the use has performed any previous illegal shutdown, if any such record is present then a warning is displayed for the user.
  - ➢ If the user has performed illegal shutdown for three consecutive times, then their account will be clicked.
  - ➢ If the system finds that any illegal user is trying to logon, then the system will be locked and can only be unlocked by the system administrator.
  - ➢ There is a validation check to see the number of times any illegal logon attempt is performed.

If the administrator has logged on, then the delete and modification option of the application will be deleted.

ELECTRONIC HOSPITAL MANAGEMENT SOFTWARE (FIG. 73.3)

Electronic hospital management software is the main dialog interface (MDI) of the application and contains the various applications that are performed in the nursing home by the operator. The MDI Form contains the various options that an operator always requires and is most frequently used in the hospital system. The MDI form contains the various sub options clicking on which various forms opens that is used for various purposes. There are following main Menu:

- ❖ File
- ❖ Main
- ❖ Patients
- ❖ Search
- ❖ Reports
- ❖ View
- ❖ Window.

Main (Fig. 73.4)

In hospitals and nursing homes, there are so many departments, e.g. accounts department, lab department, etc. If we open the lab department, first go into the main menu of "Main," select the "Main" option. It opens a "Department" option select it, you will see a dialog box appear. Similarly if we do the entry of "Doctors, Wards, Visiting Doctors, Lab, Charges, outpatient department (OPD) rooms entry, Employee record," then go to the main menu of "Main." It shows above options.

If you want Lab entry, then go the Lab option of the main menu of Main. It shows type of lab, floors (if hospital

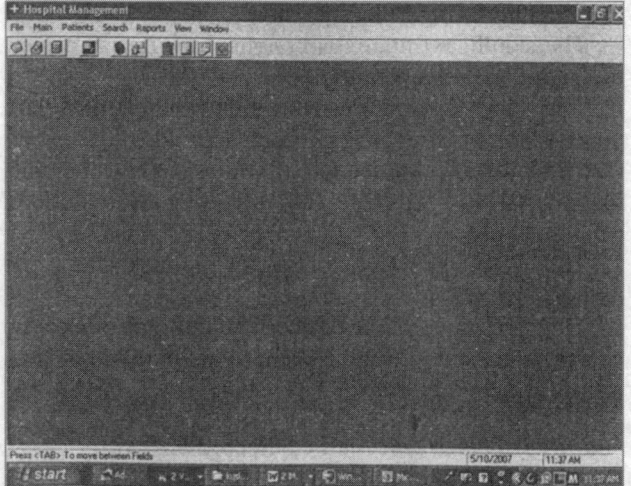

Fig. 73.3: Electronic hospital management software.

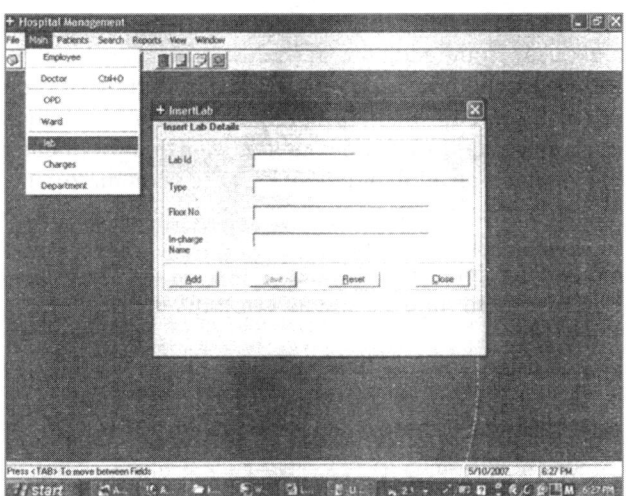

Fig. 73.4: Main.

is multistorey building, then shows first, second, or third floor), lab incharge name, etc.

Doctor's Record Entry (Fig. 73.5)

Doctor's record entry form is used to enter the details of any new doctor. The various details related about the doctor is required to be entered such as how much his/her fees, the contact number and address for emergency or keeping the records, then go to main option and select sub option Doctors.

Patient (Fig. 73.6)

The patient has the features, which are mentioned below:
- Registration form
- Generation of Treatment Sheet
- Filling Treatment Sheet on computers with the respective user ID
- Billing of admit patient
- Facilities taken by patient
- Registration of patients
- Details of the patient

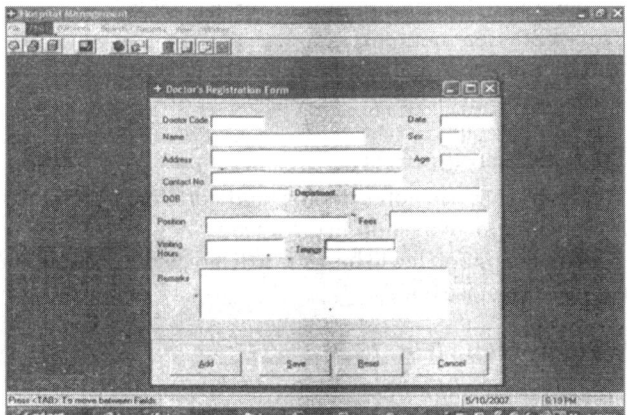

Fig. 73.5: Doctor's record entry.

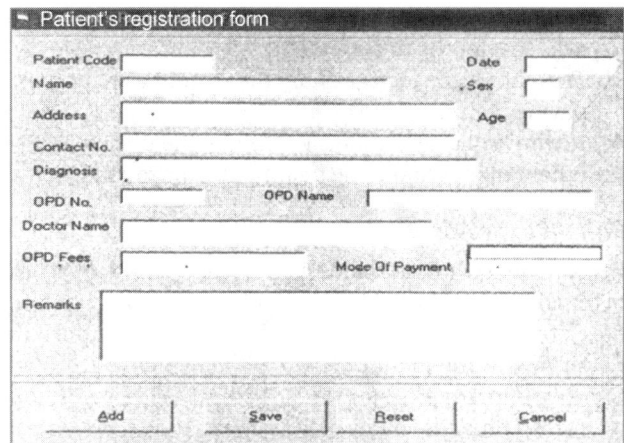

Fig. 73.6: Patient.

- Cash receipt
- Prescription of the patient
- Collection report
- Medicine given in prescription automatically goes to medical store
- Investigation given in prescription automatically goes to pathology.

In hospitals and nursing homes, there are so many patients to be admitted or come for treatment. For example, a patient comes for his/her treatment will first fill up the details of the patient. If we open the Registration Form, first go into the main menu of Patient. Select the Patient option. It opens a Registration Form option select it, you will see a dialog box appear.

Patient's Registration Form

All patient records have an identifying number, which may be called Identification number or Patient Code. This is necessary because it is the simplest way to uniquely different patient. There may be several patients with the same name so each patient is given a unique number. There is no conflict you can still find the records by the name of the patient, the program internally controls all records based on number.

While entering the details for a new patient the program automatically assigns a new number. The numerical series can be defined by the user. Hospital management takes care of maintaining complete details of patient for administrative and clinical purposes.

- ***Patient code:*** A new code number is generated and displayed. If you want to enter the panic new patient, just press "Enter."
- ***Date:*** This will show the system current date.
- ***Name:*** Enter the name of the patient.
- ***Age:*** You may enter the patient's present age.
- ***Address:*** Enter the address of the patient.
- ***Diagnosis:*** It is the same as entered in the treatment.
- ***OPD number and name:*** You will enter the OPD number, and then Name of the OPD will be displayed.

- **Doctor name:** You will have to enter the doctor's name available for the treatment.
- **Fees:** Enter the fees given by the patient and mode of payment also.
- **Remarks:** Lastly remarks written by the doctor or any other remarks about the treatment or payment.

Patient to be Admitted

Every patient who is admitted, you will enter his/her record in this form. Here the fields such as address, contact number, etc., are not entered, but we will enter more important details about the patient. That can be, which Ward, Bed number, department, etc.

- **Name:** Enter the name of the patient.
- **Sex:** You have the option of entering the sex of the patient.
- **Age:** You have the option of entering the present age of patient.
- **Admit date:** Enter the date of admit in the format DD/MM/YY as we follow the British format of date.
- **Time:** You has the option of entering the time of the patient record.
- **Referred by:** Enter the name of the referring doctor.
- **Mode of payment:** If the mode is cash you can skip the text boxes such as bank name, credit card number, date, etc.

Treatment Chart

Electronic hospital management maintains the complete treatment chart of patient records, so that it would be easy to customize the clinical enquires to meet your specific requirements for further diagnosis of the patient. While entering the details of treatment chart for a new patient the treatment chart includes the Patient Code, Patient Name, Sex, Age, Ward type, Room number, Bed number, Admit date and time. The treatment chart also includes the status of visit doctors and case history of patients and date of discharge.

Preoperation details: In the preoperation details, enter details of any allergies suffered by the patient, together with his/her biosigns and warnings. Here, you can enter the details of patient before the operation. This includes "patient code, name, allergies, height, weight, blood pressure, blood sugar, if any other details such as pregnant, breastfeeding or aged patient," etc.

Search

We can search the patient details by just entering the "Patient Code, Name, Doctor Consulted and Disease." In the same way, we also search the details of the doctors working with the hospital by entering 'Doctor Code, Name, Department, and disease' (part of the body he/she is specialized in).

Reports Menu

The report is a program prints all single-line details on a single page and each format on a separate page. Only the registered tests are printed, saving stationery and making it easier for physician to read the reports. When the reports make use of some additional reference master files program, it checks whether the patients who are admitted on a particular date are treated properly and what is the progress of the treatment. In the same way if we want to know whether the patient is an adult or not look for the adult master file. The appropriate reference; values against each test. This is possible only on a computerized system printed forms it is difficult to print all possible data.

This Main Report menu contains the following submenus:
- Lab tests
- X-rays
- Ultrasound
- Physiotherapy
- Operations
- Miscellaneous
- Ward status
- OPD patients
- Casualty patient
- Patient admitted
- Appointments
- Treatment chart
- Operation list
- Invoice.

Issuing Invoices

There are two ways to issue an invoice:
1. A practitioner can click on the "Invoice" Submenu in the Report menu at the end of a consultation.
2. A receptionist (or practitioner) can, at any time, click on the Main Form's button to open the Invoice.

In the former method, consultation times are entered automatically; in the latter, they are not. In the latter method, the name of the practitioner in whose name the invoice must be manually selected; in the former, this is automatically determined.

The following display the relevant form and instructions on how to use it:
1. Click on one of the charge for radio buttons and then complete the relevant time or service fields.
2. List the treatment taken by patient.
3. Calculate the total charge; note if paid in full.
4. Print the invoice.

View Menu (Fig. 73.7)

View menu has two option toolbar and status bar if tick mark is there in front of the option that means they are ON. If you click on the option it will become activate and if you click it again it will close (OFF).

Window Menu (Fig. 73.8)

This menu has options, which will change the windows arrangement. That means how the windows more than one are arranged.

Chapter 73: Hospital Management Information System Software

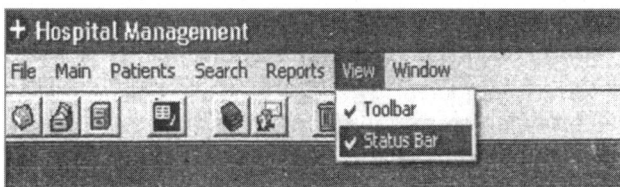

Fig. 73.7: View menu.

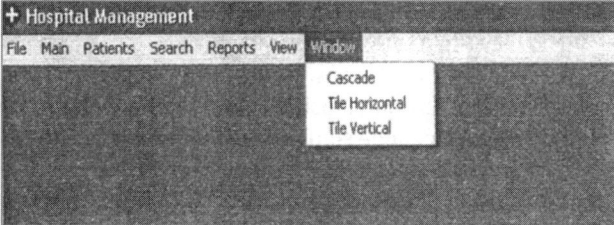

Fig. 73.8: Window menu.

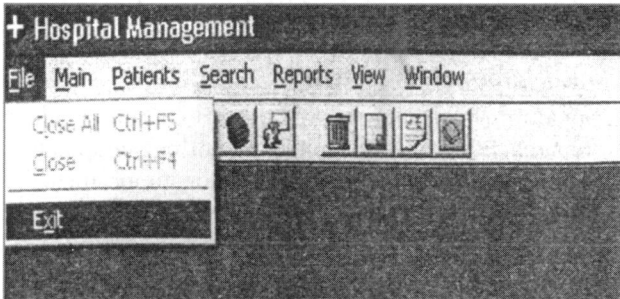

Fig. 73.9: Exit from electronic hospital management.

Exit

To exit from "Electronic Hospital Management," we have to click the Submenu "Exit" in the file main menu. Then it will display the screen shown in Figure 73.9.

COMPUTERS IN MEDICINE AND HEALTH CARE

Role of computers used in medicine, uses of computers in health care and importance of computers in medicine fields. The influence of computers is universal. Computers are used in applications ranging from running a farm, diagnosing a disease, and designing to constructing and launching a space vehicle. Many scientific computer programs serve the entire population. The links included herein relate to medicine and health care.

Resource and Patient Management System

The resource and patient management system (RPMS) is a decentralized automated information system of over 50 integrated software applications. Many RPMS applications can function in a standalone environment if necessary or appropriate. The system is designed to operate on micro- and mini-computers located in Indian health service (IHS) or tribal healthcare facilities. RPMS software modules fall into three major categories.

Administrative Applications

The RPMS administrative applications support the business of healthcare provision. Applications in this category are used to perform patient registration, collect, store, and report patient demographic information; manage the scheduling, admission, discharge and transfer of patients in inpatient facilities; create claims and handle both manual and electronic billing and accounts receivables; and electronically manage resource requests and supplies.

Clinical Applications

The RPMS clinical applications directly support the provision of healthcare programs within IHS. Applications in this category generally collect all patient related information gathered during patient contacts into one comprehensive, centralized data file to support healthcare planning, delivery, management, and research. The patient care component provides for entry of visit data that forms the core dataset used by most of the RPMS applications. Other applications in this category support patient care and include, for instance, laboratory, radiology, inpatient and outpatient pharmacy, allergy tracking, immunology, dental, women's health, etc.

Infrastructure Applications

The RPMS infrastructure applications comprise and support, environment with management, development and communication tools. The Mailman application is an electronic messaging system. VA Kernel software provides a portability layer between the underlying operating system and application code and provides a Kernel Toolkit that supplements the Kernel software package with development and quality assessment tools, capacity management tools, and system management utilities. The VA Fileman is the RPMS database management system (DBMS).

The Department of Information Resources (DIR) distributes the RPMS application suite to Headquarters and each IHS area office. The area office then releases the RPMS application suite to the healthcare facilities within its area. Different facilities use different configurations of RPMS applications, depending upon the types of services they provide.

Future Plans

The IHS plans to continue to enhance RPMS overtime adding an electronic health record, a clinical imaging, and other software modules. In addition, the IHS and the veterans' health administration plan to continue their long-standing practice of collaborating on various software development projects related to health information, exchange health informatics standards, personal health records, VistA-Office HER, and other initiatives.

HOSPITAL INFORMATION SYSTEM

A comprehensive information system dealing with all aspects of information processing in a hospital. It is an integrated computer assisted system designed to store, manipulate, and retrieve information concerned with the administrative and clinical aspects of providing services within the hospital. A HIS encompasses human information processing as well as data processing machines.

Definition

A system, which acquires, stores, processes, and delivers patient-related information in a hospital with required details in response to a query or routinely as predetermined format to those who need it is called HIS.

Benefits of Hospital Information System

- Easy access to patient data
- Helps in decision support system for the hospital authorities
- Improve monitoring of drug usage and study of effectiveness
- Efficient and accurate administration of finance diet of patient and distribution of medical aid
- Fast and reliable information storage
- Helps in improved health care delivery
- Connects people processes and data in real time across the hospital on a single platform
- Helps to force orderliness and standardization of the patient records and procedures
- It is good managerial tool and HIS
- System helps to meet management challenges
- Helps to educate patients about their disease.

Types of Hospital Information System

- Noncomputerized HIS
- Computerized HIS.

Noncomputerized HIS

Manual noncomputerized HIS consist of:
- Various documents
- Reports
- Returns
- Transmission channels
- Personnel
- Documents
- Medical records
- Admission/discharge books
- Records of laboratory tests and X-ray
- Account book
- Store ledger.

Computerized HIS

Elements in a computerized HIS are:
- A host computer
- Terminal/work station/peripherals
- Communication network
- A database
- Software
- Skin ware.

Components of HIS (Fig. 73.10)

The above framework shows how complex HIS can be advancement in computer technology and the development of information exchange standards such as Health Level-7 (HL7) and digital imaging and communication in medicine (DICOM), make the task administering and integrating such systems a little more easier. No HIS can be regarded as a success unless it has the full participation of its users. They can be easily addressed by providing adequate training education about the system.

Clinical Information System

Clinical information system (CIS) is a computer-based system that is designed for collecting storing manipulating and making available clinical information important to the health care delivery process. The CIS may extent to a single area, e.g. laboratory systems, electrocardiogram (ECG) management systems, electronic medical documentation system, radiology information system.

Business and Financial Information System

Financial information systems (FIS) are computer systems that manage the business aspect of a hospital; while healthcare organization's primary priority is to achieve

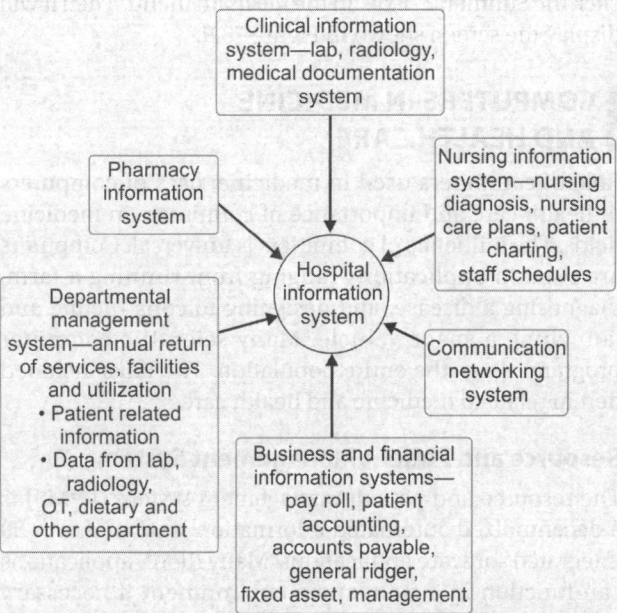

Fig. 73.10: Components of hospital information system.

maximum benefits with minimum costs. Some of the FIS are:
1. Pay roll
2. Patient accounting
3. Accounts payable
4. **General ledger:** The collection, processing, and reporting financial data generated by all transactions.
5. Fixed asset management; deals with asset data retention and depreciation forecasting.

Nursing Information System

Nursing information systems (NIS) are computer systems that manage clinical data from a variety of health care environments and made available in a timely and orderly fashion to aid nurses improving patient care.

To achieve this, most NIS are designed using database and at least one nursing classification language such as the North American Nursing Diagnosis Association (NANDA), nursing intervention classification (NIC), and nursing diagnosis extension and classification (NDEC).

Some of the features by NIS include:
- Patient charting
- Staff schedules
- Clinical data integration
- Decision support.

Benefits of NIS
- Improved workload functionality
- Better care planning
- Effective drug administration.

Pharmacy Information Systems

Pharmacy information systems (PIS) are complex computer systems that have been designed to meet the needs of a pharmacy department through this system pharmacists can supervise and have inputs on how medication is used in a hospital clinical screening, monitoring drug interactions.

Communication Networking System

Refer topic "Computerized Hospital Information System" in this chapter.

Departmental Management System

The manual noncomputerized information utilized within the departments is as follows:
- Annual return of services, facilities, and utilization
- Data from laboratory, radiology, operation theater, dietary, and other departments
- Hospital personnel data
- Financial data
- Inventory information
- Patient related information.

CONCLUSION

The HIS can be used to improve the quality of patient care, while making it more economical. These can be available from virtually any location. Clinical nurses can use their NIS to replace manual systems of data recording and to provide nursing care based on priority by referring to standard NANDA nursing approved diagnosis.

SUGGESTED READING

1. Puri B. Text Book of Computer Nursing, 1st edition. AITBS Publishers, India; 2008.
2. Neeraja KP. Textbook of Nursing Education, 1st edition. New Delhi: Jaypee Brothers Medical Publishers(p) Ltd. 2005: 41-77.
3. Polit DR, Hungler BP. Nursing Research Principles and Methods, 8th edition. New York: Lippincott; 1999
4. Jain P, Kumari N. Introduction to Computers, 3rd edition. India: PV Books; 2011.

REVIEW OF SECTION BASED QUESTIONS OF RGUHS

Long Essays
1. Explain in detail, the hospital management information system.

Short Essays
1. Use of computers in nursing profession.
   (May 2010 and Nov 2012)
2. Computer and literature search.

Annexures

Section Outline

1. Health Assessment Format
2. Community Health Assessment Format

ANNEXURE 1

Health Assessment Format

I. HISTORY TAKING

Baseline data/Biographical data

Name:

Age:

Gender:

IP No:

Address:

Contact No:

Religion: Hindu/Muslim/Christian/Any other

Marital status: Married/Unmarried

Educational status: Illiterate/Primary Education/Secondary Education/Higher Education/Graduate/Postgraduate

Occupation: Government/Private/Self-Employment/Coolie/Daily wages

Income:

Date and time of admission:

Diagnosis:

Chief C/o:
1. **Present illness:**
2. **Past illness:**
   - Past medical history: History of diabetes mellitus (DM)/hypertension (HTN)/Heart disease/tuberculosis (TB)/If allergic to any drugs
   - Past surgical history: History of any surgeries undergone
3. **Family history:** History of heart disease, HTN/DM/TB in the family and hereditary or immunologic disorders.
   - Family tree
4. **Marital history:** Duration marital life, relationships
5. **Personal history:** Appetite, rest, sleep, bowel, bladder and habits
6. **Sexual history:** Any sex-related problems
7. **Contraceptive history:** Use of oral pills/Nirodh/Rhythm method/Tubectomy/Vasectomy
8. **Psychosocial history:** Primary language/Type of employment/Economic status (Low/Middle/High)/Relationships with family/Neighbors
9. **Family history:** Good/Divorce/Separated from family/Conflicts
10. **Nutritional history:**
    - Type of diet: Veg/Mixed
    - Appetite: Good/Lack of appetite
    - 24-hour dietary recall
11. **Menstrual history:**
    - Attained menarche at the age of _____
    - Menstruation is regular/irregular
    - Flow: Normal/Excessive
    - Associated with dysmenorrhea/normal
12. **Elimination pattern:**
    - Bladder: Normal/Any hematuria/Retention of urine/Incontinence of urine/Distension of bladder
    - Bowel: Regular/Irregular/Constipation/Diarrhea/Melena
13. **Environmental history:**
    - Type of house: Kutcha/Pucca/Semi-Pucca
    - Ventilation: Adequate/Inadequate
    - Drainage: Open/Closed or no facility
    - Any breeding places for mosquitoes
    - Safe drinking water supply: Present/Absent

II. PHYSICAL EXAMINATION/ASSESSMENT

General appearance/Observation

- Body built: Well-built/Moderately built/Poor built
- Stature/Body gait
- Nutritional status
- Emotional state: Normal/Anxious/Sad/Happy
- Co-operative

Vital signs: Total peripheral resistance (TPR) and blood pressure (BP), pulse pressure, height and weight

1. **Skin and mucous membranes:**
   - Color: Normal/Pallor/Cyanosis/Jaundiced
   - Temperature: Warm/Cold/Clammy
   - Moisture: Dandruff-like scales/Fish-like scales
   - Texture: Normal/Smooth/Thin/Thick/Rough
   - Turgor: Normal/Poor
   - Vascularity: Appearance of superficial blood vessels/Petechiae
   - Edema: Pitting edema
   - Lesions: Skin tags/Senile keratosis/Ulcer/Atrophy
   - Nails: Normal/Clubbing of fingers/Capillary refill

- Shape: Koilonychia/Beau's lines(brittle)/Paronychia/Splinter hemorrhages

2. **Head:**
   - Size/Shape/Position
   - Symmetry
   - Skull deformities/Nodules or masses

3. **Hair:**
   - Color: Black/Brown/Red/Yellow
   - Distribution of hair
   - Texture: Alopecia-baldness
   - Parasites: Pediculi/Dandruff
   - Scalp lesions

4. **Face:**
   - Symmetry
   - Appearance: Pale/Flushed/Puffiness
   - Lesions
   - Facial hair
   - Periorbital edema
   - Sunken eye
   - Thinning of eyebrows

5. **Eyes:**
   - History of visual loss: Glaucoma/Cataract/Eye trauma/DM/HTN
   - History of eye pain: Photophobia/Burning/Itching/Excess tearing/Diplopia/Blurred vision
   - Visual acuity: Normal/Poor/SC (without correction)/CC (with correction)
   - Extraocular movements: Direction/Position of the eyelid/Nystagmus
   - External eye: Position/Alignment/Exophthalmos/Strabismus
   - Eyebrows: Size/Extension/Hair structure/Coarseness of hair/Ability to move
   - Eyelids/lashes: Position/Distribution/Color/Direction/Discharge/Ability to blink/Ptosis
   - Conjunctiva: Pale/Pink/Yellow/Red
   - Sclera: White/Yellow
   - Cornea: Transparent/Smooth/Shiny/Dry/Abrasion/Corneal blink reflex
   - Pupils: Size/Shape/Equality/Accommodation and reaction to light. (PERRLA: Pupils equal, round, reactive to light, and accommodation.)
   - Internal eye: Fundus-by using ophthalmoscope-red reflex/size/color/clarity of optic disc

6. **Ear:**
   - History of hearing impairment/Ear surgery/Trauma/Ear pain/Itching/Discharge/Tinnitus/Vertigo
   - Auricles: Size/Shape/Position/Color/Discharge/Cerumen/Symmetry
   - Mastoid process: Tenderness/Swelling/Nodules
   - Ear drum: Sound conduction/Auditory function-hearing loss
   - Tympanic membrane: Color/Consistency/Perforation
   - Weber test
   - Rinne Test
   - Romberg test

7. **Nose and sinuses:**
   - History of exposure to dust pollutants, or allergies, nasal obstruction, recent trauma and discharge/epistaxis/headaches/using nasal drops or sprays

External nose: Shape/Size/Skin color/Deformity
   - Nares: Symmetrical/Crust/Patency
   - Sense of smell/rhinitis
   - Septum: Alignment/Deviated nasal septum/Perforation

Internal nose: Mucosa lesions
   - Hearing acuity: Hearing loss-sensorineural/Mixed
   - Sinuses: Swollen/Frontal and maxillary sinuses—Tenderness

8. **Mouth and throat:**
   - History of dehydration, restricted intake, oral trauma, airway obstruction, change in appetite, smoking, tobacco chewing, pain or lesions in the mouth
   - Lips: Color/Texture/Hydration/Contour and lesions
   - Buccal mucosa: Color—pink, soft, moist and smooth/Lesions/leukoplakia
   - Gums and teeth: Color/Edema/Retraction/Bleeding/Lesions
   - Color: Number of teeth—32, alignment, Pearly white/brown/yellow
   - Tongue: Symmetry, moist/Coated, papillae present
   - Movement: Unilateral movement/Color
   - Gag reflex: Palpable nodule
   - Throat: Sore throat/Inflamed tonsils

9. **Neck:**

History of recent cold or infection, feels fatigue, thyroid problems, HIV infection, neck injury, taking thyroid medication and family history of thyroid disease.

Neck muscles: Symmetry/Distention of jugular veins/Controlled movements/range of motion (ROM)

Lymph nodes:
   - Size, mobility, tenderness, preauricular, poterion auricular
   - Occipital nodes at base of skull, postauricular nodes over mastoid, preauricular nodes just in front of the ear. Both sides are compared for size, shape, delination mobility consistency and tenderness
   - Deep cervical, supraclavicular nodes present or not noted
   - Any tonsillar, submental, submandibular nodes to be noted.

Thyroid: Position—Middle/Deviates 4m middle/Enlarged masses
   - Trachea: Alignment, Tracheal lings

10. **Breast:**

Personal or family history of breast disease, child after 30 age, not breastfed their infants, use of contraceptives, diuretics, digitalis, estrogen, etc.

Inspection:
   - Size and symmetry: Symmetrical/Asymmetrical
   - Contour or shape: Note masses, retraction or dimpling pendulus/conical
   - Color: Redness/Excoriation
   - Nipple and areola: size, color, shape, discharge, direction of nipple point

Palpation:

Breast tissue and lymph nodes enlargement: Present/Absent

Male breasts:
   - Nipples and areola are inspected for nodules/edema/discharge/breast enlargement/masses to be noted

11. **Respiratory system:**
    History of persistent cough, chest pain, recurrent attacks of pneumonia, TB, bronchitis, lung disease, etc.
    Inspection:
    - Respiratory rate/Rhythm/Depth
    - Shape: Normal/Barrel/Pigeon
    - Chest: Symmetrical/Asymmetrical
    - Use of accessory muscles, color/Configuration/Lesions

    Palpation:
    - Position of trachea/Palpable lumps, masses, unusual movement/Tenderness
    - Vibration: Vocal or tactile fremitus
    - Thoracic expansion

    Auscultation:
    Breath sounds: Normal—bronchovesicular and vesicular/Abnormal—rhonchi (gurgles)/Crackles (rales)/Wheeze/Pleural friction rub

    Percussion:
    - Resonance/Hyperresonance/Dullness

12. **Cardiovascular system:**
    History of hypertension, use of prescribed drugs, exercise, stressful lifestyle, chest pain, dyspnea, family history of heart disease.
    Inspection:
    - Skin color: Cyanosis and pallor
    - Edema: Present/Absent
    - Appearance of pulsations and vibrations felt over chest angle-aortic, pulmonic and Erb's point or tricuspid area
    - Jugular vein distention (JVD) with chest at 35° to 45° angle
    - Edema/swelling (grading if pitting)

    Palpation:
    - Aortic, pulmonic, Erb's, tricuspid and mitral areas
    - Peripheral pulses: Legs/Arms/Normal/Weak/Thready

    Auscultation:
    - Heart sounds S1 S2 heard
    - Murmur heard/Not heard

13. **Gastrointestinal system:**
    History of abdominal or low back pain, use of laxatives, abdominal surgery, trauma, melena, hematemesis diagnostic tests, etc.
    Inspection:
    - Skin: Color/Scar/Distension
    - Umbilicus: Position/Color
    - Contour: Round/Flat
    - Abdominal girth

    Auscultation:
    - Bowel sounds

    Percussion and **Palpation**—Four quadrants:
    - **Normal:** Flat sound (normal), tympanic sound (gas filled), dull sound (fluid filled) liver, spleen, appendix
    - Light palpation/deep
    - Tenderness
    - Consistency
    - Masses

14. **Male and female genitalia:**
    - Urinary output: Clarity/Color/Odor
    - Voiding pattern: Normal/Retention/Incontinence/Painful or burning micturition
    - Color of urine: Pale yellow/Dark yellow

    Male: Scrotum and testis—inflammation, edema, lesion masses
    Penis—Rashes, lesions, masses
    Female:
    Menstrual history
    External genitalia:
    Urethral orifice: Color/Position/Discharge/Polyps/Fistulas
    Vaginal introitus: Edema/Inflammation/Tenderness/Discharge/Lesions
    Anus: Any lesions/Hemorrhoids
    Internal genitalia: Speculum examination—use cervical brush/Spatula-cervical examination and cervical smear test

15. **Musculoskeletal system:**
    History of recent falls, trauma, lifting heavy objects, bone and joint disease/Ability to perform activities of daily living (ADL).
    Inspection:
    - Body gait/Coordination
    - Color changes: Normal/Redness/Excoriation of skin
    - Spine curvature: Normal/Kyphosis/Lordosis/Scoliosis
    - Muscle strength: ROM/Atrophied muscle-soft/Boggy
    - Movement of joints
    - Homan's sign: Positive/Negative
    - Spine: Normal curves/Positive—Kyphosis, lordosis, scoliosis/Lesions

16. **Neurological system:**
    - Level of consciousness
    - Awareness of time/Place/Person
    - Verbal responses
    - Ability to follow commands
    - Language, thinking, intellectual ability, memory and judgment
    - Long-term and short-term memory

    Sensory nerve function:
    Sensation of pain, temperature, position, vibration localized to touch.
    Cranial nerve function: Assess for all 12 nerves
    Reflexes:
    Cutaneous reflexes:
    Gluteal and abdominal reflex
    Deep tendon reflexes:
    Biceps, triceps, patellar, Achilles tendon and plantar (Babinski's reflex)

III. LAB INVESTIGATIONS

Sl. no.	Investigations	Patients value	Normal value	Remarks

IV. MEDICAL TREATMENT

Sl. no.	Name of the drug	Dose	Route	Frequency	Action

V. SURGICAL MANAGEMENT

Rehabilitation (Physiotherapy, occupational therapy).

VI. NURSING MANAGEMENT

- ❖ Nursing diagnosis according to priority
- ❖ Nursing care plan

Assessment	Nursing diagnosis	Objective	Plan of action	Rationale	Implementation	Evaluation
Subjective data:						
Objective data:						

Health Education

Conclusion

ANNEXURE 2

Community Health Assessment Format

BASELINE SURVEY DATA

1. Name of the area: Rural/Urban
2. Name of the health center
3. Name of the head of the family
4. Type of family:
    i. Nuclear
    ii. Joint
    iii. Extended
5. Religion:
    i. Hindu
    ii. Muslim
    iii. Christian
    iv. Any other
6. Housing condition:
    i. Type of house
        a. Pucca
        b. Semi-Pucca
        c. Kutcha
    ii. Rooms
        a. Number
        b. Adequate
        c. Inadequate
    iii. Occupancy
        a. Tenant
        b. Owner
        c. Monthly rent
    iv. Ventilation
        a. Adequate
        b. Inadequate
        c. No ventilation
    v. Lighting
        a. Electricity
        b. Gas lamp
        c. Oil lamp
    vi. Water Supply
        a. Tap
        b. Hand pump
        c. Well
    vii. Kitchen
        a. Separate
        b. Corner of the room
        c. Veranda
    viii. Drainage
        a. Adequate
        b. Inadequate
        c. No drainage
    ix. Lavatory
        a. Own latrine
        b. Public latrine
        c. Open air defecation
7. Family composition:

Sl. no.	Name	Relationship with head	Age in Years	Sex	Education	Occupation	Income per month in rupees
1							
2							
3							
4							
5							

   i. Total monthly income of the family in rupees
        a. Below 5,000
        b. 5,001–10,000
        c. 10,001–15,000
        d. 15,001 and above
   ii. Educational status
        a. No formal education
        b. Primary education
        c. Middle school
        d. High school
        e. PUC
        f. Graduation and above
8. Transport and communication media
    i. Transport:
        a. Own vehicle, Specify
        b. Uses BMTC/KSRTC
        c. Uses private buses
        d. Train
    ii. Communication
        a. Mobile/Landline phone
        b. Television
        c. Radio
        d. Newspaper/Magazines
        e. Post and telegraph
    iii. Language
        a. Mother tongue specify _____
        b. Known to read
            - Kannada
            - Hindi
            - English
            - Others, specify _____
        c. Known to write
            - Kannada
            - Hindi
            - English
            - Others, specify _____

9. Dietary pattern:

Sl. no.	Food available	Foods used	Food preparation and storage			
			Traditional	Ideal	Unhygienic	Hygienic
1	Rice					
2	Ragi					
3	Jowar					
4	Wheat					
5	Vegetable					
6	Fish					
7	Meat					
8	Egg					
9	Milk and Product					
10	Pulses					
11	Tubers					

10. Statement of the expenditure of the family:

Sl. no.	Item	Amount spent in rupees (approximate)	Percentage of total expenditure
1	Food		
2	Clothing		
3	Housing (rent)		
4	Medicine		
5	Children education		
6	Recreation		
7	Smoking or liquor		
8	Debt		
9	Savings		
10	Transport		
11	Others		
	Total		

11. Is there any cases of fever?   Yes/No
    If Yes, Specify the following:
    i. With rigors?
    ii. With cough?
    iii. With rash?

Sl. no.	Name	Age in years	Disease	Treatment	Remarks
1					
2					
3					

12. Does anyone have any skin disease?   Yes/No
    If Yes, specify the following:
    i. With itching?
    ii. With patch?
    iii. With rash?

Sl. no.	Name	Age in years	Disease	Treatment	Remarks
1					
2					
3					

13. Does anyone have cough for more than one week?   Yes/No
    If Yes, specify the following:

Sl. no.	Name	Age in years	Disease	Treatment	Remarks
1					
2					
3					

14. Does anyone have any other illness?   Yes/No
    If Yes, specify the following:

Sl. no.	Name	Age in years	Disease	Treatment	Remarks
1					
2					
3					

15. Is any women pregnant?   Yes/No
    If Yes, specify the following:
    1. Gravida
    2. Has she been registered?
    3. Is she getting iron and ferrous sulfate and calcium tablets?
    4. Is she is immunized with tetanus toxoid (TT)?

Sl. no.	Name	Age in years	15.1	15.2	15.3	15.4	Remarks
1							
2							
3							

16. Is there any postnatal mother within 6 weeks?   Yes/No
    If Yes, specify the following:

Sl. no.	Name	Age in years	Number of weeks	Involution	Lochia	Any breast complications/feeding problems	Remarks
1							
2							
3							

17. Vital statistics (within a year)
    1. Birth

Sl. no.	Name of the child	Name of the parents	Date of birth	Sex	Remarks
1					
2					
3					

2. Deaths

Sl. no.	Name of the person	Name of the parents	Date of death	Sex	Remarks
1					
2					
3					

3. Marriage

Sl. no.	Name of the bride	Name of the bridegroom	Age	Date of marriage	Remarks
1					
2					
3					

Annexure 2: Community Health Assessment Format

18. Is there any child below 5 years who is **not** immunized? Yes/No

    If Yes, write the following:

Sl. no.	Name	Age	Sex	BCG/Hepatitis B-0 Polio-0	Penta-1,2,3/ OPV-1,2,3/IPV-1 and 2	MR-1/Vita-min A	DPT-1/MR-2, OPVb/Vitamin A 2–9 doses	DPT-2 b	Remarks
1									
2									
3									

1. Is there any eligible couple? Yes/No
   If Yes, list them of priority.

Sl. no.	Name of the couples	Age	Sex	First priority	Second priority
1					
2					
3					

2. Family planning (FP) method

Sl. no.	Name of the couples	FP method adopted Temporary (specify)		Permanent (specify)	
		Copper T	OCP/ Condom	Tubectomy/ Lap	Vasectomy

   Family and Individual nursing care plan

3. Is there any under 5 years of age in the family who show the signs of malnutrition?
   If Yes, which of the following?

Sl. no.	Name	Age	Sex	Kwashiorkor	Marasmus	Anemia	Vitamin A deficiency	Rickets
1								
2								
3								

4. Is the sullage water being disposed off hygienically? Yes/No

   If Yes, which of the following method is followed?
   1. Drain
   2. Soak pit
   3. Kitchen garden
   If No, specify the reason _____

5. Is the rubbish being disposed off hygienically? Yes/No
   If Yes, which of the following method is followed?
   1. Composting
   2. Burning
   3. Burying
   If No, specify the reason _____

6. Are the excreta being disposed off hygienically? Yes/No
   If No, specify the reason _____

7. Are there any domestic animals? Yes/No
   If Yes, are they kept hygienically? Yes/No
   If No, specify the reason _____
   Is it housed, Separate/Not Separate

8. Is there is a well or hand pump? Yes/No
   If Yes, is it maintained in a good order?
   If No, specify the reason _____
   Is the well chlorinated?
   If Yes, date: _____
   If No, specify the reason _____

9. Whether the house is kept clean? Yes/No
   If No, specify the reason _____

10. Whether the house is sprayed? Yes/No
    If Yes, date _____
    If No, specify the reason _____

11. Is there any breeding place for insects and rodents? Yes/No

12. Are there any stray dogs in the vicinity? Yes/No
    If Yes, write the approximate number of dogs _____

13. If anyone falls ill, where do they get treatment?
    1. Hospital/Community health center
    2. Primary health center/Sub-center
    3. Private nursing home
    4. Indigenous doctor/Local Vaidya

14. Are the official health agencies services adequate? Yes/No
    If No, specify the reason _____

Individualized nursing care plan

Family oriented nursing care plan

Index

Page numbers followed by *b* refer to box, *f* refer to figure, *fc* refer to flowchart, and *t* refer to table.

A

Abdellah's nursing problems 370*b*, 370*f*
Abdellah's theory 369
   and nursing paradigm 371
   in nursing, application of 371
Abdomen 417
Abortion 198
Abraham Maslow basic human needs 484
Absentia care 161
Abuse 601
   indicators 602
   reasons for 602
Academic counseling 518
Acceptance by nursing community 358, 360, 373, 376, 379, 387, 392, 396, 399, 549
   practice 383
Accidents 107
   and injuries 26
   disease to 237*t*
   disorder to 237*t*
Accountability
   areas of 22
   role of 22
Accreditation and licensure 11
Accredited Social Health Activist 126, 127, 147
   responsibility of 145
   role of 145, 146
   selection of 145
   training of 142
Acetylcholine 252
   esterase 195
Acetylcholinesterase 194
Acquired immunodeficiency syndrome 310, 387, 493, 544, 616
Act deontologists 19
Active surveillance 241
Acupuncture 305
Acute care nurse practitioner 540
Acute grief 507
   diagnoses for 510, 511
Acute illness 260
Acute respiratory infections, control of 142
Adaptation 372, 495
   level 390
   problems 390
Adaptive coping strategies 500
Adaptive modes 390
Adaptive responses 390

Addictions 237
   nursing 542
Additional computers 642
Adequate health information, lack of 110
Administration of health services 119, 120*f*
Administrative law 24
Adolescence 486
Adolescent sexuality 492
   homosexuality 492
   masturbation 492
   sexual activity 492
Adrenocorticotropic hormone 498
Adult nurse practitioner 540
Adult sexuality 493
   early adulthood 493
   late adulthood 493
   middle adulthood 493
Advanced neonatal nurse practitioner 545
Aequorea victoria 178
Aerobic respiration 257
Affection 264
Agent, host, and environment model 567, 567*f*
Aging
   concepts of 588
   theories of 590, 590*f*, 590*t*
Aids and prosthesis, use of 603
Air pollution 106, 231, 236
Airless 314
Airway occlusion 318
Alcoholism 237
All India Blind Relief Society 131
All India Women's Conference 131
Alpha-fetoprotein analysis 194
Alternative medical system 530
Alternative medicine 529
Alternative modalities of care 529, 530
Altitude and endemic goiter 222
Alveoli 258
   structure of 258*fc*
Alzheimer's disease 494
Ambulatory care 383
Ambulatory care nurse 541
American Association of Colleges of Nursing 115
American Nurses Association 3, 43, 46, 51, 113, 327
   code of ethics 15
   model 90*f*
   purpose of 46

American Psychiatric Association 461
American Society of Human Genetics 200
Amino acids 498
Amitriptyline (elavil) 595
Amniocentesis 195, 195*f*
Amniotic sac 457
Amphetamines 253
Amygdala 250
Anaerobic respiration 257
Analytical epidemiology 212
Analyzing evidence 611
Analyzing quantitative data, tasks in 641*f*
Anaphase 172
Anaphylaxis 282
Anemia 231, 240, 597
Anesthesia 317
   general 317
   regional 317
Anganwadi
   integration with 145
   workers 126, 147
Anger and gender 576
Antenatal care 147
Antianxiety drugs 316
Anticipatory grief 507
Antidiuretic hormone 271, 272
Antiembolism stockings 315
Anxiety 314
   disorders 253
Apgar score 323*t*
Appetite suppressing drugs 279
Application service provider 643
Application to nursing 365
Appraising and synthesizing evidence 406
Appraising evidence 611
Architecture reference manual 630
Aromatherapy 530, 530*f*
   massage 530
Arteries 258
Arteriosclerosis 261
Artificial insemination 198
   by donor 197
Asphyxia 269
   diagnosis of 324
   pathophysiology of 323
Asphyxiated baby, after care of 324
Asphyxiated fetus 323
Aspirin 304
Assertiveness
   characteristics of 23
   techniques of 23

Index

Assistance under scheme, scale of 147t
Assistant District Health and Family Welfare Officer 126
Asthma, bronchial 265
Asymetrix tool book 637
Atelectasis 269, 314
Atrial fibrillation 597
Atricarium muscle relaxant 312
Attachment therapy 530
Attack rate 225
Audit 90
   committee 93
   cycle 92, 92f
   process 91, 91f
   tools 91
   types of 91
Auditors, training for 93
Auditory acuity 415
Auditory hearing 428
Auricles 414
Auscultation 412
   sounds of 412
   types of 412
Authoritarian leadership 81
Autocratic leadership 81
Autogenic training 550
Automated external defibrillator 322
Autonomic nervous system 251
Autonomy and independent practice roles 22, 558
Autonomy
   barriers of 20
   different aspects of 20
Autosomal chromosome disorders 187
Autosomal dominant inheritance 188, 189f
Autosomal recessive inheritance 189
Autosomes 183
Autotrophic nutrition 255
Auxiliary Nurse Midwife 87, 147
   Association 44
   Program started 6
   role of 145
Axilla 417
Axiomatic axioms 349
Ayurveda 532

B

Baccalaureate education 11
Bacteria 230
Bag and mask ventilation 324
Bargaining
   agent, selection of 54
   distributive 53
   integrative 53
   intra-organizational 53
   types of 53
Baroreceptors 282
Barr body determination 194
Barrel chest 416
Basal ganglia 250, 291

Basic human needs 484
Basic life support 322, 322f
Basic nursing system 383f
Basic sanitation, lack of 110
Behavior change 511
Behavior learning theories 461
Behavior modifications 279
Behavior system model 377
Behavior theories 468
Behavioral and emotional changes 421
Behind-the-ear 603
Below poverty line 147
Benzodiazepines, long-acting 595
Benztropine (cogentin) 595
Bereavement and mourning 510
Bereavement care 508
Berne's model of communication 474
Betty Neuman's system theory 384
Bhagyalakshmi scheme 148
Bharat Sevak Samaj 130
Bhore Committee 6, 10
Biliary condition 278
Biliopancreatic diversion 279
Bioelectromagnetic therapy 536
Biographical information format 443b
Biohazard symbol 331f
Bioinformatics 178
Biological theories 590, 590f
Biology-based practices 529
Biomedical waste 339, 340f
   classification of 339
   management 339
   and handling rules 342
Biopsychosocial pathology 247
Birth asphyxia 323
   management of 324
Birth, kinds of 459
Bleach solution, preparation of 333
Blinding 219
Block extension educator 126
Blood 258
   cells 258
   plasma 258
   pressure
      control of 259
      high 496
   vessels 258
Blood-borne pathogens 334
Board of Research Studies 62
Body build, types on 467
Body fluid 334
   composition of 271
   distribution of 271
   movement of 271
   regulation of 271, 271f
Body heat, sources of 288
Body image
   change 450
   disturbance, conditions with 306
   impact on 422
   stress of 306

Body language 597
Body system changes, age related 591, 591t
Body temperature
   altered 288
   conditions of increased 289
Borders district cluster project 142
Bradykinin 300
Brain 249, 250, 290, 498
   and behavior 456
   imaging 253
Brainstem 251, 291, 456
Breast 417, 505
   cancer of 240
Breathing
   deep 314
   exercises 316
   mechanism 258
Breech birth 459
Broad range theory 353
Bronchi 257
Bronchioles 257
Buccal cavity 256
Buccal mucosa 415
Budget nurse 541
Bulimia nervosa 253, 282
Bureaucratic leadership 82
Burnout 495
Business and financial information system 648

C

Calcium imbalance 276
Caloric intake 297
Canadian Nurses Association 16, 47
Cancer 280, 597
   cells 179f
Cardiac arrest 323
Cardiac care nurse 544
Cardiac massage and medication, external 324
Cardiac nurse practitioner 540
Cardiac output 282
Cardiac pump, failure of 287
Cardiogenic shock, pathophysiology of 284f
Cardiopulmonary resuscitation 320, 321f, 322, 322f
   performing 321
Cardiorespiratory status 323
Cardiovascular complications, risks of 217t
Cardiovascular disease 231, 240, 597
   risk of 500
Cardiovascular disorders 269
Cardiovascular manifestation 275
Cardiovascular problems 279
Cardiovascular system 266, 593
Care coordinator 539
Care pendulum, focus of 371f
Care plans, format for 437

Index

Career approaches, sources of 66
Career ladder 65
    model of 66, 66f
Career opportunities 65
    sources of 66
Carl Rogers self-theory 466
Carotid artery 322
Case control and cohort studies, differences between 217t
Case control studies 212, 212f
    advantages of 213
    disadvantages of 213
Catheterization laboratory nurse 542
Catheters 316
Causation of disease
    biological dynamics in 260
    concepts of 229
Causation-cardiovascular diseases, web of 231f
Celera genomics 177f
Cell
    division 170
    membrane 169, 170
    normal 179f
    organelles 170
    structure 169, 169f
Cellular division, review of 169
Central Council of Health 122
    functions of 31
Central Government Health Scheme 131
Central Government, role of 30
Central Health Education Bureau 122
Central nervous system 268
    anatomy of 290
    physiology of 290
Central sleep apnea syndrome 298
Centralized management 83
Centralized treatment facility 340
Centrosome 170
Cephalocentesis 199
Cerebellum 251, 291
Cerebral cortex 456
Cerebrovascular accident 432
Cerebrovascular disease 597
Cerebrum 291
Certification to contract 54
Certified nurse midwife 559
Certified registered nurse anesthetist 100, 542
Cesarean section 459
Cessation experiments 220
Change agent 539
Charismatic leadership 81
Charting techniques, legal aspects of 28
Chat online 638
Chelation therapy 530
Chemical disinfection 341
Chest 416
    pain, controlling 284
    posterior 416
Child development, specialists in 461

Child Health Welfare Programmes 148
Child psychiatric nurse 545, 546
Child Survival and Safe Motherhood Programme 144
Child's illness 266
Child's reaction to illness 424
Childhood illness, integrated management of 148
Chinese medicine 531
Cholera 230, 236
Chorionic villi sampling 195
Christian Medical Association 50
Christian nurses league 50
Chromosomal and genetic testing 203
Chromosomal disorders 185
Chromosomal structure, change in 186f
Chromosome 182, 183
    basic concepts of 182
    mutations 173
    number, change in 186
    ring 186
    structure, changes in 186
Chronic disease, prevention of 234, 236
Chronic grief 508
Cigarette smoking 221
Cimetidine 595
Circadian rhythm sleep disorders 299
Circulating room nurse 544
Circulatory system 258
Civil law 25
Clarify ethical dilemma 19
Clearing airway 324
Client and environment in balance 357f
Client and equipment, care of 270
Client coping skills 261, 421
Client experiencing grief and loss 310
Client seeking genetic counseling 201
Client with eating disorder 282
Client with obesity 278
Client with social isolation 311t
Client assessment 377t
Climatic conditions 232
Clinical decision-maker 538
Clinical genetics 198
Clinical information system 648
Clinical nurse
    and researcher, differences between 72
    leader 545
    researcher 79
    specialist hemophilia 545
Clinical nursing practice 388
Cloning 196
Code of ethics 7, 13, 14, 19
    for nurses 14
Code, elements of 16
Cognitive development, Piaget's stages of 465t
Cognitive psychosocial factors 587
Cohort members 215
Cohort studies 212f, 214
    advantages of 217

disadvantages of 217
elements of 214
indications for 214
prospective 214
retrospective 214
types of 214
Coital play 490
Colicky pain 302
Collaboration
    principles of 562
    types of 562
Collaborative learning unit model 563
Collaborative models within nursing 562
Collaborative partnerships, types of 562
Collaborative practice model 563f
Collective bargaining 51, 52
    advantages of 56
    characteristics of 52
    disadvantages of 56
    levels of 56, 56f
    meaning of 52
    objectives of 52
    preparation for 53
    principles of 53
    process of 53, 54f
    steps of 54, 54f
Colloids 282
Colon 238
Colonial American period 4
Color discrimination 414
Coma cocktail 293
Common causes 264f
Common diseases, treatment of 22
Common disorders 190
Common eating disorders 282
Common genetic disorders, approaches to 185
Common law 24
Common management functions 83
Commonwealth Nurses Federation 49
Communicability infectious disease 236
Communicable disease 233, 236
    prevention 574
    and control of 245
    Programs 132
Communicating nursing care plan 437
Communication 156, 157, 474f, 480, 482, 483
    and interpersonal relationships 15
    and support 202
    barriers of 473
    components of 473, 473f
    factors influencing 472
    intrapersonal 475
    levels of 475
    networking system 649
    small-group 475
    theories of 474
    types of 473

Community care
  in elderly 606
  in practice 606
Community development blocks 124
Community facilities, use of 570
Community health agency 203
Community health assessment format 657
Community Health Center 127, 151, 153
Community health nurse 223, 244, 545, 574
  in disaster
    preparedness, role of 584
    recovery, role of 585
    response, role of 584
  role of 572
Community Health Nursing, roles in 545
Community health risk assessment tools 242
Community health work 567
Community healthcare professional 129
Community nursing 383
Community participation 554
Community preparedness 584
Community psychiatric health nurse 547
Community risk assessment 243
Community-based nursing, collaboration in 563f
Comparison groups, selection of 215
Compilation and analysis of data 241
Complementary transaction 474f
Complete dentures 604
Complex nursing functions 137
Comprehensive nursing care 134, 134f
Computer networks, types of 638
Computerized hospital information system 648
Computerized nursing care plans 442
Computers, uses of 627
Conceptual framework 350, 375f, 381f
  and models, uses of 350
  development of 351, 351f
  purposes of 350
Conceptual model 350, 555t
Concrete operations 465
Concurrent parallel study designs 220
Conditions demanding resuscitation 320
Conductance regulator gene 181
Conducting physical assessment 412
Conformity assessment with standards 89
Congestive heart failure 588
Conjunctiva and sclera 414
Connective leadership 81
Consanguineous marriage 196
Conscious sedation 317
Conservation model 372
Conservational principles, concepts of 372
Constant fever 289

Constitution and Composition of Council 33
Constitutional law 24
Consumer Protection Act 25
Contextual stimuli 390
Continence nurse 545
Continuing education and career opportunities 58
Continuing Education Program 64
Continuing education
  benefits of 65
  need for 64
Continuing Nursing Education 63, 65f
  characteristics of 64
Continuing professional education 63
  evaluation of 65
Continuous positive airways pressure 298
Contract administration 55
Conversion disorder 266
Converted grief 507
Coping to nursing need, relation of 569
Cordocentesis 195f
Cordotomy 305
Coronary heart disease 190, 220, 230, 296
Corporate nurse practitioner 100
Corpus callosum 250
Corynebacterium diptheriae 230
Cotton swabs 411
Coughing 314
  performing forced 315
Counseling 513
  in nursing and education, application of 515t
  phases of 515, 515f
  skills 201
  techniques of 515
  types of 514, 515
Counselor 538
  characteristics of 513
  qualities of 513
Counter irritants 304
Craft unions 51
Created environment 385
Criminal law 25
Critical care obstetrician 560
Critique 376, 380
Critiquing theory 374
Crude death rate 225
Crystalloid 282
Cultural identity 613
Culture, concept of 613
Curanderismo therapy 535
Curative healthcare delivery system 537
Curiosity 264
Current infectious diseases 314
Current smoking, amount of 213t
Cyclical nature of theory, research, and practice 350f
Cyst, superficial 313
Cystic fibrosis 203
Cytoplasm 170

D

Daily living, activities of 377
Dais 10
Danger-incorrect disposal of sharps 334f
Dangerous Drug Act 26
Dark age (renaissance period) 4
Data collection, planning for 571
Date problems 635
Daughter cells 169
Day dreaming 471
Day-to-day stressors 496
Deaddiction nurse 546
Death and dying
  concept of 326
  issues related to 327
  responsibility for 27
  stages of 329
Death rate 225
  age specific 225
  age standardized 213t
Debbie's adaptive level, evaluation of 394
Decentralized management 83
Decision making capacity 605
Defective vision 237
Defense mechanisms 455, 469, 469t
  groups of 470
Defense medical services 131
Dehiscence 318
Dehydration 273
  risk for 595
Delegation, five rights of 84
Delivery functions 154
Delivery nursing care, functional method of 138
Dementia 598
Democratic (participative) leadership 81
Dentures 603
  and prosthesis 316
  in old age, uses of 604
Deontology 18
Deoxyribonucleic acid 169, 182, 183, 193
  basic concepts of 182
  molecule, portion of 183f
  replication 176
  technology 174
Department of Family Welfare 120
Department of Health 119
Departmental management system 649
Dependent client role 423
Depression 329, 508, 510, 511
  despair 262
Dermatological system 593
Descriptive epidemiology 211
Design and planning phase 75
Detoxification therapy 536
  benefits of 536
  contraindications for 536
  methods of 536
Developing conceptual
  definitions 74
  framework and models 351

Developing nursing care plan 440
Developing protocols for intervention 75
Development 484
    principles of 484
Developmental disability nurses 544
Dever's epidemiologic model 231
Diabetes 191, 231, 240, 261
    case of 229
    management nurse 542
    mellitus 598
Diagnostic test
    indications for 193
    role of nurse in 204
Dialysis nurse 544
Diarrhea 229
Diencephalon 291
Diet 238
    based therapy 531
Diffuse disorders 292
Diffusion 268, 271
Dimenhydrinate (gravol) 595
Diphtheria 245
Diploma education 11
Diplotene 172
Direct auscultation 412
Direct percussion 412
Directly observed treatments, short-course 228
Directorate General of Health Service 31, 121
Disability 237
    adjusted life year 227
    prevention 237
    rates 227
Disaster
    causes of 585t
    common reactions to 586
    management, phases of 583, 583f
    medical assistance teams 584
    nurse 546, 583
    preparedness, role of nurses in 585
    syndrome 585
    types of 585t
Disbelief anger 262
Discharge instructions 318
Discharge planner 539
Disease
    causation of 260
    determinants of 210
    distribution of 210
    frequency 210
    iceberg of 226, 231, 232f
    measurement of 211
    natural history of 232
    notification of 242
    registers 243
    results 234
    spectrum of 233, 233f
    types of 642
Disease causation
    pathophysiology of 249
    psychodynamics of 249
    theories of 229
Disinfection, agents used in 333
Disposal of sharps 343f
Disposal-needle destroyer/burner/cutter 334f
Distance visual acuity 414
Distorted grief 507
District Council of Health Organization 126
District Health and Family Welfare 125, 126
District level organization 125
Dobutamine 283
Doctor's record entry 645, 645f
Doctoral preparation 11
Documentation 446
    goal of 446
    purpose of 446
Dominant trait 174, 174f
Dopamine 252, 253, 284
Double blind trial 219
Double circulation 258
Down's syndrome 187, 195
Drug
    in elderly, goal of 594
    maintenance 26
    standards, control of 121
Drugs Act, misuse of 26
Dunn's high-level wellness grid 567
Dying environment 328
Dynamic ileus 318
Dynamic interacting systems 381
Dynamic interrelated phases, five 426f
Dysentery 236
Dyssomnias 298

E

Ear 414, 592
    wax 414
Early ambulation 314
Early childhood, development during 485
Early civilization, period of 4
Early morning awakening 299
Eating disorders 237, 253
Economic strikes 55
Education 156, 157, 376
Educational counseling 514
Educational preparation
    levels of 59t
    meaning of 58
Educational, vocational and personal counseling 518
Edward's syndrome 187
Effective planning machinery, lack of 109
Effective team work, obstacles to 137
Elderly abuse, types of 602t
Electrocardiography transmission 161
Electrolyte 271
    balance 271
    imbalance 274
    normal ranges of 271t
    regulation of 276t
Electromagnetic fields, effects of 536
Electronic health and telehealth 162
Electronic hospital management
    exit from 647f
    software 644, 644f
Electronic medical record software 643
    benefits of 643
    elements of 643
Embolus 314
Embryo 458f, 459f
    period of 457, 458
Emergency medical
    care 323
    system 320
Emergency obstetric care 142, 143
Emergency trauma nurse 542
Emerging environmental issues 107
Emotion 262
    characteristics of 263
    control of 265
    in health and disease, role of 265
    kinds of 262
    of pleasure 264
Emotional abuse 601
Emotional competence 570
Emotional dimension, dysfunction in 261
Emotional disturbance 266
Emotional reaction 263
Emotional stress 296
Empirical evidence, use of 356, 359, 372, 380, 394, 398
Empirical precision 358, 365, 384, 397
Employees 56
Employees State Insurance Scheme 131
Employers 56
Employment opportunities, expansion of 525
Empowers women 580
Endemic fluorosis 281
Endocrine system 593
End-of-life care 326
Endoplasmic reticulum 170
Endotracheal intubation 324
Endotracheal tube, selection of 324t
Energy
    conservation of 372
    medicine 529, 531
Enteral nutrition 281
Environment 357f, 379, 395
    (Protection) Act 342
    physical 106
    preparation of 270
    psychological 106
    social 106
Environmental field patterning 364
Environmental health
    data 243
    hazards 106

Environmental indicators 228
Environmental modification 235, 550
Environmental protection agency 107
Environmental stress 495
Environmental surveys 215
Environmental theory 106
Envy 264
Epidemiologic methods 211f
Epidemiological approach 210
Epidemiological investigation process 223, 223f
Epidemiological measurements 224fc
Epidemiological methods 211
Epidemiological triad 230f
Epidemiology
 aims of 210
 basic measurements of 224
 history of 209
 meaning of 209
 measures of preventive 239
 modern concepts of 209
 role of nurse in 245
 scope of 210
Epinephrine 593
Equipment
 common usage 379
 needed 411
 responsibility for 27
Erectile dysfunction 450
Ethic 13
 primary principles of 17
 secondary principles of 18
Ethical decision-making model dilemma 19fc
Ethical dilemma 19, 198
 common 605
 resolution of 19
Ethical issues 197, 605
Ethical philosophical theories 18
Ethical principles 17
 types of 17fc
Etiological agents, trial of 221
Eugenics, negative 196
Euthanasia 327
Euthenics 196
Evaluation 445
 principles of 445
Evaporation 289
Evidence 609
 hierarchy 406f
 types of 406
Evidence-based
 journals 610
 nursing practice 609
 practice 405
  barriers in 405
  challenges in 612
  model 405, 443
  process of 406f, 610
  users of 610
Evisceration 314

Excel 629
 mod function error 635
Excretion 259
 methods of 259b
Exercise 238, 279, 550
 and fatigue 297
Experimental epidemiology 218
Experimental studies
 advantages of 218
 aims of 218
 types of 218
Extended care facilities 537
External objects, loss of 505
Extrapyramid system 251
Extrinsic sleep disorders 299
Eye 414, 505, 592
Eyebrows 414
Eyelids 414

F

Fabiola influenced 4
Face 414
 tent 269
Facemask with reservoir bag 269
Faculty counselors 516f
Faith and prayer therapy 535
False teeth 603
Family and cultural beliefs 261
Family coping
 ability, assessment of 569
 index 569
Family dynamics, impact on 422
Family life cycle, stages of 460
Family living 570
Family nurse practitioner 540, 559
Family nursing 569
 care plan, format of 572
 diagnosis 571
 process 570
Family problems, examples of 572
Family roles, impact on 422
Family screening 198
Family surveillance 240
Family Welfare Programme 148
Family welfare services 152
 organization for 150
Fantasy 471
Fatality rate 225
Fatigue 450
Federal response plan 584
Female health supervisor training 59
Fetal death rate 225
Fetal therapy 199
Fetoscopy 196
Fetus 459f
Fever 289
 clinical manifestations of 289
 hectic 290
 irregular 290
 nursing intervention for 290
 pathophysiology of 289f

 swinging 290
 types of 289
Fiberoptic fetoscope 196
Fifth Five Year Plan 553
Filaria 239
Filenames 635
Finance committee 33
First aid 335
First interactive telemedicine system 163
First meiotic division 171
First Nurse's Registration Act 6
Fitness 238, 550
Flight nurse 100, 546
Flower essence therapy 532
Fluid 270
 and blood replacement 283
 and electrolyte balance 270
 balance 270
 imbalance 272
 intake 271
 output 272
 replacement 287
 volume
  deficit 272
  excess 272
Fluorescence in situ hybridization 186, 194
Fluorescent cDNA populations 179f
Fluorescent dyes, different 179f
Fluoxetine (prozac) 595
Focal stimulus 390
Folk medicine 532
Follicle-stimulating hormone 593
Food
 and fluids 315
 and oral fluids 318
 poisoning 229
Forensic
 nurse 543
 psychiatric nurse 547
 testing 193
Foreseeable crisis situation 571
Formal operations 465
Formatting toolbar 632
Formulated plan, preparation of 112
Formulating hypothesis 75
Framework, scope and trends 523
Free-standing surgical center 312
Frontal lobe 456
 influence 250
Frustration
 commonly occurring 496
 response to 456
Functional psychiatric disorders 249
Fungi 230
Funnel chest 416
Futuristic nursing 95

G

Gain control, attempting to 262
Gait 419

Index

Gamma amino butyric acid 252, 295, 456
Gastric hypersensitivity 265
Gastrointestinal problem 280
Gastrointestinal system 265, 593, 598
Gastrointestinal tract 272
Gate control theory 301, 302t
Gather additional data 19
Gender 575
   awareness 575
   bias 575
   considerations 160
   diversity 576
   equality 575, 580
   equity 575
   insensitive communication 576
   role 575
   sensitive issues 575
   sensitivity 576
Gene
   addition procedures 175
   basic concepts of 182
   chemistry of 183
   chips 178
   expression 179f
   mutation, sub-microscopic 173
   therapy 174, 198
      function of 175
      recent advances of 175
      types of 175
General adaptation syndrome 499
General nursing and midwifery 59
General population rates, comparison with 215
General protective measures 337
General scheme of relevant concepts 351f
Genetic 167, 185
Genetic carriers, detection of 197
Genetic computer group 178
Genetic counseling 196, 200, 202
   approach to 202
   nurse role in 203
   principles of 201
   process of 202
   prospective 200
   team 201
   types of 200
Genetic diagnosis, basis of 192
Genetic diseases 185
Genetic disorder 185, 200
   incidence of 185
   management of 191
   types of 185
Genetic engineering 205
Genetic in nursing, application of 203
Genetic makeup influences 260
Genetic mutation 173
Genetic nurse 559
Genetic predisposition, role of 190
Genetic research 199
Genetic screening
   and counseling 197
   goals of 194
Genetic services, role of administrator in 204
Genetic testing 192, 193, 203
   ethical issues in 197
   legal issues in 197
   psychosocial issues in 197
   types of 193
Genital and rectum 418
Genital and sexual system 593
Genitalia
   female 419
   male 418
Genitourinary system 599
Genome mutation 173
Genomic era 180
Genotoxic waste 341
Genotype 188
Geriatric considerations in nursing 588
Geriatric nurse
   practitioner 540
   roles of 603
Geriatric nursing 542, 547, 588, 590
   landmarks of 588
Geriatric people problems 600
Geriatric population, incidence of 589
Geriatric problems 590
Germ theory of disease 229
Gerontological nursing 547
Gerontology 588
Gestational age 324t
Glasgow coma scale 292
   assessment of 293t
Gold disk astound 637
Golgi bodies 170
Government service conduct rules 30
Governmental support, lack of 21
Grand theory 353
Graphesthesia 420
Green fluorescent protein 178
Grief
   and bereavement 506
   and depression, differences between 510t
   dysfunctional 507
   stages of 506
   symptoms of 508
   theories of 508
   therapy 509
   types of 507
Grievance
   classification of 55
   hearing 55
   process 55
Group counseling 514f
Group development, stages of 481
Group dynamic 480
   elements of 480
   objectives of 480
   principles of 480
   process 481
Groups, type of 480
Growth 484
   and development 455
      stages of 485
   of telemedicine applications 163
   principles of 484
Guidance 512
Guidance and counseling 512
   center, activity spectrum of 517f
   principles of 514
   relationship between 514
Gums and teeth 415

H

Hair 505
Hall's core care and cure model 566, 566f
Hand hygiene 331
   steps of 332f
   technique 331
Hand washing 331f
   procedure, steps in 332
Handicap 237
Handling sharps 334f
Haploid and diploid chromosomes 184
Happiness 264
Harmful waste, removal of 259
Hassles, commonly occurring 496
Hazardous period 460
Head and neck 414
Head-to-toe manner 411
Health 105, 133, 260, 369, 387, 395, 549, 561
   adjusted life expectancy 227
   alternative systems of 532
   and complimentary therapies, alternative systems of 529
   and disease-related factors 568
   and living conditions 516
   assessment 411
   assistant 126
   attitudes 570
   beliefs and practices, factors influencing 260
   conditions, knowledge of 570
   consumers, advanced roles on 69
   deficits 571
   determinants of 552
   disaster planning and preparation 244
   economics 108
   environmental influences on 106
   equilibrium, ecological model of 230f
   examination 239
   fundamental right 117
   goals 440
   hazards 339
   indicators of 130t, 144t
   informatics 234, 241
   insurance 131
   intelligence 122

Index

interventions 550
morbidity status 239
new philosophy of 564
perceived control of 549
personnel, suggested norms for 109*t*
preserve 234
professionals 30
promotional measures 196
protection 236
restoration 134
situation, analysis of 111
status indicators 228
surveillance 234, 240
team, members of 14
threats 571
Health assessment format 653
  history taking 653
  lab investigations 655
  medical treatment 655
  nursing management 656
  physical examination 653
  surgical management 656
Health belief model 401, 401*f*, 564, 564*f*
  components of 402*t*
Health care 117, 267
  agency 315
  economic
    concepts in 108
    indicators of 108
  environment 105, 106
  personnel, religion for 616
  related to dying and death, changes in 326
  resources 606
  standard for 327
Health care delivery 103, 117
  application of epidemiology in 234
  concerns 141
  indicators 227
Health care delivery system 117, 119, 132*f*, 537, 556*f*
  characters of 118
  functions of 118
  objectives of 118
  philosophy of 118
  preventive 537
  principles of 118
Health care services 117, 132
  different 128*f*
  improper utilization of 111
Health care system 326
  accessibility of 421
  barriers in 21
  history of 117
  model of 119*f*
  models 119
  stakeholders in 129
Health education 235, 245, 550
  inadequate 110
Health for all 105, 552
  concept of 551
  indicators for 552*t*

meaning of 551
nursing strategies for 555*f*
Health illness
  continuum model 566, 566*f*
  states 265
Health information
  sources of 242
  system 242
    components of 242
  uses of 242
Health Insurance Portability and Accountability Act 180
Health maintenance 134
  organizations 606
Health manpower 113
  statistics 244
Health planning 111
  process 111
Health policy
  and regulation 98
  and systems 552
  indicators 228
Health problem 235, 595, 600
  common 595
Health promoter 538
  behaviour, participation in 549
Health promotion 134, 234, 235, 267, 537, 548-550
  activities 598
  concepts of 548
  model 548, 548*f*
  nurse role in 235, 551
  selected areas of 238
Health service 606
  administration 21
  evaluation of 221
  general structure of 109
  organization of 119, 120*f*, 124, 124*f*, 125*f*
  records 243
  resources for 108
Health surveys 239
  general 239
Health system
  components of 118
  official organization of 30
  official organs of 119
Health visitors 59
  league 44
Healthy skin function 599
Hearing aids 603
  dentures 603
  indication of 603
  types of 603
  uses of 603
Heart 416, 498
  beat, irregular 323
  disease 238, 261, 508
  murmur 417
  sounds 417
Heat loss, channels of 288
Help for ships 161

Helping-trust relationship, development of 395
Hematologic systems 593
Hemorrhage 282, 318
Henderson's definition, conceptualization of 359*f*
Henderson's theory 359, 360
Hepatic disorders 278
Hepatic dysfunction 277
Hepatitis 245
  B virus 335
  C virus 335
Hereditary diseases 185
Heritable diseases 191
Heritable gene therapy 175
Heroic medicine 532
Heterotrophic nutrition 256
Heterotrophs, classification of 256
Hierarchies, types of 406
Hind Kusht Nivaran Sangh 130
Hippocampus 250, 291
Histamine 300
Hoesing and Kirk quality management model 527
Holistic client approach 385
Holistic health model 567
Holozoic nutrition 256
Home and institutional care 607
Home healthcare nurse 545, 574
Home heating system 259
Home nursing 569, 572
  general instructions for 572
Home visit
  activities during 573
  advantages of 573
  components of 573
  principles of 573
Homeopathy 533, 533*f*
Homeostasis 260, 270
  diagnostic evaluation for 260
Homeostatic mechanism 255, 259
Homozygous state 182
Hormonal regulation 272
Hospital acquired sleep disturbance 299
Hospital and nursing homes, computerization of 642
Hospital healthcare professional 129
Hospital information system 643, 648
  benefits of 648
  components of 648, 648*f*
  types of 648
Hospital management
  beginning of 644*f*
  information system software 642
  software 642, 643
Hospital policy 21
Hospital records 243
Hospital waste 339
  management, objectives of 339
  types of 339, 339*f*
Hostility 264

Index

Human behavior 455
Human beings 232, 382
Human caring theory 394, 398*f*
Human chorionic gonadotropin 195
Human chromosome 177*f*
Human development 456
Human digestive system, structure of 256
Human field patterning 364
Human genetics 169
Human genome project 169, 175
    benefits of 179
    genomic era 174
    history of 175
    limitations of 180
    mapping 176
    objectives of 176
Human growth
    and development, stages of 456
    potential for 477
Human heart 258*f*
Human immunodeficiency virus 18, 228, 333, 335, 544
    transmission, risk of 334
Human psychopathology 309*f*
Human relations, psychological aspects and 453
Human respiratory system 257, 257*f*
Human survival and health 484
Humanistic theories 466
Humor 501, 535
    therapy 535
Huntington's chorea 188
Hydrotherapy 532
Hydroxyl groups 252
Hygiene, application of principles of 570
Hyovolemic shock 283
Hypercalcemia 277
Hyperkalemia 276
Hypernatremia 274
Hyperpyrexia 289
Hypertension 229, 231, 234, 238, 261
    chronic 260
    essential 265
Hyperthermia 289
Hyperthyroidism 265
Hypocalcemia 276
    mild 276
    severe 276
Hypokalemia 275
Hyponatremia 274
Hypothalamic fever 289
Hypothalamic-pituitary
    pathway 498
    response 498
Hypothalamus 250, 251
Hypothermia 290, 323
    clinical signs of 290
Hypothesis, formulation of 212, 239
Hypothetical cigarette smoking 216*t*
Hypothyroidism 598

Hypovolemic shock 283
    care in 288
    management of 283
Hypoxemia 314, 318

I

Illegal strikes 55
Illness 260, 385
    and hospitalization, common effects of 423
    chronic 260
    client's perception of 421
    coping with 500
    family's response to 266
    general model of 500
    iceberg 266
    impact of 421
    models of 500
    multicausational concept of 265*f*
    nature of 261, 421
    perception of 261
    prevention 267
    psychological stages of 262
    specificity model of 500
    stigma of 266
    with negative progresses 266
Illness behavior 260, 420
    roles in 266
    stages of 422
    variables influencing 261, 421
Immobility 307
    conditions with 307
Immune systems 593
Immunization programme 150
Imogene king theory 380
Implementation process 443
Impulse-related disorders 253
Incidence rate 225, 226
Incinerators, types of 341
Independent practice issues 558
Indian Council for Child Welfare 130
Indian Health System Infrastructure 556
Indian Nurses Register 33
Indian Nursing Council 31, 32, 34*f*, 558
    functions of 33
    organization structure of 32
Indian Nursing Council Act 6
    amendments in 33
Indian Nursing Council Code of Ethics 14
Indian Red Cross Society 130
Individual clinicians, steps for 406
Individual counseling 515, 515*f*
Individual surveillance 240
Individualized care plan 446
Indomethacin (indocid) 595
Industrial unions 51
Infancy, characteristics of 460
Infant
    at birth, assessment of 323
    mortality rate 225

Infection 338
    chain of 336, 336*f*
    control of 335, 338
        basic principles of 331
    prevention 331
        and control of 331
Infectious agent
    control of 336
    elimination of 336
Infectious diseases 230
Influencing self-care 375*f*
Information 156, 157
Information, education and communication 156
    activity 236, 551
    objectives of 156
    tools 157
Informative counseling 514
Informed consent 198, 314, 605
Infraclavicular lymph nodes 416
Infratentorial lesions 291
Innovation
    gaining support for 621
    nature of 80
    process of 621
    steps in 619
Innovative strategies, development of 620
Inpatient surgery 313
Insomnia 298
    management of 298
Institutional care elderly 607
Instrument
    birth 459
    safety of 333
Insulin 593
Insurance companies 72
Integumentary system 413, 598
Intellectual dimension, dysfunction in 261
Intellectual energy 5
Intensive care unit 163, 442
Intentional torts 28
Interactive telemedicine services 162
Interactive therapy, preparation for 476
Intermediate nursing functions 137
Intermittent fever 290
International Council of Nurses 3, 16, 47
    activities of 48
    functions of 48
    organization chart 47*f*
International Health Regulations 242
International Health Relations and Quarantine 121
International Professional Organizations 46
International surveillance 241
Internet literatures search 638
Internet medical literature, sources of 638
Interpersonal communication 475

Interpersonal teaching-learning, promotion of 395
Interpersonal theory 464
    and nursing process 367
Inter-professionality problem 87
Intersectoral coordination 153, 153f
    advantages of 154
Interstitial fluid 271
Intestinal obstruction 313
Intestine, large 257
Intrauterine devices 151
Intrinsic sleep disorders 298
Inverse fever 290
Iodine deficiency disorders 278
Iridodiagnosis 533
Iridology 533
Irritability anger 262
Isochromosome 186
Isotonic imbalance 272
Janani Suraksha Yojana 146
    beneficiaries 147t

J

Job responsibilities 540
Johnson's behavioral model 379f
    and nursing metaparadigm 379
Johnson's behavioral system
    and nursing process 449
    application of 377
Johnson's theory 379
Joint Commission for Accreditation of Healthcare Organizations 440
Journey toward death 328
Jurisdictional strikes 55

K

Karnataka State Nursing Council 37
    functions of 37
Kashyapa Samhita 6
Kasturba Memorial Fund 131
Kelly's dimensions of profession 8
Kidney 259, 272
    diseases 240
    function, changes in 599
King's open system 381f
King's theory
    and nursing paradigm 382
    presents 383
Klinefelter syndrome XXY 188
Knowledge explosion 97
Knowledge-focused triggers 406
Known environment, loss of 505
Koch's postulates 223
Kwashiorkor 280

L

Laber's congenital amaurosis 175
Labor
    strikes, unfair 55
    unions 51

Lacrimal apparatus 414
Lady Medical Officer 126
Larynx 238, 257
Laser surgery 313
Late childhood, development during 485
Lathyrism 281
Laughter
    benefits of 535
    therapy 535
Law and ethics, distinguish between 13t
Law for nursing
    practice, sources of 24, 24f
    values of 25
Law of inheritance 174
Leader and manager 538
Leadership 81
    and management 80
        distinguish between 82
    qualities 82, 82f
    roles of 82
    styles of 81
    techniques of 83
    types of 81
Learner and teacher 538
Learning opportunities 486
Learning setting 10
Learning theories 468
Leg exercise 315
    performing 315
Legal considerations 24
Legal liability 27
Legal nurse consultant 543
Leininger's sunrise model 615f
Lens accommodation, loss of 592
Leptotene 171
Lesions 414
Levine's theory 373
Libido, decreased 450
Licensed practical nurse education 11
Life
    event stressors 496
    expectancy at births 579
    loss of 505
    process 255, 455
Lifestyle 296
    and behavioral changes 235, 550
    challenges 96
Limb 505
Limbic system 250, 250f, 291, 456
Limbus 250
Line of defense 384
Lips 415
Literacy rate 580
Liver 257
    problem 280
Living arrangements 601
Living standards 261
Living things, characteristics of 255
Local adaptation syndrome 499
Local area network 638

Local nongovernmental organizations 158
Logical form 399
Lorazepam 316
Loss 504, 506
    assessment of 506f
    categories of 505
    coping with 504, 601
    problems of 504
    profound 504
    types of 504, 505
Love 263
    deprivation of 264f
Low birth weight 235, 281
Lower extremities 419
Low-performing states 147
Lung
    cancer 216t, 238
        death rates 216t
    collapsed 314
    diseases, test for 240
    infection 314
Lymph 258
    nodes 416
Lymphatic drainage, manual 533
Lysosomes 170

M

Macronutrient deficiencies 278
Macular degeneration, age-related 599
Madilu yojane 148
Malaria 239
Male advantage 577
Malnutrition 231, 280
Management care plans 442
Management functions 83f
Manager, responsibilities of 84
Mania 266
Marasmus 280
Marital stress 495
Marriage, late 197
Masks 269
Maslow's concepts 488
Maslow's hierarchy 436
    model 565f
    of human needs 484, 484f, 565
Massachusetts general hospital 162
Maternal and child health 147
Maternal mortality rate diseases 225
Maternity clinical specialist 560
Maternity nurse practitioner 559
Maturation 484
    loss 506
Measles 245
Mediating processes 496
    appraisal 496
    coping 496
    external resources 497
    personal resources 497
Medical abuse 602
Medical asepsis 337

Index

Medical care contact 423
Medical education 122
Medical examination 215
Medical officer 147
Medical research 122
Medical sciences 62
Medical surgical nurse 544
Medical termination of pregnancy 142, 203
Medication compliance 594
Medicine
    and health care, computers in 647
    and homeopathy 121
    complementary and alternative 529
    indigenous system of 131
    integrative 533
Medicolegal case
    nurses' role in 27
    responsibility for 27
Meiosis 171
    steps of 171f
Meiotic division 172f
    stage with 173f
Men in nursing, advantages for 577
Men, misconception of 577
Mendel's first law 174
Mendel's second law 174
Mental changes 329
Mental disorders 191
Mental health problems 245
Mental illness 229-231
    psychobiology in 249
Mental retardation 237
Mentor and women 576
Menu bar 631, 631f
Meta-paradigm 349
Meta-theory 353
Metabolic disorders 292
Metabolism 594
Meta-communication 473
Metaphase 172
    stage of 194
Methyldopa 595
Microbirth plan 147t
Micronutrients deficiencies 278
Microsoft excel 633, 633f
    features of 633, 634f
Microsoft office 630
    excel 633
    part of 633
    word 630
Microsoft PowerPoint 635, 637
    presentation 636, 636f, 637f
Microsoft windows 629, 629f
    history of 629
Microwave irradiation 341
Midbrain 250
Middle adulthood, development in 487
Midwives 10, 44
Military nursing services 524
Millennium development goal indicators 228

Mind-body medicine 529
Ministry of Health and Family Welfare
    functions of 31
    services 121f, 123f
Mitochondria 170
Mitosis 170
    stages of 170f
Mobile nursing practice 524
Model nursing education, application of 368
Modification and changing health behaviors, risk factors of 267
Molecular genetics 253
Monitoring tissue perfusion 286
Monoamine oxidase inhibitors 253
Mood disorder 252, 253, 266
Morbidity indicators 226
Morbidity rates 226
Mortality and morbidity 224
Mortality rate 225
Motor system 419
Mouth and pharynx 415
MS office 629
Mucus 257
Multifactorial causation 223
    theory 230
Multifactorial disorders 190t
Multifactorial inheritance and disorders 190
Multiphasic screening 240
Multiple cause 231f
Multiple effects models 231f
Multiple sleep latency test 300
Multipurpose health
    assistants 59
    supervisors 59
Multivitamins 280
Muscle strength, tests of 420
Musculoskeletal manifestation 275
Musculoskeletal problems 280
Musculoskeletal system 593, 599
Music 501
    therapy 534
    uses of 534
Mutation 173
    and law of inheritance 169
    problems of 173
    types of 173
Myocardial infarction, prevention of 220

N

N-acetylaspartate 175
Narcolepsy 298
Narcotics 316
Narrative charting 447
Nasal cannula 269
Nasal cavity 415
Nasal speculum 411
National Development Plan 108
National Disaster Medical System 584

National Health and Family Welfare Programmes 141
National Health and Nutrition Examination Survey 243
National Health Programmes 122, 132
National League for Nursing 48, 115
National Library of Medicine 638
National Medical Library 122
National Population Policy, adoption of 142
National Professional Organizations 40
National Rural Health Mission 144
    programs, components of 141
    schemes of 145
National Staff Committee 63
National Status Indicators 227
National Strategy for Health for All 2000 552
National Students Nurses Association 43
National Surveillance 241
National Technical Committee on Child Health 142
Natural birth 459
Natural experiments 221
Natural therapy 530
Near visual acuity 414
Neck 415
Needle stick injuries, managements of 342
Neonatal and childhood illness management process, management of 149f
Neonatal mortality rate 225
Neonatal nurse
    clinician 545
    practitioner 559
Neonatal resuscitation 323, 325f
    after birth 324
Nephron 259
Nerve
    block 305
    cells 250, 456
Nervous system 599
Neuman's conceptual model 388
Neuman's model
    and nursing paradigm 386
    and nursing process 389t
    application of 388
    interpretation of 389f
Neuman's system 387-389
    model 386f, 387
Neural pathway 260
Neurectomy 305
Neuroanatomy 250
Neurodermatitis 265
Neuroendocrine response 498
Neurogenic
    fever 289
    shock 283, 285
Neurologic examination 292
Neurological system 593

Neurons 250
Neurophysiologic techniques 253
Neuropsychiatric nursing 546
Neuroregulation 252
Neurosurgical procedures 305
Neurotransmitter 252f, 253, 456
 characteristics of 456
 molecules 252
 regulation 253
New millennium nurses 100
New trends influencing health 105
Newborn
 care, essential 142
 infants, screening of 197
 screening 193
Nightingale's environmental theory 356
Nightingale's grand theory 356
Nightingale's theory 356, 357
 application of 358, 358t
 development of 356
Nitroglycerin 284
Nocturia 296
Noise 357f
 control 236
 pollution 107
Non-communicable disease programs 132
Non-governmental agencies 154
 role of 141
Non-governmental stakeholders 130
Non-heritable gene therapy 175
Non-opioids analgesics 304
Non-quantifiable information 244
Nonrapid eye movement 295
Nonsteroidal anti-inflammatory drugs 304, 594
Nonstochastic theory 590, 591
Nonverbal behaviors 513
Nonverbal communication 596
Norepinephrine 252
North American Nursing Diagnosis Association 431
Nose and sinuses 415
Nostrils 257
Numeric precision 635
Numerical rating scale 303, 303f
Nurse 130
 accountability of 20
 administration, responsibilities of 516
 administrator 22, 82
 advocate 267
 and co-workers 16
 and electoral process 115
 and midwives, training of 10
 and people 16
 and practice 16
 and profession 16
 and society 16
 anesthetist 541
 assertiveness of 20
 author 541
 autonomy of 20
  professional 21
 basic function of 380
 critical care 540
 dietician 541
 each registered 22
 economic welfare of 50
 entrepreneur 541
 extended roles of 537, 539
 for caregivers, role of 602
 functions of 539
 fundamental responsibilities of 16
 generalist 100, 526, 540
 invisibility 23
 legal responsibilities of 27
 male 10
 midwifery practitioner, independent 558
 midwives and dais 10
 monitor 267
 oncologist 543
 philosopher 541
 practice 133
 practitioner 100, 140, 526, 539, 558
 premier answerer 541
 primary 540
 provide healthcare 537
 psychopharmacologist 547
 psychotherapist 546
 qualified 60
 responsibility 270, 523
 role 404
 scope of practice for 99
 specialist 100, 140, 526, 539
 statistician 541
 visibility of 20, 23
 working in community 245
Nurse clinician 100, 140, 526
 professional advancement system for 69
Nurse educator 23, 82
 leadership qualities of 82
 role of 9
Nurse manager
 and nurse 524
 role 55
Nurse Practice Act 524
Nurse Practice Law 24
Nurse researcher 541
 roles 79
Nurse-patient relationship 360, 366, 402
Nurse-physician relationship 360
Nurse role 267, 333, 343, 422, 537, 541, 595, 612
 in termination 479
Nurses Unions and Associations 51
Nursing 3, 133, 387
 Act 380
 administration 628
 agency 375
 changing trends in 525
 coalitions, collaborating through 115
 decisions 616
 educational preparations in 58
 ethics 13
 focus of 134
 future challenges 95
 gender specific 576
 health history 429
 history of 4
 implications for 493, 494
 in 19th century 5
 in 20th century 5
 in 21st century 5
 innovations in 619
 institution collaborative relationship 563f
 institutional collaboration model 562
 management 595, 605
 men in 577, 581
 metaparadigm 357, 360, 367, 373, 399
 needs, nature of 569
 overlapping phases in 366f
 philosophy of 347
 public perception 525
 registration board 38
 regulations 48
 staff 10
 standards in 87, 89
 students, stipend for 10
 unit, system of records for 518
Nursing assessment 428
 format 443
 methods 428
 phases 428
 types of 428
Nursing audit 91, 92
 advantages of 93
 disadvantages of 93
 methods of 92
 purposes of 92
Nursing care 393
 audit 92
 collaborative approach to 564f
 concepts of 139
 delivery, patterns of 133, 134, 134f
 dimensions of 134
 evaluating quality of 445
 evaluation of 88
 managing 116
 preoperative 314
 standards, sources of 89
 visibility of 23
Nursing care plan 446
 example of 443
 formulation of 440
 individually developed 441
 sample of 450t
 sample problem of 444t
 types of 441
Nursing Council Act 37

Index

Nursing diagnosis 311, 431, 433, 435, 438
  advantages of 434
  and medical diagnosis 434
  components of 433
  limitations of 434
  risk of 433
  types of 433
  use of 431
Nursing diagnostic
  process 431
    steps of 431
  statement, formulation of 431
Nursing documentation 627
  formats for 446
Nursing education 11, 387, 620
  aims of 70
  and service 561
  challenges in 97
  committee 33
  concept of 62
  continuing 63
  counseling in 515
  development of 6
  evolution of 58
  future of 97
  levels of 58
  milestones of 6
  preceptorship in 67
  role and scope of 58, 68
  scope of 70
  trends of 97
Nursing educator 540
  in teaching, role of 70
Nursing functions
  profession of 383
  spectrum of 137
Nursing information system 649
  benefits of 649
Nursing order
  components of 438
  determining 438
Nursing practice 15, 74, 134, 521, 625
  benefits of 23
  challenges in 96
  creativity in 622
  development of 3
  evolution of 3
  governance of 40
  independent 558
  innovations in 622
  legal safeguards in 25
  scope in 523
  trends in 525
Nursing problem 369, 370
  typology of 370
Nursing process 388, 409, 426
  achievement subsystem 451
  advantages of 427
  characteristics of 427
  conceptual models of 352
  elimination subsystem 450

ingestion subsystem 450
  purposes of 427
  sexual subsystem 450
  steps of 426
  theory application in 449
  theory of 382
Nursing profession 1, 8, 86, 577
  characteristics of 7
  development of 3
  education 65
  issues of 9
  organizations 40t
  perspectives of 9
  regulatory bodies in 31t
  role of management in 83
Nursing research 71, 387
  characteristics of 72
  conceptual models in 352
  evolution of 71
  purposes of 73
Nursing Research Society 45
Nursing robot 524
  system, development of 524
Nursing roles 367
  expanded 100, 139, 526, 539, 545
Nursing standards 89, 92
  applying 437
Nursing system 375
  classifications of 375
Nursing theory 347, 356
  development of 377
  into practice, application of 449
Nutrient 255
  absorption blocking drug 279
Nutrition 238, 255, 259, 279, 280
  and diet 501
  in amoeba 256
  in humans 256
  mode of 255
  types of 255
Nutritional anemia 281
Nutritional conditions 278
Nutritional imbalanced nutrition 596
Nutritional interventions 235, 550
Nutritional problems 277

O

Observation and reporting, responsibility for 27
Obstetric care, essential 142, 143
Obstetrics and gynecological nurse practitioner 560
Obstructive pulmonary disease, chronic 598
Obstructive sleep apnea syndrome 298
Occipital lobe 250, 456
Occupational exposure
  risk of 335b
  types of 334
Occupational health nurse 524, 543, 546
Old age, development in 488

Olfactory tactility 428
Oogenesis 172
  stages of 173f
Operating room nurse 544
Operating systems of computer 629
Operation
  instrumental 313
  manual 313
  sequence of 164f
  theater 340
Opioid analgesics 304
Opioid drug addiction 252
Oral cavity 238, 592
Oral contraceptives 217t
Oral rehydration therapy 142
Orem's model, basic nursing system of 376f
Orem's theory 377
  application of 377
Organ donations 327
Organizational behaviour 482, 483
  concepts of 483
  elements of 483
  factors influencing 483
  scope of 483
Organizations, development of 5
Organize disaster drills 584, 585
Organized nursing 21
Organogenesis 458
Orientation phase, tasks of 478
Orthopedic nurse 544
Osmolar imbalance 273
Osmosis 271
Osteoarthritis 598
Ostomy 545
Otoscope 411
Otoscopic examination 415
Outpatient surgery 313
Outreach program 601
Overhydration 273
Ovum 458f
  and fertilization, meiotic divisions of 186f
Oxygen
  hazards 269
  induced apnea 269
  supplying of 284
Oxygen insufficiency 268
  diagnosis of 269
  signs of 269
  symptoms of 269
Oxygen therapy 269, 270
  equipment required for 270t
  methods of 269

P

Pachytene 172
Packaged program 641
Pain 300, 450
  acute 301, 302f
  chronic 302, 302f

duration 301
experience 301
factors influencing 302
intensity 302
location 302
management 304
modulation 301
perception 300
    assessment of 303
receptors and stimuli 300
referred 302
relief, drugs for 304
response, modify 305
scale 303f, 304f
superficial 420
transmission 300
    after 304
    pathways of 302f
    theories of 301
types of 301
Palliative care
    concepts 139
    nurse 543
Palpation 412, 417
    purpose of 412
Panchayati Raj institution 580
Pancreas 257
Pap Smear Test Facility Program 152
Pap test 221
Paradigm 349
Parasitic nutrition 256
Parasympathetic system 252
Parathyroid hormone 277, 593
Parental testing 193
Parenteral nutrition 281
Parietal lobe 250, 456
Parkinson's disease 252, 598
Parse's human becoming theory 397
Parse's theory 398t, 399
Partial dentures, removable 604
Password protection 643, 644f
Patau syndrome 187
Patient care delivery systems 625
Patient controlled analgesia 304
Patient for surgery, preparation of 314
Patient Self-determination Act 327
Patient's bill of rights 25
Patient's registration form 645
Pectus carinatum 416
Pectus excavatum 416
Pediatric critical care nurse 545
Pediatric nurse practitioner 540
Pediatric oncology care 545
Pedigree 192
    construction of 192f
    drawing 192
Pentazocine (talwin) 595
Peplau theory 368
Peplau's model
    of interpersonal process 367f
    to nursing process, application of 368f

Peplau's phases, application of 368t
Peplau's theory 366
Peptic ulcer 265
Perceived dissonance, theory of 363
Perceived health status 549
Perceived loss 505
Percutaneous umbilical blood sampling 195, 195f
Perfusion 268, 282
Perinatal mortality rate 225
Periodic limb movement disorder 299
Perioperative nurse 545
    concept of 312
Peripheral nervous system 251
Peripheral vascular disease 238
Permissive (Laissez-Faire) leadership 81
Personal conduct 13
Personal integrity, conservation of 372
Personal loss 505
Personal protective
    devices 337
    equipment 332
    use of 333
Personality
    assessment of 469
        techniques of 468
    dynamics of 462
    factors of 468
Personality development 455, 464, 485, 487
    Freud's stages of 462, 462t
Personnel in health care services 108
Pharmacy information systems 649
Pharynx 257, 415
Phenomena experienced during mourning 511t
Phenotype 188
Philanthropic foundations 155
Philosophy in nursing, doctorate of 62
Photo energy therapy 536
Physical abuse 601
Physical changes 329
Physical development 485
Physical environment 570
Physical examination 411
Physical hazards hazards 486-488
Physical illness 296
Physiological emotion responses 265
Physiological preparation 314
Piaget's cognitive development theory 465
Pie charting 447
Pigeon chest 416
Placenta 457
Planning 436
    characteristics of 111
    cycle 111f
    discharge 436
    elements of 436
    ongoing 436
    process, steps of 111

    steps in 437
    types of 436
Plants, excretion in 259
Plastic waste disinfection 341f
Platelets 258
Pneumonia 314, 598
Political action, components of 113
Political activities, restriction on 114
Political advocate 538
Political favors 113
Political focus 114
Political strategies 114
Politics
    and health policy 525
    and policy making 112
    history of 112
    role of nurse in 115
Poor environmental sanitation 230, 232
Population
    at risk 238
    attributable risk 216
    experimental 219
    screening 198
    strategy 236
    surveillance
        community 241
        local 241
    surveys 244
Portal of entry, control of 337
Portal of exit, control of 337
Positive eugenics 196
Possible nursing diagnosis 433
Postanesthesia
    care unit 316, 544
    reacting 318
Post-basic diploma courses 34
Postneonatal mortality rate 225
Postsynaptic neuron 252
Potassium imbalance 275
Powerlessness, feeling of 502
PowerPoint 629
    presentation of 637
Practice in expanded settings, challenges of 97
Practicing nurses, strategies for 78
Prasooti araike 147
Precede-proceed model 568, 568t
Preceptors, advantages of using 67
Preceptorship Preparation Program, content of 67
Preconception counseling 203
Predictive testing 193, 198
Predisease stage 232
Predominant nursing roles 537
Prehistoric period 4
Preimplantation diagnosis 196
Prenatal counseling 204
Prenatal development 457
Prenatal diagnosis 193, 197, 198
    indications for 198
Prenatal screening, indications for 193

Index

Preoperative patient admission 314
Preorientation phase, tasks of 477
Preparedness 583
Prepathogenesis stage 232
Presbyopia 592
Presymptomatic testing 193
Prevalence and incidence, relationship between 226
Prevalence rate 226
Preventive care 135
Primary health care, infrasructure of 127f
Primary Health Center 126, 126f, 127, 147, 151, 153, 552
   level, facilities at 556
Primary health prevention 235, 235t
Primary health workers, restricted use of 109
Primary healthcare 548, 551, 555t, 556
   characteristics of 553
   concept of 553f
      development of 552
   elements of 553
   goal of 403
   institutions 556
   principles of 553
   role of nurses in 555
Primary nursing
   characteristics of 139
   clinical responsibilities of 139
   concept 138
Primordial prevention 234
Princess Srinagarindra award 35
Prison nurse 538
Problem-focused triggers 406
Problem-oriented medical records 447
Problem-solving techniques 502
Profession, criteria of 8
Professional agencies, role of 155
Professional autonomy 21
   evolution of 21
Professional bodies 131
Professional conduct 13
   code of 13
   for nurses, code of 15
Professional health organizations 155
Professional nurse care provider, role of 525
Professional organization 40, 114, 115
   meaning of 40
Professional perspective barriers 80
Professional preparedness 583
Professional registered nurse 3
Professional regulatory bodies 32
Professional standards system 90
Progressive care, principal elements of 136
Progressive patient care
   benefits of 136
   concept 135
Promote research, strategies to 78

Prophylaxis
   against nutritional anemia 149
   post-exposure 333, 333f, 335
Proportionate mortality rate 225
Propranolol 595
Prospective cohort studies 214
Prostaglandins 300
Prostate disease 598
Protect public, responsibility to 27
Protein
   assays 178
   calorie malnutrition 280
   lack of 173
Psychiatric consultation liaison nurse 547
Psychiatric disorders, reaction in 266
Psychiatric illnesses 253
Psychiatric nurse educator 546
Psychiatric nursing, roles in 546
Psychiatric symptomatology 253
Psychoanalytic theory 461
Psychobiological disorders, diagnosis of 253
Psychobiological revolution 249
Psychobiology and nursing 253
Psychodynamic nursing 366
Psychological abuse 601
Psychological consequences 420
Psychological factors influencing health 261
Psychological hazards 486-488
Psychological problems 600
Psychological stressors 496
Psychological types, classification by 467
Psychology 455
   application of 455
Psychoneurosis 266
Psychosocial and sexual changes 600
Psychosocial changes 600
Psychosocial development
   Erikson's stages of 463t
   theory of 463
Psychosocial illness 265
Psychosocial rehabilitation nurse 546
Psychosomatic illness 265
Public communication 475
Public health issues, development of 243
Public health
   nurse 10
      leadership qualities of 83
   service 584
Public Health Nurse model 563, 563f
Public policy, political influence on 113
Public-Private Partnership scheme 148
Pulmonary embolus 318
Pulmonary manifestation 275
Pulse pressure 282
Pupils 414
Pyrexia 289
   low 290
   management of 290t

Q

Quality assurance 85
   concept of 86
   cycle 87f
   Donabedian model of 88f
   goals of 87
   in healthcare, models of 88t
   in nursing 85, 86
      and healthcare 86
      techniques of 90
   meaning of 85
   models of 87
   program, components of 90
   system 87
Quality care 407f
Quality control, responsibility in 27
Quality documentation, characteristics of 446
Quality management, models of 526, 528f
Quality nursing care 14
   factors affecting 93, 93f
Quality of life, indicators of 228
Quirks 634

R

Rabies 245
Randomized controlled trial 218
   design of 218f
   types of 220
Rape trauma syndrome 431
Rapid eye movement sleep 296
Real life situation 405
Recessive trait 174, 174f
Recognition strikes 55
Record keeping and reporting, responsibility for 27
Recovery room nurse 544, 545
Recruitment of students 517
Rectum 419
Red blood
   cells 173
      counts 314
   corpuscles 258
Reflex hammer 411
Reflexology 534
Registered nurse education 62
Regular exercise 500
Regulation and Prevention of Misuse Act 193
Regulatory bodies 30
   major 30
   role of 30
   vital role of 30
Regulatory law 24
Rehabilitation 197, 422, 586
   nurse 543, 545
   plan 587
   potential, evaluating 587
   process 586

Index

recovery 262
team 586, 587
Relapsing fever 290
Relaxation breathing 238, 550
Relaxation techniques 501
Relaxation therapy 550
   assisting patient with 238
   steps of 238
Relaxation/stress management 238, 550
Religious practice 616
Remedial care 135
Remittent fever 290
Remote monitoring 162
Renal system 593
Renin-angiotensin-aldosterone system 272
Reports menu 646
Reproductive and Child Health Programme 141
Reproductive system 599
   female 599
Reproductive tract infection 141
Requirement specification 164*f*
Research 72, 376
   abstract 57, 84
   barriers related to 78
   consumer 538
   in nursing profession, role of 71, 73
   leadership and management, role of 71
   process 74
   testing 193
   utilization 77
      steps in 77
      strategies for 79
Residual stimuli 390
Residual urine, catheterization for 393
Resistance, flexible lines of 385
Respiration 257, 259
Respiratory disease 296
Respiratory gases, exchange of 268
Respiratory problems 280
Respiratory support 287
Respiratory system 289, 593, 597
   anatomy of 268
   physiology of 268
Responsibility, assumption of 476
Restless leg syndrome 299
Restoration and rehabilitation 237
Restorative care 135
Restorative healthcare delivery system 537
Resuscitation 320
   kit 324
Resuscitative technique, complication of 325
Reticular activating system 291
Reticular formation 251, 291
Retirement 488
Retrolental fibroplasia 269
Retrospective cohort studies 214

Retrospective genetic counseling 200
Reversal drugs 317
Rheumatic fever, acute 230
Rheumatoid arthritis 229, 230, 265
Rhizotomy 305
Ribonucleic acid 169, 178, 193
   function of 182
   sequencing 180
Rigor 290
Rinne air and bone conduction test 415
Rising cost of health services 109
Roger's model
   abstract conceptual 363*f*, 365
   critical thinking in 364*t*
   nursing practice with 363
Rogerian framework 363
Rogers' theory 361
Romberg test 419
Routine statistics related to health 244
Roy's adaptation model 392
   evaluation in 391
Roy's adaptation theory 389
Roy's adaptive modes 390*f*
Roy's concepts, application of 391
Roy's theory and nursing metaparadigm 391
Royal British Nurses Association 46
Ruesch's theory 475
Rule deontologists 19
Ruler 632*f*
Rural areas, infrastructure norms in 152*t*
Rural Family Welfare Center 151, 153
Rural Health Services 126

S

Safe practice, guidelines for 29
Safeguarding animal rights, developing methods for 75
Safeguarding human rights, developing methods for 75
Safety and security needs 565
Safety pins 411
Salivary glands 256
Samaritan laws 25
Sample registration system 242
Saprophytes 256
Satellite telemedicine 162
Scalp and skull 414
Schizophrenia 252, 253, 266
   clients with 311
School health nurse 524, 546
   responsibility 524
Scientific process and nursing research 72
Screening health point 240
Search 646
   database 638
Second meiotic division 172
Second World War 524
Secondary health prevention 236, 236*t*

Secrete saliva 256
Sedatives 316
   and antianxiety agents 304
Seeking attention 266
Selecting nursing strategies 437
Selecting research design 75
Self-actualization needs 566
Self-assessment, areas for 476
Self-awareness 476
Self-care 403
   agency 375
   components of 403
   concept 139
   deficit 375
      theory 374
   health of people, nurses' role in 404
   in health 403
Self-catheterization, infection related to 393
Self-concept 404
   components of 404
   development of 404
Self-discharge 26
Self-esteem 404
   disturbance 502
Self-health, concept of 403
Sense of humor 535
Sensory deprivation 305
   conditions with 305
Sensory perception, lack of 305
Sensory system 420
Sentinel centers 241
Septic shock 285
   pathophysiology of 285*f*
Sequencing human genome 176
Serotonin 252, 300
Servant leadership 81
Setting priorities, fundamental principles of 436
Seven behavioral subsystem 378
Sex chromosome 183
   disorders 187
Sex ratio 579, 579*t*
Sex related problems 494
Sex role
   standards 489
   typing 486
Sex specific death rate 225
Sexual abuse 601
Sexual dysfunction 599
Sexual health 238, 489, 493, 494, 550
Sexual identity, development of 489
Sexually transmitted disease 141, 245
Shock 282, 314, 318, 422
   anaphylactic 285
   cardiogenic 283, 284
   circulatory 285
      blood volume in 286*f*
   classification of 283
   complications of 287
   distributive 285

emergency care in 288
obstructive 285
phase 585
stages of 285
vasogenic 285
Sick role 262
assumption of 423
Sickle cell anemia 173, 203
Siddha 532
medicine 532
Simple facemask 269
Simple nursing functions 137
Single blind trial 219
Single cause theory 230f
Single gene disorders 188
Single-nucleotide polymorphisms 178
Singultus 314
Sister Calista Roy's adaptation model 391f
Situational leadership 82
Situational loss 506
Skeletal muscles 498
Skills
play 485
school 485
self-help 485
social help 485
Skin
activates 272
breakdown, risk for 595
cells 195
disease 598
preparation 315
rashes, appearance of 233
texture 414
Sleep 294, 594
and arousal, physiology of 295
apnea syndrome 298
deprivation 299
disorders 298
management 298
disturbance 358t
factors affecting 296
maintenance disturbance 299
onset difficulty 299
pattern 294, 296
disturbance 295
normal 297, 297t
stages of 295
Small intestine 257
Smokers versus non-smokers, risk assessment of 217t
Smoking 426
and lung cancer, control study of 213t
cessation 238, 550
prevention 238, 550
Smooth muscle relaxants 304
Snellen chart 411
Social and mental health, indicators of 227
Social dimension, dysfunction in 261

Social hazardous wastes 107
Social integrity, conservation of 372
Social isolation 308, 311
causes of 308
characteristics of 309
deprivation model, application of 309f
different age groups 309
different conditions 310
human beings 308
nursing intervention of 311
patterns of 309
Social learning theory 468
Social sciences, statistical package for 640
Social Security Act 86
Social Security Schemes 244
Social support 421
Social system barriers 79
Social vs. therapeutic relationships 476
Societal challenges 95
Society 56
Socioeconomic indicators 228
Socioeconomic welfare 48
Sodium imbalance 274
Soft and hard palates 415
Software 643
Somatic cell 175
Somatic distress, sensation of 511
Sorrow, chronic 508
Space Nursing Society 525
Special Nutrition Program 149
Special sample survey 241
Specific death rate, cause 225
Specific health surveys 239
Specific protection 234
Specification in standards, types of 89
Speculums 411
Speech development 485
Sperm, normal 186f
Spermatogenesis 172
stages of 172f
Spermatozoa 457
Sphygmomanometer 411
Spinal cord stimulators 305
Spiritual and religious factors 261
Spiritual dimension, dysfunction in 261
Spiritual distress 435
Spiritual therapy 535
Spiritual well-being 435
Spirituality 501
and grief 509
Spontaneous birth 459
Spontaneous mutation 173
Spurious association 222
Standard safety measures 331, 335, 337
Standard toolbar 632
Standardized nursing care plans 441
State Government, role of 31
State Health Administration 122
State Health Directorate 123
State Ministry of Health 122

State Ministry of Health and Family Welfare Services 122
State Nursing Boards 38
State Nursing Councils 36
functions of 36
State of grieving, bereavement 508
State Registration Council 36, 86
Statistical analysis system 640
Statistical functions 634
Statistical package 640, 641
Statistical software packages, major 640
Statutory law 24
Stereognosis 420
Sterile procedures, performing 389
Sterilization bed scheme 152
Stethoscope 411
Stimuli by brain, interpretation of 497
Stochastic theory 590, 591
Stomach 256
Store-and-forward telemedicine 162
Strengthening referral system 143
Streptococcus 229
Stress 495, 499, 503
and adaptation 495
and immune system 499
assessment, nursing management of 501
behavioral indicator of 500
emotional indicator of 500
indicators of 500
job 495
physiologic response to 497
physiological indicators of 500
points 571
theories 499
Stressors 378, 496
affecting self-concept 404
affecting system 388f
time-related 496
types of 496
Strikes, types of 55, 55f
Stroke 597
volume 282
Structural brain lesions 291
Structural integrity, conservation of 372
Structure audit 91
Student centered teaching, emphasis on 9
Student Nurses Association 43
activities of 44
management of 43
objectives of 43
Student nursing care plans 441
Students record system 518
Students welfare, improving 517
Student-teacher relationship, authentic 10
Study designs, crossover type of 220
Study subjects, selection of 215
Subcenter level, facilities at 556
Substances, use of 616

Index

Sullivan major concepts 464
Sullivan's index 227
Sullivan's stages 464
Supratentorial lesions 291
Surgery
    purpose of 313
    to urgency, types of 313
Surgical asepsis 337
Surgical nursing, history of 312
Surgical outcomes, factors influencing 314
Surgical waiting area 317
Surveillance process 241
Survey methods, types of 244
Sustenal care 135
Sympathectomy 305
Sympathetic nervous system 498
Sympathetic-adrenal-medullary response 498
    effect of 498*t*
Sympathy strikes 55
Synaptic cleft 252
Syndrome nursing diagnosis 433
Systemic innovations 622

T

Tay Sach's disease 203
Teacher's activities, computers for 628
Teaching plans 441
Teaching skills 10
Team nursing
    benefits of 137
    composition of 137
    concept 137
Tears sobbing 264
Technical skill 5
Technical weakness 110
Technological explosion 97
Technology, challenge of 96, 97
Teeth 256, 505
Telecare 162
Telehealth 538
Telemedicine 161, 164
    benefits of 162
    technology 164
    types of 162
    uses of 162
Telenurse 161, 165, 538
Telephone triage nurse 100
Telepsychiatry 162
Teleradiology 163
Telophase 171, 172
Temperature 420
    regulation 259
Temporal association 222
Temporal lobe 250, 456
Tensions, preventing 561
Tertiary health prevention 237
Tetanus 245
    toxoid 147
        injection of 338

Thalamus 250
Thalassemia 203
Thalassotherapy 534
Thayi Bhagya Program, objectives of 145
Theophylline 595
Theoretical assertions 357, 367, 373, 379, 382, 392, 399
Theory 352
    adopting trait 461
    application of 384, 451
    characteristics of 353
    classification of 353
    components of 352, 353*f*
    model of 391
    scope of 353
    significance of 352
Therapeutic communication
    characteristics of 475
    techniques to 473
Therapeutic music 534
Therapeutic relationship
    development of 477
    phases of 477, 477*f*
Therapeutic self-care demand 375
Thermometer 411
Thrombophlebitis 314
Thrombus 314
Thyroid 416
Tibbi medicine 533
Tissues, experimental 179*f*
Title bar 630, 631*f*
Tongue 415
    depressor 411
Toolbar 632, 632*f*
Tools 631*f*
Topography of mind 461*f*
Tort 28
    types of 28*b*
Towns area committees 125
Toxic agents 107
Trachea 257, 416
Tracheostomy collar 269
Traditional beliefs about mental health 617
Traditional Chinese medicine 534
Traditional practice
    model 563, 563*f*
    status of 616
Traditional roles, variation on 99
Trained birth attendants 127
Trained *dai* 126
Trained nurses 42*fc*
Trained Nurses Association 41
    activities performed by 42
    benefits of 42
    publications of 43
Traits theory, five 468
Transactional leadership 81
Transcultural nursing 613
    goals of 614
    model 614
    role of nurse in 617

Transcutaneous electrical nerve stimulator 304
Transfer from surgery 317
Transformational leadership 81
Transmission
    control of 337
    mechanism of 189*f*
    risk of 331*f*
Transpersonal communication 475
Transplant nurse 545
Transportation 259
    in animals 258
    in plants 259
Traverse birth 459
Travi's wellness model 565, 565*f*
Treatment
    and disposal 341
    chart 646
    types of 642
Trendelenburg position 314
Triple blind trial 219
Triple X syndrome XXX 188
Trycyclic antidepressants 304
Tuberculosis 239
    nursing 544
Tuckman's stages 481
Tumor, malignant 313
Tuning fork 411
Turgor and mobility 414
Turner's syndrome 187
Twin bin 341*f*
Typhoid 236
    fever 229
Typical chromosome, parts of 183*f*

U

Ulcerative colitis 265
Ultrasonography 195
Umbilical cord 195, 457
Unani medicine 533
Unconscious 290, 294
Unconsciousness 291
    assessment of 292
    causes of 291
Uniform resource locator 639
Unintentional torts 28
Union Ministry of Health and Family Welfare 119
Unions/Labor Organization 51
United Nations Development Program 579
Universal Immunization Programs 142
Upper extremities 419
Urban Family Welfare Centers 152
Urban Revamping Scheme 152
Urinary catheterization 293
Urinary elimination 435
Urinary incontinence 595
Urinary infection
    signs of 394
    symptoms of 394

Index

Urinary manifestation 276
Urinary retention 318
Uterus 240

V

Vaginal speculum 411
Valuing human being 15
Vande Mataram Scheme 143
Vasoactive medication 284
Veins 258
Ventilation 268, 356
Ventricular fibrillation 323
Verbal descriptive scale 303
Vibration 420
Vibrio cholerae 230
View menu 646, 647f
Village Health Guides 127, 151, 242, 554
Village Health Guides Scheme 126
Village Health Post 152
Village level, facilities at 556
Virus 230
Visceral pain 302
Visibility of symptoms 421
Vision loss 599
Visual acuity, decreased 592
Visual analog scale 303, 303f
Visual basic for applications 633
Vital events, registration of 242
Vital signs 413
Vitamin 278
    A 278
        deficiency, prevention and control of 142
    B 278
    B12 278
    B2 278
    B3 278
    B6 278
    C prophylaxis 281
    D 278
    E 278
    K 278
Voice 592
    tone of 596
Voluntary agencies 154
Voluntary health agencies 131
    functions of 131

W

Waste
    accumulation and storage 340
    categories of 342, 344f
    management 343
        steps in 339
    minimization 341
    segregation of 340, 342f
    survey 340
    transportation 341
Water cure (therapy) 534
Water pollution 107, 261
Watson's carative factors, concepts of 396f
Watson's concepts, application of 397
Watson's theory 394
    and nursing metaparadigm 395
Wearing sterile gloves, techniques of 332f
Weber test 415
Weighing machine 411
Wellness 385, 432, 568
    prevention 267
Wet and dry thermal treatment 341
White blood corpuscles 258
Wide area network 638
Window menu 646, 647f
Women and political participation 580
Women empowerment 575, 578
    framework, levels of 580
    reason for 578
    strategies 580
Women health nurse practitioner 559
Women of current reality, status of 579
Women, power and politics, relationship between 115
Word 629
    window, parts of 630
World Health Organization 85, 105, 228, 229, 234, 339
World wide web 638
Wound 545
    infection 318
        signs of 394
        symptoms of 394
    management 318
Writing nursing
    care plans, guidelines for 440
    orders 438
    plan of care 440
Written care plan, purposes of 440

X

X-linked dominant inheritance 190, 190f
X-linked recessive inheritance 189, 189f
XYY syndrome 188

Y

Yoga 534, 535f

Z

Zygotene 171

Index

Urinary manifestation, 270
Uterine standard, 241
Uterus, 240

V

Vaginal speculum, 31?
Vaulting bimanual doing, 15
vandalism in schema, 117
Vasoconstriction, 289
Veins, 236
Ventilation, 306, 307
Ventricular fibrillation, 302
Verbal descriptive scale, 302
Vibration, 446
Vibrio cholerae, 230
View mount oil, 61?
Village Health Guides, 129, 151, 212, 251
Village Health Guides Scheme, 126
Village Health Post, 142
Vinegar peel medicine, 208
Virus, 236
Visceral pain, 302
Visiting day centers, 421
Vision loss, 336
Visual acuity decreased, 302
Visual analog scale, 303, 303?
Visual basic for applications, 63
Vital record registration, 242
Vitalstress, 412
Vitamin 213
A, 126
deficiency, prevention and control of, 132

W

B1, 212, 278
B6, 278
B12, 278

Waste
    accumulation and storage, 346
    categories of, 315, 314?
    management, 345
    steps in, 326
    minimization, 321
    segregation of, 316, 343
    storage, 346
    transportation, 343
Waterline Disposal, 64
WA-compliance, 107, 261
Watson's charity factor concept of, 509
Web (WWW) generic application, 61, 595
Web service theory, 594
    and nursing process and up, 393 P
Waxing, stations above a semicircle of, 327
Wee foot, 415
Watching in china, 511
Wellness, 362, 397, 368
    promotion, 367
Wet and dry method treatment, 341
Whiplash Compulsory, 158
Wide area network, 63
Window trend, 61, 61?

Women and political participation, 580
Woman empowerment, 573, 574
framework, levels of, 580
reason for, 578
strategy, 580
Women health nurse practitioner, 369
Women of reproductive status of, 579
Women power and political relationship
    between, 117
Word, 628
windows parts of, 630
World Health Organization 86, 199, 255
    266, 311, 530
World wide web, 633
Wound care
    infection, 318
    signs of, 398
    symptoms of, 368
    management, 818
    writhe nursing
        care plans, guidelines for, 330
        orders, 338
        plan of care, 330
Women care plan, purposes of, 330

X

X-linked dominant inheritance, 160
X-linked recessive inheritance, 160, 180?
XY Syndrome, 158

Y

Yoga, 556, 557?

Z

Zygotene, 171